HANDBUCH DER MEDIZINISCHEN RADIOLOGIE

ENCYCLOPEDIA OF MEDICAL RADIOLOGY

HERAUSGEGEBEN VON · EDITED BY

L. DIETHELM
MAINZ

F. HEUCK
STUTTGART

O. OLSSON
LUND

K. RANNIGER
RICHMOND

F. STRNAD
FRANKFURT/M.

H. VIETEN
DÜSSELDORF

A. ZUPPINGER
BERN

BAND/VOLUME V
TEIL/PART 6

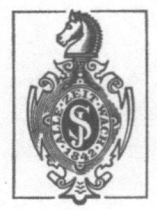

SPRINGER-VERLAG BERLIN · HEIDELBERG · NEW YORK 1977

RÖNTGENDIAGNOSTIK DER SKELETERKRANKUNGEN
TEIL 6

DISEASES OF THE SKELETAL SYSTEM
(ROENTGEN DIAGNOSIS)
PART 6

BONE TUMORS

BY

M. C. BEACHLEY · M. H. BECKER · P. A. COLLINS · K. DOI · H. F. FAUNCE
FRIEDA FELDMAN · H. FIROOZNIA · E. W. FORDHAM · H. K. GENANT
NANCY B. GENIESER · AMY GOLDMAN · G. B. GREENFIELD · H. J. GRIFFITHS
J. P. PETASNICK · P. H. PEVSNER · R. S. PINTO · P. C. RAMACHANDRAN
F. SCHAJOWICZ · I. YAGHMAI

EDITED BY
K. RANNIGER

WITH 639 FIGURES (1086 SEPARATE ILLUSTRATIONS)

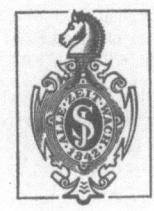

SPRINGER-VERLAG BERLIN · HEIDELBERG · NEW YORK   1977

Dr. MARY ANN TURNER

assisted Dr. RANNIGER in editing this volume and after his death acted as technical editor during the production of the volume

ISBN-13: 978-3-642-81159-3   e-ISBN-13: 978-3-642-81157-9
DOI: 10.1007/ 978-3-642-81157-9

Library of Congress Cataloging in Publication Data. Röntgendiagnostik der Skeleterkrankungen. (Handbuch der medizinischen Radiologie, Bd. 5; Encyclopedia of medical radiology, v. 5) Vol. 4, by M. Pöschl, has also special title: Juvenile Osteo-chondro-nekrosen; v. 6, by M.C. Beachley et al.: Bone tumors. In German or English. Includes bibliographies. 1. Bones—Radiography. 2. Bones—Diseases—Diagnosis. II. Althoff, Hugo. II. Title. III. Title: Diseases of the skeletal system. IV. Series: Handbuch der medizinischen Radiologie, Bd. 5. [DNLM: 1. Spine—Radiography. WM100 H236 Bd. 6 T. 1 etc.] RC78.H295 616.07′57′08s [616.7′1′0757] 68-12799

Typesetting: Universitätsdruckerei H. Stürtz AG, Würzburg

Preface

Six years ago the editors of the Encyclopedia of Medical Radiology selected two additional editors from the emerging generation of young radiologists to complete this unique compendium of radiology. Klaus Ranniger was one of them and he worked with enthusiasm and great energy at the challenge facing him. His editorial work was excellent and he succeeded in winning internationally acclaimed scientists to contribute to this volume. Their chapters have met the requirements and goals we set out to achieve in every aspect and to the highest degree.

The majority of the authors valued Klaus Ranniger not only as a fellow scientist and doctor but also as a personal friend. In America, his adopted country, he found acknowledgement of his personal achievement and scientific research. He was highly respected and admired among specialists in the field of radiology. Klaus Ranniger, our coeditor and friend, died suddenly and unexpectedly before this volume could be published. We are honored to present this volume as his legacy.

FRIEDRICH HEUCK

Vorwort

Die Herausgeber des Handbuches der medizinischen Radiologie nahmen vor sechs Jahren aus der nachfolgenden Generation von Radiologen zwei Mitarbeiter in ihren Kreis auf, um dieses im wissenschaftlichen Schrifttum der Welt einmalige Sammelwerk der Radiologie aus dem Springer-Verlag zum Abschluß zu bringen. Mit großer Tatkraft und echter Begeisterung hat Klaus RANNIGER die ihm gestellten Aufgaben übernommen. Das vorliegende Werk hat er meisterhaft vorbereitet und gestaltet. Die einzelnen Beiträge sind von international hochangesehenen Wissenschaftlern verfaßt, die Klaus RANNIGER zur Mitarbeit gewinnen konnte. Alle Autoren haben die in sie gesetzten Erwartungen und hohen Anforderungen erfüllt, ein Sammelwerk über den Stand unseres Wissens auf dem schwierigen Gebiet der Radiologie der Knochengeschwülste vorzulegen.

Die Mehrzahl der Mitarbeiter dieses Bandes war nicht nur dem Wissenschaftler und Arzt, sondern auch dem Menschen Klaus RANNIGER freundschaftlich verbunden. Er fand in dem großen Land, in das vor ihm schon viele Generationen der besten und aktiven Menschen seiner Heimat ausgezogen waren, um eine neue Zukunft zu bauen, Anerkennung durch seine persönlichen Leistungen und wissenschaftlichen Arbeiten auf zahlreichen Gebieten der Radiologie. In dem Kreis der Vertreter des Fachgebietes der medizinischen Radiologie an den Hochschulen der Vereinigten Staaten von Amerika wurde er geschätzt und geachtet. Ein unergründliches Schicksal hat unseren Mitherausgeber und Freund Klaus RANNIGER vor dem Erscheinen seines Handbuchbandes abberufen. Es war uns eine selbstverständliche Pflicht, dieses Werk als sein Vermächtnis vorzulegen.

FRIEDRICH HEUCK

Contents — Inhaltsverzeichnis

X   Contents — Inhaltsverzeichnis

XIV   Contents — Inhaltsverzeichnis

Contents — Inhaltsverzeichnis   XVII

Contributors to Volume V/6 — Mitarbeiter von Band V/6

MICHAEL C. BEACHLEY, M.D., Prof. and Chairman (1977–), Department of Radiology, Medical College of Virginia, MCV Station – Box 2, Richmond, Va. 23298, USA

MELVIN H. BECKER, M.D., Prof. of Radiology, Department of Radiology, New York University Medical Center, 560 First Avenue, New York, N.Y. 10016, USA

PHILLIP A. COLLINS, M.D., Ass. Prof., Department of Radiology, The University of Chicago, 950 East 59th Street, Chicago, Ill. 60637, USA

KUNIO DOI, Ph.D., Prof. of Radiology, University of Chicago, 950 East 59th Street, Chicago, Ill. 60637, USA

HOWARD F. FAUNCE, III, D.O., Ass. Prof. of Radiology, Department of Radiology, Medical College of Virginia, MCV Station – Box 728, Richmond, Va. 23298, USA

FRIEDA FELDMAN, M.D., Prof. of Radiology, College of Physicians and Surgeons Attending Radiologist, The Presbyterian Hospital, Columbia-Presbyterian Medical Center, 622 West 168th Street, New York, N.Y. 10032, USA

HOSSEIN FIROOZNIA, M.D., Ass. Prof. of Radiology, New York University Medical Center, University Hospital, 560 First Avenue, New York, N.Y. 10016, USA

ERNEST W. FORDHAM, M.D., Prof. and Chairman, Department of Nuclear Medicine, Presbyterian-St. Luke's Medical Center, Chicago, Ill., USA

HARRY K. GENANT, M.D., Ass. Prof., Department of Radiology, University of California, San Francisco, School of Medicine, San Francisco, Ca. 94143, USA

NANCY BRANOM GENIESER, M.D., Prof. of Radiology, New York University Medical Center, 560 First Avenue, New York, N.Y. 10016, USA

AMY GOLDMAN, M.D., Ass. Prof. of Radiology, New York University Medical Center, University Hospital, 560 First Avenue, New York, N.Y. 10016, USA

GEORGE B. GREENFIELD, M.D., Chairman, Department of Radiology, Mount Sinai Hospital Medical Center Chicago, Prof. of Diagnostic Radiology, Rush Medical College, California Avenue at 15th Street, Chicago, Ill. 60608, USA

HARRY J. GRIFFITHS, M.D., Ass. Prof. of Radiology, New England Medical Center Hospital, 171 Harrison Avenue, Boston, Mass. 02111, USA

JERRY P. PETASNICK, M.D., Director of General Radiology, Presbyterian-St. Luke's Hospital, West Congress Parkway, Chicago, Ill. 60612, USA

PAUL H. PEVSNER, M.D., Ass. Prof. of Radiology, Director, Section of Neuroradiology, Department of Radiology, Medical College of Virginia, MCV Station — Box 728, Richmond, Va. 23298, USA

RICHARD S. PINTO, M.D., Ass. Prof. of Radiology, New York University Medical Center, School of Medicine, Department of Radiology, 550 First Avenue, New York, N.Y. 10016, USA

PANOLIL C. RAMACHANDRAN, M.D., Instructor, Department of Nuclear Medicine, Rush-Presbyterian-St. Luke's Medical Center, 1753 West Congress Parkway, Chicago, Ill. 60612, USA

KLAUS RANNIGER, M.D., Prof. and Chairman (1972–1976), Department of Radiology, Medical College of Virginia, MCV Station — Box 2, Richmond, Va. 23298, USA

FRITZ SCHAJOWICZ, M.D., Prof., World Health Organization, Osteo-Articular Pathology Center, Hospital Italiano, Gascon 450, Buenos Aires, Argentina

ISSA YAGHMAI, M.D., Ass. Prof. of Radiology, Director, Bone and Joint Radiology, Department of Radiology, Medical College of Virginia, MCV Station — Box 728, Richmond, Va. 23298, USA

Diagnosis, Classification, and Nomenclature of Bone Tumors

by

Fritz Schajowicz

A. Introduction

There is still a great deal of confusion regarding the interpretation of bone tumors and a considerable diversity of opinion regarding the histogenesis, nomenclature, classification, and treatment of bone tumors and tumorlike conditions. This is partly due to their relative rarity, and to the difficulty in accumulating an appreciable number of cases with a good standard of technical preparation of the material.

The study of bone tumors should be approached from a dynamic standpoint, the pathologist working in close collaboration with the radiologist and clinician and wherever possible, making comparative radiographic and pathologic studies (Figs. 1 and 2).

The application of modern methods such as histochemical studies, microangiography, autoradiography, in vitro tissue cultures, genetic studies, fluorescent microscopy, and electron-microscopy has facilitated the study of the vital processes of bone tissue. These processes consist principally in formation and destruction of bone (apposition and resorption) which, throughout life proceed in a harmonious manner, but which are profoundly disturbed under pathologic conditions.

B. Diagnosis of Bone Tumors

There are three main ways of diagnosing a bone lesion: (1) clinical examination, (2) radiology, and (3) pathologic procedures. These methods should always be used in combination and, whenever necessary, complemented by biochemical and hematologic studies. Biochemical and hematologic methods, however, have, at present, only a limited role in most cases of bone tumors and should not be regarded as essential information except in special circumstances. Serum calcium, phosphorus, alkaline phosphatase, and acid phosphatase are important in some conditions (hyperparathyroidism, Paget's disease, metastatic carcinoma, myeloma). Plasma and urinary proteins, catecholamines in the urine, and bone marrow cytology are important in myeloma and metastatic neuroblastoma, respectively. Hematologic investigation is essential in malignant lymphomas and leukemia with involvement of bone.

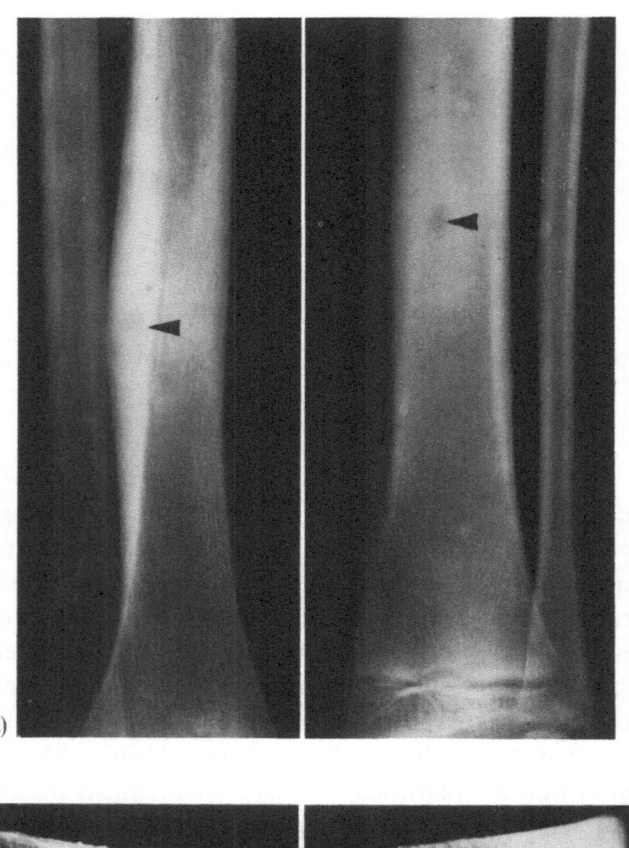

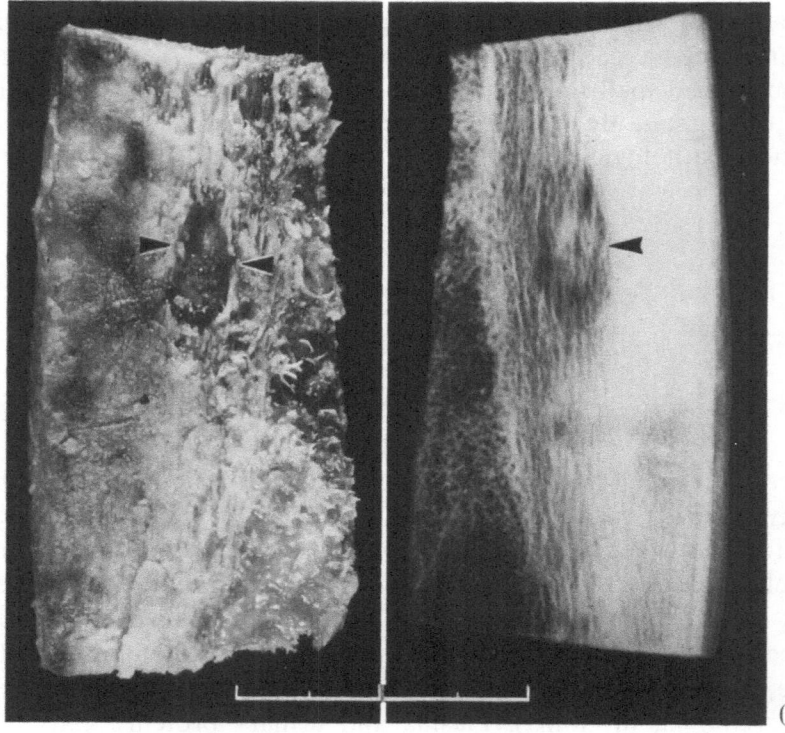

Fig. 1a–c. Osteoid osteoma. Male, 9 years old, shaft of tibia. (a) Lateral and anterior-posterior radiographs showing typical small "nidus," surrounded by reactive bone sclerosis. (b) photograph of specimen showing hyperemic aspect of "nidus". (c) radiograph of slab, 5 mm thick, of specimen showing a dense calcified zone in the center of the radiolucent "nidus"

C. Radiologic Examination

Radiology in the diagnosis of bone tumors is of great importance. Radiographs should always be available to the pathologist, who should never make a definite diagnosis on bone tumors without knowing the radiologic features. The following rules might be followed to record the radiographic aspect of bone lesions.

1. Whether the lesion is monostotic or polyostotic.
2. The type of bone affected (tubular or flat).
3. The site of the lesion with reference to the epiphysis, growth plate, metaphysis, or diaphysis and with reference to its medullary, cortical, or juxtacortical location.
4. An estimate of how much of the total length and circumference of the bone is affected.
5. The presence or absence of adjoining soft-tissue changes with particular mention of fascial planes, tumor tissue, etc.
6. The nature of any bone changes present (destructive, proliferative, or mixed).
7. The character of the bony margins of the lesion (sharp, ill-defined, thick, thin, increased density, or decreased density).
8. The nature of any cortical bone changes, such as the involvement of medullary or periosteal surfaces, cortical invasion, pressure atrophy, etc.
9. The density of tumor tissue, with particular regard to the presence of calcification and its roentgen characteristics (solid, punctate, smoky).
10. The character of periosteal reaction (laminated, solid, or sunburst).

Radiographic techniques may vary in accordance with the nature of bone destruction or proliferation as well as the presence or absence of perifocal soft-tissue changes.

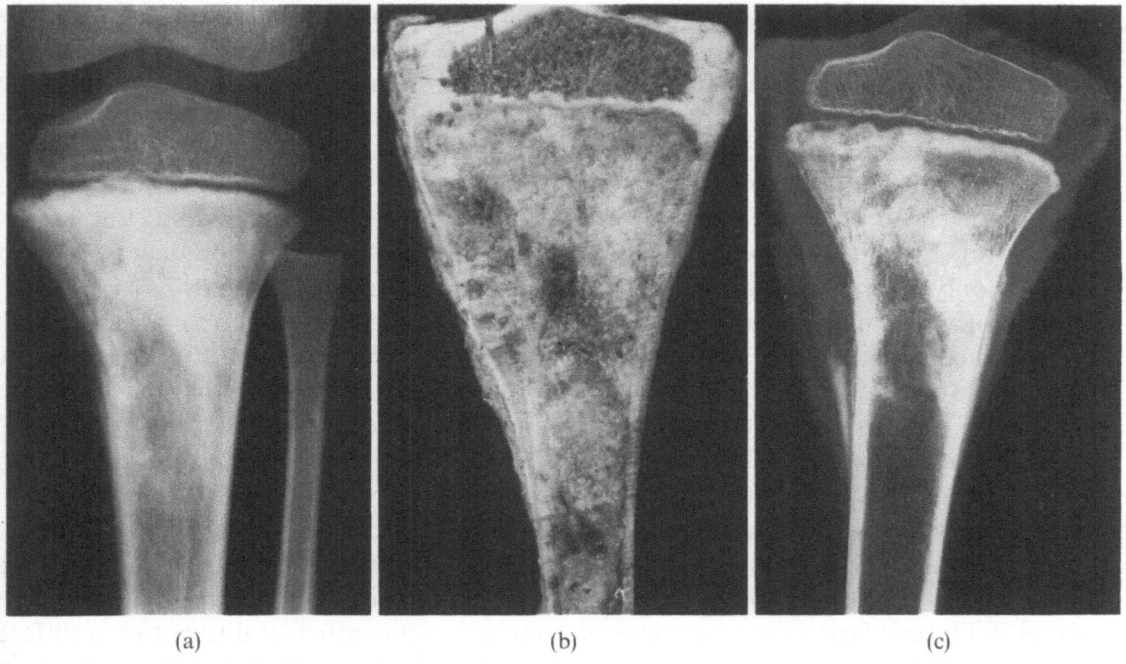

(a)   (b)   (c)

Fig. 2a–c. Osteosarcoma (osteogenic sarcoma). Male, 5 years old, upper metaphysis of tibia. (a) Radiograph showing predominantly sclerotic lesion. (b) photograph of specimen. (c) radiograph of slab, 5 mm thick, of specimen, showing typical Codman's spur, not clearly visible in clinical radiograph

Body-section radiography (tomography), magnification techniques, angiography, the use of subtraction techniques, and other methods must be employed whenever routine roentgen exposures fail to reveal adequately the roentgen characteristics of the bony- or soft-tissue abnormality.

D. Pathologic Examination

Biopsy should be systematically carried out in all cases since it is impossible to assure the precise nature of the affection by the other methods. It should not be omitted in any case in which radical surgery or radiotherapy is contemplated.

Biopsy can be carried out in two ways: (1) by open surgical biopsy (incisional or excisional) and (2) by needle biopsy (aspiration or trocar). In most cases it is most important for the pathologist to be familiar with the clinical and the radiologic picture and to know the exact origin of the material submitted.

I. Surgical Biopsy

There has been much discussion of the possible danger of surgical biopsy leading to an increase in the growth or dissemination of the tumor. Most authors maintain that surgical biopsy carried out by a competent surgeon under the necessary conditions of asepsis and with the correct technique does not involve any great danger. However, in cartilaginous lesions an incisional biopsy may result in implantation making adequate further surgery often impossible. The major source of errors in diagnosis is inadequate tissue due to a defective technique when the specimen submitted is from only the periphery or is taken from zones of reactive bone formation or areas of necrosis.

With the material obtained by open surgical biopsy, two possibilities present themselves: (1) an immediate histologic examination, during the operation, by means of frozen sections or (2) to close the wound and await the results after embedding the material in paraffin. Frozen sections (of fresh- or formalin-fixed material) for diagnosis should be done only where surgical treatment is to be immediately carried out.

One of the main advantages of frozen sections is that the surgeon can judge immediately whether the specimen is adequate and can verify that he has not taken edematous, necrotic tissue or adjacent healthy tissue. However, only few pathologists have sufficient experience with frozen sections of bone tumors to give immediate opinion when the possibility of amputation has to be considered. Many prefer to imbed the material in paraffin as they maintain that frozen sections do not always permit recognition of the necessary histologic details, particularly in giant cell tumors, in cartilaginous tumors, and in "round cell" tumors. They feel that such new growths as chondroma, chondrosarcoma, Ewing's sarcoma, primary reticulosarcoma of bone, multiple myeloma, metastasis of undifferentiated carcinoma, or neuroblastoma, present sufficient difficulties in differential diagnosis even with paraffin sections and reason that the difficulties are even greater in the case of frozen sections. Indeed, local conditions and experience and the degree of mutual confidence of clinicians and pathologists must necessarily control the practice adopted in any institution.

II. Needle or Aspiration Biopsy

There has been much discussion of the value of this method of diagnosing bone lesions, one of the main objections being the relative degree of confidence inspired by a diagnosis based on very small particles of tissue.

Experimental work and daily practice in thousands of cases have shown the method to be harmless and the results highly satisfactory in experienced hands and under x-ray control (SCHAJOWICZ and DERQUI, 1968).

E. Value and Limitations of Histochemistry in the Study of Bone Tumors

The study of the histochemical distribution of different substances, including a large number of enzymes, has been intensified during the last years. Nevertheless, its application is still limited, and a huge field remains open for future investigations.

The histochemical studies have been very important in helping to resolve some histogenetic problems, more specifically the high enzymatic activity of osteoclasts, and to show the identical histochemical behavior of giant cells in osteoclastoma, in other giant-cell lesions of bone (so-called variants of giant-cell tumor), and in normal osteoclasts, thus establishing a histogenetic relationship between these histologic elements.

The study of the polysaccharide glycogen also permitted the demonstration of similar behavior for the tumor cells in epiphyseal (benign) chondroblastoma and in chondromyxoid fibroma. The cells from both are rich in this substance.

Not only has histochemistry contributed to our understanding of normal and pathologic ossification, but the *diagnostic value* of some of these more sophisticated procedures cannot be overemphasized. The discovery of abundant cytoplasmic glycogen granules in Ewing's sarcoma and their absence in primary reticulum cell sarcoma of bone (SCHAJOWICZ, 1959) provides an important and simple method of differential diagnosis; the presence of obvious alkaline phosphatase activity makes it possible to detect foci of osteogenesis (osteoblastic activity) which otherwise are difficult to demonstrate with the ordinary technique; in this way hyalinized connective tissue and cartilage can be differentiated from osteoid. Chordomas and mucous-secreting carcinomas are often very difficult to differentiate with H & E stains; the use of a simple PAS stain permits an easy differential diagnosis showing the presence of abundant cytoplasmatic glycogen granules in chordoma and the existence of mucoproteins resistent to ptyalin digestion in metastic mucous-secreting carcinomas.

F. Electron Microscopy

Although electron microscopy has been helpful in resolving some histogenetic problems, at present its routine use in the diagnosis of tumors has been of little practical value. Sometimes it may help with the decision in cases of a difficult diagnosis—for example, in "round cell" sarcomas, by easily showing abundant cytoplasmic glycogen in Ewing's sarcoma and its absence in reticulosarcoma and metastatic neuroblastoma, and the presence of neurofilaments and intracellulary catecholamines in neuroblastoma. Electron microscopy has been of value, too, in establishing the nature of some tumors, confirming identical ultrastructural features of giant-cells in giant-cell tumors and osteoclasts, the notochordal origin of chordoma, and that at least some "adamantinomas" of long bones are of epithelial origin. It is possible that further advances may resolve other still disputed problems in this difficult field of bone pathology.

G. Classification and Nomenclature of Bone Tumors

One of the main reasons for the prevailing confusion and difficulties in understanding skeletal tumors is the lack of a common terminology and, above all, of a classification that is sufficiently complete to cover the different histologic types and, at the same time, simple enough to be easily applied and understood by clinicians and pathologists. This is largely due to the inadequacy of our knowledge of the embryology and histogenesis of normal bone tissue and its possible blastomatous anomalies.

For this reason nearly all authors proposing new classifications admit that they must be considered provisional until new biologic and clinical knowledge confirms or modifies the ideas on which they are based. The classifications proposed and used in the various scientific centers are extremely numerous. There is hardly a country which has not adopted and proposed one or more classifications of its own based on the various possible criteria.

Some schemes for the classification of bone tumors have been based on histogenetic or embryogenetic concepts (Geschickter and Copeland, Jaffe, Lichtenstein, Lent Johnson, and others), despite the fact that the knowledge of the histogenesis, as stated above, is incomplete and possibly misleading. The other criteria, with a view to practical utility, and which, in our opinion, is more simple, is based on the application of morphohistologic features, particularly the type of differentiation showed by the tumor cells and the type of intercellular material that they produce.

The World Health Organization, interested in the establishment of internationally accepted classifications which would enable cancer workers in all parts of the world to compare their findings and which would facilitate collaboration among them, organized since 1958 more than 20 International Reference Centers covering almost all different tumor types.

The WHO International Reference Center (IRC) for the Histological Definition and Classification of Bone Tumors was established in 1963 at the Osteo-Articular Pathology Center, Italian Hospital, Buenos Aires, Argentina. Under my direction the IRC prepared and distributed material (clinical information, radiographs, and microscopic slides) from selected cases to seven Collaborating Centers for histologic typing according to a tentative classification previously established by a group of experts at a meeting in Geneva in 1963.

In all, 350 cases were thus studied by these centers and were reviewed at meetings held in 1967 and 1969 and attended by the heads of the centers. The classification was later reviewed by eight other pathologists who had been designated by WHO, and the final version was then adopted. This classification, and the definitions and explanatory notes that accompany it with color photographs and radiographs, was published in 1972 by WHO (Histological Typing of Bone Tumors). It is based, as stated above, simply on histologic criteria, that is, on the recognizable product of the proliferating cells, because it allows a useful degree of prediction of the properties and behavior of the tumor concerned.

In most instances the tumors apparently arise from the type of tissue they produce, but such an assumption cannot always be proved as there are some neoplasms which are highly undifferentiated without showing any kind of tissue production, as, for example, Ewing's sarcoma, and which can only be classified by the site of its most probable origin, i.e., in the bone marrow.

The classification includes benign and malignant neoplasms primary in bone together with certain "tumorlike" lesions that are included because of their frequent clinical and histologic similarity to bone tumors, and because of uncertainty with regard to the neoplastic or nonneoplastic nature of some of them.

H. Histological Typing of Primary Bone Tumors and Tumorlike Lesions (WHO)

I. *Bone-Forming Tumors*
  A. Benign
    1. Osteoma
    2. Osteoid osteoma and osteoblastoma (benign osteoblastoma)
  B. Malignant
    1. Osteosarcoma (osteogenic sarcoma)
    2. Juxtacortical osteosarcoma (parosteal osteosarcoma)

II. *Cartilage-Forming Tumors*
  A. Benign
    1. Chondroma
    2. Osteochondroma (osteocartilaginous exostosis)
    3. Chondroblastoma (benign chondroblastoma, epiphyseal chondroblastoma)
    4. Chondromyxoid fibroma
  B. Malignant
    1. Chondrosarcoma
    2. Juxtacortical chondrosarcoma
    3. Mesenchymal chondrosarcoma

III. *Giant-Cell Tumor (Osteoclastoma)*

IV. *Marrow Tumors*
    1. Ewing's sarcoma
    2. Reticulosarcoma of bone
    3. Lymphosarcoma of bone
    4. Myeloma

V. *Vascular Tumors*
  A. Benign
    1. Hemangioma
    2. Lymphangioma
    3. Glomus tumor (glomangioma)
  B. Intermediate or Indeterminate
    1. Hemangioendothelioma
    2. Hemangiopericytoma
  C. Malignant
    1. Angiosarcoma

VI. *Other Connective Tissue Tumors*
  A. Benign
    1. Desmoplastic fibroma
    2. Lipoma
  B. Malignant
    1. Fibrosarcoma
    2. Liposarcoma
    3. Malignant mesenchymoma
    4. Undifferentiated sarcoma

VII. *Other Tumors*
    1. Chordoma
    2. "Adamantinoma" of long bones
    3. Neurilemmoma (schwannoma, neurinoma)
    4. Neurofibroma

VIII. *Unclassified Tumors*

IX. *Tumorlike Lesions*
    1. Solitary bone cyst (simple or unicameral bone cyst)
    2. Aneurysmal bone cyst
    3. Juxta-articular bone cyst (intraosseous ganglion)
    4. Metaphyseal fibrous defect (nonossifying fibroma)
    5. Eosinophilic granuloma
    6. Fibrous dysplasia
    7. "Myositis ossificans"
    8. "Brown tumor" of hyperparathyroidism

References

Bone-Forming Tumors
(Benign and Malignant)

Barry, H.C.: Paget's disease of bone. Edinburgh: E.&S. Livinstone, 1969

Byers, P.D.: Solitary benign osteoblastic lesions of bone — Osteoid osteoma and benign osteoblastoma. Cancer (Philad.) **22**, 43–57 (1968)

Collins, D.H.: Paget's disease of bone. Incidence and subclinical forms. Lancet **2**, 51–57 (1956)

Dahlin, D.C., Coventry, M.B.: Osteogenic sarcoma; a study of six hundred cases. J. Bone Jt Surg. **49A**, 101–110 (1967)

Dahlin, D.C., Johnson, E.W., Jr.: Giant osteoid osteoma. J. Bone Jt Surg. **36A**, 559–572 (1954)

D'Aubigné, R.M., Meary, R., Mazabraud, A.: Sarcome osteogenique juxtacortical. Rev. Chir. orthop. **45**, 873–884 (1959)

Davidson, J.W., Chacha, P.B., James, W.: Multiple osteosarcomata. J. Bone Jt Surg. **47B**, 537–541 (1965)

Dwinnell, L.A., Dahlin, D.C., Ghormley, R.K.: Parosteal (Juxtacortical) osteogenic sarcoma. J. Bone Jt Surg. **36A**, 732–744 (1954)

Fine, G., Stout, A.P.: Osteogenic sarcoma of the extraskeletal soft tissues. Cancer (Philad.) **9**, 1027–1043 (1956)

Fitzgerald, D.D., Dahlin, D.C., Sim, M.D.: Metachronous osteogenic sarcoma. Report of twelve cases with two long-term survivors. J. Bone Jt Surg. **55-A**, No. 3, 595–605, 1973

Freiberger, R.H., Loitman, B.S., Halpern, M., Thompson, T.C.: Osteoid osteoma. A report of 80 cases. Amer. J. Roentgenol. **82**, 194–205 (1959)

Jaffe, H.L.: Osteoid osteoma: A benign osteoblastic tumor composed of osteoid and atypical bone. Arch. Surg. (Chicago) **31**, 709–728 (1935)

Jaffe, H.L.: Benign osteoblastoma. Bull. Hosp. Jt Dis. (N.Y.) **17**, 141–151 (1956)

Lichtenstein, L., Sawyer, W.R.: Benign osteoblastoma. Further observations and report of 20 additional cases. J. Bone Jt Surg. **46A**, 755–765 (1964)

Lindbom, A., Söderberg, G., Spjut, H.L.: Osteosarcoma. Review of 96 cases. Acta radiol. (Stockh.) **56**, 1–19 (1961)

McKenna, R.J., Schwinn, C.P., Soong, K.Y., Higinbotham, N.L.: Osteogenic sarcoma arising in Paget's disease. Cancer (Philad.) **17**, 42–66 (1964)

McKenna, R.J., Schwinn, C.P., Soong, K.Y., Higinbotham, N.L.: Sarcomata of the osteogenic series (osteosarcoma, fibrosarcoma, chondrosarcoma, parosteal osteogenic sarcoma, and sarcomata arising in abnormal bone): An analysis of 552 cases. J. Bone Jt Surg. **48A**, 1–26 (1966)

O'Hara, J.M., Hutter, R.P.V., Foote, F.W., Miller, T., Woodard, H.Q.: An analysis of thirty patients surviving longer than ten years after treatment from osteogenic sarcoma. J. Bone Jt Surg. **50A**, 335–354 (1968)

Porretta, C.A., Dahlin, D.C., James, J.M.: Sarcoma in Paget's disease of bone. J. Bone Jt Surg. **39A**, 1314–1329 (1957)

Price, C.H.G.: The prognosis of osteosarcoma. Brit. J. Radiol. **39**, 181 (1966)

Price, C.H.G., Goldie, W.: Paget's sarcoma of bone: A study of 80 cases. J. Bone Jt Surg. **51B**, 205–224 (1969)

Scaglietti, O., Calandriello, B.: Ossifying parosteal sarcoma: parosteal osteoma or juxtacortical osteogenic sarcoma. J. Bone Jt Surg. **44A**, 635–647 (1962)

Schajowicz, F., Lemos, C.: Osteoid osteoma and osteoblastoma closely related entities of osteoblastic derivation. Acta orthop. scand. **41**, 272–291 (1970)

Schajowicz, F., Slullitel, I.: Giant cell tumor associated with Paget's disease. J. Bone Jt Surg. **48A**, 1340–1349 (1966)

Schajowicz, F., Lemos, C.: Malignant osteoblastoma. J. Bone Jt. Surg. **58B**, 202–211 (1976)

Sim, F., Cupps, R., Dahlin, D., Ivins, J.M.D.: Postradiation sarcoma of bone. J. Bone Jt Surg. **54-A**, 1479–1489 (1972)

Sweetnam, R.M.D.: Amputation in osteosarcoma. J. Bone Jt Surg. **55-B**, 189–192 (1973)

Cartlage-Forming Tumors
(Benign and Malignant)

Barnes, R., Catto, M.: Chondrosarcoma of bone. J. Bone Jt Surg. **48B**, 729–764 (1966)

Bethge, J.F.J.: Hereditäre multiple Exostosen und ihre pathogenetische Deutung. Arch. orthop. Unfall-Chir. **54**, 667–696 (1963)

Codman, E.A.: Epiphyseal chondromatous giant cell tumors of the upper end of the humerus. Surg. Gynec. Obstet. **52**, 543–548 (1931)

Dahlin, D.C.: Chondromyxoid fibroma of bone with emphasis on its morphological relationship to benign chondroblastoma. Cancer (Philad.) **9**, 195–203 (1956)

Dahlin, D.C., Henderson, E.D.: Mesenchymal chondrosarcoma: further observations on a new entity. Cancer (Philad.) **15**, 410–417 (1962)

Ehrenfried, A.: Multiple cartilaginous exostoses, hereditary deforming chondrodysplasia. J. Amer. med. Ass. **64**, 1642–1646 (1915)

Fairbank, H.A.T.: Dyschondroplasia. Synonyms: Ollier's disease, multiple enchondroma. J. Bone Jt Surg. **30B**, 689–708 (1948)

Goldman, R.L.: Mesenchymal chondrosarcoma, a rare malignant chondroid tumor usually primary in bone. Report of a case arising in extraskeletal soft tissue. Cancer (Philad.), vol. 20, 1494–1498 (1967)

HENDERSON, E.D., DAHLIN, D.C.: Chondrosarcoma of bone. A study of two hundred and eighty-eight cases. J. Bone Jt Surg. 45A, 1450–1458 (1963)

HUVOS, A., MARCOVE, R., ERLANDSON, R., MIKE, M.D.: Chondroblastoma of bone. Cancer (Philad.) 29, No. 3, 760–771 (1972)

JAFFE, H.H.: Juxtacortical chondroma. Bull Hosp. Jt Dis. (N.Y.) 17, 20–29 (1956)

JAFFE, H.L.: Hereditary multiple exostosis. Arch. Path. (Chicago) 36, 335–357 (1943)

JAFFE, H.L., LICHTENSTEIN, L.: Benign chondroblastoma of bone: A reinterpretation of the so-called calcifying or chondromatous giant cell tumor. Amer. J. Path. 18, 969–992 (1942)

JAFFE, H.L., LICHTENSTEIN, L.: Chondromyxoid fibroma of bone: A distinctive benign tumor, likely to be mistaken especially for chondrosarcoma. Arch. Path. (Chicago) 45, 541–551 (1948)

KAHN, L.B., WOOD, F.M., ACKERMAN, L.V.: Malignant chondroblastoma. Report of two cases and review of the literature. Arch. Path. (Chicago) 88, 371–376 (1969)

LEVINE, G., BENSCH, K.M.D.: Chondroblastoma — the nature of the basic cell. A study by means of histochemistry, tissue culture, electron microscopy and autoradiography. Cancer (Philad.) 29, 1546–1562 (1972)

LICHTENSTEIN, L., HALL, J.E.: Periosteal chondroma: A distinctive benign cartilage tumor. J. Bone Jt Surg. 34A, 691–697 (1952)

LICHTENSTEIN, L., BERNSTEIN, D.: Unusual benign and malignant chondroid tumors of bone. Cancer (Philad.) 12, 1142–1157 (1959)

MARCOVE, R.C., KAMBOLIS, C., BULLOUGH, P.G., JAFFE, H.L.: Fibromyxoma of bone. A report of three cases. Cancer (Philad.) 17, 1209–1213 (1964)

MERLINO, A.F., NIXON, J.E.: Periosteal chondroma. Amer. J. Surg. 107, 773–776 (1964)

NOSANCHUC, J.K., KAUFER, H.: Recurrent periosteal chondroma. Report of two cases and review of the literature. J. Bone Jt Surg. 51A, 375–380 (1969)

RALPH, L.L.: Chondromyxoid fibroma of bone. J. Bone Jt Surg. 44B, 7–24 (1962)

ROCKWELL, M., SAITER, E., ENNEKING, W.M.D.,: Periosteal chondroma. J. Bone Jt Surg. 54A, 102–108 (1972)

SCHAJOWICZ, F., GALLARDO, H.: Epiphyseal chondroblastoma of bone. A clinico-pathological study of 69 cases. J. Bone Jt Surg. 52B, 205–226 (1970)

SCHAJOWICZ, F., GALLARDO, H.: Chondromyxoid fibroma (fibromyxoid chondroma) of bone. Clinico-pathological study of 32 cases. J. Bone Jt Surg. 53B, 198–216 (1971)

TAKIGAWA, K.M.D.: Chondroma of the bones of the hand. A review of 110 cases. J. Bone Jt Surg. 53A, 1591–1600 (1971)

TIWISINA, T.: Dyschondroplasia (Ollier) mit multiplen Hämangiomen und örtlicher maligner Entartung (Chondrosarkom). Beitr. klin. Chir. 88, 8–15 (1954)

Giant Cell Tumor
(Osteoclastoma)

DAHLIN, D.C., CUPPS, R.E., JOHNSON, E.W., JR.: Giant cell tumor. A study of 195 cases. Cancer (Philad.) 25, 1061 (1970)

HUTTER, R.V.P., WORCESTER, J.N., JR., FRANCIS, K.C., FOOTE, F.W., JR., STEWART, F.W.: Benign and malignant giant cell tumors of bone. A clinicopathological analysis of the natural history of the disease. Cancer (Philad.) 15, 653–690 (1962)

JAFFE, H.L., LICHTENSTEIN, L., PORTIS, R.B.: Giant cell tumor of bone: Its pathologic appearance, grading, supposed variants, and treatment. Arch. Path. (Chicago) 30, 993–1031 (1940)

JEWELL, J.H., BUSH, L.F.: Benign giant cell tumor of bone with a solitary pulmonary metastasis. A case report. J. Bone Jt Surg. 46A, 848–852 (1964)

MNAYMNEH, W.A., DUDLEY, H.R., MNAYMENH, L.G.: Giant cell tumor of bone: An analysis and follow-up study of the forty-one cases observed at the Massachusetts General Hospital between 1925 and 1960. J. Bone Jt Surg. 46A, 63–75 (1964)

MURPHY, W.R., ACKERMAN, L.V.: Benign and malignant giant-cell tumors of bone. A clinical-pathological evaluation of thirty-one cases. Cancer (Philad.) 9, 317–339 (1956)

PAN, P., DAHLIN, D.C., LIPSCOMB, P.R., BERNATZ, P.E.: Benign giant cell tumor of the radius with pulmonary metastasis. Proc. Mayo Clin. 39, 344–349 (1964)

SCHAJOWICZ, F.: Giant-cell tumors of bone (Osteoclastoma). A pathological and histochemical study. J. Bone Jt Surg. 43A, 1–29 (1961)

THOMSON, A.D., TURNER-WARWICK, R.T.: Skeletal sarcomata and giant-cell tumour. J. Bone Jt Surg. 37B, 226–303 (1955)

Marrow Tumors

BERGSAGELD, E.M.D.: Plasma cell myeloma. An interpretative review. Cancer (Philad.) 30, No. 6, 1588–1594 (1972)

BETHGE, J.F.J.: Die Ewingtumoren oder Omoblastome des Knochens. Differentialdiagnostische und kritische Erörterungen. Ergebn. Chir. Orthop. 39, 327–425 (1955)

BROWN, T.S., PATERSON, C.R., M.D.: Osteosclerosis in myeloma. J. Bone Jt Surg. 55-B, 621–623 (1973)

CARSON, C.P., ACKERMAN, L.V., MALTBY, J.D.: Plasma cell myeloma: A clinical, pathologic, and roentgenologic review of 90 cases. Amer. J. clin. Path. 25, 849–888 (1955)

DAHLIN, D.C., DOCKERTY, M.B.: Amyloid and myeloma. Amer. J. Path. 26, 581–593 (1950)

DAHLIN, D.C., COVENTRY, M.D., SCANLON, P.W.:

Ewing's sarcoma. A critical analysis of 165 cases. J. Bone Jt Surg. **43A**, 185–192 (1961)

EDEIKEN, J., HODES, P.J.: Reticulum cell sarcoma (primary of bone). In: Roentgen diagnosis of diseases of bone, pp. 605–615. Baltimore: The Williams & Wilkins Company, 1967

FRANCIS, K.C., HIGINBOTHAM, N.L., COLEY, B.L.: Primary reticulum cell sarcoma of bone; Report of 44 cases. Surg. Gynec. Obstet. **99**, 143–146 (1954)

FRIEDMAN, B., HANOAKA, H.: Round cell sarcoma of bone. A light and electron microscopic study. J. Bone Jt Surg. **53A**, 1118–1136 (1971)

GITLOW, S.E., BERTANI, L.M., RAUSEN, A., GRIBETZ, D., DZIEDZIG, S.W.: Diagnosis of neuroblastoma by qualitative and quantitative determination of catecholamine metabolites in urine. Cancer (Philad.) **25**, 1377–1383 (1970)

HOU-JENSEN, K., PRIORI, E., DMOCHOWSKI, L.: Studies on ultrastructure of Ewing's sarcoma of bone. Cancer (Philad.) **29**, No. 2, 280–286 (1972)

IVINS, J.C., DAHLIN, D.C.: Malignant lymphoma (reticulum cell sarcoma) of bone. Proc. Mayo Clin. **38**, 375–385 (1963)

McCORMACK, L.J., IVINS, J.C., DAHLIN, D.C., JOHNSON, E.W., JR.: Primary reticulum-cell sarcoma of bone. Cancer (Philad.) **5**, 1182–1192 (1952)

OSSERMAN, E.F., TAKATSUI, K.: Plasma cell myeloma: Gamma globulin synthesis and structure. A review of biochemical and clinical data, with description of a newly recognized and related syndrome. "H-Gamma-2-Chain (Franklin's) disease." Medicine **42**, 385 (1963)

PARKER, F., JR., JACKSON, H., JR.: Primary reticulum cell sarcoma of bone. Surg. Gynec. Obstet. **68**, 45–53 (1939)

PASMANTIER, M.W., AZAR, H.A.: Extraskeletal spread in multiple myeloma. A review of 57 autopsied cases. Cancer (Philad.) **23**, 167–174 (1969)

SCHAJOWICZ, F.: Ewing's sarcoma and reticulum cell sarcoma of bone: with special reference to the histochemical demonstration of glycogen as an aid to differential diagnosis. J. Bone Jt Surg. **41A**, 349–356 (1959)

SHOJI, H., MILLER, T.M.D.: Primary reticulum cell sarcoma of bone. Cancer (Philad.) **8**, 1234–1244 (1971)

SNAPPER, I., TURNER, L.B., MOSCOVITZ, H.L.: Multiple myeloma. New York: Grune and Stratten 1953

STEINER, P.E.: Hodgkin's disease; the incidence, distribution, nature and possible significance of the lymphogranulomatous lesions in the bone marrow. Arch. Path. (Chicago) **36**, 627–637 (1943)

UEHLINGER, E., BOTSZTEJN, CH., SCHINZ, H.R.: Ewingsarkom und Knochenretikulosarkom: Klinik, Diagnose und Differentialdiagnose. Oncologia (Basel) **1**, 193–245 (1948)

VALDERRAMA, J.A., BULLOUGH, P.C.: Solitary myeloma of the spine. J. Bone Jt Surg. **50B**, 82–90 (1968)

WALDENSTROM, J.: The incidence and cytology of different myeloma types. Lancet **1**, 1147 (1961)

WRIGHT, C.J.: Long survival in solitary plasmocytoma of bone. J. Bone Jt Surg. **43B**, 467 (1961)

Vascular Tumors
(Benign and Malignant)

COHEN, J., CRAIG, J.M.: Multiple lymphangiectases of bone. J. Bone Jt Surg. **37A**, 585–596 (1955)

DORFMAN, H.D., STEINER, G.C., JAFFE, H.L.: Vascular tumors of bone. Hum. Path. **2**, 349–376 (1971)

FALKMER, S., TILLING, G.: Primary lymphangioma of bone. Acta orthop. scand. **26**, 99 (1956)

GOIDANICH, I.F., CAMPANACCI, M.: Vascular hamartomata and infantile angioectatic osteohyperplasia of the extremites. A study of 94 cases. J. Bone Jt Surg. **44A**, 815 (1962)

GORHAM, L.W., STOUT, A.P.: Massive osteolysis (acute spontaneous absorption of bone, phantom bone, disappearing bone). Its relation to hemangiomatosis. J. Bone Jt Surg. **37A**, 985–1004 (1955)

HARTMANN, W.H., STEWART, F.W.: Hemangioendothelioma of bone. Unusual tumor characterized by indolent course. Cancer (Philad.) **15**, 846–854 (1962)

LATTES, R., BULL, D.C.: A case of glomus tumor with primary involvement of bone. Ann. Surg. **127**, 187–191 (1948)

LIDHOLM, S.O., LINDBOM, A., SPJUT, H.J.: Multiple capillary hemangiomas of the bones of the foot. Acta path. **51**, 9–16 (1961)

MARCIAL ROJAS, R.A.: Primary hemangiopericytoma of bone. Review of the literature and report of the first case with metastases. Cancer (Philad.) **13**, 308–313 (1960)

MORGENSTERN, P., WESTING, S.W.: Malignant hemangioendothelioma of bone. Cancer (Philad.) **23**, 221–224 (1969)

OTIS, J., HUNTER, R.V.P., FOOTE, F.W., MARCOVE, R.C., STEWARTT, W.: Haemangioendothelioma of bone. Surg. Gynec. Obstet. **127**, 295–305 (1968)

ROSENQUIST, C.J., WOLFE, D.C.: Lymphangioma of bone. J. Bone Jt Surg. **50A**, 158–162 (1968)

SECKLER, S.G., RUBIN, H., RABINOWITZ, J.G.: Systemic cystic angiomatosis. Amer. J. Med. **37**, 976–986 (1964)

SHERMAN, R.S., WILNER, D.: The roentgen diagnosis of hemangioma of bone. Amer. J. Roentgenol. **86**, 1146–1159 (1961)

THOMAS, A.: Vascular tumors of bone: A pathological and clinical study of 27 cases. Surg. Gynec. Obstet. **74**, 777–795 (1942)

UNNI, K.K., IVINS, J.C., BEABOUT, J.W., DAHLIN, D.C.: Hemangioma, hemangiopericytoma and hemangioendothelioma of bone. Cancer (Philad.) **27**, 1403–1414 (1971)

Other Connective Tissue Tumors (Benign and Malignant)

CATTO, M., STEVENS, J.: Liposarcoma of bone. J. Path. Bact. **86**, 248–253 (1963)

CUNNINGHAM, M.P., ARLEN, MYRON: Medullary fibrosarcoma of bone. Cancer (Philad.) **21**, 31–37 (1968)

DAHLIN, D.C., HOOVER, N.W.: Desmoplastic fibroma of bone. Report of two cases. J. Amer. med. Ass. **188**, 685–687 (1964)

DAHLIN, D.C., IVES, J.C.: Fibrosarcoma of bone. A study of 114 cases. Cancer (Philad.) **23**, 35–41 (1969)

DAWSON, E.K.: Liposarcoma of bone. J. Path. Bact. **70**, 513 (1955)

EYRE-BROOK, A.L., PRICE, C.H.G.: Fibrosarcoma of bone. Review of 50 consecutive cases from the Bristol bone tumor registry. J. Bone Jt Surg. **51B**, 20–37 (1969)

GILMER, W.S., JR., MACEWVEN, G.D.: Central (medullary) fibrosarcoma of bone. J. Bone Jt Surg. **40A**, 121 (1958)

GOLDMAN, R.L.: Primary liposarcoma of bone. Report of a case. Amer. J. clin. Path. **42**, 503–508 (1964)

HART, J.M.D.: Intraosseous lipoma. J. Bone Jt Surg. **55-B**, 624–632 (1973)

HUTTER, R.V.P., FOOTE, F.W., FRANCIS, K.C., SHERMAN, R.S.: Primitive multipotential primary sarcoma of bone. Cancer (Philad.) **19**, 1–25 (1966)

RABHAN, W.N., ROSAI, J.: Desmoplastic fibroma. Report of 10 cases and review of the literature. J. Bone Jt Surg. **50A**, 487–502 (1968)

RETZ, L.D.: Primary liposarcoma of bone. Report of a case and review of the literature. J. Bone Jt Surg. **43A**, 123–129 (1961)

ROSS, O.F., HADFIELD, G.: Primary osteo-liposarcoma of bone (Malignant mesenchymoma). Report of a case. J. Bone Jt Surg. **50B**, 639–643 (1968)

SCHAJOWICZ, F., CUEVILLAS, A.R., SILBERMAN, F.S.: Primary malignant mesenchymoma of bone. Cancer (Philad.) **19**, 1423–1428 (1966)

SMITH, W.E., FIENBERG, R.: Intraosseous lipoma of bone. Cancer (Philad.) **10**, 1151–1152 (1957)

Neurogenic Tumors

DESANTO, D.A., BURGESS, E.: Primary and secondary neurilemmoma of bone. Surg. Gynec. Obstet. **71**, 454–461 (1940)

GROSS, P., BAILEY, F.R., JACOX, H.W.: Primary intramedullary neurofibroma of the humerus. Arch. Path. (Chicago) **28**, 716–718 (1939)

HART, M.S., BASCOM, W.C.: Neurilemmoma involving bone. J. Bone Jt Surg. **40A**, 465–468 (1958)

SAMTER, T.G., VELLIOS, F., SHAFER, W.G.: Neurilemmoma of bone. Report of 3 cases with a review of the literature. Radiology **75**, 215–222 (1960)

Other Tumors

CHANGUS, G.W., SPEED, J.S., STEWART, F.W.: Malignant angioblastoma of bone. A reappraisal of adamantinoma of long bone. Cancer (Philad.) **10**, 540–559 (1957)

DAHLIN, D.C., MACCARTY, C.S.: Chordoma: a study of fifty-nine cases. Cancer (Philad.) **5**, 1170–1178 (1952)

GLOOR, F.: Das sogenannte Adamantinom der langen Röhrenknochen. Virchows Arch. path. Anat. **336**, 489–502 (1963)

HEFFELFINGER, J., DAHLIN, D., MACCARTY, C.S., BEABUT, M.D.: Chordomas and cartilaginous tumors at the skull base. Cancer (Philad.) **32**, No. 2, 410–420 (1973)

HICKS, J.D.: Synovial sarcoma of tibia. J. Path. Bact. **67**, 151 (1954)

HIGINBOTHAM, N.L., PHILLIPS, R.F., HOLLON, F.W., HUSTU, H.O.: Chordoma. Thirty-five year study at Memorial Hospital. Cancer (Philad.) **20**, 1841–1850 (1967)

LEDERER, H., SINCLAIR, A.J.: Malignant synovioma simulating adamantinoma of the tibia. J. Path. Bact. **67**, 167–168 (1954)

MACCARTY, C.S., WAUGH, J.M., COVENTRY, M.B., O'SULLIVAN, D.C.: Sacrococcygeal chordomas. Surg. Gynec. Obstet. **113**, 551–554 (1961)

MOON, N.E.: Adamantinoma of the appendicular skeleton. Clin. Orthop. **43**, 189–213 (1965)

OTTOLENGHI, C.E., SCHAJOWICZ, F., RAFFA, D.: Le kyste osseus essentiel uniloculaire. Etude clinique et anatompathologique de 123 cas. Rev. Chir. orthop. **55**, 287–303 (1964)

SCHAJOWICZ, F., SLULLITEL, J.: Eosinophilic granuloma of bone and its relationship to Hand-Schuller-Christian and Letterer-Siwe syndromes. J. Bone Jt Surg. **55-B**, No. 3, 545–565 (1973)

TILLMAN, B.P., DAHLIN, D.C., LIPSCOMB, P.R., STEWART, J.R.: Aneurysmal bone cyst: An analysis of 95 cases. Mayo Clin. Proc. **43**, 478–495 (1968)

Electron Microscopy

ALBORES-SAAVEDRA, J., DIAZ-GUTIERREZ, D., ALTAMIRANO-DIMAS, M.: Adamantinoma de la Tibia. Observaciones Ultraestructurales. Rev. med. Hosp. gen. Mex. **31**, 241–252 (1968)

FRIEDMAN, B., GOLD, H.: Ultrastructure of Ewing's sarcoma of bone. Cancer (Philad.) **22**, 307–322 (1968)

GHADIALLY, F.N., MEHTA, P.N.: Ultrastructure of osteogenic sarcoma. Cancer (Philad.), **25**, 1457–1467 (1970)

HANOAKA, H., FRIEDMAN, B., MACK, R.P.: Ultrastructure and histogenesis of giant cell tumor of bone. Cancer (Philad.), **19**, 1408–1423 (1970)

Kempson, R.L.: Ossifying fibroma of the long bones. A light and electron microscopic study. Arch. Path. (Chicago) **82**, 218–233 (1966)

Maldonado, J.E., Brown, A.L., Jr., Bayrd, E.D., Pease, G.L.: Ultrastructure of the myeloma cell. Cancer (Philad.) **19**, 1613–1627 (1966)

Murad, T.M., Narasimha Murthy, M.S.: Ultrastructure of a chordoma. Cancer (Philad.) **25**, 1204 (1970)

Rosai, J.: Adamantinoma of the tibia. Amer. J. clin. Path. **51**, 786–792 (1969)

Schajowicz, F., Cabrini, R.L., Simes, R.J., Klein-Szanto, A.J.P.: Ultrastructure of Chondrosarcoma. Clinical Orthopaedics and Related Research **100**, 378–386 (1974)

Spjut, H.J., Luse, S.A.: Chordoma: An electron microscopic study. Cancer (Philad.) **17**, 643–656 (1964)

Ueno, L.: Electron microscopic observations of giant cell tumors of bone. J. Jap. orthop. Ass. **38**, 724–725 (1964)

Wellmann, K.E.: Chondroblastoma of the scapula. A case report with ultrastructural observations. Cancer (Philad.) **24**, 408–416 (1969)

Welsh, R.A., Meyer, A.T.: A histogenetic study of chondroblastoma. Cancer (Philad.) **17**, 578–584 (1964)

General References

Aegerter, E., Kirkpatrick, J.A., Jr.: Orthopedic, diseases, physiology, pathology, radiology. 3rd ed., W.B. Saunders Co., Philadelphia 1968

Coley, B.L.: Neoplasms of bone and related conditions: Their etiology, pathogenesis, diagnosis, and treatment. New York: Paul B. Hoeber, Inc. 1949

Dahlin, D.C.: Bone tumors, 2nd Ed., Springfield, Ill., Charles C Thomas 1967

Dominok, G.W., Knoch, H.G.: Knochengeschwülste und geschwulstähnliche Knochenerkrankungen. Jena: VEB Gustav Fischer 1971

Fairbanks, T.: An atlas of general affections of the skeleton. Edinburgh: E. & S. Livingstone, Ltd. 1951

Jaffe, H.L.: Tumors and tumorous conditions of the bones and joints. Philadelphia: Lea and Febiger 1958

Jeffree, G.M., Price, C.H.G.: Bone tumors and their enzymes. J. Bone Jt Surg. **47B**, 120 (1965)

Johnson, L.C.: A general theory of bone tumors. Bull. N.Y. Acad. Med. **29**, 164–171 (1953)

Lichtenstein, L.: Bone tumors. 4th Ed., Saint Louis: C.V. Mosby 1971

Mayer, L.: Malignant degeneration of so-called benign osteoblastoma. Bull. Hosp. Jt. Dis. **28**, 4–13 (1967)

Netherlands Committee on Bone Tumours: Radiological atlas of bone tumours, **1**. Baltimore: The Williams and Wilkins Co. 1966

Ottolenghi, C.E.: Diagnosis of orthopaedic lesions by aspiration biopsy. Results of 1,061 punctures. J. Bone Jt Surg. **37A**, 443–464 (1955)

Price, C.H.G., Ross, F.G.M.: Bone, certain aspects of neuplasia, Proceedings of the 24th Symposium of the Colston Research Society. London: Butterworths 1973

Radiological Atlas of Bone Tumours, Vol. I and II, Netherlands Committee on Bone Tumours (ed.). The Hague: Mouton & Co 1966 and 1973

Schajowicz, F., Ackerman, L.V., Sissons, H.A.: Histological typing of bone tumours. International histological classification of tumours. No. 6, World Health Organization, Geneva, 1972 (Bibliography)

Schajowicz, F., Cabrini, R.L.: Histochemical studies of bone in normal and pathological conditions (with special reference to alkaline phosphatase, glycogen and mucopolysaccharides. J. Bone Jt Surg. **36B**, 474 (1954)

Schajowicz, F., Derqui, J.C.: Puncture biopsy in lesions of the locomotor system; review of results in 4,050 cases, including 941 vertebral punctures. Cancer (Philad.) **21**, 531–548 (1968)

Schreyvogel, R.: Benignes Osteoblastom. Schweiz. med. Wschr. **98**, 1009–1013 (1968)

Spjut, H.J., Dorfman, H.D., Fechner, R.E., Ackerman, L.V.: Tumors of bone cartilage, Washington, D.C., Armed Forces Institute of Pathology (Atlas of Tumor Pathology, 2* series, fascicle 5) 1971

Uehlinger, E.: Die pathologische Anatomie der Knochengeschwülste. Helv. Chir. Acta **20**, 597 (1959); **40**, 5 (1973)

Uehlinger, E.: Pathologische Anatomie der Knochengeschwülste (unter besonderer Berücksichtigung der semimalignen Formen). Chirurg **45**, 62 (1974)

Radiologic Approach to Bone Tumors

by

George B. Greenfield

There are multiple factors to analyze and evaluate in approaching the diagnosis of bone tumors. The probability of the presence of a given lesion will depend upon the probability of these factors being associated with the given lesion, modified by the incidence of the given lesions at large (LODWICK, 1966). These factors, sometimes described as predictor variables, are as follows:

A. Location

The location of a lesion is of diagnostic significance with respect to which bone is involved, which portion is involved (epiphysis, metaphysis, diaphysis), and whether the lesion is central or eccentric, or involves the medulla, cortex, or periosteum.

Most primary tumors of bone, which occur during the adolescent growth spurt, have some predilection for the knee. These would involve the distal femur or proximal tibia. This could be explained by the theory of Lent C. Johnson. A tumor of a specific cell type tends to originate in the field of maximal activity of homologous normal cells (JOHNSON, 1953).

The location of the various tumors with respect to which bone is involved has been tabulated by DAHLIN for 3987 cases. The figures for tumors of osseous origin are reproduced (Figs. 1, 2, and 3) (DAHLIN, 1967).

Table 1. Preferential location of various tumors of bone

Epiphysis	Chondroblastoma
	Giant cell tumor, after fusion of growth plate
Metaphysis	Osteogenic sarcoma
	Parosteal sarcoma
	Chondrosarcoma
	Fibrosarcoma
	Nonossifying fibroma
	Giant cell tumor prior to fusion of growth plate
	Unicameral bone cyst (nonneoplastic)
Diaphysis	Myeloma
	Ewing's tumor
	Reticulum cell sarcoma

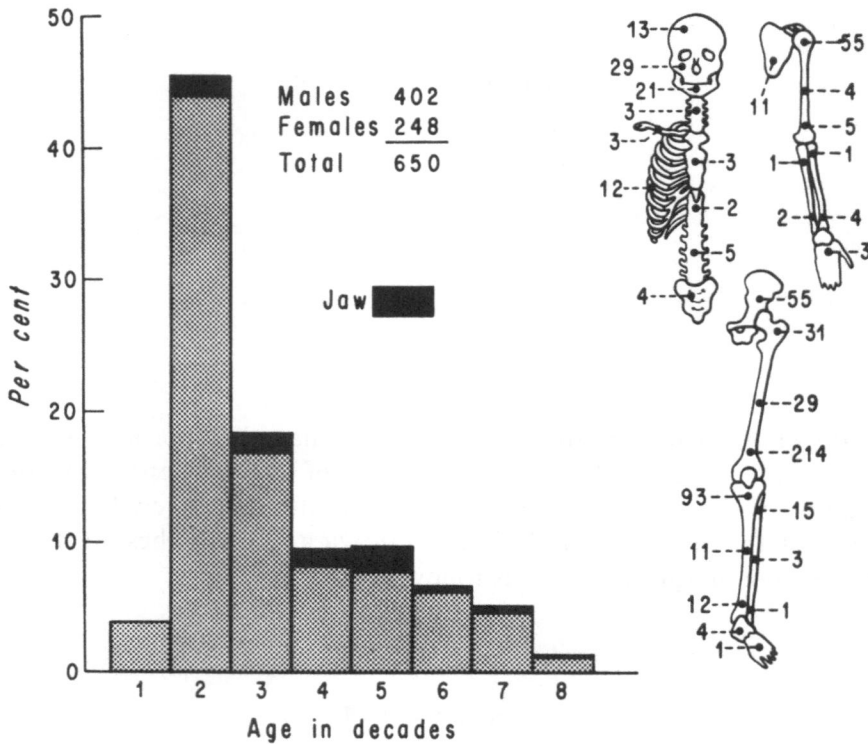

Fig. 1. Osteogenic sarcoma. (From DAHLIN, DAVID, C., Bone Tumors 2nd ed., 1967. Courtesy of CHARLES, C THOMAS, publisher, Springfield; Illinois)

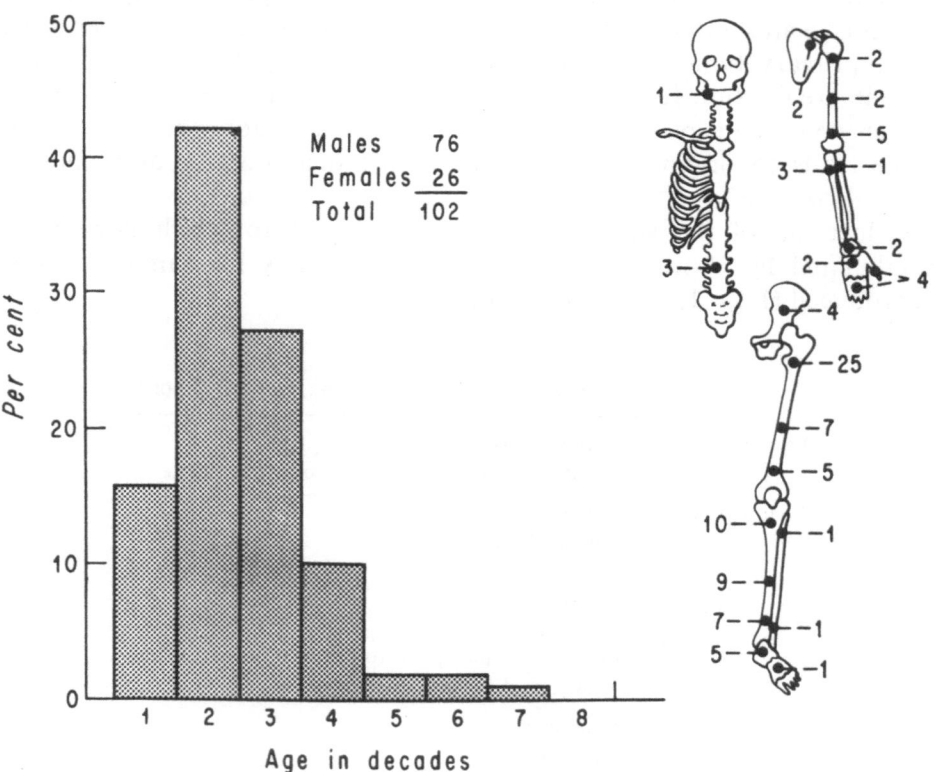

Fig. 2. Osteoid osteoma. (From DAHLIN, DAVID, C., Bone Tumors 2nd ed., 1967. Courtesy of CHARLES, C THOMAS, publisher, Springfield; Illinois)

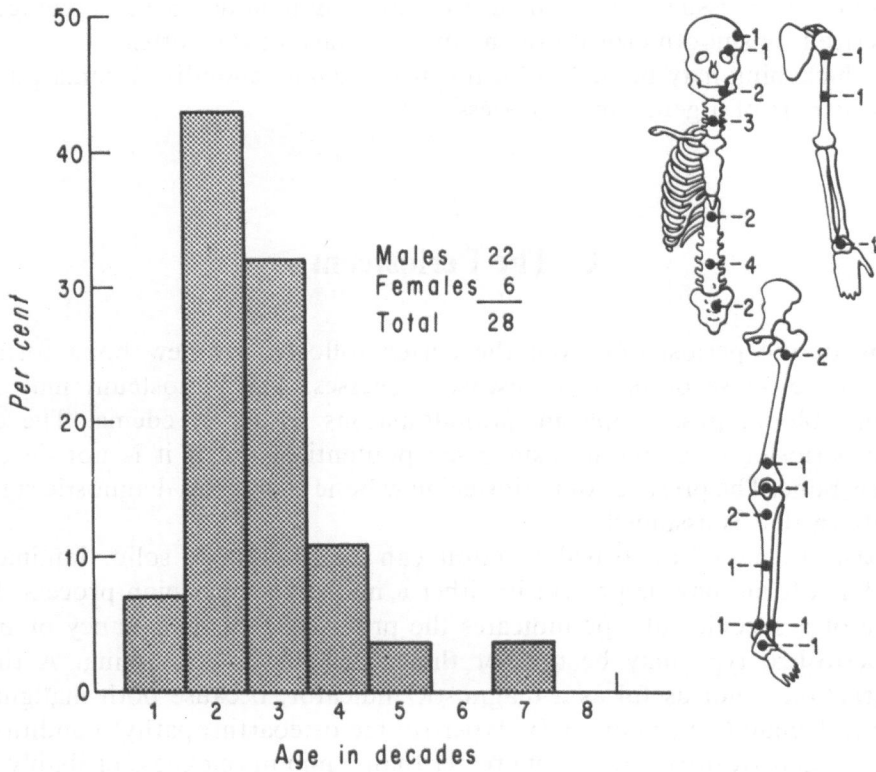

Fig. 3. Benign osteoblastoma. (From DAHLIN, DAVID, C., Bone Tumors 2nd ed., 1967. Courtesy of CHARLES, C THOMAS, publisher, Springfield; Illinois)

The location is also important with respect to which portion of a tubular bone is involved. The common tumors, with respect to typical epiphyseal, metaphyseal, or diaphyseal location are summarized in Table 1 (GREENFIELD, 1969).

The location of the lesion with respect to the central axis of bone is also of diagnostic significance. An osteosarcoma, other than a parosteal sarcoma, is typically centrally located. If the origin of the tumor can be localized to the periosteum, cortex, or medulla, another helpful parameter is introduced. An osteoid osteoma, for example, can originate at any of the above three sites. The roentgen picture is slightly different for each.

B. Cortex

The salient cortical changes with respect to bone lesions are destruction, erosion, and thickening.

Destruction of the cortex may be total or segmental in the area of involvement. A malignant tumor usually sweeps away the entire area of cortex, while a process such as osteomyelitis may leave intact segments in/between destroyed areas. An exception to this rule is Ewing's tumor. A very aggressive process may cause permeative cortical destruction.

Erosion of the cortex may be external or internal. External erosion results from pressure from a soft-tissue tumor, aneurysm, or lymph node. Several benign lesions are characterized by smooth erosion of the inner surface of the cortex.

Cortical thickening may be due to local causes such as chondrosarcoma and osteoid osteoma, or as part of a generalized process.

C. The Periosteum

Elevation of the periosteum from the cortex followed by new bone formation is a fundamental response of bone to disease processes. The periosteum may be lifted by any agent; blood, pus, neoplasm, granulomatous tissue, or edema. The cambium layer of the periosteum retains its osteogenic pontential, and if it is not destroyed, it will form new bone. The presence of periosteal new bone is of lesser diagnostic significance than the pattern that is assumed.

Three basic forms of periosteal reaction can be discerned: solid, laminated, and spiculated. Each form may be present in either a malignant or benign process, however, the presence of a specific subtype indicates the probability of malignancy or benignity. The solid periosteal type may be thin or thick, straight or undulating. A thin, solid periosteal reaction is not useful as a diagnostic indicator, because both malignant (e.g., leukemia) and benign (e.g., pulmonary hypertrophic osteoarthropathy) conditions cause this finding. Solid periosteal reaction of greater than 1 mm in thickness probably indicates a benign process (EDEIKEN and HODES, 1967). Thick, undulating periosteal reaction, commonly seen in venous stasis, also is an indication of benignity.

Laminated or "onion-skin" periosteal reactions occur in malignant tumors and in benign conditions such as pulmonary hypertrophic osteoarthropathy or osteomyelitis. It is, however, most commonly associated with Ewing's tumor. The laminations are delicate in Ewing's tumor.

Spiculated periosteal reaction is due to a disturbance in the reparative stage that follows periosteal elevation. The spicules are said not to be tumor bone. Tumor cells or other agents prevent the filling in of the subperiosteal space with bone. Spicules then form along the stretched periosteal vessels and the extensions of Sharpey's fibers. Another theory relates spicule formations to electrical fields from piezoelectric effects of bone crystal.

This picture represents a rapid, aggressive process, that can be either malignant or benign. Several localized primary malignant tumors of bone, metastases, osteomyelitis and lues, thyroid acropachy, hemangiomas, and anemias may cause a spiculated appearance. LODWICK (1966) has divided spiculation into three roentgen patterns: the sunburst, or radiating from a central point (typically osteogenic sarcoma); the hair-on-end or parallel, involving a long segment (typically Ewing's); and velvet, or low and slanting (typically chondrosarcoma). Malignant spicules tend to be long and slender, while benign spicules tend to be short and squat.

When periosteum is locally elevated and destruction of the apex of the formed triangle occurs at a rate that exceeds the osteogenic potential, a periosteal cuff is seen at the margin of the lesion that is called Codman's triangle. This may be formed in both malignant and benign processes.

The absence of periosteal new bone formation is also of diagnostic significance, particularly in localized lesions. The so-called fibrocystic lesions of bone are characterized by this absence.

D. Destruction of Bone

A basic response of bone to injury is destruction. Loss of bone substance may occur by resorption through the action of osteoclasts, osteocytes, or direct destruction of trabeculae by metastatic tumor cells (JAFFE, 1958). Tissue culture studies with time-lapse motion pictures have shown dissolution of bone before an advancing osteoclastic front. Osteoclasts, by virtue of their secretory activity, lyse both mineral and organic matrix of bone. Osteocytes have also been shown to have osteolytic properties. Halisteresis, or the concept of decalcification of bone with a residual normal matrix, is no longer considered valid, except on a minor scale. Hyperemia is said to facilitate osteolysis.

Early bone destruction may be recognized radiologically as a subtle alteration of bone texture or a barely perceptible decrease in bone density. There is a latent period between the onset of a destructive process, such as osteomyelitis, and roentgen demonstrability that is about 10 days, and may be much longer in the case of a slow process in rarefied bone.

Several factors are involved in the radiographic visibility of a destructive focal lesion. The ratio of volume of bone destroyed to the density of adjacent uninvolved bone is of prime importance. A destructive focus is more apparent in cortex than in medulla, and more readily seen in bone of normal density than in osteoporotic bone. The margination of the lesion is significant. A sharply circumscribed lesion with a narrow zone of transition has much greater visibility than one in which the edges fade off into imperceptibility. Radiographic technique is important. Attention should be paid to obtaining an exposure to give proper density (MAS) and contrast (KV), as well as maximum sharpness (small focal spot, nonscreen films) and limitation of scattered radiation (collimation and grid).

Bone destruction has a wide spectrum of roentgen appearance, and several patterns along this spectrum can be discerned. The simplest and the most benign in appearance are cystlike dissolutions. These represent small areas of well-marginated radiolucencies most commonly seen subchondrally or marginally in the arthritides. These may contain synovial fluid or fibrous or granulation tissue. The radiologic term "cyst" does not necessarily connote a fluid-filled cavity. A larger solitary focus may be seen, representing a lesion that grows slowly enough to destroy all of the bone in the involved area before progressing. This circumscribed lysis has been termed "geographic" by LODWICK (1966).

Another pattern, the result of multiple smaller excavations, appears as many moderate-sized radiolucencies that tend to become confluent and represent a more active lesion. This regional invasive pattern has been termed moth-eaten (LODWICK, 1966).

A larger endosteal destructive area appears as a punched-out lesion.

The most aggressive and infiltrative lesions tunnel in the cortex and cause a myriad of tiny radiolucencies with no definite border between the involved area and normal bone. This diffuse invasive pattern is termed permeative.

Permeative bone destruction results from very rapid growth, high infiltrativeness, and rapid spread. This does not allow time for the total regional destruction of bone. In permeative bone destruction, the cortex may apparently be intact although diminished in density. A large component of soft tissue invasion may be present without gross cortical destruction.

E. Margination or Zone of Transition

The margin or zone of transition between normal bone and a lesion is an indication of its aggressiveness and of the reparative response that is evoked. The margins may be ill-defined or sharply defined, partially or completely surrounding the lesion. There may be irregular, smooth, or scalloped edges. There may be no wall, a fine thin wall, or a thick sclerotic wall surrounding the lesion. A permeative destructive process has a wide zone of transition. An expansile lesion may have a narrow zone of transition. An osteogenic sarcoma has characteristically a wide zone of transition. A tumor with a narrow zone of transition should be scrutinized very carefully about its perimeter for widening and indistinctness of its margin. This may indicate a spurious initial impression or secondary malignant change, such as an enchondroma transforming into a chondrosarcoma.

Some lesions, such as a nonossifying fibroma, characteristically have a thin sclerotic scalloped rim, while others such as enchondroma or chondrosarcoma may evoke a thick sclerotic marginal response.

F. Increase in Bone Density

Increase in bone density can be due to several different etiologies. One means is the failure of primary spongiosa to be resorbed in the metaphysis during the process of enchondral bone formation. There may also be errors of internal modeling of compacta and spongiosa. Certain lesions can stimulate normal osteoblasts to form excessive new bone, at times as a reparative process. The periosteum, cortex, or endosteum may each respond singly or in combination.

Periosteal new bone formation assumes a variety of patterns that are of great diagnostic significance. The osteoblastic response of the compacta is somewhat limited, as space for the addition of new bone is not present. The major response causing bone sclerosis is that of endosteal osteoblasts depositing new bone on the surface of trabeculae in the spongiosa. New bone in the intertrabecular spaces is also formed. The reason that certain lesions consistently evoke an osteoblastic response while others do not is unknown; however, these tendencies can be utilized for roentgen diagnosis.

An increase in bone density can also be caused by tumor new bone formation in the osteogenic and cartilaginous types of tumors. An osteogenic sarcoma forms tumor osteoid. This osteoid may or may not be calcified. Thus the tumor may range from a sclerotic appearance to a purely osteolytic appearance.

Another mechanism of new bone formation is by metaplasia to osteoblasts, the best example of which is myositis ossificans. New bone formation, both intra- and extraosseous, must be differentiated from calcification. Mature bone shows organization into cortex and trabeculae, in contrast to the amorphous clumps of varying size seen in calcification. Immature and early bone formation can be seen as an ill-defined cloud of increased density with few if any dense conglomerations. Many diseases are characterized by widespread increase in density of the spongiosa.

A soft tissue osteogenic sarcoma may show a pattern of streaky calcification or ossification.

G. Matrix Calcification

Calcification or ossification within the tumor matrix (as opposed to reactive bone sclerosis) indicates the osteogenic or chondrogenic series of tumors, if calcification is not in necrotic tissue.

Calcification in an enchondroma characteristically takes the form of amorphous clumps or a punctate pattern. Calcification in a medullary bone infarct shows either a serpiginous pattern or is well-demarcated by a calcific rim.

In the soft tissues, calcification in a hemagioma takes the familiar form of phleboliths. A chondrosarcoma may show amorphous spotty or streaky calcification.

H. Expansion of the Cortex

Expansion is related to the slow rate of growth or enlargement of a lesion with respect to the rate of bone repair. It only indicates a slow growing lesion, and is not a valid criterion of malignancy or benignity. The expanded area may be centrally or eccentrically located. The more common causes of bone expansion are summarized in Table 2.

Table 2. Causes of bone expansion

I. Primary benign tumors of bone	III. Primary malignant tumors of bone
1. Giant cell tumor	1. Multiple myeloma
2. Enchondroma	2. Malignant giant cell tumor
3. Benign chondroblastoma	3. Chondrosarcoma
4. Chondromyxoid fibroma	4. Fibrosarcoma
5. Desmoplastic fibroma	5. Adamantinoma (long bone)
6. Lipoma of bone	6. Osteogenic sarcoma (rare feature)
II. Tumorlike processes	IV. Metastatic tumors of bone
1. Unicameral bone cyst	1. Carcinoma of kidney
2. Fibrous dysplasia	2. Carcinoma of thyroid
3. Aneurysmal bone cyst	3. Treated metastases
4. Eosinophilic granuloma	
5. Dermoid inclusion cyst	

I. Trabeculation

Trabeculation refers to the apparent septa that are seen in a radiolucent bone lesion. These septa are ridges in the wall of the lesion, and are due to uneven involvement. Trabeculation may be seen in malignant lesions, e.g., expansile form of multiple myeloma, or benign lesions, e.g., brown tumor of hyperparathyroidism. A lesion may be heavily trabeculated or lightly trabeculated, e.g., giant cell tumor. An osteogenic sarcoma is not expected to show trabeculation.

J. Size

The size of a lesion is an important consideration. Most malignant tumors are larger than 6 cm in diameter when first seen, although benign tumors may also be larger than 6 cm. Benign lesions that characteristically are of very small size are fibrous cortical defects and the nidus of an osteoid osteoma.

K. Shape

The shape of a solitary lesion is also to be considered. A rapidly growing tumor can be expected to have a roundish shape. The sclerotic lesions of tuberous sclerosis sometimes have an ovoid shape. The moth-eaten destructive lesions of a reticulum-cell sarcoma sometimes have an ovoid shape with the long axis parallel to the long axis of the bone. An unicameral bone cyst characteristically has the shape of a truncated pyramid.

L. The Joint Space

Articular and intervertebral cartilage form an effective barrier to the spread of neoplasms, until the late stages of the disease. An infective process, because of the presence of proteolytic enzymes, can involve cartilage, or cross a joint in early stages.

This is particularly important in the spine. An inflammatory disease, such as Pott's disease, will involve the intervertebral disc while a metastatic or primary tumor will not, except in very rare instances.

A tumor involving the end of a bone may, however, cause a severe osteoporosis in the adjacent bone across a joint. This is not to be confused with invasion.

M. The Age of the Patient

The age of the patient is one of the most important factors in the diagnosis of a bone lesion.

The various primary bone tumors, as well as cysts occur in the younger age groups. The lymphomas are frequent in adulthood. Giant cell tumor occurs most frequently in the 20–40 year bracket.

In the older age groups metastatic tumors, multiple myeloma, and primary bone tumors arising in abnormal bone are most frequent. The age of maximum incidence of the various primary bone tumors are tabulated in Table 3.

Table 3. The Incidence of the Various Tumors

Tumor	Age of maximum incidence (decades)
Osteogenic sarcoma	2, 3 (smaller peak at 7)
Parosteal sarcoma	4, 5
Chondrosarcoma	4, 5, 6
Fibrosarcoma	4
Giant cell tumor	3, 4
Ewing's tumor	2
Reticulum cell sarcoma of bone	3, 4
Multiple myeloma	5, 6, 7
Benign chondroblastoma	2
Chondromyxoid fibroma	2, 3
Nonossifying fibroma	2
Osteoid osteoma	2, 3
Nonneoplastic Lesions	
Solitary bone cyst	1, 2
Aneurysmal bone cyst	2, 3

N. The Incidence of the Various Tumors

If one considers roentgen diagnosis as the prediction of the histology of a given lesion, then one must be influenced by the relative incidence of the various tumors at large. It goes without saying that the rarer tumors occur less frequently, and that uncommon manifestations of commoner tumors are sometimes more probable.

A table of incidence of various bone tumors, based on extensive data, has been developed by LODWICK and is used in computer systems (LODWICK, 1966).

References

see p. 67 (Chapter "General Concepts and Pathology of Tumors of Osseous Origin")

General Concepts and Pathology of Tumors of Osseous Origin

by

George B. Greenfield

It is of little advantage to the radiologist to be partisan to the discussions of the histogenesis and classification of bone tumors that concern the research pathologist. Within the vast spectrum of possible histologic types and subtypes of neoplasms, there are condensations of a finite number of definite clinicopathologic entities. JAFFE (1958) states that this concept should be the basis of classification, rather than the listings in which the various tumors were compared solely on the basis of fundamental cell type. The listing by tissue de-emphasizes the fundamental radiologic and clinical essentials, and subordinates these pictures to the basic tissue.

I. Osteoma

A true osteoma is a benign tumor that contains only osseous tissue. AEGERTER believes that these lesions represent hemartomas (AEGERTER and KIRKPATRICK, 1968). It arises in intramembranous bone and may be multiple.

II. Osteoid Osteoma

Osteoid osteoma is generally considered to be a benign tumor of bone. The actual lesion, called the nidus, is 1 cm or less in size. The nidus initially is uncalcified, but on maturity may develop calcification. This may vary from small flecks to calcification of the major portion. Another component of the lesion is reactive sclerosis, cortical thickening, and periosteal reaction. The degree of this reactive new bone formation varies considerably and is influenced by the location of the nidus. The nidus may be intramedullary, intracortical, or subperiosteal. The roentgen appearances of all three are dissimilar. In addition, an intracapsular osteoid osteoma in the femoral neck provokes a minimum of reactive sclerosis because of the low bone-producing capability of the intracapsular periosteum.

Microscopically, the nidus consists of osteoid and osseous tissue within a highly vascular stroma. Giant cells are present. The nidus is sharply demarcated from the surrounding reactive sclerosis.

III. Benign Osteoblastoma

Benign osteoblastoma is an uncommon neoplasm characterized histologically by the presence of osteoblasts and giant cells in a vascular connective tissue stroma. This lesion is similar to osteoid osteoma in microscopic appearance and in age incidence but differs in size, location, and roentgen appearance.

IV. Osteogenic Sarcoma or Osteosarcoma

Osteogenic sarcoma is a primary malignant tumor of bone in which osteoid is formed directly from sarcomatous tissue. Osteoid may also be formed from cartilaginous tissue, which can be present in abundance. This is an entity distinct from fibrosarcoma of bone, which does not give rise to osteogenesis, and chondrosarcoma, which is a malignant tumor of cartilage.

Osteogenic sarcoma may be grouped by location as central, parosteal (juxtacortical sarcoma), multiple osteogenic sarcomatosis, and soft tissue osteogenic sarcoma. The clinical picture and prognosis is different for each, emphasizing that the clinicopathologic entity rather than the cell type is the important conceptual consideration.

Microscopically, the typical appearance consists of osteoid arising directly from neoplastic cells. The amount and calcification of this osteoid may vary greatly, along with the amount of cartilage that may be present. The lesion may be highly vascular. Tumor cells of great variability in degree of anaplasia are present as well as giant cells.

The varied calcification of osteoid leads to a radiologic spectrum of purely sclerotic to purely osteolytic. The type and prognosis is the same, only the roentgen pattern differs.

A. Benign Tumors of Osseous Origin

I. Osteoma

Osteoma is an uncommon benign tumor containing only osseous tissue. Malignant change is said not to occur. They arise only in membranous bone; they most commonly involve the external table of the calvarium, although they may occur in the internal table. The frontal and the ethmoid paranasal sinuses are the sinuses most commonly involved (Figs. 1, 2). They may also occur in the other paranasal sinuses and in the mandible. Osteoma of the nasal bones has also been reported (BADRAWY, 1967). A common complication is obstruction of the ostium of a paranasal sinus. Proptosis has also been reported. Radiologically, a characteristic, extremely dense, radiopaque, structureless, well-circumscribed mass is seen which may be round or ovoid (Figs. 3, 4). They are usually less than 2 cm in diameter but may attain larger size (Fig. 5). If a large size tumor is in a paranasal sinus, it may cause expansion of the sinus wall (Figs. 6a, b, Fig. 7). Complications of frontal sinus osteomas include reversible blindness (GÜTTICH and MÜLLER, 1967) and recurrent intracranial neurologic problems (BARTLETT, 1971), as well as recurrent pyogenic meningitis reported due to frontal and ethmoidal osteomas (SIEGLER, 1964).

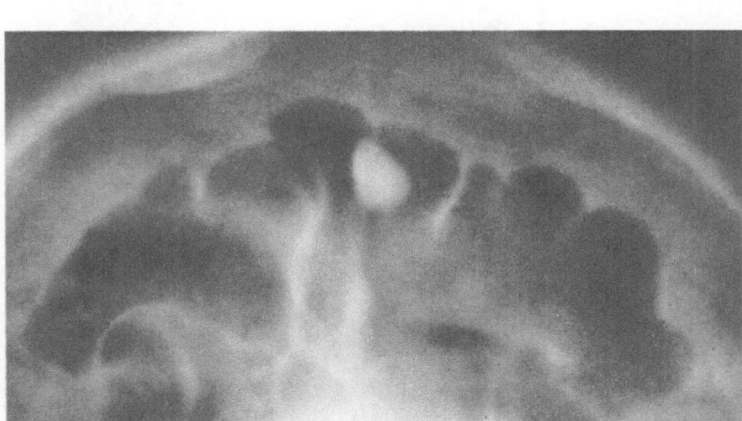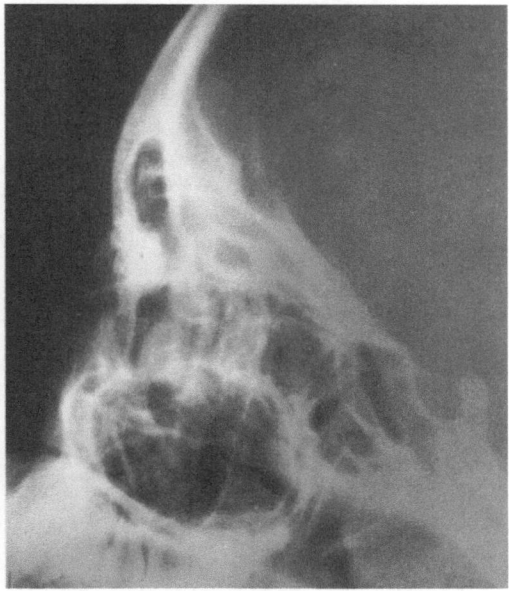

Fig. 1   Fig. 2

Fig. 1. Osteoma of frontal sinus. A small, dense, structureless bony condensation in frontal sinus is noted. (From GREENFIELD, 1969. Courtesy of J.B. Lippincott Company, Publisher, Philadelphia, Pa.)

Fig. 2. Osteoma of frontal sinus. Lateral view demonstrates a well-circumscribed structureless mass within frontal sinus

Fig. 3. Osteoma of frontal sinus. A roundish, well-circumscribed, dense, structureless lesion is seen in left frontal sinus. (From GREENFIELD, 1969. Courtesy of J.B. Lippincott Company, Publisher, Philadelphia, Pa.)

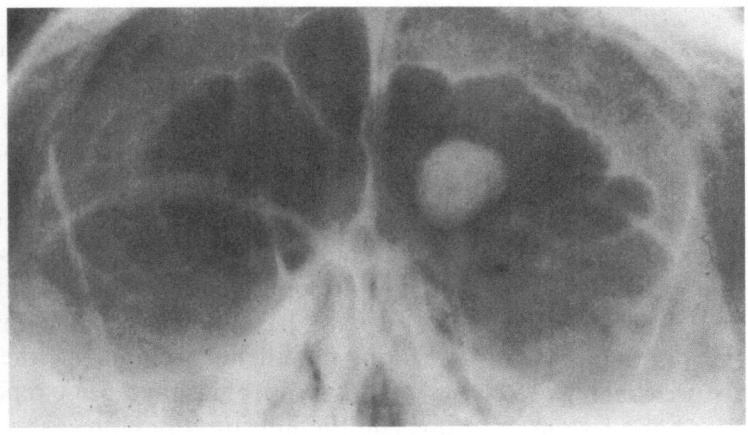

In the differential diagnosis it should be remembered that these lesions only arise from membranous bone. A lesion with the appearance of an osteoma in a long bone may be a bone island, a focus of fibrous dysplasia. Osteoma-like bone response to tropical ulcer has been reported (KOLAWOLE and BOHRER, 1970).

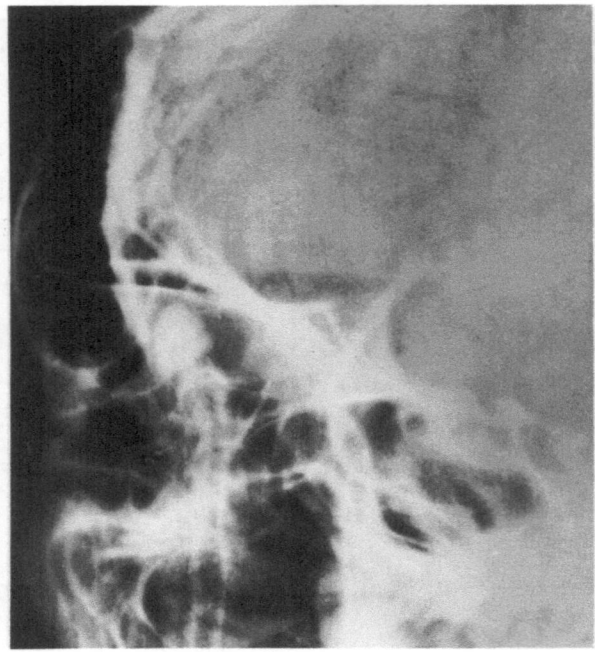
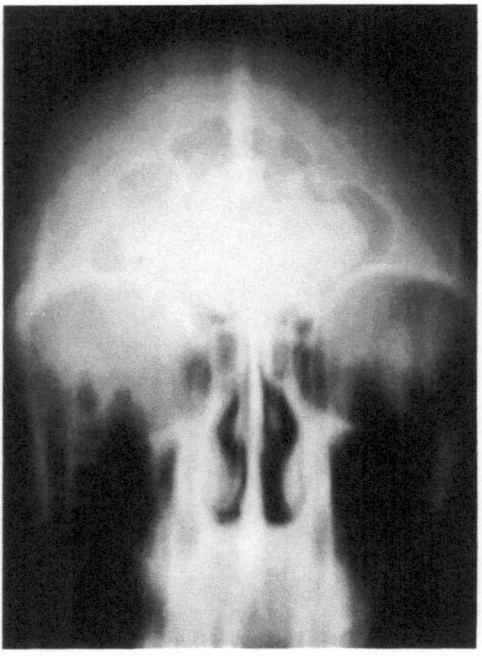

Fig. 4   Fig. 5

Fig. 4. Osteoma of frontal sinus. Lateral view demonstrates well-circumscribed, small, dense, structureless mass at posterior aspect of hypertrophied frontal sinuses. Hyperostosis frontalis interna is incidentally noted

Fig. 5. Osteoma of frontal sinus measuring 4 × 7 cm. Laminograph. A dense, structureless, irregularly outlined, ossific mass is present. (From GREENFIELD, 1969. Courtesy of J.B. Lippincott Company, Publisher, Philadelphia, Pa.)

If an osteoma arises from the inner table of the calvarium, it should be differentiated from hyperostosis resulting from a meningeoma, or from hyperostosis frontalis interna. Soft tissue osteomas in the tongue (GOLDBERG et al., 1970), and in the kidney (CALDERON et al., 1965), have also been reported. A partially pneumatized osteoma has also been reported (WEBER, 1963).

Gardner's syndrome is a familial disease consisting of osteomata, soft tissue tumors, and polyposis chiefly of the colon (GARDNER, 1962). It is transmitted as an autosomal dominant. The colonic polyps are premalignant, and a colonic carcinoma may be present at the time of diagnosis (Figs. 8a, b). Polyposis of the gastrointestinal tract may rarely be present outside of the colon, and adenocarcinoma of the duodenum has been reported. Approximately 150 cases of this syndrome have been reported in the literature to date. The bone lesions may precede the intestinal polyposis.

Leiomyomas of the gastrointestinal tract and retroperitoneum have been noted as well as carcinoid tumors and lymphoid polyps of the ileum. Mesenteric and retroperitoneal fibromatoses, desmoid tumors, incisional fibromas, and excessive development of peritoneal adhesions postoperatively are associated findings in some patients.

Radiologically, the bone abnormalities are benign osteomas consisting of dense bony proliferation ranging from slight cortical thickening to large masses. All parts of the skeleton may be involved. In the skull, dense osteomas in the calvarium may be seen as well as osteomas in the paranasal sinuses. The mandible characteristically shows

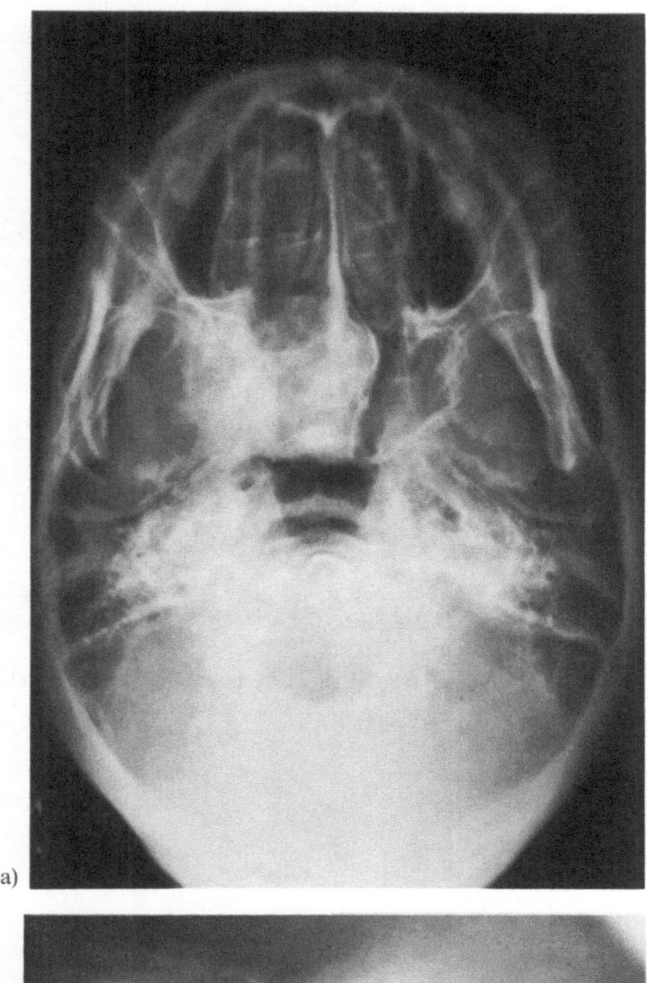

(a)

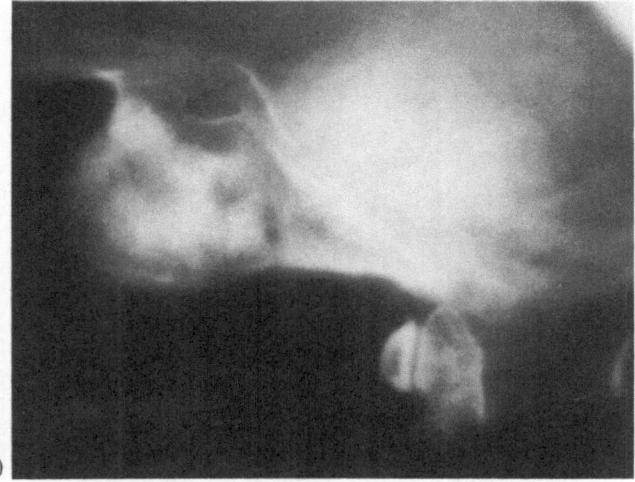

(b)

Fig. 6a and b. Osteoma of sphenoid sinus. Basal view of skull and lateral laminogram of the sphenoid sinus reveal a dense, structureless mass which has expanded the sphenoid sinus

lobulated osteomas arising from the cortex of the mandibular angle. The central portions of the mandible may also be involved with patches of eburnation near the roots of the teeth. Dental abnormalities may also be present. The tubular bones may show dense pedunculated exostoses, and localized cortical thickening which may be wavy. The ribs and pelvis may be involved with localized cortical thickening. The bone lesions are said not to undergo malignant change.

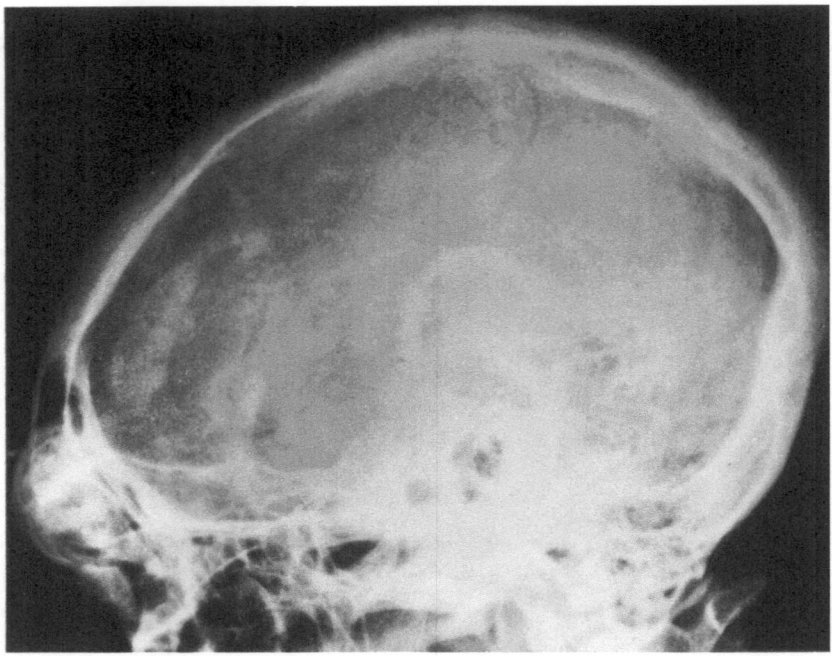

Fig. 7. Osteoma of frontal sinus. A large, dense, structureless mass seen expanding frontal sinus is present

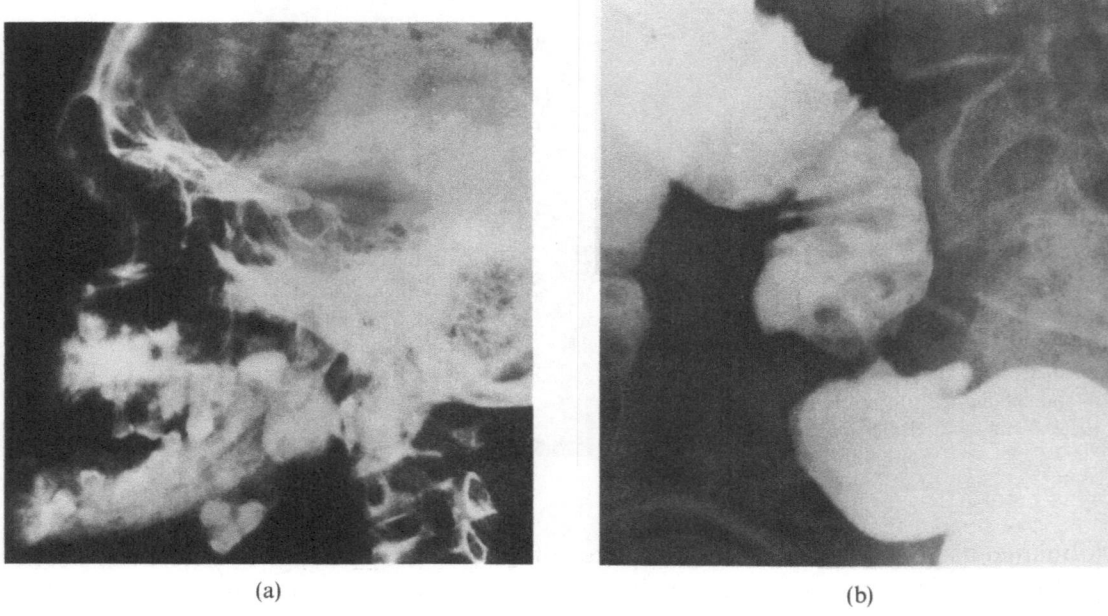

(a)   (b)

Fig. 8a and b. Gardner's syndrome. (a) Skull and mandible show dense osteomas. Large osteomas near angle of mandible are seen. (b) Same patient as in A. An annular constricting carcinoma in sigmoid colon is present

II. Osteoid Osteoma

Osteoid osteoma is a common benign lesion of bone, considered to represent a neoplasm. The sex incidence is 3:1 predominance in males. The majority of patients are in the 5–20 year age group, with a range of 17 months to 56 years. There are reports of untreated osteoid osteomas becoming clinically inactive (VICKERS et al., 1959). As the lesion heals, the nidus becomes less radiolucent, but the cortical reaction does not resolve. This lesion is characterized clinically by pain, and is typically relieved by salicylates, at least in the early stages. Incomplete removal results in persistant or recurrent pain (MORRESAN et al., 1950). Neurologic symptoms in osteoid osteoma include muscle atrophy and diminution of activity of muscle stretch reflexes (RUSHTON et al., 1955).

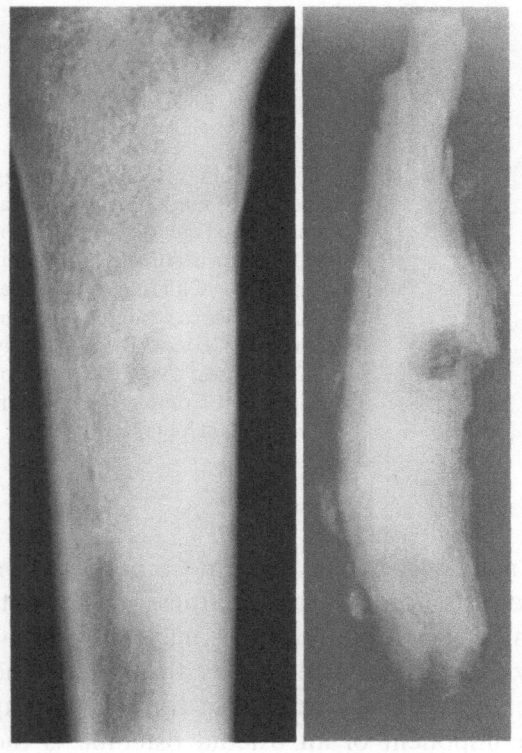

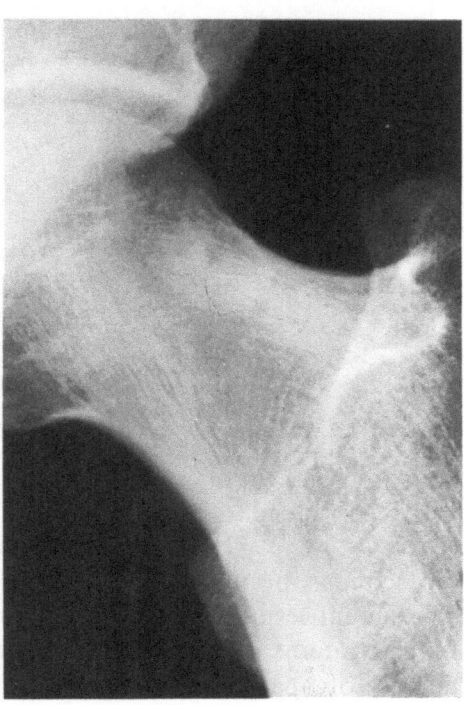

Fig. 9a   Fig. 9b   Fig. 10

Fig. 9a and b. Osteoid osteoma. (a) Dense cortical thickening with radiolucent nidus is seen. (b) Radiograph of resected specimen of osteoid osteoma. Actual lesion is 7 mm-round radiolucency called nidus. Surrounding reactive and sclerotic bone is present. A small amount of calcification within nidus is present in this specimen due to calcification of lesional osteoid. (From GREENFIELD, 1969. Courtesy of J.B. Lippincott Company, Publisher, Philadelphia, Pa.)

Fig. 10. Osteoid osteoma. Femoral neck. Very little bone sclerosis is present. A small radiolucent nidus at the outer aspect of the femoral neck can be seen. (From GREENFIELD, 1969. Courtesy of J.B. Lippincott Company, Publisher, Philadelphia, Pa.)

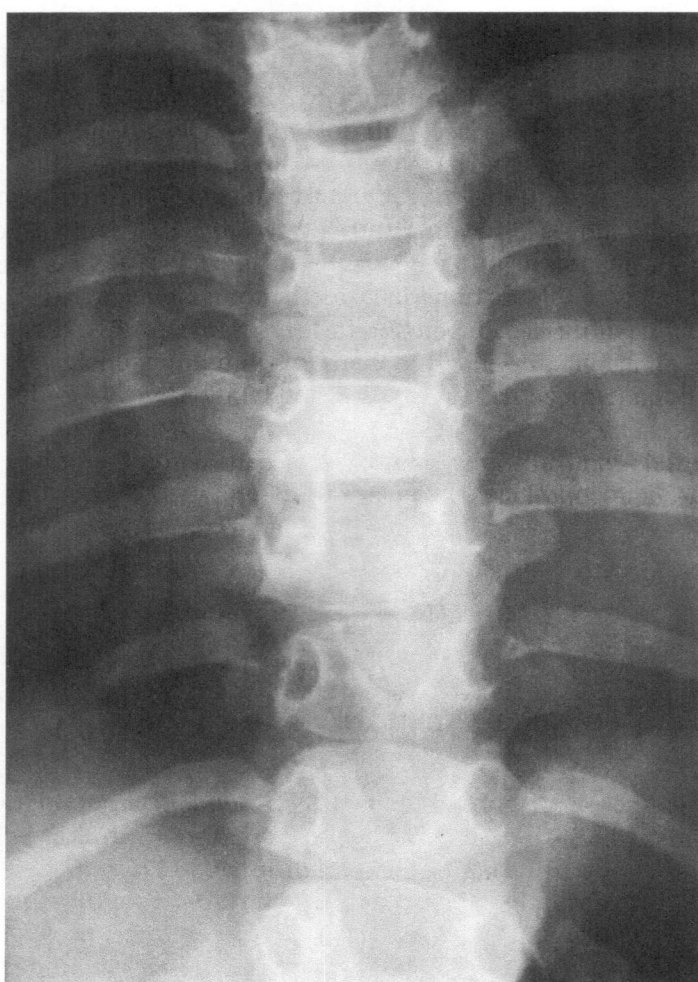

Fig. 11. Osteoid osteoma involving right pedicle of ninth dorsal vertebra. There is marked enlargement of pedicle with sclerosis. (Courtesy of Dr. Harven White, Children's Memorial Hospital, Chicago, Illinois.) (From GREENFIELD, GEORGE B., Radiology of bone diseases, 1969, Courtesy of J.B. Lippincott Company, Publisher, Philadelphia, Pa.)

Cervical radicular pain as well as torticollis may occur in a cervical spinal location (SCOTT et al., 1971). Elsewhere in the spine, scoliosis, lordosis, and stiffness may result. No scoliosis occurs in a spinous process lesion. Hypertrophic changes may be present. The actual lesion is small, 1 cm or less in size, and is referred to as the nidus. The nidus contains osteoid which may or may not be calcified, accounting for the varying degrees of opacity radiologically. The second component of an osteoid osteoma is the dense surrounding sclerotic reaction. This can be quite extensive, particularly if the lesion is located intracortically (Figs. 9a, b).

The nidus in a long bone may be intracortical, intramedullary, or subperiosteal. Each has a characteristic roentgen appearance. The lesion is seen more commonly in the femur and the tibia (Fig. 10). About half of all cases will show involvement in either of these two bones. Other areas include the other long bones, the vertebrae, particularly the neural arch or a vertebral process, ribs, pelvis, elbow, hip, and almost any other bone (Fig. 11). Lesions in the skull, mandibular condyle, the metacarpals and metatarsals, and the distal phalanges have been reported. Painless osteoid osteomas have also been reported (LAWRIE et al., 1970).

Radiologically, in the typical intracortical osteoid osteoma, there is a very small

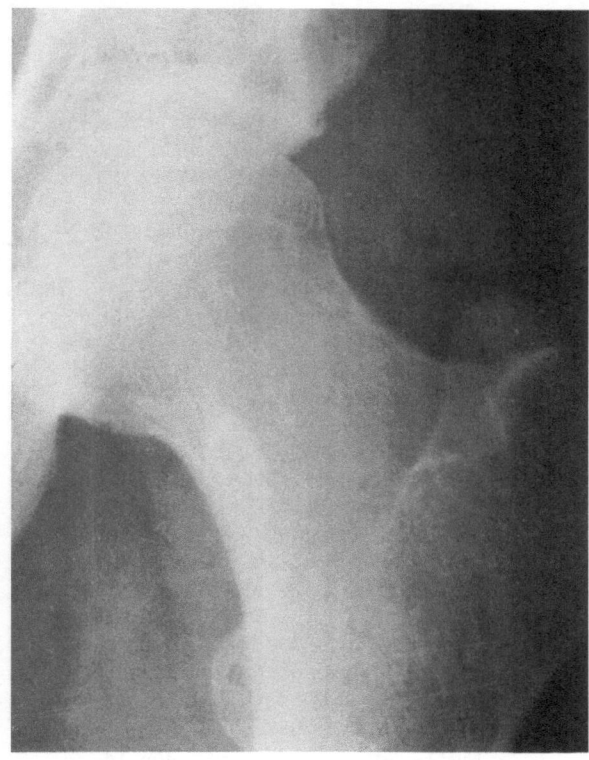

Fig. 12. Osteoid osteoma of the femoral neck. Localized density at the medial portion of the femoral neck is noted with a central radiolucency. Excessive sclerotic change in bone is not present. (Courtesy of Dr. Antonio Pizarro, Hines Veteran Administration Hospital, Hines, Illinois)

radiolucent nidus, less than 1 cm in diameter (Fig. 12). This is surrounded by a large dense sclerotic zone of cortical thickening. Periosteal reaction, usually of the solid type, but sometimes of the laminated type, may also be seen (Fig. 13). The nidus may be centrally calcified resulting in a ringlike radiolucency (Fig. 14). The nidus may be entirely calcified, or the dense sclerotic reaction may obscure the nidus, causing some difficulty in the roentgen diagnosis (Fig. 15). The nidus need not be centrally located within the area of sclerosis but may be eccentrically placed.

An intramedullary nidus typically shows very little reactive sclerosis. This may cause internal cortical thickening (Fig. 16). A not uncommon location for an intramedullary osteoid osteoma is the neck of the femur, which sometimes may be associated with osteoporosis of the femoral head and neck (Figs. 17a, b, Fig. 18). Severe growth disturbances associated with lesions in this location have been reported (GIUSTRA and FREIBERGER, 1970). Lymphofollicular synovitis in association with intra-articular osteoid osteoma has also been described (SNARR et al., 1973). The roentgen findings include uniform narrowing of the interosseous space, subperiosteal bone apposition involving the affected bone as well as adjacent bones. Lymphofollicular inflammation in the adjacent soft tissues is reported to be a consistent finding in intraarticular osteoid osteoma. Differentiation must be made from rheumatoid arthritis.

A less common location for the nidus is subperiosteally (Figs. 19a, b). This may manifest itself as a small bulge of the contour of the bone (Fig. 20). A radiolucency in the peripheral-most portion, and a thin shell of margination, associated with some thickening of the cortex is characteristically seen.

Synovitis in an adjacent joint not involving an intracapsular osteoid osteoma may also be present. The neural arch and spinous and transverse processes are more commonly

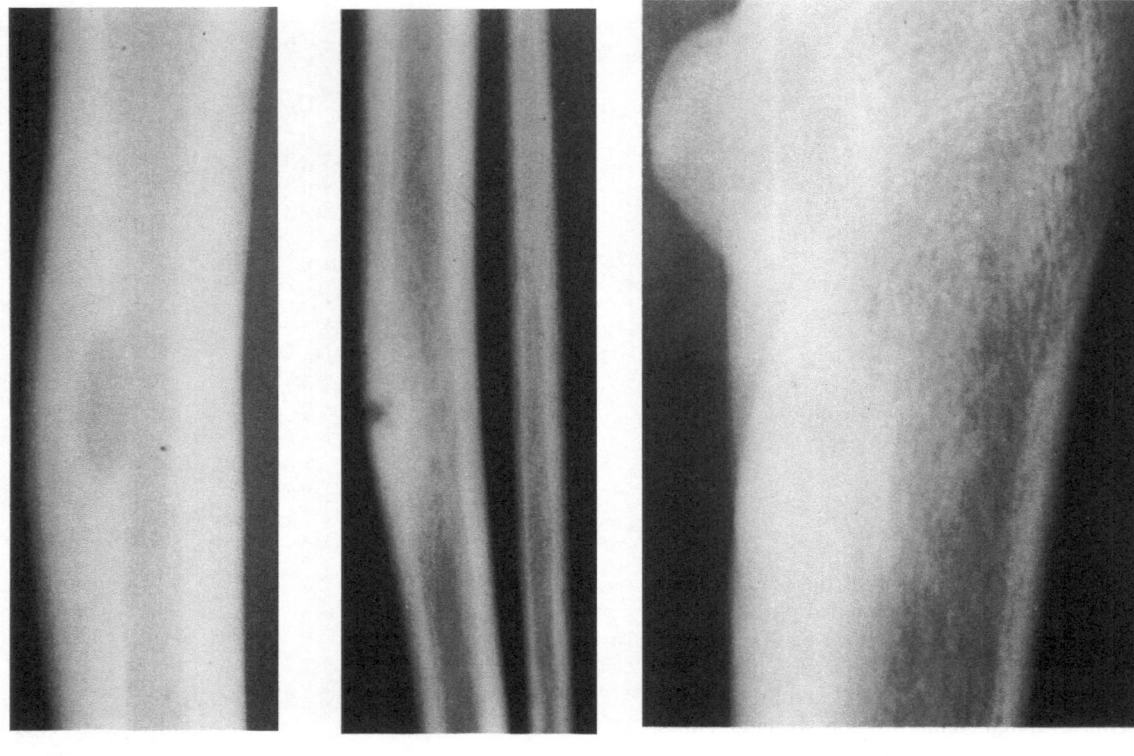

Fig. 13   Fig. 14   Fig. 15

Fig. 13. Laminogram of osteoid osteoma. There is a cortical location within endosteal abutment. An ovoid radiolucent nidus with no areas of calcification is present. A fusiform cortical thickening with periosteal new bone formation is seen. (From GREENFIELD, GEORGE B., Radiology of bone diseases, 1969, Courtesy of J.B. Lippincott Company, Publisher, Philadelphia, Pa.)

Fig. 14. Osteoid osteoma. A small radiolucent nidus is seen at anterior aspect of tibia, which has caused moderate amount of cortical sclerosis and thickening

Fig. 15. Osteoid osteoma. Dense cortical thickening is noted at proximal medial femoral shaft which almost completely obscures small radiolucent nidus. (From GREENFIELD, GEORGE B., Radiology of bone diseases, 1969, Courtesy of J.B. Lippincott Company, Publisher, Philadelphia, Pa.)

involved than the bodies in the vertebral column. Enlargement of the adjacent transverse processes in cases of laminar involvement may also occur. This leads to scoliosis of the spine.

If the nidus is not readily apparent from conventional radiographs, over-penetrated films or body section radiography are required for demonstration. Osteoid osteoma with a multicentric nidus has been reported (GLYNN and LICHTENSTEIN, 1973).

In the differential diagnosis we have to consider an intracortical abscess. Arteriography may show a vascular flush in osteoid osteoma, while the abscess cavity would not show this finding (LINDBOM et al., 1960). In the event the nidus is not visible, the differentiation from osteogenic sarcoma or Garré's sclerosing osteomyelitis would have to be made. There is no spiculated periosteal reaction, as is commonly associated with osteogenic sarcoma. The location need not be metaphyseal, and the bone may have an expanded appearance because of cortical thickening, which is not expected in osteogenic sarcoma. Garré's osteomyelitis would be more difficult to differentiate. Intracapsular osteoid os-

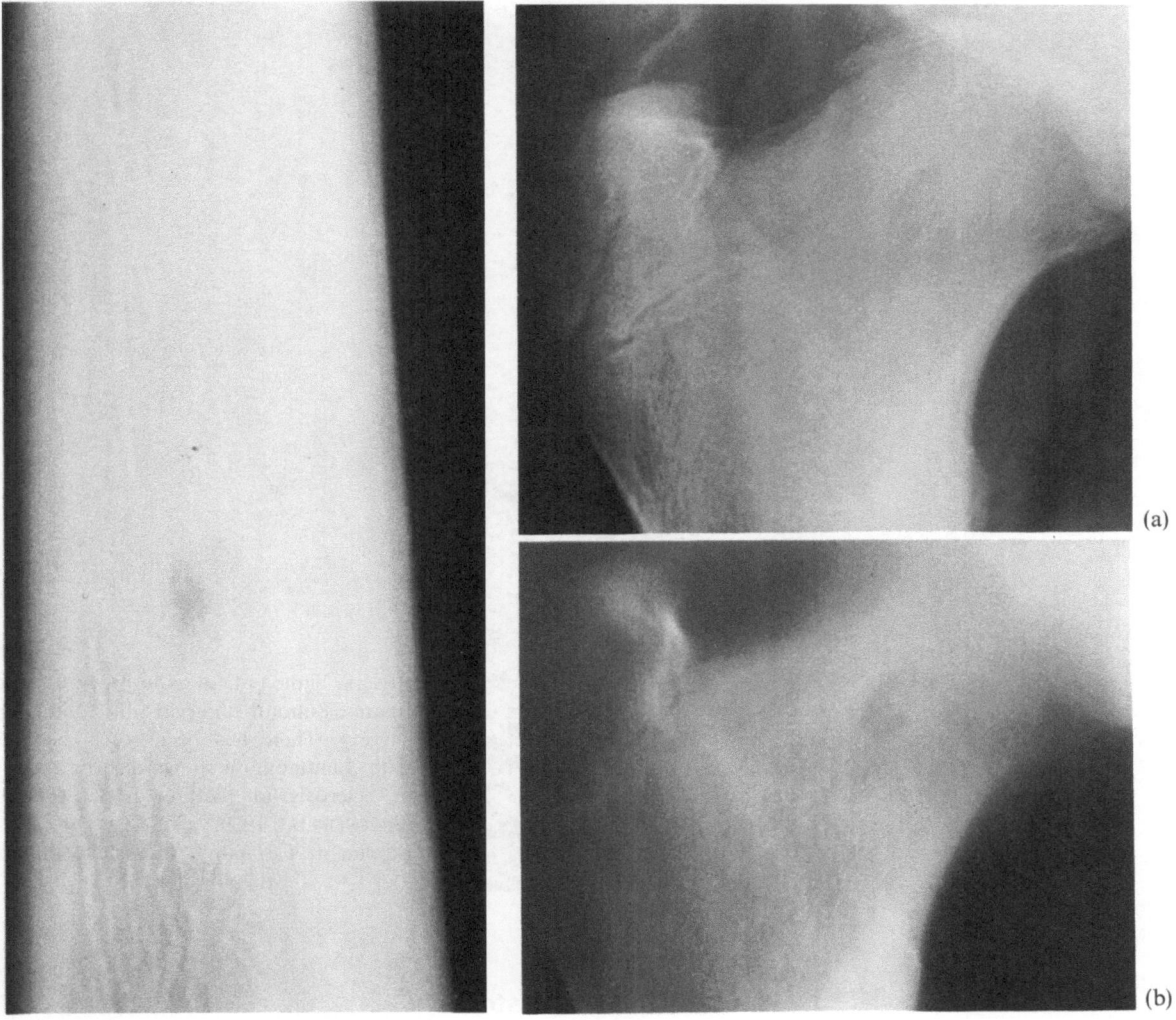

Fig. 16   Fig. 17

Fig. 16. Intramedullary osteoid osteoma. A small radiolucent nidus is seen with very little surrounding reactive bone sclerosis. This finding is characteristic of intramedullary location of nidus. There is no appreciable cortical thickening. (From GREENFIELD, GEORGE B., Radiology of bone diseases, 1969, Courtesy of J.B. Lippincott Company, Publisher, Philadelphia, Pa.)

Fig. 17a and b. (a) Osteoid osteoma of femoral neck. A small radiolucent nidus in femoral neck is noted without significant reactive bone sclerosis. (b) Laminograph: There is good demonstration of nidus containing small central calcification without reactive bone sclerosis. (From GREENFIELD, GEORGE B., Radiography of bone diseases, 1969, Courtesy of J.B. Lippincott Company, Publisher, Philadelphia, Pa.)

teoma involving a joint with lymphofollicular synovitis and osteoporosis should be differentiated from involvement with rheumatoid arthritis.

A solitary enostosis would also have to be differentiated, but this is a well-defined condensation of bone in the medulla, with sharp margins and is clinically asymptomatic. There is no reactive bone sclerosis or cortical thickening. Tuberculous bone abscess, syphilitic osteitis with periostitis, hyperostosis, and destructive areas, as well as fibrous dysplasia should be considered in the differential diagnosis.

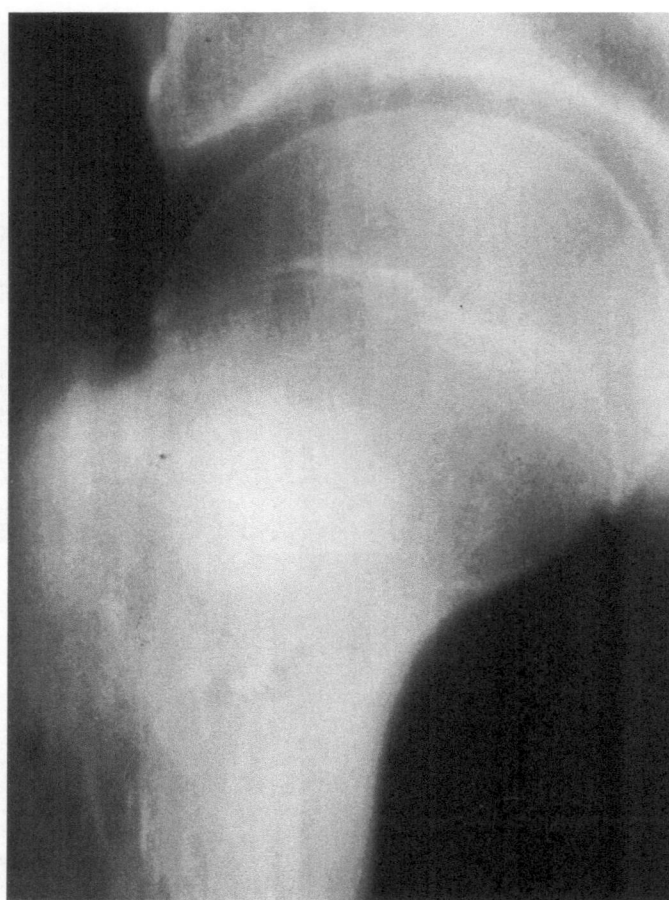

Fig. 18. Same patient as in previous two figures. 8-month interval film following surgery. There has been recurrence of pain. Laminogram shows recurrent area of sclerosis in femoral neck. (From GREENFIELD, 1969. Courtesy of J.B. Lippincott Company, Publisher, Philadelphia, Pa.)

III. Osteoblastoma

Osteoblastoma is a rare neoplasm primary in bone representing a vascular osteoid and bone-forming benign tumor. It was described by JAFFE and MAYER (1932) under the title "An Osteoblastic Osteoid Tissue Forming Tumor of a Metacarpal Bone." Other names referring to this entity in the literature have been osteogenic fibroma of bone, and giant osteoid-osteoma by DAHLIN and JOHNSON (1954). It is also commonly known as benign osteoblastoma.

The peak age incidence is between 7 and 20 years with a reported range between 5 and 78 years. Males are more frequently involved than females. This is a painful lesion but not as severe as osteoid osteoma. Neurologic symptoms with spinal involvement have been reported.

Radiologically the lesion presents with a wide variety of patterns. The most common location is in the vertebral column, principally in the transverse and spinous processes, but the vertebral bodies may also be involved (Fig. 21). Approximately half of the cases affect the spine. The sacrum may also be involved. Other areas of involvement are the carpals and tarsals, the calvarium, the long bones, the scapula, ribs, patella, maxilla (JENT et al., 1969), mandible, and pelvis (Fig. 22).

The size of the lesion may vary from 2 to 12 cm in diameter. There is usually an expansile bone lesion that is well-outlined and well-circumscribed, particularly when

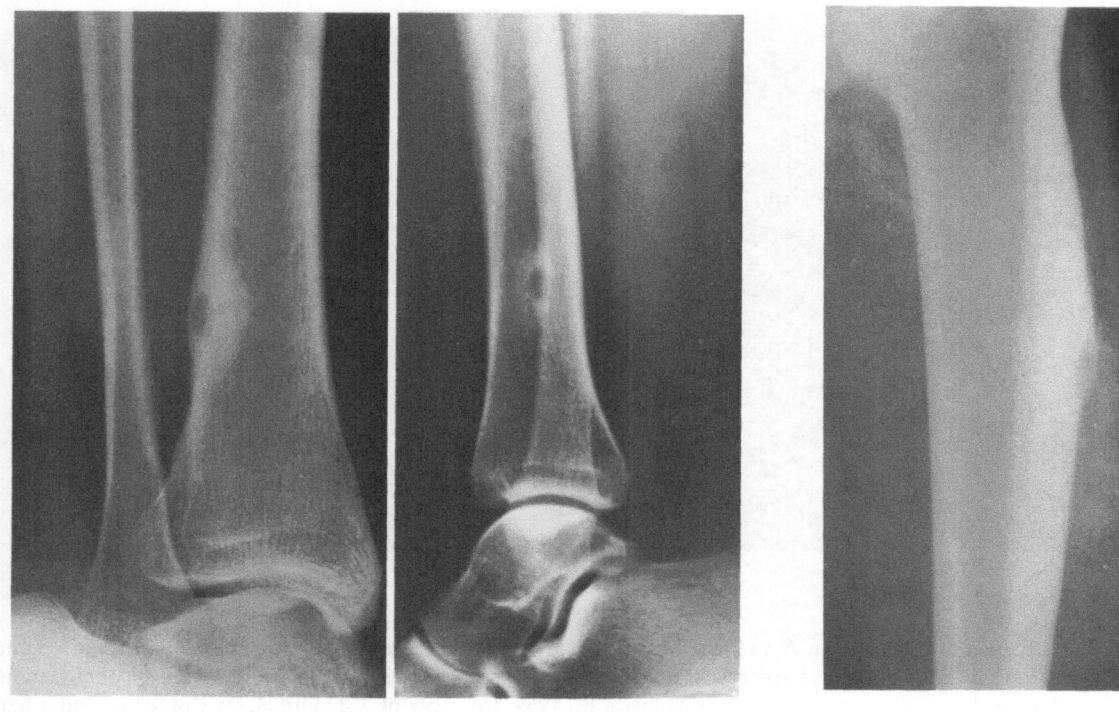

Fig. 19a   Fig. 19b   Fig. 20

Fig. 19a and b. Osteoid osteoma, subperiosteal type. Radiolucent lesion, or nidus, is causing slight bulge of contour of distal tibia. A small amount of reactive sclerosis is seen

Fig. 20. Subperiosteal osteoid osteoma. Bulging of periosteum by nidus is seen as well as cortical thickening. (From GREENFIELD, 1969. Courtesy of J.B. Lippincott Company, Publisher, Philadelphia, Pa.)

the neural arch is involved. The tumor may break through the cortex and result in a well-defined, soft tissue mass, which may show a thin calcific margination. The matrix of the tumor contains a variable amount of calcification. This may range from radiolucent, with small spotty calcific areas, to a dense radiopacity, particularly following radiation therapy. Rapid growth and pathologic fractures may occur. Although periosteal new bone formation is not characteristic, a sparse amount of reactive solid type of periosteal new bone formation may be present. The surrounding reactive bone sclerosis, commonly seen in osteoid osteoma is not usually present. The lesions in the small tubular bones may be eccentric and are usually metaphyseal or diaphyseal, but not epiphyseal. Rarely, a cuboid bone may be involved with reactive sclerosis and periosteal new bone formation, which would be difficult to differentiate from an osteogenic sarcoma. Malignant degeneration has, to 1967, only been reported in one case (MAYER, 1967).

In the differential diagnosis, the chief consideration is the ossifying character of the lesion. Expansion of bone with a thin marginal calcific shell and the usual lack of periosteal new bone formation would help to differentiate most lesions from an osteogenic sarcoma. The lesion does not have the dense reactive sclerosis commonly seen in an intracortical osteoid osteoma, and the "nidus" is much larger. Differentiation from cartilaginous tumors can be made by the lack of clumps of amorphous calcification, usually seen in the latter. Differentiation from giant cell tumor can be made by ossification of the matrix, and the fact that the epiphysis usually is not involved.

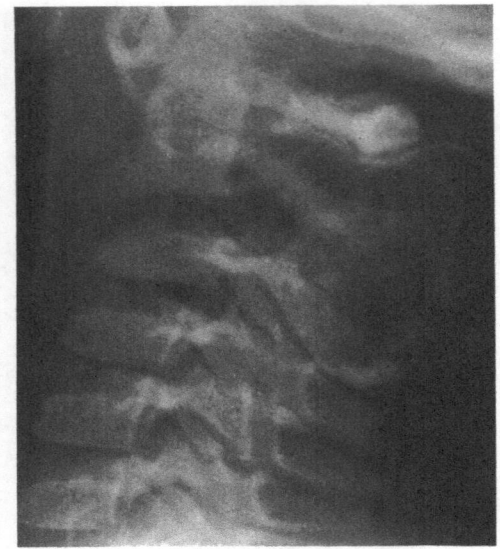 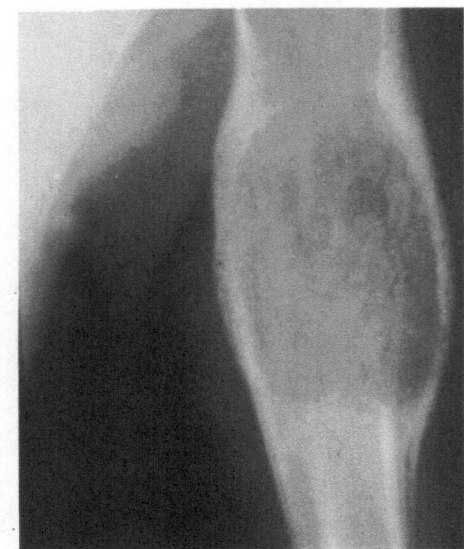

Fig. 21   Fig. 22

Fig. 21. Benign osteoblastoma. A well-circumscribed expansile lesion originating at spinous process of second cervical vertebra and involving spinous process of third cervical vertebra is noted. (Previously published in Radiology of bones diseases, GREENFIELD, GEORGE B., 1969. Courtesy of J.B. Lippincott Company, Publisher, Philadelphia, Pa. Originally contributed by Dr. Harvey White, Children's Memorial Hospital, Chicago, Illinois)

Fig. 22. Benign osteoblastoma. Note expansile lesion with thick cortical shell in proximal humeral diaphysis. Extensive ossification of matrix is present. A minimal amount of periosteal new bone formation, which has laminated appearance, may be seen at distal aspect of lesion, forming a buttress. There is no periosteal new bone formation about periphery of lesion. (From GREENFIELD, 1969. Courtesy of J.B. Lippincott Company, Publisher, Philadelphia, Pa. Originally contributed by Dr. Harvey White, Children's Memorial Hospital, Chicago, Illinois)

B. Malignant Tumors of Osseous Origin

I. Osteogenic Sarcoma (Osteosarcoma, Central Osteosarcoma)

Osteogenic sarcoma is the second most common primary sarcoma of bone component tissue (multiple myeloma is the first). The ratio of involvement of males to females is about 2:1. The majority of these tumors arise in the 10–25 year age bracket. A smaller peak incidence occurs in older age groups. Osteosarcomas in the older age groups may be associated with Paget's disease, post-irradiated bone, or osteochondromas. Other associated reported conditions include fibrous dysplasia and osteogenesis imperfecta, in younger patients.

Radiation-induced osteosarcomas can be due to teletherapy or ingested radium and mesothorium, or following injection of thorotrast. Common instances in which radium was ingested in the past are watch dial painters (MARTLAND, 1929) and those patients who were administered therapeutic radium water.

In the younger patient, osteosarcoma most often involves the tubular bones. When it occurs in an older patient, the flat bones are often involved.

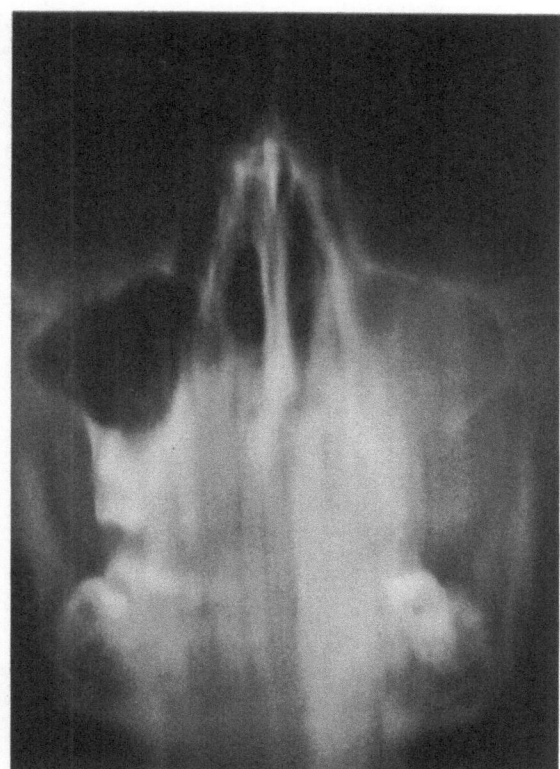

Fig. 23. Osteogenic sarcoma originating in left zygoma. Tomogram in Water's view. Clouding of left maxillary antrum and partial destruction of inferior wall of antrum is present. Superior margin of left orbit is also destroyed

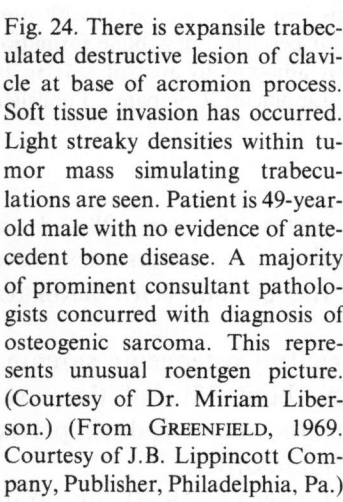
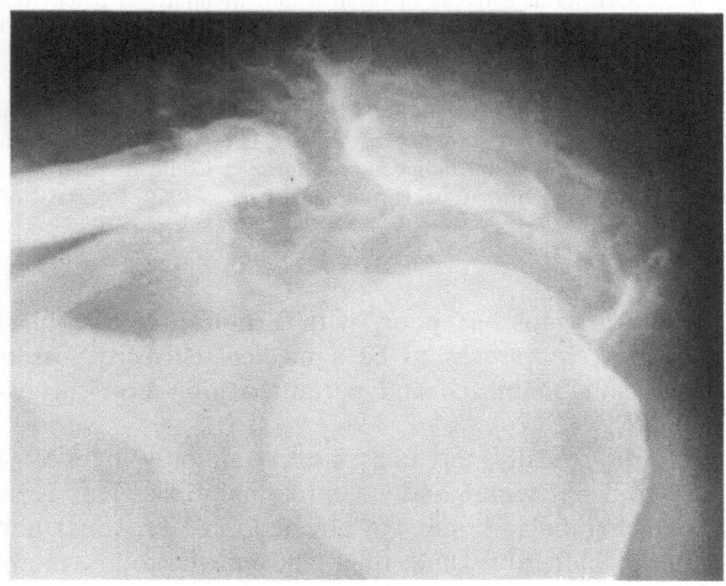

Fig. 24. There is expansile trabeculated destructive lesion of clavicle at base of acromion process. Soft tissue invasion has occurred. Light streaky densities within tumor mass simulating trabeculations are seen. Patient is 49-year-old male with no evidence of antecedent bone disease. A majority of prominent consultant pathologists concurred with diagnosis of osteogenic sarcoma. This represents unusual roentgen picture. (Courtesy of Dr. Miriam Liberson.) (From GREENFIELD, 1969. Courtesy of J.B. Lippincott Company, Publisher, Philadelphia, Pa.)

The chief clinical symptom prior to metastasis is pain at the tumor site. The pain begins insidiously and intermittently and progresses to severe constancy. A palpable mass develops, with associated inflammatory signs and local venous dilatation. Effusion in a contiguous joint is common. Pathologic fractures may occur. Systemic symptoms then follow. The duration of symptoms prior to diagnosis averages several months. The serum alkaline phosphatase is usually slightly elevated in the presence of a large lesion.

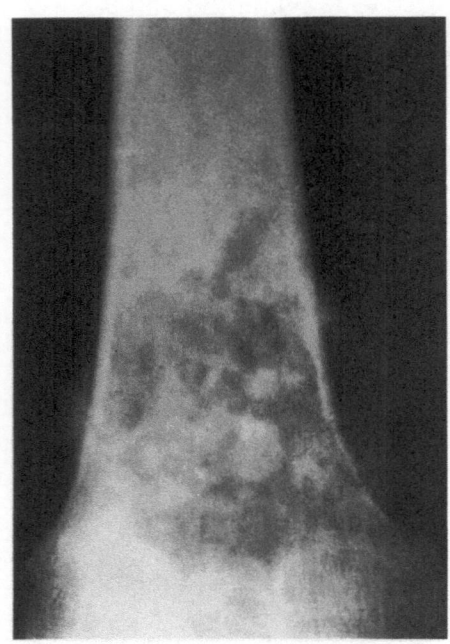

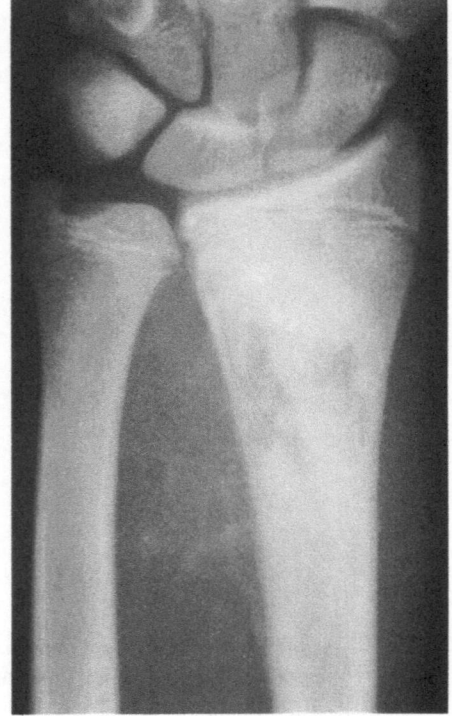

Fig. 25   Fig. 26

Fig. 25. Osteogenic sarcoma of distal femur. Metaphyseal patchy destructive changes are noted interspersed with patchy sclerotic areas. Codman's triangle and periosteal new bone formation is seen. There is wide zone of transition of lesion

Fig. 26. Osteogenic sarcoma. Distal radius. An area of sclerosis in metaphysis is seen. The epiphyseal ossification center is not involved. Radiolucency represents biopsy site. A small amount of periosteal new bone formation at ulnar aspect of distal radius is seen forming Codman's triangle which is adjacent to area of soft tissue tumor new bone formation. (From GREENFIELD, 1969. Courtesy of J.B. Lippincott Company, Publisher, Philadelphia, Pa.)

The prognosis is poor, with a mortality rate in some series of over 90%. In a few cases, so rare as to be a medical curiosity, osseous pulmonary metastases have inexplicably stabilized and permitted long-term survival of the patient (GOLDENBERG, 1957).

Radiologically, the areas most commonly involved with central osteogenic sarcoma are the distal femur and the proximal tibia. This is seen in about 75% of the cases in which tubular bones are affected. The proximal humerus, the distal radius, pelvis, femoral shaft, ribs, skull, tibia, and maxilla follow in approximate order.

There may be involvement of the sternum, spine, hand (CARROLL, 1957), or rarely almost any bone in the body, including the patella (Figs. 23, 24) (GOODWIN, 1961).

In the tubular bones, the tumor is characteristically of metaphyseal origin (Fig. 25). If the epiphysis has not as yet fused to the shaft, then the epiphyseal cartilage plate serves as a barrier to spread to the epiphysis (Fig. 26). After epiphyseal fusion, the end of the bone is commonly involved. The joint forms an effective barrier against transarticular spread. In late stages of the disease, the tumor may cross both the epiphyseal cartilage and the joint (Figs. 27, 28, 29a, b). Regional osteoporosis of a contiguous bone may simulate involvement. Rarely, the tumor may originate in the diaphysis

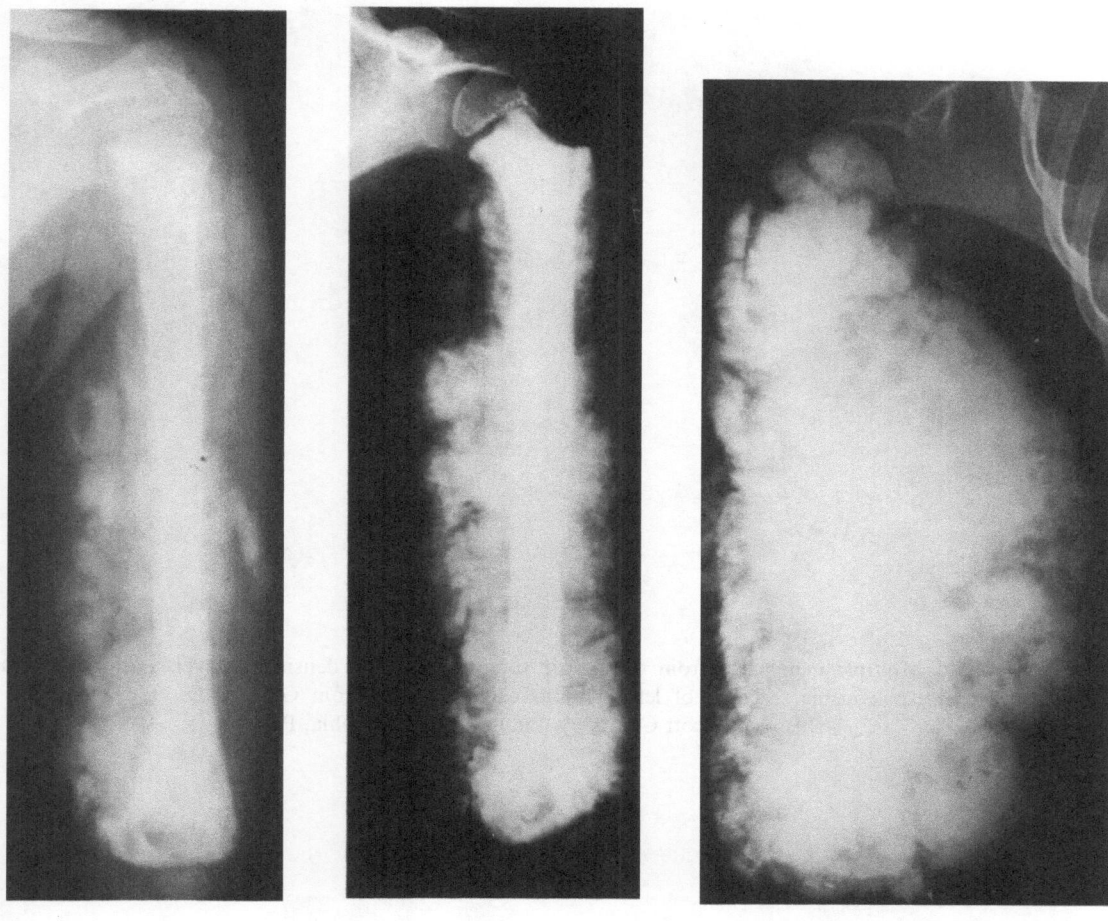

Fig. 27   Fig. 28   Fig. 29a

Fig. 27. Osteogenic sarcoma. There is involvement of entire diaphysis. Epiphyses at both ends of humerus are spared. Soft tissue involvement with extensive soft tissue tumor bone formation as well as spiculated periosteal new bone formation is seen. (From GREENFIELD, 1969. Courtesy of J.B. Lippincott Company, Publisher, Philadelphia, Pa.)

Fig. 28. Same patient as in Fig. 27. 1 month interval film. Osteogenic sarcoma. Involvement of humerus and soft tissues have progressed. In addition, beginning invasion of epiphyseal ossification centers at their bases are seen. (From GREENFIELD, 1969. Courtesy of J.B. Lippincott Company, Publisher, Philadelphia, Pa.)

Fig. 29a. Same patient as in previous two figures. 4 month interval since Fig. 28. There is now extreme soft tissue ossification. Involvement of epiphyseal ossification centers is now complete. There has been no spread accross joints. The chest film of this patient is seen in Fig. 29b. (From GREENFIELD, 1969. Courtesy of J.B. Lippincott Company, Publisher, Philadelphia, Pa.)

(Figs. 30, 31). The size of the tumor is frequently larger than 6 cm when first seen, and extends from the metaphysis downward to the shaft.

It must be understood that the term osteogenic sarcoma refers to the histological production of osteoid and not to the roentgen appearance of sclerosis. In about 50% of cases, a dense sclerotic appearance is seen on the radiograph (Fig. 32). The remainder range in density from moderately sclerosing, to mixed productive and destructive, to purely osteolytic (Figs. 33a and b, 34, 35). These variations in density depend upon

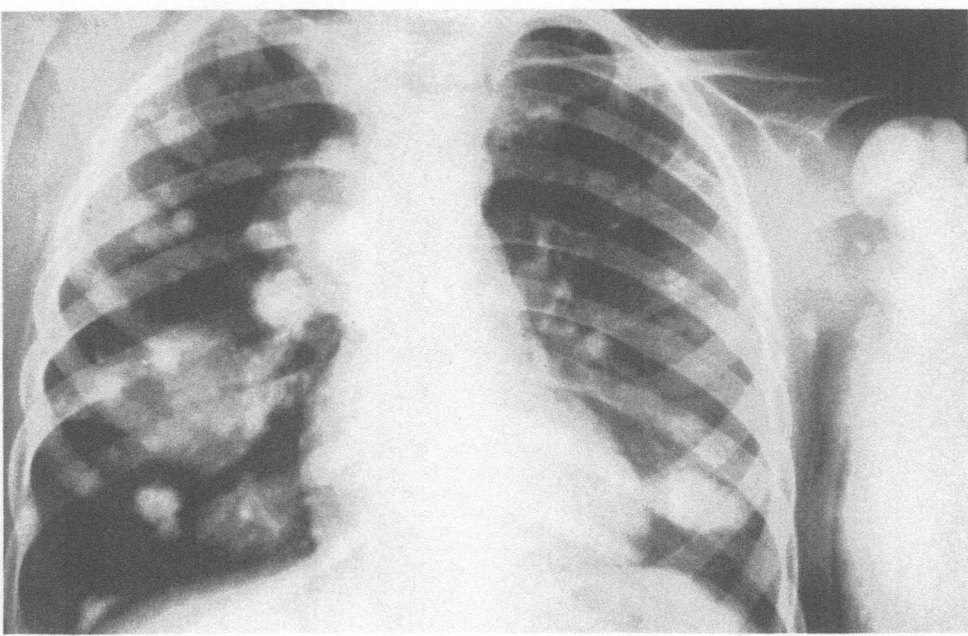

Fig. 29 b. Chest. Multiple metastases from osteogenic sarcoma. Calcific density of several of metastases is present. Extensive osteogenic sarcoma of left humerus can be seen. (From GREENFIELD, 1969. Courtesy of J.B. Lippincott Company, Publisher, Philadelphia, Pa.)

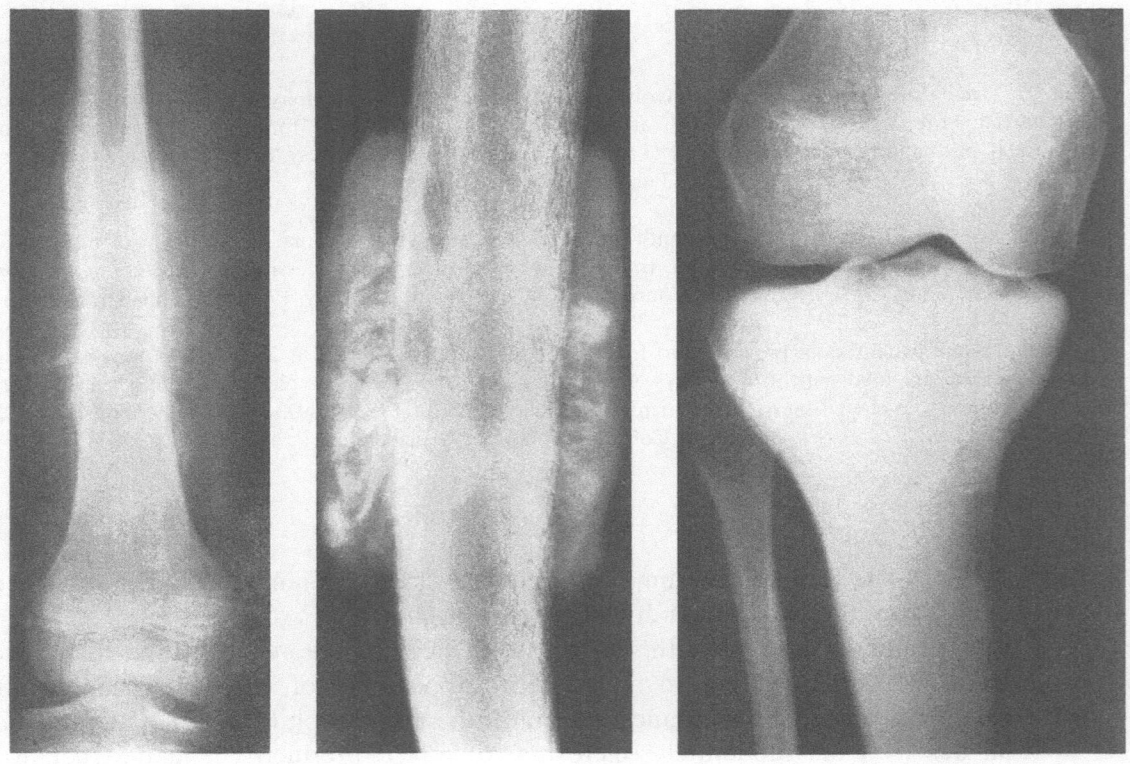

Fig. 30   Fig. 31   Fig. 32

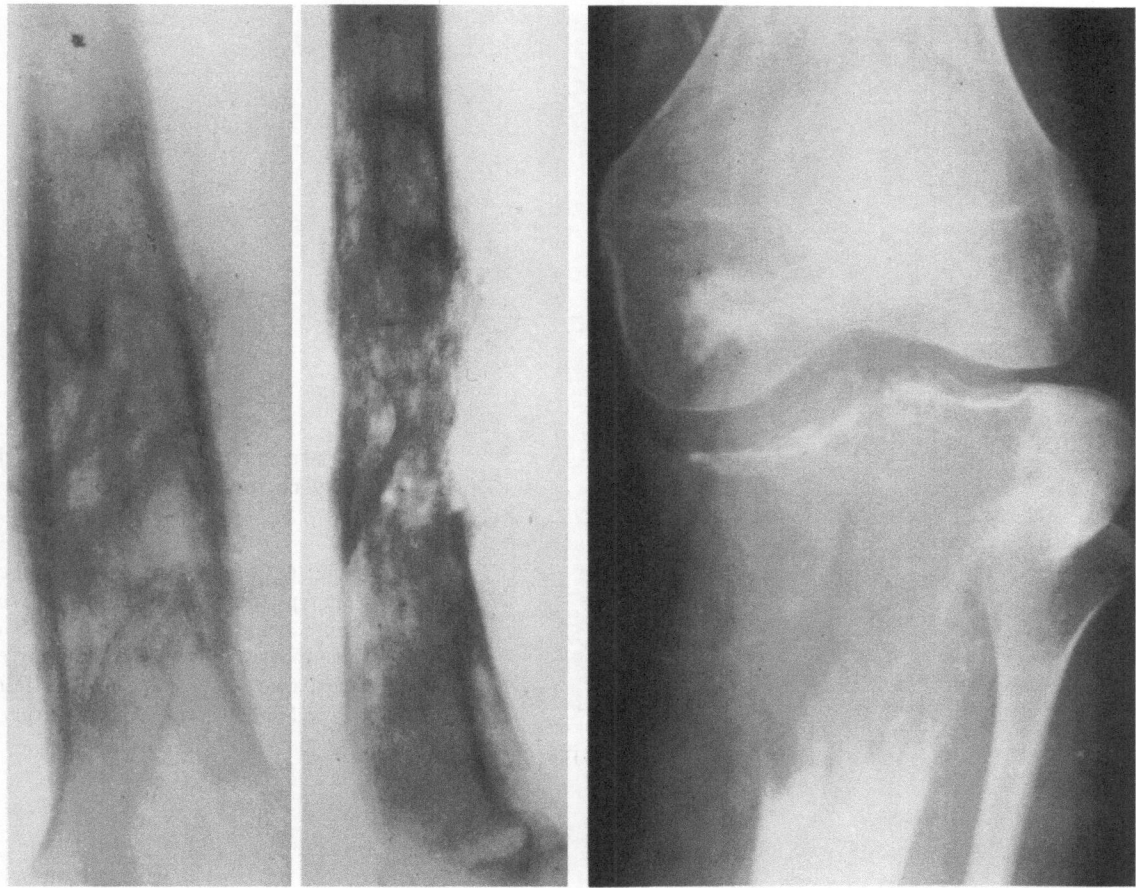

Fig. 33a   Fig. 33b   Fig. 34

Fig. 33a and b. Osteogenic sarcoma of distal femur. A large area of alternating sclerotic and radiolucent patches is seen with cortical destruction and spiculated periosteal new bone formation. There is very wide zone of transition. (Courtesy of Drs. ANTONIO PIZARRO and JAMES F. KURTZ, Hines Veteran Administration Hospital, Hines, Illinois)

Fig. 34. 17-year-old female. Osteogenic sarcoma. A purely destructive lesion of proximal tibia is seen. Margin of the destroyed area is irregular, and several moth-eaten areas of destruction are seen extending down the shaft. There is no expansion of bone. The latter two findings differentiate this from giant cell tumor. Osteoporosis of distal femur is present causing a radiolucent appearance which is not due to an invasion by tumor. (From GREENFIELD, 1969. Courtesy of J.B. Lippincott Company, Publisher, Philadelphia, Pa.)

Fig. 30. Osteogenic sarcoma. Femur. Diaphyseal origin. Long spiculated new bone formation is seen in involved area. This associated with more solid type of periosteal new bone. (From GREENFIELD, 1969. Courtesy of J.B. Lippincott Company, Publisher, Philadelphia, Pa.)

Fig. 31. Radiograph of amputation specimen of humerus with diaphyseal osteogenic sarcoma. Destructive cortical changes are seen. There is associated soft tissue mass showing spiculated type of periosteal new bone formation

Fig. 32. Osteogenic sarcoma. Proximal tibia. Sclerotic dense appearance of epiphysis and upper shaft is seen. Epiphyseal fusion has already occurred. Area of radiolucency at medial aspect of tibia is biopsy site. There is no evidence of periosteal reaction or new bone formation. No destructive areas are seen. This is a purely sclerotic osteogenic sarcoma. (From GREENFIELD, 1969. Courtesy of J.B. Lippincott Company, Publisher, Philadelphia, Pa.)

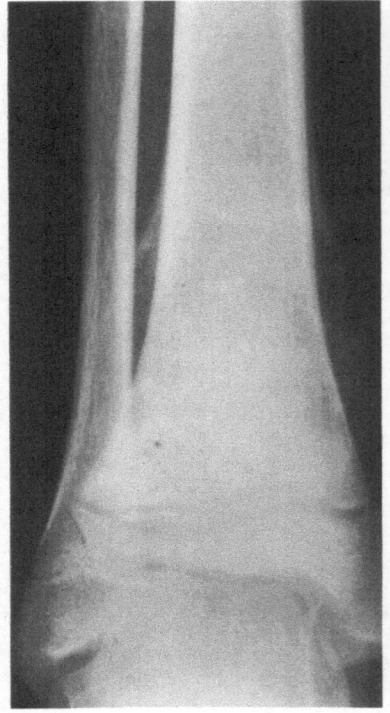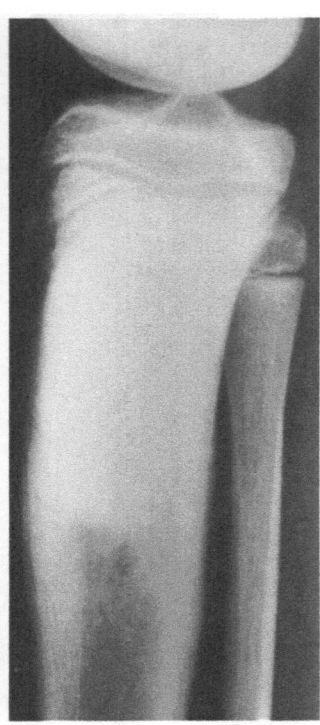

Fig. 35   Fig. 36

Fig. 35. Osteogenic sarcoma (distal tibial metaphysis). Codman's triangles may be seen at proximal aspect of lesion

Fig. 36. Osteogenic sarcoma, sclerosing type (proximal tibial metaphysis). Note dense sclerotic area involving metaphysis, limited by epiphyseal cartilage plate and showing fairly well-circumscribed distal margin

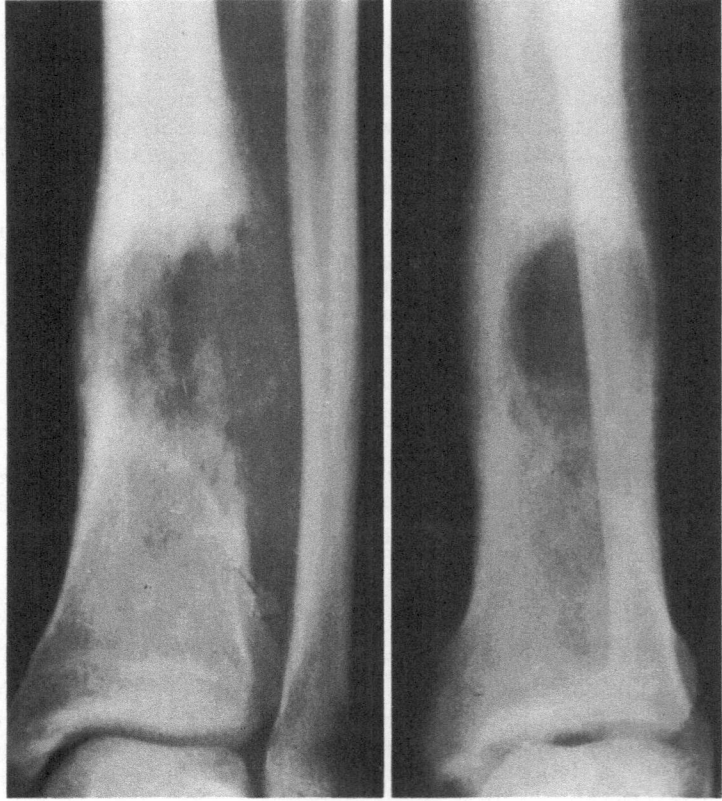

Fig. 37. Osteogenic sarcoma of distal tibia. Osteolytic type. There is large destructive area with very wide zone of transition. Periosteal new bone formation and a Codman's triangle are present. There is destruction of cortex on lateral side in entire area of involvement. (Courtesy of Dr. ANTONIO PIZARRO, Hines Veteran Administration Hospital, Hines, Illinois)

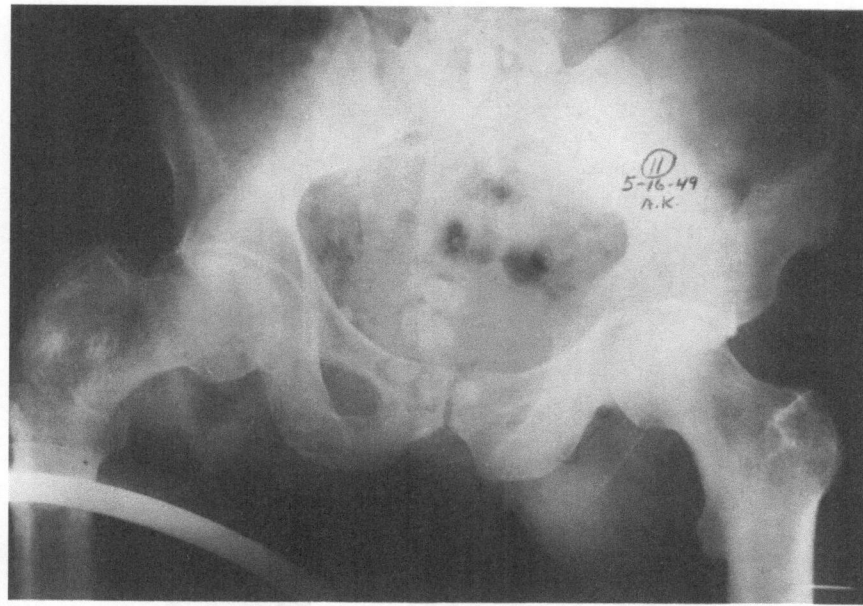

Fig. 38. Radiograph showing destructive area in intertrochanteric region of right femur with wide zone of transition, and a pathologic fracture in subtrochanteric region. A small amount of periosteal new bone formation at the upper outer aspect of femur is also noted. Other bony structures visualized appear normal

the amount of calcified osteoid present as well as the vascularity, and do not represent basic differences in type of tumor.

The bone in the lesion may be extremely sclerotic (Fig. 36). Dense sclerosis per se is not pathognomonic of osteogenic sarcoma as other conditions can be equally dense, e.g., sclerosing or Garre's osteomyelitis, Charcot's joint, and osteoid osteoma.

When the lesion is mixed or osteolytic, the destructive patterns may be permeative, moth-eaten, or rarely geographic. The most significant roentgen feature in this respect is a wide zone of transition (Figs. 37, 38, 39). The lesion has ill-defined margins which blend imperceptibly with normal bone.

The periosteal appearance is the most popularized feature of this lesion. Classically, long, thin, filiform spicules of periosteal new bone radiate from a projected central point to give the "sunburst" pattern (Figs. 40, 41a, b, c, and 42). A long segment pattern of periosteal parallel spicules may also be present. Spiculated periosteal reaction is not exclusively seen in osteogenic sarcoma, nor only in malignant tumors. Benign conditions, such as osteomyelitis or thyroid acropachy may also show spicules, but these tend to be short and squat. Rarely, the tumor may present with laminated periosteal reaction or no periosteal reaction. When the tumor aggressively destroys the periosteum or newly formed bone, then the zone of transition between intact periosteum and the destroyed area forms a cuff called Codman's triangle (Fig. 43). This is not pathognomonic of osteogenic sarcoma, and can even be seen in aggressive benign conditions, e.g., hemophilic pseudotumor.

In the flat bones, the basic aspects of the tumor are similar (Fig. 44). There may be dense sclerosis or extensive destruction. Spiculated periosteal new bone formation may be present. A wide zone of transition is also characteristic here. Rarely, an osteogenic sarcoma in a flat bone may present as an expansile lesion showing some of the other features which distinguish this lesion.

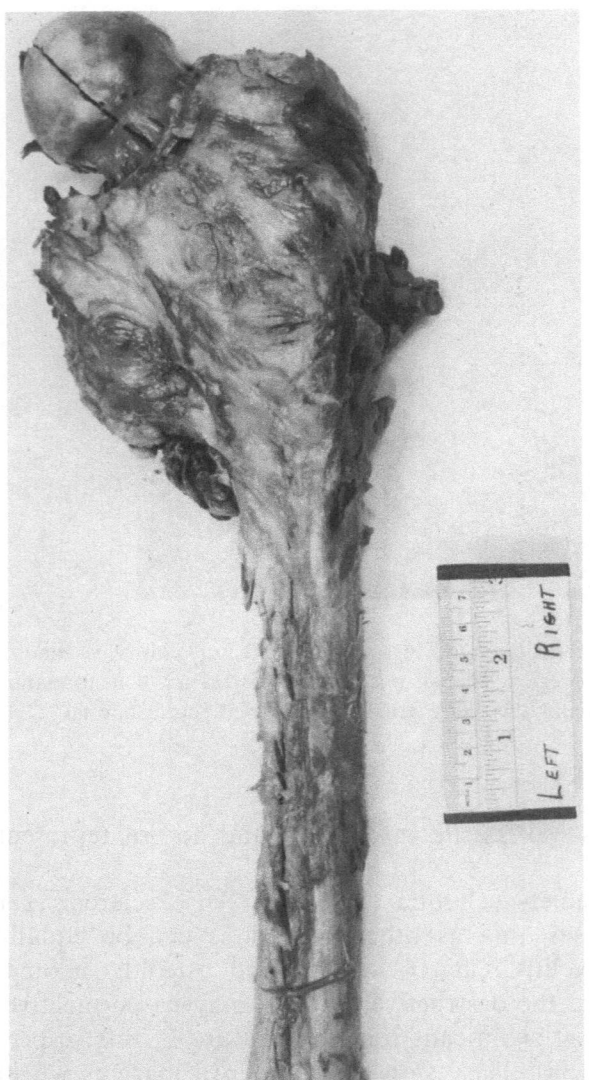

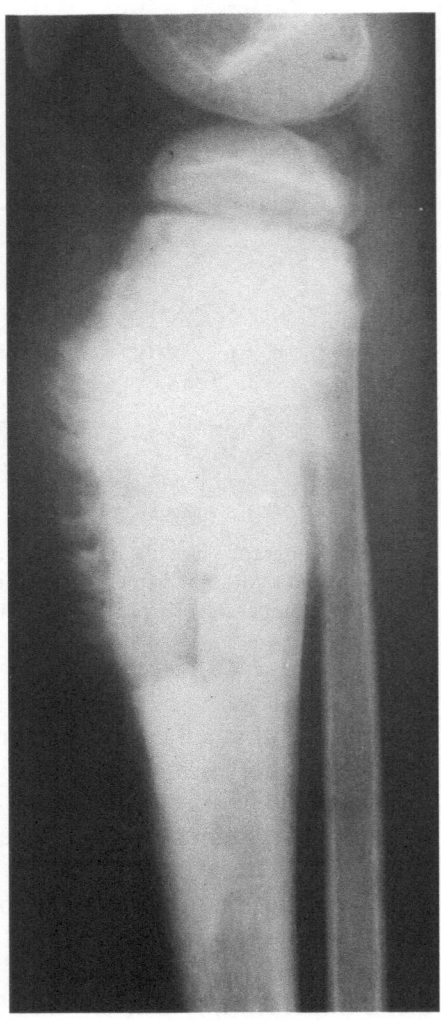

Fig. 39   Fig. 40

Fig. 39. Amputation specimen showing tumor extension in inter- and subtrochanteric regions. This represented an osteogenic sarcoma. (Courtesy of Drs. Antonio Pizarro, and James F. Kurtz, Hines Veteran Administration Hospital, Hines, Illinois)

Fig. 40. Osteogenic sarcoma. Proximal tibia. Perpendicular spiculated periosteal new bone formation or "sunburst" pattern is present. There is dense sclerosis of metaphysis extending down toward shaft. Epiphysis is not involved. A biopsy site is also noted. Soft tissue swelling is present. (From Greenfield, 1969. Courtesy of J.B. Lippincott Company, Publisher, Philadelphia, Pa.)

Fig. 41 a and b. Osteogenic sarcoma of the distal tibia. There is an area of dense sclerosis involving metaphyses and extending into epiphyseal region. Lateral view demonstrates spiculated "sunburst" type of periosteal new bone formation posteriorly. There is very wide zone of transition about the lesion. (Courtesy of Antonio Pizarro, M.D., Hines Veteran Administration Hospital, Hines, Illinois)

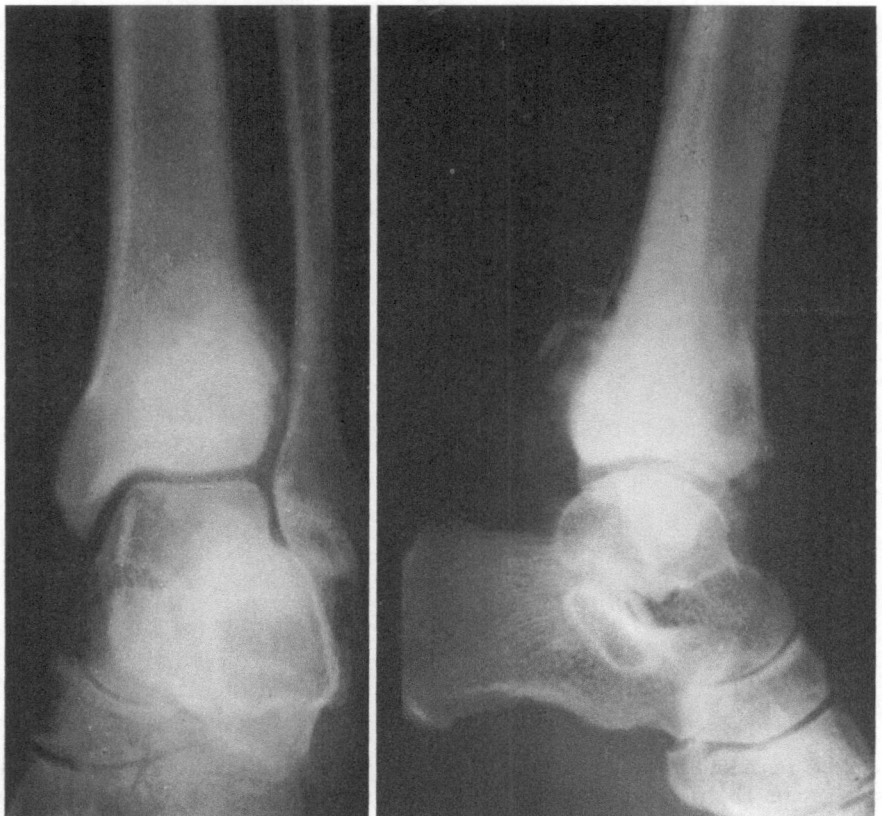

Fig. 41a   Fig. 41b

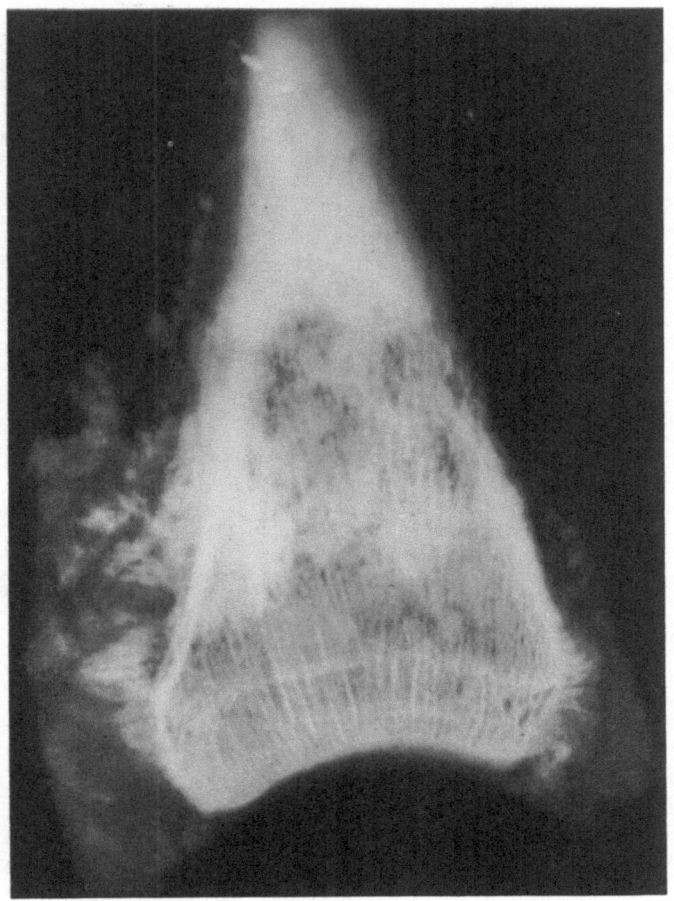

Fig. 41c. Amputation specimen showing
details of sclerotic area. Scattered destructive areas are also apparent. Note
bilateral spiculated type of periosteal
new bone formation as well as calcific
debris in soft tissues

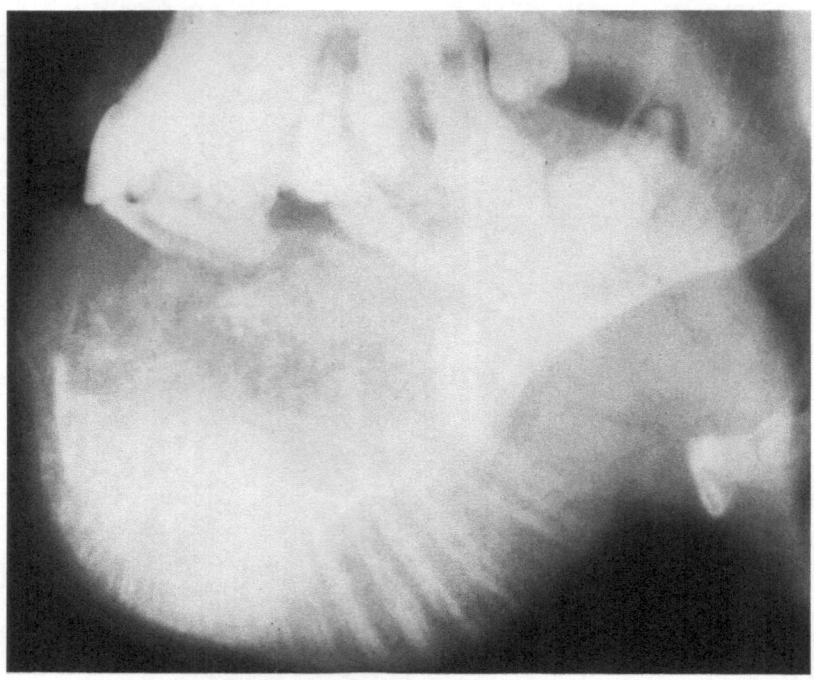

Fig. 42. Osteogenic sarcoma involving mandible with long slender spiculated periosteal new bone formation, or "sunburst" pattern. Destructive and sclerotic changes in mandible are also present, representing a mixed type of osteosarcoma. (From GREENFIELD, 1969. Courtesy of J.B. Lippincott Company, Publisher, Philadelphia, Pa.)

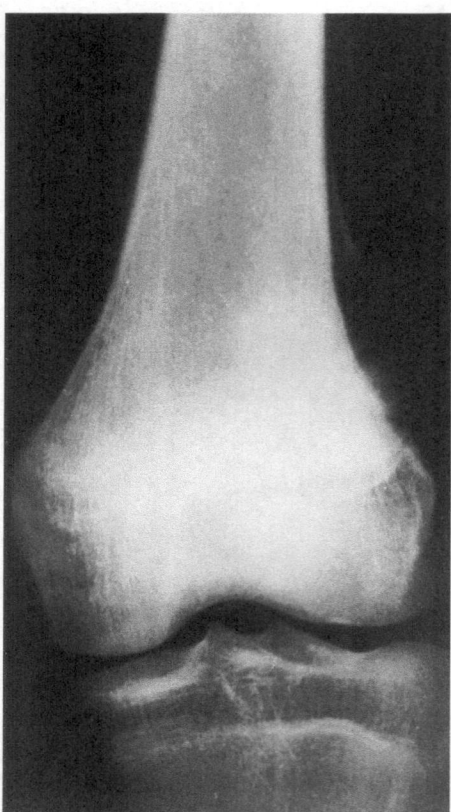

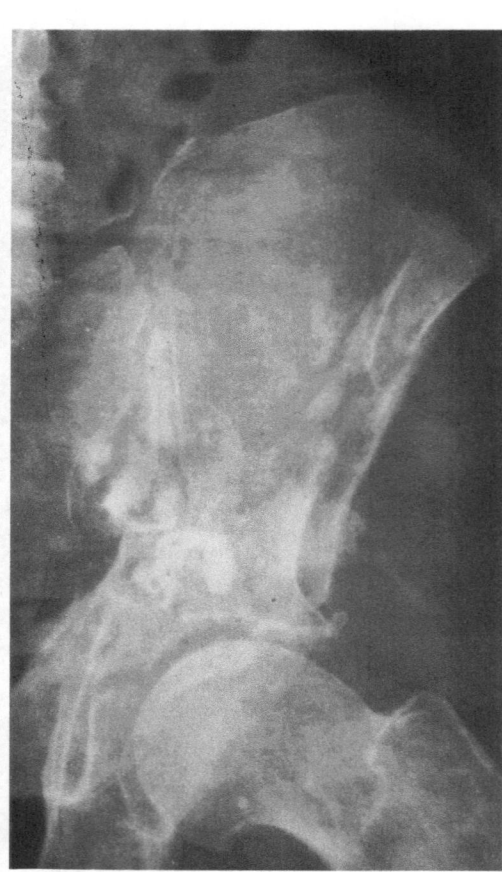

Fig. 43   Fig. 44

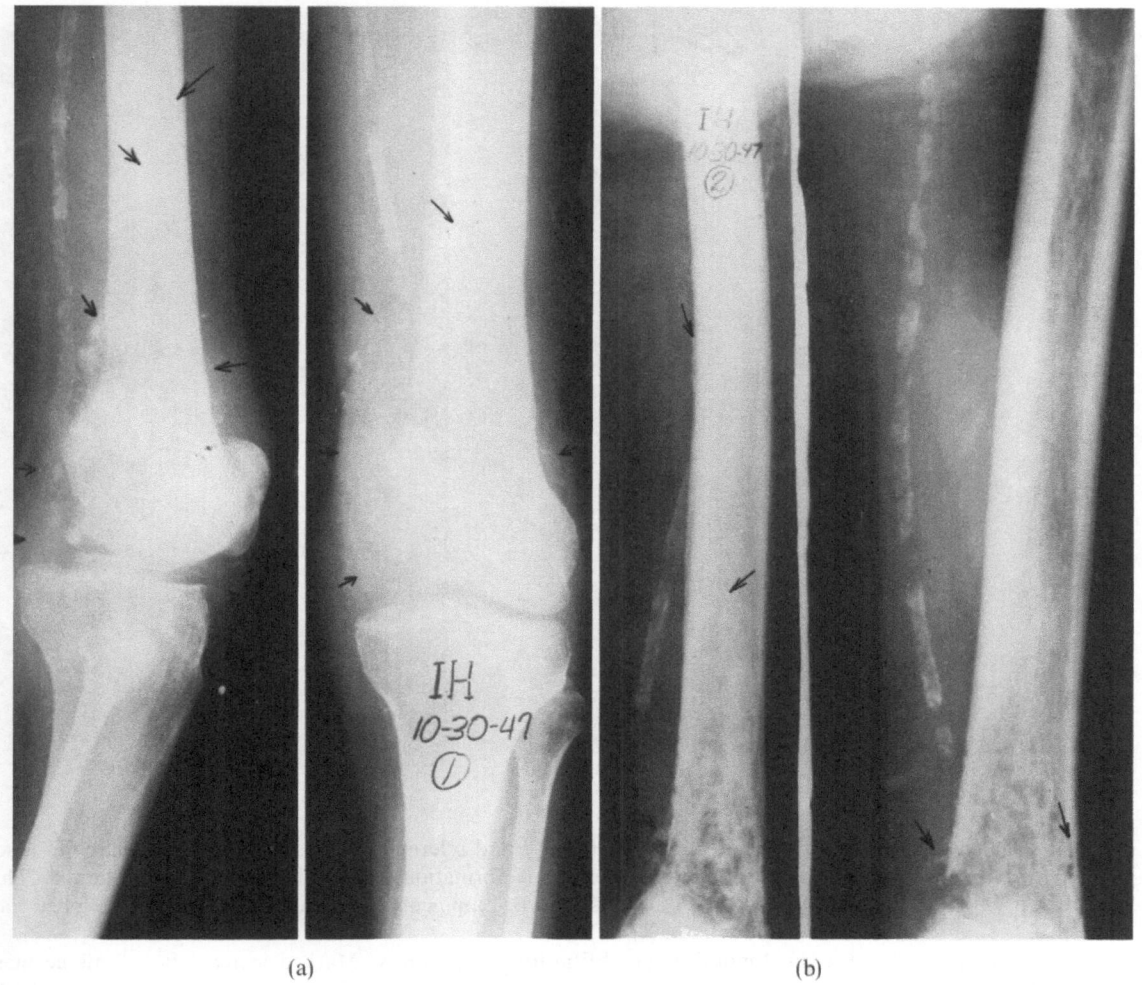

(a)   (b)

Fig. 45a and b. Osteogenic sarcoma of distal femur. Destructive changes with very wide zone of transition are noted at distal femoral metaphysis. A sparse amount of periosteal new bone formation is also noted. There is cortical destruction and invasion of soft tissues with definitive soft tissue mass. Incidental dense vascular calcification is also noted. (Courtesy of Drs. ANTONIO PIZARRO and JAMES F. KURTZ, Hines Veteran Administration Hospital, Hines, Illinois)

Fig. 43. Osteogenic sarcoma, distal femur. A densely sclerosing area in metaphysis with wide zone of transition is seen. Spiculated periosteal new bone formation as well as Codman's triangle is present on medial side

Fig. 44. Osteogenic sarcoma involving pelvis. Patchy sclerotic areas ill-defined, are seen in ilium extending into base of pubis. There is cortical destruction of pelvic rim. Articular cartilage and femoral head are intact. (Courtesy of Dr. ANTONIO PIZARRO, Hines Veteran Administration Hospital, Hines, Illinois)

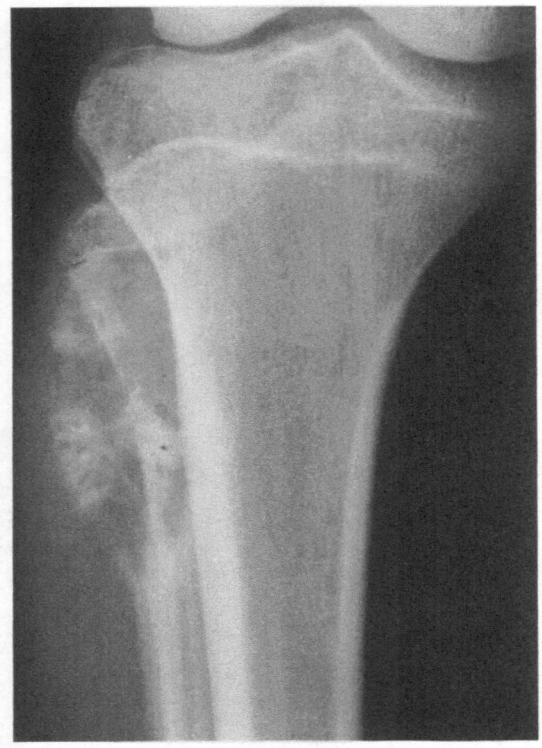

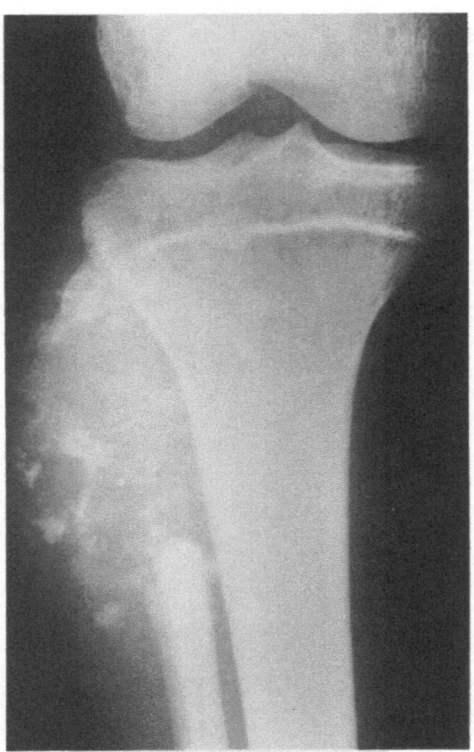

Fig. 46   Fig. 47

Fig. 46. Osteogenic sarcoma. Proximal fibula. Destructive and sclerotic changes of proximal fibula with associated soft tissue, mass, periosteal and tumor new bone formation and Codman's triangle is noted. This is prebiopsy film. (From GREENFIELD, 1969. Courtesy of J.B. Lippincott Company, Publisher, Philadelphia, Pa.)

Fig. 47. Same patient as Fig. 46. 1 month interval film following biopsy. Marked increase in soft tissue mass and increase in tumor new bone formation within mass is seen. (From GREENFIELD, 1969. Courtesy of J.B. Lippincott Company, Publisher, Philadelphia, Pa.)

Another characteristic finding in osteogenic sarcoma is destruction of the cortex with invasion of the soft tissues (Figs. 45a, b, 46, 47, 48). The cortex is usually destroyed in the entirety of its involvement. The soft tissue tumor mass may calcify, showing amorphous calcification or ossification (Fig. 49). There may be an alignment of calcific densities radiating outward from the central tumor. The mass may be very large and very dense, sometimes exceeding the size and density of the central tumor. Pathologic fractures are common (Fig. 50).

These tumors metastasize commonly via the blood stream, and more rarely by way of the lymphatics. In the vast majority of instances, the tumor metastasizes early by way of the bloodstream. Hematogenous metastases are often present at the time of diagnosis (Fig. 51). The pulmonary lesions may present as well-defined soft tissue nodules. They may also present as calcified or ossified masses, sometimes simulating calcified granulomas (Fig. 52). Another characteristic manifestation is cavitation in the lesions (Fig. 53). These may have thick or thin walls (ROTTE, 1969). Pneumothorax may result (KEW, 1966). The lesions may progress to coalescence, extensive involvement, and pleural effusion. Pulmonary hypertrophic osteoarthropathy, with generalized periosteal reaction and clubbing of the fingers, may develop in consequence (Figs. 54a, b, 55).

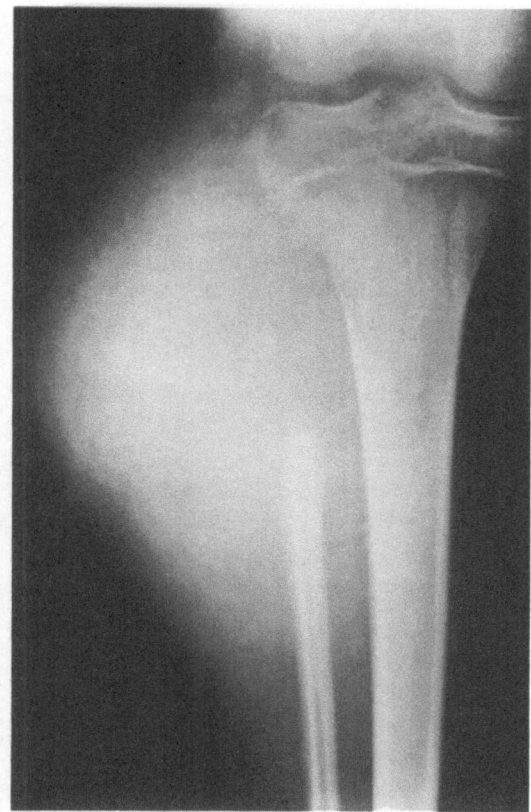

Fig. 48. Same patient as in previous two figures. 1 month interval film since Fig. 47. Very marked increase in size of soft mass is noted. (From GREENFIELD, 1969. Courtesy of J.B. Lippincott Company, Publisher, Philadelphia, Pa.)

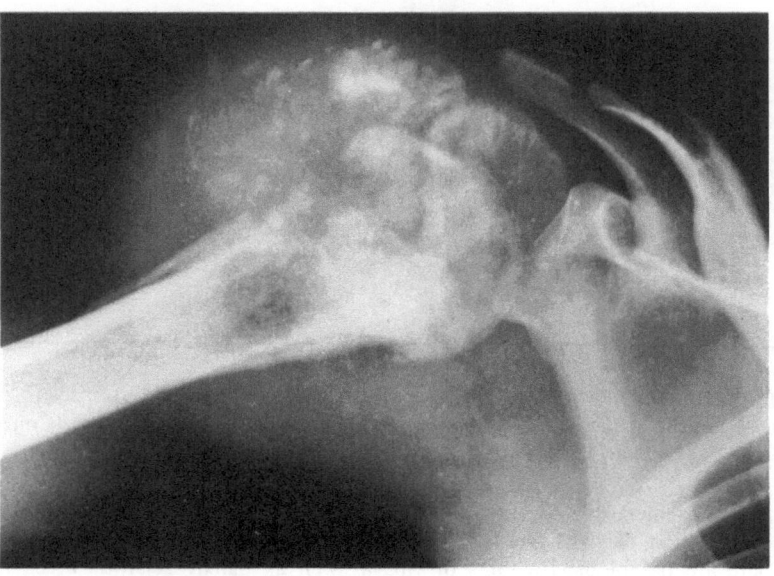

Fig. 49. Osteogenic sarcoma. Proximal humerus. Epiphyseal end of bone is involved in mixed sclerotic and lytic type of lesion. There is large soft tissue mass following breakthrough of cortex at outer aspect of upper humerus. Marked tumor new bone formation within mass is seen as well as periosteal elevation at distal aspect of tumor. Note solid nature of this periosteal new bone formation, particularly at medial side. (From GREENFIELD, 1969. Courtesy of J.B. Lippincott Company, Publisher, Philadelphia, Pa.)

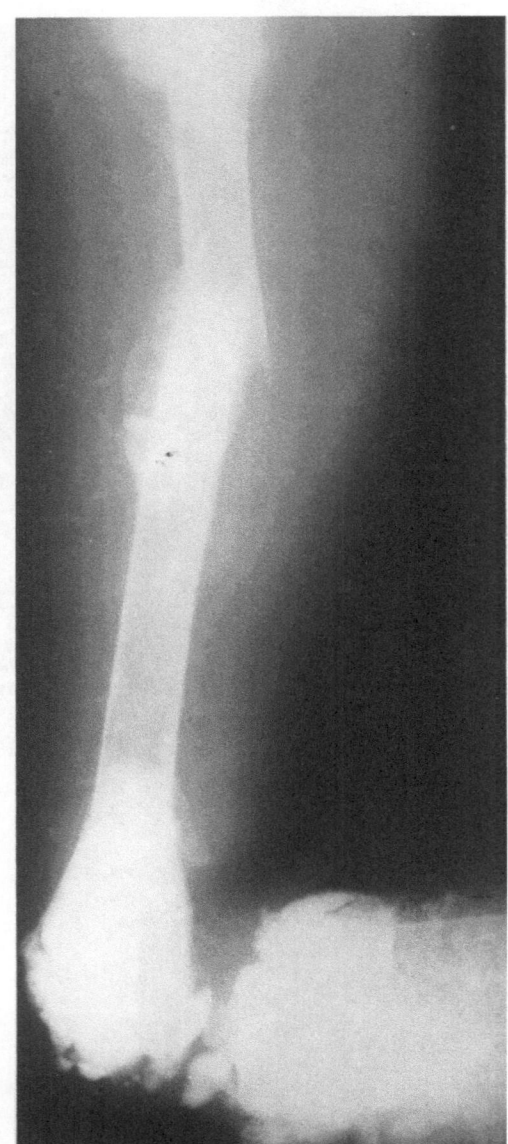

Fig. 50. Advanced osteogenic sarcoma. Involvement of knee with sclerosis of all bones is seen as well as pathologic fracture of femoral shaft and sclerosis at proximal femur. (From GREENFIELD, GEORGE B., Radiology of bone diseases, 1969, Courtesy of J.B. Lippincott Company, Publisher, Philadelphia, Pa.)

Fig. 51. Osteogenic sarcoma involving scapula with pulmonary metastases. Dense sclerosis of scapula is noted with large area of periosteal new bone formation. Pulmonary metastases are seen. (Courtesy of Dr. ANTONIO PIZARRO, Hines Veteran Administration Hospital, Hines, Illinois)

Fig. 52. Hematogenous metastases from osteogenic sarcoma to lungs and skeletal system. Female, age 55, with previous amputation of right femur for primary osteogenic sarcoma. Calcified metastatic deposits in lung noted. There are pathologic fractures of ribs as well as patchy sclerotic areas in left humeral head and shaft

Fig. 53. Thin-walled cavitating metastases from osteogenic sarcoma. These lesions eventually progressed to spontanous pneumothorax. Nodular densities in remainder of lung fields are present. (From GREENFIELD, GEORGE B., Radiology of bone diseases, 1969, Courtesy of J.B. Lippincott Company, Publisher, Philadelphia, Pa.)

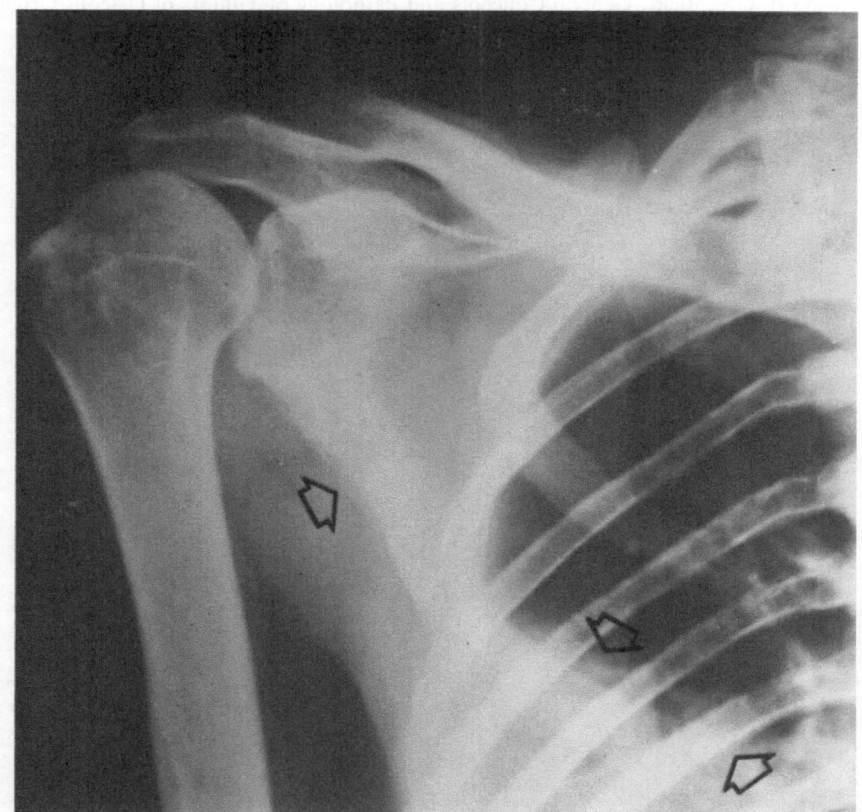

Fig. 51

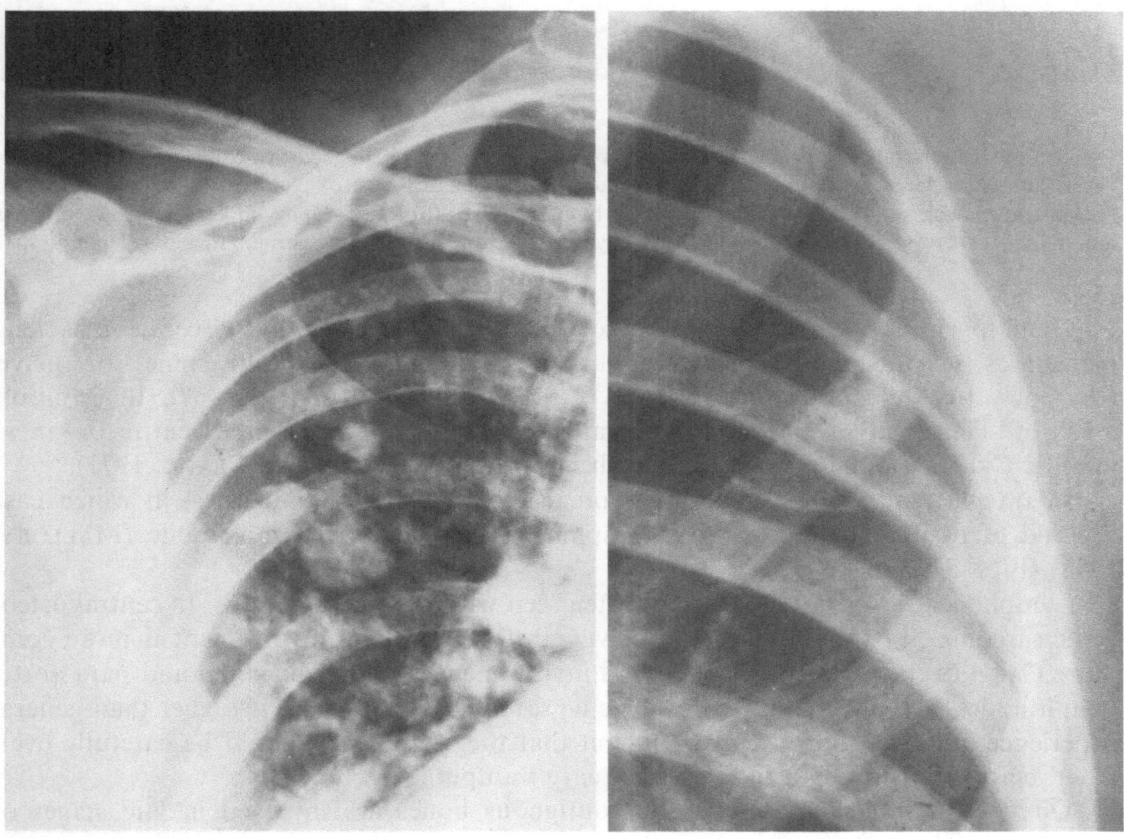

Fig. 52

Fig. 53

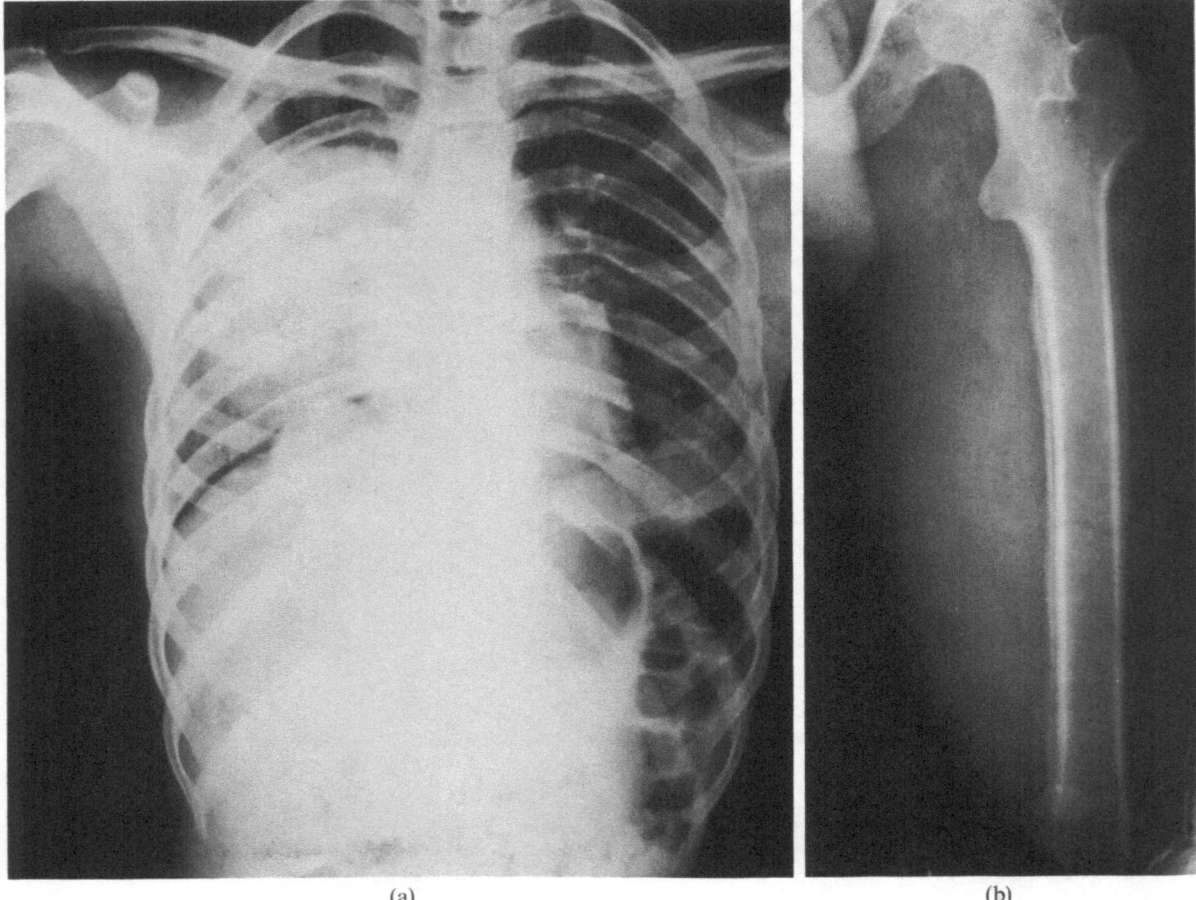

(a)   (b)

Fig. 54a and b. Metastatic osteogenic sarcoma with pulmonary hypertrophic osteoarthropathy. (a) Posteroanterior chest film shows large metastatic mass in right lung with laminated type of periosteal new bone formation seen in the clavicle and at the outer margins of both scapulae. (b) Radiography of left leg shows previous amputation. There is bilateral dense laminated type of periosteal new bone formation along femoral shaft

Hematogenous metastases to other organs occur. Occasionally, visceral or skeletal metastases may be seen, the latter usually involving the skull, spine, or pelvis (Figs. 56a, b). Metastases to distal parts of the skeleton are rare (Figs. 57a, b). Multiple areas of skeletal involvement are generally considered to be of multicentric origin in infants. Calcified renal metastases have been reported (NELSON and CLARK, 1971).

In rare instances, metastases may spread by way of the lymphatics, in which case a cloud of ossification is seen radiographically in a regional lymph node (MALLORY, 1941) (Figs. 58, 59).

Lymphogenous metastases are not often seen with peripheral lesions. In central osteogenic sarcomas, of the shoulder and pelvic girdles, lymphatic involvement is more common. CACERES et al. (1969) reported 11% involvement of the mediastinal and para-aortic lymph nodes in centrally located osteogenic sarcomas. This figure is higher than general experience indicates, but it does point out that the lymphatics should be carefully evaluated before performing a fore or hindquarter amputation.

Direct extension is common. The contiguous bones are involved in late stages of the disease. The soft tissues adjacent to the lesion are commonly invaded, and a very large soft tissue mass commonly develops, which may calcify or ossify (Fig. 60).

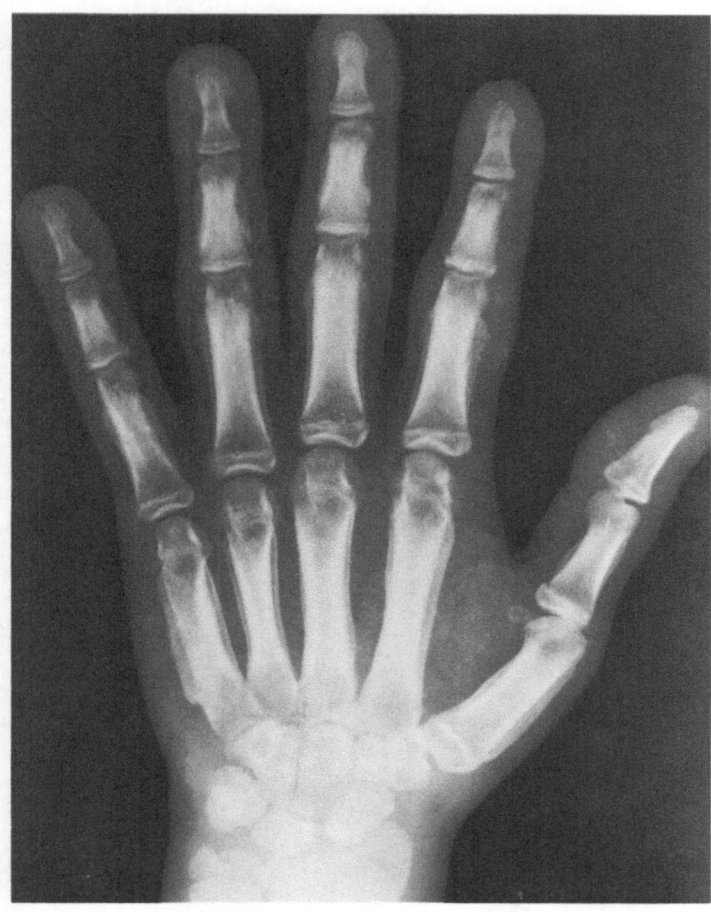

Fig. 55. Pulmonary hypertrophic osteoarthropathy secondary to pulmonary metastases from osteogenic
sarcoma. A dense solid type of periosteal new bone formation involving
metacarpals, proximal, and middle
phalanges is seen. Periosteal new
bone formation only involves diaphyses. Clubbing of soft tissues of fingers is also present

The differential diagnosis should include solitary aggressive lesions with wide zone
of transition. Osteolytic, mixed, and sclerotic lesions should be considered. In many
instances, radiologic appearance of a tumor may be atypical, and histologic appearance
may be indeterminate. It is not uncommon to have differing opinions from various
prominent consulting pathologists.

The list of differential diagnostic possibilities are summarized in Table 1.

Table 1. Differential diagnosis of osteogenic sarcoma

1. Ewing's sarcoma	6. Benign osteoblastoma
2. Chondrosarcoma	7. Garre's osteomyelitis
3. Giant cell tumor	8. Charcot's joint
4. Fibrosarcoma	9. Osteoblastic metastases
5. Parosteal sarcoma	

Ewing's sarcoma is a primary malignant neoplasm considered by some to be derived
from immature reticulum cells of the bone marrow. This tumor occurs less frequently
than osteogenic sarcoma. The peak age incidence is 15 years, with a range of 5–30 years.
This range overlaps that of osteogenic sarcoma, except in the older age groups. The
distribution varies according to the age of the patient, owing to the different locations
of red marrow at different ages. In the younger patient, the tubular bones are likely

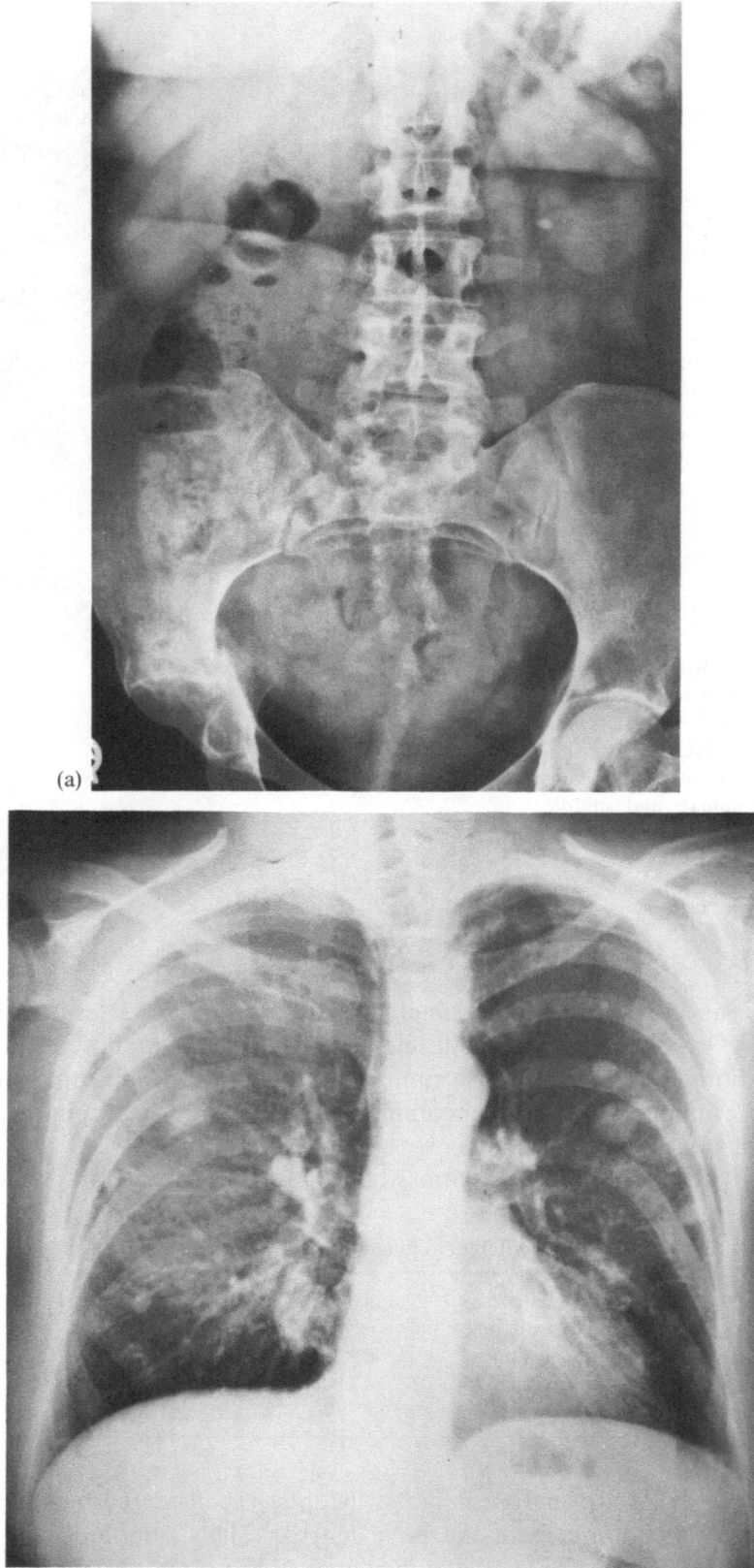

Fig. 56a and b. Metastatic osteogenic sarcoma following disarticulation at right hip for primary osteogenic sarcoma. (a) Destructive areas and pathologic fracture at right acetabulum are seen. In addition, two distinct small ossific densities in left upper quadrant are present. (b) Posteroanterior chest film shows multiple nodular calcified metastases. Pathologic rib fractures are also present

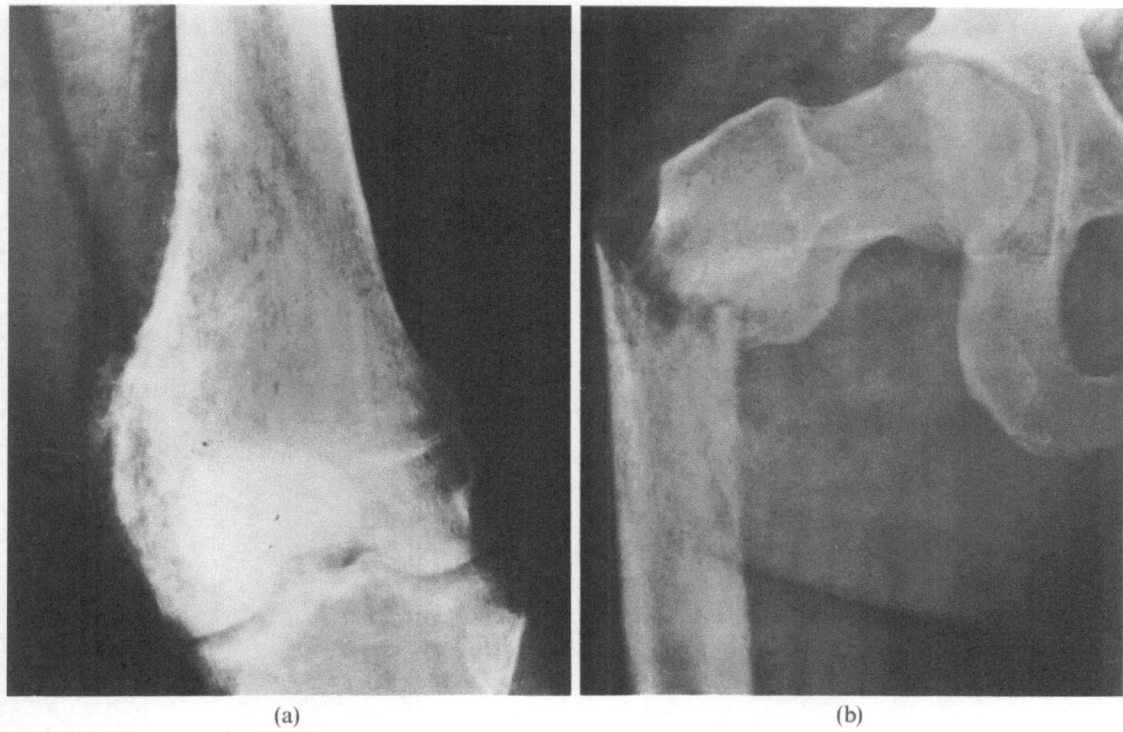

(a)   (b)

Fig. 57a and b. Osteogenic sarcoma in distal right femur, with metastases to proximal right femur, progressing to pathologic fracture. Male. Age 32. (a) An area of permeative destructive change at distal femur with very wide zone of transition, and showing "sunburst" and solid type of periosteal new bone formation, with Codman's triangle at medial aspect of femur is seen. (b) 9 months later destructive area with pathologic fracture of left femur is present

to be involved, while in a patient over 20 years of age, the flat bones tend to be involved. The femur, tibia, os calcis, and innominate bone are common sites.

In the flat and cuboidal bones, there is a characteristic roentgen appearance of mottled destruction and patchy reactive bone sclerosis, all with a wide zone of transition.

A "classic" appearance in the long bones is described, which occurs in less than half of the cases. This comprises an ill-defined permeative area of bone destruction involving a large central portion of the mid-shaft. This is in contrast to osteogenic sarcoma which characteristically involves the metaphysis. There is a fusiform configuration associated with a fine, delicate lamellated periosteal new bone response. Osteogenic sarcoma typically shows a "sunburst" spiculated type of periosteal new bone response. In Ewing's tumor, the tumor cells permeate through the Haversian canals and invade the soft tissues, leaving an intact cortex, cortical sequestration, or a cortex only segmentally destroyed. This is similar to what may be seen in osteomyelitis. In contrast, an osteogenic sarcoma sweeps away the cortex in the entire area of involvement. Because the tumor forms no osteoid or chondroid, the soft tissue mass, which may be large, is free of calcifications except for periosteal new bone formation or debris. An osteogenic sarcoma may show a very heavily calcified or ossified soft tissue mass.

No neoplastic new bone is formed, only reactive sclerosis. The dense sclerosis seen in the sclerotic forms of osteogenic sarcoma is not seen in Ewing's tumor. A spiculated type of periosteal response is sometimes seen in Ewing's tumor, but this is of the long-segment type in contrast to the "sunburst" pattern typical of osteogenic sarcoma. When the ribs are involved, an expansile lesion with an associated extrapleural soft tissue mass is sometimes seen, an appearance that would be rare for osteogenic sarcoma.

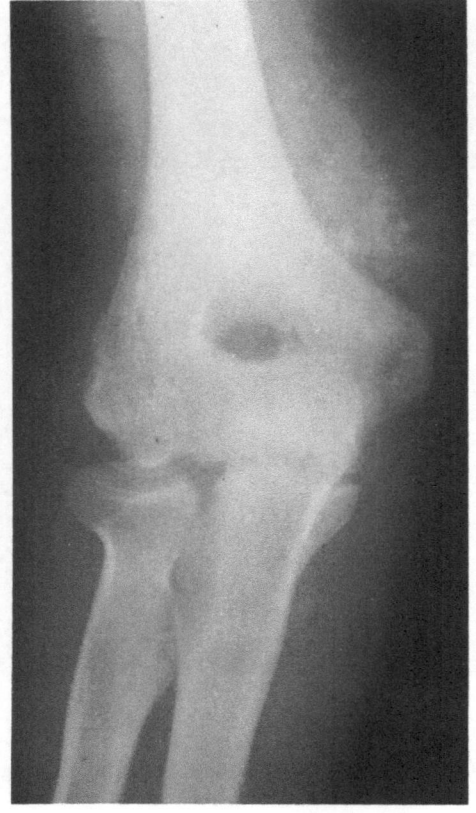

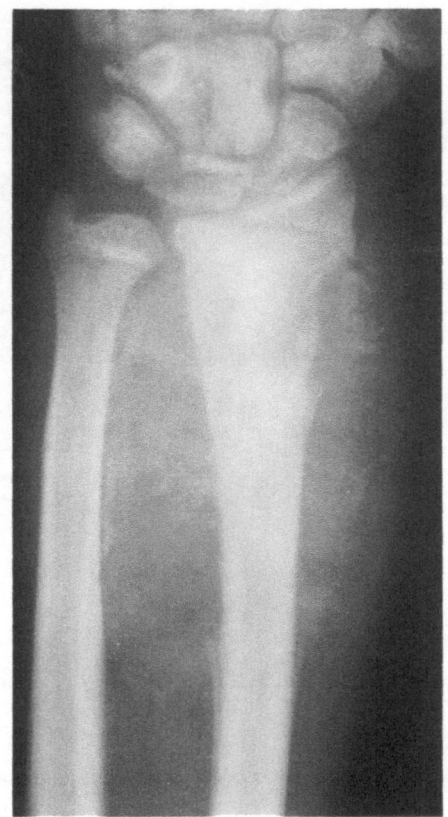

Fig. 58   Fig. 59

Fig. 58. Osteogenic sarcoma metastatic to supratrochlear lymph node. Soft tissue swelling containing streaky calcific densities is seen. (From GREENFIELD, 1969. Courtesy of J.B. Lippincott Company, Publisher, Philadelphia, Pa.)

Fig. 59. Same patient and same extremity as Fig. 58. Osteogenic sarcoma of distal radius which has metastasized to supratrochlear lymph node. An area of sclerosis at distal radius involving metaphysis and diaphysis but not epiphysis is seen. Radiolucency is secondary to biopsy. Large soft tissue mass, perpendicular striated periosteal new bone formation, and Codman's triangle are noted. (From GREENFIELD, 1969. Courtesy of J.B. Lippincott Company, Publisher, Philadelphia, Pa.)

The afore mentioned appearances only describe the typical forms. An atypical lesion may prove to be a diagnostic challenge indeed.

Chondrosarcoma is a malignant tumor of cartilaginous origin that remains essentially cartilaginous throughout its development. Chondrosarcoma may originate within the bone, where it is called central, or outside of the confines of the cortex, where it is referred to as peripheral or juxtacortical. It may originate de novo, or it may arise in a pre-existing cartilaginous lesion, such as osteocartilaginous exostoses or enchondromas.

There is a wide range of age distribution, with more than 50% of the patients older than 40 years. The age distribution only marginally overlaps that of osteogenic sarcoma.

Radiologically, in central chondrosarcoma, the most common sites are the femur and proximal humerus. The tibia, ribs, ilium, scapula, or sternum may also be involved.

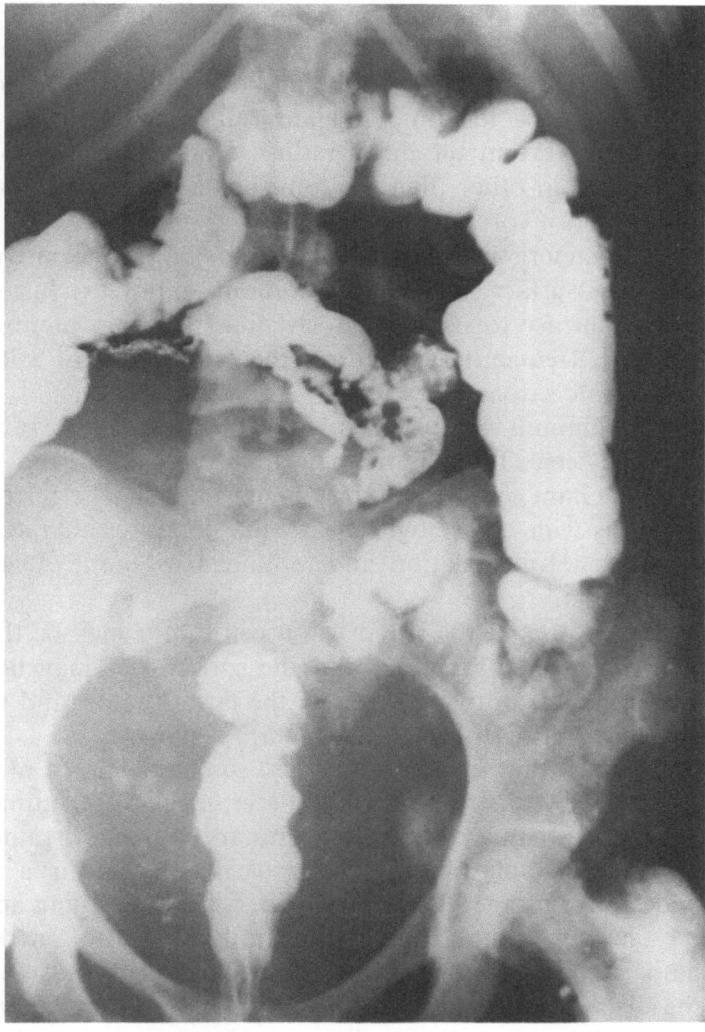

Fig. 60. Osteogenic sarcoma primary in greater trochanter of left femur which has involved soft tissues of pelvis. A large soft tissue mass is seen with streaky tumor new bone formation. Tumor has metastisized to bony pelvis as well. Soft tissue mass is seen displacing barium-filled colon and ilium. (From GREENFIELD, 1969. Courtesy of J.B. Lippincott Company, Publisher, Philadelphia, Pa.)

The lesion has a metaphyseal predilection, in common with osteogenic sarcoma. The tumor forms cartilage, which is readily recognized by amorphous, punctate, small, flocculent, dense, irregular calcifications, which may range from sparse to heavy. Neoplastic new bone is not formed directly, but dense reactive sclerosis may be present.

Chondrosarcoma may present as an osteolytic expansile lesion, well marginated, with either endosteal cortical thickening or thinning. This appearance is not consistent with that of osteogenic sarcoma.

There may be simple periosteal new bone formation, long segment fine spiculation, or even rarely lamination. The tumor may develop a wide zone of transition and almost the entire diaphysis of a long bone may be involved. The lesion may destroy the cortex and invade the soft tissues, where dense calcifications in a large tumor mass may be seen. This appearance may be very difficult to differentiate from an osteogenic sarcoma. The different age distributions, the "sunburst" periosteal reaction, the metaphyseal location, the dense tumor new bone formation, and the lack of an expansile picture seen in osteogenic sarcoma would help in the differential diagnosis.

Giant cell tumor is an uncommon tumor derived from skeletal connective tissues.

The incidence of malignancy is estimated at approximately 20%. It is not possible to predict on histologic or radiologic grounds the future behavior of the majority of these lesions (JAFFE, 1958). Three-quarters of cases occur in the 20–40 years age bracket, thus only marginally overlapping the age distribution of osteogenic sarcoma.

The classic location of giant cell tumor is in the distal femur or proximal tibia, to a lesser extent the distal radius, and has been reported in almost all tubular bones. Locations in other than the long bones are encountered in 15% of cases. Mandibular and spinal involvement is rare.

Characteristically the tumor, in a long bone, involves the end of the bone to the articular surface in patients in whom epiphyseal fusions has already taken place. This is in contrast to osteogenic sarcoma which is predominantly metaphyseal. Giant cell tumor is frequently located off the central axis of a long bone, in contrast to a central osteogenic sarcoma.

In common with the osteolytic type of osteogenic sarcoma, a large area of radiolucency may be seen. There is no new bone formation and reactive bone sclerosis is usually sparse. Giant cell tumor typically does not show a sclerotic rim but the zone of transition is not as wide as osteogenic sarcoma. Features characteristic of giant cell tumor include expansion, trabeculation, and a round shape, none of which are typically seen in osteogenic sarcoma.

The cortex at the site of giant cell tumor may be thinned and destroyed, in common with osteogenic sarcoma, and the soft tissues may be invaded. The extent of the soft tissue mass is not as great as in the latter tumor, and the calcifications and ossifications so typical of osteogenic sarcoma are lacking.

Finally, the periosteal response so characteristic of osteogenic sarcoma is completely lacking, and this response is not seen in giant-cell tumor even after pathologic fracture.

Fibrosarcoma of bone is a primary malignant tumor of fibroblastic tissue that does not form neoplastic osteoid or cartilage. This is a rare tumor of bone. There is a wide range of age distribution with a peak in young adulthood.

The tumor may originate centrally, or less often periosteally, where it is sometimes associated with a large soft tissue mass. The most common sites of involvement are the distal femur and proximal tibia. Other sites of involvement are the mandible, long bones of the upper limbs, ribs, scapula, sacrum, or pelvis. The origin is usually metaphyseal, but may extend into the epiphysis.

The chief roentgen feature, in common with the osteolytic type of osteogenic sarcoma, is a large bony destructive lesion that may assume many patterns. In contrast to osteogenic sarcoma, there is no neoplastic new bone formation, nor can flocculent calcifications be seen within the radiolucent areas. A unique feature among neoplasms is the tendency toward bone sequestration in fibrosarcoma. There may be thinning, expansion, or destruction of the cortex. Massive expansion simulating an aneurysmal bone cyst may be seen. Reactive bone sclerosis and periosteal new bone formation are sparse. The spiculated "sunburst" type of periosteal new bone formation is not seen in fibrosarcoma. A wide zone of transition may be present.

The soft tissues may be invaded, but the calcification and ossification so frequently seen in osteogenic sarcoma is not present.

Parosteal sarcoma, or juxtacortical osteogenic sarcoma is a distinct entity separate from osteogenic sarcoma. The tumor originates from the periosteum or immediate parosteal connective tissue. It is a rare tumor with a wide range of age incidence, but the majority occurring in patients over 30 years. The prognosis is better than in central osteogenic sarcoma. The tumor usually originates at the metaphysis, in the parosteal region. About half of the cases occur in the lower femur. The proximal femur, humerus, and tibia are other sites. There is considerable variation in size of the tumor. The density of the mass may be homogeneously ossified or more rarely may show scattered areas of calcification. One characteristic radiologic finding is a distinct radiolucent line of demarcation between the tumor and the cortex of bone, the line representing the periosteum or fibrotic capsule. The tumor may invade the bone or completely surround it without invasion. In common with osteogenic sarcoma dense bone formation may be present, however, the large extraosseous component with minimal invasiveness, and in early stages the radiolucent line of demarcation serve to differentiate this lesion from central osteogenic sarcoma.

Benign osteoblastoma is another primary tumor of bone which in common with osteogenic sarcoma shows ossification of the matrix. It is a rare neoplasm, similar histologically to osteoid osteoma. The most common location is in the vertebral arch. About half of the cases have vertebral involvement. The tubular and long bones may also be involved. The lesions in the long bones may be located in the metaphysis or the diaphysis. Roentgenologically the lesion typically presents as an expansile, well-circumscribed lesion. Extensive ossification of the matrix may be present although this is not necessarily so. The size of the tumor is variable. There may even be cortical breakthrough and a soft tissue component. A cortical shell from expansion may be present but there is characteristically sparse periosteal new bone formation. The typical spiculated or "sunburst" type of periosteal new bone formation so common in osteogenic sarcoma is not seen. The lesion is characterized by a narrow zone of transition, in contrast to an osteogenic sarcoma that has a wide zone of transition. The dense reactive sclerosis that is commonly seen in osteoid osteoma is not present in this lesion.

Garre's osteomyelitis, or chronic sclerosing osteomyelitis is a low grade chronic infection causing sclerotic reaction without destruction or sequestration. The involved area may be a portion or all of the bone. The increase in density can be as intense as that seen in osteogenic sarcoma (Fig. 61). Characteristically there is no periosteal new bone response and no spiculated periosteal reaction. The soft tissues are not invaded and there is no cortical destruction as in osteogenic sarcoma. The zone of transition may be wide in common with the latter tumor.

Charcot's joint may cause reactive sclerosis that is as intense as the increased density seen in osteogenic sarcoma. The sclerosis may affect the bones on both sides of the joint, unlike in osteogenic sarcoma. In addition, there is joint space destruction, which is not seen in osteogenic sarcoma. Charcot's joint is also characterized by fragmentation and soft tissue debris, which can be differentiated from the ossification and calcification in the soft tissue mass of osteogenic sarcoma by the cortex, the angular fragments, and the organization of the osseous fragments in Charcot's joint. No periosteal new bone formation nor "sunburst" type of periosteal reaction is present in Charcot's joint, in contrast to osteogenic sarcoma.

Osteoblastic metastases also present a picture that is locally similar to the radiographic appearance of osteogenic sarcoma (Figs. 62a, b, c). Osteoblastic metastases may occur in the younger age groups secondary to cerebellar medulloblastoma, particularly after surgery. Hodgkin's disease may present as an osteosclerotic lesion. In the older age groups, carcinoma of the breast, particularly after treatment, and in the male, carcinoma of the prostate, commonly give osteoblastic metastases. Osteoblastic metastases especially secondary to the latter may be associated with a marked degree of spiculated periosteal reaction, sometimes of the sunburst pattern (LEHRER et al., 1970). Although the roentgen appearance may be similar, the older age of the patient, and the fact that the lesion is seen in bone which is not obviously involved with Paget's disease, should lead the observer to consider carcinoma of the prostate.

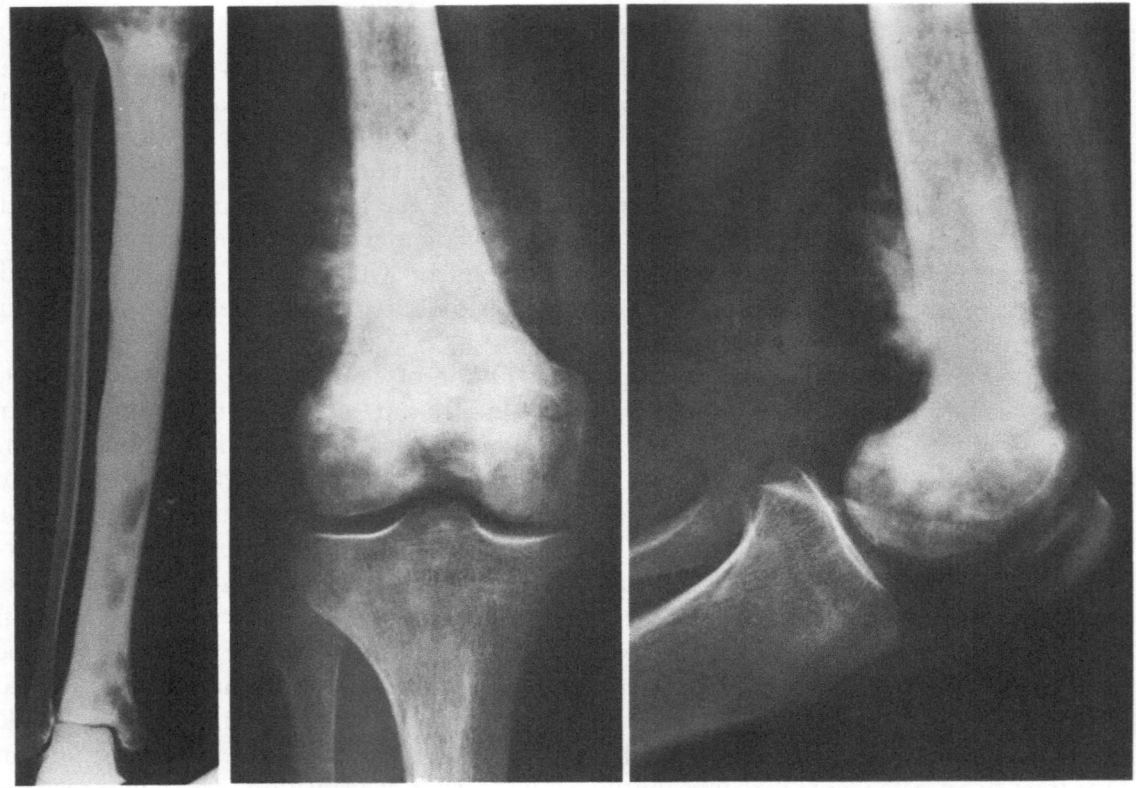

Fig. 61   Fig. 62a   Fig. 62b

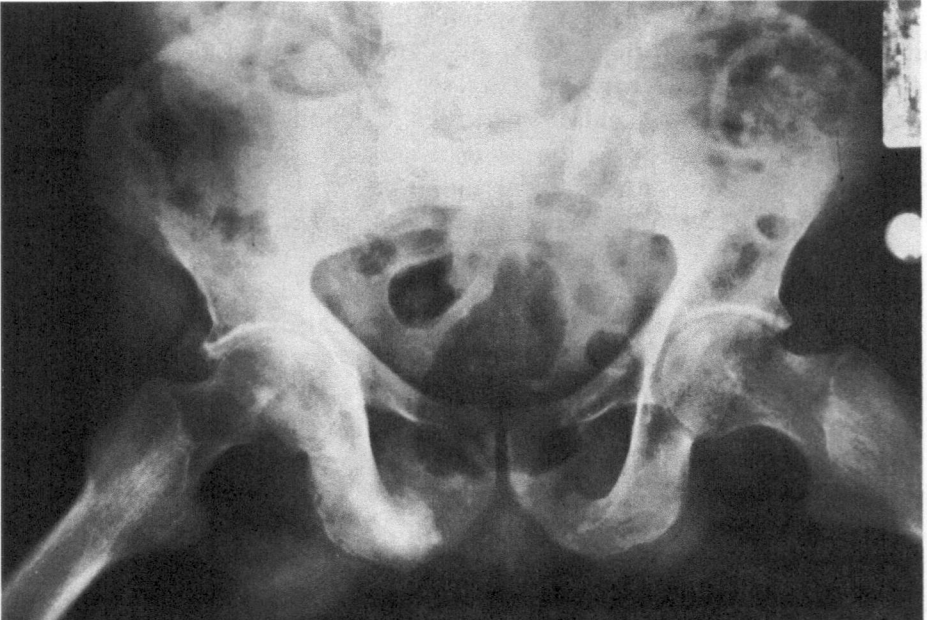

Fig. 62c

Fig. 61. Garre's sclerosing osteomyelitis. Dense sclerosis of the shaft of tibia is seen. Distal tibia shows irregular residual areas of normal bone. There is no cortical destruction nor is there periosteal new bone formation

Fig. 62a–c. Osteoblastic metastases from carcinoma of prostate simulating osteogenic sarcoma. (a) and (b) The distal femur shows dense area of sclerosis with spiculated "sunburst" type of periosteal new bone formation, cortical destruction, and large soft tissue mass. (c) Pelvis contains sclerotic and destructive changes in left ischium and pubis. Patient is a 79-year-old male with proven carcinoma of prostate. Biopsy revealed prostatic metastases

II. Primary Multicentric Osteogenic Sarcoma

Multiple osteogenic sarcomatosis is generally thought to represent primary multicentric development of osteogenic sarcomas. Several opinions to the contrary have been published, but the general appearance of bilateral and symmetrical areas of involvement, which are all approximately of the same size tend to confirm the body of former opinion. This represents a distinct clinical entity.

Cases have been reported of extensive skeletal metastases from a primary osteogenic sarcoma, but the later development of smaller metastatic foci distinguish this condition. Multicentric osteogenic sarcomatosis is a rare disease occurring principally in childhood. It may occur in infants, adolescents, young adults, and has been reported in a 50-year-old male. The disease runs a rapidly fatal course. Pulmonary metastases occur early. Multicentric osteogenic sarcomas in Paget's disease may also occur. The serum alkaline phosphatase level is elevated, and the serum calcium and phosphate levels are usually normal.

Radiologically the lesions are characterized by simultaneously appearing radiopaque densities in the metaphyses of the long bones adjacent to the epiphyseal cartilage plate. They are all approximately the same size. The lesions are distributed symmetrically bilaterally. They can vary from a few bones being involved to very extensive bony involvement. The long bones as well as the pelvis, spine, ribs, sternum, and clavicle may be involved.

In the tubular bones, the epiphysis may be invaded. The short tubular bones and the bones of the carpus and the tarsus may also be involved. Spiculated periosteal new bone formation and soft tissue invasion may occur, similar in appearance to solitary osteogenic sarcoma.

In the differential diagnosis, one must consider primary osteogenic sarcoma that has metastasized to the skeletal system. In this event we would expect to find a single larger tumor and multiple smaller areas, without necessarily the bilateral symmetrical distribution of uniform sized densities found in this disease.

Metaphyseal densities from multiple bone islands or osteopoikilosis have a characteristic appearance of multiple punctate areas of increased density clustered about the metaphyseal regions in the long bones, and in the pelvis.

Recently giant bone islands have been described. These are very well-circumscribed and do not conform to a bilateral symmetrical distribution. Metaphyseal densities secondary to heavy metal or phosphorus intoxication can be differentiated from multicentric osteosarcoma by their linear character.

III. Osteogenic Sarcoma Developing in Abnormal Bone

Although osteogenic sarcoma may develop de novo in the older age groups, the consideration of an underlying bone abnormality as a precursor must be entertained. One possibility is the malignant transformation of a previously benign tumor, such as osteochondroma or enchondroma. Other than local transformation of a benign tumor, the development of osteogenic sarcoma in bone involved with Paget's disease, or in bone that had been previously radiated is not uncommon. Osteogenic sarcoma rarely develops in fibrous dysplasia. In an area of chronic osteomyelitis with long standing discharge of a sinus, the skin may be involved with a squamous cell carcinoma. This causes a destructive pattern in bone, and is to be differentiated from sarcomatous degeneration. Development of fibrosarcoma has also been reported.

IV. Osteogenic Sarcoma as a Complication of Paget's Disease

Paget's disease is a common disease in the northern sections of the United States, England, and the Western European plain. It is a disease of unproven etiology characterized by destructive and reparative changes in bone. Malignant transformation has been estimated to occur from 3 to 14% of patients. The Paget's disease may be quite limited and still be a site of sarcoma. Paget's sarcoma only originates in involved bone (Fig. 63).

Clinically, the alkaline phosphatase is usually elevated in Paget's disease. With the development of an osteosarcoma the alkaline phosphatase value tends to become yet higher.

The type of sarcoma developing in Paget's disease, in approximately 50% of cases, is osteogenic sarcoma, 25% being fibrosarcoma, with anaplastic sarcoma, giant-celled sarcoma, and reticulosarcoma following. Giant cell tumor has also been described in association with Paget's disease (RUSSELL, 1949).

The mean age is 67.6 years, for England (PRICE and GOLDIE, 1969). The mean age for the United States is 55 years. The age ranges from 46 to 91 years. The ratio of males to females is 2:1. There is a high incidence of pathologic fractures.

Radiologically, the areas involved are not limited. The pelvis, humerus, and femur are frequently involved, while the calvarium, scapula, mandible, calcaneous, vertebral column, and the other long bones may also be involved (Fig. 64). An area of bone destruction with ill-defined margins and a wide zone of transition is usually seen. Areas of increased density resembling ordinary osteogenic sarcoma may rarely be seen. Spiculated periosteal new bone response may be present, and increased density in the soft tissues may also be seen due to soft tissue invasion (Fig. 65). The osteolytic form tends

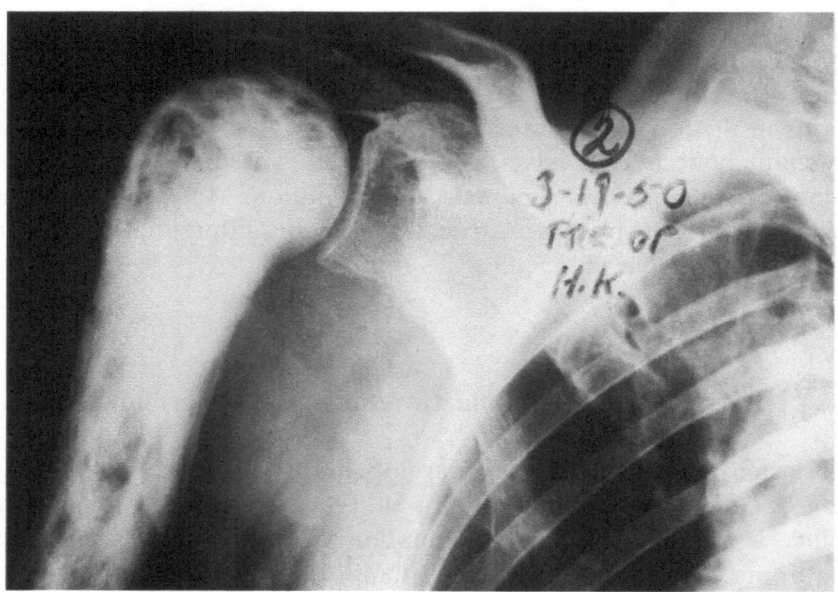

Fig. 63. Osteogenic sarcoma complicating Paget's disease. Changes of Paget's disease including cortical thickening, and coarsening of trabecular pattern are noted in proximal humerus. In addition, a dense area of sclerosis with a very wide zone of transition is noted, principally in humeral neck, extending into head and toward shaft. There is no evidence of cortical destruction. A minimal amount of spiculated periosteal new bone formation is seen at medial aspect of humerus. This proved to be an osteogenic sarcoma. (Courtesy of Drs. ANTONIO PIZARRO and JAMES F. KURTZ, Hines Veteran Administration Hospital, Hines, Illinois)

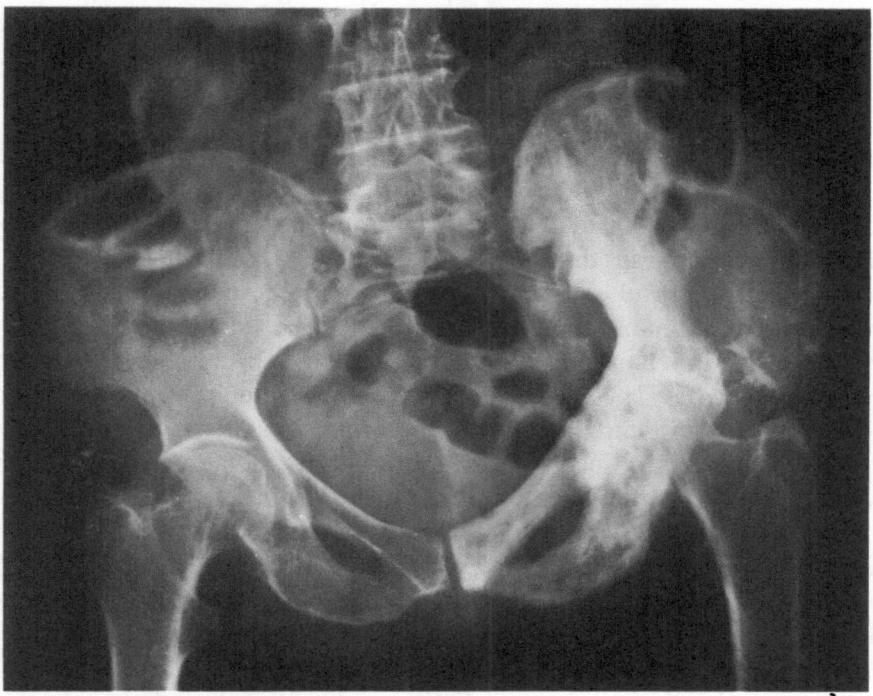

Fig. 64. Paget's disease of pelvis with malignant transformation. Paget's disease of left side of pelvis is seen with enlargement of contour of bone, cortical thickening, and increase in trabecular pattern. There is a large destructive area of left ilium with a small amount of spiculated periosteal new bone formation

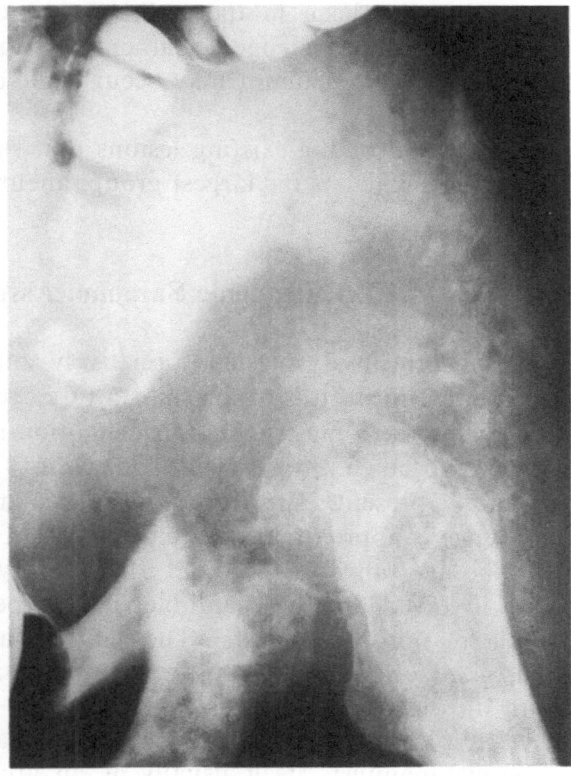

Fig. 65. Osteogenic sarcoma of pelvis associated with Paget's disease. An extensive destructive area in acetabulum and ilium is seen. New bone formation in tumor mass is noted. The tumor does not cross articular surface and femoral head is spared. Changes of Paget's disease in ischium and pubis are noted. Associated soft tissue mass is seen to cause displacement of barium-filled colon. This represents the radiologically osteolytic picture of osteogenic sarcoma. (From GREENFIELD, 1969. Courtesy of J.B. Lippincott Company, Publisher, Philadelphia, Pa.)

to predominate. The lesions may be multiple suggesting multifocal origin (DERMAN et al., 1951). The tumor usually spreads by the hematogenous route, but lymphogenous metastases may also occur (MANEY, 1952; GRININGER and RIGLER, 1965).

V. Osteogenic Sarcoma Arising in Previously Irradiated Bone

Ionizing radiation may lead to the formation of malignant tumors, changes from which the cellular structural components of bone are not immune.

These changes may result either from internal or external radiation sources. Internal radiation effects of humans are well documented by MARTLAND (1929), who called attention to watch dial painters who had ingested radium and mesothorium during the course of their work. These individuals developed anemia, bone necrosis, osteomyelitis, pathologic fractures, carcinomas of the paranasal sinuses, and mastoids, and bone sarcomas. The ingested radioactive substances were metabolized in the body in the same manner as calcium, and were deposited in bone. Other "bone-seeking" radioactive isotopes may also have the same effect, particularly radiostrontium.

External radiation, when a skeletal part is in a radiation treatment field, can cause radiation osteitis of bone, destructive areas, pathologic fractures, sclerosis, and local inhibition of bone growth. The development of sarcoma is in a low percentage of patients, and after a relatively long latent period, precise dosage data is lacking.

The percentage incidence of postradiation sarcoma in long-term survivors of breast cancer has been reported as being between 0.07 and 0.22%. Approximately 200 cases of sarcoma arising in bone following external irradiation have been reported in the English literature to date. Osteogenic sarcoma following thorotrast injection has also been reported (ALTNER et al., 1972).

The latent period ranges from 3 to 42 years. Sarcoma may develop either in normal bone that has been in the radiation treatment field or at the site of a pre-existing irradiated lesion. Osteogenic sarcoma or fibrosarcoma are the usual types. Chondrosarcoma and Ewing's tumor may occur while other tumors may show a complex histologic picture.

Radiation of pre-existing lesions that show sarcomatous development include giant cell tumor, which is the largest group, aneurysmal bone cyst, osteoblastoma, and fibrous dysplasia.

VI. Osteogenic Sarcoma Associated with Fibrous Dysplasia

While fibrous dysplasia is a relatively common lesion of the skeleton, the development of sarcoma in fibrous dysplasia is a rare event. ELMSLIE (1914) and COLEY and STEWART (1945) described malignant transformation in this condition. Many new cases have since been reported, both following and without prior irradiation. Albright's syndrome may be rarely present. The fibrous dysplasia may be polyostotic or monostotic. The sex incidence is approximately equal.

The age range at the onset of discovery of the sarcoma is from 11 to 54 years. The sites involved are the mandible, femur, pelvis, scapula, humerus, tibia, maxilla, and fibula in approximate order. The cell types are osteogenic sarcoma, fibrosarcoma, spindle cell, giant cell, or chondrosarcoma. The sarcomas arise in that bone that is affected with fibrous dysplasia.

Radiologically, the well-documented changes of fibrous dysplasia are apparent. The sarcoma manifests itself usually as an area of destruction. Areas of rarefaction and cortical destruction may be present. There may be an expansile or trabeculated lesion. Marked bone sclerosis and a "sunburst" type of periosteal reaction may be present manifesting an osteogenic sarcoma.

VII. Osteogenic Sarcoma in Osteogenesis Imperfecta

Osteogenesis imperfecta may rarely show a large soft tissue mass containing dense ossification. This is usually due to hyperplastic callus formation, which has been described as simulating a sarcoma (BANTA et al., 1971). Very rarely the simulator is simulated, and a true osteogenic sarcoma is found.

VIII. Soft Tissue Osteogenic Sarcoma

Osteogenic sarcoma arising in the soft tissues is a very rare but well-documented entity. It may arise de novo or it may occur as a late complication of radiation therapy (BOYER and NAVIN, 1965). It has been reported as arising in the heart, lungs (NOSANCHUCK and WEATHERBEE, 1969), pulmonary artery (McCONNELL, 1970), pleura (COHN and HALL, 1968), breast (AUBREY and ANDREWS, 1971), uterus (KARPER and MERENDINO, 1964), retroperitoneum, and in the soft tissues of the neck (JUSSAWALLA and DESAI, 1964), extremities, or trunk (Fig. 66).

The age group tends to be older than in osteogenic sarcoma of bone, with a reported age range from 8 to 80 years, but rare in the first two decades of life. The site of involvement is 90% in the extremities, most commonly in the lower extremity.

Radiologically a soft tissue mass is seen, which may attain a size of up to 10 centimeters. Varying amounts of streaky radiopacity may be seen. The opacification may be fuzzy and show some spiculation at its periphery (Fig. 67).

The adjacent bone may be secondarily invaded. This can be differentiated from an osteogenic sarcoma of bone invading the soft tissues, by a saucerized cortical defect indicating an external origin. At this stage, differentiation from a parosteal sarcoma radiologically may be difficult.

In the differential diagnosis several entities must be considered. A soft tissue density showing radiopacity should be classified into lesions showing calcification or lesions showing ossification. Ossification can be determined by the recognition of organization into cortex and trabecular pattern, although in early stages and in undifferentiated lesions this may be very difficult.

Calcifications would include metastatic calcification, calcinosis, and dystrophic calcification.

Of the lesions that show true ossification, a pseudomalignant osseous soft tissue tumor should be considered. This represents a lesion that was described by FINE and STOUT (1956), and ANGERVALL et al. (1969). This is a rare lesion that occurs in a younger age group than soft tissue osteogenic sarcoma. A soft tissue mass is present which shows a zone phenomenon. Peripheral mature bone and an immature center is reflected in the roentgen picture as an ossified rim around a centrally more radiolucent area. The prognosis with this tumor is relatively good. The tumor usually obtains a size of not larger than 3 cm. Females are more often involved than males.

Myositis ossificans is also to be considered in the differential diagnosis. This represents a condition of soft tissue heterotopic bone formation. The lesion often occurs post-traumatically, although a neurologic etiology has also been implicated. It does not necessarily

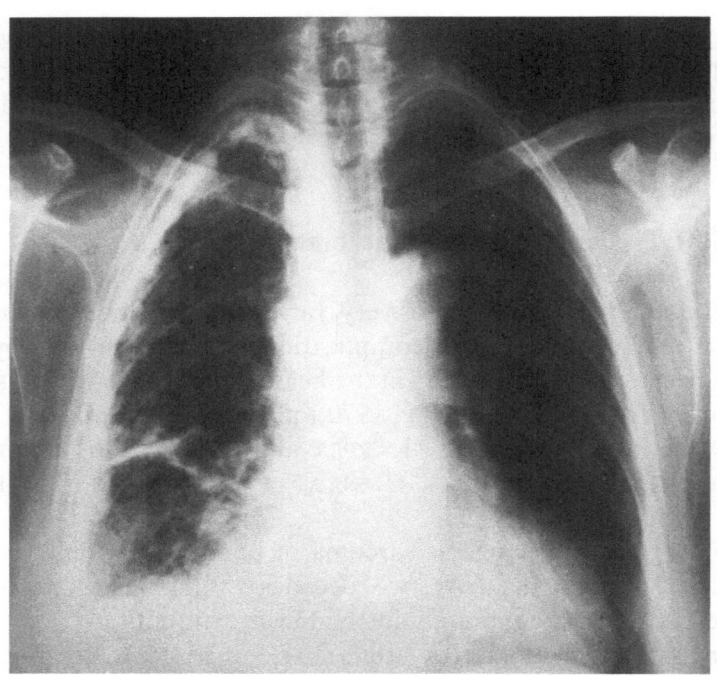
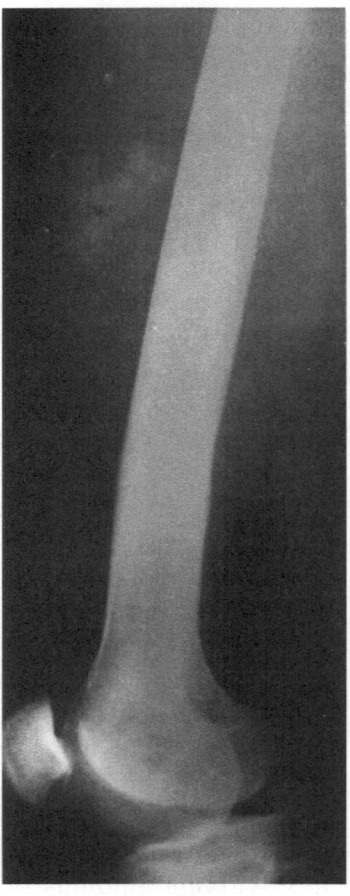

Fig. 66   Fig. 67

Fig. 66. Osteogenic sarcoma primary in right pleura. Female, age 51 with history of right-sided chest pain, shortness of breath, and dry cough. A^{18}F bone scan showed dense localization of fluorine to entire right hemithorax. Thoracotomy and biopsy reveal osteogenic sarcoma. Posteroanterior chest film shows dense pleural thickening with calcification on right, as well as parenchymal infiltrations. (Courtesy of EDWIN J. LIEBNER, M.D., Professor of Radiology, University of Illinois, Abraham Lincoln School of Medicine, Chicago, Illinois)

Fig. 67. Soft tissue osteogenic sarcoma of thigh. A mass containing multiple calcific densities is noted in thigh. A thin calcific rim inferiorly is seen, but major density extends throughout lesion. Bone is not involved. (Courtesy of Drs. ANTONIO PIZARRO and JAMES F. KURTZ, Hines Veteran Administration Hospital, Hines, Illinois.) (From GREENFIELD, 1969. Courtesy of J.B. Lippincott Company, Publisher, Philadelphia, Pa.)

have a circumscribed form and may occur about joints. There is a typical roentgen picture of an initial cloudlike density which, in a relatively short period of time, shows differentiation into well-defined ossific structure. This is self-limiting. It may blend with the cortex of bone. It does not continuously progress. Other soft tissue tumors may also contain osseous elements including malignant mesenchymoma, giant cell tumor of the soft tissues, pariosteal osteoma, fibrosarcoma, soft tissue osteoma, and lipoma. Synovioma, which shows calcification, should also be considered, as should pseudosarcomatous fasciitis. The latter is a clinically benign, rare, soft tissue lesion histologically resembling a sarcoma. The roentgen findings are of a soft tissue mass without sharp demarcation. A small percentage of cases show calcification or ossification.

References

ACKERMAN, L.V., SPJUT, H.J.: Tumors of bone and cartilage. Atlas of tumor pathology, section II, fascicle 4, Armed Forces Institute of Pathology, Washington, D.C.: National Research Council 82–97 (1962)

AEGERTER, E., KIRKPATRICK, J.A.: Orthopedic diseases. 3rd ed. pp. 554–560. Philadelphia: W.B. Saunders Co. 1968

ALBERTINI, A. VON: Über Sarkombildung auf dem Boden der Ostitis deformans Paget. (Kasuistischer Beitrag). Virchows Arch. path. Anat. 268, 259–273 (1928)

ALLAN, C.J., SOULE, E.A.: Osteogenic sarcoma of the somatic soft tissues. Clinicopathologic study of 26 cases and review of literature. Cancer (Philad.) 27, 1121–1133 (1971)

ALTNER, P.C., SIMMONS, D.J., LUCAS, H.F., CUMMINS, H.: Osteogenic sarcoma in a patient injected with thorotrast. J. Bone Jt Surg. 54A, 670–675 (1972)

AMSTUTZ, H.C.: Multiple osteogenic sarcomata-metastatic or multicentric? Report of two cases and review of literature. Cancer (Philad.) 24, 923–931 (1969)

ANGERVALL, L., STENER, B., STENER, I., AHREN, C.: Pseudomalignant osseous tumour of soft tissue. A clinical, radiological and pathological study of five cases. J. Bone Jt Surg. 51B, 654–663 (1969)

APPALANARASAYYA, K., MURTHY, A.S.R., VISWANATH, C.K., DEVI, O.B.: Osteoma involving the orbit. Case report and review of literature. Int. Surg. 54, 449–453 (1970)

AUB, J.C., EVANS, R.D., HEMPELMANN, L.H., MARTLAND, H.S.: The late effects of internally-deposited radioactive materials in man. Medicine 31, 221 (1952)

AUBE, L., ROY, L., LESSARD, R.: Osteoid osteoma of the distal phalanges. Canad. med. Ass. J. 98, 455–458 (1968)

AUBREY, D.A., ANDREWS, G.S.: Mammary osteogenic sarcoma. Brit. J. Surg. 58, 472–474 (1971)

BACON, G.A., MOE, J.H.: Primary bone tumor study 1940–1956. Univ. Minn. med. Bull. 32, 312–319 (1961)

BADRAWY, R.: Bilateral ivory osteoma of the nasal bones. (First case recorded). Ann. Otol. (St. Louis) 76, 216–219 (1967)

BANTA, J.V., SCHREIBER, R.R., KULIK, W.J.: Hyperplastic callus formation in osteogenesis imperfecta simulating osteosarcoma. J. Bone Jt Surg. 53-A, 115–122 (1971)

BARTLETT, J.R.: Intracranial neurological complications of frontal and ethmoidal osteomas. Brit. J. Surg. 58, 607–613 (1971)

BLOCH, C.: Postradiation osteogenic sarcoma. Report of a case and review of literature. Amer. J. Roentgenol. 87, 1157–1162 (1962)

BONILLA-COLON, J.: Multicentric osteogenic sarcoma. Bol. Assoc. méd. P. Rico 58, 392–396 (1966)

BOYER, C.W., NAVIN, J.J.: Extraskeletal osteogenic sarcoma; a late complication of radiation therapy. Cancer (Philad.) 18, 628–633 (1965)

BRAGG, D.G., SHIDNIA, H., CHU, F.C.H., HIGINBOTHAM, N.L.: The clinical and radiographic aspects of radiation osteitis. Radiology 97, 103–111 (1970)

BREGEAT, P., HAMARD, H.: Une exophtalmie par ostéome. A propos d'une observation du syndrôme de Devic, Bussy, Gardner. Arch. Ophtal. 28, 247–252 (1968)

BRODER, M.S., LEONIDAS, J.C., MITTY, H.A.: Pseudosarcomatous fasciitis: An unusual cause of soft-tissue calcification. Radiology 107, 173–174 (1973)

BRODY, G.L., FRY, L.R.: Osteogenic sarcoma: experience at The University of Michigan. Univ. Mich. med. Bull. 29, 80–87 (1963)

BÜCHELER, E., HEYMER, B.: Kalzifizierte Lungenmetastasen eines osteogenen Sarkoms des Os ilium. Fortschr. Roentgenstr. 105, 418–421 (1966)

BUFFAT, J.D.: A propos des ostéoblastomes vertébraux. Helv. chir. Acta 34, 141–144 (1967)

BULLOUGH, P.G.: Ivory exostosis of the skull. Postgrad. med. J. 41, 277–281 (1965)

BYERS, P.D.: Solitary benign osteoblastic lesions of bone. Osteoid osteoma and benign osteoblastoma. Cancer (Philad.) 22, 43–57 (1968)

CACERES, E., ZAHARIA, M., TANTALEAN, E.: Lymph node metastasis in osteogenic sarcoma. Surgery 65, 421–422 (1969)

CADE, S.: Osteogenic sarcoma: A study based on 133 patients. J. roy. Coll. Surg. Edinb. 1, 79–111 (1955)

CALDERON, D.O., MUSA, H.E., OTERO, G.O.: Renal osteoma. J. Urol. (Baltimore) 93, 350–352 (1965)

CALDICOTT, W.J.H.: Diagnosis of spinal osteoid osteoma. Radiology 92, 1192–1195 (1969)

CARROL, R.E.: Osteoid osteoma of the hand. J. Bone Jt Surg. 35A, 888–893 (1953)

CARROLL, R.F.: Osteogenic sarcoma in the hand. J. Bone Jt Surg. 39A, 325–331 (1957)

CASTLE, W.B., DRINKER, K.R., DRINKER, C.K.: Necrosis of the jaw in workers employed in applying a luminous paint containing radium. J. industr. Hyg. 7, 371–384 (1925)

CATALDO, E., SAVAGE, M., SHKLAR, G.: Osteogenic sarcoma of femur metastatic to mandible. Report of a case. Oral Surg. 19, 86–92 (1965)

CHANG, C.H., PIATT, E.D., THOMAS, K.E., WATNE, A.L.: Bone abnormalities in Gardner's syndrome. Amer. J. Roentgenol. 103, 645–652 (1968)

CHANDLER, F.A., KAEL, H.I.: Osteoid osteoma. Arch. Surg. (Chicago) 60, 294–304 (1950)

COHN, L., HALL, A.D.: Extraosseous osteogenic sarcoma of the pleura. Ann. thorac. Surg. 5, 545–549 (1968)

COLE, A.R.C., DARTE, J.M.M.: Osteochondromata after irradiation in children. Pediatrics 32, 285–288 (1963)

COLEY, B.L., SHARP, G.S.: Paget's Disease: A predisposing factor to osteogenic sarcoma. Arch. Surg. (Chicago) 23, 918–936 (1931)

COLEY, B.L., STEWART, F.W.: Bone Sarcoma in Polyostotic Fibrous Dysplasia. Ann. Surg. 121, 872 (1945)

COVENTRY, M.B., DAHLIN, D.C.: Osteogenic sarcoma. J. Bone Jt Surg., 39A, 741–758 (1957a)

COVENTRY, M.B., DAHLIN, D.C.: Osteogenic sarcoma: Critical analysis of 430 cases. J. Bone Jt Surg. 39A, 741–757 (1957b)

CRABBE, W.A., WARDILL, J.C.: Benign osteoblastoma of the spine. Brit. J. Surg. 50, 571–575 (1963)

CRUZ, M., COLLEY, B.L., STEWART, F.W.: Postradiation bone sarcoma: Report of eleven cases. Cancer (Philad.) 10, 72–88 (1957)

DAHLIN, D.C.: Bone tumors: general aspects and data on 3987 cases. Springfield, Illinois: C.C. Thomas 1967

DAHLIN, D.C., JOHNSON, E.W., JR.: Giant osteoid osteoma. J. Bone Jt Surg. 36A, 559–572 (1954)

DAVIDSON, J.W., CHACHA, P.B., JAMES, W.: Multiple osteosarcomata. Report of a case. J. Bone Jt Surg. 47B, 537–541 (1965)

DERMAN, H., PIZZOLATO, P., ZISKING, J.: Multicentric osteogenic sarcoma in Paget's disease with cerebral extension. Amer. J. Roentgenol. 65, 221–226 (1951)

DEVAS, M.B.: Malignant change in chronic osteomyelitis. Brit. J. Surg. 40, 140–142 (1952)

DOCKERTY, M.B., GHORMLEY, R.K., JACKSON, A.E.: Osteoid osteoma: A clinicopathologic study of 20 cases. Ann. Surg. 133, 77–89 (1951)

DOMINOK, G.W., KNOCH, H.G.: Knochengeschwülste und geschwulstähnliche Knochenerkrankungen. Jena: VEB Gustav Fischer 1971

DORFMAN, H.D., MICHAELS, G.L.: Cardiac metastasis in osteogenic sarcoma. Bull. Hosp. Jt Dis. (N.Y.) 27, 1–8 (1966)

DUGGAR, G.E.: Subungual osteoma. J. Amer. Podiatry Ass. 60, 324–325 (1970)

DUNLOP, J.A.Y., MORTON, K.S., ELLIOTT, G.B.: Recurrent osteoid osteoma. Report of a case with a review of the literature. J. Bone Jt Surg. 52B, 128–133 (1970)

EDEIKEN, J., HODES, P.J.: Roentgen diagnosis of diseases of bone. Baltimore: The Williams & Wilkins Co. 1967

EDEIKEN, J., DePALMA, A.F., HODES, P.J.: Osteoid osteoma. (Roentgenographic emphasis). Clin. Orthop. 49, 201–206 (1966)

EWING, J.: Radiation osteitis. Acta radiol. (Stockh.) 6, 399–412 (1926)

FINE, G., STOUT, A.P.: Osteogenic sarcoma of the extraskeletal soft tissues. Cancer (Philad.) 9, 1027–1043 (1956)

FINLAYSON, R.: Osteogenic sarcoma with multiple skeletal tumours. J. Path. Bact. 66, 223–229 (1953)

FLAHERTY, R.A., PUGH, D.G., DOCKERTY, M.B.: Osteoid Osteoma. Amer. J. Roentgenol. 76, 1041–1051 (1956)

FOWLES, S.J.: Osteoid osteoma. Brit. J. Radiol. 37, 245–252 (1964)

FREIBERGER, R.H.: Osteoid osteoma of the spine. A cause of backache and scoliosis in children and young adults. Radiology 75, 232–236 (1960)

FREIBERGER, R.H., LOITMAN, B.S., HALPERN, M., THOMPSON, T.C.: Osteoid osteoma, a report on 80 cases. Amer. J. Roentgenol. 82, 194–205 (1959)

GARDNER, E.J.: Follow-up study of family group exhibiting dominant inheritance for a syndrome including intestinal polyps, osteomas, fibromas, and epidermal cysts. Amer. J. hum. Genet. 14, 376–390 (1962)

GESCHICKTER, C.F., COPELAND, M.M.: Tumors of bone. 3rd ed. Philadelphia: J.B. Lippincott Co. 1949

GILLIS, L., LEE, S.: Cancer as a sequel to war wounds. J. Bone Jt Surg. 33B, 167–179 (1951)

GIUSTRA, P.E., FREIBERGER, R.H.: Severe growth disturbance with osteoid osteoma. A report of two cases involving the femoral neck. Radiology 96, 285–288 (1970)

GLYNN, J.J., LICHTENSTEIN, L.: Osteoid-osteoma with multicentric nidus. J. Bone Jt Surg. 55A, 855–858 (1973)

GOIDANICH, I.F., BATTAGLIA, L.: Osteoblastoma (Fibroma osteogenetico). Neoplasia benigna di tessuto osteoblastico. Studio clinico, radiografico ed anatomopatologico di 14 casi. Chir. Organi Mov. 46, 353–388 (1958)

GOLDBERG, A.F., SKUBLE, D.F., LATRONICA, R.J.: Osteoma of the tongue: report of case. J. oral Surg. 28, 457 (1970)

GOLDENBERG, R.R.: Osteogenic sarcoma of the tibia with pulmonary metastasis. Report of a case with ten-year survival. J. Bone Jt Surg. 39A, 1191–1197 (1957)

GOLDING, J.S.R., SISSONS, H.A.: Osteogenic fibroma of bone: A report of two cases. J. Bone Jt Surg. 36-B, 428–435 (1954)

GOODWIN, M.A.: Primary osteosarcoma of the patella. case report. J. Bone Jt Surg. 43B, 338–341 (1961)

GRATZEK, F.R., HOLMSTROM, E.G., RIGLER, L.G.: Post irradiation changes. Amer. J. Roentgenol. 53, 62–76 (1945)

GREENFIELD, G.B.: Radiology of bone diseases. Philadelphia: J.B. Lippincott Co. 1969

GRININGER, D.R., RIGLER, R.G.: Lymphatic metastases from Paget's sarcoma. Geriatrics 23, 97–101 (1965)

GÜTTICH, H., MÜLLER, E.S.: Großes Stirnhöhlenosteom und reversible Blindheit. Hals-, Nasen- u. Ohrenarzt 15, 155–158 (1967)

HALLBERG, O.E., BEGLEY, J.W., JR.: Origin and treatment of osteomas of the paranasal sinuses. Arch. Otolaryng. (Chicago) 51, 750–760 (1950)

HALPERT, B., RUSSO, P.E., HACKNEY, V.C.: Osteogenic sarcoma with multiple skeletal and visceral involvement. Cancer (Philad.) 2, 789–792 (1949)

HAMILTON, J.G.: The metabolism of the fission products and the heaviest elements. Radiology **49**, 325–343 (1947)

HATCHER, C.H.: The development of sarcoma in bone subjected to roentgen or radium irradiation. J. Bone Jt Surg. **27**, 179–195 (1945)

HAYLES, A.B., DAHLIN, D.C., COVENTRY, M.B.: Osteogenic sarcoma in children. J. Amer. med. Ass. **174**, 1174–1177 (1960)

HEUL, R.O. VAN DER: (Pseudo-osteoblastoma extraossale). Ned. T. Geneesk. **107**, 1061–1063 (1963)

HILTON, G.: Osteoclastoma associated with generalized bone disease. Brit. J. Radiol. **23**, 437–439 (1950)

HOFFMAN, R.R., CAMPBELL, R.E.: Roentgenologic bone-island instability in hyperparathyroidism. Radiology **103**, 307–308 (1972)

HUVOS, A.G., HIGINBOTHAM, N.L., MILLER, T.R.: Bone sarcomas arising in fibrous dysplasia. J. Bone Jt Surg. **54A**, 1047–1056 (1972)

JAFFE, H.L.: Osteoid osteoma: A benign osteoblastic tumor composed of osteoid and atypical bone. Arch. Surg. (Chicago) **31**, 709–728 (1935)

JAFFE, H.L.: Osteoid osteoma of bone. Radiology **45**, 319–334 (1945)

JAFFE, H.L.: Benign osteoblastoma. Bull. Hosp. Jt Dis. (N.Y.) **17**, 141–151 (1956a)

JAFFE, H.L.: Osteogenic sarcoma of bone. Clin. Orthop. **7**, 27–40 (1956b)

JAFFE, H.L.: Tumors and tumorous conditions of the bones and joints. Philadelphia: Lea and Febiger 1958

JAFFE, H.L., BODANSKY, A.: Diagnostic significance of serum alkaline and acid phosphatase values in relation to bone disease. Bull. N.Y. Acad. Med. **19**, 831–848 (1943)

JAFFE, H.L., LICHTENSTEIN, L.: Osteoid osteoma: Further experience with this benign tumor of bone: With special reference to cases showing the lesion in relation to shaft cortices and commonly misclassified as instances of sclerosing non-suppurative osteomyelitis or cortical-bone abscess. J. Bone Jt Surg., **22**, 645–682 (1940)

JAFFE, H.L., MAYER, L.: An osteoblastic osteoid tissue-forming tumor of a metacarpal bone. Arch. Surg. (Chicago) **24**, 550–564 (1932)

JEFFREYS, T.E., STILES, P.J.: Pseudomalignant osseous tumour of soft tissue. J. Bone Jt Surg. **48-B**, 488–492 (1966)

JENT, J.N., CASTRO, H.F., GIROTTI, W.R.: Benign osteoblastoma of the maxilla. Case report and review of the literature. Oral Surg. **27**, 209–219 (1969)

JOHNSON, L.C.: A general theory of bone tumors. Bull. N.Y. Acad. Med. **29**, 164–171 (1953)

JOHNSTON, A.D.: Clinical problems in osteoid osteoma. Evidence of osteoclastic aversion to osteoid. Bull. Hosp. Jt Dis. (N.Y.) **23**, 80–94 (1961)

JONES, E.L., CORNELL, E.D.: Gardner's syndrome; review of the literature and report on a family. Arch. Surg. (Chicago) **92**, 287–300 (1966)

JUSSAWALLA, D.J., DESAI, J.G.: Primary osteogenic sarcoma arising in extraskeletal soft tissues of the neck. Brit. J. Surg. **51**, 504–505 (1964)

KALLIO, E.: Osteoid osteoma of the metacarpal and metatarsal bones. Acta orthop. scand. **33**, 246–252 (1963)

KARLEN, A.: Osteogenic Sarcomatosis or Multifocal Osteogenic Sarcoma. Acta Path. Microbiol. Scand. **55**, 1–7 (1962)

KARPER, C.M., MERENDINO, V.J.: Uterine osteogenic sarcoma: histochemical studies and report of a case. Obstet. Gynec. **24**, 629–633 (1964)

KAUFFMAN, S.L., STOUT, A.P.: Extraskeletal osteogenic sarcomas and chondrosarcomas in children. Cancer (Philad.) **16**, 432–439 (1963)

KEW, M.C.: Cavitating pulmonary metastasis associated with spontaneous pneumothorax. Lancet **86**, 571–574 (1966)

KLENERMAN, L., OCKENDEN, B.G.: Osteosarcoma occurring in osteogenesis imperfecta. Report of two cases. J. Bone Jt Surg. **49B**, 314–323 (1967)

KOLAWOLE, T.M., BOHRER, S.P.: Ulcer osteoma-bone response to tropical ulcer. Amer. J. Roentgenol. **109**, 611–618 (1970)

KOPP, W.K.: Benign osteoblastoma of the coronoid process of the mandible: report of a case. J. med. Genet. **27**, 653–655 (1969)

KRAGH, L.V., DAHLIN, D.C., ERICH, J.B.: Osteogenic sarcoma of the jaws and facial bones. Amer. J. Surg. **96**, 496–505 (1958)

KRAMER, H.S.: Benign osteoblastoma of the mandible. Report of a case. Oral Surg. **24**, 842–851 (1967)

LAURENT, L.E., SALENIOUS, P.: Hyperplastic callus formation in osteogenesis imperfecta. Report of a case simulating sarcoma. Acta orthop. scand. **38**, 280–289 (1967)

LAWRIE, T.R., ATERMAN, K., PATH, F.C., SINCLAIR, A.M.: Painless osteoid osteoma. A report of two cases. J. Bone Jt Surg., **52A**, 1357–1363 (1970)

LEGIER, J.F., TAUBER, L.N.: Solitary metastasis of occult prostatic carcinoma simulating osteogenic sarcoma. Cancer (Philad.) **22**, 168–172 (1968)

LEHRER, H.Z., MAXFIELD, W.S., NICE, C.M.: The periosteal "sunburst" pattern in metastatic bone tumors. Am. J. Roentgenology **108**, 154–161 (1970)

LICHTENSTEIN, L.: Bone tumors. 3rd ed. pp. 202–228. St. Louis: The C.V. Mosby Company 1965

LICHTENSTEIN, L., SAWYER, W.R.: Benign osteoblastoma. Further observations and report of twenty additional cases. J. Bone Jt Surg. **46A**, 755–765 (1964)

LIEDBERG, G., LINDHOLM, K., LINDSTEDT, E., LINDSTET, G.: Gardner's syndrome. Report of a family. Acta chir. scand. **136**, 81–84 (1970)

LIND, O., MILLERSTROM, K.: Osteoid osteoma in the mandibular condyle: case report and survey of the literature. Acta oto-laryng. (Stockh.) **57**, 467–474 (1964)

LINDBOM, A., LINDUALL, N., SÖDERBERG, G., SPJUT, H.: Angiography in osteoid osteoma. Acta radiol. (Stockh.) **54**, 327–333 (1960)

LINDBOM, A., SÖDERBERG, G., SPJUT, H.J.: Osteosarcoma. A review of 96 cases. Acta radiol. (Stockh.) **56**, 1–19 (1961)

LODWICK, G.S.: Solitary malignant tumors of bone: the application of predictor variables in diagnosis. Semin. Roentgenol. **1**, 293–313 (1966)

LODWICK, G.S.: The bones and joints. Chicago: Year Book Med. Publ. 1971

LOONEY, W.B.: Late effects (twenty-five to forty years) of the early medical and industrial use of radioactive materials. Their relation to the more accurate establishment of maximum permissible amounts of radioactive elements in the body. J. Bone Jt Surg. **37A**, 1169–1187 (1955); **38A**, 175–218 (1956); and **38-A**, 392–406 (1956)

LOWRY, K., JR., HAYNES, C.D.: Osteogenic sarcoma of extraskeletal soft tissues: a case report. Amer. Surg. **30**, 97–100 (1964)

LUCAS, H.F., ROWLAND, R.E., MILLER, C.E., HOLTZMAN, R.B., HASTERLIK, R.J., FINKERL, A.J.: An unusual case of radium toxicity. Amer. J. Roentgenol. **90**, 1042–1052 (1963)

MACLELLAN, D.I., WILSON, F.C.: Osteoid osteoma of the spine. A review of the literature and report of six new cases. J. Bone Jt Surg. **49A**, 111–121 (1967)

MALLORY, T.B.: Case records of the Massachusetts General Hospital (Osteogenic sarcoma of humerus, with ossifying metastases in the regional nodes). New Engl. J. Med. **225**, 953–958 (1941)

MANEY, A.W.: Lymphatic dissemination of a sarcoma superimposed on Paget's disease of the os calcis. Brit. J. Surg. **40**, 84–87 (1952)

MARCOVE, R.C., FREIBERGER, R.H.: Osteoid osteoma of the elbow—a diagnostic problem. Report of four cases. J. Bone Jt Surg. **48A**, 1185–1190 (1966)

MARCOVE, R.C., MIKE, V., HAJEK, J.V., LEVIN, A.G., HUTTER, R.V.P.: Osteogenic sarcoma under the age of twenty-one. A review of one hundred and forty-five operative cases. J. Bone Jt Surg. **52A**, 411–423 (1970)

MARSH, H.O., CHOI, C.B.: Primary osteogenic sarcoma of the cervical spine originally mistaken for benign osteoblastoma. A case report. J. Bone Jt Surg. **52A**, 1467–1471 (1970)

MARTEL, A.J., BONANNO, C.A.: Multiple polyposis of the gastrointestinal tract with osteoma and soft tissue tumors. Amer. J. dig. Dis. **13**, 588–591 (1968)

MARTLAND, H.S.: Occupational poisoning in manufacture of luminous watch dials. J. Amer. med. Ass. **92**, 466–473 (1929)

MAYER, L.: Malignant degeneration of so-called benign osteoblastoma. Bull. Hosp. Jt Dis. (N.Y.) **28**, 4–13 (1967)

MAYNARD, J.H., FONE, D.J.: Haemochromatosis with osteogenic sarcoma in the liver. Med. J. Aust. **2**, 1260–1263 (1969)

MCANALLY, A.K., DOCKERTY, M.B.: Carcinoma developing in chronic γraining dutaneous sinuses and fistulas. Surg. Gynec. Obstet. **88**, 87–96 (1949)

MCCONNELL, T.H.: Bony and cartillaginous tumors of the heart and great vessels. Report of an osteosarcoma of the pulmonary artery. Cancer (Philad.) **25**, 611–617 (1970)

MCKENNA, R.J., SCHWINN, C.P., SOONG, K.Y., HIGINBOTHAM, N.L.: Osteogenic sarcoma arising in Paget's disease. Cancer (Philad.) **17**, 42–66 (1964)

MCKENNA, R.J., SCHWINN, C.P., SOONG, K.Y., HIGINBOTHAM, N.L.: Sarcomata of the osteogenic series (osteosarcoma, fibrosarcoma, chondrosarcoma, parosteal osteogenic sarcoma, and sarcomata arising in abnormal bone): an analysis of 552 cases. J. Bone Jt Surg. **48A**, 1–26 (1966)

MOBERG, E.: The natural course of osteoid osteoma. J. Bone Jt Surg., **33-A**, 166–170 (1951)

MOOKHERJEE, P.K.: A case of osteogenic sarcoma invading a paired bone. Brit. J. Radiol. **44**, 393–395 (1971)

MORRESAN, G.M., HAWES, L.E., SACCO, J.J.: Incomplete removal of osteoid osteoma. Amer. J. Surg. **80**, 476–481 (1950)

MORSE, D., JR., REED, J.O., BERNSTEIN, J.: Sclerosing osteogenic sarcoma. Amer. J. Roentgenol. **88**, 491–495 (1962)

MORTON, K.S., BARTLETT, L.H.: Benign osteoblastic change resembling osteoid osteoma. Three cases with unusual radiological features. J. Bone Jt Surg. **48 B**, 478–484 (1966)

MOSELEY, J.E., BASS, M.H.: Sclerosing osteogenic sarcomatosis. Radiology **66**, 41–45 (1956)

MURRAY, R.O., JACOBSON, H.G.: The radiology of skeletal disorders. Baltimore: Williams & Wilkins 1971

NELSON, J.A., CLARK, R.E., PALUBINSKAS, A.J.: Osteogenic sarcoma with calcified renal metastases. Brit. J. Radiol. **44**, 802–804 (1971)

NEUHAUSER, E.B.: Sickle cell trait and osteogenic sarcoma. Postgrad. Med. **45**, 67–69 (1969)

NIEBAUER, J.J.: Development of squamous-cell carcinomata in the sinus tracts of chronic osteomyelitis. J. Bone Jt Surg. **28**, 280–285 (1946)

NOSANCHUK, J.S., WEATHERBEE, L.: Primary osteogenic sarcoma in lung. Report of a case. J. thorac. cardiovasc. Surg. **58**, 242–247 (1969)

PEARSON, K.D., RUBIN, D., SZEMES, G.C., PREGER, L.: Extraosseous osteogenic sarcoma of the chest. Brit. J. Dis. Chest **63**, 231–234 (1969)

PLATT, H.: Sarcoma in abnormal bones. Brit. J. Surg. **34**, 232–239 (1947)

PLATT, H.: Survival in bone sarcoma. Acta orthop. scand. **32**, 267–280 (1962)

POULSEN, J.O.: Osteoid osteoma. Acta orthop. scand. **40**, 198–204 (1969)

PORETTA, C.A., DAHLIN, D.C., JAMES, J.M.: Sarcoma in Paget's disease of bone. J. Bone Jt Surg. **39-A**, 1314–1329 (1957)

PRABHAKAR, B., REDDY, D.R., DAYANANDA, B., RAO, G.R.: Osteoid osteoma of the skull. J. Bone Jt Surg. **54 B**, 146–148 (1972)

PRICE, C.G.H.: Osteogenic Sarcoma, an Analysis of

the Age and Sex Incidence. Brit. J. Cancer **9**, 558–574 (1955)

PRICE, C.H.G., GOLDIE, W.: Paget's sarcoma of bone. A study of eighty cases from the Bristol and the Leeds bone tumour registries. J. Bone Jt Surg. **51 B**, 205–224 (1969)

PRICE, C.H.G., ROSS, F.G.M.: Bone, certain Aspects of Neoplasia. Proceedings of the 24th Symposium of the Colston Research Society. London: Butterworths 1973

PRICE, C.H.G., TRUSCOTT, D.E.: Multifocal osteogenic sarcoma. J. Bone Jt Surg. **38 B**, 524–533 (1957)

PRITCHARD, J.E., MCKAY, J.W.: Osteoid osteoma. Can. med. Ass. J. **58**, 567–575 (1948)

PROWLER, J.R.: Osteogenic sarcoma of the maxilla. Report of a case. Oral Surg. **28**, 141–148 (1969)

PURCELL, H.M., MILLS, S.D., LIPSCOMB, P.R.: Osteoid osteoma in childhood. Pediatrics **9**, 295–303 (1952)

Radiological Atlas of Bone Tumours, Vol. II and II, Netherlands Committee on Bone Tumours (ed.). The Hague: Mouton & Co 1966 and 1973

RAYNE, J.: Gardner's syndrome. Brit. J. oral Surg. **6**, 11–17 (1968)

RIDDELL, D.M.: Malignant change in fibrous dysplasia; report of a case. J. Bone Jt Surg. **46 B**, 251–255 (1964)

ROCA, A.N., SMITH, J.L., BAO-SHAN, J.: Osteosarcoma and parosteal osteogenic sarcoma of the maxilla and mandible: study of 20 cases. Amer. J. clin. Path. **54**, 625–636 (1970)

ROCKWELL, M.A., ENNEKING, W.F.: Osteosarcoma developing in solitary enchondroma of the tibia. J. Bone Jt Surg. **53 A**, 341–344 (1971)

RONNEN, J.R. VON: Bösartige primäre Knochentumoren. Arch. Chir. Neerl. **17**, 23–54 (1965)

RONNEN, J.R. VON: Histological and Radiographical Classification of Osteosarcoma in Relation to Therapy. A Review of 245 Cases Located in the Extremities. J. Belge de Rad. **51**, 215–221 (1968)

RONNEN, J.R. VON, HEUL, R.O. VAN DER: On the Roentgenological Diagnosis and Differential Diagnosis of Bone Sarcomas. Colston Papers, **24**, 97–112 (1973)

ROSBOROUGH, D.: Osteoid osteoma. Report of a lesion in the terminal phalanx of a finger. J. Bone Jt Surg. **48 B**, 485–487 (1966)

ROSENMERTZ, S.K., SCHARE, H.J.: Osteogenic sarcoma arising in Paget's disease of the mandible. Review of the literature and report of a case. Oral Surg. **28**, 304–309 (1969)

ROSENSWEIG, J., PINTARK, K., MIKAIL, M., MAYMAN, A.: Benign osteoblastoma (giant osteoma): report of an unusual rib tumor and review of the literature. Canad. med. Ass. J. **89**, 1189–1192 (1963)

ROSS, F.G.: Osteogenic sarcoma. Brit. J. Radiol. **37**, 259–276 (1964)

ROSS, P.: Gardner's syndrome. Amer. J. Roentgenol. **96**, 298–301 (1966)

ROTTE, K.H.: Höhlenbildende Lungenmetastasen. Arch. Geschwulstforsch. **33**, 275–282 (1969)

RUSHTON, J.G., MULDER, D.W., LIPSCOMB, P.R.: Neurologic symptoms with osteoid osteoma. Neurology (Minneap.) **5**, 794–797 (1955)

RUSSELL, D.S.: Malignant osteoclastoma and the association of malignant ostoclastoma with Paget's osteitis deformans. J. Bone Jt Surg. **31 B**, 281–290 (1949)

RYAN, J.: A case of multiple osteosarcoma. J. Coll. Radiol. Aust. **7**, 93–96 (1963)

SABANAS, A.O., DAHLIN, D.C., CHILDS, D.S., JR., IVINS, J.C.: Postradiation sarcoma of bone. Cancer (Philad.) **9**, 528–542 (1956)

SABANAS, A.O., BICKEL, W.H., MOE, J.H.: The natural history of osteoid osteoma of the spine, review of the literature and report of three cases. Amer. J. Surg. **91**, 880–889 (1956)

SALZER, M., SALZER-KUNTSCHIK, M.: Das benigne Osteoblastom. Langenbecks Arch. klin. Chir. **302**, 755–778 (1963)

SAMY, L.L., MOSTAFA, H.: Osteomata of the nose and paranasal sinuses with a report of twenty one cases. J. Laryngol. **85**, 449–469 (1971)

SCHMORL, G.: Über Ostitis deformans Paget. Virchows Arch. path. Anat. **283**, 694–751 (1932)

SCHREYVOGEL, R.: Benignes Osteoblastom. Schweiz. med. Wschr. **98**, 1009–1015 (1968)

SCHULMAN, L., DORFMAN, H.D.: Nerve fibers in osteoid osteoma. J. Bone Jt Surg. **52 A**, 1351–1356 (1970)

SCOTT, M., LIGNELLI, G.J., SHEA, F.J.: Cervical radicular pain secondary to osteoid osteoma of spine. J. Amer. med. Ass. **217**, 964–965 (1971)

SHERMAN, M.S.: Osteoid osteoma: Review of the literature and report of thirty cases. J. Bone Jt Surg. **29**, 918–930 (1947a)

SHERMAN, M.S.: Osteoid osteoma associated with changes in adjacent joint. Report of two cases. J. Bone Jt Surg. **29**, 483–490 (1947b)

SIEGLER, J.: Recurrent pyogenic meningitis due to an osteoma of the frontal sinus. J. Laryng. **78**, 226–228 (1964)

SILBERMAN, W.W.: Osteoid osteoma. J. int. Coll. Surg. **38**, 53–66 (1962)

SIM, F.H., CUPPS, R.E., DAHLIN, D.C., IVINS, J.C.: Postradiation sarcoma of bone. J. Bone Jt Surg. **54 A**, 1479–1489 (1972)

SINGH, A.D., SCUDDER, I.B.: Multiple osteogenic sarcomas: report of a case. J. Bone Jt Surg. **47 B**, 542–547 (1965)

SINGLETON, E.B., ROSENBERG, H.S., DODD, G.D., DOLAN, P.A.: Sclerosing sarcomatosis. Amer. J. Roentgenol. **88**, 483–490 (1962)

SMITH, J.: Giant bone islands. Radiology **107**, 35–36 (1973)

SNARR, J.W., ABELL, M.R., MARTEL, W.: Lymphofollicular synovitis with osteoid osteoma. Radiology **106**, 557–560 (1973)

STEINER, G.C.: Postradiation sarcoma of bone. Cancer (Philad.) **18**, 603–612 (1965)

STERN, W.E.: Malignant "degeneration" (osteogenic

sarcoma) occurring in preexisting Paget's disease of the skull. A new case report with supplemental tabulation of recent cases. Bull. Los Angeles neurol. Soc. **34**, 221–232 (1969)

SUMMEY, T.J., PRESSLY, C.L.: Sarcoma complicating Paget's disease of bone. Ann. Surg. **123**, 135–153 (1946)

SWEETNAM, R.: Osteosarcoma. Ann. roy. Coll. Surg. Engl. **44**, 38–58 (1969)

TANNER, H.C., DAHLIN, D.C., CHILDS, D.S.: Sarcoma complicating fibrous dysplasia. Oral Surg. **14**, 837–846 (1961)

TARKKANEN, J., PALJAKKA, P., HOLOPAINEN, E.: Die Osteome der Nasennebenhöhlen. Mschr. Ohrenheilk. **102**, 320–325 (1968)

TULLOH, H.P., HARRY, D.: Osteoblastoma in a rib in childhood. Clin. Radiol. **20**, 337–338 (1969)

UEHLINGER, E.: Die pathologische Anatomie der Knochengeschwülste. Helv. Chir. Acta **20**, 597 (1959); **40**, 5 (1973)

UEHLINGER, E.: Pathologische Anatomie der Knochengeschwülste (unter besonderer Berücksichtigung der semimalignen Formen). Chirurg **45**, 62 (1974)

VICKERS, C.W., PUGH, D.C., IVINS, J.C.: Osteoid osteoma, a 15 year follow-up of an untreated patient. J. Bone Jt Surg. **41-A**, 357–358 (1959)

VOGELSANG, H., WEIDENMANN, O.: Angiographische Befunde bei einem Riesenzelltumor und einem benignen Osteoblastom der Halswirbelsäule. Fortschr. Röntgenstr. **110**, 843–851 (1969)

VAN WAY, C.W., LAWLER, M.R.: Osteogenic sarcoma-
tous emboli to the femoral arteries. Amer. J. Surg. **117**, 745–747 (1969)

WEBER, W.: Einzigartiges, teilpneumatisiertes, großes Osteom der Schläfenschuppe. Hals-, Nasen- u. Ohrenarzt **11**, 349–351 (1963)

WEINFELD, F.S., DUDLEY, R.D., JR.: Osteogenic sarcoma. J. Bone Jt Surg. **44-A**, 269–276 (1962)

WENDE, S.: Sarkom der Schädelkalotte nach Röntgentherapie. Fortschr. Röntgenstr. **96**, 278–282 (1962)

WET DE, I.S.: Osteoid osteomata. Review of the literature with a report of five cases. S. Afr. J. Surg. **5**, 13–24 (1967)

WILNER, D., SHERMAN, R.S.: Bone sarcoma associated with Paget's disease. Cancer (Philad.) **16**, 238–244 (1966)

WOODRUFT, M.: The challenge of osteosarcoma. Ann. roy. Coll. Surg. Engl. **44**, 299–307 (1969)

YAGHMAI, I., ABDOLMAHMOUD, S.Z., SHAMS, S., AFSHARI, R.: Value of arteriography in the diagnosis of benign and malignant bone lesions. Cancer (Philad.) **27**, 1134–1147 (1971)

YANNOPOULOS, K., BOM, A.F., GRIFFITHS, C.O., CRIKELAIR, G.F.: Osteosarcoma arising in dysplasia of the facial bones: case report and review of the literature. Amer. J. Surg. **107**, 556–564 (1964)

YONEYAMA, T., GREENLAW, R.H.: Osteogenic sarcoma following radiotherapy for retinoblastoma. Radiology **93**, 1185–1186 (1969)

ZITER, F.M., JR.: Roentgenographic findings in Gardner's syndrome. J. Amer. med. Ass. **192**, 1000–1002 (1965)

Parosteal Osteosarcoma*

by

Issa Yaghmai

Parosteal osteosarcoma is a malignant tumor arising in the juxtacortical portion of long bones, and because of its location, rarity, and histopathologic appearance, it has different synonyms: parosteal osteoma (GESCHICKTER and COPELAND, 1951); juxtacortical osteosarcoma (JAFFE and SELIN, 1952); juxtacortical osteogenic sarcoma (DWINNELL et al., 1954); ossifying parosteal sarcoma (SCAGLIETTI and CALANDRIELLO, 1955); parosteal osteogenic sarcoma (DAHLIN, 1967); and parosteal osteoid sarcoma (RANNIGER and ALTNER, 1966). The term parosteal osteosarcoma has been used more frequently than other synonyms, and we believe it is the best term for this lesion.

This lesion was described by MÜLLER as early as 1843, but it was not until 1947 that it was recognized as a distinct and separate entity by HATCHER. The term parosteal osteoma was used for the first time by GESCHICKTER and COPELAND (1951). These tumors are rare and comprise only 1.7% of all benign and malignant tumors of bone (ACKERMAN and SPJUT, 1971), and less than 1% of malignant tumors of bone (DAHLIN, 1967). This tumor is considered separately from true osteosarcoma because of its distinctly less malignant behavior and better prognosis. COPELAND and GESCHICKTER (1959) reported 15 cases and believed that parosteal osteosarcoma occurs in both malignant and benign forms, with the malignant form being the most common. They believed that the initial lesion is most frequently a benign proliferation of ossifying fibrous tissue, which results in a round bony mass projecting from the shaft of a long bone, and that these tumors show a tendency to progressive growth and to ultimate malignant change. They also hold that the malignant phase of the process is akin, in its histology, to sclerosing osteosarcoma or fibrosarcoma, and that evolution from benign to malignant form is gradual and extends over a number of years. But the majority of pathologists do not agree with this theory and believe that these lesions are malignant from the beginning and can be considered as low-grade osteosarcomas.

A. Clinical Features

I. Age and Sex

The occurrence of parosteal osteosarcoma is commonly seen in the third, fourth, and fifth decades of life. The majority of patients are over 23 years of age, with the average age around 35 years. Females are more commonly involved than males.

---

* With cases contributed by KLAUS RANNIGER, M.D.

II. Localization

The posterior portion of the metaphysis of the distal femur is the most common site of parosteal osteosarcoma, and 72% of cases reported by DAHLIN (1967) appeared at this site. Other sites include the tibia, fibula, humerus, radius, and ulna, and it is usually the metaphyseal portion of these cylindrical bones which is involved (Fig. 1). Vertebral, scapular, and phalangeal parosteal osteosarcoma has been reported by JACOBSON (1958) and a case of mandibular involvement by SOM and PEIMER (1961).

III. Symptoms

Soft tissue swelling and pain are the main complaints of the patients. Local tenderness and a slowly growing mass of several months or years duration have been reported. Some of these patients have been seen after previous operations and the presence of previous surgery provides suspicion of parosteal osteosarcoma.

The tumor usually presents as a palpable hard mass which does not adhere to the skin. It is frequently associated with mild pain on palpation and occasionally limitation of motion of the adjacent joint due to the enormous size of the lesion. This tumor

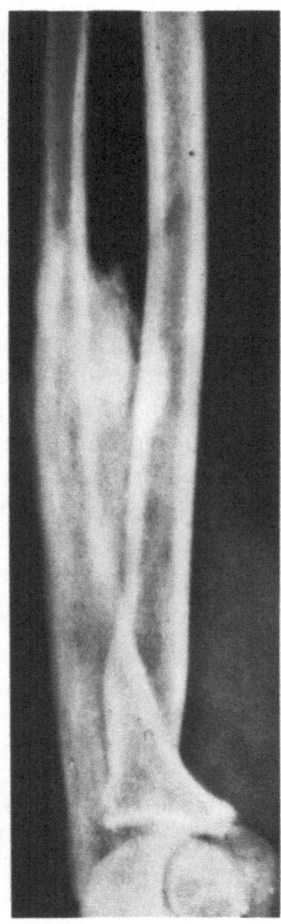

Fig. 1. Parosteal osteosarcoma
of midshaft of ulna

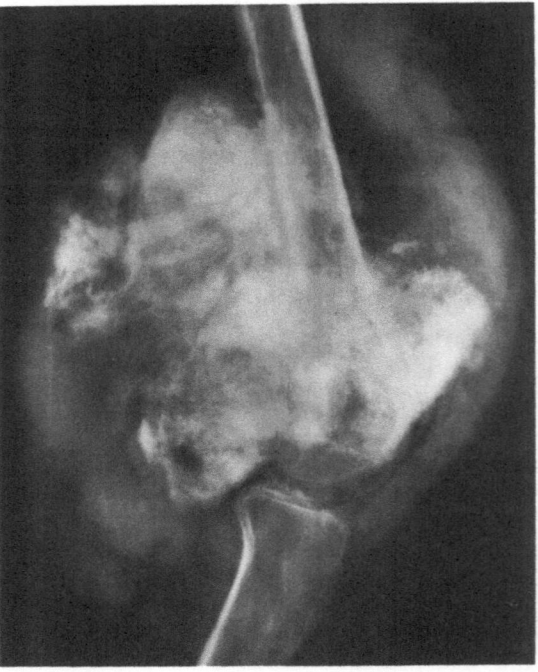

Fig. 2. Parosteal osteosarcoma involving distal shaft of femur, which reveals amorphous ossification of tumor that encircles the bone. Cortex of distal femur is clearly seen through bulk of the tumor which apparently seems intact

has a relatively better prognosis. They rarely develop metastases, though in some cases metastases have occurred up to 15 years following resection.

IV. Roentgenographic Features

In plain roentgenograms, the tumor appears as a partially ossified mass arising in the vicinity of the periosteum and extending to the soft tissue in a mushroom fashion. The tumor is seen to be juxtacortical and in most instances has a tendency to encircle the shaft of cylindrical bones. It is seen firmly attached to the cortex along its broad base (Fig. 2). In most cases, there is a partially free space of varying length and 1–3 mm in thickness between the tumor and cortex of underlying bone (Fig. 3a, b). In the majority of cases, the tumor is lobular in outline and, as a rule, sharply delineated; however, angular projections sometimes extend into the surrounding soft tissues. More than 80% of reported cases reveal evidence of marked amorphous ossification, but occasionally true osseous trabeculation may be observed. The density of the shadow is not uniform as a rule. The greatest density is usually found at the base of the tumor, this density

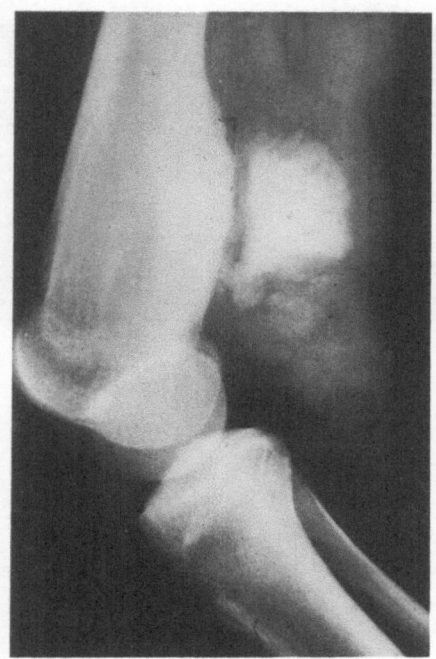

(a)

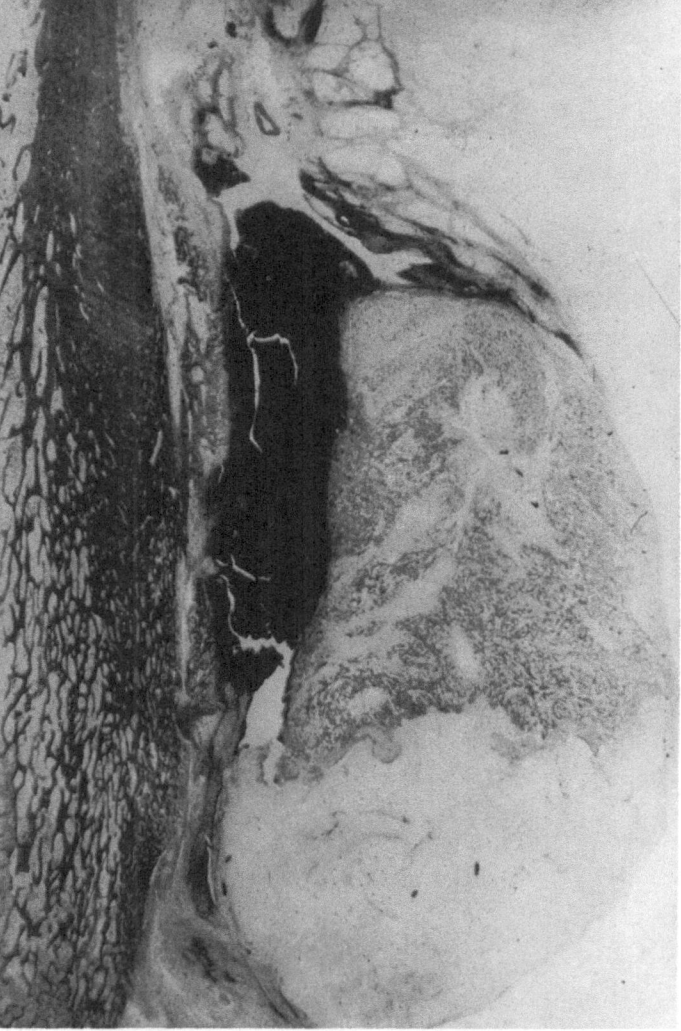

(b)

Fig. 3a and b. Parosteal osteosarcoma of lower portion of shaft of the femur posteriorly. There is a free space measuring 3 mm in thickness between tumor and relatively thickened cortex of distal end of femur. Amorphous ossification is noted in plain roentgenogram (a) and a section of gross specimen (b)

being equal to that of the normal bone cortex and of the adjacent spongiosa. The periphery of the tumor is typically less ossified than its base, and osseous trabeculation is seen more easily in these regions due to relatively less thickness of tumor at its periphery. High kv Bucky films also may help to demonstrate osseous trabeculation in some of the lesions. Numerous poorly defined and irregular radiolucent areas are

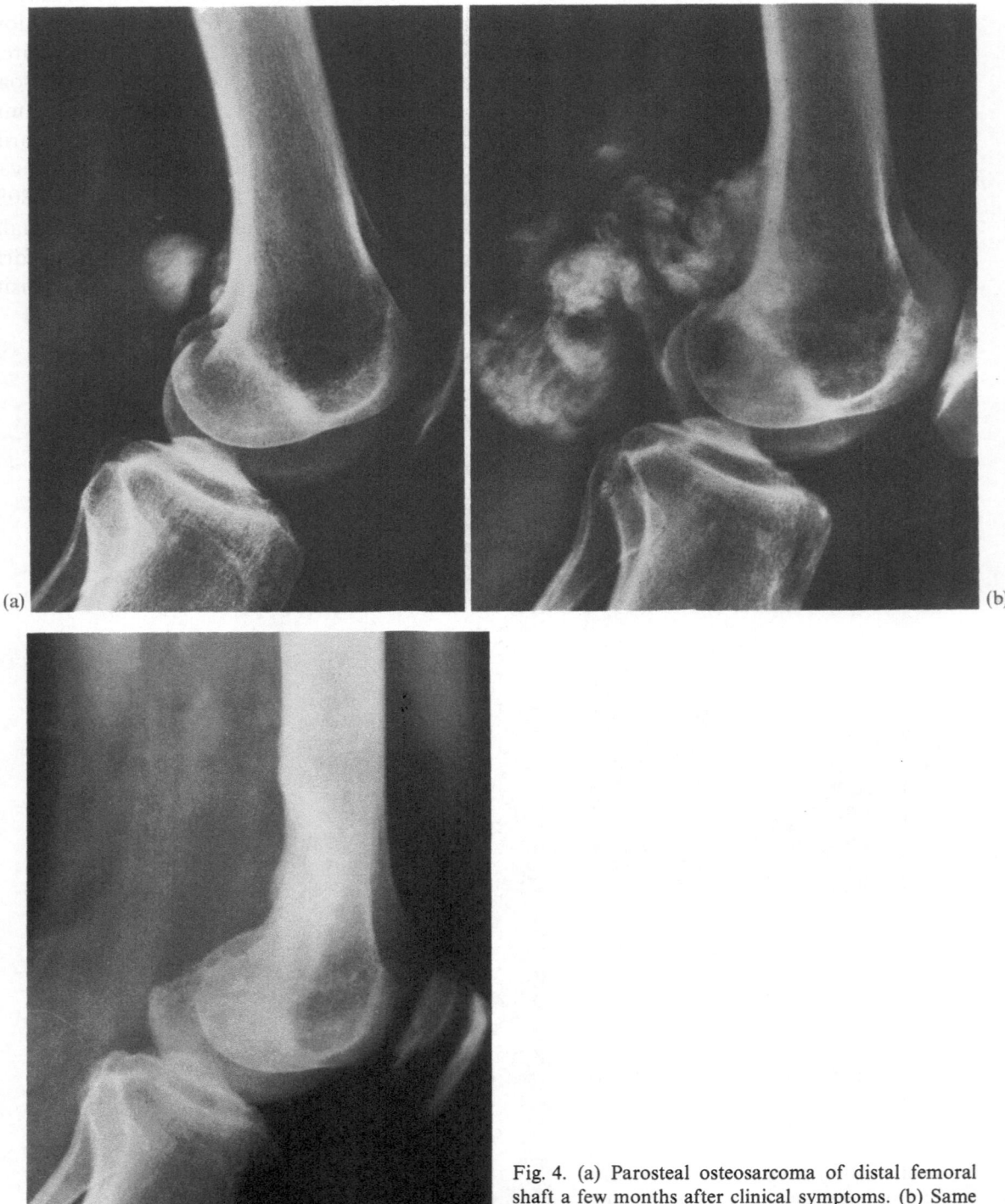

(a)

(b)

(c)

Fig. 4. (a) Parosteal osteosarcoma of distal femoral shaft a few months after clinical symptoms. (b) Same tumor, untreated, 4 years later. (c) Same patient 3 years after local resection. (With permission of Radiology)

seen in the substance of some cases, related to the zone of cartilage or fibromatous tissue (Figs. 2, 3, 4).

The more dense and uniform the ossification, the less the tendency of the tumor for rapid and infiltrating growth, and metastasis. One outstanding feature is the lack of periosteal elevation. Erosion of the cortex is rarely seen, and then only in the early stage of the disease. Medullary involvement is noted only in very long-standing tumors or in tumors that have been previously operated. In the neighborhood of the tumor, small radiopacities may be present, with no apparent relation to the main mass of the tumor. These areas, if not removed along with the main tumor, may give rise to recurrence. Usually recurrences have the appearance of scattered radiopacities of varied size which may become confluent later.

V. Angiographic Features

Simple radiographic examination is usually conclusively diagnostic, although there are some cases of parosteal osteosarcoma which are more malignant than others, and differentiation of these lesions on the basis of plain films is impossible. The same difficulty exists in the differentiation of true osteosarcoma from parosteal osteosarcoma. A biopsy is a valuable adjunct in confirming the diagnosis. Certain limitations, however, are imposed on the decision. The amount of tissue received in the specimen may not clearly delineate the character of the lesion. In addition, the specimen represents only a part

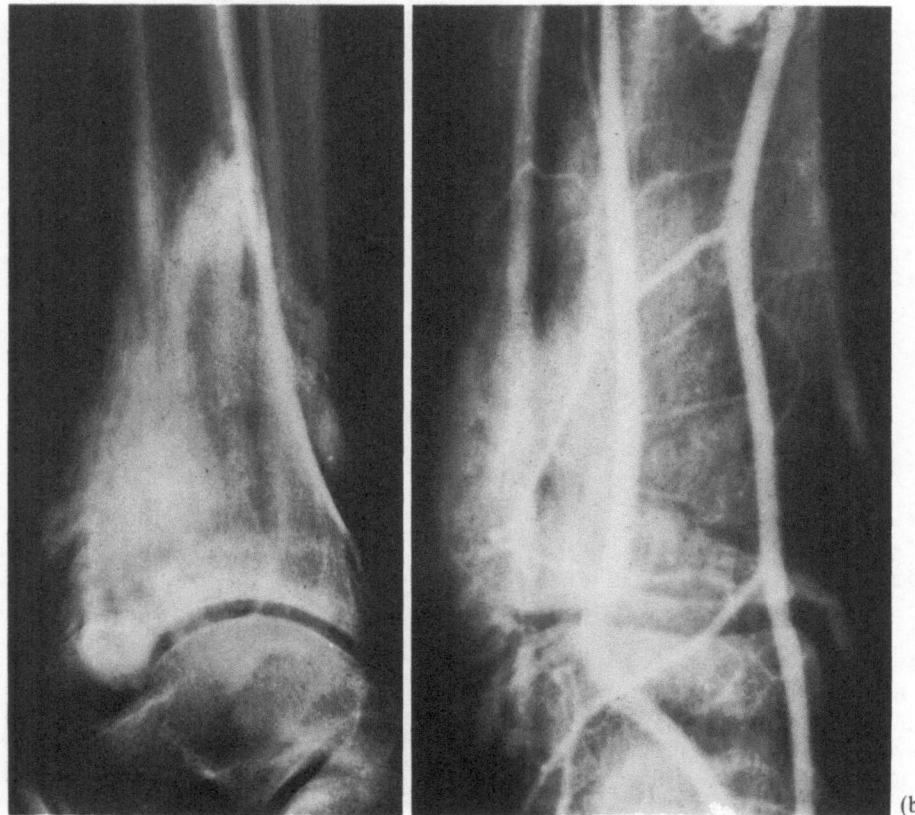

(a)   (b)

Fig. 5a and b. Parosteal osteosarcoma of distal tibia (a). Arteriogram reveals only a few vessels in tumor area, mainly in surface of the tumor (b)

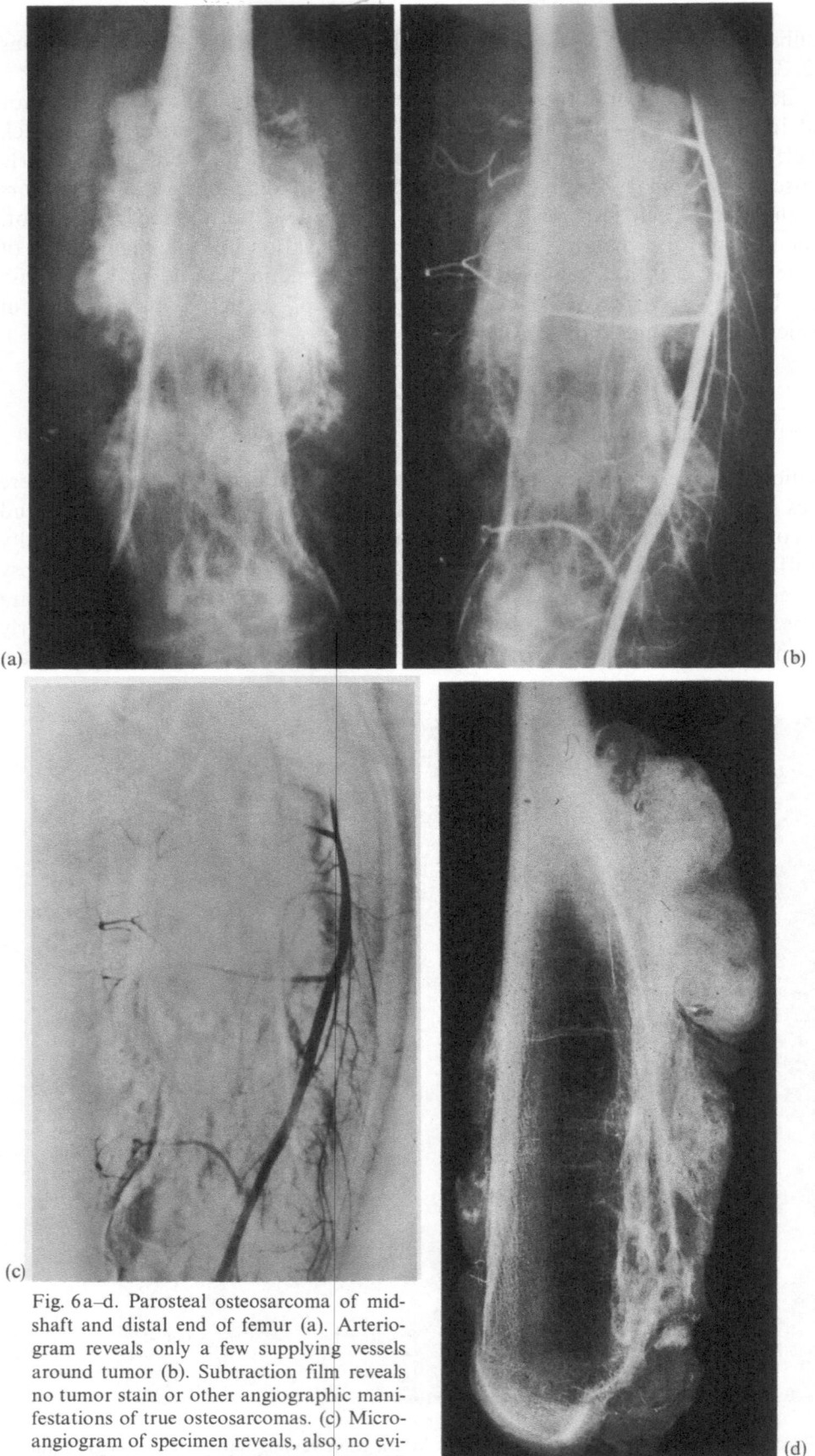

Fig. 6a–d. Parosteal osteosarcoma of mid-shaft and distal end of femur (a). Arteriogram reveals only a few supplying vessels around tumor (b). Subtraction film reveals no tumor stain or other angiographic manifestations of true osteosarcomas. (c) Micro-angiogram of specimen reveals, also, no evidence of hypervascularity in tumor area (d)

of the tumor, making the determination of malignant activity difficult. In these doubtful cases, angiography will be of help in the differential diagnosis.

A true osteosarcoma, regardless of its osteolytic, sclerotic, and mixed roentgenographic pattern, is a hypervascular tumor (refer to chapter on angiography), with the presence of numerous pathologic vessels. Their heavy tumor stain and large abnormal veins and presence of venous and arterial invasion are typical for a rapidly growing malignant tumor. The angiographic appearance of parosteal osteosarcoma is quite different. In our experience, these lesions are not vascular or are only slightly vascular, with very faint or no tumor stain. There is a close relation between the number of vessels in these lesions, the degree of differentiation of the cells, and the degree of the malignancy. The least-vascular lesions are the most differentiated tumor, and vice versa. The least-differentiated tumors, which are the most vascular, we believe are true osteosarcomas. There are some cases with moderate degrees of vascularity which could explain the variety of clinical behavior of these lesions. In our experience there was a very close relation between the number of vessels in a tumor and the degree of their malignancy. We believe the vascular channels are the main route for fast spread of the tumor cells, and the more vessels there are in a malignant tumor, the greater the chance of earlier and faster spread of the disease, and the poorer the prognosis (Figs. 5, 6).

VI. Differential Diagnosis

Plain roentgenograms are important in the differential diagnosis of the lesions. There are several other lesions which could roentgenographically simulate this lesion.

Myositis ossificans. The heterotopic bone seen in myositis ossificans circumscripta can sometimes be confused with parosteal osteosarcoma, especially in cases of traumatic or idiopathic myositis ossificans which show a sessile base and attachment of the ossifications to the shaft of a long bone.

The bone mass in myositis ossificans often shows a clear-cut trabecular pattern. The border of the lesion is often angular, and when its base is sessile, periosteal elevation may be present as the result of subperiosteal hematoma. The density of the mass shadow is greatest in its peripheral parts, the reverse of parosteal osteosarcoma. A careful study will show that it does not have the characteristic broad base of parosteal osteosarcoma.

Osteochondroma. Osteochondroma can ordinarily be easily differentiated from parosteal osteosarcoma from a roentgenographic standpoint. The continuity of bony cortex and spongiosa into the base of the tumor with the pedunculated or sessile base of an exostosis is absent in parosteal osteosarcoma. In osteochondroma, cartilaginous inclusions containing areas of calcification are found; the ossification in osteochondroma is less extensive and dense than in parosteal osteosarcoma. Furthermore, these benign lesions do not usually encircle the shaft of the bone, and a small clear zone between tumor and shaft is not present.

Osteosarcoma. The presence of cortical destruction, extensive medullary involvement, periosteal reaction, ill-defined border, and Codman's triangle on conventional radiographs easily make the differential diagnosis between this tumor and parosteal osteosarcoma.

VII. Histopathologic Features

Gross pathology. Parosteal osteosarcoma usually forms a large, lobulated, hard mass with bony density adherent to the periosteum and cortex (Fig. 7). This tumor usually

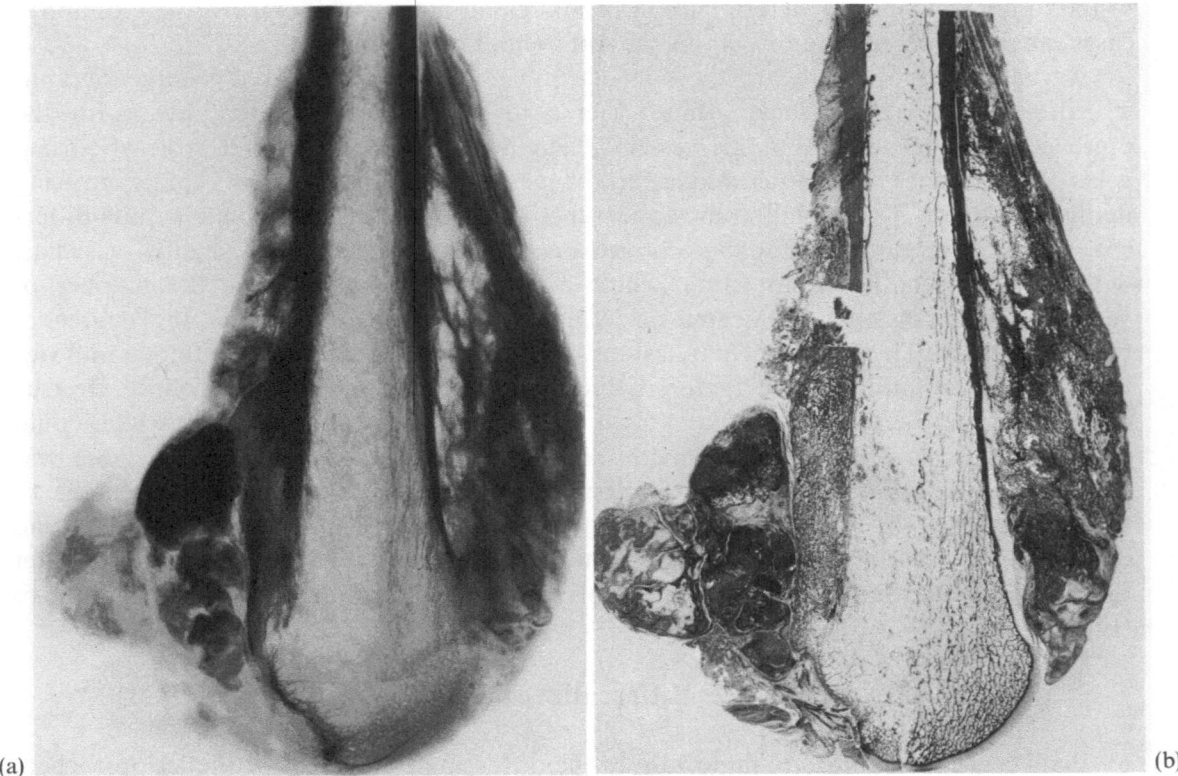

(a)   (b)

Fig. 7a and b. Parosteal osteosarcoma of distal shaft of femur (a). A section of gross specimen reveals intact cortex in anterior and posterior surface and clear zone anteriorly (b)

does not disrupt the cortex until late in the course of the disease, or after inadequate repeated surgical therapy. The tumors are predominately ossified, accounting for the roentgenographic density; however, in cut surfaces, occasionally fibrous tissue is seen between the ossified tissue. These zones are the ones most likely to show histologic evidence of malignancy. In some instances there are small foci of cartilage tissue. The degree of ossification or sclerosis is considerably less in cases with a higher degree of malignancy. Myositis ossificans, which is usually considered in the differential diagnosis, is often completely separated from the cortex, and does not produce as extensive a broad base as is seen in parosteal osteosarcoma.

Histopathology. The diagnosis of parosteal osteosarcoma is often difficult from the biopsy specimen alone because the biopsy may be from zones in which the bone and osteoid are well developed and closely resemble normal bone. Biopsy material is almost inscrutable, making it necessary for the pathologist to review the case with the orthopedist or radiologist (ACKERMAN and SPJUT, 1971). Multiple biopsies from different parts of a tumor, especially from the least densely ossified area, are needed to evaluate the malignant potentiality of the tumor. Pre-biopsy angiography in these cases is helpful for selecting the proper site or sites for biopsy. The most vascular part of the tumor will usually be the most informative part for diagnosis in these cases. Osteoblasts may show little or no indication of their malignancy. The stroma may be poorly cellular, but usually there are areas of moderate cellularity. Between the more or less normal trabeculae are atypical proliferating spindle-shaped cells in which one finds occasional, or sometimes fairly numerous, mitotic figures. Evidence of malignancy may be found only in small foci, making it necessary to study multiple sections for an accurate diagnosis.

Islands of normal or atypical fibromatous or chondromatous tissues are commonly seen in these tumors. At the periphery, the growths are more apt to show increased cellularity and, occasionally, the features of an osteosarcoma or fibrosarcoma. The recurrent tumors may reveal an increase in an atypical cellular form, with an accompanying increased growth potential.

Differentiation between myositis ossificans and parosteal osteosarcoma is difficult. An important microscopic differential feature is the ossification and maturation, which are usually found in the central portion of the parosteal osteosarcoma and peripherally in myostitis ossificans.

B. Treatment

The appropriate surgical treatment for patients with parosteal osteosarcoma must be evaluated with the knowledge of the potential degree of malignancy. Therefore, the main effort should be directed toward obtaining histopathologic proof of the sarcoma by biopsy. Accurate assessment of a large tumor with considerable variability of its cell composition is difficult by performing a single, blind biopsy. Pre-biopsy angiograms in these cases can help to evaluate the relation of the tumor to surrounding arteries and veins, as well as directing the biopsy site to the most vascular part of the tumor.

If the tumor has definite histologic evidence of malignancy, amputation is the treatment of choice. For small or very well-differentiated tumors, wide resection of the tumor and underlying cortex will be feasible.

However, in the majority of cases reported in the literature, recurrence was seen at the site of previous surgery, after segmental resection. The majority of reported cases after excision of a recurrence finally ended in a second recurrence. There were 17 recurrences in 6 patients reported by VAN DER HEUL et al. (1967). Of these 17 recurrences, 13 were demonstrated by clinical or roentgenographic examination within 3 years after the last treatment, 10 within 2 years, and 5 within 1 year. In only 1 case was a recurrence noted after 9 years. The histology of the recurrent tumor was more malignant than the original tumor. There was more cellularity, marked pleomorphism, and greater numbers of mitosis than in the primary tumor. Amputation, therefore, is considered as the best treatment for recurrence of parosteal osteosarcoma.

With proper treatment, cure can be obtained in the majority of patients. In those where metastases appear, long periods of survival can be anticipated. An average of 8–20 years survival for those patients with metastasis has been reported in the larger reported series. Removal of a single lung metastasis may cure the patient, or at least prolong survival. Tumor growth, both in primary neoplasms and recurrences, was not affected by radiotherapy.

References

AAKHUS, T., EIDE, O., STOKKE, T.: Parosteal osteogenic sarcoma. Acta radiol. (Stockh.) **54**, 29–40 (1960)

ACKERMAN, L.V.: Extra-osseous localized non-neoplastic bone and cartilage formation (so-called myositis ossificans). J. Bone Jt Surg. **40A**, 279–298 (1958)

ACKERMAN, L.V., SPJUT, H.J.: Tumors of bone and cartilage. In: Atlas of tumor pathology, 2nd Series, Fasc. 5. Washington, D.C.: Armed Forces Institute of Pathology (1971)

ARENA, F., CINGANO, A.: Osteoma parosteal. Bol. Soc. argent. Ortop. Traum. **18**, 149–151 (1953)

CALANDRIELLO, B.: Anoora sul sarcoma parostele ossificante. Arch. Putti Chir. Organi mor. **9**, 371–382
(1957)

COLEY, B.L.: Atypical forms of bone sarcoma. Bull.
Hosp. Jt Dis. (N.Y.) **12**, 148–173 (1951)

COPELAND, M.M., GESCHICKTER, C.F.: The treatment
of parosteal osteoma of bone. Surg. Gynec. Obstet.
108, 537–548 (1959)

DAHLIN, D.C.: Bone tumors. 2nd ed. Springfield, Ill.:
Charles C. Thomas 1967

DWINNELL, L.A., DAHLIN, D.C., GHORMLEY, R.K.:
Parosteal (juxtacortical) osteogenic sarcoma. J.
Bone Jt Surg. **36A**, 732–734 (1954)

GESCHICKTER, C.F., COPELAND, M.M.: Parosteal osteosarcoma of bone: A new entity. Ann. Surg. **133**,
790–806 (1951)

HALPERN, M., FREIBERGER, R.H.: Arteriography in
orthopedics. Amer. J. Roentgenol. **94**, 194–206
(1965)

HARKESS, J.W.: Parosteal osteosarcoma. Amer. Surg.
30, 730–736 (1964)

HATCHER, C.H.: Extraskeletal ossification simulating
sarcoma. J. Bone Jt Surg. **29**, 542 (1947)

HEUL, R.O., VAN DER, VON RONNEN, J.R.: Juxtacortical osteosarcoma, diagnosis, differential diagnosis,
treatment, and an analysis of 80 cases. J. Bone
Jt Surg. **49A**, 415–439 (1967)

JACOBSON, S.A.: Early juxtacortical osteosarcoma (parosteal osteoma). J. Bone Jt Surg. **40-A**, 1310–1328
(1958)

JAFFE, H.L.: Tumors and tumorous conditions in
bone and joints. Philadelphia: Lea and Febiger
1958

JAFFE, H.L., SELIN, G.: Tumors of bones and joints,
New York Academy of Medicine. A symposium
in the musculoskeletal system: pp. 338–339. New
York: the MacMillan Company (1952)

MATHIAS, P.F., SUBRAHMANYAM, C.S.V., RAO, B.O.P.:
Juxtacortical osteogenic sarcoma. Indian J. Radiol.
17, 1–4 (1963)

MÜLLER, J.: Über ossificierende Schwämme oder Osteo-
id-Geschwülste. Arch. Anat. Physiol. wiss. Med.
396–442 (1843)

NORMAN, A., DORFMAN, H.: Juxtacortical circumscribed myositis ossificans: Evaluation and radiologic features. Radiology **96**, 301–306 (1970)

PACK, G.T., BRAUND, R.R.: Development of sarcoma
in myositis ossificans. J. Amer. med. Ass. **119**,
776–779 (1942)

RANNIGER, K., ALTNER, P.C.: Parosteal osteoid sarcoma. Radiology **86**, 648–651 (1966)

RATTI, A.: L'arteriografia e l'osteomedullografia nella
diagnosi dei tumori delle ossa. Radiol. clin. **28**,
263–275 (1959)

RATTI, A.: Die Osteomedullographie der Knochenerkrankungen mit besonderer Rücksicht auf die Tumoren. Röntgenblätter **14**, 241–247 (1961)

SAMMONS, B.P., SARKISIAN, S.S., KREPELA, M.C.: Juxtacortical osteogenic sarcoma. Amer. J. Roentgenol. **79**, 592–597 (1958)

SCAGLIETTI, O., CALANDRIELLO, B.: Sarcoma parostale
ossificante. Arch. Putti Chir. Organi mov. **6**, 9–37
(1955)

SCAGLIETTI, O., CALANDRIELLO, B.: Ossifying parosteal
sarcoma; parosteal osteoma or juxtacortical osteogenic sarcoma. J. Bone Jt Surg. **44A**, 635–647
(1962)

SIRSAT, M.V., DOCTOR, V.M.: Parosteal (juxtacortical)
osteogenic sarcoma. J. postgrad. Med. **11**, 191–197
(1965)

SOM, M., PEIMER, R.: Juxtacortical osteogenic sarcoma
of mandible. Amer. med. Ass. Arch. Otol. **74**,
532–536 (1961)

STEVENS, G.M., PUGH, D.G., DAHLIN, D.C.: Roentgenographic recognition and differentiation of
parosteal osteogenic sarcoma. Amer. J. Roentgenol. **78**, 1–12 (1957)

STRICKLAND, B.: The value of arteriography in the
diagnosis of bone tumors. Brit. J. Radiol. **32**,
705–713 (1959)

TAVERNIER, L., ROUSSELIN, L.: Ostéosarcomes ossifi-
cants, limités, à évolution lente, improprement dits
ostéomes. Lyon chir. **45**, 741–744 (1950)

WESTON, W.J., REID, J.D., SAUNDERS, J.H.: Parosteal
osteogenic sarcoma of bone. J. Bone Jt Surg. **40B**,
722–729 (1958)

WOLFEL, D.A., CARTER, P.R.: Parosteal osteosarcoma.
Amer. J. Roentgenol. **105**, 142–146 (1969)

YAGHMAI, I., SHAMSA, A.Z., SHARIAT, S., AFSHARI, R.:
Value of arteriography in the diagnosis of benign
and malignant bone lesions. Cancer (Philad.) **27**,
1134–1147 (1971)

Cartilaginous Tumors and Cartilage-Forming Tumor-like Conditions of the Bones and Soft Tissues

by

Frieda Feldman

A. Introduction

Cartilaginous lesions are important because, as a group, they constitute the most prevalent form of bone tumor in some series. At the same time, however, they paradoxically present a difficult challenge for even the most experienced pathologists since the line between the benign and malignant counterparts of these lesions frequently cannot be finely drawn. The pathologist may be particularly insecure in the separation of the benign lesions from the so-called low grade or well-differentiated chondrosarcomas. This constitutes a crucial conflict, since the majority of chondrosarcomas are well-, or moderately well-differentiated.

The distinction between benign and malignant is of additional importance within this family of lesions, since a greater potential exists for cure if malignant members are recognized early and treated definitively. The doubling time of well-differentiated chondrosarcoma, however, is long, with estimates of one year or longer. Extrapolations have indicated that many of these lesions have been present for years. It has further been suggested that the rare chondrosarcoma occurring in the young individual may have been present at birth (SPRATT, 1965). This slow evolution gives clinicians, surgeons, and radiologists a false sense of security, leading to prolonged observation and less than adequate resection until a time when tumors have reached unmanageable proportions in inaccessible locations, sometimes after years of slow, subtle growth. This "too little-too late" approach in the management of early chondrosarcoma may mean the difference between cure and ultimate fatality. O'NEAL and ACKERMAN (1952), too, emphasize that the poor results in low grade chondrosarcomas, in spite of their favorable nature and generally more favorable location, have usually been due to underdiagnosis, inadequate resection, and resulting recurrences, which may take on a progressively aggressive character.

Another difficulty lies in the recognition of the less common, poorly differentiated chondrosarcoma which may have a rapid clinical evolution as well as several recently recognized variants, which may have intermediate histologic characteristics. The potential of the latter group is even more poorly understood. In general, however, the so-called classic chondrosarcoma has been misdiagnosed and underread as a benign neoplasm more than any other bone tumor.

At the other end of the spectrum lies a hazard with equally grim repercussions, i.e., that of "overdiagnosing" and "overtreating" the benign counterparts of this family of lesions. Furthermore, a lack of knowledge of the high risk of local seeding of cartilagi-

Table 1. Tumors of cartilaginous origin (location and classification)

		Benign		Malignant
Peripheral	Metaphysis and/or Diaphysis	Osteochondroma	Solitary Multiple	Chondrosarcoma primary, Chondrosarcoma secondary
	Epiphysis	Juxtacortical chondroma Dysplasia epiphysealis hemimelica	Solitary Multiple	
Central	Metaphysis	Enchondroma	Solitary Multiple	Chondrosarcoma primary, Chondrosarcoma secondary
	Epiphysis	Chondromyxoid fibroma[a] Chondroblastoma	—	

[a] Rarely cortical in location.

Table 2. Nomenclature of Cartilaginous Tumors

Prefered Terminology	Synonyms
Solitary osteochondroma	Exostosis Enchondroma Osteocartilaginous exostosis
Multiple osteochondromatosis	Hereditary multiple exostoses Metaphyseal aclasis Diaphyseal aclasis Dyschondroplasia[a] Hereditary deforming dyschondroplasia[a]
Dysplasia epiphysealis hemimelica	Tarsoepiphyseal aclasis Benign epiphyseal osteochondroma Intra-articular osteochondroma of astragalus Carpal osteochondroma
Solitary enchondromas	Chondroma
Multiple enchondromatosis	Ollier's disease Dyschondroplasia[a] Hereditary deforming dyschondroplasia[a]
Juxtacortical chondroma	Paraosteal chondroma Periosteal chondroma Subperiosteal chondroma Eccentric chondroma
Chondroblastoma	Benign chondroblastoma Epiphyseal chondroblastoma Codman's tumor[b] Calcified giant cell tumor[b] Epiphyseal chondromatous giant cell tumor[b]
Chondromyxoid fibroma	Fibromyxoid chondroma

[a] Same name in use for both entities. [b] Terminology no longer in use.

nous tumors, benign as well as malignant, frequently in the course of biopsy, leads to additional difficulty in terms of recurrence and future treatment.

Lastly, the location and multiplicity of the lesions, as well as the age of the patient, play an inordinately important role in the classification of these lesions. Thus, difficulties in histologic interpretation and a poorly understood potential combine with a classically slow evolution to make cartilage lesions a difficult group to manage. More than most neoplasms, therefore, cartilaginous tumors of bone require the close cooperation of the pathologist, the surgeon, and the radiologist in achieving adequate treatment, and less of a tendency exists to rely solely on one discipline for definitive interpretation and/or evaluation.

The chief emphasis of this review, however, will be on roentgenology, both in terms of its basic role in the initial diagnostic approach to these lesions, and its complementary role in their further characterization, once their cartilaginous nature has been established. Emphasis will also be placed on the significance and clinical implications of particular roentgen features.

In keeping with a primarily roentgenographic orientation, the simplest classification of a chondrogenic series of tumors has been adopted, based on their biologic behavior, i.e. benign vs. malignant, presumed pathogenesis, i.e. primary vs. secondary, and location with relation to a particular bone, i.e. central, eccentric, or peripheral as outlined in Table 1. Table 2 contains a number of pseudonyms which have been employed for these lesions. Preferred nomenclature will be placed first.

B. Solitary Osteochondroma

A solitary osteochondroma is a cancellous bony projection with a cartilage cap, most frequently located in the metaphysis and occasionally in the diaphysis of a tubular bone. It may, however, be associated with any bone that is preformed in cartilage.

Osteochondromas are the commonest cartilaginous neoplasms as well as the commonest benign neoplasms of bone (SPJUT et al., 1971). Solitary and multiple osteochondromas constituted 45% of 1025 benign bone tumors and 12% of all bone tumors studied by DAHLIN (1967). Nearly 90% were solitary lesions.

I. Pathogenesis

Although generally held to be noninherited hamartomatous malformations, their genesis is disputed. VIRCHOW's postulate (1879), that a fragment of growth plate cartilage separated, rotated 90° and grew transversely to the shaft's long axis, has received support from experiments where epiphyseal cartilage transplanted to adjacent metaphyses of young rabbits has produced osteochondroma-like lesions (D'AMBROSIA and FERGUSON, 1968). Others postulated perverted activity of the periosteum (MÜLLER, 1914) with formation of cartilaginous nodules by its cambium layer; the presence of cartilage rests in the periosteum or within tendinous attachments to bone which subsequently become activated; or the presence of a periosteal defect which allowed a segment of growth plate to herniate through it during embryologic development (MÜLLER, 1914; WEIL,

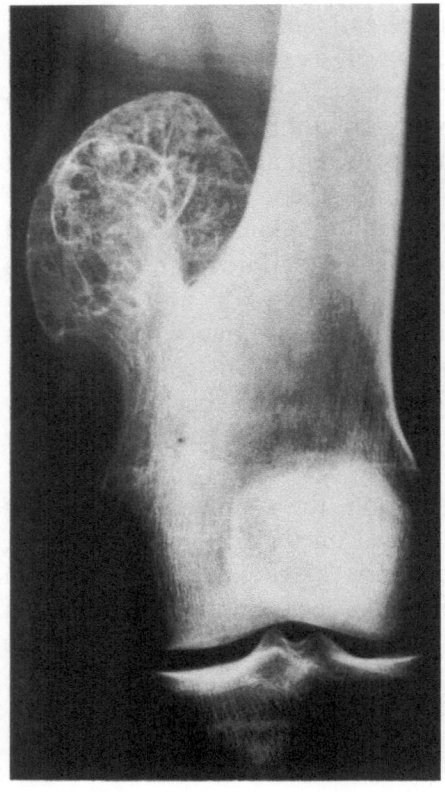

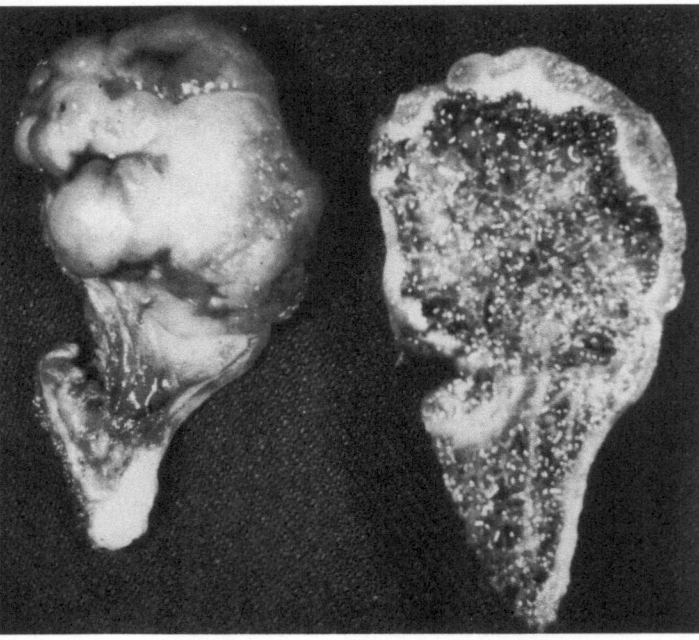

Fig. 1   Fig. 2

Fig. 1. Solitary benign osteochondroma: 30-year-old male with 15 year history of painless mass in left thigh. Exostosis extends beyond otherwise normally contoured femur. Note that cortex of base of exostosis blends with that of main shaft. Trabeculae of host bone also extend into and blend with that of exostosis. Latter simulates pedunculated polyp on narrow bony stalk. Exostoses most commonly point away from epiphysis and joint. Although bulbous periphery of exostosis appeared smooth and sharply demarcated, its large size prompted excision

Fig. 2. Pedunculated osteochondroma. Left, gross specimen, surface view: Irregular, smooth glistening cartilage cap covers bulbous end of stalked exostosis. Narrow neck is seen inferiorly. Entire external surface of sessile tumor may be capped by cartilage. Right, cut section: Note fatty, cancellous bone with spongiosa extending into neck of stalk. Cartilage cap is seen superiorly

1957). The process of enchondral ossification was then thought to continue at an angle to the shaft with the cartilaginous cap of the exostosis constituting a new aberrant growth plate. Indeed, the continuity of the trabeculae, cortex, and periosteum of the exostosis with that of the main shaft and often at varying angles to the main shaft is evident, both roentgenographically (Fig. 1) and pathologically (Fig. 2). KEITH (1920), in addition to favoring an origin from the cartilaginous growth plate, proposed that diaphyseal aclasis, i.e., defective modeling, contributes to the broad appearance of the diametaphyseal region of the affected bone. This failure of modeling with a flaring of the shaft particularly at the level of the exostosis is always apparent on the roentgeno-gram and serves as an aid to diagnosis particularly in cases with small and/or fairly sessile projections (Fig. 3). Osteochondromata have also developed after radiation therapy in the young (COHEN and D'ANGIO, 1961; MURPHY and BLOUNT, 1962; PEREZ et al., 1967).

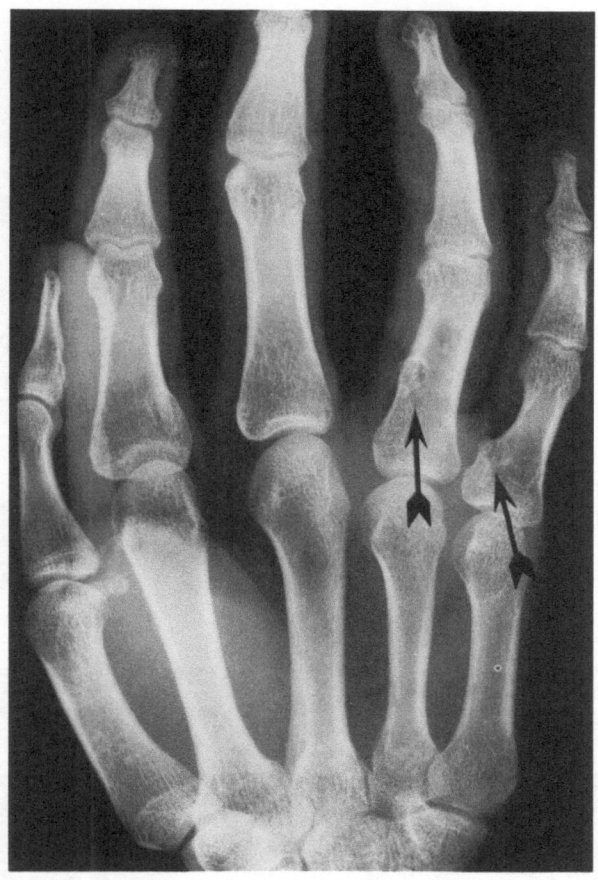

Fig. 3. Osteochondroma: Note small nubbin-like exostoses with flaring of proximal shafts of proximal phalanges (arrows). Modeling deformity is usually noted at level of exostosis

II. Site

An osteochondroma may be related to any bone that develops by enchondral ossification including the base of the skull (Fig. 4). Long bones are predilected. The commonest locations are the lower femoral and upper tibial metaphyses with an incidence of 36% at the knee, 50% including the knee and proximal humerus (DAHLIN, 1967) and 95% including all bones of the extremities (SPJUT et al., 1971). The flat bones, including the scapula (PRATT et al., 1958; WOUTERS et al., 1974), ilium, clavicle (PRATT et al., 1958), sternum, spinous process of the vertebral body, the remainder of the vertebral column (GOKAY and BUCEY, 1955; ILGENFRITZ, 1951; JAFFE, 1968; MEYERDING, 1927; PECK, 1964) and the small tubular bones of the hands and feet are less frequent loci (Figs. 3, 5). They are rarely associated with either the carpal (HEIPLE, 1961) or tarsal bones (MILCH, 1954). Solitary osteochondromas of the distal phalanx of the first toe have been related to trauma and are not included in some series (DAHLIN, 1956), despite the fact that they have similar radiologic and pathologic features (Fig. 6). On occasion, they are subungual and may be associated with considerable discomfort (Fig. 7).

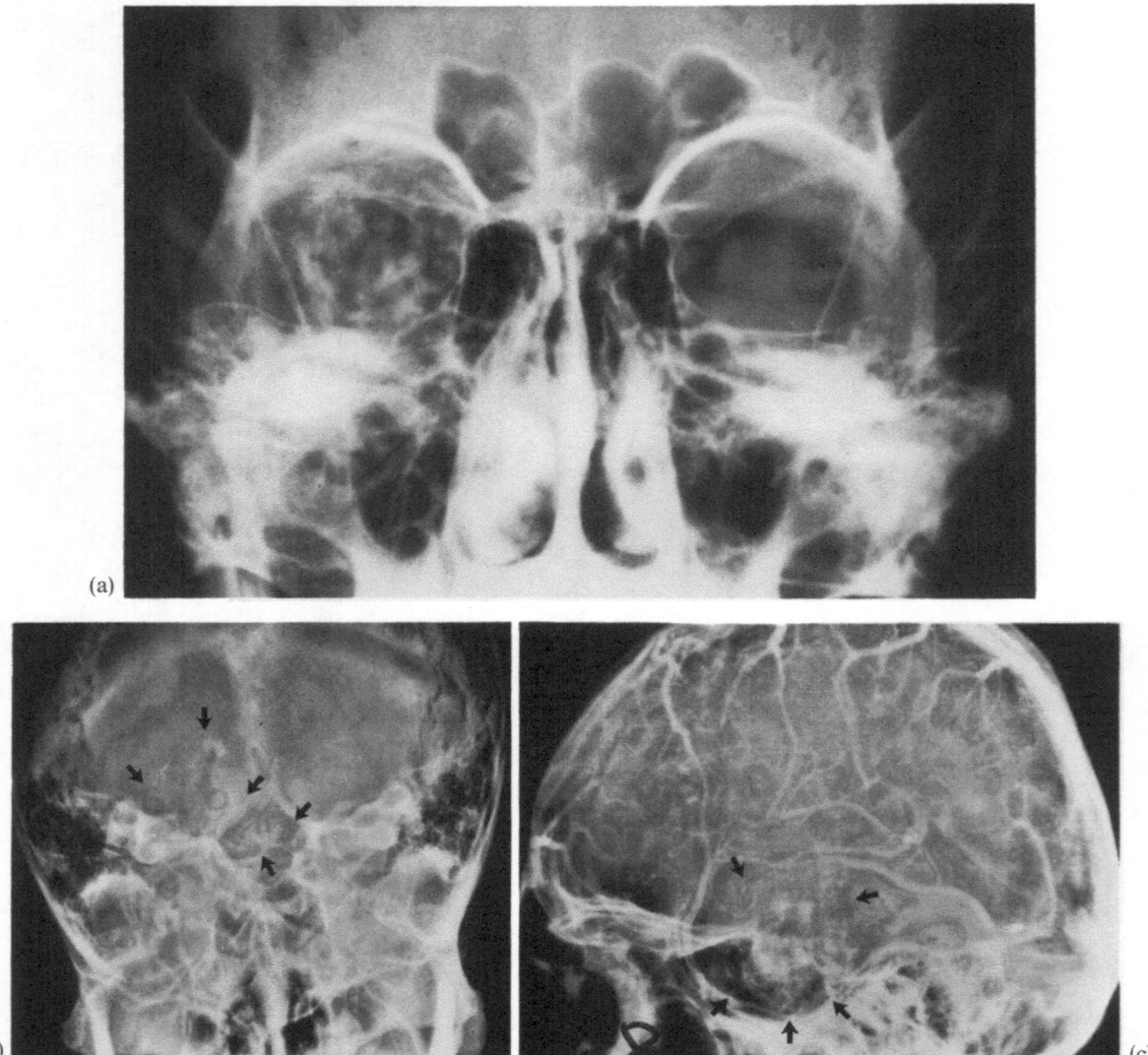

Fig. 4a–c. Solitary osteochondroma, base of skull: Although osteochondromas may involve any bone that develops by enchondral ossification, they are more commonly seen in this location in cases with multiple osteochondromatosis. (a) Calcified cartilage cap is seen through right orbit. (b) Townes view shows extent of lesion and its origin from skull base. (c) Carotid arteriogram, lateral view: Defines peripheral margins of relatively avascular lesion. Its superior and inferior portions projected above and below sella turcica (arrows) (Courtesy of Dr. Richard Taxin)

Fig. 6. Exostosis, terminal phalanx of first toe: Spur-like appearance together with continuity of cortex and trabeculae with that of host phalanx establish diagnosis. Exostoses involving distal phalanges have been related to trauma with or without superimposed infection and are therefore not included in statistical compilations of most series. They possess many of roentgenologic and pathologic features of classic osteocartilaginous exostosis

Fig. 7. Subungual exostosis, foot: These are not included in benign tumor statistics of most series. When situated under nail, they rarely measure more than 1 cm in diameter. Proliferating fibrocartilaginous tissue capping growing subungual exostosis resembles callous in its morphologic gradations while maturing on trabeculae, further supporting likelihood of lesion representing response to injury. Ulceration and infection may coexist

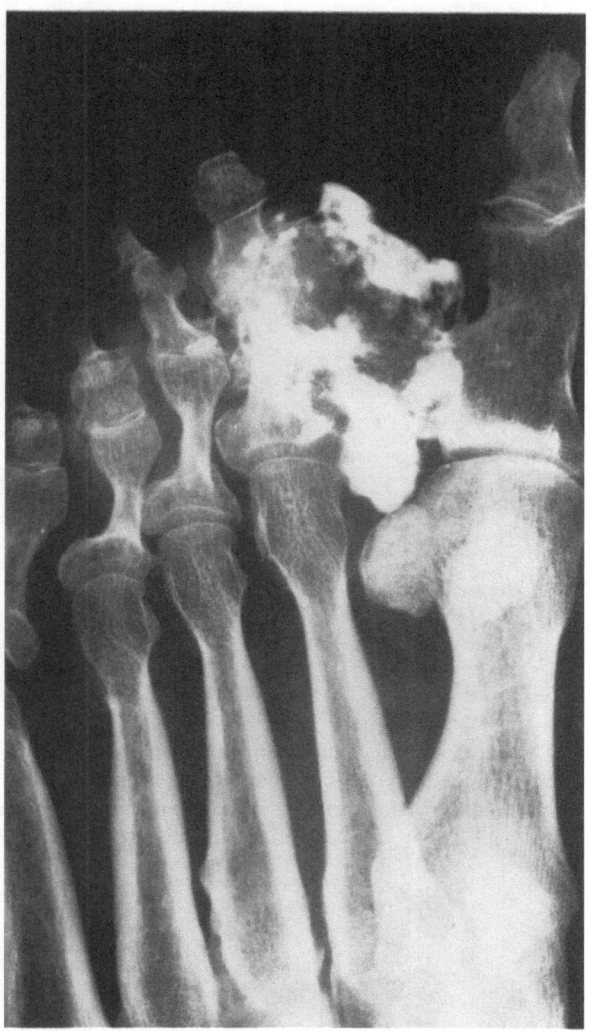

Fig. 5. Osteochondroma, foot: Well-defined narrow neck projects laterally from proximal portion of proximal phalanx. Although this benign lesion had not increased in size for more than 10 years, discomfort necessitated its removal

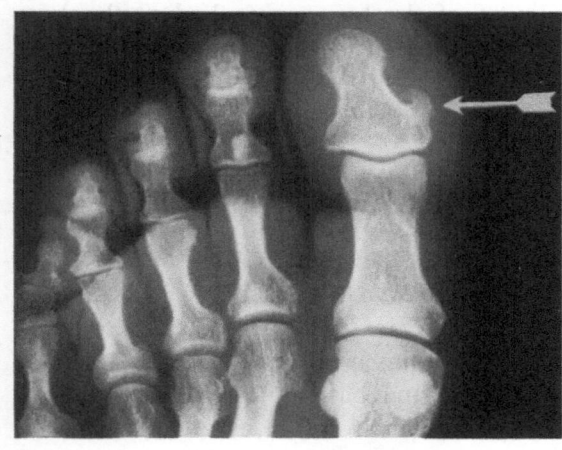

Fig. 6

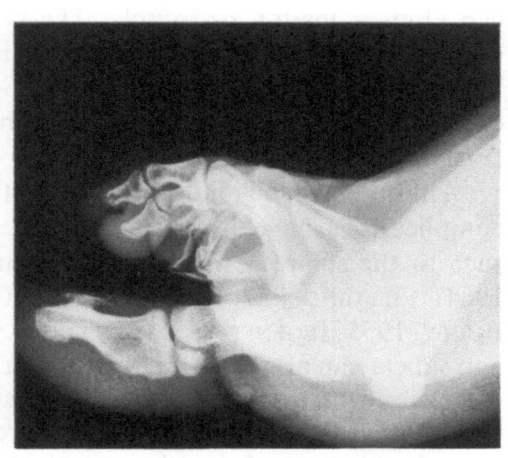

Fig. 7

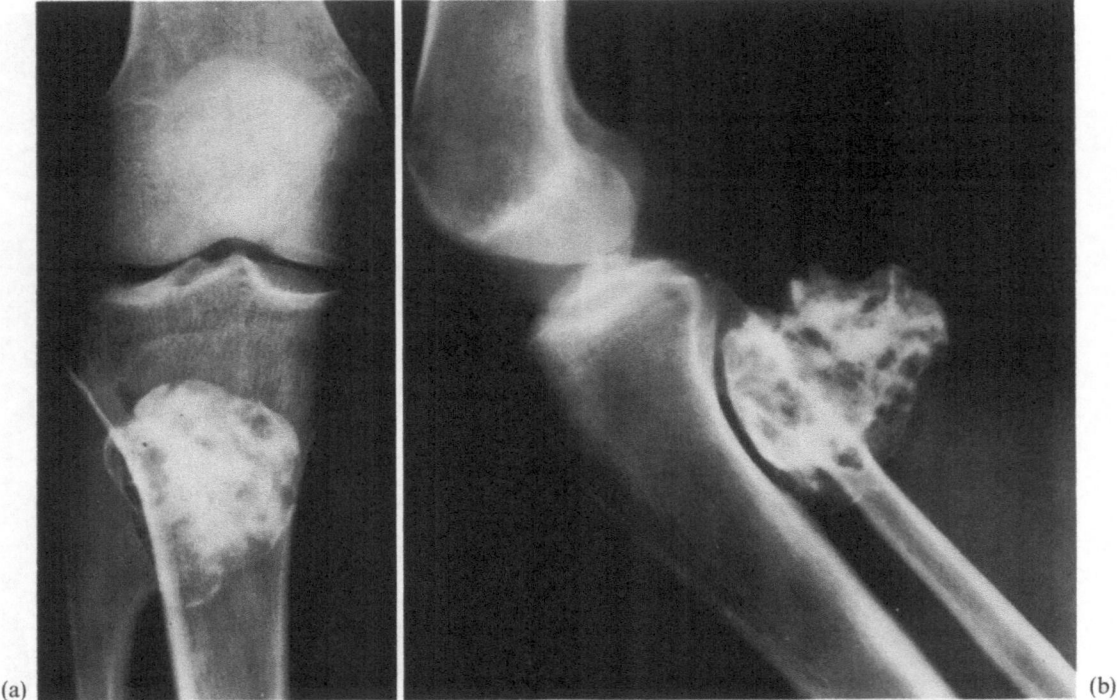

(a)   (b)

Fig. 8a and b. Osteochondroma, fibula: (a) AP view—large cauliflower-sized lesion arises from fibula by means of medially directed narrow neck. Latter is partially obscured by tibia, resulting in simulation of tibial lesion. (b) Lateral view—Both base and periphery of exostosis were sharply demarcated. Erosion of posterior tibial cortex is related to extrinsic mechanical pressure

III. Clinical

No significant sex predilection has been noted in some series (Spjut et al., 1971). In others (Dahlin, 1967) males predominate in a 3:2 ratio. The lesion has most commonly been discovered as a painless lump usually between 2–21 years of age. Symptoms may be due to impingement on neighboring bones (Figs. 8a and b, 9), nerves or blood vessels, or can be related to the irritation of a bursa which may develop if the cartilaginous cap abuts a tendon or muscle. The synovial lining of the bursa, attached at the base of the exostosis, may rarely be accompanied by false aneurysm formation in a neighboring blood vessel (Anastasi et al., 1963; Schoene et al., 1973). Accelerated growth of an exostosis with or without accompanying pain has also been related to trauma (Figs. 10a, b).

Although osteochondromata are infrequently noted in the vertebral column, serious complications have been encountered due to the proximity of important structures, such as the spinal cord, nerve roots, and cauda equina (Chiurco, 1970; Cohen et al., 1964; Fielding and Ratzan, 1973; Geschickter and Copeland, 1949; Gokay and Bucey, 1955; Ilgenfritz, 1951; Thomas and Andress, 1971). Compression of the carotid and subclavian arteries with obstruction of venous return has been reported. An odontoid osteochondroma was responsible for sudden death in one patient (Rose and Feketa, 1964). Other unusual complications were those of cyanosis in an infant, related to bilateral osteochondromas of the ribs and diaphragm (Hopkins and Freitag, 1965). Osteochondromata are commonly removed for cosmetic reasons or when symptoms become mani-

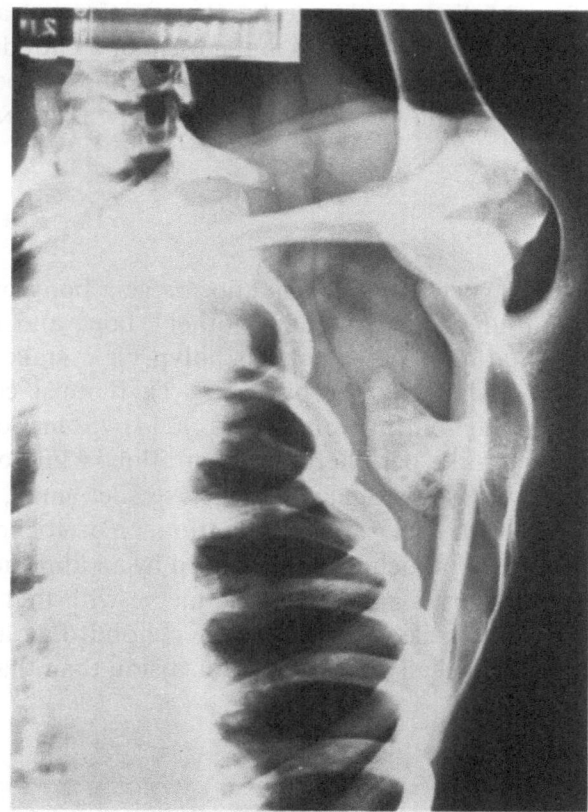

Fig. 9. Osteochondroma, scapula. Tangential view
—large, sharply defined osteochondroma is seen in
profile directly abutting rib cage

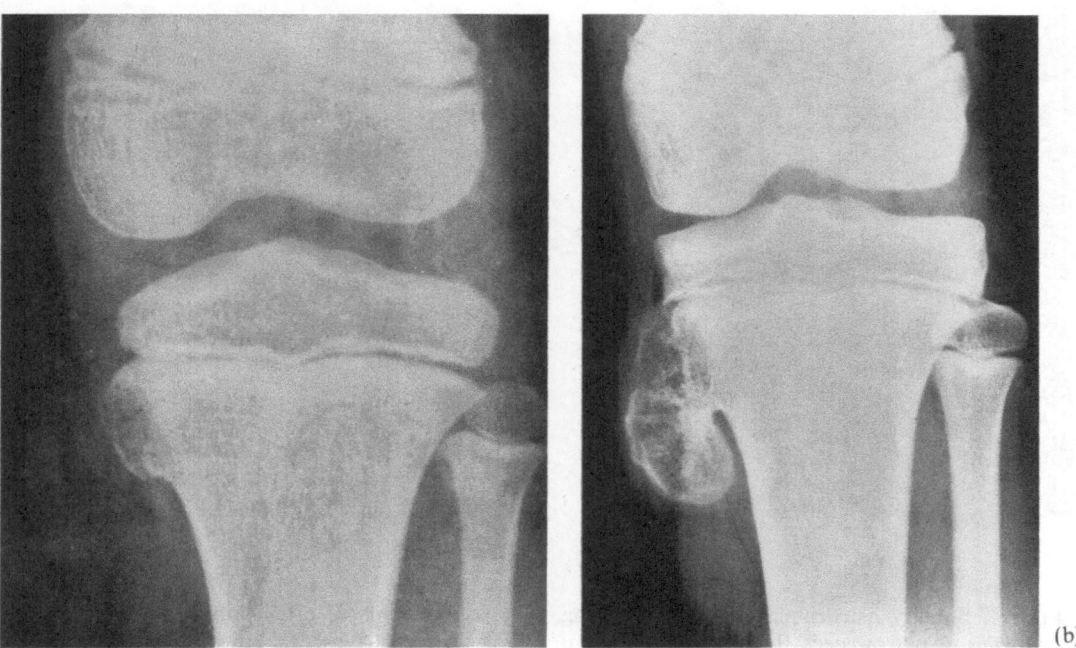

Fig. 10a. Osteochondroma, tibia: This medially directed broad based exostosis was incidental finding on
2/15/71. (b) 7/26/73: Exostosis is now directed away from joint space and increased in size in this actively
growing child. Exostoses often become quiescent after growth plate closure

fest. Malignant change has been estimated as occurring in less than 1% of cases and most commonly occurs in the form of a chondrosarcoma. Osteogenic sarcoma (SLULITTEL et al., 1971) as well as other sarcomas appear to be exceptional with the exact type often not universally agreed upon (ANDERSON et al., 1969).

IV. Roentgen

The osteochondroma appears as a bony protruberance extending beyond the cortical contour of the host or "mother" bone and is usually attached to it by a narrow neck simulating a pedunculated polyp on a stalk (Fig. 11). Its trabeculae blend with those of the shaft via the base (Fig. 1). It most commonly points away from the epiphysis and neighboring joint (Figs. 1, 11). Some osteochondromas are broad-based with a plateau-like peripheral configuration, while others taper more sharply (Figs. 12, 13, 14, 22a, b). Occasionally they are sessile, small, or near nubbin-like excrescences (Fig. 3). Even with the latter configuration, an osteochondroma is always suspect due to a localized failure of modeling, as evidenced by an abnormally wide shaft at the level of the exostosis, whose cortex and trabeculae merge with that of the host bone.

The cartilage cap of the osteochondroma may not be apparent unless it is mineralized, but it is usually of a larger dimension than that appreciated on a roentgenogram, particu-

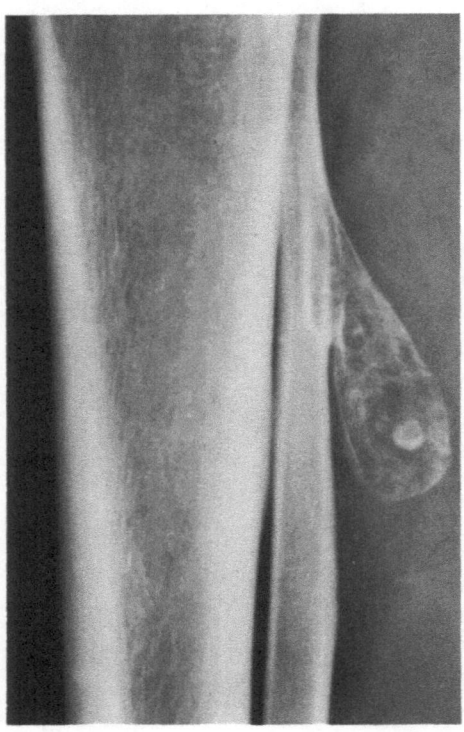

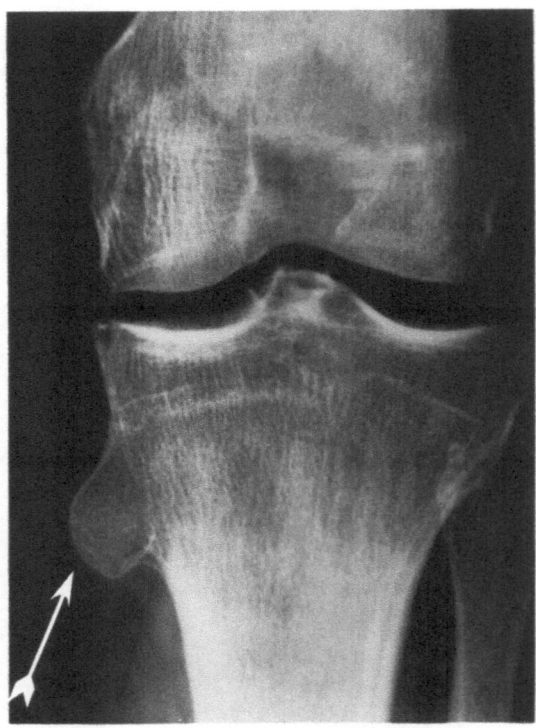

Fig. 11   Fig. 12

Fig. 11. Solitary osteochondroma, fibula: Long, slender pedunculated osteochondroma projects from tibia by means of narrow neck. Its thick cartilage cap is rimmed by sharp calcific border. Rounded ossific density superimposed on inferior portion of exostosis was situated within adjacent bursa

Fig. 12. Solitary osteochondroma, tibia: Note broad-based neck and plateau-like periphery. Exostosis is still directed away from joint space

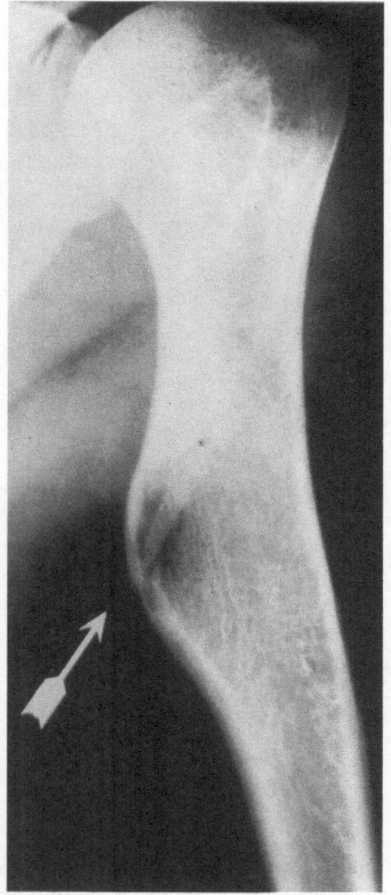

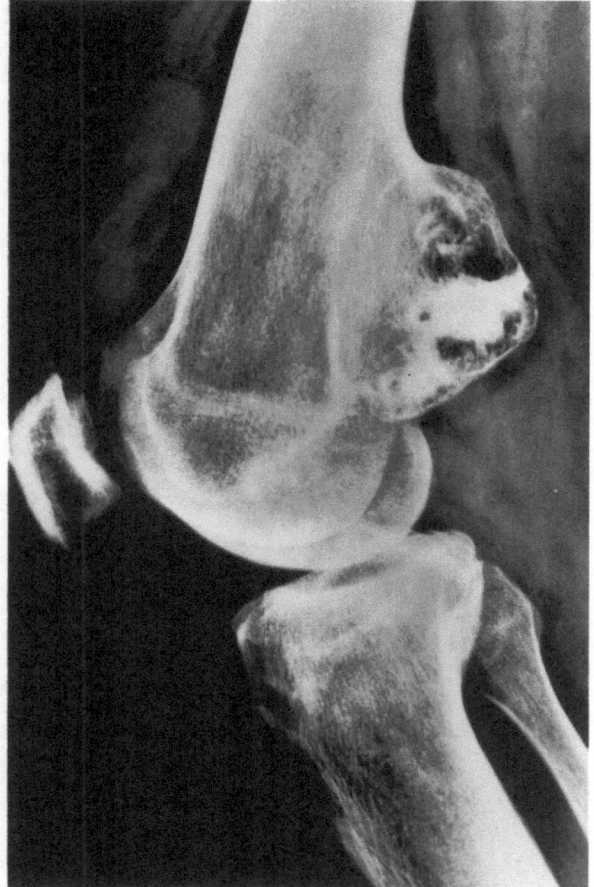

Fig. 13   Fig. 14

Fig. 13. Solitary osteochondroma, humerus: Incidental finding of diaphyseal osteochondroma of sessile variety. Though flat, its cortex is still continuous with that of underlying bone. Note abnormal width of bone at level of osteochondroma owing to failure of normal tubulation. Cartilaginous cap covered major portion of external surface of this sessile tumor

Fig. 14. Osteochondroma, femur: This broad-based, sharply circumscribed and heavily mineralized projection was discovered as result of symptoms related to impingement on neighboring structures

larly in children. Since the cartilage cap becomes inactive, with cessation of bone growth, it should be thin or atrophied in the adult. An unusually thick or growing cap may indicate malignancy in an adult, while mineral irregularly deposited along its periphery, or a sudden spurt in growth suggests malignancy in both young and old. Xerography may aid in visualizing the extent of the unmineralized portion of the cartilaginous cap.

The visualized bony exostoses vary in overall size from less than 1 cm to over 10 cm. In adults, lesions over 8 cm are regarded with suspicion and should be carefully analyzed for the presence of chondrosarcoma (Spjut et al., 1971).

When seen "en face" the exostosis may mimic a central medullary lesion with a sclerotic rim (Figs. 14a, b). The latter reflects the cortex of the exostosis. The calcifications within the cap may be projected onto the center of this "pseudo medullary" shadow further simulating an enchondroma or even a central chondrosarcoma (Fig. 24c). An osteochondroma related to a rib may likewise be visualized "en face" and simulate

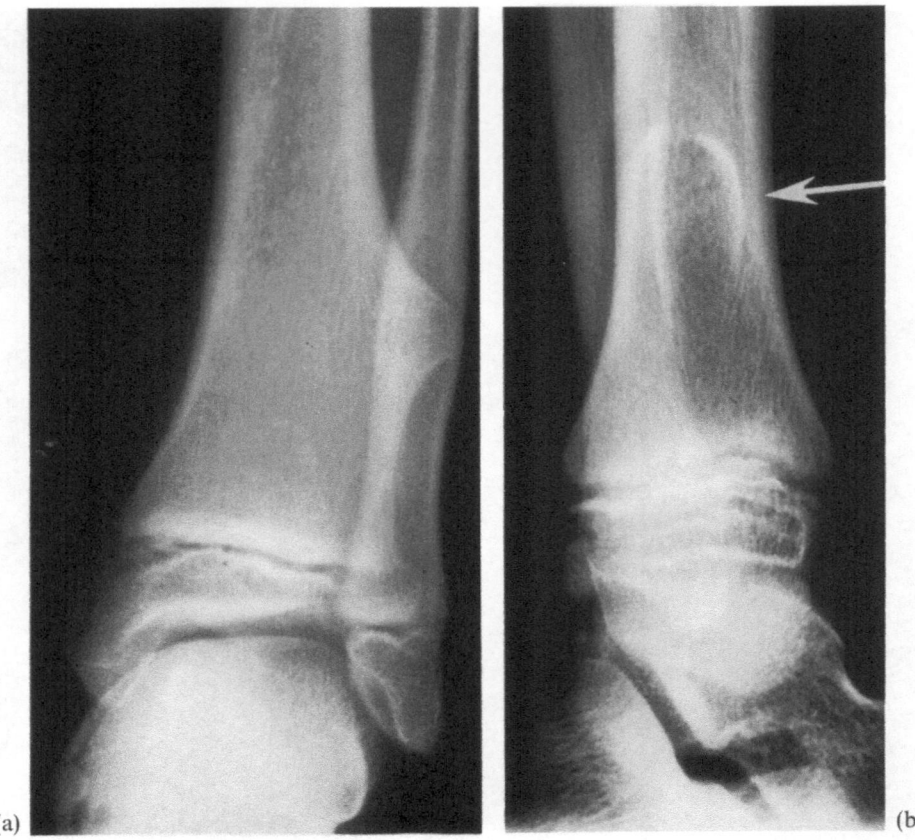

(a)   (b)

Fig. 15a and b. Solitary osteochondroma, tibia: (a) AP view. Smooth lateral projection is partially obscured by fibula. (b) Lateral view. Exostosis superimposed on tibial shaft simulates intramedullary lesion. Note ring-like density cast by cortex of exostosis seen on end (arrow)

an intrapulmonary or intrathoracic lesion (Figs. 15a, b, 24c). An exostosis associated with the vertebral column, particularly when accompanied by neurologic symptoms, should be evaluated by a combination of plain films and myelography. On the latter study, the osteochondroma may appear as a circumscribed extradural mass indenting the pantopaque column with occasional compression and/or displacement of the spinal cord or cauda equina (CHIURCO, 1970; ROSE and FEKETA, 1964; THOMAS and ANDRESS, 1971). The size and location of the tumor can best be determined by tangential views which also best serve to define the base of the lesion.

V. Histology

1. Gross

Whatever its size and shape, the exostosis is encased by a periosteum that covers and adheres closely to the irregular surface of the hyaline cartilage cap and is continuous with the periosteum of the adjacent cortical bone. It is usually thick but may be delicate. If enchondral ossification is still in progress, a thin yellowish growth zone or plate can be identified on the undersurface of the cartilage cap (Fig. 2). The spongy bone which blends with that of the shaft is seen immediately beneath the growth plate (Figs. 16, 17).

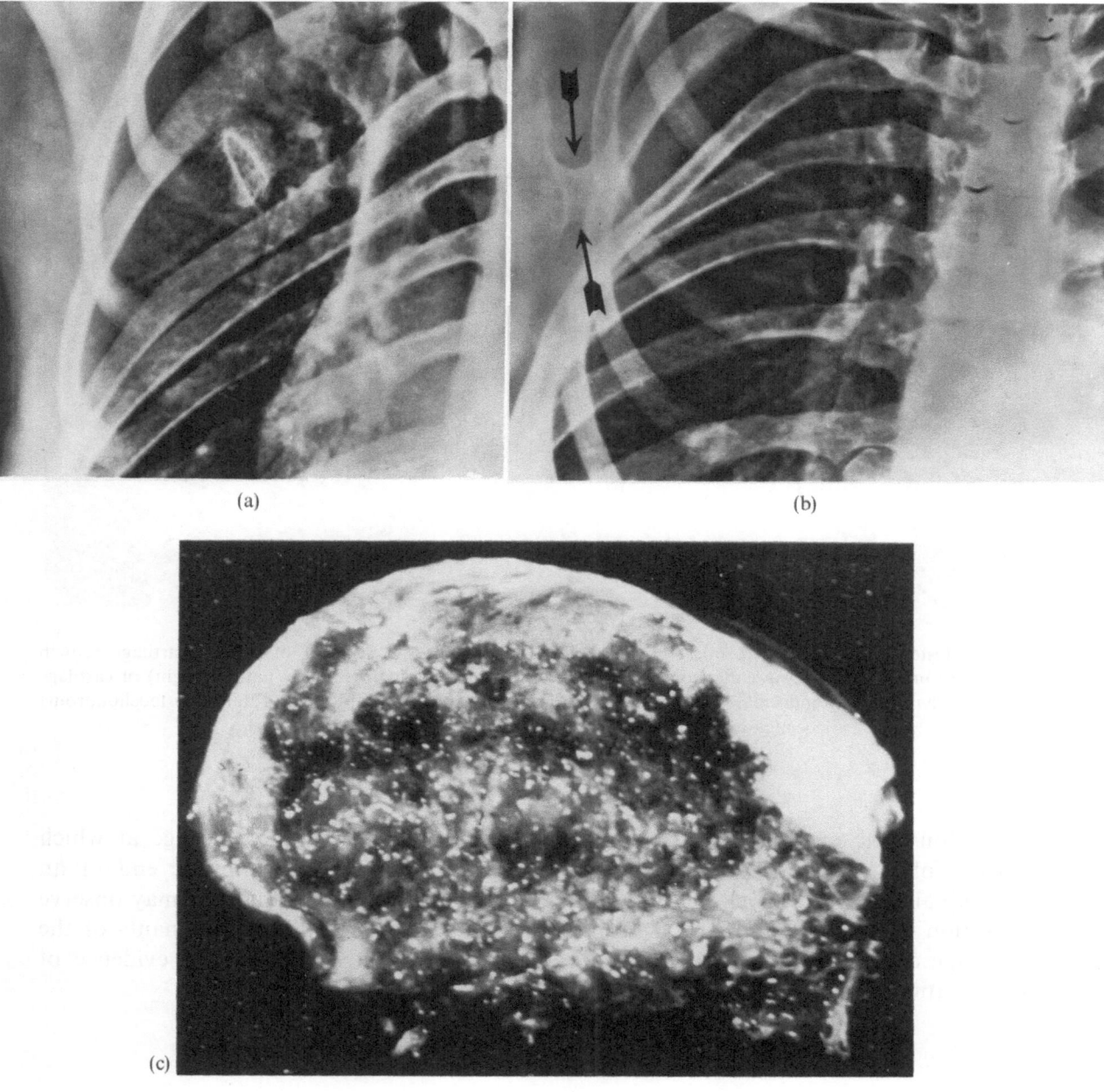

(a)

(b)

(c)

Fig. 16a–c. Solitary osteochondroma, scapula: (a) Chest—oblique view. Scapular exostosis seen on end simulates intrapulmonary lesion on oblique view. Separation of ribs suggests diagnosis. (b) Chest—PA view silhouettes scapula. Exostosis is now visualized in profile and its relationship to right hemithorax is clarified. (c) Osteochondroma, gross specimen, cut surface. Note cancellous bone covered by partly calcified hyaline cartilage cap superiorly

The younger the patient, the more prominent will be the cartilage cap, which varies from 1–3 mm and may be as large as 6 mm. LICHTENSTEIN (1965) has noted that if the cartilage cap measures 1 cm or more in thickness the possibility of chondrosarcoma should be seriously considered.

Since an exostosis grows by enchondral ossification of its proliferating cartilage, its enlargement should cease at puberty when this growth zone becomes closed off

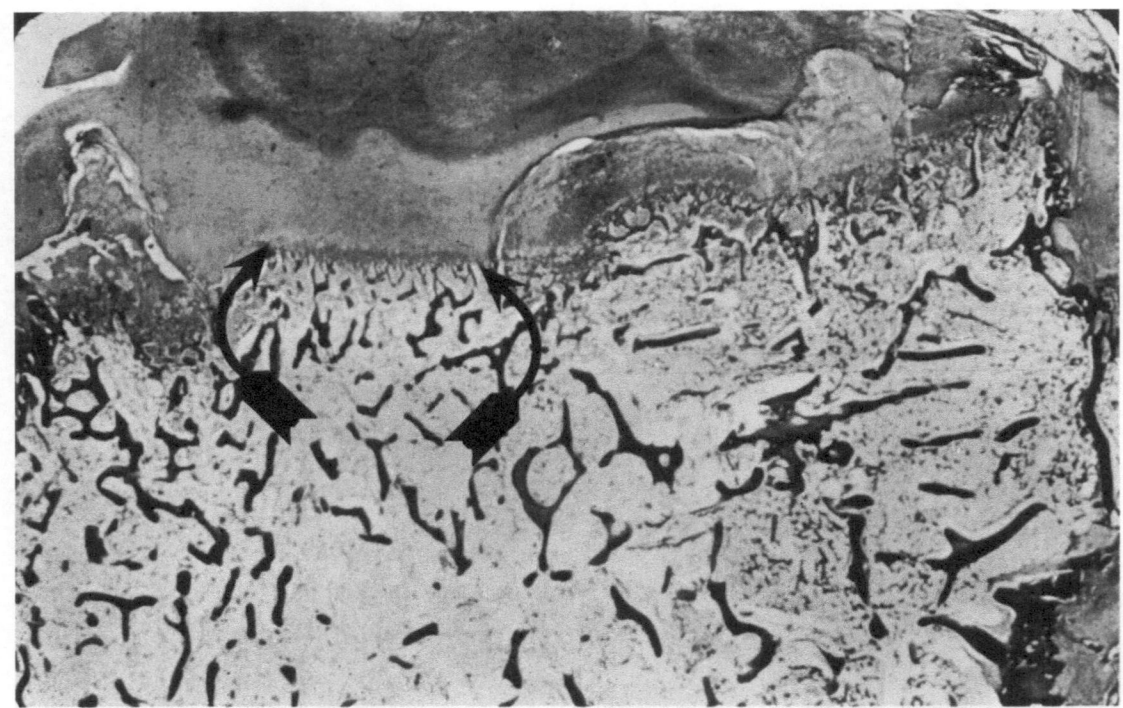

Fig. 17. Osteochondroma, tibia, microscopic section: Arrows bracket segment of normal cartilage growth plate with orderly growth via endochondral ossification. Note adjoining disorderly pattern (right) of cartilage cap of evolving osteochondroma. Cancellous bone and fatty marrow of metaphysis and stalk of osteochondroma occupy lower part of field. (Courtesy Dr. AUSTIN D. JOHNSTON)

by a thin plate of bone. The cartilage cap then tends to involute. The age at which growth of an exostosis ceases is variable but roughly coincides with the end of an individual's growth period, and often precedes it by several years. Thus, one may observe cessation of growth in specimens from adolescents or even children. Remnants of the cartilage cap, however, may persist into the fourth or fifth decades with evidence of calcification and other regressive changes.

2. Microscopic

The cartilage cells of the cap are arranged in a manner similar to that seen in a normal growth plate with the underlying trabeculae usually exhibiting foci of cartilage derived from enchondral ossification (Fig. 18). These foci may occasionally be seen in adults even though the cap is atrophied or absent. They may retain a latent capacity for growth and some have postulated that such reactivation affords an explanation for the occasional chondrosarcomatous degeneration of a solitary exostosis in later life.

It has been estimated that less than 1% of solitary osteochondromas undergo malignant transformation, but this figure is difficult to document (DAHLIN, 1967; DORFMAN, 1973; SPJUT, 1973; SPJUT et al., 1971). Of the malignant lesions considered to have arisen from solitary osteochondromas, the majority are chondrosarcomas. Two osteogenic sarcomas (DAHLIN, 1967; DAHLIN and COVENTRY, 1967) and one sarcoma which was variously classified as an osteogenic sarcoma and/or a fibrosarcoma by several consultants, have also been reported (ANDERSON et al., 1969).

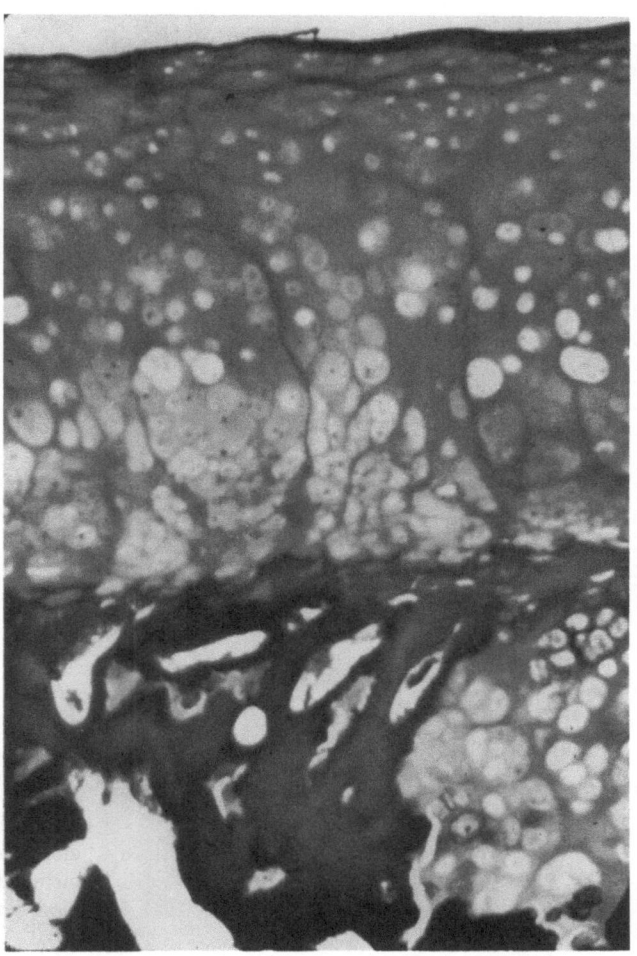

Fig. 18. Cartilaginous cap of osteochondroma, selected microscopic field shows cartilaginous cells superiorly. Note bony end plate and ossification inferiorly. Strip of periosteum may overly cartilage cap

No factor such as bone formation, calcification, long duration, or slow growth with increasing rate of growth, has proved to be absolutely reliable in determining malignant evolution from benign tumors. The evidence is always presumptive that the tumor was originally benign (O'NEAL and ACKERMAN, 1952).

C. Radiation-Induced Osteochondromas

Benign exostoses may form following radiation therapy for a variety of pre-existing lesions, utilizing a variety of media, including external radiation with orthovoltage and 22 MeV supervoltage roentgen rays, radon seed implantations, and systemically administered radioactive substances (Thorium X) (SPIESS, 1957). Doses have ranged from less than 1000 R to over 6000 R (ARKIN and SIMON, 1950; BERDON et al., 1965; COLE and DARTE, 1963; KATZMAN et al., 1969; MURPHY and BLOUNT, 1962; PEREZ et al., 1967; RUBIN et al., 1959). Patients were usually children less than 3 years of age when the radiotherapy was administered.

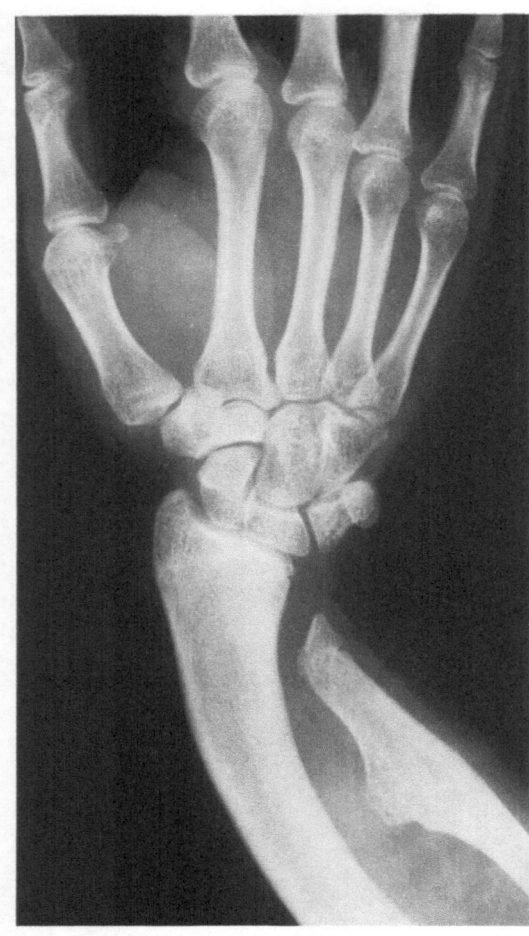

Fig. 19. Radiation-induced osteochondroma: 16-year-old male treated with radium implants for soft tissue hemangioma at 1 year of age. Subsequent growth deformities included bowing and early asymmetric epiphyseal closure. Note similarity to diaphyseal aclasis (Fig. 21 d and e, 22 e)

Radiation-induced exostoses have most commonly been described in patients who were treated for malignant childhood tumors and in patients who have received radiotherapy for hemangiomas (Fig. 19) and/or lymphangiomas (Fig. 20 a, b, c, d) (FANCONI and ILLIG, 1959; MURPHY and BLOUNT, 1962).

In a review of 31 children who had received radiation therapy for malignant (Wilms' tumor, neuroblastoma, and retinoblastoma) as well as for benign disease (hemangiolymphangioma, hemangioma), 5 patients developed exostoses within the field of treatment. Two exostoses were located in the scapula, one each in the clavicle, the humerus, the 12th rib, the distal femur, and the proximal tibia. Multiple sites were noted in 2 patients. Radiotherapy was given with orthovoltage, i.e. 200 kV and 250 kV with a half-value layer of between 0.9–1 mm copper. The average tumor dose was 2850 R and the range was from 1400–4284 R. Treatment periods ranged from 15–180 days, with an average of 28 days. The pathologic diagnosis in two osteochondromas which were excised was that of benign osteochondroma. Radiologically and histologically the exostoses had the appearance of lesions arising de novo.

Other recorded radiation doses have ranged from less than 1000 R to over 6000 R with the interval between radiation and diagnosis of exostoses ranging from 17 months to more than 15 years. Radiation-induced sarcomas of bone, in general, are most commonly osteosarcomas (CAHAN et al., 1948). A rare combination of chondrosarcoma in a radiation-induced exostosis has been reported in one case (PEREZ et al., 1967).

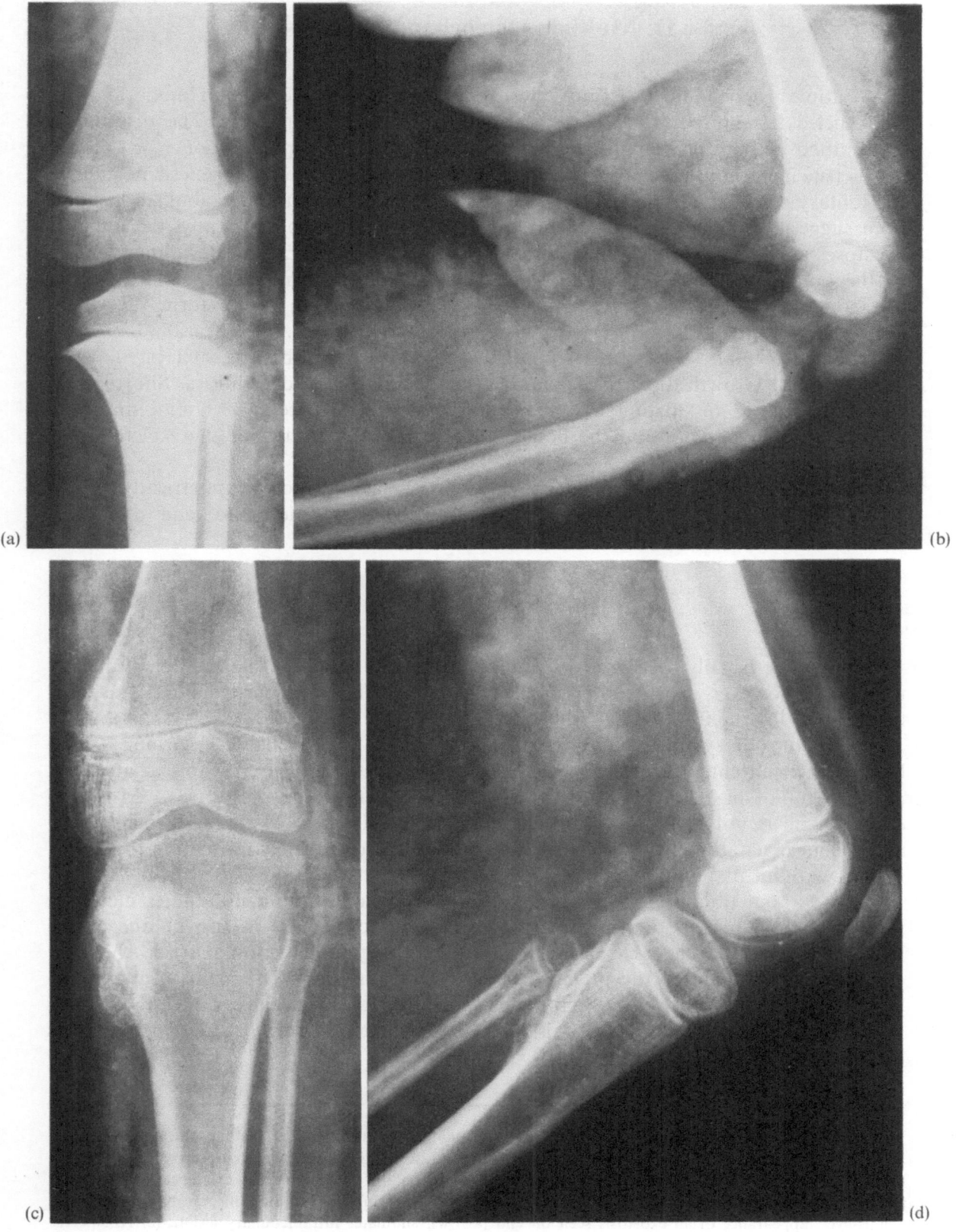

Fig. 20a–d. Radiation-induced osteochondromas. (a) and (b) AP and lateral left leg 1954. This infant received external radiation therapy for congenital hemangiolymphangioma October, 1954. (c) and (d) AP and lateral left leg approximately 5 years later. Multiple exostoses now project from distal femur and proximal tibia. Latter exostosis appears to be ridging adjacent fibula

D. Multiple Osteochondromatosis

Multiple osteochondromas are inherited as an autosomal dominant mode and are transmitted to approximately half the offspring of affected parents. The disorder is transmitted by both parents. In some series it has a 2:1, M:F predilection.

Its true incidence and cause are unknown. In addition to the pathogenesis postulated for solitary osteochondromas, disordered acid mucopolysaccharide metabolism has also been suggested (SOLOMON, 1964). Pathologically and roentgenographically, the multiple exostoses are similar to the solitary osteochondromas; however, a greater circumference of the bone is usually involved and less common sites are more apt to be involved (LARSON et al., 1957; WRONSKI et al., 1964) (Figs. 21 a, b). In severe forms all bones preformed in cartilage are affected to some degree (Fig. 21 c). Diaphyseal (diaphyseal aclasis) and metaphyseal exostoses (metaphyseal aclasis) may be present (KEITH, 1920) (Figs. 21 d, e). Growth disturbances are reflected in dramatic deformities. Shortness of the bones due to dissipation of the longitudinal growth force in a lateral direction, accompanied by curvature of the bones, adds to the "dwarfing" of the skeleton. The skull is rarely involved.

The lesions of multiple osteochondromatosis are generally more symmetrically distributed than those of multiple enchondromatosis which, though widespread, tend to predominate unilaterally, particularly in the extremities.

I. Clinical

Lesions are usually first discovered at about 2 years of age. Most are detected prior to puberty, however, exostoses, particularly in cases with multiple osteochondromatosis, may appear for the first time in adult life.

The dating of symptoms is often inexact. Pain is not a reliable criterion. It may be mild, intermittent, and insidious, not disturbing the patient sufficiently to seek attention until the tumor has reached considerable and often inoperable proportions. Most frequently pain is not severe or persistent but occasionally it may gradually increase so as to be incapacitating. On the other hand, pain may occur acutely in relation to trauma with or without pathologic fracture.

Pain without fracture should arouse suspicion. Periodic follow-up studies including roentgenograms may be indicated. A slow but definite increase in size of one of the bony swellings after the end of the normal skeletal growth period may be the only clinical feature heralding the presence of an osteochondroma. Often this growth is so gradual that it may take years before the patient seeks advice unless pressure and/or impingement on neighboring soft tissue structures such as vessels and nerves causes discomfort.

Fig. 21 a–c. Multiple osteochondromatosis: A 50-year-old male with a 9 year history of multiple masses about right knee and wrist, and 3 year history of pain and swelling. (a) AP view knees. Exostoses project from practically entire girth of bone with marked loss of modeling. Most exostoses are directed away from joints. (b) Lateral view, right knee. Bone ends are bulbous and club-shaped. Lucent sharply circumscribed "bulls-eye" appearance of an exostosis seen on end (arrow), simulates intramedullary lesion. (c) AP, pelvis. Deformed pelvis is studded with numerous small osteochondromas particularly about pubic rami (arrow). Typically widened, foreshortened femoral necks result from failure of normal tubulation. Discrepancy in leg length is due to pelvic abnormality as well as coexisting growth discrepancy between two femora. Note bilateral varus deformities

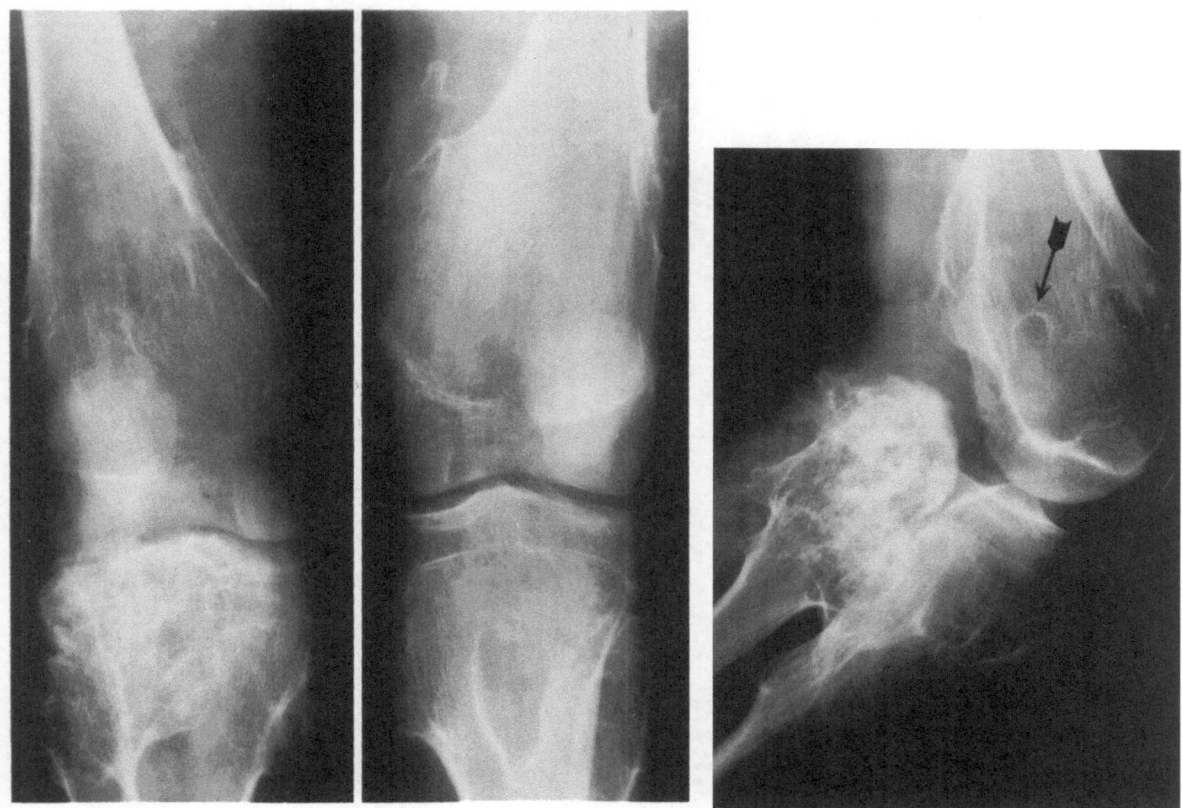

Fig. 21a   Fig. 21b

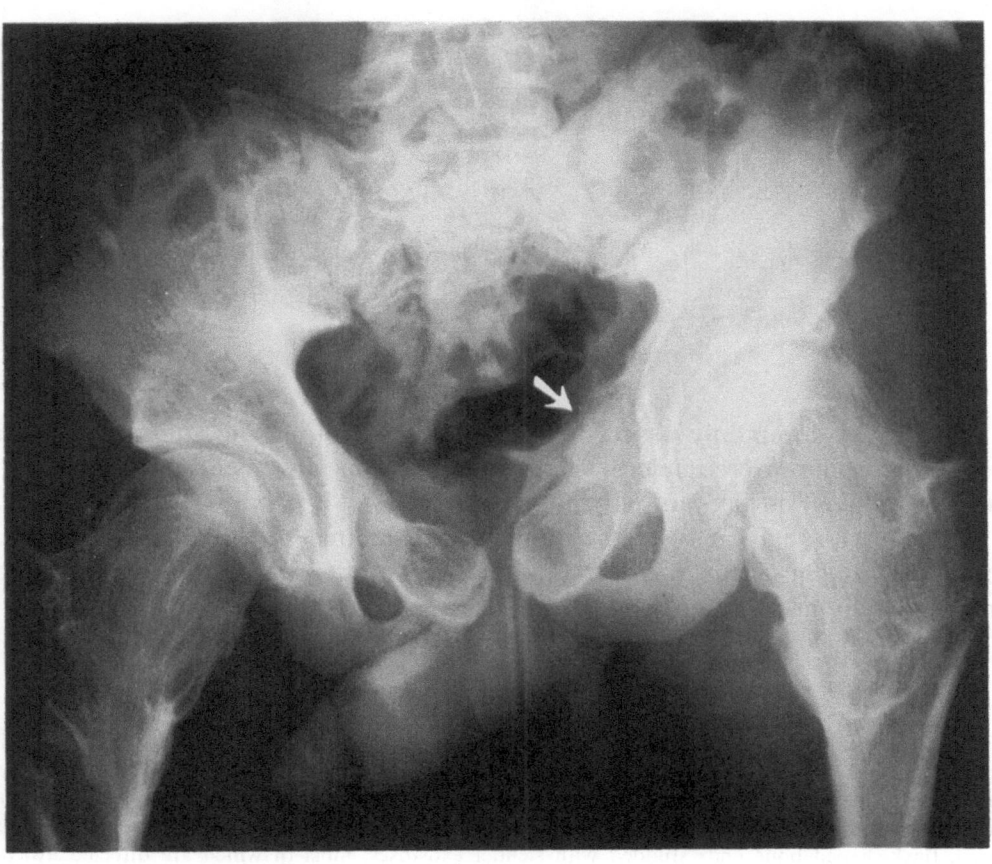

Fig. 21c

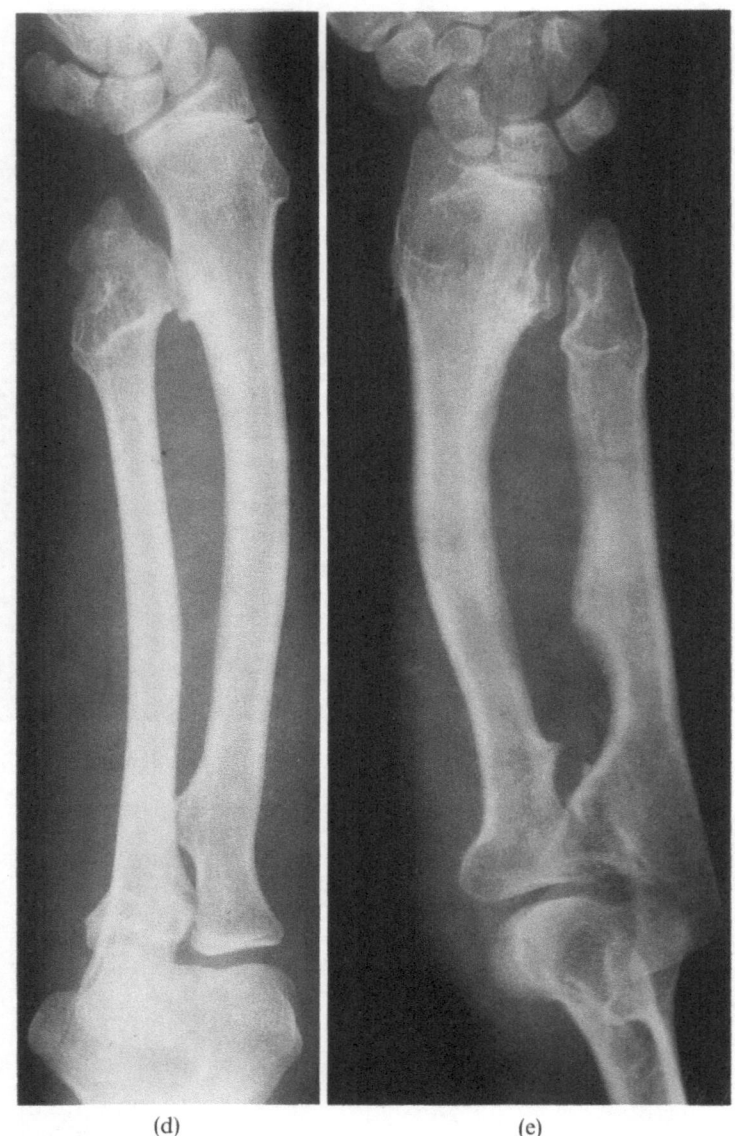

(d)   (e)

Fig. 21d and e. Diaphyseal aclasis. Both forearms are affected. Note shortened ulnae with bowing and early growth plate closure of right radius. Diaphyseal as well as metaphyseal exostoses are present

Other less commonly associated signs and symptoms in addition to pain and/or a mass or swelling were tenderness, stiffness, pain on movement, elevated local temperature, and a neighboring joint effusion.

In general, a mass may be the only clinical finding. Asymptomatic tumors are most commonly diagnosed on physical examination, or they may be discovered incidentally on a roentgenogram taken for an unrelated reason.

Fig. 22a–c. Multiple osteochondromatosis: (a) Right thoracic rib cage detail from PA chest film. Note sharply defined tent-like appearance of osteochondroma partially hidden by rib cage. (b) Tangential view scapula. Exostosis is larger than anticipated on basis of PA chest film. Second lesion is also demonstrated (arrow). (c) AP view knees. Confirm widespread involvement and presence of multiple osteochondromatosis. Note flared, flask-shaped bone ends studded with slender exostoses, most of which are directed away from joint space. Cartilaginous caps are not mineralized and therefore not visualized

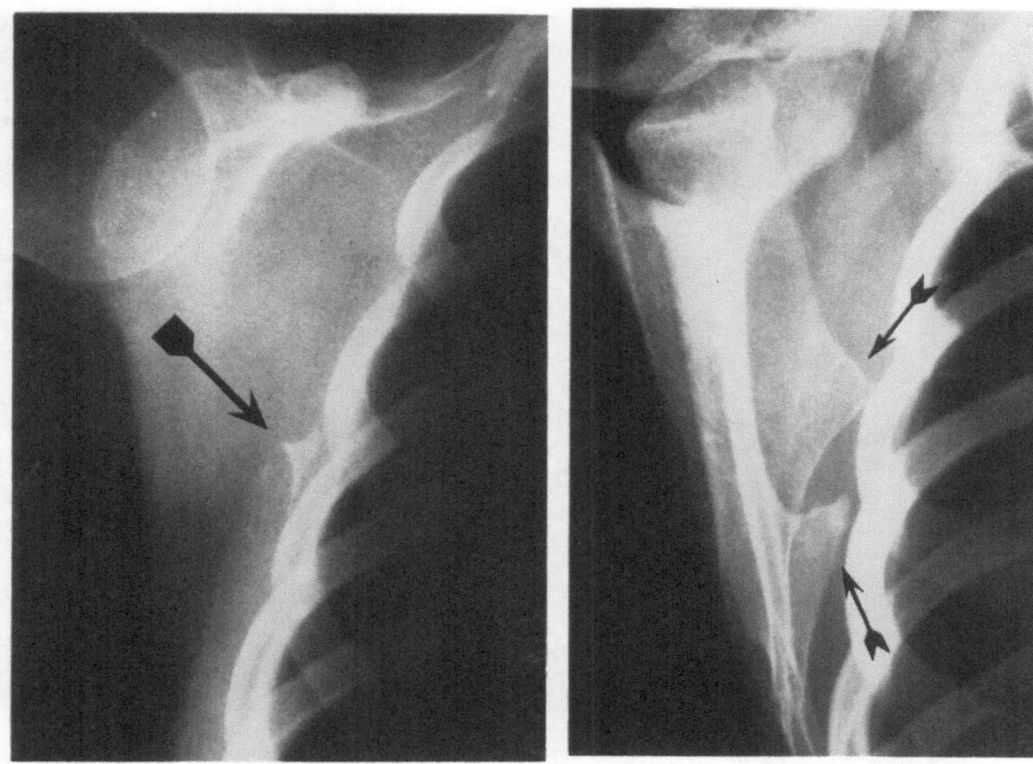

Fig. 22a   Fig. 22b

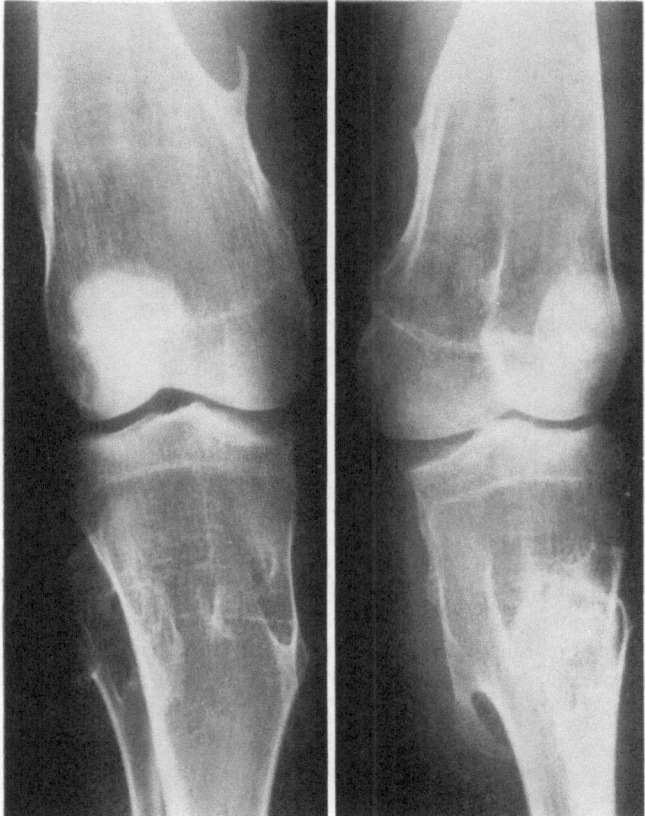

Fig. 22c

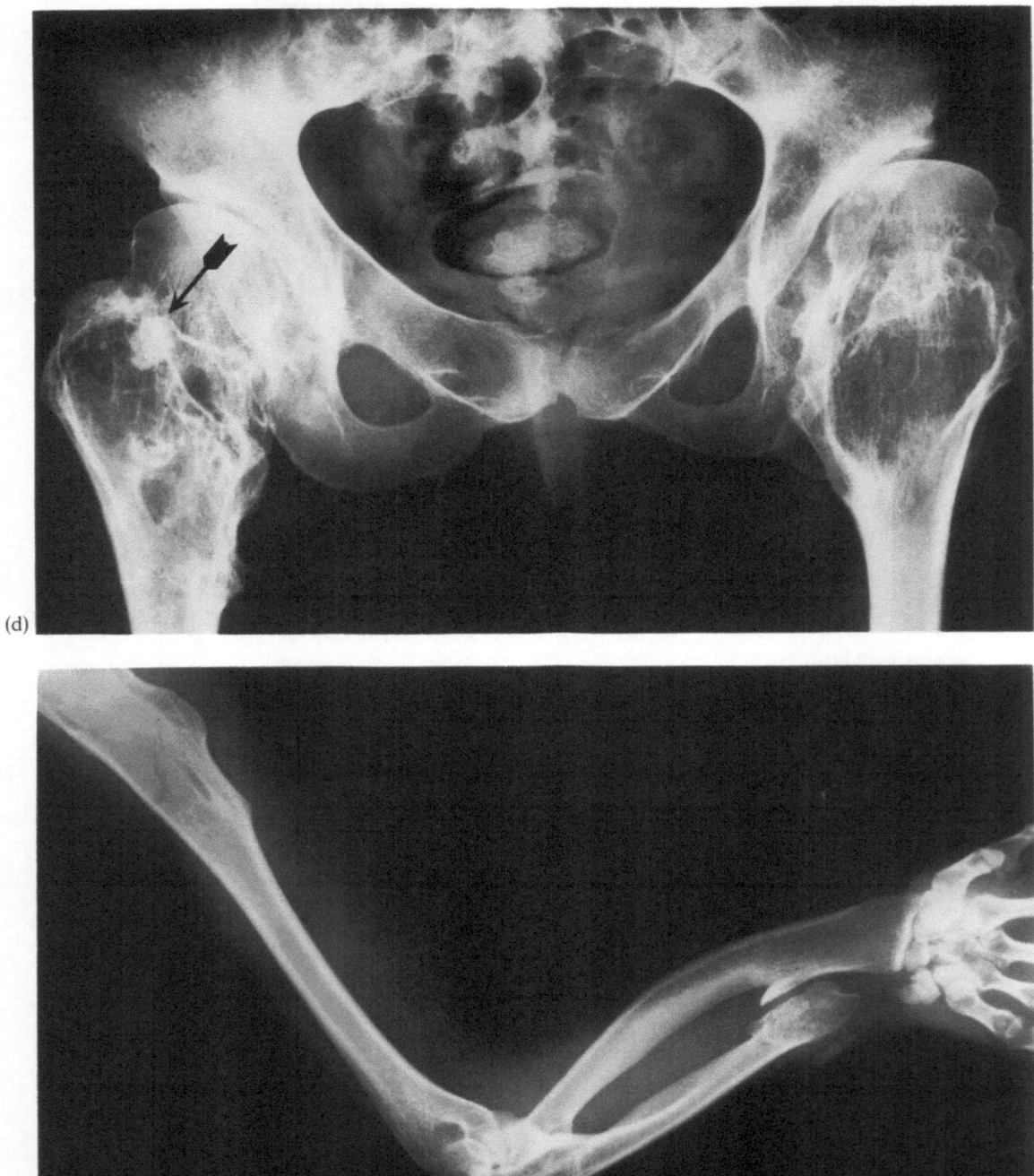

Fig. 22d and e. AP view pelvis. Note abnormally and asymmetrically modeled pubic bone with shallow acetabulae, flattened femoral heads, short, squat femoral necks partially obscured by bulbous greater trochanters, and bilateral valgus deformities. Right-sided calcified exostosis seen on end simulates intramedullary enchondroma (arrow). (e) Right forearm. Bowed radius, foreshortened ulna, and multiple exostoses are typical of diaphyseal aclasis. Note associated deformity of proximal humeral shaft. Other arm was similarly affected

II. Roentgen Features

Frequently the first site of involvement noted is that of a rib (JOSEPH and FONKALSRUD, 1972) or the vertebral margin of the scapula since both areas are visualized on routine films of the chest (Figs. 22a, b). Occasionally an incidentally included proximal humeral shaft may furnish further corroborative evidence of multiple lesions. Since the bones about the knees are the most frequently involved, they should be examined when a diagnosis of multiple osteochondromatosis is considered on the basis of finding a single lesion elsewhere (Fig. 22c).

Once the diagnosis is made, more proximally located exostoses should be sought in view of their greater predilection for sarcomatous transformation. Pelvic exostoses

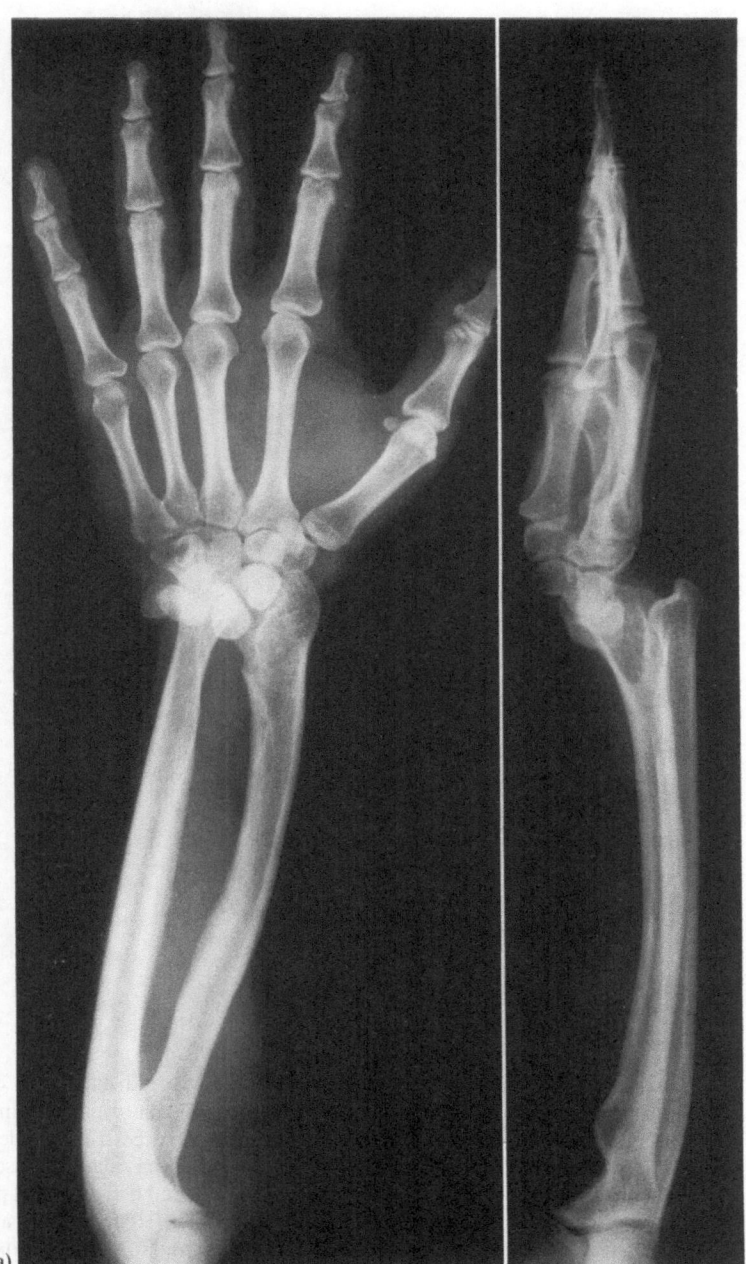

Fig. 23a and b. Madelung's deformity: 48-year-old female with deformed arms since birth with chief complaint of restricted motion of wrist. (a) AP view left forearm. Note V-shaped configuration of carpal bones, sloped radial, and ulnar articular surfaces, dorsal dislocation of distal ulna and slight radial bowing. (b) Lateral view. Dorsal dislocation of distal ulna is present simulating bayonette configuration. Deformities were bilateral. There were no associated endocrine abnormalities or any other abnormal clinical or laboratory findings

(a)   (b)

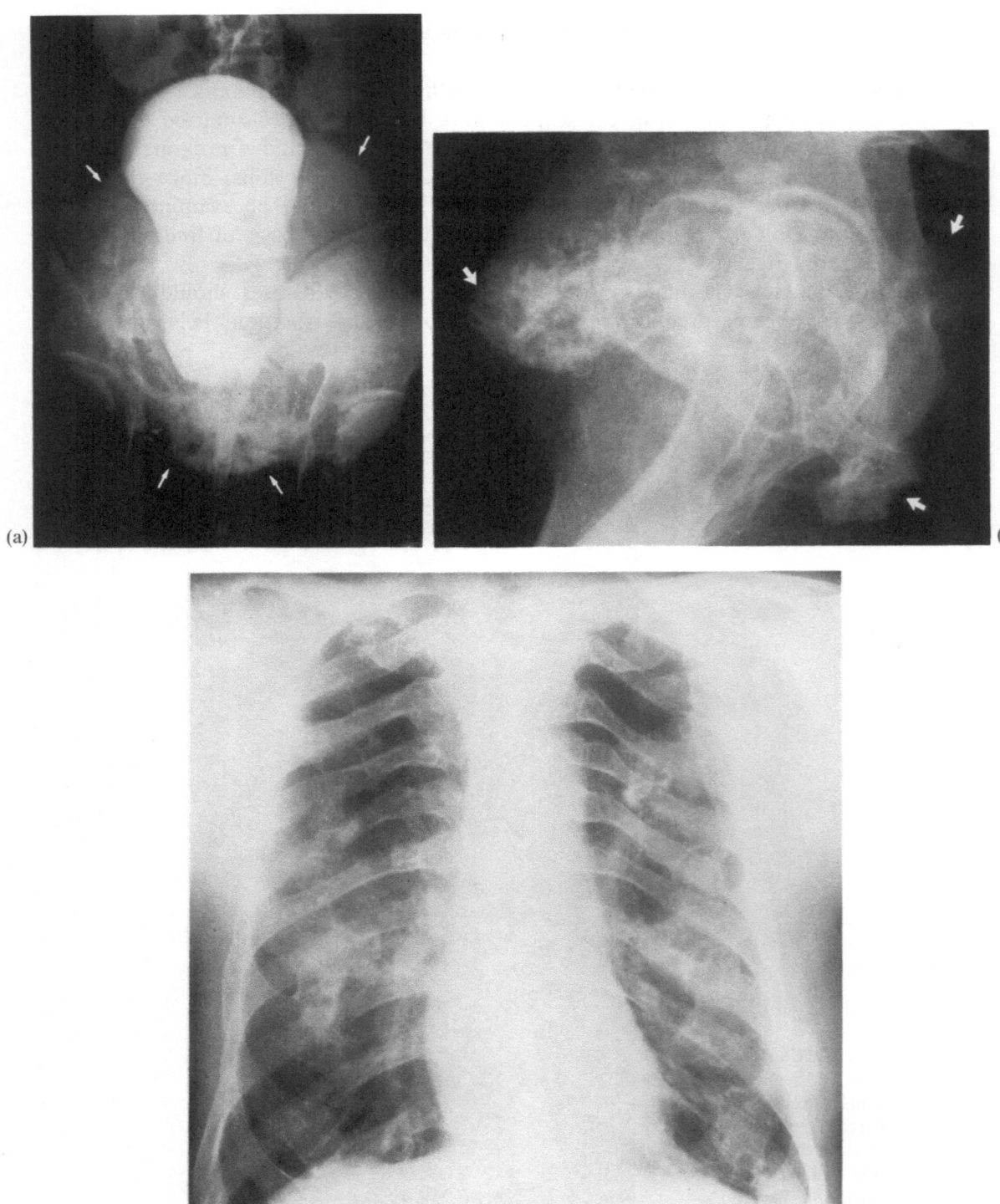

Fig. 24a–c. Multiple osteochondromatosis: 37-year-old male with chief complaint of changing bowel habits. (a) AP abdomen. Huge abdominal mass (arrow) is seen originating in pelvis compressing and elevating opacified urinary bladder. Subsequent barium enema was successful in solely filling rectum. (b) Lateral view pelvis. Numerous cauliflower-shaped exostoses arising from iliac and ischial bones (arrows). Anterior pubic rim lesion had undergone sarcomatous transformation and had extended posteriorly, displacing pelvic and abdominal contents. Partial pelvectomy afforded marked relief. Patient was alive and well 8 years later. (c) PA chest. Thorax is deformed by multiple exostoses arising from both proximal humeri and multiple ribs. Some of osteochondromas simulate pulmonary parenchymal lesions as well as enchondromas

are frequently prominent about the iliac surfaces in the region of the superior apophyseal attachments, and along the pubic rami and ischia (Fig. 22d).

Growth disturbances in the form of skeletal shortening and bowing are dramatically reflected about the wrists and forearms (Fig. 22e). When both the radius and the ulna are involved, the latter will grow disproportionately less, accounting for ulnar deviation of the hand in 30% of patients. Posterior dislocation of the radial head may also result from the disproportionate length of the radius. This should not be confused with the classic Madelung deformity (Figs. 23a, b), which has a bayonet-like configuration of the wrist on the lateral roentgenogram, due to the dorsal dislocation of the distal ulna. The latter is apparently increased rather than decreased in length as is common in multiple exostosis.

The lesions are individually similar to solitary osteochondromas. However, several projections often appear in the same bone at approximately the same level. Most of the exostoses are discovered during the first decade of life with their most prominent growth taking place prior to skeletal maturation. The cartilage caps most commonly atrophy by the early 20's and may eventually disappear. Therefore, roentgen documentation of renewed growth of an exostosis suggests malignant transformation, while a new exostosis appearing for the first time after skeletal maturity should also arouse suspicion.

Calcifications within the cartilaginous cap are generally more widespread in malignant lesions, more patchy, streaky, irregular, and of more variable density at the periphery of the tumor. In a benign exostosis, however, the visualized mineral of the cartilage cap is frequently well-defined and it may additionally be peripherally deposited in the form of a calcific or an ossific shell (Fig. 14). Xerography may serve to better define the nonmineralized portions of the lesions. Comparison of successive radiographs may show a gradual, often subtle, increase in the size of the tumor. This, in itself, is highly suspicious of an aggressive lesion, since the cap should grow smaller rather than larger with advancing age. Any change in the cartilage cap in terms of size, irregularity of its contours, or new mineral deposition beyond its previously roentgenographically documented contours, suggests malignant transformation (Figs. 24a, b, c). When accompanied by signs of bone destruction with progressive invasion of the neck or base, the diagnosis of malignancy is certain. This evidence of roentgen change is extremely helpful.

III. Course

The occurrence of malignant degeneration in an exostosis which has previously been asymptomatic or which has been regarded as a benign lesion is a difficult histologic diagnosis to make. The malignant lesion may have obliterated all traces of the benign precursor and serial biopsies are usually not available. Even the latter may be unreliable since they solely reflect small areas of these frequently bulky neoplasms. Comparison of the integrity of the base of the exostosis on serial roentgenograms may serve to demonstrate what may be an exceedingly slow transition and may serve to bolster a "borderline" histologic diagnosis.

Secondary chondrosarcomas have developed over a wider age range than the primary lesions. This is related to the younger population at risk which includes cases with multiple enchondromatosis as well as those with multiple osteochondromatosis.

The incidence of chondrosarcomatous transformation in multiple osteochondromatosis which earlier had been estimated at 5% (EHRENFRIED, 1915) and then at 11% (JAFFE, 1943, 1968) is now considered to be closer to 20% (DAHLIN, 1968; JAFFE, 1943). This is still thought to be low, however, in view of the fact that many patients in various series were children who might subsequently have developed sarcomas. The increased incidence of chondrosarcomatous transformation is not solely attributed to the greater number of exostoses at risk, but rather to the fact that these tumors are intrinsically more liable to the development of a sarcoma.

It is unusual to find this complication in more than one member of an affected family (CROWELL and WEPSIC, 1972; SOLOMON, 1974). Knight (1960) reported three brothers so affected, but in two of them the diagnosis was based entirely on verbal evidence. In three cases the malignant change followed soon after a pregnancy (BOYER, 1814; DREVON et al., 1950; GARDNER, 1937). However, a real causal relationship is extremely doubtful. Another questionable role has been assigned to trauma which antedated a change in the character of several recorded cases.

E. Solitary Enchondromas

These benign cartilaginous neoplasms of bone are most frequently located within the medullary cavity and have no sex predilection. They are less common than exostoses and comprised just over 10% of 1025 benign bone tumors in DAHLIN's (1969) series. This figure includes solitary and multiple enchondromas.

I. Pathogenesis

The lesion, composed of hyaline cartilage, has been thought to be of hamartomatous origin (LEVY et al., 1946) or to originate from cartilage cell rests which were not normally ossified and were subsequently contained within the metaphysis of a normal bone. SCHERER's (1928) findings appear to support this theory, since sectioning of 1125 right femurs revealed 20 cartilaginous rests in the upper femur, 2 in the lower femur, and 1 apparently active enchondroma. All were found in patients more than 25 years old. The rests were small, often calcified or ossified, and none had expanded the cortex. O'NEAL and ACKERMAN (1952) have suggested that perhaps those lesions that do not become quiescent at puberty or at the time of bone maturation may be dangerous in terms of future aggressive behavior.

II. Site

More than 50% of all enchondromas are found in the small bones of the hands and feet (Figs. 25, 26, 27, 28, 29, 30); of these, 90% are in the hands (DAHLIN, 1967; SPJUT et al., 1971). Not infrequently a large limb bone, such as the humerus, femur, and occasionally the tibia is involved (Fig. 31). Central chondromas of the ribs (Fig. 32), sternum, and scapula are less common. The patella and vertebral column are rare sites (HERNDON and COHEN, 1970; LAMMOT, 1968; RAY, 1905; STEPHENSON, 1953) since cartilage tissue from the normal growth centers and intervertebral discs of the spine, as well as from the notochord may be found throughout the developing vertebral column (BICK and COPEL, 1950; COHEN et al., 1956, 1964; COHEN and D'ANGIO, 1961; REICHMAN and THORD, 1969). Therefore, theoretically, a tumor from a cartilage rest could develop anywhere in the spine, as it may in the long bones. NAG and FALCONER (1966) reviewed

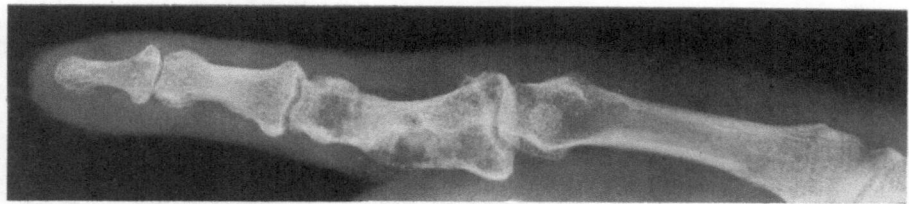

Fig. 25. Solitary enchondroma, phalanx: Lucent highlights represent multiple intramedullary foci of cartilage resulting in marked modeling deformity. Endosteal thinning and medullary expansion distinguish this enchondroma from peripherally situated osteochondroma

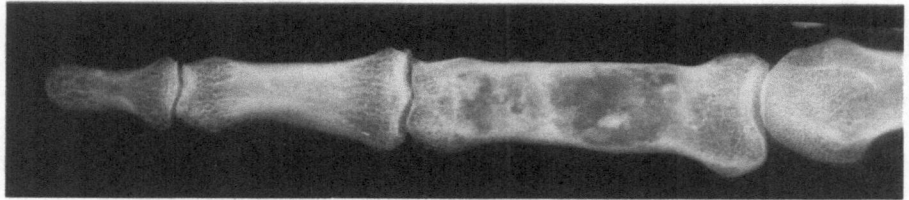

Fig. 26. Enchondroma, phalanx — hand: Sole site. Metaphyseal and diaphyseal lucent lesions represent cartilaginous foci, associated with coarsened central calcific deposits and focal endosteal scalloping resulting in hourglass configuration

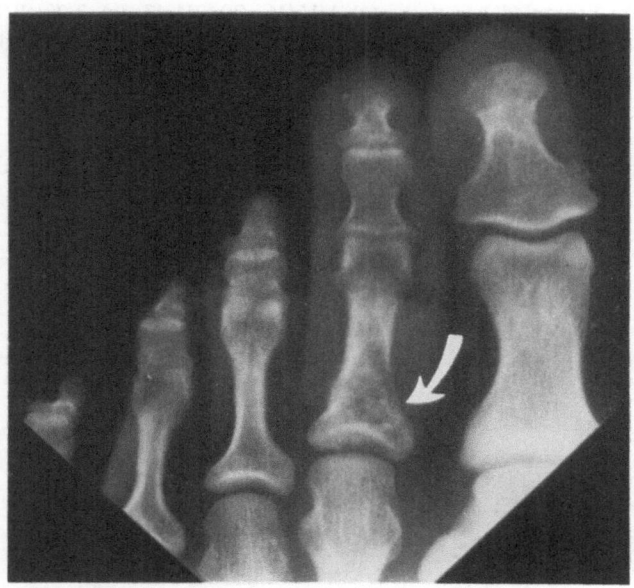

Fig. 27. Enchondroma, phalanx — toe: Solitary lytic lesion in proximal phalanx of second toe contains mineral in form of pinpoint calcific deposits. Latter are indicative of cartilaginous lesion

the world literature and found only 80 reported cases of benign cartilaginous tumors of the spine. Most of these chondromas were of the spinous process, lamina, transverse process, or pedicle (BELL, 1971; NAG and FALCONER, 1966). Only 16 cases of vertebral body chondromas were recorded up to 1966. Since then RAND (1963) has published a case report, bringing the total to 17. LICHTENSTEIN (1965) has stated that many "so-called enchondromas of the vertebral column appear actually to represent instances in which herniated intervertebral disc tissue was mistaken for neoplastic cartilage."

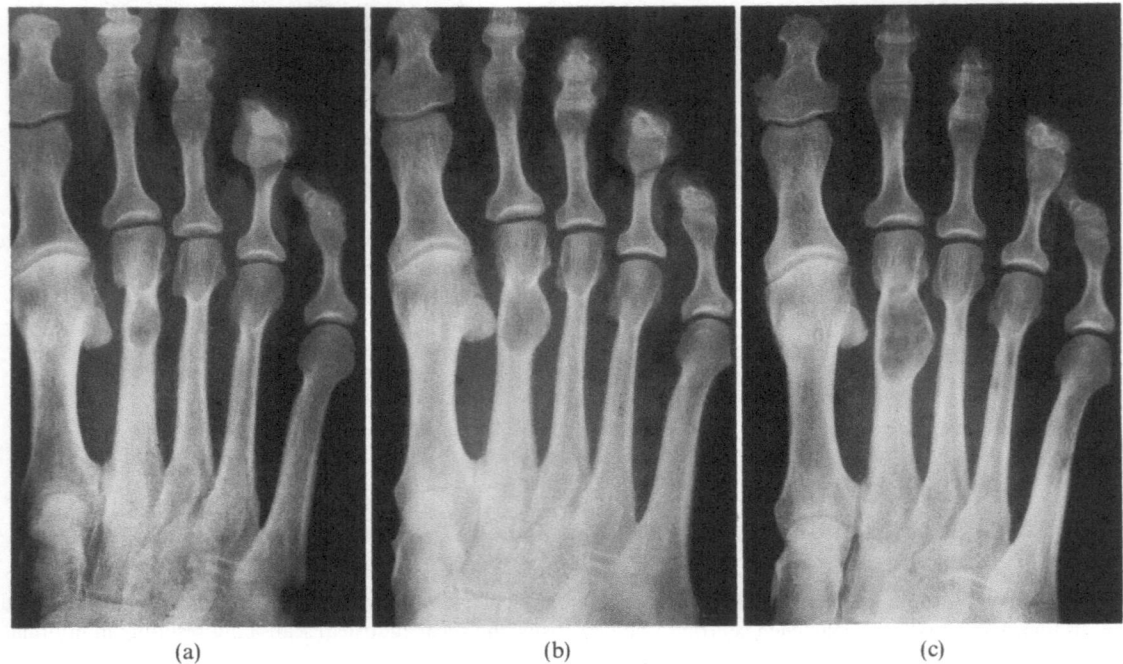

(a)   (b)   (c)

Fig. 28a–c. Growing enchondroma: 62-year-old male with benign enchondroma of second metatarsal. Lesion's gradual increase in size prompted curettage. (a) 1/16/46, (b) 2/4/47, (c) 2/20/48. Note eccentric expansion of persistently well-demarcated lesion. Outer cortex remains well-defined and preserved

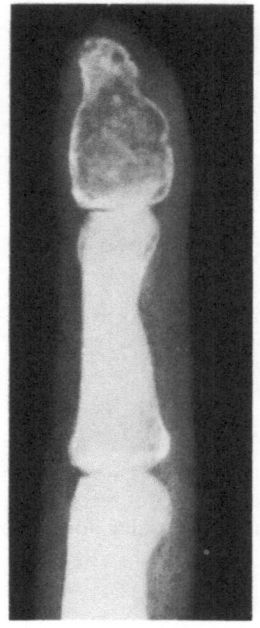

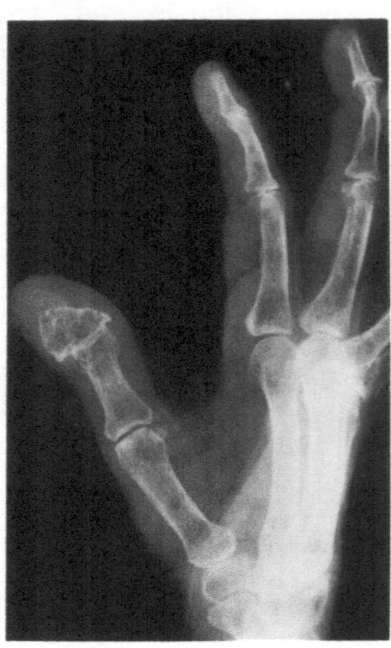

Fig. 29   Fig. 30

Fig. 29. Enchondroma, phalanx—hand: 40-year-old female with chief complaint of painful digit. Distal phalanx is uncommon location for enchondroma. However, stippled calcification with fusiform cortical thinning and expansion aid in its identification. Small volar fracture is evident

Fig. 30. Enchondroma, phalanx—hand: This hazy expansile lucent lesion of distal phalanx had no roentgen evidence of mineral within it. Two fracture lines traverse lesion. Amputation of distal phalanx revealed benign enchondroma. (Courtesy of Dr. HARVEY HECHT)

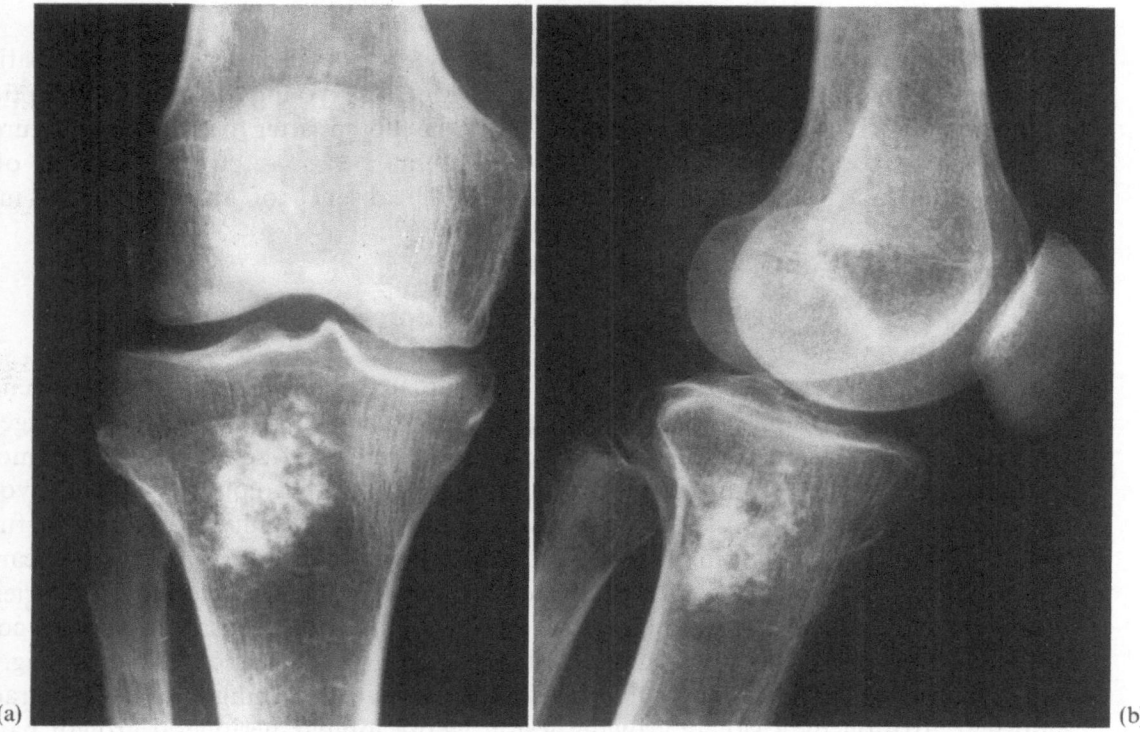

(a)   (b)

Fig. 31a and b. Enchondroma, tibia: (a) AP view. 58-year-old asymptomatic female had this rounded, heavily mineralized, centrally located metaphyseal lesion, (b) lateral view further defines coarse flocculant calcifications scattered uniformly throughout lesion. Normal trabeculae abut its somewhat irregular contours. Curettage yielded normal cartilage tissue

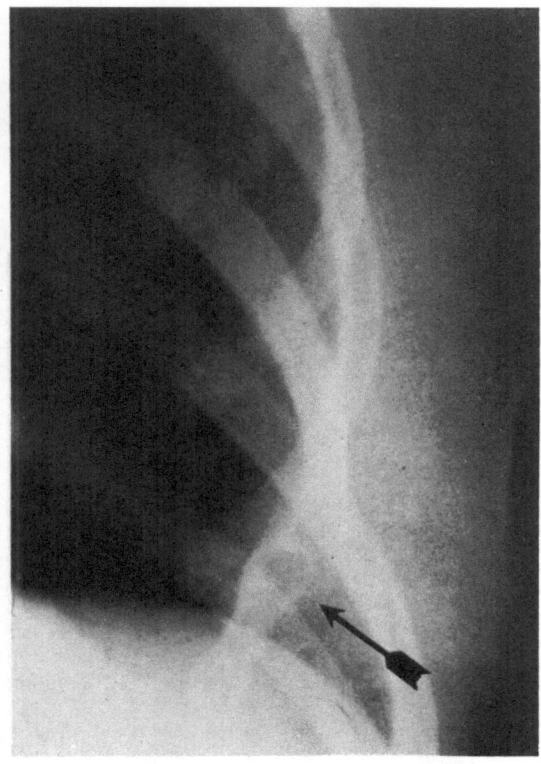

Fig. 32. Enchondroma, rib: This small, solitary, central, well-demarcated, slightly expansile, lytic lesion was discovered as incidental finding on routine chest film

III. Clinical Features

Enchondromas are most frequently incidentally discovered in asymptomatic patients in the second to fifth decades. Their observation in very young children is exceptional (LICHTENSTEIN, 1965). Pain and swelling, may be noted after pathologic fracture of an attenuated cortex, and occasionally after trauma per se. Activated growth of an enchondroma may be responsible for pain in the absence of any antecedent injury (Figs. 28a, b, c).

IV. Roentgen Features

Enchondromas most often appear as well-demarcated, round, or ovoid radiolucencies, centrally situated within the metaphysis of the middle and/or proximal phalanges of the hands or feet (Figs. 25, 26, 27, 28). Diaphyseal lesions may be seen, most commonly, as a result of extension from a metaphyseal locus (Fig. 26). The epiphysis is not involved in the presence of an unfused growth plate and is usually not affected after fusion (JAFFE, 1968). Essentially similar roentgen findings may be noted in the metacarpals and metatarsals where the lesion tends to be more distally located but still oriented to the growth plate. The distal phalanges are rarely affected (Figs. 29, 30). The cortex is usually expanded in a symmetric, fusiform fashion by the enchondroma (Fig. 26), but, eccentric expansion may occur (Figs. 25, 28). Cortical thinning is related to gradual endosteal attrition by a slowly growing lesion whose lobular peripheral growth pattern contributes to an occasional hourglass or multilobulated configuration. The frequently cloudy or hazy appearance of the area of rarefaction serves as a clue to its chondroid composition, as well as to its mineral content. The latter is not always identifiable roentgenographically.

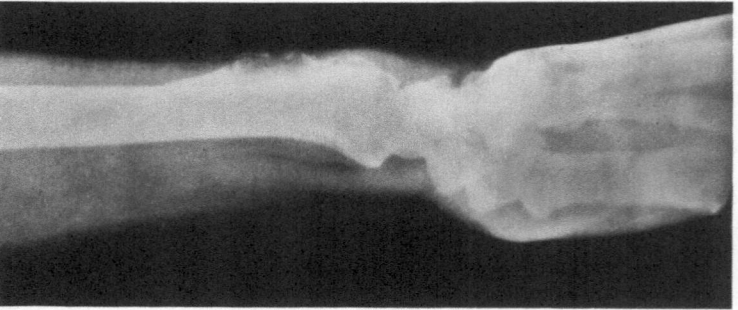

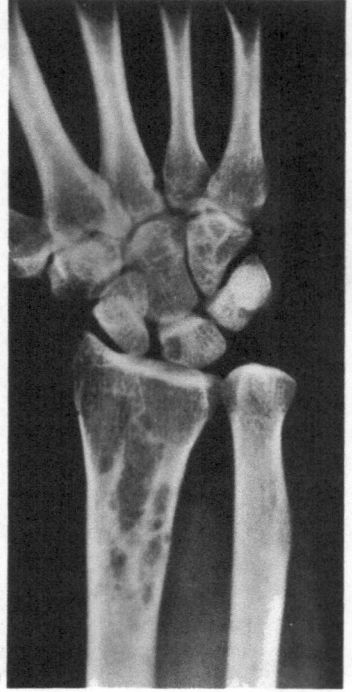

(a)

(b)

Fig. 33a and b. Enchondroma, radius: 29-year-old female nurse noted swelling along dorsum of distal forearm. (a) PA view. Several well-defined columnar-shaped radiolucencies are seen within medullary cavity. Hazy matrix contained no definitely roentgenographically definable mineral. (b) Lateral view. Expanding lesion has thinned overlying radial cortex dorsally

When detectable, mineral deposits may assume various patterns. Small discrete calcific or ossific foci scattered throughout the lesion often create a finely stippled "snowfall" effect (Fig. 29), while larger or coarser conglomerates occasionally described as flocculent or "popcorn ball" in appearance may mask the rarefied portion of the lesion (Fig. 31). The more heavily mineralized lesions are usually seen within the medullary cavities of long limb bones, where they may abut normal appearing cancellous bone or be bordered by a sharply defined dense rim of reactive sclerosis. There is usually no associated periosteal reaction. Similarly, periosteal reactions rarely occur in association with enchondromas of the small bones of the hands or feet in the absence of a fracture.

Enchondromas in the long limb bones may be extensive and, at times, a considerable portion of the shaft (Figs. 33a, b) or even the entire shaft may be involved. The cortex in these long bones is frequently relatively dense and thick and may not appear to be significantly expanded. If the outer cortical contour does bulge or flare slightly, the expansion is likely to be localized (Fig. 33b).

The endosteal surface, too, may be ridged or grooved. Gradual erosion from pressure of the adjacent lobulated periphery of the lesion may result in localized defects having an hourglass configuration. Larger lesions may be identified by longer segments of endosteal ridging with a resultant waffle-iron or washboard appearance. Either one or both endosteal surfaces may appear scalloped.

V. Differential Diagnosis

An enchondroma with conspicuous cortical expansion may be mistaken for an osteochondroma just as an exostosis which is seen on end through the shaft of an affected bone may simulate an enchondroma. Analysis of the bones interior and its external contour by means of multiple views, as well as the distribution of the visualized mineral within the lesion will aid in distinguishing the two entities.

Enchondromas may occasionally bulge or project some distance from the remainder of the shaft contour and resemble osteochondromas, but they have no stalk or neck at the junction of their base with the shaft, may be mineralized throughout their extent rather than in the region of a peripheral cartilaginous cap, as in an exostosis, and they do not usually point away from a joint, as an exostosis frequently does.

Giant cell tumors involve the epiphyses or the ends of bones, contain no calcifications and are infrequent in the phalanges, which are the commonest sites for enchondromas (JAFFE, 1968). Solitary bone cysts are also unusual in the phalanges. They are more radiolucent, contain no mineral, and are usually larger than enchondromas. If fractured, small cortical fragments may be displaced into the cyst and callus formation is often evident. Epidermoid inclusion cysts occur almost exclusively in the distal phalanges, a rare site for enchondromas. They rarely calcify. Fibrous dysplasia is a much less common phalangeal lesion, which, however, may be associated with small areas of calcification as well as modeling deformities. However, typical involvement of other bones, including the skull, and clinical stigmata, such as skin lesions and precocious puberty in females, aid in its distinction. Infarcts, especially in the long bones, may mimic enchondromas. However, infarcts are usually elongated and more heavily calcified at their periphery where healing is initiated (Fig. 34). This peripheral fibro-osseous wall has been identified in approximately 50% of roentgenograms in cases of bone infarction (MURRAY and JACOBSON, 1971). Mineral deposits in enchondromas tend to be more centrally distributed as well as more fluffy, flocculent, or stippled in appearance. The radiopacity in a bone infarct is related to calcium deposition in necrotic marrow and

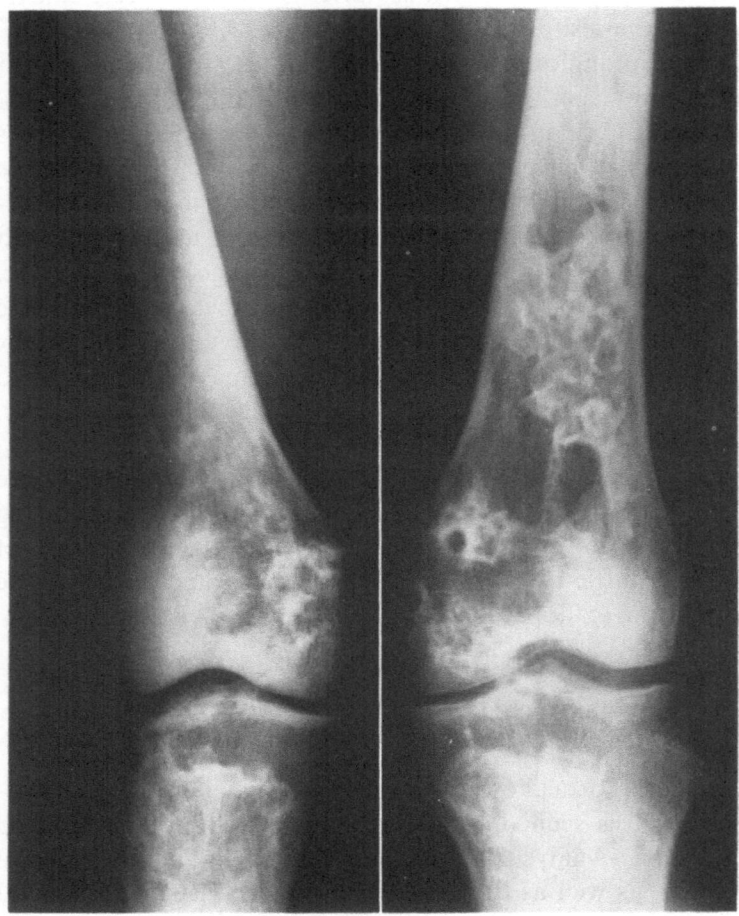

Fig. 34. Bone infarction: Underwater construction worker complained of intermittent pain in both legs. Note multiple mottled lesions diffusely distributed throughout medullary cavities of both femora and tibiae. Epiphyseal, diaphyseal, and metaphyseal areas are all involved. Lesions are long and sharply marginated with relatively radiolucent centers. They are most heavily mineralized at their peripheries, i.e. note sclerotic borders. Only few lesions contain discrete calcific deposits. Note normal bone contours with no associated thickening or thinning of regional cortices or loss of tubulation as in multiple enchondromatosis (see Fig. 40). (Courtesy of Dr. RUBEN POCHACZEVSKY)

disintegrating osseous tissue, while mineral within cartilaginous lesions, in addition to being deposited in poorly nourished or necrotic areas, usually within the deeper regions of the lesion, is commonly associated with enchondral bone formation. Bone infarcts are frequently multiple and are usually not associated with modeling deformity of the involved shaft, unless engrafted on a process such as sickle cell anemia. Modeling deformities and growth disturbances, however, are invariably present in multiple enchondromatosis as in multiple osteochondromatosis.

Although the presence of characteristic calcification establishes the cartilaginous nature of a lesion, a larger enchondroma occurring within a long bone may be difficult, if not impossible, to differentiate from a slowly growing or low grade chondrosarcoma (Figs. 35a, b). Malignant transformation of a benign enchondroma may also be impossible to distinguish on the basis of a single film.

The early chondrosarcoma per se, notwithstanding whether it arose de novo or via the transformation of a benign lesion, may be distinguished from an enchondroma by a generalized or localized lack of marginal definition, cortical disruption with or without pathologic fracture and periosteal reaction. The latter may be localized or involve a long segment of the shaft and can be thick and flared. Prominent fusiform widening or "bulging" of the shaft with or without cortical thickening and sclerosis is an ominous feature (Figs. 35a, b).

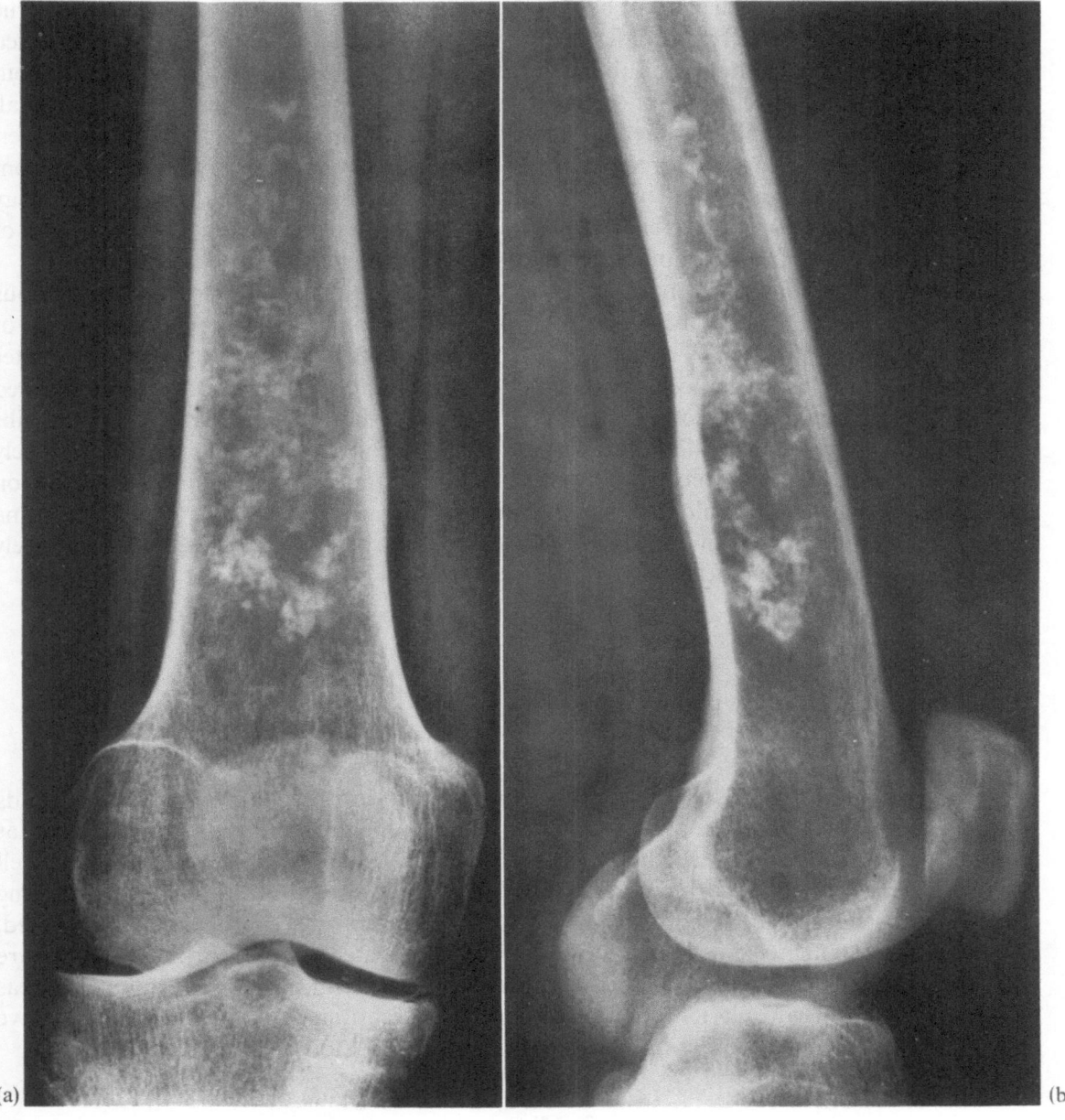

Fig. 35a and b. Enchondroma, femur: Stippled, flocculant "popcorn-ball" arrangement within this long cartilaginous lesion differs from medullary calcification associated with bone infarcts of Figure 34. Central portions of enchondroma are as heavily mineralized as peripheral portions. Endosteal erosion as well as subtle localized bulging of external cortical contour of distal femur create medullary deformity in form of hourglass configuration. (a) AP view, (b) lateral view

Although the evaluation of a primary chondrosarcoma per se and/or the reputed evolution of a chondrosarcoma from a benign enchondroma may be a slow process, serial roentgenograms, when available, may be of inestimable value in confirming a change in the character or aggressive nature of a lesion. Any centrally located cartilaginous lesion, and particularly one situated within a long bone close to the trunk, that exhibits a sudden or gradual change in its size, configuration or margination, perforates the cortex or appears to have its mineral content gradually dissipated or "eaten away," should be suspected of being or having become malignant. This is particularly true if the lesion is harbored by an older individual complaining of pain. It has been stated that enchondromas of the large tubular bones that show flocculent calcification without a lytic component rarely are or rarely become malignant and therefore, in general, lesions which are partially rarefied should be regarded with greater suspicion. However, mineralization per se does not preclude the presence of a chondrosarcoma. JAFFE additionally states that a central chondrosarcoma and/or chondrosarcomatous degeneration may be roentgenographically appreciated on the basis of a reduction or disappearance of the radiopacity within the lesion, particularly around the periphery.

Size has occasionally been used as a criterion for malignancy with cartilaginous lesions larger than 3–4 cm being suspect. This suspicion is enforced as the locus of the tumor approaches the body axis. The closer the lesion is to the trunk, the greater is the degree of inherent biologic malignancy. Therefore, chondromatous lesions situated within the proximal shafts of long bones, the pelvis, thoracic cage (including the ribs and sternum), larger than 3–4 cm should be regarded with particular suspicion. Conversely site, as identified radiographically, may also be of importance in confirming an impression of benignity, since, as a rule, both malignant degeneration of a solitary enchondroma and primary chondrosarcoma in the phalanges, metacarpals, or metatarsals per se rarely occur (SHELLITO and DOCKERTY, 1948).

VI. Histology

1. Gross

Since the majority of solitary enchondromas occur in the small bones of the hands and feet and since most are treated by curettage, enchondromas are rarely seen as intact specimens. Lesions which have been removed intact are most commonly well delimited, with the neighboring cortical bone generally thinned or attenuated. Grooving of the endosteal surface, frequently in a lobular fashion, may be grossly appreciated.

Curetted fragments consist of lobules of bluish-white hyaline cartilage which are usually firm, but may be soft and even somewhat myxoid in places. Intermingled areas of yellowish tissue most often contain areas of calcification or ossification which have been considered as an expression of aging or regression (LICHTENSTEIN, 1965).

2. Microscopic

The tumor tissue is divided into facets or lobules of varying size by interlobular bands of connective tissue in which most of the blood vessels are found. It is in the vicinity of these blood vessels that calcification and/or ossification of cartilage is usually initiated.

Enchondromas exhibit varying degrees of cellularity. Some are rich in cells, while others are sparsely cellular. Therefore, the degree of cellularity, as well as the extent of calcification and ossification, and the character of the matrix are of no practical significance in evaluating the benignity or malignancy of cartilaginous lesions. However, the cell nuclei per se are most important in their appraisal. In benign enchondromas the nuclei are most commonly single, uniform in size, and consistently small, not plump. Occasional binucleate cells may be noted but these, too, are small and not found regularly in all fields (Fig. 36).

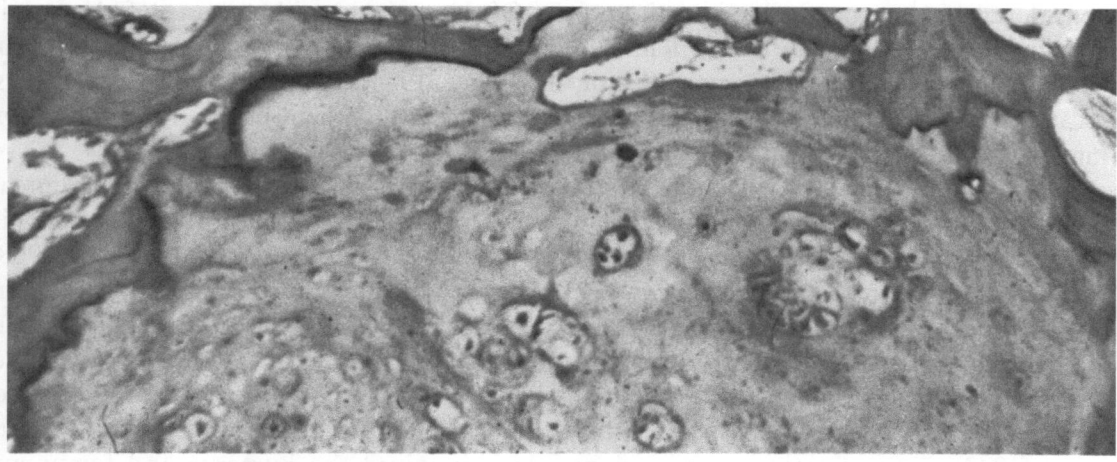

Fig. 36. Benign enchondroma, photomicrograph (× 100): Cells occupy individual lacunae in background of hyaline cartilage matrix. They are mononuclear, though sometimes distributed in clones or clusters. Nuclei are small. Many lacunae are empty, signifying cell death

In general, the lesions of younger patients show a greater degree of cellularity despite their benignity. This is particularly true of biopsies from phalangeal enchondromas and those from cases of multiple enchondromatosis at any age and from any site. Therefore, the age of the patient and the site of the lesion from which the biopsy was obtained are important in the histologic evaluation of cartilage tumors. Generally speaking, primary chondrosarcomas of the skeleton are uncommon in the young, while primary chondrosarcomas of the small bones of the extremities are rare at any age. Secondary chondrosarcomas deriving from solitary enchondromas of the small bones are even rarer, with some authorities claiming never to have seen a case which was not malignant de novo (ACKERMAN and SPJUT, 1962; DAHLIN, 1967). Both malignant degeneration of solitary enchondromas as well as primary chondrosarcomas are more frequent in the long bones, and more frequent in adults.

VII. Treatment and Course

Curettage is the accepted treatment for enchondromas of the small bones of the hands and feet. Surgical therapy is invariably successful for benign lesions with a generally low recurrence rate. Chemical cautery has occasionally been used in conjunction with curettage. Radiation has no place in the treatment of enchondromas.

Block excision, when feasible, is most commonly recommended. This is especially true when dealing with the more proximally situated enchondromas, particularly in view of the ongoing controversy concerning the possibility of malignant degeneration of these lesions.

In general, central cartilaginous lesions in long bones, even though solitary, and particularly when large, are regarded by the pathologist with great suspicion, which, as with an exostosis, is proportionately heightened as the lesion approaches the trunk. Different anatomic sites all have their particular problem. It is felt by some authorities that cartilaginous tumors of the ribs, clavicle, scapula, sternum, and vertebrae are either actually or potentially malignant in such a high percentage of cases that all should be treated by wide excision when first seen. Local excision may fail, too, in tumors considered benign, particularly in the pelvis. Of 40 patients with tumors of the pelvis, considered benign at the Mayo Clinic, 9 (22.5%) were reported as having died and 8 (20%) were living with recurrence (GHORMLEY et al., 1946). Recurrences in most of these locations are often beyond the limit of curability despite their benignity, and tumors may go on to compromise the function of normal neighboring structures.

PLATT (1931), and COLEY and SANTORA (1947) were early exponents of malignant transformation of enchondromas. JAFFE and LICHTENSTEIN also support this view while AEGERTER (1970) refers to chondrosarcoma superimposed on enchondroma. JAFFE (1968), however, has warned of a tendency to exaggerate the malignant potential of solitary enchondromas in long bones, while others (SPJUT et al., 1971) also note that malignant transformation even of solitary enchondromas in long bones is not always well documented and not always able to be documented. The possibility of pathologic error is illustrated by an early paper on solitary benign enchondromas by JAFFE and LICHTEN-STEIN (1943). Two of eight central lesions which involved the humerus and femur and were diagnosed as enchondromas were rediagnosed as chondrosarcomas within a year. In view of the long natural history of chondrosarcoma and the difficulty in evaluating all parts of the lesion on the basis of limited biopsy material, it is tempting to postulate that many of the benign enchondromas that reputedly have undergone malignant transformation were probably chondrosarcoma de novo. In commenting on their series of benign enchondromas of the large bones, O'NEAL and ACKERMAN (1952) noted that all had a slight but definitely higher incidence of abnormal nuclei than did the cartilage of the benign osteochondromas (O'NEAL and ACKERMAN, 1952). Cytologically they assumed a position between the definitely benign tumors and the low grade chondrosarcomas. This frequently "borderline" histologic appearance has resulted in the rendering of conflicting opinions by several pathologists evaluating the same biopsy material or biopsy material taken from a different portion of the lesion at the same time or after a short interval of time.

Although O'NEAL and ACKERMAN (1952), as well as ACKERMAN and SPJUT (1962), regard as suspect any intramedullary cartilaginous tumor of a long bone, "particularly as its site of origin approaches the body axis," where its inherent biologic malignancy is purportedly greater, the latter also state that, "we have seen no example in our material of a chondrosarcoma arising from a pre-existing enchondroma which could be proved pathologically."

HENDERSON and DAHLIN (1963) also emphasize that the number of chondrosarcomas of central origin which began in benign precursors cannot be known with certainty and state that, "Unequivocal histologic evidence of pre-existing enchondroma has been exceedingly rare in our experience." Therefore, the concept of malignant transformation of solitary enchondromas is not universally supported. SPJUT et al. (1971) further graphically illustrate the nature of the problem in noting that, of the 13 cases of malignant degeneration of benign lesions reported by COLEY and HIGGENBOTHAM (1940), 7 were incorrectly diagnosed. Of the remaining 6, 4 had had known lesions for 2 years or less. In only 2 cases, i.e., one 10 years after and one 30 years after the original diagnosis of a benign enchondroma was made, did a reasonable possibility exist that chondrosarcomatous transformation had occurred (SPJUT et al., 1971). This histologic controversy regarding the proper documentation of the malignant potential of solitary enchondromas further emphasizes the importance of roentgenographic evaluation of the lesion, particularly in terms of its temporal development. Serial roentgenograms, when available, may be of inestimable value in confirming the current nature of, or in confirming a progressive change in, a particular lesion. The radiologist must therefore work in close concert with the pathologist as well as the orthopedist for the proper evaluation of these lesions.

F. Multiple Enchondromatosis

Multiple enchondromatosis is a rare abnormality. Unlike multiple osteochondromatosis, no hereditary or familial influence has been demonstrated. In contrast to a solitary enchondroma, it represents a widespread anomaly of skeletal development and was referred to as a dyschondroplasia by OLLIER (1900).

Specifically, it is a cartilage dysplasia of bone, characterized by a failure of normal enchondral ossification with production of tumefactive cartilaginous masses in multiple metaphyses and their adjacent shafts. As the name implies, much of the proliferating cartilage originates within the bone. It may, however, also develop beneath the periosteum and extend into the bone (Fig. 37). As with solitary enchondromas, lesions occur in bones which are preformed in cartilage, but the facial bones, skull, spine, carpal, and tarsal bones are rarely affected.

Widespread involvement with a tendency to unilaterality, most pronounced in the distal extremities, is known as OLLIER's Disease (1900) (Figs. 38, 39a, b).

I. Pathogenesis

The question of the source of the cartilage in the interior of the bones in skeletal enchondromatosis is unsettled. SPEISER (1925) postulated that the periosteum, by means

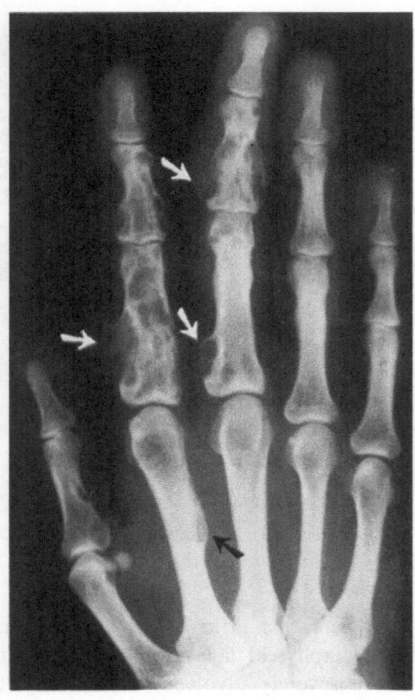

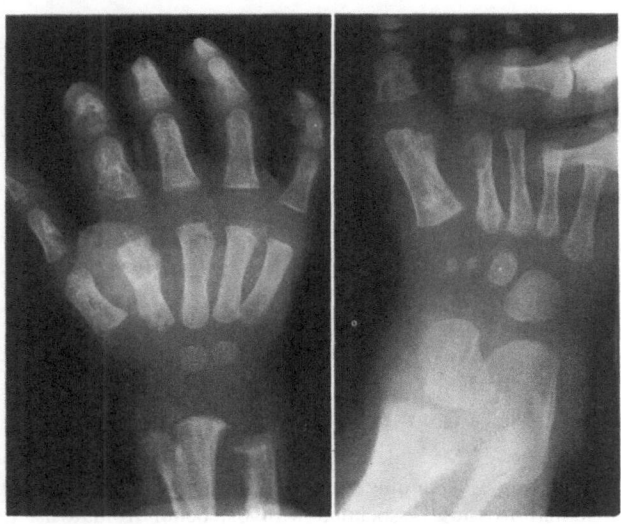

Fig. 37   Fig. 38a   Fig. 38b

Fig. 37. Multiple enchondromatosis—hand: Only three fingers of one hand are affected. Multiple lesions may be confined solely to one area, one extremity, or one bone. Note cortical (arrows) as well as medullary distribution of lesions resulting in modeling deformities of affected phalanges

Fig. 38a and b. Multiple enchondromatosis: Widespread metaphyseal deformities exist as result of numerous expanding lesions at multiple sites including distal radius, ulna, tibia, and fibula of this young child

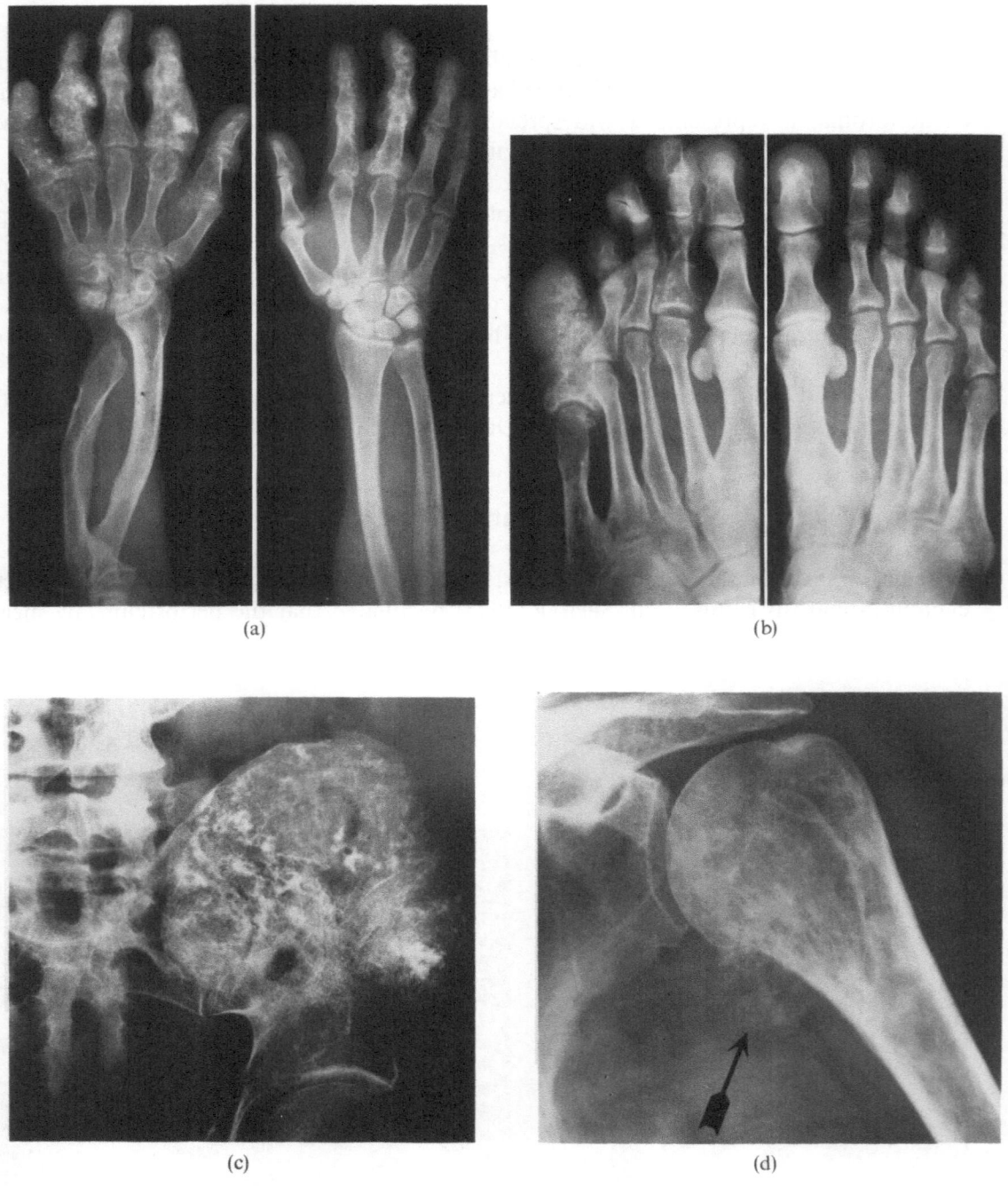

Fig. 39a–d. Multiple enchondromatosis: (a) PA view both hands and forearms. Marked deformities due to multiple expanding heavily mineralized lesions in both hands. Note diaphyseal aclasis. Deformities are similar to those associated with osteochondromatosis. Left side is more severely involved. Note complete disruption of lateral cortical contour of both proximal and mid phalanges of left 5th finger. Cartilaginous mass had proceeded to grow beyond confines of cortex, as noted by new calcific deposits as well as cortical disruption. A chondrosarcoma was resected from left 5th finger. (b) Left foot with multiple site involvement. Chondrosarcomatous transformation in left 5th toe was surgically documented. Right foot was normal. (c) Left hemipelvis. Area was grossly deformed with widespread cartilaginous calcification. Note typical fan-like, columnar arrangement of cartilage in this location. Major portion of ilium was involved. Acetabular region was spared. (d) Left humerus. Chondrosarcomatous transformation occurred in left humerus (arrow). *All chondrosarcomas in this patient developed on left*

of its cambium layer, and the cartilage growth plates give rise to the enchondromas or central cartilage nests. VIRCHOW (1875) maintained that the growth plates are the sole source of the enchondromas.

II. Clinical

The appearance of multiple enchondromata in early childhood is followed by progressive skeletal deformity resulting from the failure of normal enchondral ossification. In some cases skeletal involvement becomes stabilized after puberty. In others it is progressive with the development of monstrous deformities.

Early recognition generally parallels widespread involvement. The condition usually becomes evident at about 2 years of age (Fig. 38). Phalangeal swelling, bowing of the long bones, growth discrepancies between the radius, and ulna associated with restricted

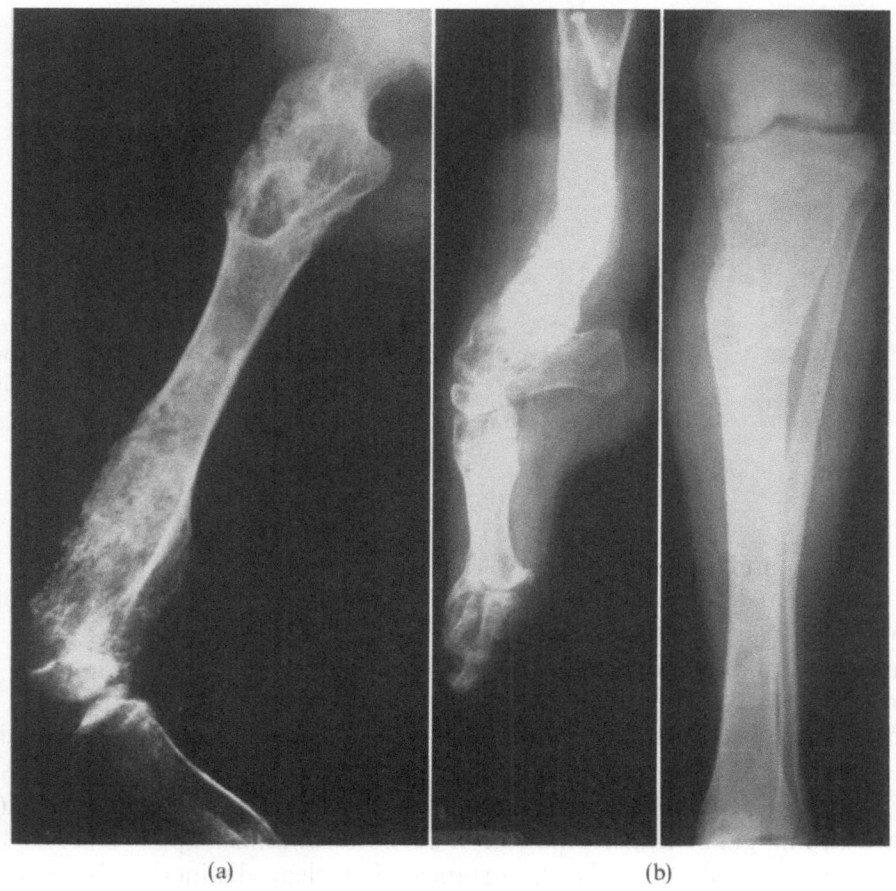

(a)   (b)

Fig. 40a and b. Multiple enchondromatosis: Teenage patient with chief complaint of recently increasing leg length disparity. Marked shortening of right lower extremity was noted at early age. (a) Right femur: Club-shaped expansion of distal and proximal femur is due to multiple medullary enchondromas. Heavy mineralization is seen with cartilaginous lesions contained within medullary cavity. Mineral is therefore contained within confines of medullary cavity rather than external to it. This contrasts with peripheral mineralization are seen in cartilaginous caps of osteochondromas. (b) Note marked disparity in leg length with deformity of contralateral left proximal tibia

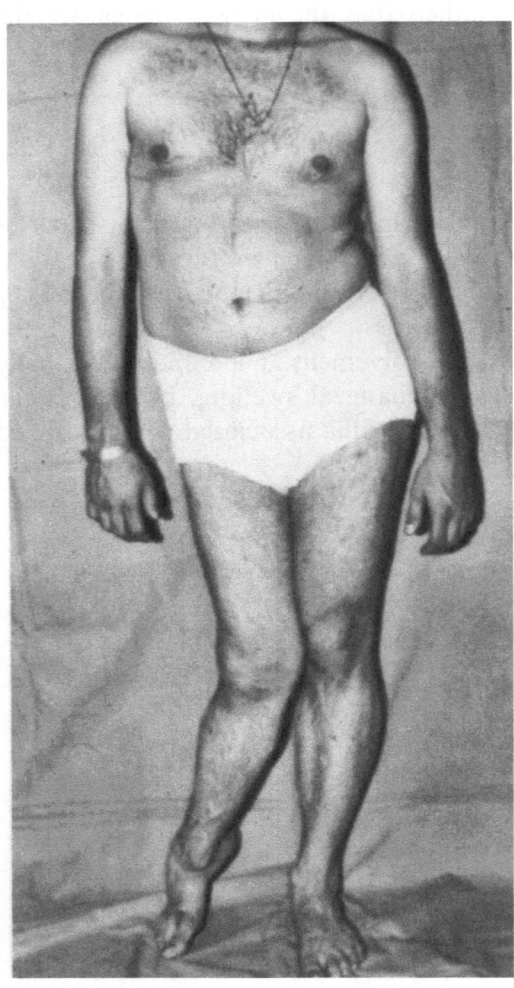

Fig. 40c. Photograph of patient with multiple enchondro-matosis emphasizing markedly retarded growth of right lower extremity, sharp pelvic tilt and resulting compensatory scoliosis

forearm motion, and ulnar deviation of the hand may be noted early (Fig. 39a). The forearm and wrist deformities are similar to those present in many cases of multiple osteochondromatosis, and both entities have been referred to by a common name, i.e. hereditary deforming chondrodysplasia.

Retarded growth of the lower extremities may be striking, particularly when one lower limb is more heavily affected (Fig. 40a, b). At the age of 2 or 3 years the discrepancy in lower limb length may approach 2–4 cm and in young adults may be as much as 25 cm (Fig. 40b). A compensatory scoliosis and sharp pelvic tilt are frequent (Fig. 40c). The hazard of malignant transformation in enchondromatosis approaches 50% in some series. This again emphasizes the importance of a clear distinction between instances of skeletal enchondromatosis and multiple osteochondromatosis in which the purported risk is considerably less. The malignant tumors are overwhelmingly chondrosarcomas (COWAN, 1965; JAFFE, 1968; LICHTENSTEIN, 1965). One example of an osteosarcoma developing in a 68-year-old man with enchondromatosis has been reported by BRADDOCK and HADLOW (1966). The lesion metastasized to the lungs. Necropsy revealed several intercostal and retroperitoneal hemangiomata, together with angiomatous changes in the aortic lymph nodes.

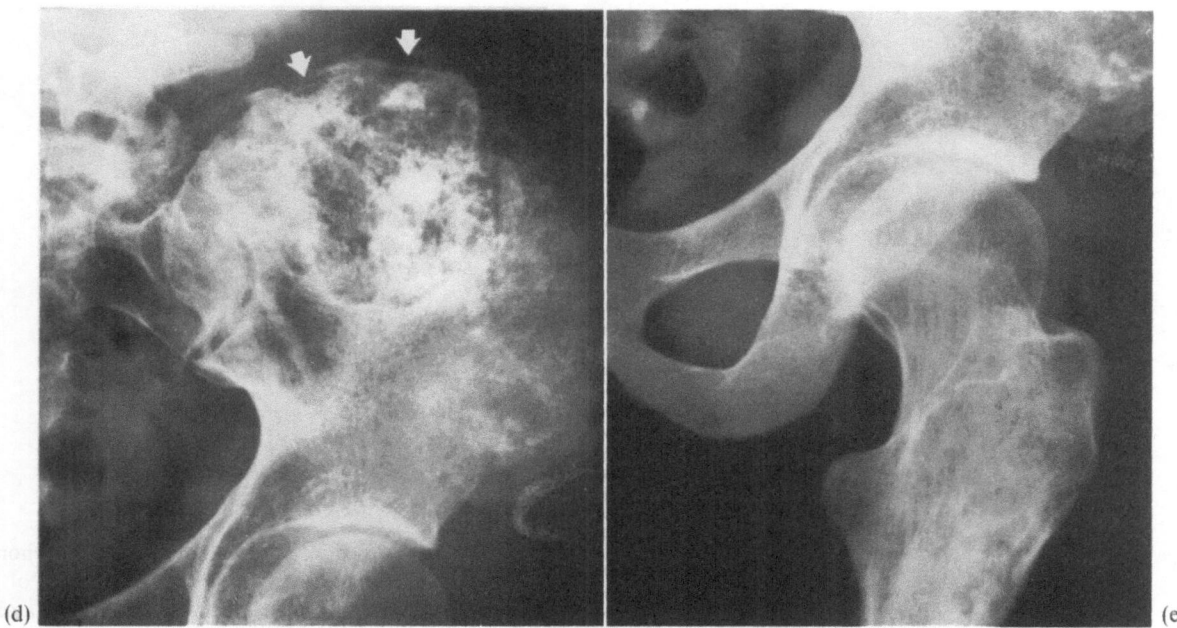

(d)   (e)

Fig. 40d and e. Left ilium. Detail view shows heavy calcification and ossification within this large cartilaginous locus. Recent pain prompted examination. Interrupted superior iliac cortex (arrows) prompted surgical extirpation. Low grade chondrosarcoma was found. (e) Enchondromas involved proximal left femoral shaft as well as lower leg

Multiple enchondromatosis may be associated with skin and soft tissue anomalies, including vitiligo, multiple pigmented nevi, hemangiomas, lymphangiomas, and phlebectasia. The chance association of multiple enchondromas and hemangiomas of the soft tissues is known as Maffucci's syndrome (Fig. 41). Associated mucous membrane and visceral involvement by hemangiomas may also be included in this syndrome. Although the abnormal soft tissue component in Maffucci's syndrome most often consisted of cavernous or capillary hemangiomas or phlebectasia (i.e. 96 of 103 reviewed by LEWIS et al., 1973), 2 cases were associated with lymphangiomas alone and 5 cases had venous plus lymphatic lesions. They were all considered to be examples of Maffucci's syndrome (LODWICK, 1965). It is of interest that the case of osteosarcoma in enchondromatosis described by BRADDOCK and HADLOW (1966) which was associated with hemangiomata was not classified as Maffucci's syndrome on the mistaken premise that "hemangiomata in this case were seen in the subcutaneous tissues but not in the skin, as in Maffucci syndrome." Therefore, the recently quoted figure of 105 cases of Maffucci's syndrome found by LEWIS and KETCHAM (1973), after a review of the literature, could probably be increased if all the essential features of the syndrome were recognized. MAFFUCCI, in 1881, 18 years before Ollier described multiple enchondromatosis, documented all the essential features of the syndrome noted today. Indeed, the features noted by MAFFUCCI at the time of his first description of the syndrome included multiple enchondromas and subcutaneous hemangiomas. It is believed to be congenital but not hereditary, with no racial or sex predeliction (ALBORES-SAAVEDRA et al., 1964; ANDRÉN et al., 1963). The average age at which symptoms were first noted in 105 cases was 5 years; 25% had symptoms at birth or in the first year of life, 45% before the age of 6 and 78% before puberty. The presenting abnormality may be skeletal or vascular (BEAN, 1958; BERENBAUM and TZAMOURANIS, 1958). Skeletal deformity will often become stable at

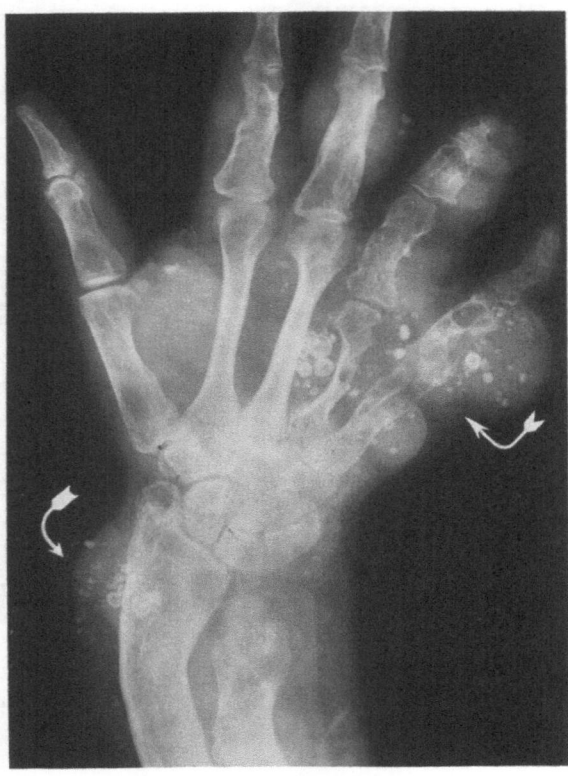

Fig. 41. Maffucci's syndrome: Multiple enchondro-matosis associated with hemangiomas of soft tissues. Widely distributed enchondromas and soft tissue hemangiomas containing phleboliths coexist with haphazard and random distribution. Note marked shortening of some fingers and overgrowth of others, i.e. additional influence of vascular malformation. Aclasis, as seen in multiple enchondromatosis alone, is present

puberty but progression may continue after skeletal growth has ceased. This is particularly important in view of the fact that malignant transformation of the associated enchondromas to chondrosarcomas occurs as with multiple enchondromatosis alone (ANDERSON, 1965; SPJUT et al., 1971). Sarcomatous transformation of an enchondroma was reported in 15.2% of 105 cases. This figure is somewhat lower than that generally cited (ANDERSON, 1965; ELMORE and CANTRELL, 1966). Sarcomatous transformation of both hemangiomas and lymphangiomas (NARDELL, 1950) has been reported. The risk, however, is greater for the skeletal component. It is difficult to prove whether other benign and malignant ·tumors which have been reported in association with Maffucci's syndrome occurred coincidentally, i.e. a cerebral glioma, fibrosarcoma, pancreatic adenocarcinoma, and ovarian teratoma. It is of interest, however, that almost all of the tumors were of mesodermal origin. Tumors derived from other germ layers do not occur with increased frequency. The overall incidence of malignant tumors in Maffucci's syndrome is 23%.

Maffucci's syndrome is not the result of a gross chromosomal aberration. Karyotyping was performed in 10 cases and yielded a normal pattern in all instances. Mental retardation is not associated with the syndrome. Maffucci's syndrome is therefore characterized by dyschondroplasia and vascular and/or lymphatic mesodermal dysplasia, most commonly in the form of cavernous or capillary hemangiomas or phlebectasia. There is no direct relationship between the bony and vascular lesions. Vascular and cartilaginous lesions need not necessarily occur in the same extremity to be considered as Maffucci's syndrome, and may, in fact, be distributed at random. Phlebectasia may be clinically evident in the form of soft, easily compressible blue-tinged serpiginous masses, while hemangiomas may also visibly involve any portion of the skin surface. Visceral hemangiomas have been described.

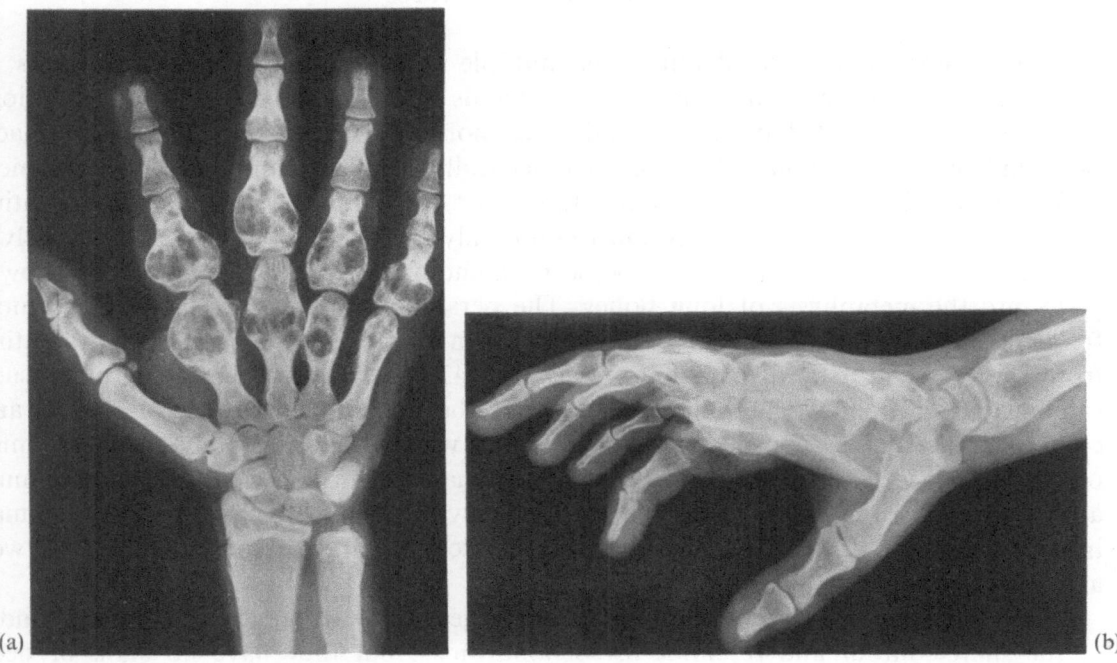

(a)   (b)

Fig. 42a and b. Multiple enchondromatosis—Ollier's disease. Hand: (a) AP view, (b) lateral view. Numerous radiolucent, poorly mineralized cartilaginous lesions have caused marked general deformity as well as overall shortening of this heavily affected limb. Lesions are most often rounded or ovoid. Bone ends tend to become bulbous due to failure of normal modeling. (Courtesy of Dr. JOSEPH WALTER)

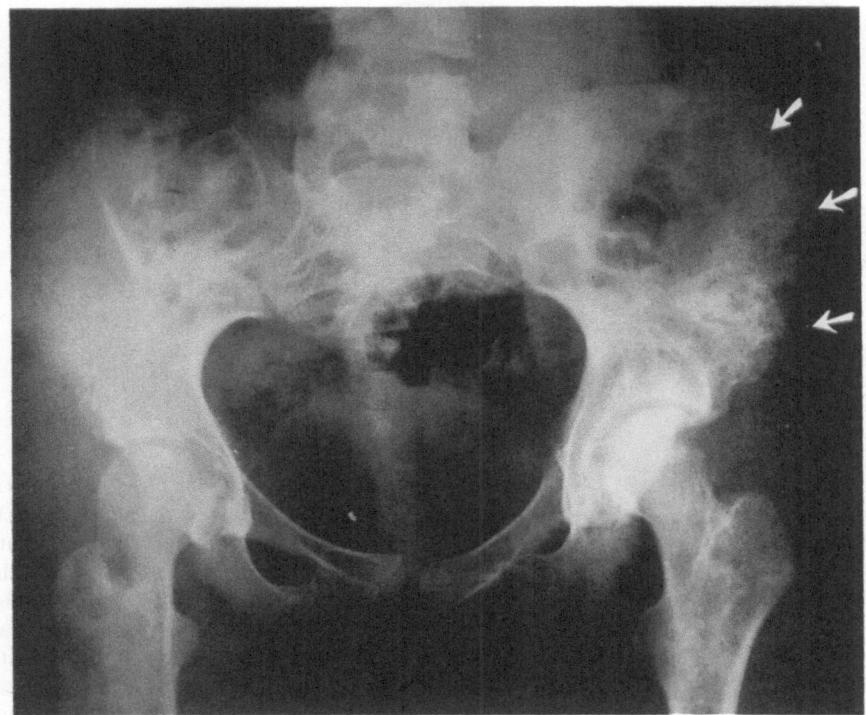

Fig. 43. AP view, pelvis. Note linear radiolucencies within left iliac wing representing columns or islands of poorly mineralized cartilage arranged in typical radial or fan-like fashion. Note obvious deformity of hips and abnormal femora with predominant right-sided involvement

III. Roentgen Features

The enchondromas are identified as multiple rarefactions involving the shafts of the tubular bones, including those of the hands and feet (Figs. 37–41). The lesions are most often rounded or ovoid, and since normal modeling does not take place, bone ends become bulbous (Fig. 42), asymmetrically expanded, and generally deformed. Affected limb bones are always short. Linear or rounded radiolucencies representing columns of islands of cartilage are most commonly seen in the flat bones of the pelvis, but radiolucent columns may also be seen extending from the region of the growth plate into the metaphysis of long bones. The persistent columns of cartilage are most frequently seen in the innominate bones in the form of linear radiolucent bands radiating from the crests in a fan-like manner (Figs. 39c, 43). As the subjects grow older such radiolucent striping may occur in the ends of the long bones as well. Punctate and conglomerate calcific deposits are frequently seen within the linear radiolucent columns of cartilage, as well as within the other enchondromas. Expansile lesions, cortical thinning and cortical disruption are more frequent than with solitary enchondromas and may involve less common sites, such as the clavicle, scapula and base of the skull, as well as the sternum and rib cage.

Enchondromas may occasionally bulge or project some distance from the remainder of the shaft contour and resemble osteochondromas, but they have no stalk or neck at the junction of their base with the shaft, may be mineralized throughout their extent

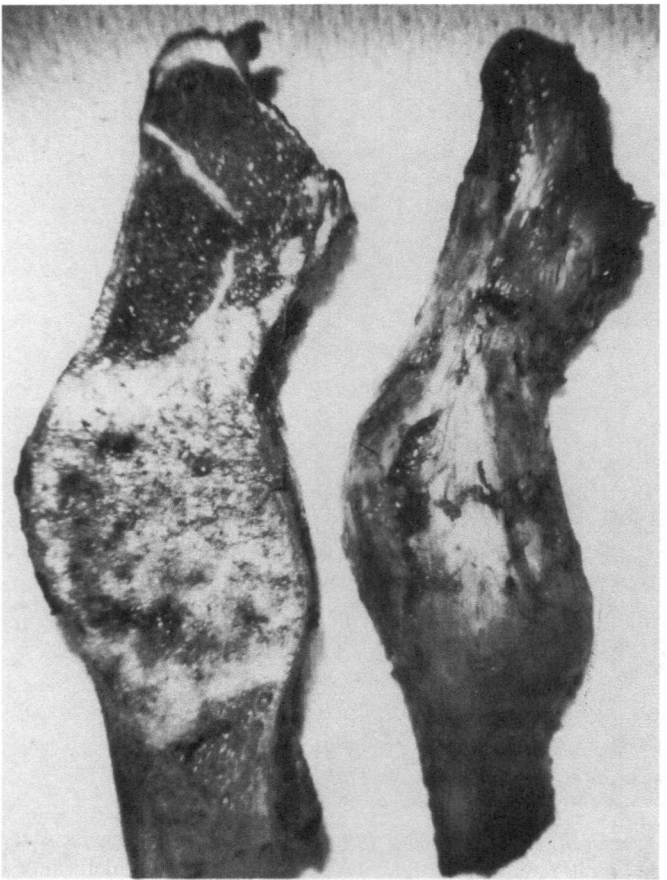

Fig. 44. Gross specimen: Fibula of patient with multiple enchondromatosis. (Left) Cut section. (Right) Surface view. Central medullary partially calcified cartilaginous lesion expands cortex asymmetrically. Note endosteal scalloping on left, predominantly metaphyseal location, and resultant localized external bulging of surface of bone at this level. (Right) Bowed cortex is not grossly disrupted. Note overall deformity and abnormal modeling

rather than in the region of a peripheral cartilaginous cap, as in an exostosis, and they do not usually point away from a joint, as an exostosis frequently does (Figs. 42, 44).

Chondrosarcomatous transformation has most frequently occurred in middle age and may or may not be heralded by pain. Roentgenographically one looks for a sudden change in size, configuration, or cortical contour, as well as extension of the lesion beyond cortical confines. Growth and/or invasion of neighboring soft tissue parts may be evidenced by an extension of mineral deposits particularly as compared with previous studies. Pain is most often associated with the more aggressive lesions (Figs. 39a, b, d, 40d).

IV. Histology

A specimen originating from one of the sites of multiple enchondromatosis may be distinguished histologically from one originating in a solitary enchondroma. A biopsy from the former usually reveals cartilage that is more cellular. The cells are more variable in shape, their nuclei are larger, and double nuclei are more frequent with less calcium impregnation of the cartilage matrix (JAFFE, 1968; LICHTENSTEIN, 1965; LICHTENSTEIN and JAFFE, 1943).

These findings are compatible with the persistent cartilage proliferation in this disorder, which has led many to characterize the lesional tissue of multiple skeletal enchondromatosis as being in a precancerous state (Figs. 45, 46). LICHTENSTEIN has noted, in examining amputated limbs from such patients, that it is not unusual to find evidence of chondrosarcomatous change developing in two or more tumor sites simultaneously

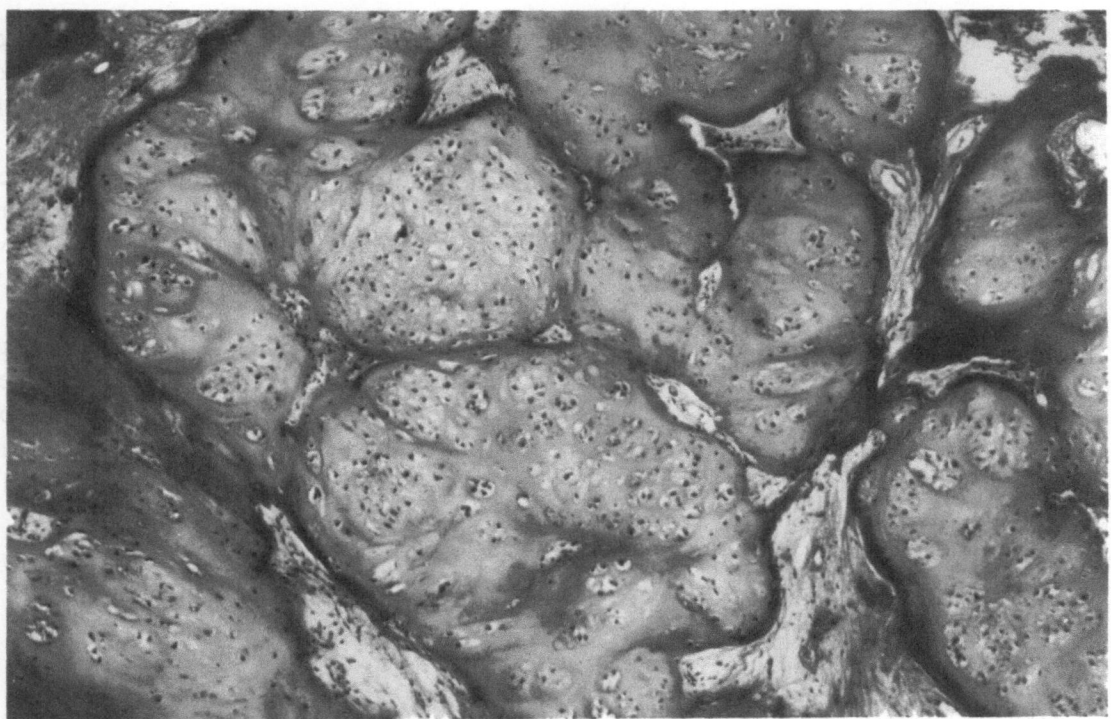

Fig. 45. Ollier's disease: Histologic section (×75) of biopsy material from patient in Fig. 40c. This is lobular arrangement of hypercellular hypertrophic cells which creates some difficulty in differentiating Ollier's disease from chondrosarcoma

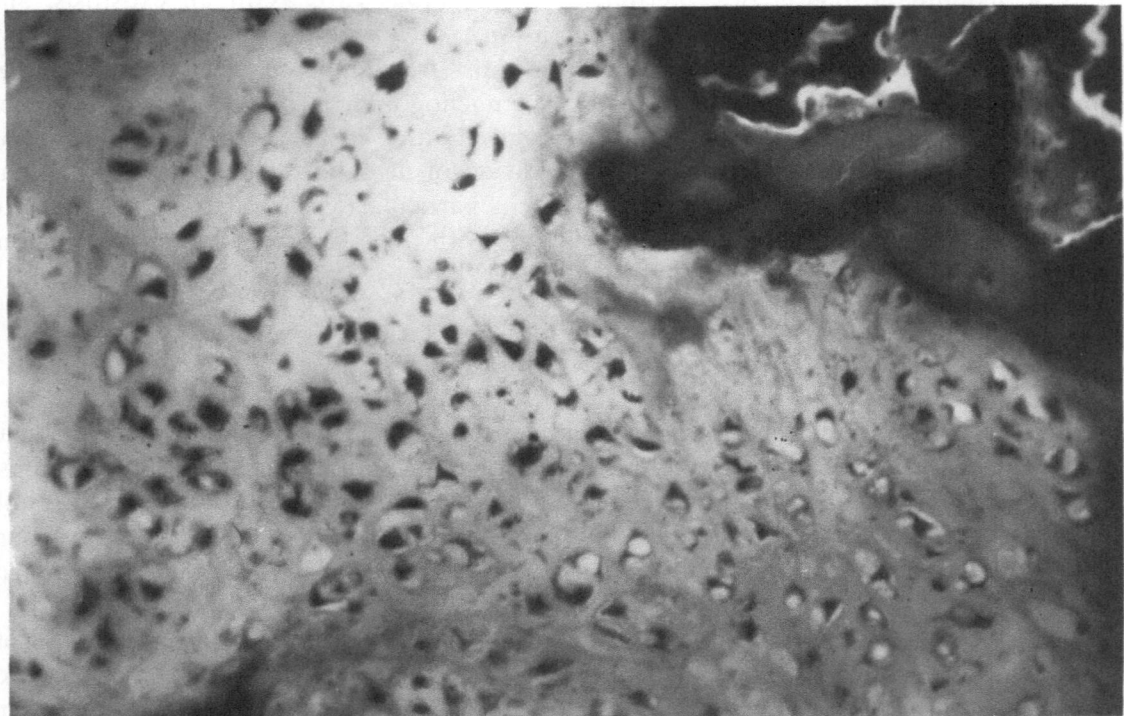

Fig. 46. Low-grade chondrosarcoma in Ollier's disease (×150): Note cells with large dark and sometimes multiple nuclei. Dark zone in upper right field represents appositional new bone

(Fig. 39). The development of chondrosarcoma is not confined to the pronounced cases (COWAN, 1965). Chondrosarcomatous transformation occurring in one or more bones is a common complication with a risk as high as 50% (JAFFE, 1968). Prognosis is usually worse than in chondrosarcoma arising from an exostosis.

A 15% incidence of sarcomatous transformation in the enchondromas associated with Maffucci's syndrome has recently been noted (LEWIS and KETCHAM, 1973). This figure is somewhat lower than that generally cited. Only two 5-year survivals have been reported following amputation for secondary chondrosarcoma in this syndrome (LEWIS and KETCHAM, 1973).

In two large series with multiple enchondromas, including Ollier's disease and Maffucci's syndrome, DAHLIN's incidence for chondrosarcoma transformation was noted as 20–30% of cases, and JAFFE's as 50%. Hence, one-third to one-half of cases develop one or more secondary chondrosarcomas. Rarely osteosarcoma is reported as a complication of enchondromas (BRADDOCK and HADLOW, 1966; ROCKWELL and ENNEKING, 1971).

G. Dysplasia Epiphysealis Hemimelica

This developmental disorder has most often been described as an asymmetric cartilaginous overgrowth of one side of one epiphysis or of a carpal or tarsal bone. FAIRBANK (1956) used the term hemimelica to graphically describe the limited locus of the lesions. They are, however, not always hemimelic or solitary. KETTLEKAMP's et al. (1966) study of 167 lesions in 57 patients revealed multiple lesions in more than two-thirds of the cases. The entire femoral capital epiphysis was affected in three patients, while multiple bones were involved in several others. However, though more than one epiphysis may be involved, they are usually situated on one extremity.

Dysplasia epiphysealis hemimelica is distinct from the epiphyseal hypoplasias since it is a disorder of excessive growth and it, therefore, shares much in common with hyperplasias of other segments, i.e. enchondromatosis and osteochondromatosis. Its limited distribution, however, precludes its being classified as a true bone dysplasia (RUBIN, 1964).

I. Pathogenesis

The etiology is unknown. There was no instance in which siblings or parents were similarly affected in KETTELKAMP's et al. series of 57 patients. It was therefore stated that the condition was neither familial nor hereditary. A recent report, however, noted the unusual occurrence of a variety of benign cartilage tumors which appeared in two generations of the same family (HENSINGER et al., 1974). Various combinations included dysplasia epiphysealis hemimelica, intracapsular chondromas, extraskeletal osteochondromas, and typical osteochondromas among the seven affected family members. Six were affected by dysplasia epiphysealis hemimelica, 3 by intracapsular chondromas, 3 by extraskeletal osteochondromas, and 2 by typical osteochondromas. With the exception of the osteochondromas, the conditions are exceedingly rare, with a collective reported incidence of less than 75 cases. The condition was found to be autosomal dominant with a variable expressivity. Thus it would appear that this family is unique in that they displayed a multiplicity of rare cartilage lesions as well as an hereditary tendency for their development (HENSINGER et al., 1974). Many of these tumors were asymptomatic.

II. Site

Distribution is characteristically on one side of the limb and most commonly in the lower limb (Figs. 47, 48). The talus and distal femoral and tibial epiphyses are the most common sites (KEATS, 1957; TREVOR, 1950). Upper limb involvement has also been reported (FAIRBANK, 1956; KETTELKAMP et al., 1966). The medial side is affected twice as often as the lateral. Multiple lesions are usually confined to one extremity.

III. Clinical

Pain is not a prominent feature. It is most often related to restricted motion due to the presence of the local cartilaginous growth, or to occasional fracture, as in multiple osteochondromatosis or multiple enchondromatosis. Locking or catching of the knee joint rarely occurs (KETTELKAMP et al., 1966). Growth appears to be unaffected and shortening of the limb is unusual.

IV. Roentgen

The only apparent abnormality in infancy may be metaphyseal widening or deformity. Ossification centers of affected bones usually appear prematurely. Later, numerous and

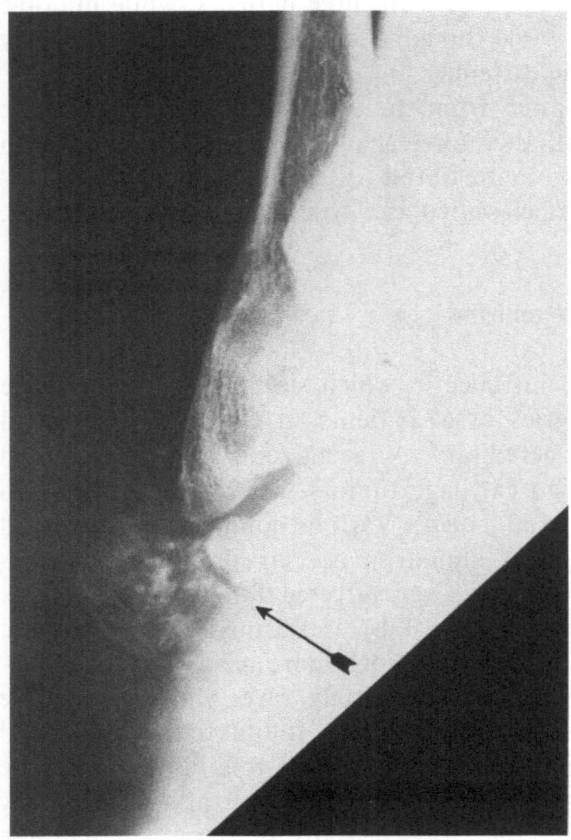
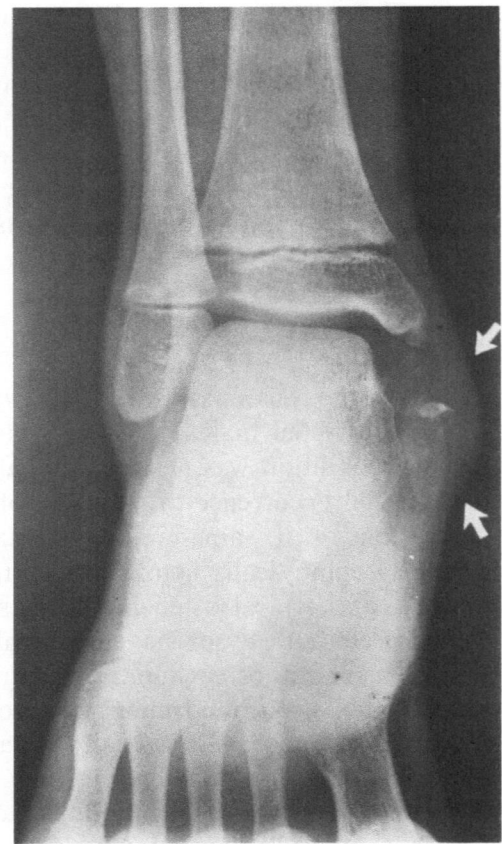

Fig. 47   Fig. 48

Fig. 47. Dysplasia epiphysealis hemimelica, tarsus: Detail view. Note large irregularly contoured calcified lesion adjacent to talus. Thin lucent line of demarcation denotes incomplete ossification of cartilage (arrow)

Fig. 48. Dysplasia epiphysealis hemimelica in 10-year-old male: Lesion is associated with medial aspect of talus which is affected twice as often as lateral aspect. Note multiple irregular radiopacities which appear to be separate from talus itself. As lesion matures, however, cartilaginous mass continues to ossify and will eventually fuse and blend with neighboring bone. Final appearance may be that of exostosis (Fig. 49)

irregular multicentric radiopacities may occur adjacent to one side of, but not necessarily connected to, the affected bone. Therefore, an irregularly shaped, mineralized mass may be noted, which appears isolated from the main epiphysis of a long bone or from an ossification center of a carpus or tarsus (Figs. 47, 48). As the lesion matures, the mass fuses and blends with the texture of the affected neighboring bone. The final appearance is similar to that of an exostosis. In view of its epiphyseal location a chondroblastoma may occasionally mimic this developmental disorder (Fig. 49). The lesions are readily distinguishable on a histologic basis.

The direction of the projection is haphazard. When the bulk of the mass impinges on an articular surface, a malalignment of the joint may occur. Massive enlargement of the body of the talus has also been observed (FAIRBANK, 1956; KETTELKAMP et al., 1966). No other growth disturbances occur and the metaphysis and diaphysis of the affected bone are normal in caliber and shape.

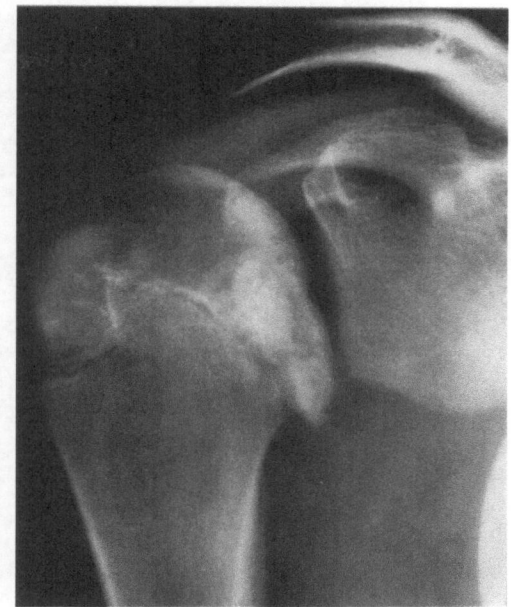

Fig. 49. Chondroblastoma, humerus: 14-year-old male with chief complaint of pain and limited motion of right shoulder. This lesion was thought to be example of dysplasia epiphysealis hemimelica on basis of initial biopsy. Note overall hazy amorphous appearance of lesion due to its heavy mineral content. Definitive surgery several months later established diagnosis of chondroblastoma

V. Histology

The basic process is the result of an abnormal growth of cartilage related to an epiphysis or to a tarsal or carpal bone with associated endochondral ossification. This results in an exostosis which, with the exception of its location, is indistinguishable from an osteocartilaginous exostoses. The lesions have, in fact, been called epiphyseal osteochondromas. Some retain their ability to grow in the adult by cartilaginous proliferation in a manner similar to that described in metaphyseal and diaphyseal exostoses.

Grossly, the lesion may appear as a pedunculated mass with a cartilaginous cap or as a slightly irregular enlarged articular surface not clearly distinguishable from the remainder of the epiphysis. Prior to complete ossification, a cleavage area of cartilage may be observed between the ossification center of the lesion and the epiphysis, which corresponds to its occasionally apparent discontinuity on radiographs.

It is histologically indistinguishable from an osteocartilaginous exostosis, with a base of normal bone and a cap of hyaline cartilage most often encountered. Bone formation occurs by enchondral ossification.

VI. Course

The course of the disease in adult life has not been entirely clarified. Most patients are discovered because they experience pain due to rapid growth of the lesion. Tissue sections from some of these cases showed active cartilage proliferation. However, follow-up and clinical observation from 9–31 years have confirmed the benign nature of the lesion. Malignant degeneration has not yet been reported (KETTELKAMP et al., 1966).

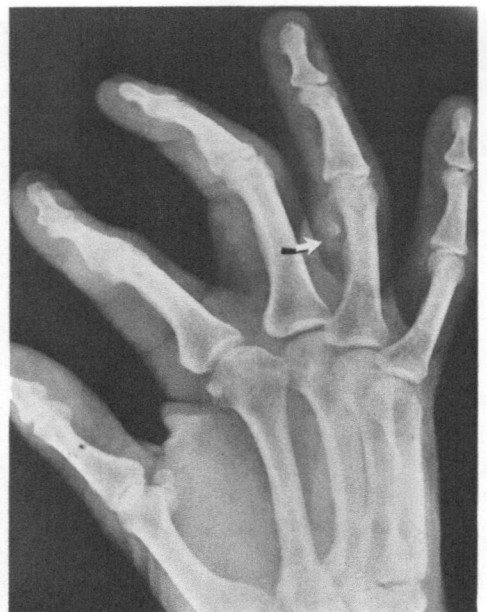 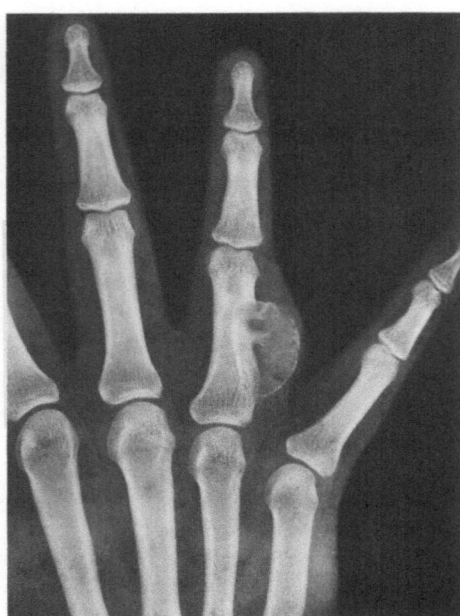

Fig. 50   Fig. 51

Fig. 50. Juxtacortical (periosteal) chondroma—hand: Note shallow cortical indentation along lateral volar aspect of proximal phalanx of 4th finger. Only small portion of cartilaginous mass is mineralized (arrow)

Fig. 51. Juxtacortical (periosteal) chondroma—hand: Lesion again involves common site, i.e. phalanx of hand. Eccentric, cortically oriented, cartilaginous mass is well-circumscribed both medially and laterally. A well-marginated sclerotic base separates cortically oriented lesion from medullary cavity. Cartilaginous mass is peripherally defined by thin radiopaque calcific shell

H. Juxtacortical (periosteal) Chondroma

Juxtacortical chondromas are usually solitary, benign cartilage lesions which develop in the periosteum and/or immediate paraosteal connective tissue of a bone. They characteristically erode their underlying cortical bed, forming a depression or declivity in the underlying cortex. The latter is not penetrated and serves to separate the lesion from the medullary cavity. LICHTENSTEIN and HALL (1952) classified this lesion as a distinctive, benign, cartilaginous tumor in 1952 on the basis of six cases, all but one of which were observed within a period of a year.

I. Clinical

They are most frequently found in young or middle aged adults, have no sex predilection and occur most frequently in the phalanges (Figs. 50, 51) of the hands and feet (LICHTENSTEIN and HALL, 1952; MEYER, 1958). The carpal navicular bone and the upper shaft of the tibia and humerus accounted for three of the six sites in the original paper (LICHTENSTEIN and HALL, 1952). Clinical symptoms are not striking with histories of variable pain and swelling ranging from months to years (JAFFE, 1956). In one instance where the tumor involved an index finger, the patient had been aware of a gradual swelling for 10 years before he sought treatment.

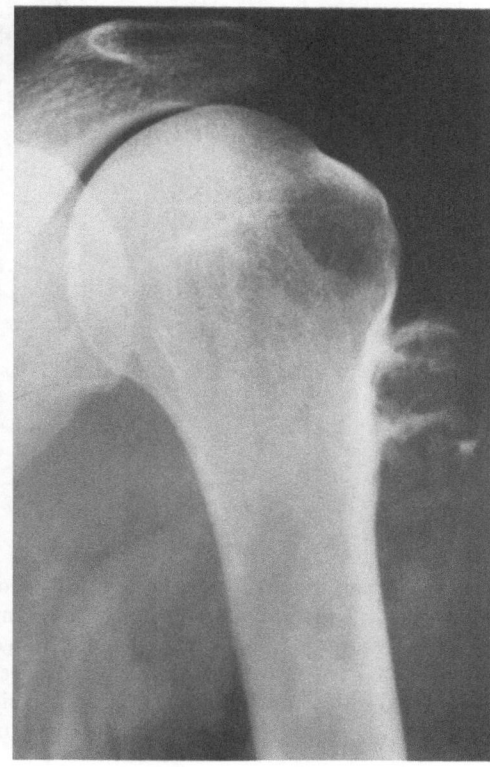

Fig. 52. Juxtacortical (periosteal) chondroma, humerus: 35-year-old male with chief complaint of aching arm of 1 year's duration. Saucer-shaped depression along lateral cortex of proximal humerus has sclerotic base which confines lesion to cortex. Calcification is present within central portions of tumor mass. Peripheral or lateral extent of lesion was not defined. At surgery lesion was entirely within cortical confines and did not extend into medullary cavity. Its lateral border was confined by periosteum

II. Roentgen

They present as an eccentric, semilunar, cortically oriented radiolucency which appears to have eroded the cortex from without. The erosion which has a well-marginated sclerotic base, separating it from the medullary cavity, has a crater or cup-like configuration (Figs. 52, 53). A buttress of periosteal new bone may be present, particularly at the proximal end of the defect (JAFFE, 1968) (Fig. 53b). They usually are 1 or 2 cm and rarely exceed 3 or 5 cm in their greatest dimension. Occasionally, merely a subtle shallow cortical indentation is identified (JAFFE, 1956).

Its peripheral cartilaginous component may be ill-defined or not roentgenographically visible. However, it may be sprinkled with fluffy or coarse granular calcifications (Figs. 52, 53b). Occasionally, and particularly if the cartilaginous mass is large, it may be outlined by a thin radiopaque shell representing a calcified or ossified capsule (Fig. 51). The latter may develop about the periphery of the cartilage through a process of metaplasia (JAFFE, 1968). If not visualized in profile by means of multiple views, a juxtacortical chondroma may occasionally simulate a central medullary lesion and be misdiagnosed as an enchondroma (Fig. 53).

III. Differential Diagnosis

A fibrous cortical defect most often occurs in the distal femoral metaphysis in an otherwise normal young child. Cortical defects have usually disappeared spontaneously post puberty, a time when juxtacortical chondromas are frequently discovered. Fibrous cortical defects usually have well-defined, medial margins, but they are frequently

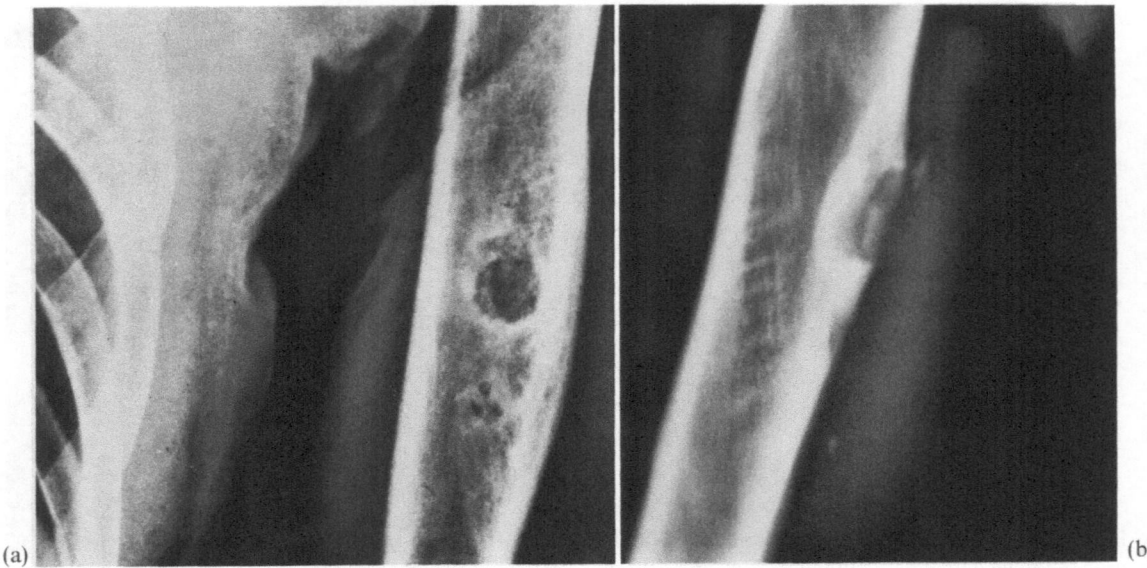

(a)   (b)

Fig. 53a and b. Juxtacortical (periosteal) chondroma, humerus: (a) AP view. If not visualized tangentially, juxtacortical chondroma may occasionally simulate central medullary lesion and be misdiagnosed as enchondroma or central chondrosarcoma, (b) Tangential view establishes intracortical location of lesion which is separated from medullary cavity by thickened sclerotic hypertrophied cortical bed. Two cartilaginous nidi are noted within cortex. Lateral confines of lesion could not be definitely identified. Cortex assumes buttress-like configuration proximal to lesion. (COURTESY of Dr. RICHARD TAXIN)

scalloped internally and may extend into the medullary cavity, where they are referred to as nonossifying fibromas. The fibrous lesion is clearly encompassed by bone along its lateral or external contour. Though it may expand or balloon the cortex, the latter is still preserved and distinguishable, whereas the external boundary of the juxtacortical chondroma is often not distinguishable or else is defined by a thin mineralized shell at a distance from the external boundaries of the remainder of the shaft. Juxtacortical chondromas frequently contain mineral within the tumor mass. Fibrous cortical defects are rarely mineralized and are unusual in the hands and feet, which are favored sites for juxtacortical chondromas. Histologically they are distinctive lesions.

Villonodular synovitis of the tendon sheath (giant cell tumor or fibrous xanthoma of the tendon sheath) may occasionally erode the cortex of an adjacent bone, which is most commonly a phalanx, but the associated soft tissue mass does not contain calcific foci. Glomus tumors also do not contain calcific foci and are most commonly related to the distal phalanges in the subungual region.

Neurofibromatosis may also occasionally be associated with localized bony erosions or undulating bony contours; however, other stigmata, including skin lesions and typical widespread skeletal deformities, including discrepancies in growth, aid in differentiation.

IV. Histology

1. Gross

The subperiosteal juxtacortial chondroma is seen to be a lobulated growth which is well-circumscribed over its convexity by investing periosteal connective tissue. It is occasionally flattened, rounded, or ovoid in contour and the cartilaginous mass has ranged from about 1.5–3.5 cm in greatest dimension (LICHTENSTEIN and HALL, 1952). It is often firm or rubbery and of a whitish or bluish color commonly identified with cartilaginous growths. Although the mass is imbedded in the cortex, the medullary cavity of the underlying bone is seldom involved (SPJUT et al., 1971). The cup-shaped or semilunar cortical hollow is apparently created by gradual pressure erosion. In instances in which the growth was "shelled out of its bed" it was observed that the base of the hollow was composed of smooth, hard, sclerotized cortical bone, such as is visualized on the roentgenogram.

2. Microscopic

Though microscopically similar to benign enchondromas, these lesions may exhibit a considerable degree of cellularity, binucleate cells, and nuclear atypism, to a greater degree than would be expected in a benign cartilaginous tumor. Although its cartilage is usually less cellular than that of a solitary enchondroma of a long bone, it is generally more cellular than the cartilage taken from a distally situated solitary enchondroma, e.g. in a phalanx. Therefore, histologic sections of juxtacortical chondroma, reviewed without the benefit of knowing their source, may be misinterpreted as low grade chondrosarcoma.

This is particularly true if tissue from the periphery of the lobules is examined. Cells with large nuclei may abound at the edge or periphery of a juxtacortical chondroma so that if taken from an intramedullary location, the same section could satisfy the criteria of a low-grade chondrosarcoma. On the other hand, tissue taken from the center tends to be less bizarre and more mature. The cartilage of a juxtacortical chondroma, therefore, may differ not only from other benign cartilage lesions, but may exhibit

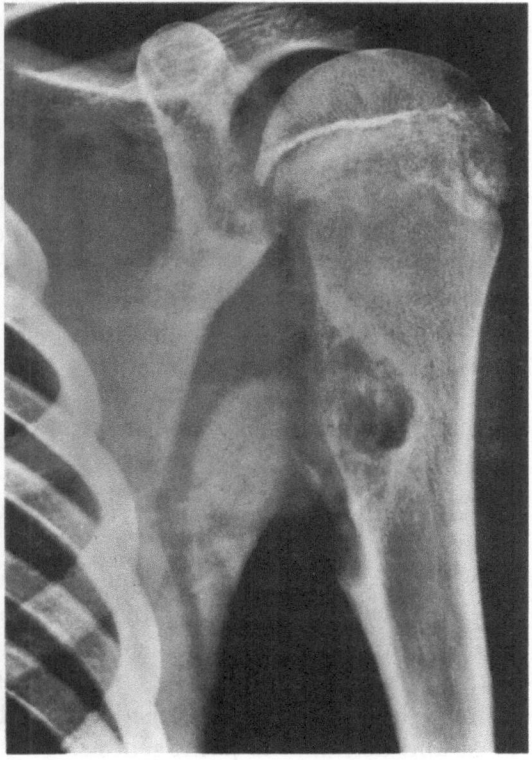

Fig. 54. Chondrosarcoma: This large eccentric lesion with hazy ill-defined and faintly calcified matrix in 14-year-old male was diagnosed as cartilaginous lesion. However, in view of its large size and medullary cavity involvement, diagnosis of juxtacortical chondroma was not tenable. Initial biopsy was interpreted chondromyxoid fibroma. Subsequent biopsies and partial resection revealed well-differentiated chondrosarcoma, unusual lesion in this age group

cellular variations within its own substance. A large, eccentric, or extraosseous cartilaginous lesion suggests malignancy, so that large size may be just as important a criterion of malignancy as high cellularity in certain locations (Fig. 54).

The pathologist must, therefore, be apprised of the orientation of the biopsy and the orientation of the lesion. This knowledge, together with the radiographic identification of a juxtacortical location and a smooth sclerotic base, is important to the histologist.

V. Course

Juxtacortical chondromas, like other benign cartilaginous tumors, may recur if incompletely excised (NOSANCHUK and KAUFER, 1969). Nests of cartilage cells within the periosteum and adjacent sclerotic bone several millimeters from the main mass have been observed. Since they, too, may serve as nidi for recurrence, en bloc resection is usually attempted.

Neither malignant transformation nor metastases has occurred, in JAFFE's (1956, 1968) experience. It is of additional interest that of 288 chondrosarcomas reviewed by HENDERSON and DAHLIN (1963), 13 arose in the periosteal region. However, these were chondrosarcomas de novo.

I. Chondroblastoma

The lesion was given its present name and first regarded as an independent clinico-pathologic entity by JAFFE and LICHTENSTEIN (1942). The presence of multilobulated giant cells within chondroblastomas had led to considerable confusion in the semantics of this lesion. It had been referred to as a "cartilage containing giant cell tumor" by KOLODNY (1927), as a "calcifying giant cell tumor" by EWING (1928) and as an "epiphyseal chondromatous giant cell tumor" by CODMAN (1931), who described nine cases from the bone tumor registry, all of which involved the humeral epiphysis. Since CODMAN was an orthopedic surgeon with a special interest in the shoulder, the lesion was, for a while, thought to be restricted to the humerus. It is now known to have a wider distribution occurring in the epiphysis of any long bone as well as in flat bones. The tumor has often been referred to as CODMAN's tumor since he was generally mistakenly credited with its initial description.

I. Pathogenesis

The pathogenesis is unsettled. The term chondroblastoma, as originally employed by JAFFE and LICHTENSTEIN (1942), was used to connote a benign lesion whose tumor cells were cartilaginous in origin with the suffix "blast" serving to indicate that mature cartilage was not produced by the lesion. On the basis of light microscopy, the basic proliferating cells of benign chondroblastoma have been thought to be chondroblasts that produce a chondroid or chondroid-like substance which may vary in amount from lesion to lesion. However, considerable difficulty exists in further categorizing the chondroblast and defining its pathogenesis.

A cartilage germ cell origin was originally postulated by JAFFE and LICHTENSTEIN, and an origin from cells of the enchondral plate by LEVY et al. (1946), while AEGERTER and KIRKPATRICK (1968) stated that chondroblastomas contained embryonic cartilage. A derivation from cartilage forming connective tissue occurring as a perversion or acceleration of normal endochondral growth has recently been suggested by LICHTENSTEIN. SCHAJOWICZ and GALLARDO (1971) and VALLS et al. (1955), however, have proposed that the tumor cell is reticulohistiocytic in origin with chondroblastic differentiation. The features they list as favoring a histiocytic origin include reticulin production, metalophilia, and the nature of cell growth in tissue culture. They demonstrated reticulin fibers surrounding individual cells and groups of cells by the use of silver stains. However, it has been noted that metalophilia and reticulin production may be a feature of cartilaginous tumors, as well as of reticulohistiocytic cells. The silver reaction is, therefore, nonspecific.

Electron microscopic studies have tended to support JAFFE and LICHTENSTEIN's original contention of a cartilage germ cell origin with certain variations. LEVINE and BENSCH (1972) in comparing the ultrastructure of chondroblastoma cells with fetal and adult cartilage cells, thought that they showed features of both. However, while they agreed that the chondroblastoma is truly cartilaginous in origin, they questioned the contention that it is made up of embryonic cells. They postulated that the focally cellular areas in chondroblastoma may merely represent less well-differentiated neoplastic tissue rather than truly embryonic cells and therefore suggested that the name chondroblastoma may be a misnomer. WELSH and MEYER (1964), comparing the ultrastructure of two chondroblastomas, fetal cartilage, chondrosarcoma, and tissue cultures of normal human cartilage, dismissed any similarity between chondroblastoma cells and fetal cartilage cells, and concluded that chondroblastomas probably arise as a result of the reaction of normal cartilage cells towards an altered local environment, rather than as a result of an intrinsic alteration of the cartilage cells per se. WELSH and MEYER's (1964) views that the tumor cells resembled normal epiphyseal cartilage cells growing in tissue cultures served to support LICHTENSTEIN's (1965) recently suggested hypothesis of an origin from an anomalous or accessory epiphyseal cartilage center whose growth was stimulated at the time of puberty by sex hormones or unknown factors. WELLMAN (1969), after an electron microscopic study of one scapular lesion, noted that the tumor originated from "cartilage forming matrix cells," while HUVOS et al. (1972), after studying two benign chondroblastomas, wrote that the cells are "most likely immature chondrocytes." They suggested that rapid replication and lack of differentiation may preclude the formation of lacunae and "normal" cartilaginous matrix. These considerations and the fact that bone is a dynamic organ (JOHNSON, 1953; SPJUT et al., 1971) emphasize the problems involved in categorizing the basic tumor cell population and in defining the pathogenesis of chondroblastoma. A continuum appears to exist in the transition of a chondroblast to a mature cell so that it is difficult to define at what point a chondroblast becomes a chondrocyte. Generally, ultrastructural studies support the view, as does the usual occurrence of chondroblastoma in epiphyseal regions, that the tumor cells have a truly cartilaginous rather than a reticulocytic origin and the term chondroblastoma continues to be used to designate this neoplasm of bone that is quite distinct from chondroma or chondrosarcoma.

II. Prevalence and Site

Chondroblastomas comprise approximately 1% of benign primary bone tumors in several reported series (DAHLIN, 1967; DAHLIN and IVINS, 1972; HUVOS and MARCOVE,

Table 3. Chondroblastoma. Sites of 692 lesions

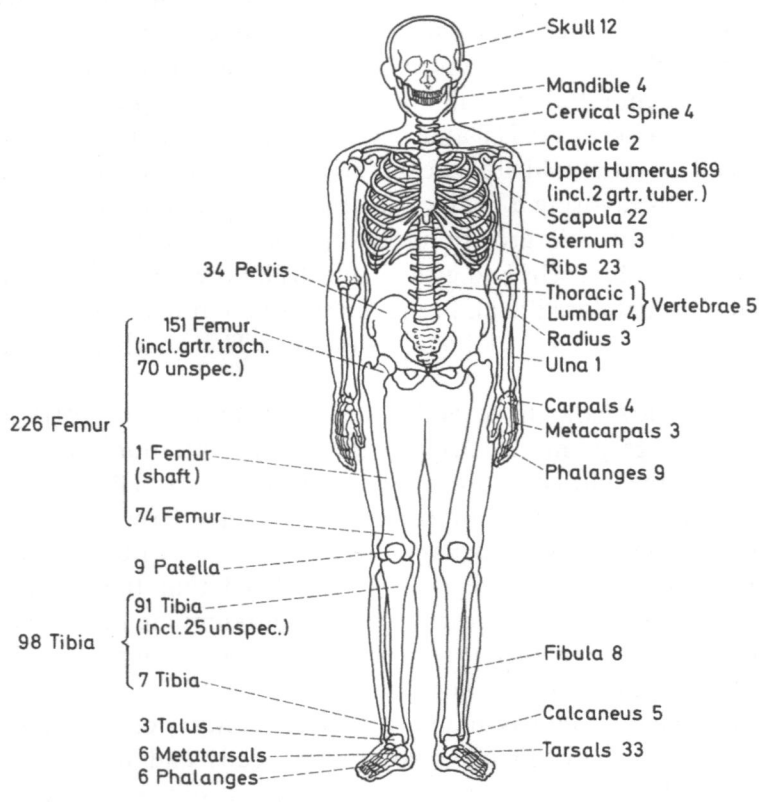

Anterior view of human skeleton
692 Lesions in 691 Cases (1 case had 2 sites)

Data from BURACZEWSKI et al., 1957; CARES, 1971; COLEMAN, 1966; DAHLIN and IVINS, 1972; FECHNER and WILDE, 1974; GARAVANIS and GIANSANTI, 1971; HUVOS and MARCOVE, 1973; LEVINE and BENSCH, 1972; McBRYDE and GOLDNER, 1970; MANGINI, 1964; NETHERLANDS COMMITTEE ON BONE TUMORS, 1966; NEVIASER and WILSON, 1972; OPPENHEIM and BOAL, 1965; PIEPGRAS et al., 1972; BALZER et al., 1968; SCHAJOWICZ and GALLARDO, 1970; SHERMAN and UZEL, 1956; SPJUT et al., 1971; SUNDARAM, 1966; TANGHE and MARTENS, 1969; VARMA and GUPTA, 1972; WELLMAN, 1969; WIESNIEWSKI et al., 1973; WITWICKI et al., 1969

1973; KUNKEL et al., 1956; SCHAJOWICZ and GALLARDO, 1970; SPJUT et al., 1971). Mote than 500 cases have been reported in the world literature, many of which are single case reports or small series of cases. It comprised less than 1% of 2900 primary bone tumors at the Mayo Clinic (DAHLIN, 1967; DAHLIN and IVINS, 1972).

Table 3 documents the sites of predilection derived from several large series. Chondroblastoma is primarily a tumor of the skeleton. DAHLIN and IVINS (1972) in referring to a case reported as "the first recorded example of primary extraskeletal chondroblastoma" (KINGSLEY and MARKEL, 1971) noted that the example was not altogether convincing. In the skeleton, the femur, humerus, tibia, and tarsal bones in descending order harbor nearly 70% of the tumors (DAHLIN and IVINS, 1972). The talus and os calcis were the most commonly affected tarsal bones (DAHLIN and IVINS, 1972; TANGHE and MARTENS, 1969). Discrepancies as to site may arise because the correct diagnosis often is not made when lesions appear in uncommon or atypical sites (ASSOR, 1973; BURACZEWSKI et al., 1957; CARES, 1971; DENKO and KRAUEL, 1955; LATTES, 1964; MANGINI, 1964; NEVIASER and WILSON, 1972; TANGHE and MARTENS, 1969; VANDENBERG and COLEY,

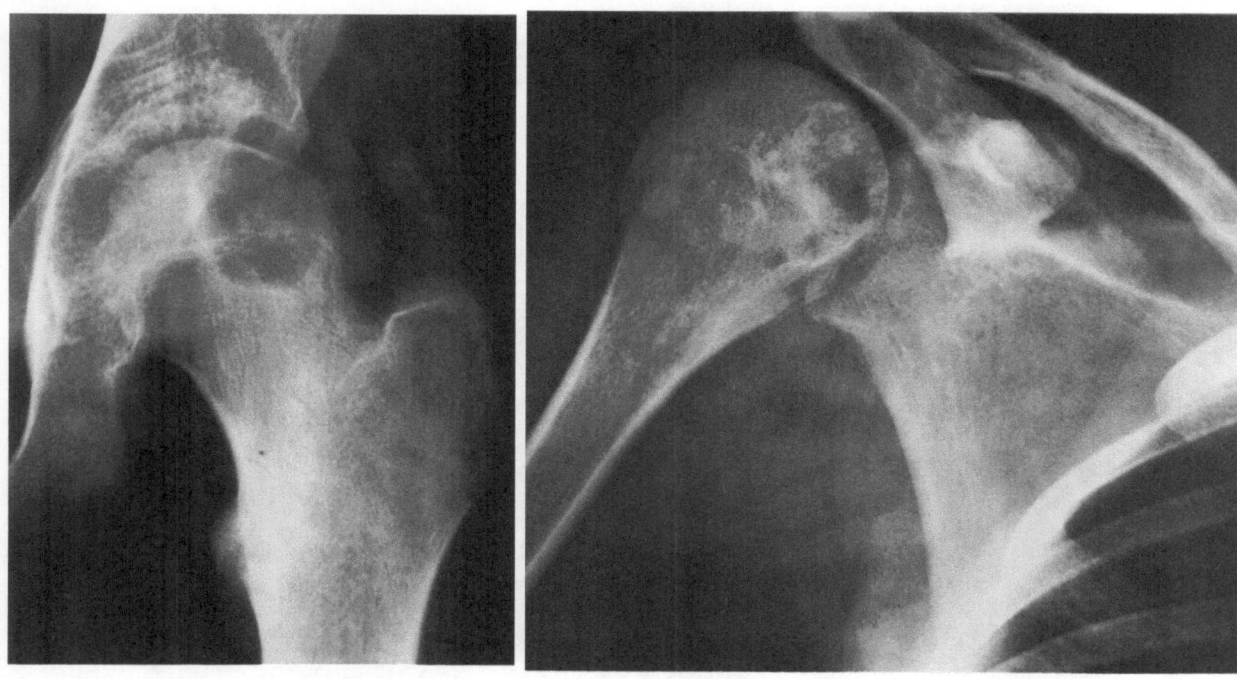

Fig. 55   Fig. 56

Fig. 55. Chondroblastoma, femur: 15-year-old limping female with 1 year history of painful left hip, previously treated with antituberculous drugs. Lytic lesion of left femoral head is sharply demarcated, confined to epiphysis and has stippled calcification within it

Fig. 56. Chondroblastoma, humerus: 15-year-old female admitted with painful left shoulder. Note rounded, well-defined, eccentric, well-marginated, radiolucent lesion with coarser mineral deposits within it. Tumor is separated from adjacent spongiosa by rim of bony condensation

1950; WISNIEWSKI et al., 1973; WRIGHT and SHERMAN, 1964), and because of the lack of precise statistical evidence in papers and books (JAFFE, 1968; LICHTENSTEIN, 1965) (Figs. 55, 56, 57a, b, 58a, b).

Long bone lesions affect the epiphysis in the overwhelming majority of cases, although lesions may extend into the adjacent metaphyses (Fig. 59a). The apophyses or secondary centers of ossification, such as those for the humeral tubercle, the femoral lesser and greater trochanter (Fig. 60), and the acromion constitute occasional sites (WRIGHT and SHERMAN, 1964). The lesion is rarely solely metaphyseal. The metaphyses of the lower tibia and the distal femur provided the sites of origin for two of DAHLIN and IVINS (1972) cases. A few other primarily metaphyseal chondroblastomas (DAHLIN and IVINS, 1972; FECHNER and WILDE, 1974; HATCHER and CAMPBELL, 1951; SALZER et al., 1968; SCHAJOWICZ and GALLARDO, 1970; SHERMAN and UZEL, 1956) and one of a tibial diaphysis (SALZER et al., 1968), have been recorded (Table 4). With few exceptions (CARES, 1971; DENKO and KRAUEL, 1955), the sites of occurrence were related to either primary or secondary centers of enchondral ossification and thus could have been derived from the cartilage of the neighboring growth plates (DAHLIN and IVINS, 1972; HUVOS and MARCOVE, 1972).

Costal tumors may occur at either end or in the mid portion of the rib (ASSOR, 1973; GOLDEN, 1971; LATTES, 1964; TANGHE and MARTENS, 1969), while tumors of the scapulae and innominate bones usually involve the glenoid or acetabular regions.

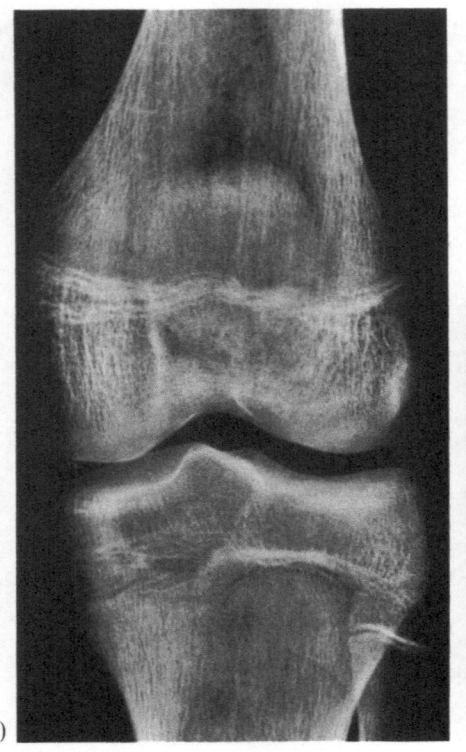
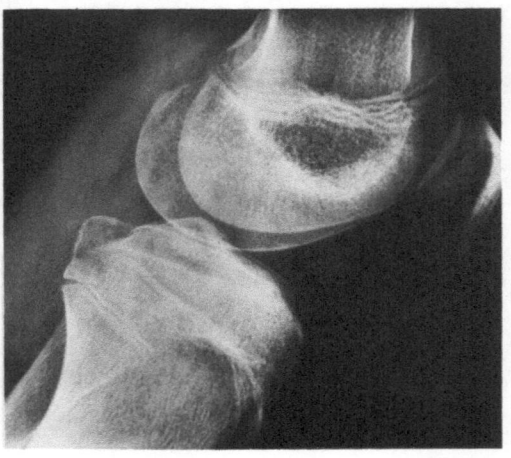

(a)   (b)

Fig. 57a and b. Chondroblastoma, tibia: $15^1/_2$-year-old male with knee pain. (a) Note subchondral rounded radiolucent lesion within tibial epiphysis extending down to growth plate. Although lesion abuts articular cartilage it does not disrupt it. Fractures are unusual in chondroblastomas. Tomograms revealed no evidence of mineral within lesion. (b) Lateral view. Lesion involves posterior superior aspect of medial tibial epiphysis. At surgery, it was found in contact with unfused growth plate

Table 4. Chondroblastomas. Rare sites

Author	Sex/age	No. of cases	Bone	Site
DAHLIN and IVINS (1972)	Not spec.	2	Distal tibia Distal femur	Metaphysis Metaphysis
FECHNER and WILDE (1974)	F/13	1	Proximal femur	Metaphysis
HATCHER and CAMPBELL (1951)	M/8	1	Proximal tibia	Metaphysis
SALZER et al. (1968)	M/18	1	Distal tibia	Diaphysis
SCHAJOWICZ and GALLARDO (1970)	F/13 M/32 M/15	3	Lower femur Proximal femur Lower femur	Metaphysis Neck Metaphysis
SHERMAN and UZEL (1956)	F/9	1	Proximal tibia	Metaphysis
ARONSOHN et al. (1976)[a]	M/18	1	Femoral neck	Metaphysis
	Total	10		

[a] ARONSOHN, R.S., HART, W.R. and MARTEL, W.: Metaphyseal chondroblastoma of bone. Am. J. Roentgenol. 127:686–688, 1976

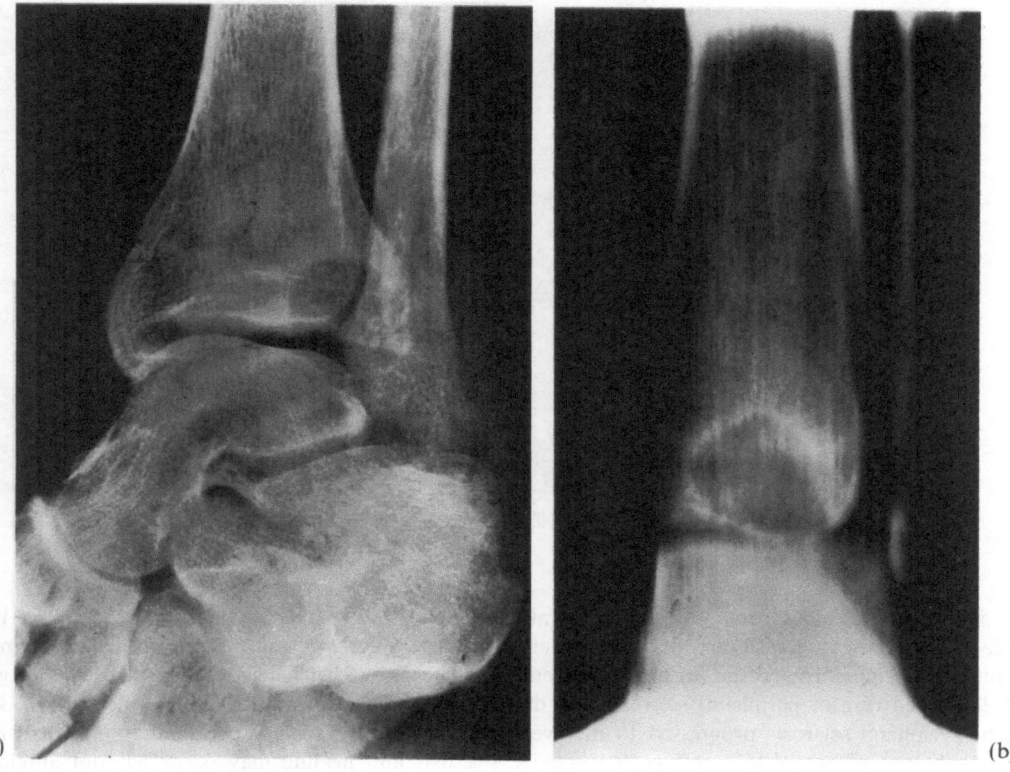

(a)

(b)

Fig. 58a and b. Chondroblastoma, tibia: 29-year-old male with ankle swelling. (a) Lesion abuts articular surface, is uniformly rounded, and well-defined, (b) Laminagrams reveal marginal bony condensation with convex ballooning of inferior subarticular margin of lesion. Articular surface was preserved. Mineral could not be roentgenographically detected within lesion

Chondroblastomas in unusual sites tended to involve older people (WRIGHT and SHERMAN, 1964). Of 11 patients with rib lesions, 7 were more than 30 years old, the oldest being 59 years. Four patients with temporal bone tumors studied by DAHLIN and IVINS (1972) were 30–56 years of age.

III. Age and Sex Distribution

There is an approximate 2:1 male to female ratio in several large series 81:42 (DAHLIN and IVINS, 1972), 44:25 (SCHAJOWICZ and GALLARDO, 1970), 116:48 (SALZER et al., 1968), 33:23, 15:10 (HUVOS and MARCOVE, 1973), with ages varying from 3–73 years. Chondroblastoma rarely occurs over the age of 30 (DAHLIN and IVINS, 1972). More than 60% of patients were in their second decade at the time of diagnosis. In SCHAJOWICZ and GALLARDO'S (1970) series, 75.3% were in the second decade of life and 88.5% were 5–25 years. In the NETHERLANDS COMMITTEE (1966) series, 95% were 5–25 years, while SALZER et al. (1968) noted 71% of 171 patients in the second decade. It has been suggested that the occasional cases in older people (Fig. 61) could represent instances of long evolution which may have started in adolescence and remained unchanged or symptomless for many years (MCBRYDE and GOLDNER, 1970). A case report of a congenital atypical benign chondroblastoma of a rib (KADELL et al., 1970) noted at birth and

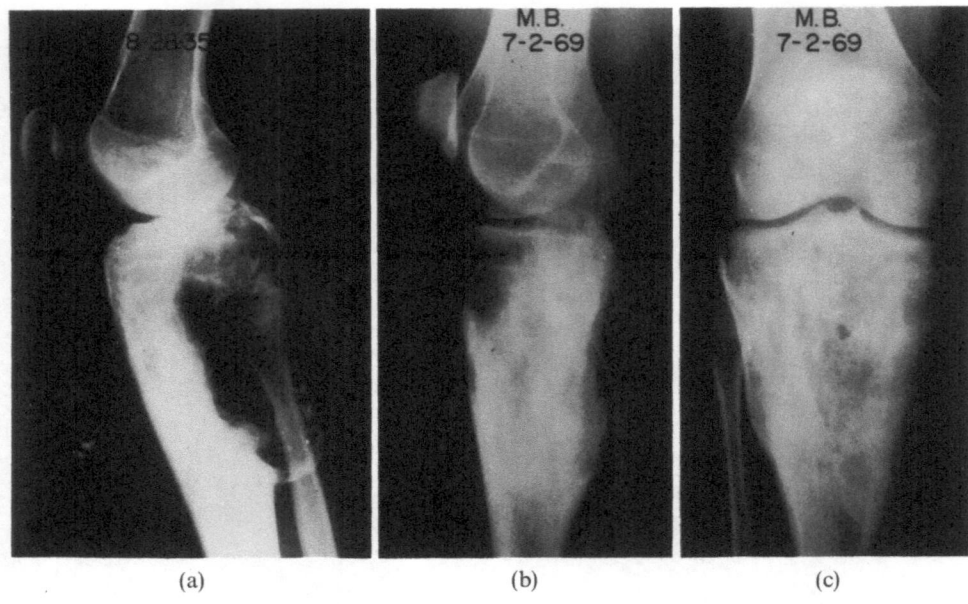

(a)   (b)   (c)

Fig. 59a–c. Chondroblastoma, tibia: (a) Lateral view 8/28/35. Expanded lytic chondroblastoma involving epiphysis and metaphysis with early peripheral sclerosis. Clinically early or recurrent lesions may be characterized by minimal peripheral sclerosis. (b) and (c) Lateral and AP views 7/2/69. Lesion may then expand gradually with thickened ring of peripheral sclerosis and development of central mottled fluffy calcification. In above patient peripheral sclerosis progressed to involve entire lesion over 35-year period. Lesions frequently heal even in absence of complete curettage. Progressive sclerosis and healing may occur without application of bone chips. This tendency toward centripetal healing is of clinical and roentgenographic importance. If lytic defect does not develop peripheral sclerosis, it may serve as warning of recurrence, particularly if coupled with recrudescence of pain and tenderness at site. (Figure courtesy of A.G. Huvos, M.D., R.C. Marcove, M.D., R.A. Erlandson, Ph.D. and V. Miké, Ph.D.)

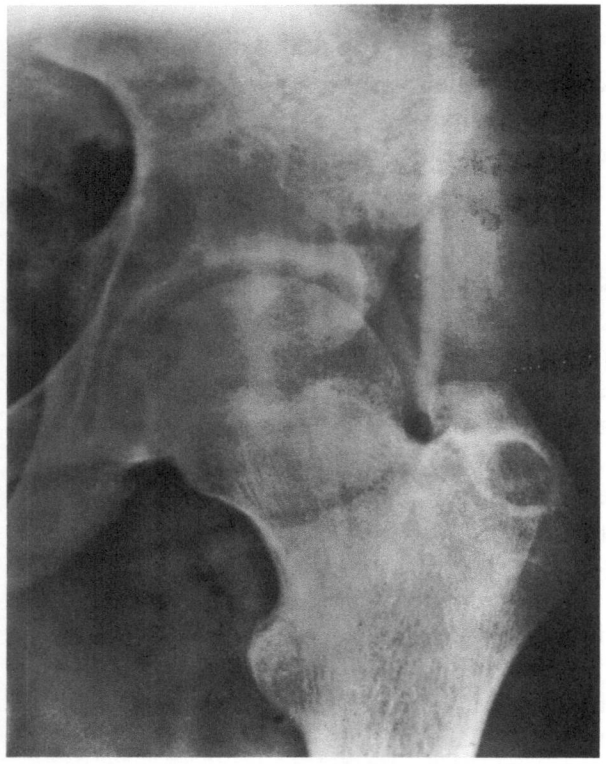

Fig. 60. Chondroblastoma in secondary center of ossification: Apophysis of greater trochanter is site of this rounded lucent lesion bounded by well-defined sclerotic border

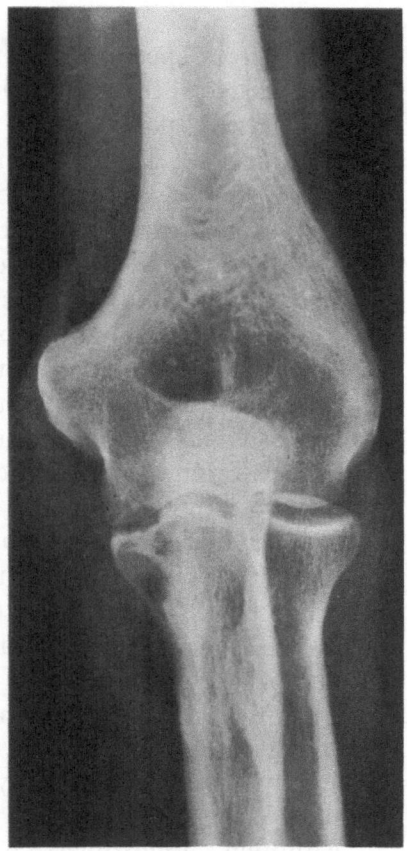

Fig. 61. Chondroblastoma, left ulna: This lucent, subchondral, well-defined lesion occurred in 58-year-old male with vague symptoms of 2 years duration. Uncommon sites tend to be involved in older people

removed at 6 months of age was considered so complex histologically by DAHLIN and IVINS (1972) that it was not considered acceptable and, therefore, not included in their review.

IV. Symptoms

The symptoms are nonspecific. Pain is the most characteristic complaint, generally of a few months' duration, but in some instances noted for 1–8 years (DAHLIN and IVINS, 1972). Local swelling, ordinarily of a few months' duration, was noted by approximately 10% of patients, usually in areas not obscured by a great deal of overlying soft tissue. Stiffness or limitation of motion of the adjacent joint were occasionally experienced. However, associated effusion described in 21 of the 69 cases of SCHAJOWICZ and GALLARDO (1970) was rarely recorded in the Mayo Clinic Series (DAHLIN and IVINS, 1972). Examinations often revealed tenderness on pressure over the lesion and, sometimes, a mass. Muscular wasting of the involved extremity was occasionally noted. In three cases in the Mayo Clinic series, articular symptoms necessitated arthrotomy a few months prior to the discovery of the tumors. Menisectomy had been performed in two of these cases without effect after clinical and laboratory studies had provided no diagnostic clues. A similar case has recently been described by Dr. Colin Alexander in a proximal tibia (personal communication). Pathologic fracture as a primary presentation is exceedingly rare (DAHLIN and IVINS, 1972; HUVOS and MARCOVE, 1973; SPJUT et al., 1971).

V. Roentgen Findings in Chondroblastoma

Since gross specimens showing an entire tumor in its setting are seldom available, our knowledge of the tumor's in situ appearance, development, and effect on surrounding bone is largely gleaned from roentgenograms. The characteristic roentgen appearance is that of a small, i.e., less than 4 cm in greatest diameter, round, or ovoid, well-defined, eccentric, epiphyseal rarefaction most commonly involving the epiphysis of a long bone (DAHLIN and IVINS, 1972; HUVOS and MARCOVE, 1973; MCLEOD and BEABOUT, 1973; PLUM and PUGH, 1958; SHERMAN and UZEL, 1956; SPJUT et al., 1971) (Figs. 55–58).

The epiphyseal tumor is usually separated from the adjacent spongiosa by a sclerotic rim or well-defined margin of bony condensation (Figs. 56, 60, 62). In the majority of lesions the size of the central defect has ranged from 1.5–4 cm and the epiphyseal line was most commonly open. However, central lucent foci not much larger than an osteoid osteoma and lesions as large as 7 cm have been described (LICHTENSTEIN, 1967). They may originate in a secondary ossification center such as the apophysis of the greater trochanter or greater tuberosity of the humerus with metaphyseal extension. Stippled calcification has been noted in 50% of some series (EDEIKEN and HODES, 1967) and in 25% of others (MCLEOD and BEABOUT, 1973). The so-called densified tumor described by JAFFE and LICHTENSTEIN (1942) with an indistinct border was occasionally observed. However, gross examination of the resected specimen usually revealed that the tumor was well-delimited from the surrounding bone by a fixed sclerotic margin with central and/or peripheral radiopaque stippled or fluffy calcification. Flocculent calcific densities (Figs. 56, 62) often described as "fluffy or popcorn ball" in appearance frequently produced a streaky or overall mottled effect. Such mottling was noted on roentgenograms of more than half of SCHAJOWICZ and GALLARDO's (1970) cases.

Although chondroblastomas abut the articular cartilage, it is unusual for them to disrupt it. However, extension of a mass into the adjacent joint or soft tissues as well as active periosteal new bone formation have been rarely reported manifestations (CASE RECORDS OF MASSACHUSETTS GENERAL HOSPITAL, 1964; COLEMAN, 1966; PLUM and PUGH, 1958) (Fig. 63). Larger lesions, in addition to extending into the adjacent metaphyses (Fig. 59) may expand laterally as well and may occasionally erode the overlying cortex (Fig. 64), producing a rounded extraosseous soft tissue mass (DAHLIN and IVINS, 1972). Xerography and/or angiography may serve to better define or identify any associated soft tissue component. Angiography may also help to identify the occasional highly vascular component of chondroblastoma. Chondroblastomas may histologically mimic an aneurysmal bone cyst in certain microscopic fields.

The clinically early or recurrent lesions of HUVOS and MARCOVE (1973) were characterized radiographically by slight peripheral sclerosis. It is of interest that these early lesions, when observed on serial roentgenograms, were seen to expand slowly with the gradual development of a sclerotic peripheral boundary as well as central calcific deposits. At still later stages the peripheral sclerosis became thicker and more pronounced with increasing central mottling and opacification (Fig. 63). Lesions were observed to heal frequently even after incomplete curettage, with progressive calcification developing peripherally at first and later centrally. This roentgen finding of progressive sclerosis and centripetal healing was demonstrated even without the application of bone chips, and was felt by HUVOS and MARCOVE to be of clinical importance. The failure of this peripheral and gradual centripetal sclerosis to develop within a postoperative lytic defect proved to be of definite value in diagnosing a recurrence. This was particularly true if coupled with a clinical recrudescence of pain and tenderness in the lytic area (HUVOS and MARCOVE, 1973).

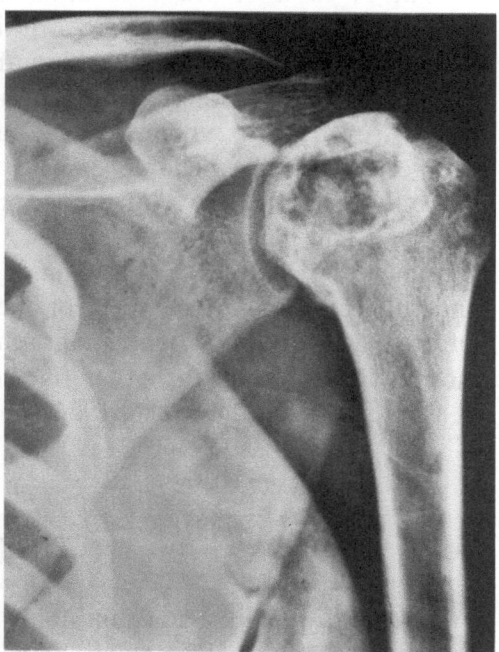

Fig. 62. Chondroblastoma, left humerus: Rounded, well-defined area of rarefaction in epiphysis is separated from adjacent spongiosa by sclerotic rim. Central calcific densities produce overall mottled effect and represent mineral deposition within chondroid matrix

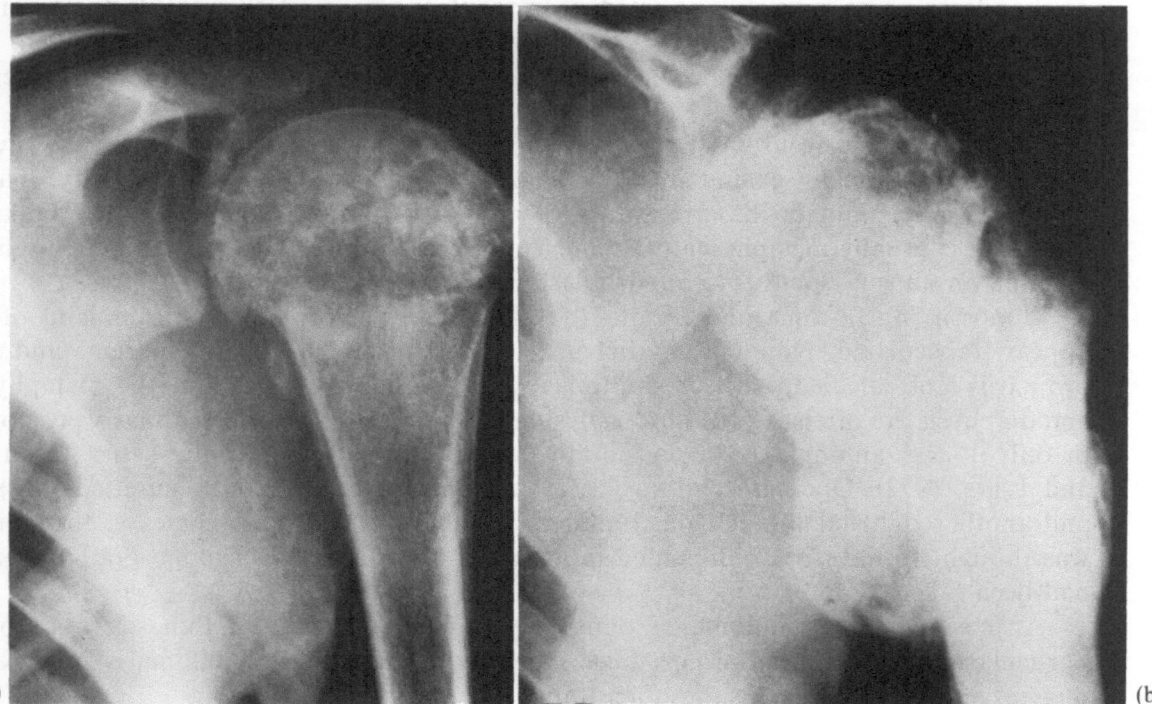

(a)   (b)

Fig. 63a and b. Recurrent chondroblastoma: (a) (Left) 3/5/66 Recurrent lesion of humerus showing expansion and periosteal new bone formation despite two curettages. (b) (Right) 1/5/70 Radiopacity developed peripherally and then centrally with fluffy small opacities developing during 4 year period following 1966 cryosurgery. Lesion has remained clinically inactive. Early recurrent lesions may be characterized by minimal peripheral sclerosis, gradual expansion, and development of central fluffy calcifications, as in Fig. 59. (Courtesy of A.G. HUVOS, M.D., R.C. MARCOVE, M.D., R.A. ERLANDSON, Ph.D. and V. MIKÉ, Ph.D.)

The 11 cases of SHERMAN and UZEL (1956) were evidently all of medullary origin, being largely or wholly contained within the bone but they showed considerable variability in the location of the lesion within the epiphysis, which was closed in some cases but remained open in others. The lesion was in contact with or touching the epiphyseal line in seven cases while it was totally confined within the epiphysis in three cases. In another case the metaphysis held the entire process which contacted the epiphyseal line only superiorly. Five of the lesions showed varying degrees of involvement of both epiphysis and metaphysis.

The cortex in the area of the tumor showed various effects, i.e., destruction, expansion, and thinning—along that part of the margin next to any soft tissue tumor extension. Of six cases followed roentgenographically, 1 revealed no apparent change after a 16-month period, while the other five observed 1–7 months all revealed a slight increase in size (SHERMAN and UZEL, 1956).

VI. Differential Diagnosis

Enchondromas are less commonly situated in the long bones and are most commonly metaphyseal rather than epiphyseal in location. Chondrosarcomas, too, are predominantly metaphyseal within the long bones, uncommonly extend to the ends of the bones and are uncommonly noted in the age group that chondroblastomas favor. Dense conglomerate calcification of the degree often seen in association with an enchondroma or chondrosarcoma is usually not evident in roentgenograms of chondroblastomas prior to treatment (PLUM and PUGH, 1958). There is also a close correlation between the lack of a mottled appearance on the roentgenogram and a dearth of microscopic evidence of calcification.

Osteoblastomas occur in the metaphysis when they involve long bones, however, they may occasionally extend into the epiphyseal area and frequently calcify. They, therefore, may simulate the appearance of a chondroblastoma. However, the bulk of the lesion is usually metaphyseal. Osteoblastomas most commonly involve the vertebral column, an unusual locus for chondroblastoma (POCHACZEVSKY et al., 1960).

Nonossifying fibroma and fibrous dysplasia rarely involve the epiphysis and often appear trabeculated. Nonossifying fibromas have scalloped medullary margins and are ordinarily not calcified, while a multiplicity of lesions involving both the metaphysis and diaphysis are often seen in fibrous dysplasia. Multiple chondroblastomas were noted in only 1 case among the 88 consultative cases of the Mayo Clinic series (DAHLIN and IVINS, 1972). One case had two lesions. A left talar lesion was curetted in 1964 and another right tarsal navicular tumor in October, 1967. In another case, the tumor was thought to have been implanted in a distant area from which bone graft material had been taken.

An eosinophilic granuloma of bone may be surrounded by a thin sclerotic zone, particularly after radiation or curettage. However, eosinophilic granuloma is rarely epiphyseal and multiple lesions are often found.

Malignant tumors, either primary, such as a lytic form of osteosarcoma, or metastatic are less commonly epiphyseal. The patient's age, the absence of a primary tumor, and the singleness of the lesion, as well as its epiphyseal location, all ordinarily serve to direct one away from a diagnosis of metastatic cancer. Metastases are generally less common below the knees and elbows, while chondroblastoma frequently favors the proximal tibia. Although the possibility of an osteolytic osteosarcoma could be entertained, the usual spherical or ovoid shape of the chondroblastoma, its epiphyseal location, its fairly distinct borders, the absence of any marked degree of cortical thinning and expansion, the paucity of periosteal reaction, and the relatively small size of the lesion all mitigate against a diagnosis of osteosarcoma.

Several reports from countries where bone tuberculosis is common note that chondroblastomas, particularly when occurring at the knee and particularly when associated with a certain amount of periosteal reaction, may mimic tuberculous osteoarthritis (VARMA and GUPTA, 1972; WITWICKI et al., 1969). However, the absence of dependable evidence of a synovitis or joint effusion, the lack of marked deossification at the joint, and the failure to note any joint changes such as narrowing or areas of articular cartilage destruction should arbit against a diagnosis of tuberculosis. Other infections and particularly a Brodie's abscess and/or cystic osteomyelitis would tend to be excluded on similar grounds. Cystic osteomyelitis is rarely confined to the epiphysis and is most commonly situated within the metaphysis.

Giant cell tumor must be considered in the differential diagnosis of chondroblastoma, particularly when long bones are involved. However, giant cell tumor occurs most commonly after the growth plate has closed, and favors the 20–40-year-old age group. The untreated giant cell tumor, unlike most chondroblastomas, does not have a sharply defined sclerotic margin delimiting it from the normal medullary bone, but rather tends to fade imperceptibly into the neighboring bone with irregular, ill-defined boundaries, particularly in the flat bones. Giant cell tumor is roentgenographically visualized as a predominantly lytic lesion and does not have the hazy, mottled appearance so often associated with a chondroid or calcified matrix.

Intraosseous ganglia, though well-defined and subchondral in location, do not calcify.

Aneurysmal bone cysts are most frequently metaphyseal, but may involve the epiphysis, usually after growth plate fusion. They are less well-demarcated, more expansile, do not contain mineral, and are therefore more radiolucent than chondroblastomas, unless fracture with subsequent repair has occurred. Chondroblastomas rarely fracture, however, some chondroblastomas may contain extremely vascular areas which are histologically similar to those seen in aneurysmal bone cysts. These chondroblastomas, unlike most cartilaginous tumors, may be extremely vascular on angiography, leading some authorities to suggest that the vascular component may represent a secondary change engrafted on the pre-existing tumor. Such foci further serve to illustrate the occasional histologic overlap of lesions (JAFFE, 1968).

Another such overlap occurs with chondromyxoid fibroma. Chondromyxoid fibroma is primarily a metaphyseal lesion which infrequently involves the epiphysis. When it does, the bulk of the lesion is seen to be metaphyseal. It usually does not have the mottled or hazy appearance that is so characteristic of a chondroblastoma since chondromyxoid fibromas rarely calcify.

The characteristic roentgen features of a chondroblastoma, therefore, include an eccentric area of bone destruction which is sharply delimited from the surrounding normal bone usually by a thin margin of increased density. There may or may not be an appearance of mottling within the radiolucent area, which is a reflection of its chondroid matrix, with or without associated calcification and/or ossification (Figs. 56, 62). Trabeculation and active periosteal reaction are rarely seen (Fig. 63). The tumor, when it involves the long bones, almost always affects the epiphysis but may extend to the adjacent metaphysis (Figs. 59, 63, 64). Rarely will the shaft be solely involved, when it is, the tumor will usually abut the epiphyseal plate. A smooth well-outlined soft tissue mass is occasionally discernible in association with large tumors which have destroyed the overlying cortical bone by pressure erosion.

VII. Pathologic Findings

1. Gross Features

Amputations or segmental resections are rarely performed for chondroblastomas and therefore intact lesions are rarely studied (Figs. 64, 65). Occasionally published examples of resected specimens have shown good demarcation from surrounding bone (Huvos and Marcove, 1973). Areas of hemorrhage, cysts, and necrosis may be seen (Figs. 65a, b). When present, cysts usually comprise a small proportion of the lesion, tend to be peripherally located and measure less than 1 cm in diameter (Jaffe and Lichtenstein, 1948). Rarely a chondroblastoma may be predominantly cystic with the tumor presenting as a gritty mass at one pole (Oppenheim and Boal, 1955; Spjut et al., 1971). Rarely, large tumors may thin the cortex and/or extend into the adjacent joint space, but it is unusual for the tumor to transgress the articular cartilage.

Large tumors in Dahlin and Ivins (1972) series had a maximum diameter of 15 cm and were clinically of long duration. In 6 of their 125 cases, cystic changes were noted by the surgeon to be so extensive that a simple cyst was simulated. The neoplastic element in these cases was chiefly confined to small peripheral foci. Two of the large cystic neoplasms contained blood (Dahlin and Ivins, 1972). Of the 25 patients of Huvos and Marcove (1973), 6 (24%) were found to have aneurysmal bone cysts associated with primary chondroblastomas. Among 9 recurrent lesions, 5 or 56% had demonstrable aneurysmal bone cysts, including all 3 with multiple recurrences (Huvos et al., 1972).

Bone is an uncommon component within the tumor, although the bone surrounding may be slightly sclerotic (Gravanis and Giansanti, 1971).

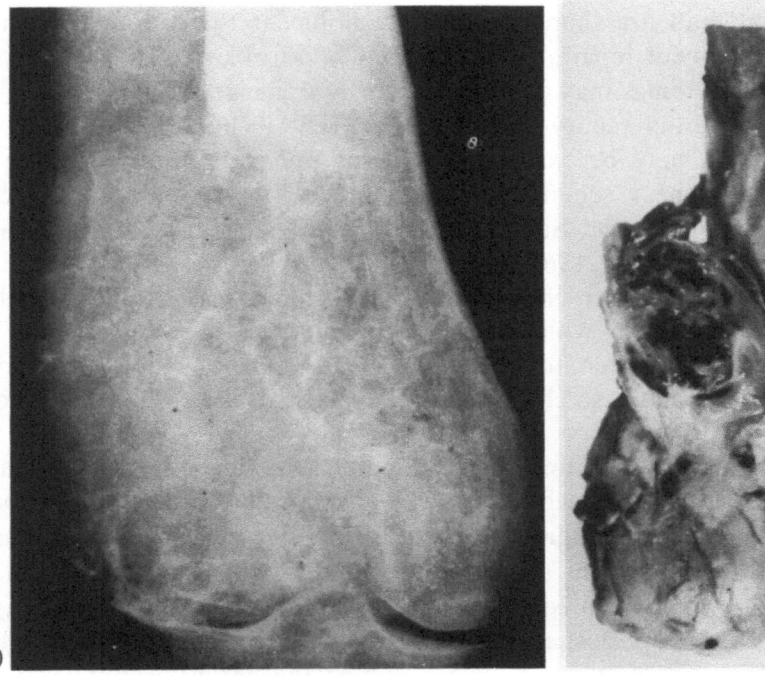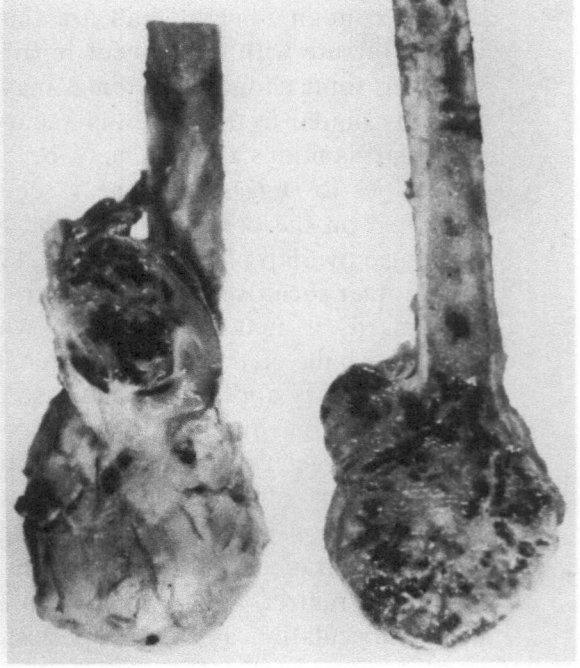

(a)   (b)

Fig. 64a and b. Chondroblastoma, femur: Roentgenogram (a) and hemisection (b) of 32-year-old woman with extensive epiphyseal and metaphyseal involvement. Expansion and destruction of cortical bone together with cystic and hemorrhagic necrosis are grossly evident. (Courtesy of A.G. Huvos, M.D., R.C. Marcove, M.D., R.A. Erlandson, Ph.D. and V. Miké, Ph.D.)

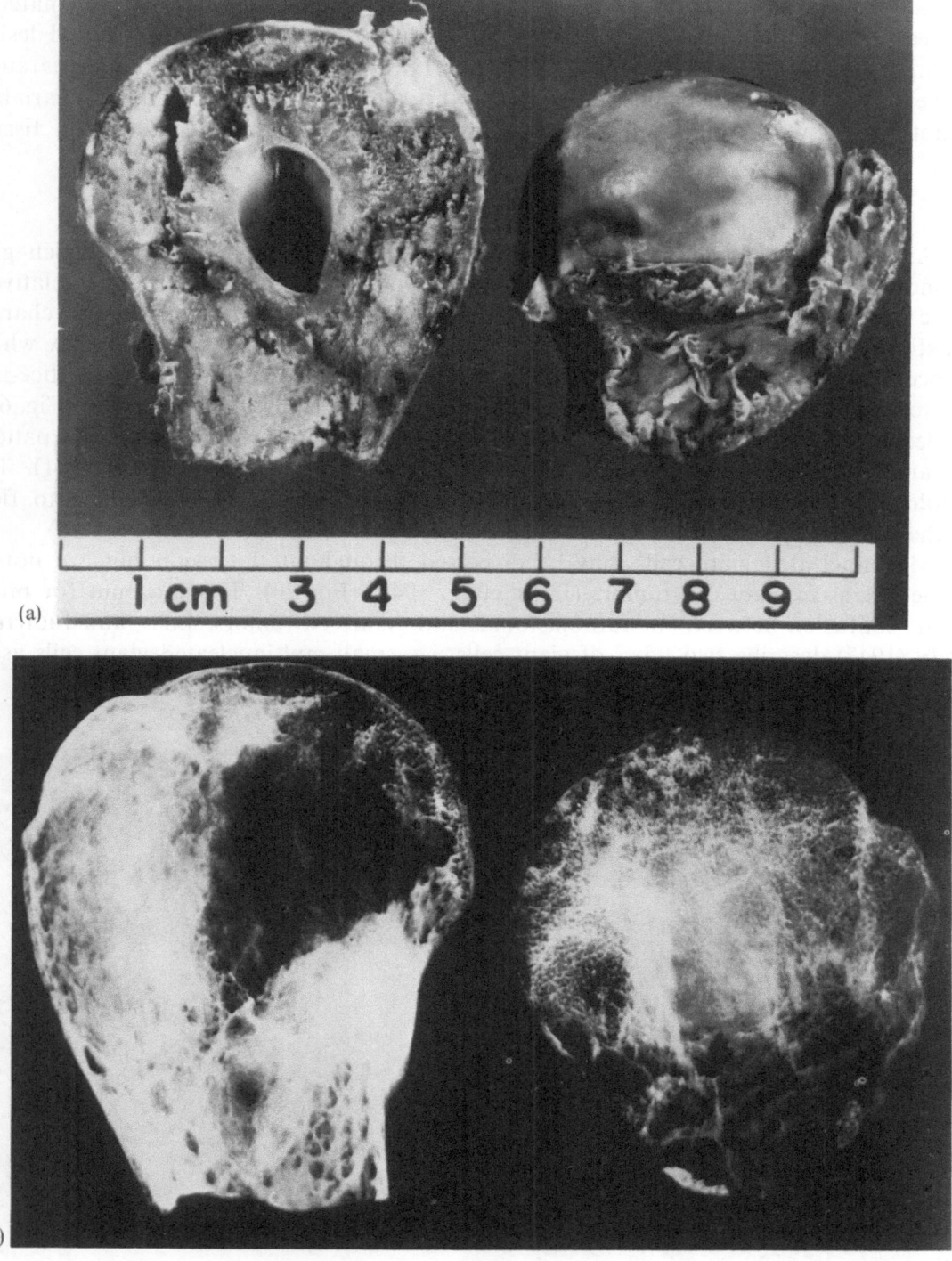

Fig. 65a and b. Chondroblastoma, humerus: Gross hemisection (a) and roentgenogram (b) of resected specimen of humeral head of 33-year-old woman. Central chondrification and cyst formation are noted. (Courtesy of A.G. Huvos, M.D., R.C. Marcove, M.D., R.A. Erlandson, Ph.D., and V. Miké, Ph.D.)

The characteristic consistency of curettings vary from soft to gritty, depending upon the amount of calcification or ossification present. Flecks of gritty calcific material or recognizable bluish-grey cartilaginous fragments coming from an epiphyseal lesion strongly suggest chondroblastoma (DAHLIN and IVINS, 1972). A cartilaginous appearance, however, may be inconspicuous or absent and the calcific component is similarly variable. Curettings may be friable and red or grey or brown, simulating granulation tissue.

2. Microscopic

As seen by light microscopy, the cells considered to be chondroblasts, which give chondroblastoma its distinctiveness, are usually polygonal or rounded with a relatively large nucleus. Nucleoli are common. The cells are commonly polyhedral in shape, characteristically uniform, closely packed, and separated by a scanty interstitial matrix which is occasionally frankly chondroid in its makeup (Figs. 66–68). A delicate lattice-like intercellular calcification resembling a picket fence or chicken wire may be seen (Fig. 69). A clearly defined cell membrane is an aid to diagnosis. However, since the cell pattern is varied, the cell membranes are not viewed in every field (SPJUT et al., 1971). The cytologic pattern not only varies from specimen to specimen but from field to field in the same specimen, reflecting the evolutionary cycle of the lesion (Figs. 69, 70).

Multinucleated giant cells may be dispersed throughout the lesion but are not as numerous as in giant cell tumors (JAFFE et al., 1940) (Fig. 70). They account for much of the confusion between chondroblastomas and giant cell tumors. JAFFE and LICHTEN-STEIN (1942) describe two types of giant cells, i.e. small multinucleated giant cells asso-

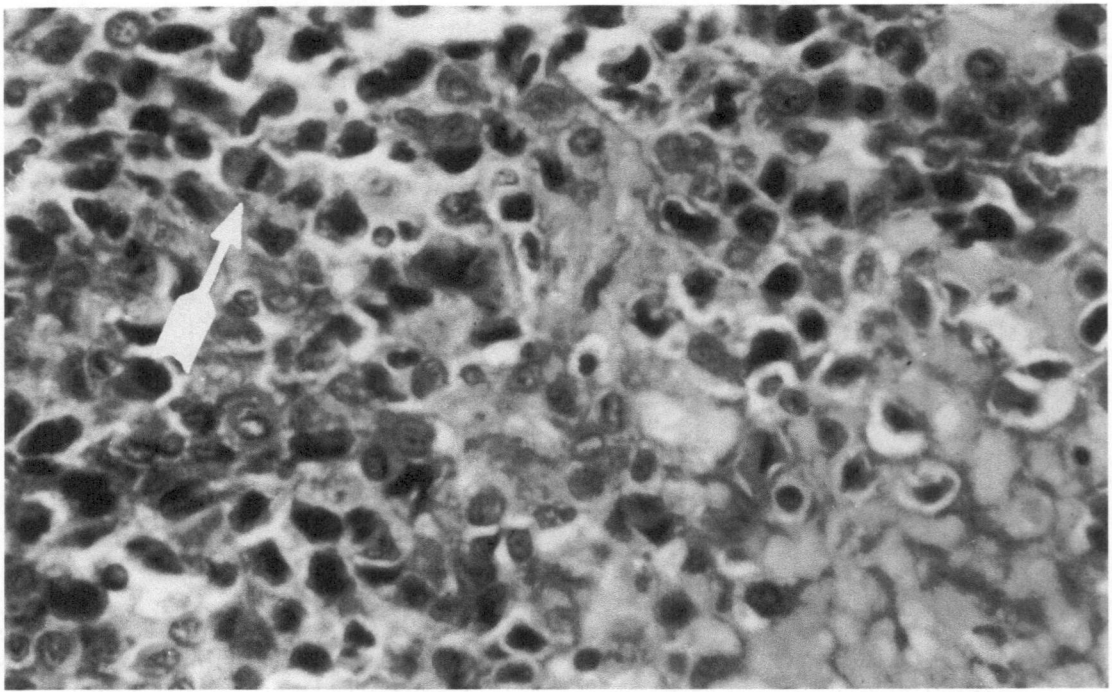

Fig. 66. Chondroblastoma photomicrograph (× 50): Note chondroid matrix in lower right. Some cells have disappeared. Viable cells are polyhedral and remain individually distinct. Mitotic figure is seen above left (arrow). There is sufficient atypism to raise histologic suspicion of malignancy. Lesion was biologically benign. (Courtesy AUSTIN D. JOHNSTON, M.D.)

ciated with the tumor component and reactive, foreign body type giant cells, which are larger, multinucleated and which they regard as multinucleated macrophages seen in association with areas of hemorrhagic necrosis. GRAVANIS and GIANSANTI (1971) also state that the giant cells seen in chondroblastomas are not derived from chondroblastic cells but rather represent osteoclasts or foreign body giant cells.

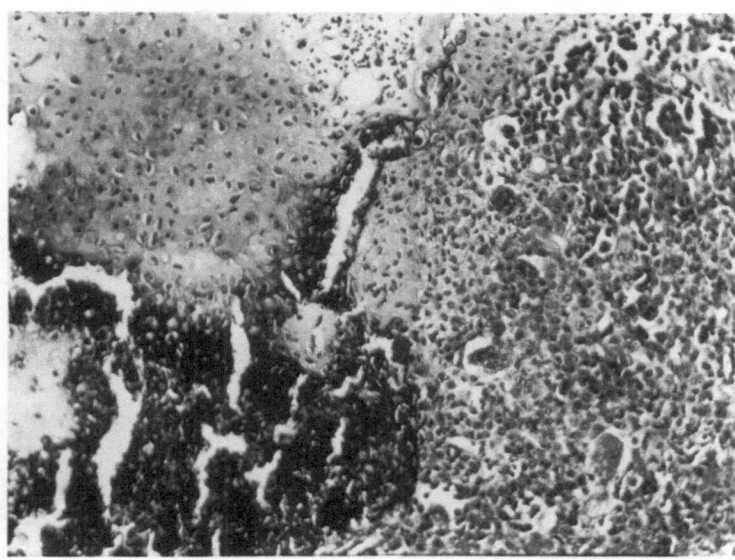

Fig. 67. Chondroblastoma (×150): Typical histological appearance with chondroid matrix in upper half and dark zone of calcification below. (Courtesy of DAVID D. DAHLIN, M.D.)

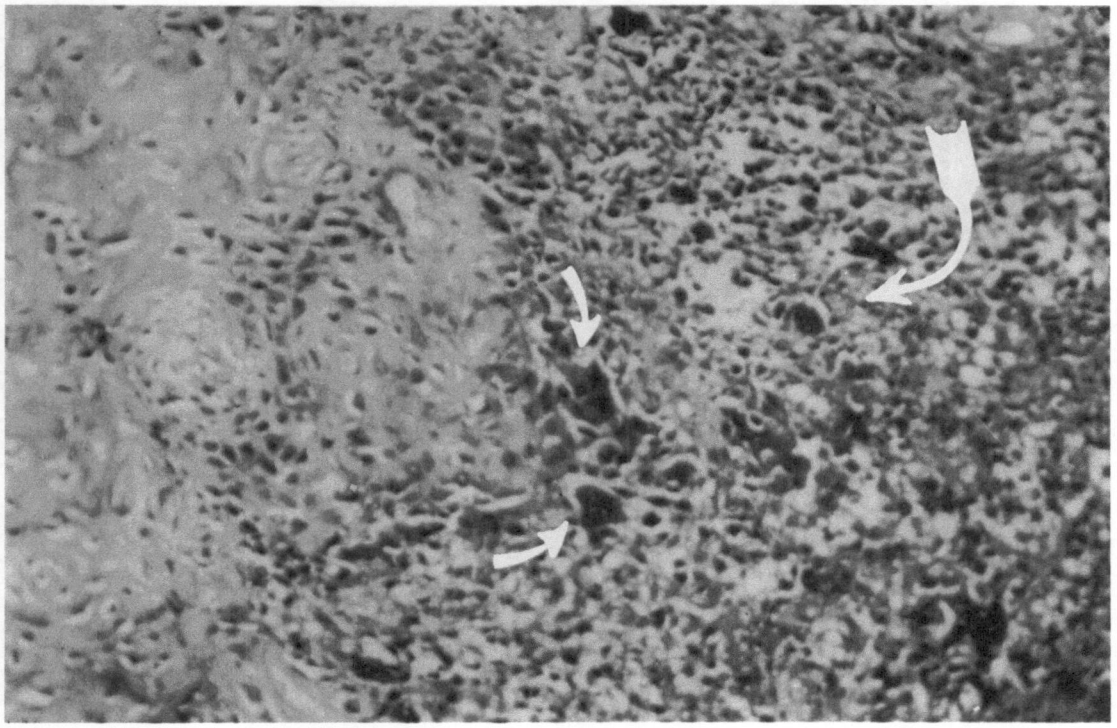

Fig. 68. Recurrent chondroblastoma, photomicrograph (×75): Interface between chondroid matrix (left) and cellular portions of tumor (right) is often delineated by giant cells resembling osteoclasts (small arrows, left) and differing from tumor giant cells (large arrow, right). (Courtesy of AUSTIN D. JOHNSTON, M.D.)

Large aneurysmally dilated blood vessels may be seen at the periphery of the tumor (Fig. 71). They were observed in 24% of 25 cases of Huvos and Marcove (1973) who felt that they were associated with an increased propensity for recurrence (Huvos et al., 1972). Dahlin and Ivins (1972) noted cystic changes in 20 of their tumors. In many instances the "cystic" spaces contained much blood. These lesions tended to bleed

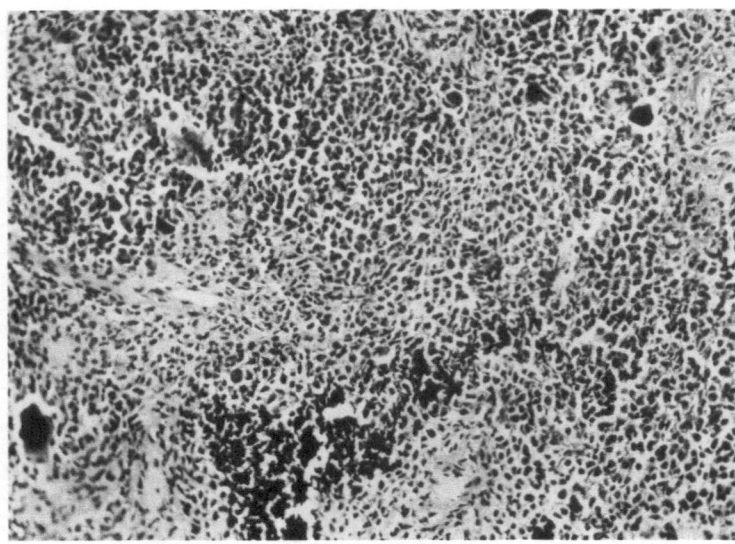

Fig. 69. Chondroblastoma, photomicrograph (×160): Scattered multinucleated giant cells, focal areas of calcification, and scanty interstitial matrix are typical constituents of this lesion. Calcific deposits in matrix frequently outline empty lacunae, producing a "lace-like" or "chicken-wire" configuration that is highly characteristic of this tumor. Clumps of mineralized material (upper field) are occasionally seen. (Courtesy of David C. Dahlin, M.D.)

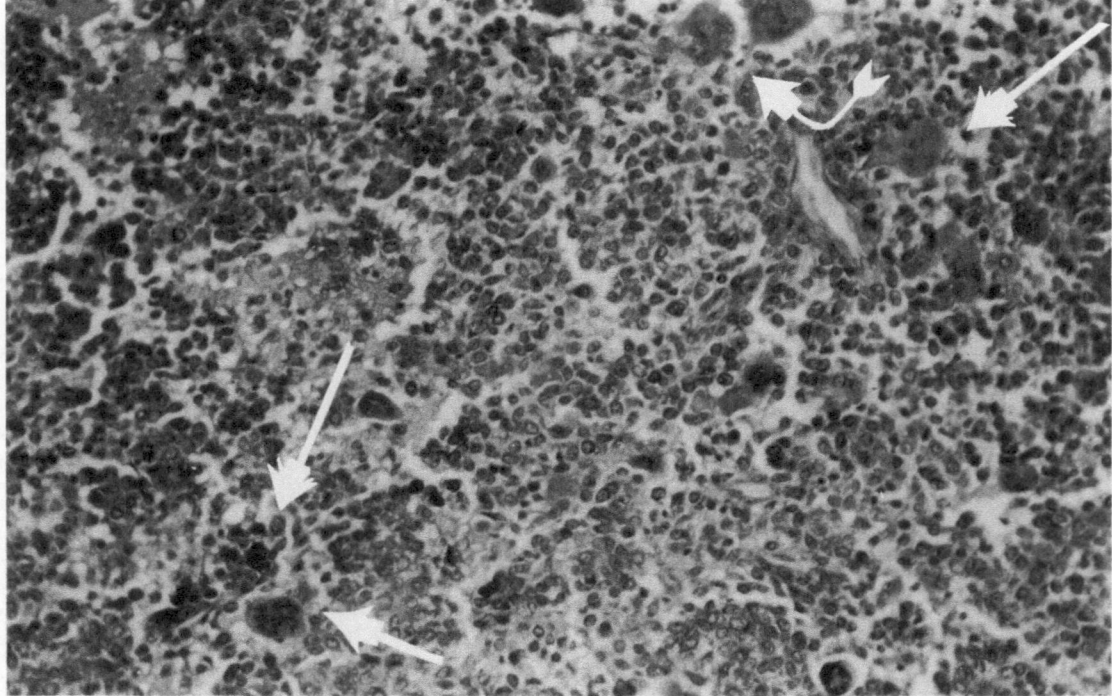

Fig. 70. Chondroblastoma, photomicrograph (×75): Some chondroblastomas contain zones markedly similar to those found in giant cell tumors, but mononuclear cells remain discrete and not pseudo-syncytial as in giant cell tumor. Note numerous multinucleated giant cells dispersed throughout lesion (arrows). (Courtesy of Austin D. Johnston, M.D.)

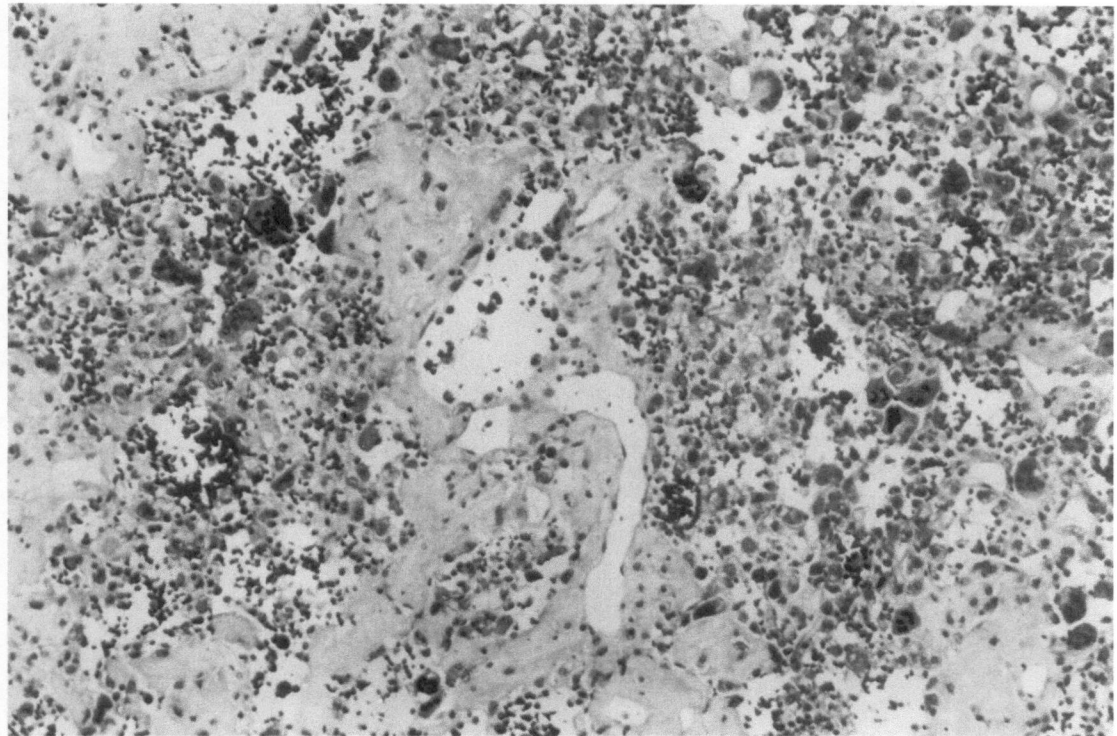

Fig. 71. Chondroblastoma with associated aneurysmal bone cyst formation. Photomicrograph (× 100): Chondro-blastomas may contain zones indistinguishable from aneurysmal bone cyst. While some authorities have included such lesions among their aneurysmal bone cysts, most prefer to designate lesion according to well-established underlying process, in this case chondroblastoma. (Courtesy of A.G. Huvos, M.D. and R.C. Marcove, M.D.)

heavily at the time of surgery. Although some have included such lesions among their aneurysmal bone cysts, others refer to them merely as cystic chondroblastomas (Dahlin and Ivins, 1972; Shajowicz and Gallardo, 1970). Fibrous tissue or less often bands of neoplastic cells may form the walls of partitions of such cystic spaces and Dahlin and Ivins (1972) prefer to designate the lesion according to the underlying process, i.e. as a chondroblastoma. They make note of the hypervascularity as a secondary phenomenon. Other lesions such as giant cell tumors, fibrous dysplasias, giant cell repara-tive granulomas, and simple cysts may often contain such zones, which in themselves are indistinguishable from aneurysmal bone cysts (Fig. 71).

The designation of a tumor as a chondroblastoma depends on the finding of foci of typically rounded cells in a chondroid matrix. These foci, however, may be sparse and not evident in every section of the tumor, or they may be so numerous as to dominate the histologic findings to such an extent that large portions of the tumor resemble chondromas or chondrosarcomas. The constituent cartilage cells of chondrosar-coma are often binucleate and hyperchromatic and set in a well-defined intracellular matrix. The rounded or polyhedral cells or so-called chondroblasts have been considered by some to be cytologically specific for chondroblastoma, but Dahlin and Ivins have seen morphologically identical cells in a few other lesions, and particularly in benign giant cell tumors. Therefore, prominent zones where these cells are arranged in sheets and particularly those without cartilage, may closely mimic giant cell tumors (Vanden-berg and Coley, 1950). Mitotic figures are sparse.

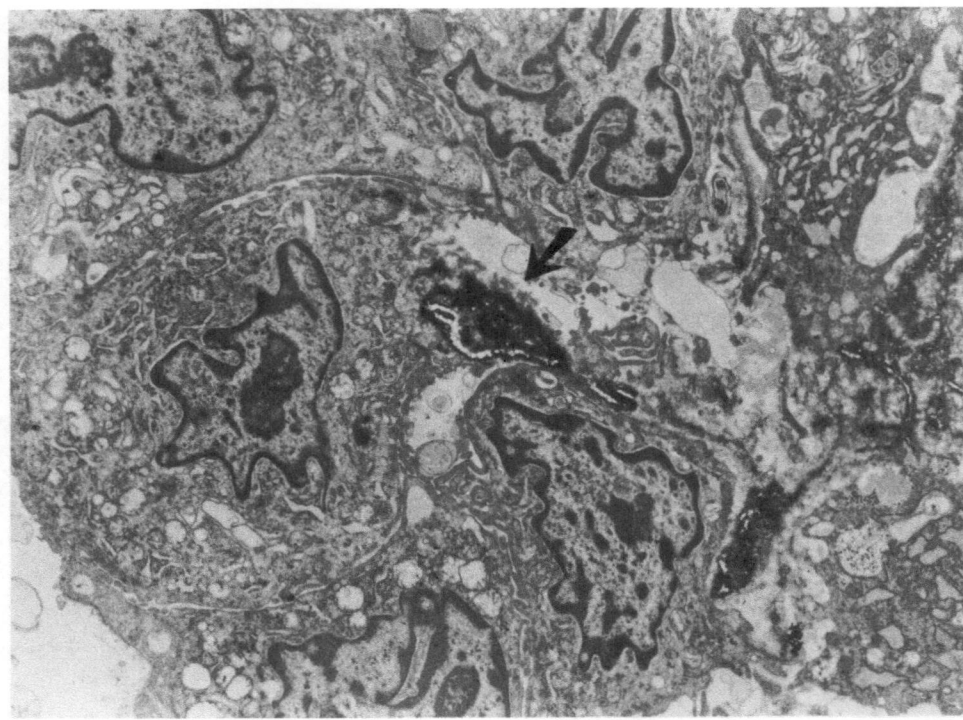

Fig. 72. Chondroblastoma, electron microscopic section (×6300): Atypical chondroblasts surround focus of calcification (arrow). Note highly indented nuclei. (Courtesy of A.G. Huvos, M.D., R.C. Marcove, M.D., R.A. Erlandson, Ph.D., and V. Miké, M.D.)

Calcification is an outstanding histologic feature of chondroblastoma (Figs. 67, 72). It is invariably present in the cellular areas of the tumor both within and between the cells. Whenever this calcification is particularly heavy, the tumor cells swell and undergo degeneration and necrosis like cartilage cells undergoing calcification preparatory to osseous transformation. Jaffe and Lichtenstein (1948) noted that this calcification is primary and that accompanying tumor necrosis is secondary to it. In the wake of the latter, and as part of the reparative process which includes resorption of calcific detritus and organization of hemorrhage, connective tissue replacement of necrotic fields may be seen. This connective tissue may assume the form of collagenous plaques sometimes resembling chondroid or osteoid matrix. The latter may go on to active osseous transformation.

Dystrophic calcification in cartilage islands was observed in two-thirds of the 125 cases of Dahlin and Ivins (1972). The calcific deposits in the matrix ordinarily outlined empty lacunae, producing what they also describe as a lace-like or chicken-wire pattern that is highly characteristic of this tumor (Dahlin and Ivins, 1972; Huvos and Marcove, 1973) (Fig. 69). Occasionally amorphous clumps of mineralized material are seen.

Ossification not associated with dystrophic tissue, but contained within cartilage islands, may also be seen in some cases. Such ossification may cause chondroblastomas to be confused with primary osteoblastic lesions including osteosarcomas. Sections from the periphery of the tumors also often show new bone formation, especially in relation to the surrounding cancellous trabeculae.

Another "histologic overlap" has been advocated by Dahlin (1956, 1967) who has noted that, "Chondromyxoid fibroma-like zones are seen in a few chondroblastomas, while chondroblastoma-like islands are not uncommon especially in the interlobular portions of chondromyxoid fibromas." He has postulated that a relationship exists between benign chondroblastoma and chondromyxoid fibroma, and has suggested that both lesions have their origins in cells of the growth plate (TURCOTTE et al., 1962). However, only in the rare case is it difficult to decide in which category a tumor belongs.

JAFFE (1948) has stressed the distinction between the two lesions, emphasizing that chondroblastoma originates in the epiphysis, that it is predominantly epiphyseal in location, that metaphyseal involvement is secondary, i.e. rarely has the bulk of a chondroblastoma been centered in the metaphysis, and that microscopic evidence of calcification is common in chondroblastomas and unusual in chondromyxoid fibromas.

It is therefore possible to histologically confuse benign chondroblastomas with a number of other lesions, including malignant neoplasms, such as chondrosarcoma and osteosarcoma, as well as with benign chondroma, giant cell tumor, and chondromyxoid fibroma. As noted by DAHLIN and IVINS (1972), "Mistaking benign chondroblastoma for a malignant tumor, especially a chondrosarcoma or an osteosarcoma is still possible. This occurred in two of the early cases in the Mayo Clinic series." However, an awareness of the histologic range of this tumor should obviate this problem, for all but the very rare atypical lesions.

3. Electron Microscopic Findings

Similar electron microscopic findings have been described when studying cells taken from different chondroblastomas (HUVOS et al., 1972; WELLMAN, 1969; WELSH and MEYER, 1964). Chondroblasts are larger, more spherical, and have a greater nucleus to cytoplasmic ratio than chondrocytes seen in normal human cartilage, and they are smaller, less differentiated and generally not as irregularly shaped as the cells seen in chondrosarcoma. In chondrosarcomas, many tumor cells were still contained within well-defined lacunae, and resembled chondroma cells and normal chondrocytes more closely than chondroblasts.

Other ultrastructural features of chondroblastoma cells include cytoplasmic-blunted microvillous processes, continuous dense bands of nuclear substance along the inner nuclear membrane, the frequent occurrence of multilobed nuclei, and large nucleoli. Glycogen particles, as well as small bundles of cytoplasmic filaments, characterize the cytoplasm of the tumor cells (Figs. 72, 73).

VIII. Treatment and Results

Since in the vast majority of cases chondroblastoma exhibits a benign clinical behavior, conservative therapy has usually been advocated. Curettage, with or without bone grafting, or local excision, preferably en bloc, together with an uninvolved zone of normal tissue as appropriate to the size and site of the lesion, or curettage combined with radiation therapy, have all been employed (AEGERTER and KIRKPATRICK, 1968; DAHLIN and IVINS, 1972; HUVOS and MARCOVE, 1973; HUVOS et al., 1972). Some authorities stress that radiation should not be employed in view of its inherent risk and the generally good results obtained with conservative therapy. Radiation has been advocated when a surgical approach is impossible, after local aggressive recurrence, and when implantation has occurred within the joint space (DAHLIN and IVINS, 1972; SCHAUWECKER et al., 1969).

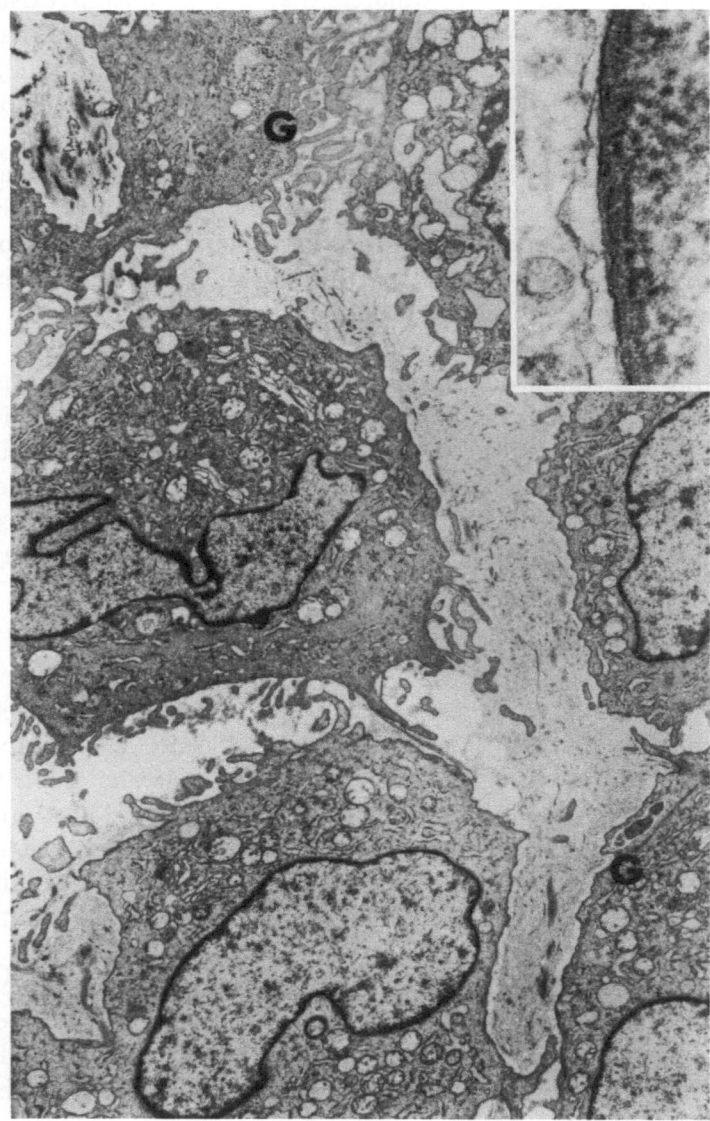

Fig. 73. Chondroblastoma, electron microscopic section (× 8000): Typical chondroblasts surrounded by matrix. Glycogen (*G*). Insert (upper right) shows fibrous lamina at high magnification (× 90,000). (Courtesy of A.G. Huvos, M.D., R.C. Marcove, M.D., R.A. Erlandson, Ph.D. and V. Miké, Ph.D.)

Several case reports (Case Records of Massachusetts General Hospital, 1964; Dahlin and Ivins, 1972; Huvos and Marcove, 1973; Huvos et al., 1972) document aggressive recurrence with neighboring soft tissue involvement. This is felt to be related to spillage and seeding of tumor cells during the course of the initial surgical intervention. This eventuality may even necessitate amputation despite the fact that true malignant transformation has not occurred (Kahn et al., 1969; Sundaram, 1966).

Huvos et al. (1972) reported recurrence rates among 25 patients treated with different modalities (excluding amputation, block excision, and irradiation) on a 3 year basis, since all but one of the recurrences occurred within 3 years of treatment (Fig. 63). A 25% recurrence rate for curettage plus packing with bone chips, as opposed to a rate of 60% with curettage alone, suggested that bone packing was beneficial. Patients treated by cryosurgery also had a lower recurrence rate than those who had curettage alone, but the difference was not statistically significant due to the small number of cases in each group. They also noted that chondroblastoma without associated aneurysmal bone cysts yielded a 20% 3-year postoperative recurrence rate, while patients in whom chondroblastoma was associated with an aneurysmal bone cyst had a 100% recurrence rate. The overall recurrence rate for chondroblastoma was 38%, a higher figure than that reported in other series. This was explained by the fact that several patients had been referred with clinically evident recurrent lesions.

Curettage effected cure in about 90% of 125 cases of benign chondroblastoma reviewed by the Mayo Clinic (DAHLIN and IVINS, 1972). Good results were obtained by conservative means in all cases involving the extermities. Treatment consisted chiefly of curettage with or without bone grafting in the Mayo Clinic patients, i.e. 38 of the 125 cases reviewed. A large number of lesions occurred in the pelvic bones (18%), again possibly the result of selection of difficult cases for referral. Their favorite therapy for chondroblastoma in expendable bones or portions of bones was en bloc resection when feasible. In other sites, wide exteriorization was recommended, so that complete excision by curettage and cautery could be accomplished under direct vision. Conservative surgery for recurrence, even with neighboring soft tissue implants, was favored over amputation "since the risk of metastases is negligible unless sarcomatous change has occurred" (DAHLIN and IVINS, 1972).

Although chondroblastoma generally has an essentially benign clinical behavior, a few cases with a more aggressive or malignant course have been documented. Several of these, however, share a common denominator of previous radiotherapy. The case of HATCHER and CAMPBELL (1951) developed chondrosarcoma in an area previously diagnosed as a chondroblastoma of the upper humerus. The malignancy, however, occurred 4 years post radiation therapy and was considered to be radiation produced. STEINER (1965) also documented a sarcoma that occurred at the site of irradiation and another post radiation sarcoma was mentioned by RAVAULT et al. (1969). A chondroblastoma of the pelvis in the Mayo Clinic series was felt to have possibly become malignant after biopsy and irradiation. It is, therefore, felt by some authorities that these lesions are more properly classified as radiation induced sarcomas (DAHLIN and IVINS, 1972; HATCHER and CAMPBELL, 1951; KAHN et al., 1969; RAVAULT et al., 1969; STEINER, 1965).

The NETHERLANDS COMMITTEE ON BONE TUMORS (1966) noted the development of metastasizing and fatal fibrosarcoma 14 years after apparently successful curettage of a benign chondroblastoma. No irradiation had been employed. Undifferentiated sarcoma developed in another case nearly 6 years after the first of three conservative operations and no irradiation, as noted by SIRSAT and DOCTOR (1970). This case is included in the series of SCHAJOWICZ and GALLARDO (1970), as well as a case in which they could not prove that the tumor was not an atypical primary malignant cartilage tumor de novo. Therefore, of the seven cases noted above, four had a previous history of radiotherapy employed in the treatment of a primary benign chondroblastoma, one developed a fibrosarcoma 14 years later which could have developed de novo, and one developed an undifferentiated sarcoma 6 years after conservative treatment for an apparently benign chondroblastoma.

Other instances of so-called malignant transformation of benign chondroblastoma may have been diagnosed as a result of local soft tissue recurrence or extension which is probably related to tumor spillage during surgical intervention, without necessarily representing a true malignant transformation of an underlying benign neoplasm. This misinterpretation is even more likely to be made if there is more than one recurrence. Benign chondroblastomas may also be mistaken for other primary malignant tumors, especially chondrosarcomas or osteosarcomas, as occurred in two of the early cases in the Mayo Clinic series. Conversely, they also made note of four primary sarcomas in which the histologic appearance strongly suggested chondroblastoma on initial study.

Actual metastases from benign chondroblastoma have been documented with actual autopsy findings in one case (KAHN et al., 1969) 15 years after the first of four ineffectual curettages and partial resections of a primary tumor in the pelvic bone.

Metastases involved the lung, pleura, diaphragm, liver, and subcutaneous tissues. The metastatic nodules had the typical microscopic features of a chondroblastoma. Another case reported in the same article (KAHN et al., 1969) was that of a 14-year-old girl with a distal femoral lesion which was twice treated by curettage and bone grafting. A midthigh amputation was done 19 months later due to local lymphatic dissemination. There were no metastases after 18 months. The former case, as well as several others (COPELAND and GESCHICKTER, 1949) have been considered by some to have been chondrosarcoma from the outset (SHERMAN and SHERMAN, 1971). Another metastasizing chondroblastoma reported by SWEETNAM and ROSS (1967) has not generally been accepted since it was not described histologically nor was it illustrated. COPELAND and GESCHICKTER (1949) recognized two types of chondroblastoma, i.e. benign and "malignant" chondroblastomas, implying that they have a common origin and possibly transitions and reported that 15 of their 25 cases of chondroblastoma were malignant. Such a high percentage of malignant cases is quite contrary to the experience of all others who have dealt with this lesion and their evidence in the form of three published photomicrographs was felt to be unconvincing by some authorities (COLEMAN, 1966; KAHN et al., 1969). LICHTENSTEIN (1965), in commenting on the concept of COPELAND and GESCHICKTER, noted that "their malignant chondroblastomas so-called are actually frank chondrosarcomas readily distinguishable from benign chondroblastomas." LICHTENSTEIN and BERNSTEIN (1959) have recently observed a small number of neoplasms that they have classified as "atypical chondroblastomas" which behaved in an aggressive fashion (VARMA and GUPTA, 1972).

In general, chondroblastoma is felt by most authorities to be an essentially benign bone tumor. Atypical sarcomas, especially chondrosarcomas, may mimic chondroblastoma in rare instances but there is no convincing evidence for a primary malignant chondroblastoma. Conservative surgical removal is nearly always effective. It is recommended that the patient be followed so that recurrences which are occasionally aggressive may be detected early. The tumor may respond favorably to radiation therapy and may be cured by it. However, radiotherapy should be employed only for surgically inaccessible lesions. Late sarcomatous change has been reported in a few cases, whether radiation therapy was employed or not. The two metastasizing benign chondroblastomas that were documented are pathologic rarities.

J. Chondromyxoid Fibroma

This benign tumor of bone was established as an entity in 1948 when it was first described by JAFFE and LICHTENSTEIN. It occurs less frequently than chondroblastoma. It constitutes approximately 2% of benign bone tumors and less than 1% of all benign plus malignant bone tumors (DAHLIN, 1956, 1967; FELDMAN et al., 1970; GOLDANICH, 1957; IWATA and COLEY, 1958; RAHIMI et al., 1972; SCHAJOWICZ and GALLARDO, 1971). The incidence in SCHAJOWICZ and GALLARDO's (1971) series was somewhat lower than

1% for all tumoral and tumor-like lesions and somewhat less than half of all chondroblastomas observed in the same time period. Recent additions to our previous tabulation of 207 cases in 1970 (FELDMAN et al., 1970) include 32 cases from 10 Latin American countries (SCHAJOWICZ and GALLARDO, 1971), 11 cases reported by the NETHERLANDS COMMITTEE ON BONE TUMORS (1966), 41 by the BONE TUMOR COMMITTEE of the JAPANESE ORTHOPEDIC ASSOCIATION, NATIONAL CANCER CENTER (1966), and 4 cases from the Mayo Clinic included in a study of 76 cases, most of which had previously been tabulated (RAHIMI et al., 1972). There have been several scattered case reports (RYALL, 1970; SACHDEVA et al., 1969).

Most authors have emphasized the distinct histologic characteristics as well as the benign clinical behavior of this lesion, despite recurrences (DAHLIN, 1956; FRANK and ROCKWOOD, 1969; JAFFE and LICHTENSTEIN, 1948; SCHAJOWICZ and GALLARDO, 1976; SPJUT et al., 1971; TURCOTTE et al., 1962) a more aggressive course in the young (RALPH, 1962; SCAGLIETTI and STRINGA, 1961) and a few reports of malignant transformation (AEGERTER and KIRKPATRICK, 1968; IWATA and COLEY, 1958), some of which have not been universally accepted. Others have separated off histologic subgroups from chondromyxoid fibroma such as myxoma of bone (BAUER and HARRELL, 1954; SCAGLIETTI and STRINGA, 1961) and fibromyxoma of bone (MARCOVE et al., 1964), which have also not been universally accepted.

An interrelationship between chondromyxoid fibroma and chondroblastoma (DAHLIN, 1956; RALPH, 1962; WILLIS, 1967) has also been postulated with both tumors presumably arising from epiphyseal plate cells; one lesion growing towards the metaphysis and the other towards the epiphysis. Individual cases with microscopy reminiscent of both lesions have been cited. JAFFE (1965, 1968), however, did not accept this as evidence for a morphologic interrelationship, stating that "although one may encounter sporadic microscopic fields in some chondromyxoid fibromas in which groups of cells resemble those of benign chondroblastoma, one does not see spotty calcification within these tissue fields, such as are characteristic of benign chondroblastoma."

Recently, LICHTENSTEIN and BERNSTEIN (1959) reported several unusual chondroid tumors of bone noting a number of solitary, well-localized, benign bone tumors which defied precise diagnosis and displayed a considerable range of structure. They described seven cases of chondromyxoid fibroma with histologic variations such as indistinct lobulation, greater cellularity, and fields of undifferentiated cells, which led them to be designated as atypical chondromyxoid fibroma. Four of these seven contained focal calcification, reminiscent of benign chondroblastoma. LICHTENSTEIN and BERNSTEIN, however, also emphasized, as JAFFE (1965, 1968) did, that the histologic diagnosis of any bone tumor should be based on its predominant tissue pattern and reiterated that these two lesions should be viewed as distinct clinical pathologic entities. In the vast majority of cases most experienced bone pathologists recognize chondromyxoid fibroma as a lesion with distinct characteristics and assert their ability to distinguish typical examples from chondroblastoma (DAHLIN, 1967; LICHTENSTEIN and GOLDMAN, 1964). Its complex histologic range, however, has, on occasion, been the source of confusion, not only with chondroblastoma, but with chondrosarcoma and particularly chondrosarcoma with myxomatous degeneration, with resultant unduly aggressive management. Chondrosarcoma, however, is a diagnosis which is particularly suspect in the young and is an unusual lesion in the age group which chondromyxoid fibroma tends to favor.

A small number of cases of chondromyxoid fibroma have reputedly undergone malignant transformation. However, a review of the original biopsy material by other authorities has not always supported this contention. It is of interest in this regard that four cases included in DAHLIN'S (1956) review had previously been reported as malignant tumors, while three of JAFFE and LICHTENSTEIN's (1948) original eight cases of chondromyxoid fibroma had been carried as chondrosarcomas in their files prior to their identification of this entity in 1948. Recently, LICHTENSTEIN (1965) has described a small number of atypical chondromyxoid fibromas as well as chondroblastomas which have behaved in a more aggressive fashion locally. However, DAHLIN has noted that the evidence overwhelmingly indicates that the risk of malignant transformation of "bona fide chondromyxoid fibroma," unless radiation is employed, is so slight that radical treatment is unnecessary (RAHIMI et al., 1972).

Recognition of this uncommon lesion is, therefore, important not only from the standpoint of its histologic and clinical features, which on occasion may be misleading and ominous, but from a roentgen standpoint, since it is one of those bone lesions in which the roentgenogram may be decisive in tempering a histologic impression of malignancy.

I. Age and Sex

Ages of patients have reputedly ranged from 4–79 years (SALZER et al., 1968). LICHTENSTEIN has seen only a single case in a child below the age of 10. 57% of patients, were less than 30 years old. It is believed (SALZER et al., 1968) that a slow clinical evolution and a subtle unappreciated onset of symptoms account for the lesions discovered in older people. As opposed to chondroblastoma, which has a male predominance, chondromyxoid fibroma has shown no significant sex predilection.

II. Clinical Features

Complaints were nonspecific. In the majority of cases, pain, most often mild, local, and intermittent had been present from months to years prior to consultation. Most were aware of swelling and/or a mass, in view of the lesion's commonly peripheral location, i.e. about the knee. Occasional tenderness to palpation, limp, and slight limitation of motion were also noted. However, in one series of five children, 5–10 years of age, pain, swelling, and restricted motion developed within 3–6 weeks, leading to speculation that the lesion may be more aggressive in the young (SCAGLIETTI and STRINGA, 1961).

Asymptomatic lesions have been discovered on roentgenograms taken routinely or because of a history of trauma. Trauma does not seem to be related to the pathologic process. Pathologic fracture, per se, was a rarity. It was noted in one case in our experience (FELDMAN et al., 1970) and in nine other cases (HERFARTH, 1932; LETTIN, 1963; SETH and RAO, 1964; SIDEMAN et al., 1960–61; TURCOTTE et al., 1962). Four pathologic fractures are mentioned in the recent Mayo Clinic review which may have been included in our previous compilation (RAHIMI et al., 1972). Therefore, either 10 or 14 pathologic fractures have been noted among 295 cases, an incidence of 3–4%.

The duration of pain among 76 patients in the Mayo Clinic series (RAHIMI et al., 1972) ranged from 2 weeks to 132 months. Its onset coincided with pathologic fracture in 3 cases. Swelling was recognized by a minority of patients, from 2–72 months with an average of 10 months prior to consultation. Six lesions, i.e. two costal, two in the ilium, one in the ischium, and one in the occiput were asymptomatic and found incidentally on roentgenograms in their series. A few were known to have been present for several years prior to treatment.

Table 5. Chondromyxoid fibroma. Sites of 363 cases

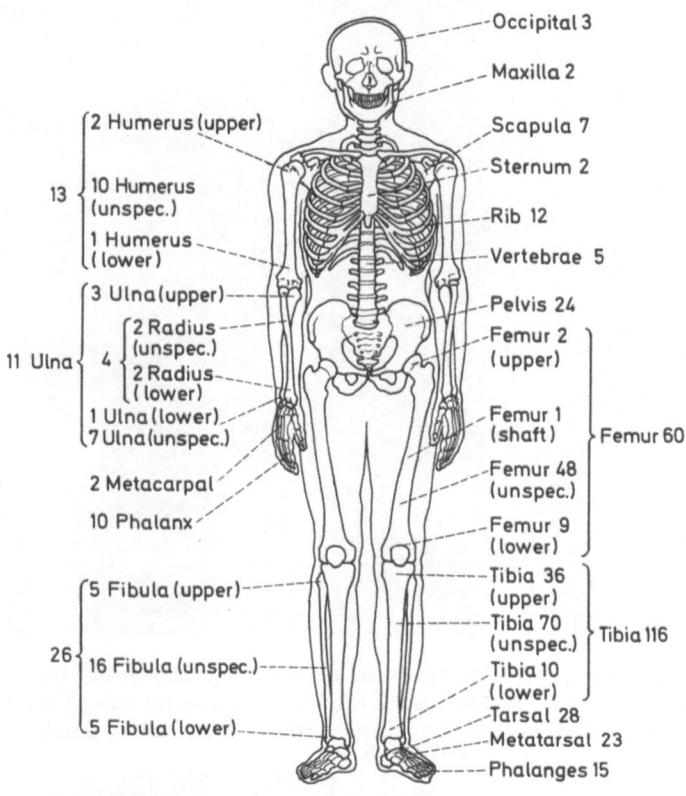

Anterior view of human skeleton
Anterior view of human skeleton

Data from DUTT et al., 1969; FELDMAN et al., 1970; FRANK and ROCKWOOD, 1969; MIKULOWSKI and ÖSTBERG, 1971; MURPHY and PRICE, 1971; Netherlands Committe on Bone Tumors, 1966; PISAR, 1969; RAHIMI et al., 1972; RAMINI, 1974; RYALL, 1970; SCHAJOWICZ and GALLARDO, 1971; SCHUTT and FROST, 1971, SPJUT et al., 1971

III. Sites of Localization

Sites of localization as noted in several major series are shown in Table 5. A chondromyxoid fibroma is most commonly located in the metaphyseal region of a large tubular bone of a lower limb at a variable distance from the epiphyseal line and often in contact with it (Figs. 74a, b). The preferred site appears to be the upper tibia. It is of interest that SCHAJOWICZ and GALLARDO (1971) had no case involving the distal femur, a frequent site in most series. This tumor has only recently been recognized in such sites as the mandible (SCHUTT and FROST), sternum (TEITELBAUM and BESSONE, 1969), rib, (GOORWITCH, 1951; RAMINI, 1974), and vertebral column (BENSON and BASS, 1955; RAMINI, 1974; SCHAJOWICZ and GALLARDO, 1971). We are including a third lesion in the vertebral column (Figs. 75a, b). This was responsible for spinal cord compression as in a previous case involving the spine (BENSON and BASS, 1955) and one of a rib (RAMINI, 1974). The rib lesion occurred in a 44-year-old man. A case reported as a giant chondromyxoid fibroma of the sternum which included an illustration of the histology was not acceptable to RAHIMI et al. (1972) who felt that the histology was suggestive of a chondrosarcoma. A chondromyxoid fibroma of the occipital bone in RAHIMI's series was noted to be the first recorded example of such a lesion in the skull. No report of carpal bone involvement has been noted.

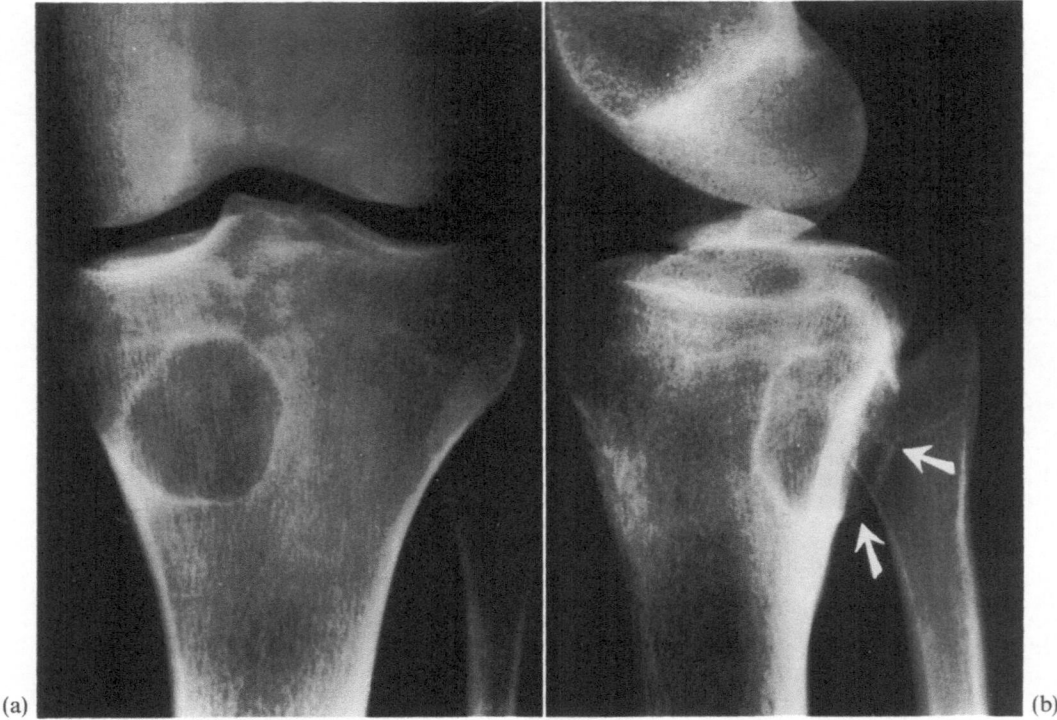

(a)

(b)

Fig. 74a and b. Chondromyxoid fibroma, tibia: (a) AP view. 21-year-old female with chief complaint of 4 months of pain and 2 weeks of swelling of left knee. (b) Lateral view. Clearly demarcated metaphyseal lesion expands and exquisitely thins cortex (arrows). Note lack of intralesional mineralization

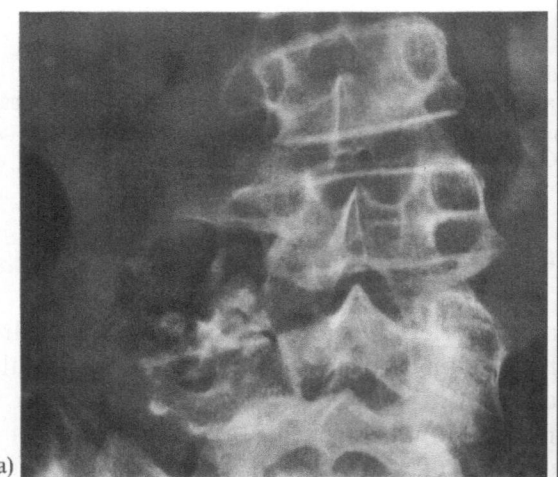

(a)

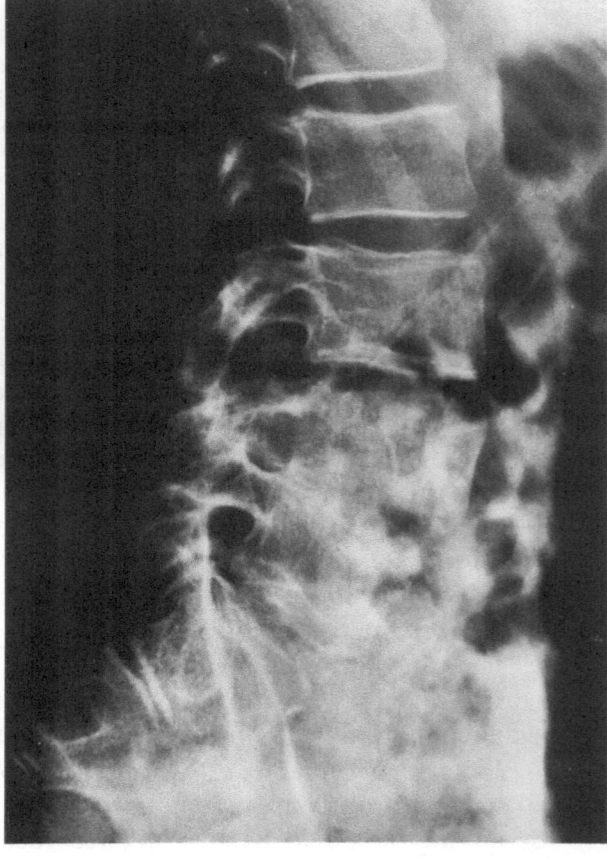

(b)

Fig. 75. Chondromyxoid fibroma, lumbar spine: This 14-year-old male had 2 year history of low back pain with radiation to right hip. (a) AP and (b) lateral views reveal large lytic expanding lesion which has partially destroyed vertebral body and right posterior elements at L-4 level. Small bony densities within confines of lesion are due to fragmentation postbiopsy. Lesion had infringed on spinal canal

IV. Roentgenographic Features

Roentgenograms most commonly suggest a benign lesion whose appearance varies depending on whether a long, small tubular or flat bone is involved (Figs. 74, 76–78) (FELDMAN et al., 1970; MURPHY and PRICE, 1971; RAMINI, 1974). In a long tubular bone, the lesion typically appears as a round or oval (Figs. 74a and b) metaphyseal

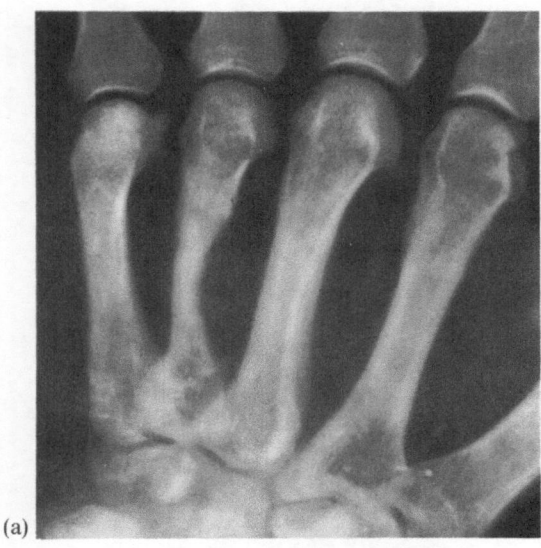 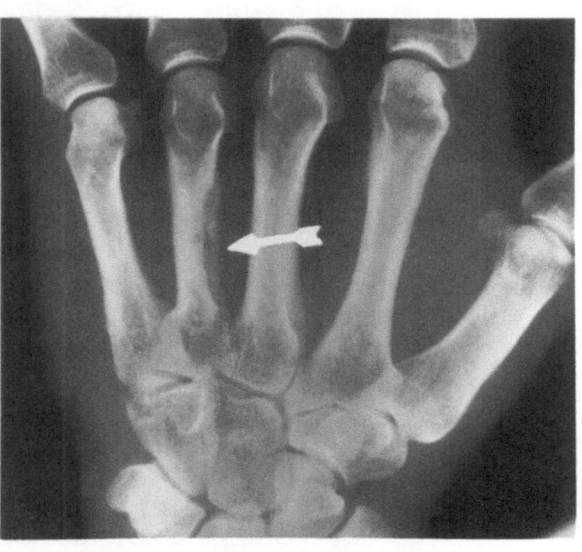

(a)　　　　　　　　　　　　　　　　　　　　　　　　　　　　(b)

Fig. 76a and b. Chondromyxoid fibroma, metacarpal: (a) PA view of left hand—eccentric lesion 3 cm in length and 0.5 cm in width erodes lateral aspect of 4th metacarpal. Thin, barely discernible shell of cortex demarcates lesion laterally. Note reactive sclerosis medially, (b) $5^{1}/_{2}$ months post surgery. Metacarpal is remodeling with apposition of new cortical bone. Residual scalloped defect measures 2.3×0.3 cm

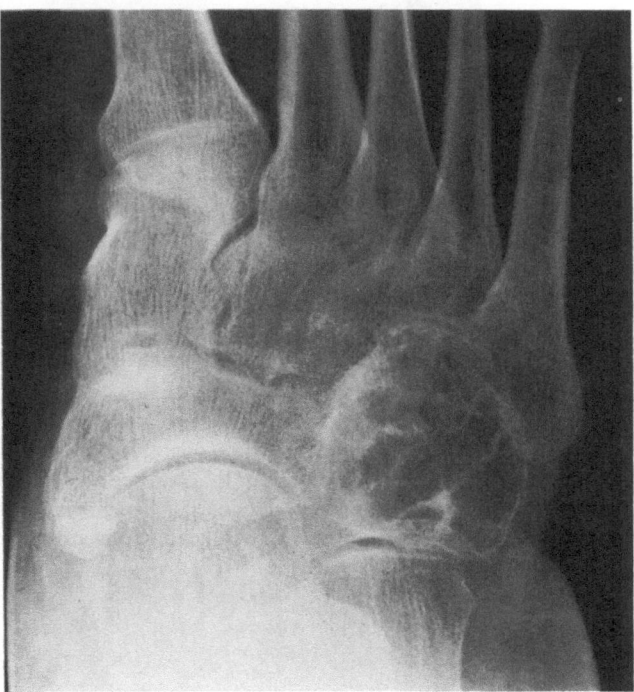

Fig. 77. Chondromyxoid fibroma, cuboid: Oblique view. Entire body of cuboid is re-placed by expanding lucent lesion. Lateral cortex is markedly thinned

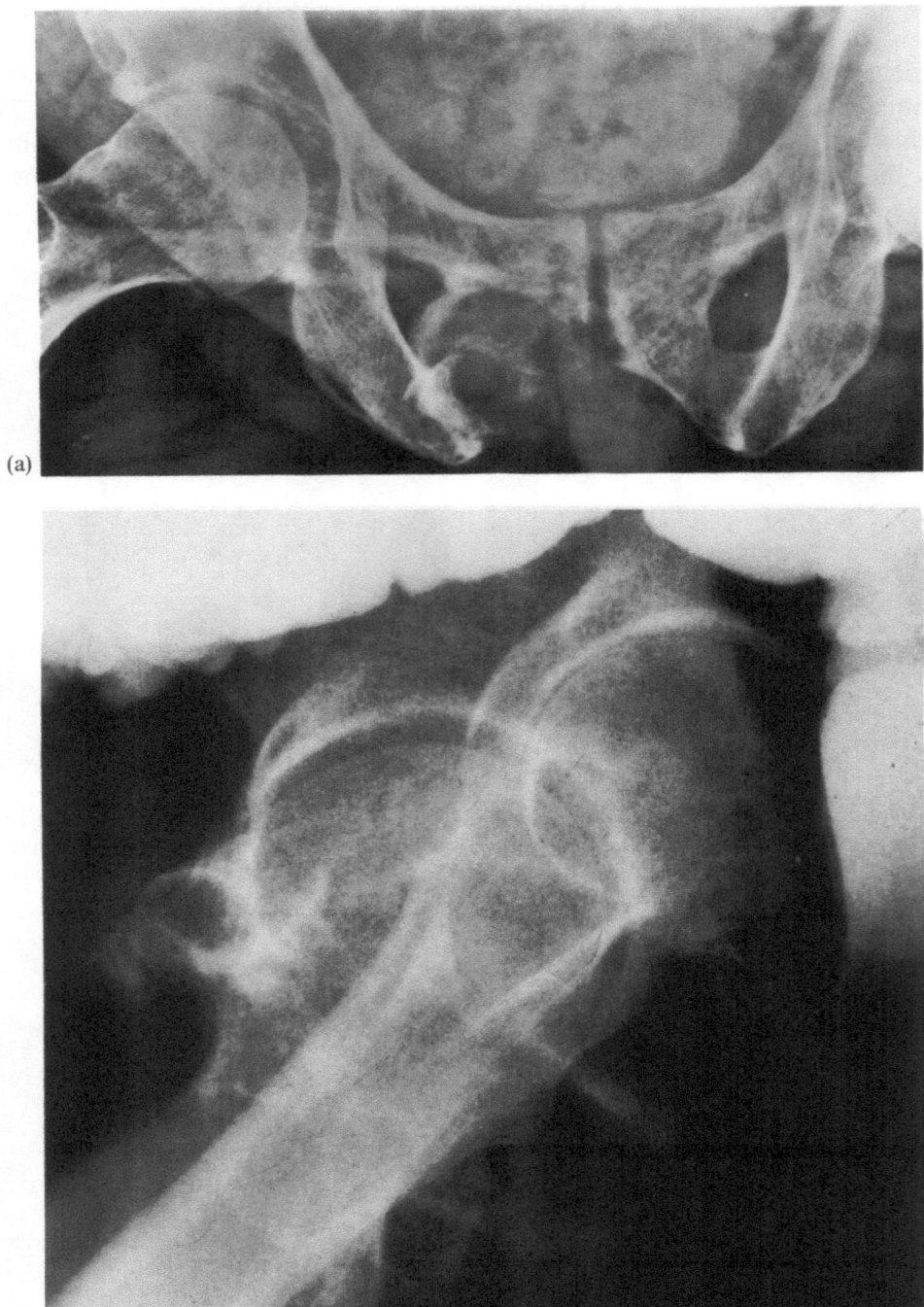

Fig. 78a and b. Chondromyxoid fibroma, pelvis: (a) AP view. Rounded lucent lesion involves right ischio-pubic area. Inferior cortical margin has been disrupted by previous biopsy. Note "pseudo-trabeculae" in center of lesion. These bony ridges reflect lobular peripheral growth of lesion, which has grooved its posterior cortical confines. (b) Lateral view. Lesion has expanded and thinned overlying anterior cortex. It is radiolucent with no roentgenographically detectable mineral within it

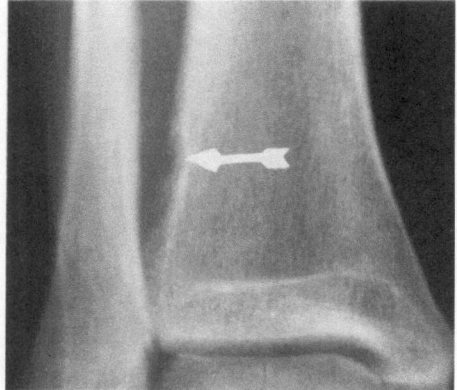

Fig. 79

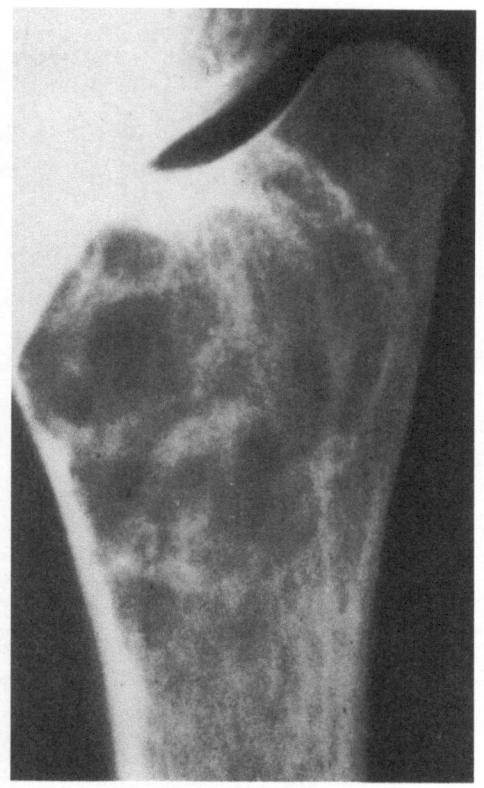

Fig. 79. Chondromyxoid fibroma, tibia: 27-year-old male had pain along lateral aspect of ankle for $1^1/_2$ years with swelling and night pain for 6 months. 1 cm long, 0.4 cm wide, and 0.6 cm in AP diameter lucent lesion expands and thins lateral tibial cortex. Lesion was entirely intracortical and had not involved medullary canal. Because of unusual location of lesion, possibility of chondromyxoid fibroma was not considered

Fig. 80. Chondromyxoid fibroma, fibula: 48-year-old female had 1 year history of lateral right knee pain, increasing in severity for 4 months. The 2×2.5 cm defect in fibular head and neck occupies practically entire width of narrow tubular bone. Note pseudo-trabeculae and sclerotic superior rim

Fig. 80

radiolucency whose long axis is directed along the axis of the bone. They have ranged in size from 1–10 cm but in long bones are most commonly $3 \times 2 \times 2$ cm (Fig. 79). When the lesion involved a small tubular bone (Fig. 80), it generally occupied its entire width. In flat bones the tumor has the same generally benign features but tends to be larger (DUTT et al., 1969; FELDMAN et al., 1970; PISAR, 1969; RAHIMI et al., 1972). The largest lesion in our series (Fig. 81) was in an iliac bone and measured 11.5×13 cm (FELDMAN et al., 1970). Another tumor in an iliac bone measured $12 \times 8 \times 6$ cm (RAHIMI et al., 1972).

Only rarely, and in advanced lesions, does the tumor cross the unfused growth plate. In RAHIMI'S (1972) series, 12 of 76 lesions abutted the growth plate. The lesion occasionally abuts the adjacent diaphysis but (TURCOTTE et al., 1962) a solely diaphyseal location is rarely observed, i.e., in 3 of 207 cases in our series (Fig. 82). Three tumors were noted as having a "definite diaphyseal location" in the review of RAHIMI et al. (1972) but it is not stated whether these lesions abutted the metaphysis. Presumably these 3 lesions were found among their 76 cases rather than among the total of 297 which they reviewed in the literature.

The eccentrically situated defect is typically well-demarcated along its internal border. Frequently, a rim of sclerotic bone, which may be pronounced, separates the lesion from the remainder of the marrow cavity. An osteomyelitis was reputedly simulated in one case (VIX and FAHMY, 1969). Occasionally a scalloped internal border simulates the curvilinear medial margin most often associated with nonossifying fibroma. The outer cortical surface may be expanded in a fusiform manner but it is usually well-defined. However, the expansion may be so marked that the lesion is externally delimited

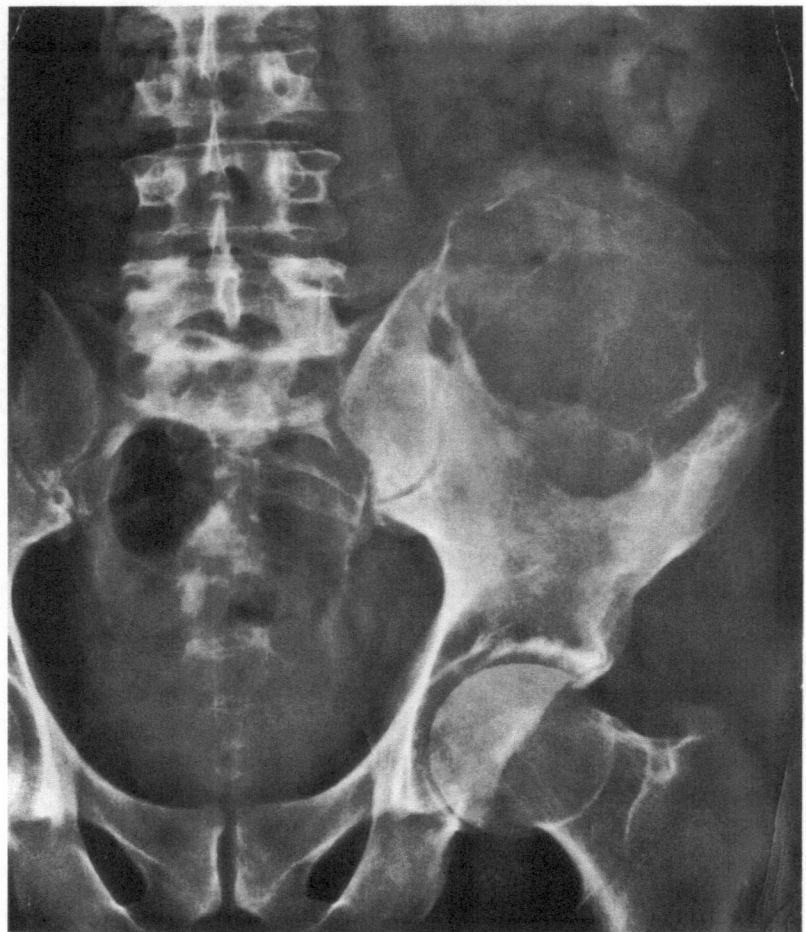

Fig. 81a

Fig. 81a and b. Chondromyxoid fibroma, pelvis: (a) AP view. Large lytic lesion literally balloons superior iliac cortex which appears interrupted superior-medially. Periosteum, however, was preserved at surgery. Note sharp inferior demarcation of tumor. No mineral was noted within lesion either roentgenographically or pathologically. (b) Gross specimen of partially resected ilium. Ovoid lobulated mass excised en bloc measured 12.5 × 12.7 cm. On cross section (above) it was yellow, moderately firm and not very mucinous with incomplete lobular pattern. Note central areas of myxomatous degeneration and cavitation

by an attenuated exquisitely thinned cortex which is barely discernible (Figs. 74, 76A, 81). Although this apparent lack of external margination or "bite out of bone" appearance is localized, it may on occasion mimic an aneurysmal bone cyst or a malignant tumor (RALPH, 1962). Rarely prominent projections into surrounding soft tissues may enforce this latter view (FELDMAN et al., 1970; RAHIMI et al., 1972). The peripheral part of the tumor abutting the soft tissues may also contain remnants of a partially preserved cortex which has been pushed away from the bone. In a case of HUTCHINSON and PARK (1960), cortical erosion with extension of the process into the soft tissues suggested malignancy. At surgery the tumor had extruded through a cortical defect and extended upward to the joint line beneath the deep fascia. The neighboring soft tissues, however, were otherwise unaffected. At surgery the tumor is generally well delimited externally by a thin shell of newly formed periosteal bone or directly by the periosteum (SCHAJOWICZ and GALLARDO, 1971).

Cortical layering or other evidence of active periosteal new bone formation as well

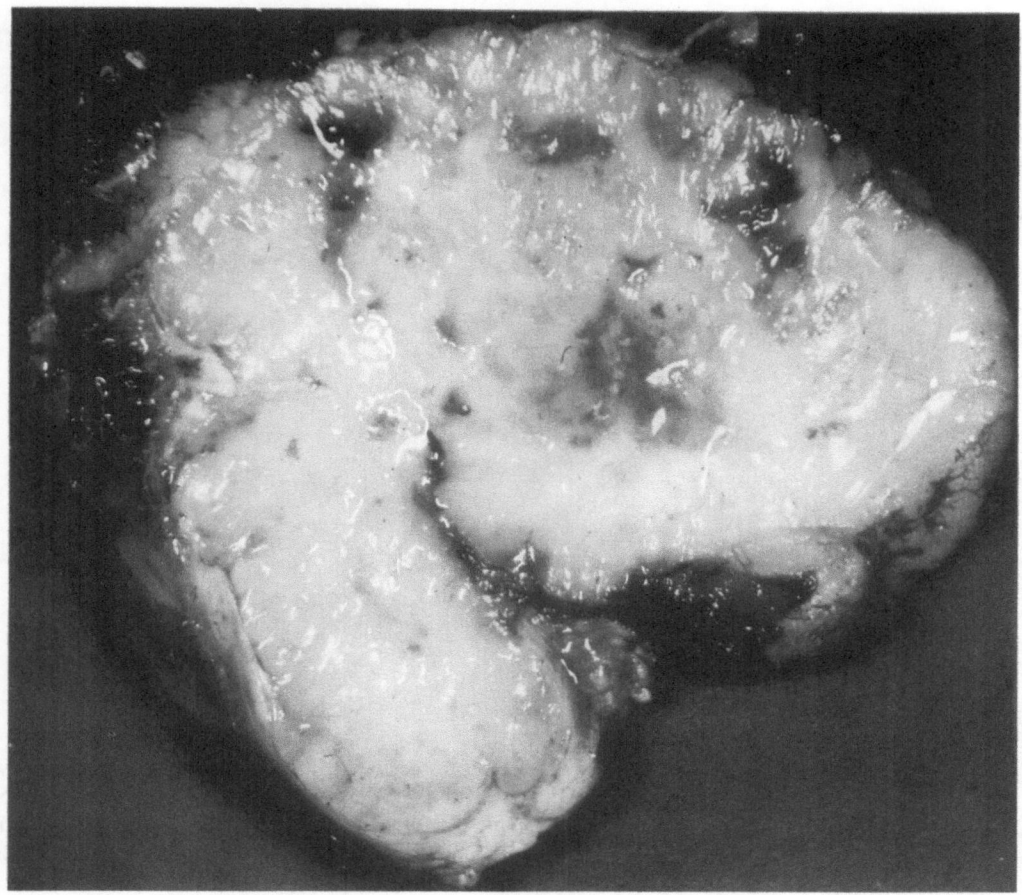

Fig. 81 b

as a Codman's triangle is unusual (FELDMAN et al., 1970; RAHIMI et al., 1972; SALZER et al., 1968). SPJUT et al. (1971) note that periosteal reaction is not seen unless a fracture is present (Fig. 82). Rarely, apparently uninvolved bone, a short distance beyond the visible confines of the lesion, may show cortical thickening. The usual benign roentgen features of the tumor, therefore, vary in bones of different size and types.

Although the lesion has frequently been described as having a soap-bubble appearance (Fig. 80) or as being trabeculated, in most instances the roentgenographic impression of trabeculation is a false or misleading one. The bony septa which appear to be compartmentalizing or dividing the lesion are in fact "pseudo-trabeculae" which do not traverse the tumor, but are a reflection of its lobulated periphery grooving the cortex with which it comes in contact. Therefore, intralesional trabeculae are simulated by the ridged or corrugated endosteal bone seen on end through the usually radiolucent, unmineralized lesion (Fig. 78a). If one were to tomograph a particular lesion, no bony septa would be delineated within the tumor substance.

In our previous study (FELDMAN et al., 1970), it was noted that tumoral calcification has rarely been observed either roentgenographically (i.e. 5 of 207 cases − 2%), or microscopically (i.e., 14 of 207 cases with 2 said to show concomitant ossification). SCHAJOWICZ and GALLARDO (1971) reported only one case in which areas of spotty calcification were radiographically visible. In a recent review of 76 cases, RAHIMI et al. (1972) affirmed the rarity of roentgenographically visible calcification by adding a single case. However,

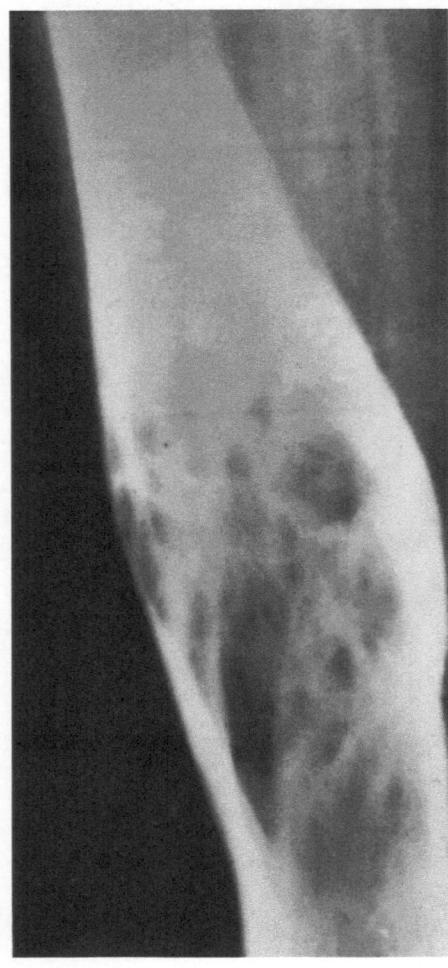

Fig. 82. Chondromyxoid fibroma, humerus: This lesion was associated with two unusual features—diaphyseal location and pathologic fracture after trauma. Callus from previous fracture is still evident medially with cortical thinning laterally. Expanding lesion is 10 cm long. Note satellite defects. Satellite lesions are most often seen in association with recurrence and are most often due to residual tumor remnants. This patient had no previous surgery

they noted microscopic evidence of calcification in 27%, an unusually high figure. JAFFE and LICHTENSTEIN, however, in their original report on this lesion (1948) and LICHTENSTEIN (1965) more recently, continue to emphasize that microscopically evident calcification or ossification is only an occasional and inconspicuous feature.

V. Differential Diagnosis

In the majority of cases the roentgen appearance is that of a nonmalignant process and the differential diagnosis must be made from among benign lesions such as enchondroma, chondroblastoma, osteoblastoma, nonossifying fibroma, aneurysmal bone cyst, simple bone cyst, and giant cell tumor. The lack of roentgenographically discernible intralesional calcification is a helpful feature, since mineral is frequently present and roentgenographically identifiable in both benign chondroblastoma and enchondroma.

Benign chondroblastomas are distinguished by their epiphyseal location, only occasionally abutting the metaphysis. They may, in addition, show evidence of lesional calcification and periosteal reaction. Both are exceptional findings in chondromyxoid fibroma.

Enchondromas are usually centrally located and contain calcifications which are fine or coarse and which may be scattered throughout the lesion in a stippled pattern.

They are most commonly located in the small cylindrical bones of the hands and feet and may be multiple.

Giant cell tumors are epiphyseal in location and are rarely seen under the age of 20 years or prior to growth plate closure (JAFFE et al., 1940). They most commonly have ill-defined bony landmarks and are poorly demarcated from the neighboring medullary cavity. They invariably extend to the end of the bone and often involve the entire width of the bone, while chondromyxoid fibroma is eccentrically situated within a long bone from which it is usually well-demarcated internally, frequently by a sclerotic rim. Although chondromyxoid fibroma may secondarily involve the epiphysis, the bulk of the lesion is predominantly metaphyseal and it most frequently occurs in patients younger than those with giant cell tumor.

Benign osteoblastomas, too, may show an intense sclerotic reaction along their periphery, as well as internally, particularly in long bones, but the lesion's center is usually seen as a hazier density on the roentgenogram. Its greater degree of opacity reflects its osteoid matrix which may be made additionally opaque by mineral deposits finely distributed throughout the lesion (POCHACZEVSKY et al., 1960). A soft tissue mass is more frequently associated with benign osteoblastomas and they most commonly involve the vertebral column, a rare locus for chondromyxoid fibroma (Fig. 75). A nonosteogenic fibroma may also appear as a small eccentric radiolucent defect well-demarcated internally. However, it frequently extends into the diaphyses, frequently has a scalloped internal border and is not usually as expansile as chondromyxoid fibroma. The lesions of fibrous dysplasia may be central or eccentric and are commonly characterized by a "ground glass" hazy translucency. Associated modeling deformities may be pronounced and polyostotic involvement is not infrequent. The aneurysmal bone cyst exhibits more marked cortical expansion with occasional "blow-out" fractures which are uncommon in chondromyxoid fibroma. It's medullary border may be hazy and ill-defined. Aneurysmal bone cysts, too, often occur in the spine where their aggressive nature may lead them to involve more than one vertebral level.

Unicameral bone cysts usually affect the metaphysis prior to epiphyseal closure and are infrequent after 20 years of age. They are usually centrally located causing fusiform symmetric cortical expansion. Pathologic fracture is a frequent occurrence in bone cysts and a rare one in chondromyxoid fibroma.

While chondromyxoid fibroma is not a particularly common tumor, its recognition is of importance in that pathologically it may be mistaken for a chondrosarcoma, a myxosarcoma, and occasionally even a fibrosarcoma and, as such, treated more radically than necessary. Conversely, as noted by DAHLIN (1956) because of the fear of unnecessarily radical treatment for benign tumors, pathologists have often considered or made the diagnosis of chondromyxoid fibroma when the lesion in question was actually a chondrosarcoma with disastrously inadequate treatment resulting (RAHIMI et al., 1972). Therefore, despite its clinically benign behavior, due to its complex histologic range, distinction from other tumors may occasionally be a problem. The roentgenogram may, therefore, be of prime importance in confirming the diagnosis.

VI. Pathologic Findings

1. Gross Features

All morphologic considerations of chondromyxoid fibroma are dominated by the problem of distinguishing it from chondrosarcoma. It is generally pale, or flesh-colored, rubbery, and resilient with a smooth, bosselated outer surface (Fig. 81 b). It is incompletely lobulated and unlike chondrosarcoma, it is usually confined by an intact periosteum, even in those areas in which a cortex is not evident roentgenographically (Jaffe and Lichtenstein, 1948). It is usually firm, reflecting its fibrous component, and its mucinous content varies so that it is never as "slimy" as a chondrosarcoma or a myxoma. Only rarely are fragments as soft and myxoid as the histology suggests (Lichtenstein, 1965). Some lesions have a bluish-hue with localized areas of yellow-grey or brown discoloration. While its appearance may suggest cartilage tumor tissue on casual inspection, it lacks the faceted pattern and blue-white luster of an enchondroma, neither does it have the semitranslucent blue-white lobular pattern of chondrosarcoma (Spjut et al., 1971).

2. Microscopic

The basic microscopic pattern is that of areas of spindle-shaped, ovoid, or stellate cells, without cytoplasmic borders, loosely dispersed within a myxoid and occasionally chondroid intercellular matrix (Figs. 83, 84). The myxoid character of the matrix has been attributed to its aqueous content rather than mucin (Lichtenstein, 1965) since special stains fail to demonstrate the latter.

The lesion tends to be demarcated into pseudolobules by narrow vascularized curving bands of more compact tumor cells. It is the increased concentration of cells at the periphery of the lobules that is of extreme importance in identifying this neoplasm (Figs. 85a and b). At the more cellular periphery, the cells are often spindle-shaped and fibroblastic and occasional mitotic figures may serve to simulate fibrosarcoma.

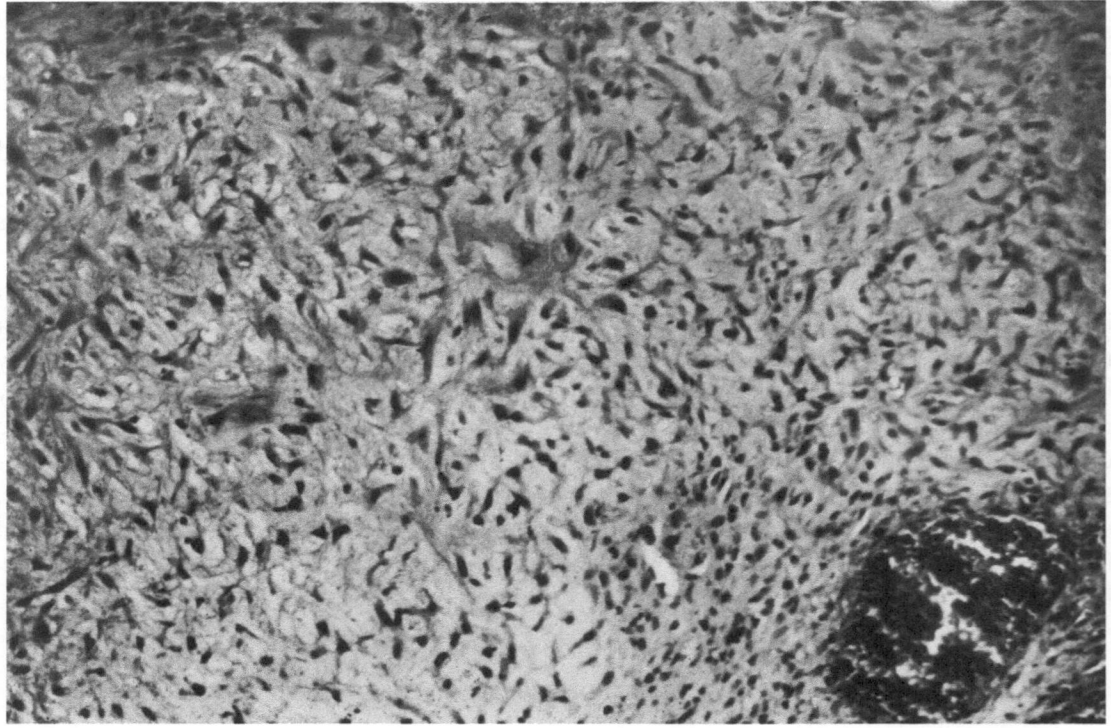

Fig. 83. Chondromyxoid fibroma, photomicrography (×150): Basic microscopic pattern is that of spindle-shaped, ovoid, or stellate cells without cytoplasmic borders, usually dispersed within myxoid or chondroid, finely fibrillar intercellular matrix. Cells close to blood vessel at lower right tend to be fibroblastic, while those at upper left at some distance from blood vessel are more chondroid in character

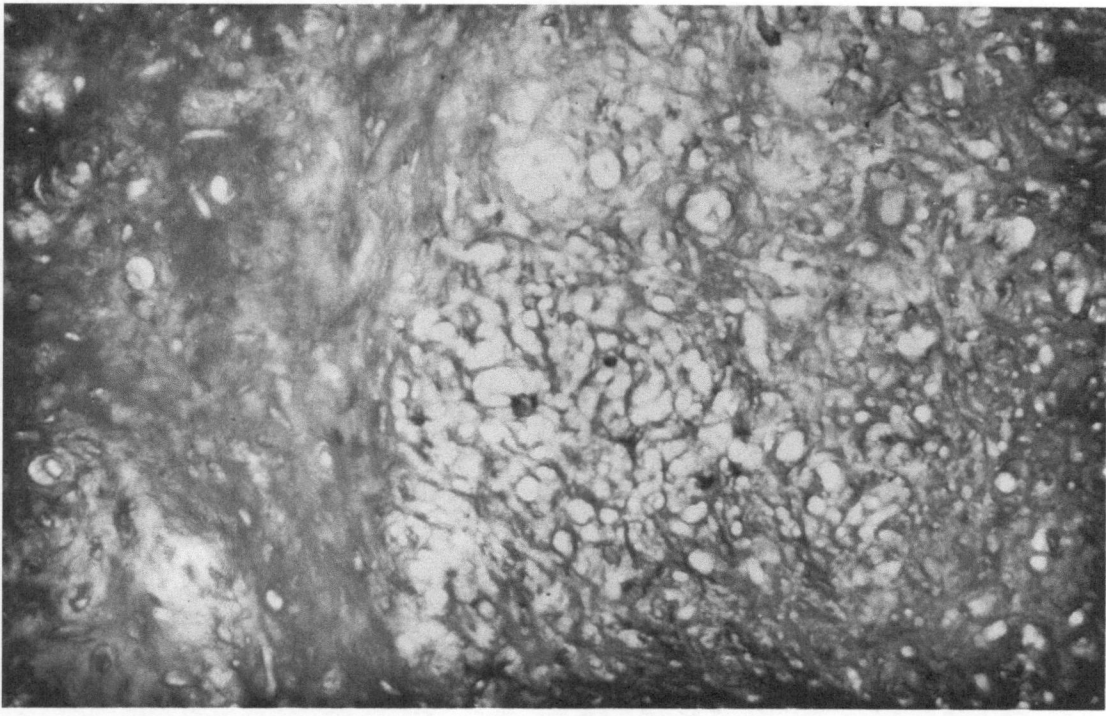

Fig. 84. Chondromyxoid fibroma, photomicrograph (× 150): Matrix on left belongs to fibroblastic component and stains like hyaluronic acid. That on right stains like acid mucopolysaccharide (chondroitin sulphate) of chondroid matrix. (Courtesy of Dr. Austin D. Johnston)

The peripheral tumor cells are also more compact with prominent nuclei, some of which may be plump, atypically large, double, multiple, or hyperchromatic, creating an unduly ominous appearance. It is the central portion of the lobules that tends to be more myxoid. The central myxoid cells are elongated or multipolar with fairly distinct cytoplasmic borders.

The cytology varies somewhat with the age or degree of maturation of the lesion. Increasing maturity appears to be reflected in progressive collagenization of the intracellular matrix. In the older tumors, many of the cells come to lie in lacunae and the matrix takes on a chondroid appearance. This chondroid appearance considered in conjunction with tumor cells with prominent hyperchromatic nuclei and cells with two or more nuclei, accounts for the fact that chondromyxoid fibroma is often mistaken for chondrosarcoma by pathologists unfamiliar with the lesion. Rahimi et al. (1972) also note the possible confusion of chondromyxoid fibroma with chondrosarcoma which is further exaggerated by the fact that large nuclei are present in about one-third of chondromyxoid fibromas. They additionally emphasize that though myxoid areas may be prominent in chondrosarcomas, they also have a more distinct hyaline cartilage quality together with a lack of the characteristic admixture of fibromatous elements so prominent in chondromyxoid fibroma (Fig. 83). Chondrosarcomas also lack the abrupt boundaries of chondromyxoid fibroma (Fig. 85).

The possible relation of chondromyxoid fibroma to so-called myxoma of bone has been difficult to evaluate since the existence of a true myxoma of bone outside of the jaw bone, analogous to myxoma or myxosarcoma of skeletal soft parts, has not been firmly established (Enzinger and Shiraki, 1972). In commenting on Bloodgood's

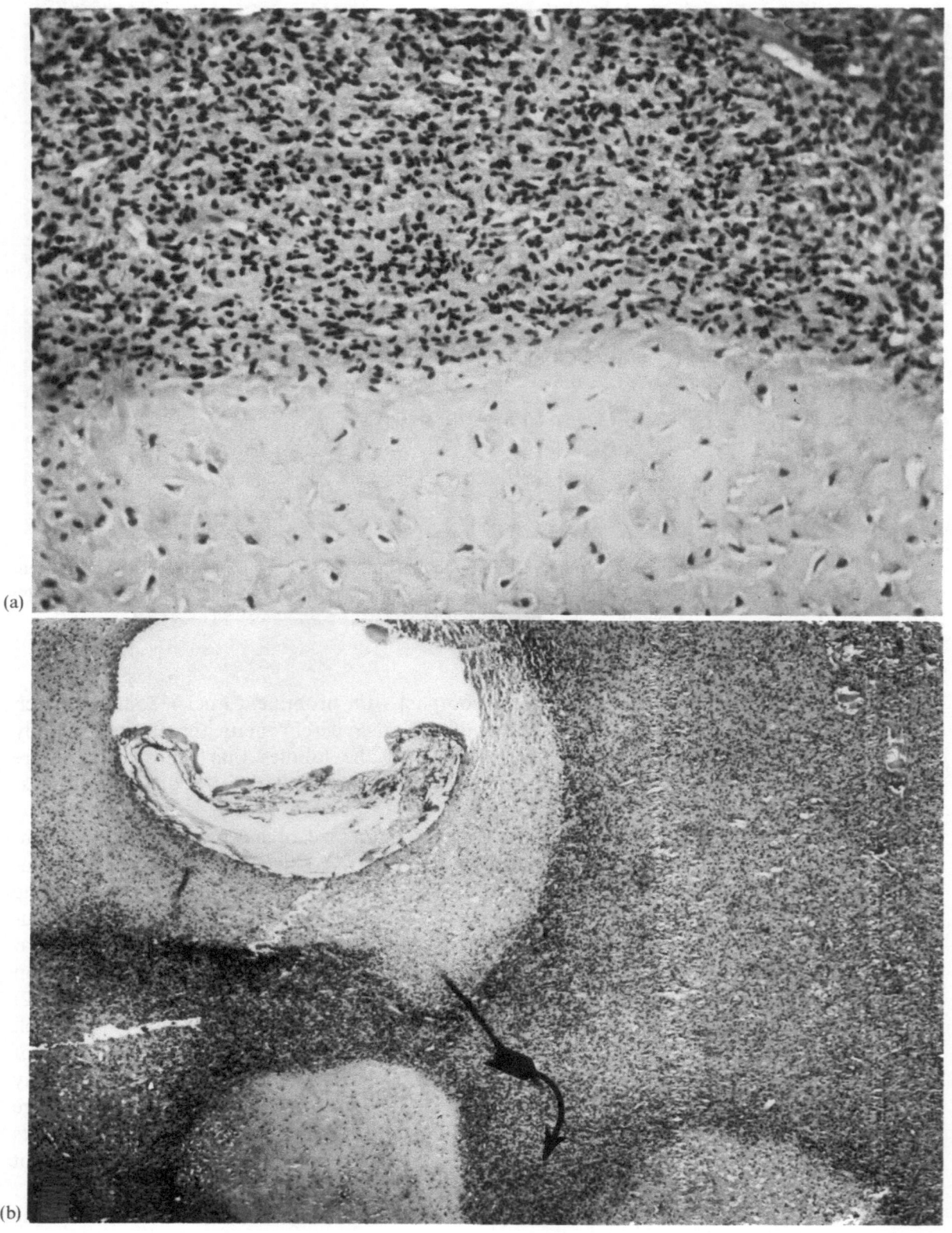

Fig. 85. (a) Chondromyxoid fibroma, photomicrograph (× 150): Shows cellular peripheral area (top) and chondroid area (bottom). (b) Photomicrograph (× 150) shows two adjacent areas of chondroid tissue inferiorly divided into characteristic lobules (arrow). Lesions tend to be demarcated into pseudolobules by narrow vascularized curving bands of compact tumor cells. Note blood vessels in upper field

paper (1924) which ostensibly dealt with "myxoma of bone" LICHTENSTEIN (1965) notes that, "It is impossible to determine precisely what the tumors described actually represent. The more aggressive ones may well have been chondrosarcomas exhibiting secondary myxoid change." He also notes that if one defines myxoma as "a mesenchymal connective tissue neoplasm of soft slimy appearance containing abundant mucin within its ground substance, then chondromyxoid fibroma fails to meet these criteria." If one further compares chondromyxoid fibroma tissue with that of an umbilical cord, one finds little resemblance between them. Nevertheless, chondromyxoid fibroma is sometimes misdiagnosed as a myxoma of bone. LICHTENSTEIN states that the tumors reported by BLOODGOOD (1924) and by BAUER and HARRELL (1954) are cases in point, while the five cases reported by SCAGLIETTI and STRINGA (1961) of "myxoma of bone" in children appear to represent instances of chondromyxoid fibroma which grew rapidly and had a greater tendency to recur. In discussing this problem, RAHIMI et al. (1972), too, note that, in their experience, more mucinous appearing chondromyxoid fibromas tend to occur in the younger patients and have a greater capacity for recurrence and that they cannot distinguish a pattern in the cases of BAUER and HARRELL (1954) and SCAGLIETTI and STRINGA (1961) reported as myxomas or in those of MARCOVE et al. (1964), reported as fibromyxomas that is sufficiently distinctive histologically to warrant a separate designation. They felt that all these lesions fell into the range of histologic variation of chondromyxoid fibromas. They further state that rare myxomas such as one described by PEROU et al. (1967), and STOUT (1948) are extremely unusual in bone and do not have the pattern of chondromyxoid fibroma, whereas the myxomatous tumors of the jaw are almost certainly of odontogenic derivation and are also not related to chondromyxoid fibroma.

Prominent foci resembling those of chondroblastoma were found in one-quarter of the tumors in the Mayo Clinic series (RAHIMI et al., 1972). The closely packed cells located at the periphery of the chondromyxoid fibroma lobules, are sometimes round or polygonal and contain nuclei that are round or oval and often indented. These cells were felt to resemble those of benign chondroblastoma and were intermingled with fibroblasts and multinucleated giant cells (DAHLIN, 1956; RAHIMI et al., 1972). Multinucleated giant cells and hemosiderin-laden macrophages may be seen in the vicinity of extravasated blood as well as around blood vessels which travel within the tracts of supporting connective tissue. The presence of multinuclear cells within the connective tissue framework may cause the lesion to be mistaken for a giant cell tumor (DAHLIN, 1956; RAHIMI et al., 1972). The giant cells contain acid phosphatase, as is true of those in giant cell tumors (KUHLMAN and McNAMEE, 1970; SCHAJOWICZ and GALLARDO, 1971).

Quantitative microchemical studies by KUHLMAN and McNAMEE (1970) of several neoplasms, including giant cell tumor, and chondroblastoma, as well as chondromyxoid fibroma, showed that very high levels of acid phosphatase were present in the giant cell tumor and the chondroblastoma with moderate activity noted in the chondromyxoid fibroma. The latter finding had been unexpected, since chondromyxoid fibromas are ordinarily not thought to contain giant cells. It is of interest in this regard that osteoclast giant cells were found in 40% of the tumors in the Mayo Clinic series (RAHIMI et al., 1972). However, not only may giant cells be found in many chondromyxoid fibromas but probably in some areas of all chondromyxoid fibromas. This would serve to explain KUHLMAN and McNAMEE's findings (1970). They further noted that alkaline phosphatase activity was very low in all three tumors as opposed to the osteosarcomas analyzed. The low levels of alkaline phosphatase present in giant cell tumor, chondroblastoma, and chondromyxoid fibroma may be related to their small propensity to produce collagen. Inorganic pyelophosphatases were very active in the giant cell tumor and osteosarcoma and considerably less active in the chondromyxoid fibromas, chondroblasts and chondro-

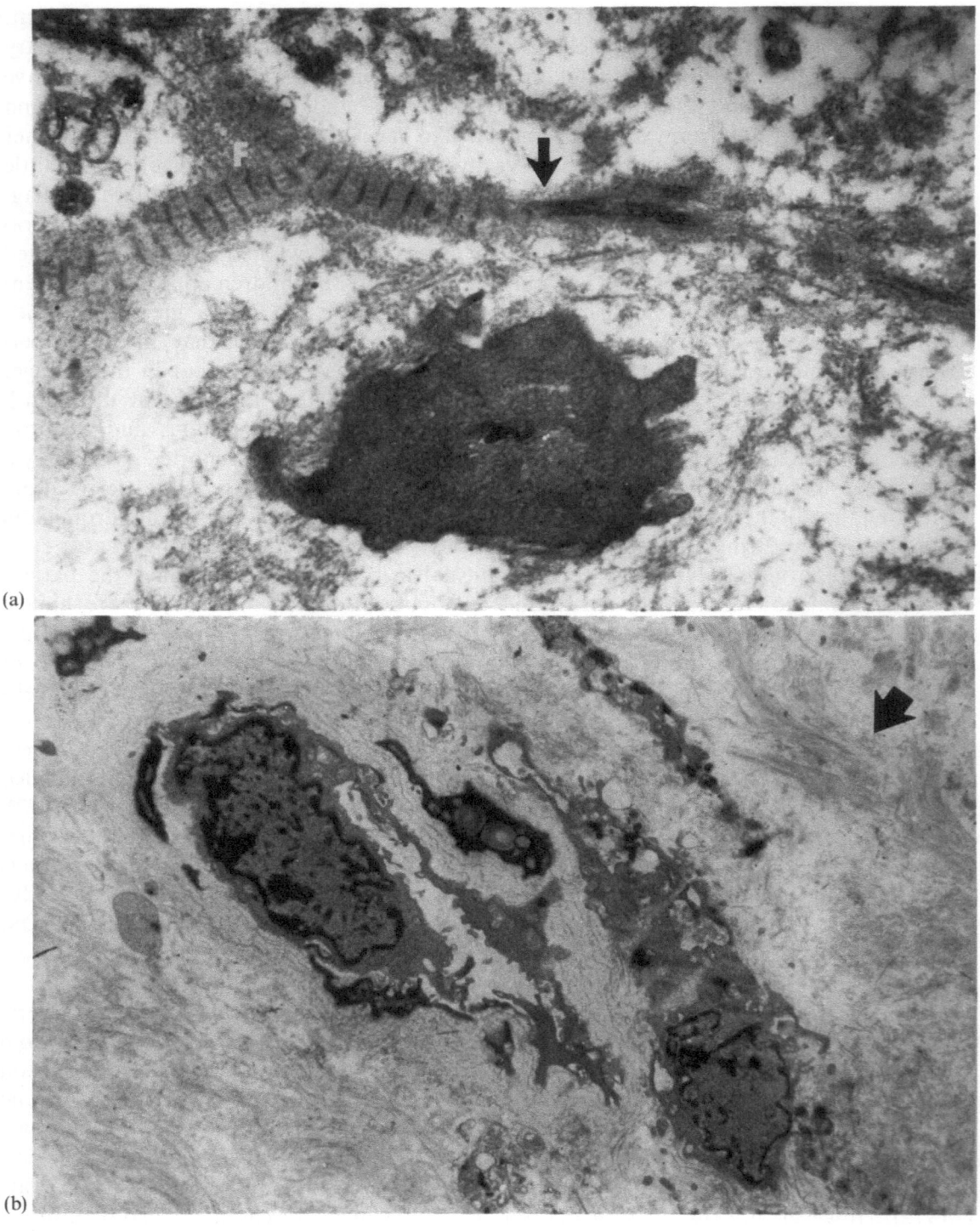

Fig. 86. (a) Chondromyxoid fibroma, electron micrograph (×30,000): Collagenous fiber bundle (F) having distinctive major banding periodicity of 973 A is seen in intercellular matrix. Intraperiod bands are also visible in many of these structures and loose aggregations of fibril 100–200 A in diameter (arrow) are also present. (b) Electron micrograph (×5500): Cells from fibrous component. Note collagen fibrils in upper right field (arrow). (Courtesy of AUSTIN D. JOHNSTON, M.D.)

blastoma. In general, the highest levels of inorganic pyelophosphatases were found in the most rapidly growing tumors. The pattern of an aneurysmal bone cyst may also be simulated in certain microscopic fields by narrow spaces between tumor lobules and adjacent bone which are usually occupied by loose, richly vascularized, nonneoplastic connective tissue, and occasional extravasated blood (RAHIMI et al., 1972).

Focal calcification is uncommon in most series as previously noted but was seen in 21 tumors or 27% of the Mayo Clinic series with necrotic foci within lobules present in 11% of the tumors (RAHIMI et al., 1972). It was somewhat more common in the tumors of older patients. The calcified material was seen in the chondroid portion of the lesions or the fibroblastic or collagenized tissue at the periphery or within tumor lobules. Osteoid and fine bone trabeculae were described by BENEDETTI et al. (1962). They were found in seven tumors. No bone trabeculae crossed the tumor mass.

Therefore, in addition to the problematic overlap between the two benign lesions of chondroblastoma and chondromyxoid fibroma, and the small number of atypical chondromyxoid fibromas reported, chondromyxoid fibroma per se may also be confused histologically with chondrosarcoma, myxosarcoma, myxoma, giant cell tumor, and chondroblastoma. In view of the broad spectrum of histologic features with which it may be associated, roentgenograms take on added significance in diagnosing this tumor and particularly where "problem cases" are concerned. The ultrastructure of chondromyxoid fibroma has just begun to be documented (TORNBERG et al., 1973) (Figs. 86a, b).

VII. Treatment, Recurrence, Malignant Transformation

The treatment of choice is complete excision, when practical, with curettage and packing with bone chips as an alternative. JAFFE and LICHTENSTEIN (1948) originally knew of no recurrence and noted that "even with incomplete removal, spontaneous regression of the remnants follow." In our review of 207 cases, 17 of 26 recurrences were attributed to incomplete tumor removal (FELDMAN et al., 1970). Among the 24 cases diagnosed and treated at the Mayo Clinic and separated from the 52 seen in consultation, curettage was the initial therapy in 15 tumors, 6 of which recurred (RAHIMI et al., 1972). Four recurred within 2 years, one within 6.5 years, and one at 9 years post curettage. Various combinations of cautery, grafting, and irradiation employed as adjuncts did not obviate recurrence. Of the 14 recurrences which developed among the entire group of 76 patients, 11 occurred within 2 years, 2 after 3 years and 1 after 6 years. Soft tissue involvement by lobules of tumor contiguous with or adjacent to recurrent lesions in bone were seen in a few cases. In one case, a nodule of recurrent chondromyxoid fibroma was removed from the subcutaneous tissue before a recurrence in the underlying os calcis became manifest (RAHIMI et al., 1972). Another recurrent chondromyxoid fibroma of MIKULOWSKI and ÖSTBERG (1971) was of interest in that a tumor was removed from the soft tissues, apparently without connection to the neighboring bone, approximately 19 years after the original excision of a chondromyxoid fibroma from the medial malleolus of a tibia. Actually, the patient had noticed a gradually enlarging lump at the site of the operative wound for 10 years, i.e., 9 years after the original surgery. The histologic picture was largely the same in both preparations. The tumor was noted to have grown in the soft tissues apparently without connection to bone. This again emphasizes the fact that the cartilage family of lesions have a propensity to cellular implantation and subsequent growth within soft tissues. In SCHAJOWICZ and GALLARDO'S (1971) series, only 1 among 32 lesions recurred 2 years after tibial curettage. A segmental resection was then performed. No case received radiotherapy. They commented that their low recurrence rate was possibly due to the use of wide excision or block resection as the initial treatment in 42.3% of their cases. They also commented that the higher incidence of recurrence reported in the literature ranging from 12.5–25% (RALPH, 1962; DAHLIN, 1967) could be a consequence of the preference for curettage as the initial treatment.

The tendency to local recurrence after curettage seems to be higher in young children (RALPH, 1962; SCAGLIETTI and STRINGA, 1961). It has been postulated that the thin cortex and spongiosa in children offer less resistance to tumor growth. RAHIMI et al. (1972), also emphasized that age had a significant bearing on recurrence. Of 14 recurrences among the 76 patients they reviewed, 11 developed in cases less than 15 years old. In discussing the relationship of histologic appearance to recurrence they noted that 12 of the 14 recurrences were in patients who originally had the most mucinous appearing lesions. Furthermore, 14 of the 19 predominantly mucinous tumors arose in patients who were 5–14 years old. Correlating the presence of large or atypical nuclei with recurrence, they found that all but one of the recurrences came from among the group of 31 tumors with such nuclei. Here, too, 17 of the patients whose tumors contained atypical nuclei were less than 15 years old. Hence, the tumors that are most myxoid and have large nuclei are found more often in younger patients, i.e. the ones who are most likely to develop recurrence after curettage (RAHIMI et al., 1972).

Although the tumor is usually easily separated from the surrounding bone, its lobulated periphery and friability may contribute to its incomplete removal. A small lobule extending from the main mass into a groove or pocket of bone may be overlooked and may serve as a nidus for future recurrence, This circumstance, rather than the natural tendency for the tumor to recur, could also explain the recurrences with apparent multicentric foci (DAHLIN, 1956; FELDMAN et al., 1970). The presence of small tumor lobules in the spongiosa separated from the bulk of the tumor by a rim of sclerotic bone impedes an adequate and complete extirpation of the lesion by curettage.

The role of radiation therapy was difficult to evaluate or assess, since it was most often used as an auxiliary postoperative measure. Although 12 cases had received radiotherapy in the Mayo Clinic series, details as to tumor dose, timing, equipment used, or quality of radiation were unknown in 5 cases (RAHIMI et al., 1970). The value of radiotherapy to a predominantly benign lesion composed of tissue unlikely to be radiosensitive has been questioned and is generally felt to be contraindicated for surgically accessible lesions in view of the risk of inducing sarcoma. Radiation therapy was noted to have probably contributed to two serious complications in the Mayo Clinic consultative group of cases. One patient developed fibrosarcoma of an irradiated tibia 6 years after an estimated dose of 5000 R. Death with evidence of metastases resulted a year later despite amputation for the sarcoma. Another patient developed radionecrosis and chronic osteomyelitis after curettage and radiation therapy for a tibial tumor, requiring skin grafting and crutches 8 years after the initial treatment. It is, therefore, the general opinion that radiation therapy for this tumor is contraindicated with the possible exception of surgically inaccessible lesions. No case received radiotherapy in SCHAJOWICZ and GALLARDO's (1971) series.

The malignant potential for chondromyxoid fibroma has been contested in the literature. RAHIMI et al. (1972) noted that, "malignant transformation is extremely improbable and we have found no case in which malignant change has been convincingly documented." SCHAJOWICZ and GALLARDO (1971) had no case in their series and also note that, "It appears to be very exceptionable."

Nevertheless, isolated cases have been reported. Three of these (FILIPPONE, 1966; SETH and RAO, 1964; WITWICKI and DZIAK, 1967) were felt by RAHIMI and DAHLIN to contain insufficient documentation or none at all. Another case (GILMEN et al., 1963), too, was open to question, since recurrence and malignant chondrosarcomatous degeneration were postulated 5 months after curettage. The case of IWATA and COLEY (1958) in which two pathologists diagnosed chondromyxoid fibroma, apparently required amputation 17 months post original surgery, at which time a "chondrosarcoma" was diagnosed. There were no accompanying photomicrographs. A case reported by LEVY et al. (1946) was of interest not only from the standpoint of malignant alteration, but from the standpoint of distant metastases ascribed to this tumor. A lesion in the femur was surgically removed in November, 1960. Rebiopsy in July, 1962 at the same site was said to exhibit elements of fibrosarcoma, chondrosarcoma, and osteosarcoma. A nodular density in the right pulmonary apex and clinical evidence of spinal cord metastases were reported. No autopsy was performed. DAHLIN (RAHIMI et al., 1972) in commenting on this case, noted that a review of the original material revealed histologic changes that the regarded as characteristic of chondrosarcoma. In the series of RAHIMI et al. (1972), the only case in which malignant evolution was observed was in a patient who developed an anaplastic fibrosarcoma at the site 6 years after radiation therapy for chondromyxoid fibroma. They felt, that, "All evidence indicates that the risk of malignant transformation of bona fide chondromyxoid fibroma, unless radiation is employed, is so slight that it need not lead to unnecessary radical treatment." They also point out that "paradoxically because of the fear of unnecessary radical treatment for benign tumors, pathologists have often considered, or made the diagnosis of chondromyxoid fibroma when the lesion in question was actually a chondrosarcoma, with disastrously inadequate treatment resulting" (RAHIMI et al., 1972).

The majority of recorded cases have responded well to simple operative measures. However, most authorities agree that complete removal by a resection that includes the tumor bed is necessary to prevent the relatively high rate of recurrence seen after curettage alone. The efficacy of complete resection has been documented by SCHAJOWICZ and GALLARDO (1971) and is also attested to by the success of such treatment in recurrent tumors.

K. Chondrosarcoma

Chondrosarcoma is a malignant tumor derived from cartilage cells. It maintains its essential cartilaginous nature throughout its evolution, though associated areas of spindle cell dedifferentiation, myxomatous degeneration, and ossification may be seen. Myxomatous stroma, particularly in the center of large nodules, may be the result of avascular degeneration, while the intercellular matrix produced by tumor cartilage may undergo calcification or ossification by means of enchondral bone formation (Figs. 87a, b). However, even if small areas of neoplastic osteoid are found evolving from sarcomatous stroma, the diagnosis must be osteosarcoma rather than chondrosarcoma, even though the bulk of the lesion may be cartilaginous. Conversely, while some osteogenic sarcomas contain cartilage, it is cartilage formed in the course of osteogenesis from primitive mesenchyme. Chondrosarcoma develops from full-fledged cartilage (though not necessarily hyaline cartilage), and one never sees tumorous osteoid tissue or bone evolving from sarcomatous stroma directly; an event which one always sees somewhere in an osteogenic sarcoma, no matter how much cartilage it contains (LICHTENSTEIN, 1965). The distinction deserves emphasis. It is of the utmost clinical importance

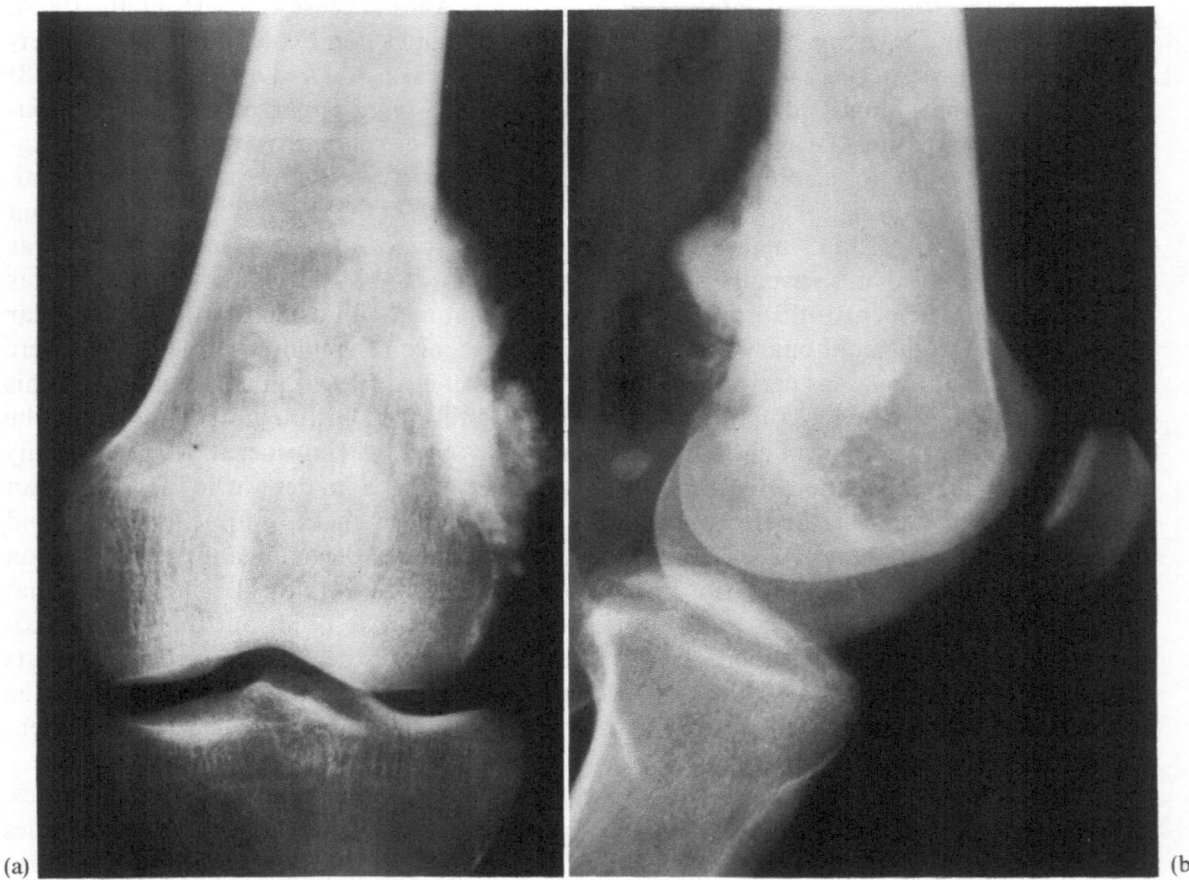

(a)   (b)

Fig. 87a and b. Chondrosarcoma, femur: 38-year-old female with known painless, enlarging mass for 1 year, knee pain of 2 months, and numbness of right 4th and 5th toes of 2 weeks' duration. (a) AP view: Lesion appears eccentric. Intense reactive sclerosis simulates paraosteal osteogenic sarcoma. Biopsy revealed chondrosarcoma with extensive metaplastic bone formation, as result of enchondral ossification, as well as cartilage calcification. (b) Lateral view: Faint stippled mineralization is seen within soft tissue mass extending beyond normal femoral contour. No evidence of recurrence was noted $5^1/_2$ years post amputation

in view of the generally slower course and more favorable prognosis of chondrosarcoma in both skeletal and extraskeletal sites.

Chondrosarcomas have been classified as central or peripheral and primary or secondary. If development begins in the bone's interior, the lesions are called central chondrosarcomas; if in relation to the bone's surface or through malignant degeneration of the cartilaginous cap of an osteochondroma, they are designated as peripheral chondrosarcomas.

Both central and peripheral lesions may be primary or secondary chondrosarcomas. The majority of chondrosarcomas arise de novo and are called primary, while secondary chondrosarcomas are those developing from pre-existing benign cartilaginous lesions. It is commonly difficult to satisfactorily demonstrate the latter event. Secondary central chondrosarcomas may have evolved from a pre-existing enchondroma (most commonly in patients with multiple skeletal enchondromatosis) while peripheral chondrosarcomas may occur as a result of malignant degeneration of an osteochondroma (most commonly in patients with hereditary multiple exostosis). Chondrosarcoma has been infrequently associated with Paget's disease (LICHTENSTEIN, 1965; PORRETTA et al., 1957), fibrous dysplasia (FEINTUCH, 1973; HUVOS et al., 1972), bone infarct, and unicameral bone cyst (GRABIAS and MANKIN, 1974; LICHTENSTEIN, 1965). Rarely chondrosarcoma, as well as osteosarcoma or fibrosarcoma, may develop as a sequal to radiotherapy (COHEN and D'ANGIO, 1961; HATCHER and CAMBELL, 1951; LICHTENSTEIN, 1965). One case of chondrosarcoma developed in a rib of an 11-year-old girl approximately 8 years post radiotherapy for Ewing's sarcoma, while another appeared in a distal femur 6 years after irradiation of another Ewing's tumor (LICHTENSTEIN, 1965). Chondrosarcoma has also been experimentally induced by the intravenous injection of beryllium compound in rabbits and successfully transplanted into the anterior chamber of the eye (HIGGINS et al., 1964).

I. Incidence

Chondrosarcoma is less common than osteogenic sarcoma, appears at a later age, and has a much slower course (DAHLIN, 1967; JAFFE, 1968; LICHTENSTEIN, 1965; MCKENNA et al., 1966; SALIB, 1966–67; SPJUT et al., 1971). JAFFE (1968) estimated that chondrosarcomas constitute about 10% of cases in a representative series of bone tumors. While it represented 7.6% of the primary malignant bone tumors in an early compilation of the Bone Sarcoma Registry of the American College of Surgeons, it comprised 22% of malignant bone tumors in a later review by ACKERMAN and SPJUT (1967), i.e. 91 of 410 cases. It was the second most common primary malignant bone tumor at the Mayo Clinic (DAHLIN, 1967), i.e. 334 of 1918 cases (17%).

Central chondrosarcomas predominate in some series (JAFFE, 1968; LICHTENSTEIN and JAFFE, 1943; LINDBOM et al., 1961), and peripheral chondrosarcomas in others (O'NEAL and ACKERMAN, 1952). Of O'NEAL and ACKERMAN's (1952) 40 cases, 25 were peripheral, 10 central, and 5 unclassifiable. A comparative incidence of 88 osteosarcomas and fibrosarcomas of bone was given. There were 20 central tumors, 13 peripheral, and 6 of uncertain origin among the 25 male and 14 female patients of LINDBOM et al. (1961).

II. Age and Sex

Males predominate in ordinary chondrosarcoma in most series with ratios ranging from 5.3:1 (DAHLIN, 1967; LINDBOM et al., 1961; O'NEAL and ACKERMAN, 1952) to 1.5:1. Males predominate in both types of lesions (peripheral and/or central). In O'NEAL and ACKERMAN's (1952) review, 19 of 25 peripheral chondrosarcomas (76%) and 7 of 10 central lesions (70%) occurred in males. The majority of patients have reached adult life, i.e. between 30 and 60 years. The average age of onset of symptoms was 36 years for women and 51 years for men in one series of 39 cases (LINDBOM et al., 1961). Its uncommon occurrence in children and adolescents makes the diagnosis of chondrosarcoma suspect in a child, particularly if not engrafted on multiple enchondromatosis or multiple osteochondromatosis (Figs. 24, 39). In the young, these tumors are most often osteosarcomas, which incidentally contain malignant cartilage. However, in the young, those tumors which, on careful analysis, are entirely cartilaginous, have a prognosis which is frequently that of osteosarcoma (BARNES and CATTO, 1966; COLEY and HIGINBOTHAM, 1954; GILMEN et al., 1963; TALERMAN et al., 1967). Only 10 of 288 cases of chondrosarcoma studied by HENDERSON and DAHLIN (1963) were under 20 years of age (Figs. 54, 88). In secondary chondrosarcoma, however, peak ages are, on the average, 10 years younger, but even these patients are older than those with osteosarcoma (BARNES and CATTO, 1966). In O'NEAL and ACKERMAN's series (1952) the ages

180 F. FELDMAN: Cartilaginous Tumors and Tumor-like Conditions

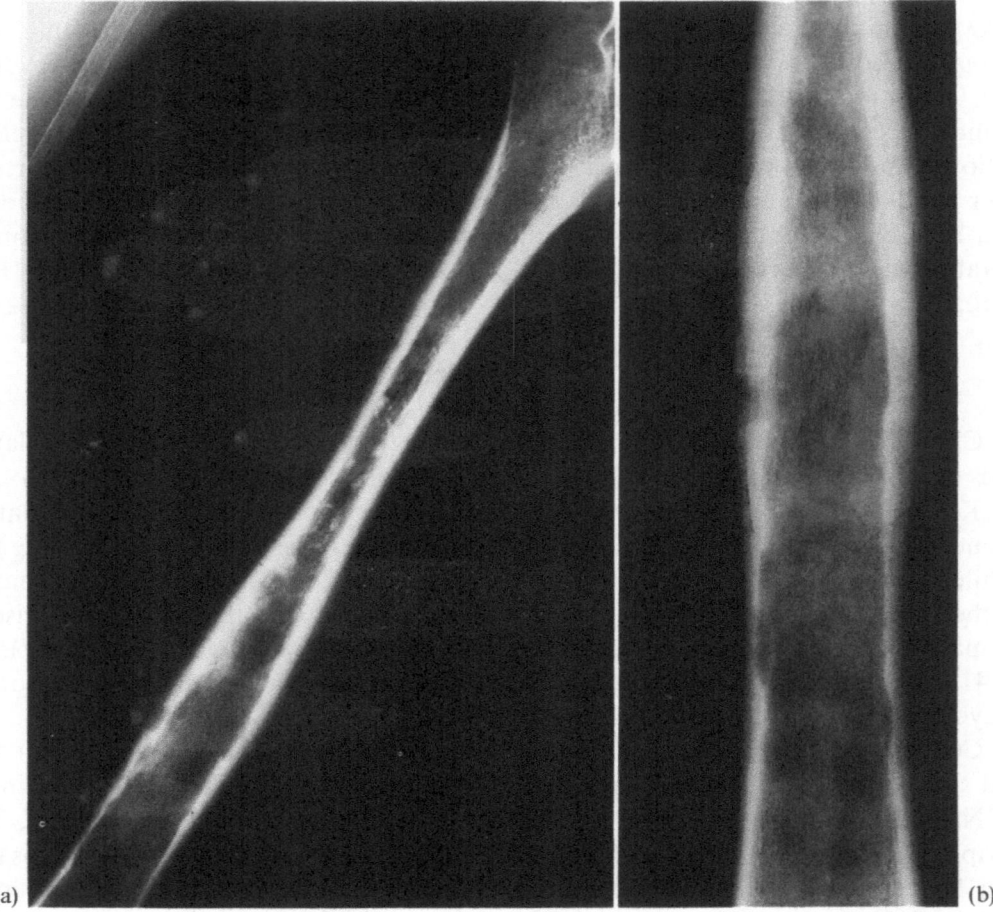

Fig. 88a and b. Chondrosarcoma, femur: 21-year-old female complaining of leg pain. (a) AP view: Note diaphyseal flaring, marked disproportionate localized cortical thickening, and endosteal scalloping caused by this slowly growing tumor. Coarse, granular calcifications are evident in proximal tumor bed. (b) Magnification view, distal femur: No discrete mineral deposits are noted in this area but poor definition of internal trabecular architecture and hazy quality of medullary cavity suggests a chondroid matrix. Note internal scalloping caused by lobular pattern of growth of this slowly expanding tumor. Lateral cortical defect represents a biopsy site

at which 14 peripheral chondrosarcomas were diagnosed ranged from 11–60 years with an average of 32.8 years. An average age of onset of 49.9 years was noted in the 10 tumors regarded as arising centrally.

III. Clinical

The dating of the onset of symptoms is problematic and is often inexact. The age at onset of symptoms was considered by O'NEAL and ACKERMAN (1952) to be reliably contemporaneous with the onset of the neoplasm in cases with peripheral lesions in accessible sites. It was considered not to be reliable in peripheral intrapelvic tumors or tumors presenting in the thoracic cavity. In their experience the onset or appearance of intramedullary lesions antedated their associated symptomatology by a long interval. The marked calcification noted in many of their central lesions despite a brief clinical history was felt to represent indirect evidence of long standing. LICHTENSTEIN (1965), however, has noted an opposite experience with longer clinical histories in cases with peripheral chondrosarcomas than in those with central lesions. Very short histories associated with a rapidly fatal clinical course are exceptional in most series.

From a clinical point of view, the onset of pain in a cartilaginous growth that has previously been dormant or asymptomatic is an ominous sign suggesting malignancy. Pain, however, is commonly not a disabling or even prominent feature. It may be subliminal, intermittent, associated with periods of well being, and exacerbation or entirely absent, with the patient presenting with a mass of huge proportions. Pain, in general, is more apt to be associated with aggressive central lesions that expand and disrupt the cortex, or with peripheral lesions which impinge on sensitive neighboring structures, such as nerves, blood vessels, and occasionally bones (Fig. 87). Pain may additionally result from a pathologic fracture (Figs. 89a, b) or a sudden spurt of growth. It is the appearance of a mass, however, often of prominent proportions, which may be particularly evident in peripheral locations, that most frequently causes patients to seek treatment. In O'NEAL and ACKERMAN's series (1952), the presence of a tumor was the first symptom in 14 of 25 peripheral chondrosarcomas (56%), while pain was the initial symptom in 9 (36%). Conversely, pain was the first symptom in 7 of 10 central chondrosarcomas, only 3 of which developed a palpable tumor by the time of admission.

Occasionally, patients may date the onset either of pain and/or of a visible mass from the time of trauma which may be trivial. LICHTENSTEIN (1965), in commenting that one must be critical of the role of trauma in relation to bone tumors in general, was nevertheless impressed by the frequency with which an injury was followed, after a reasonable interval, by malignant manifestations.

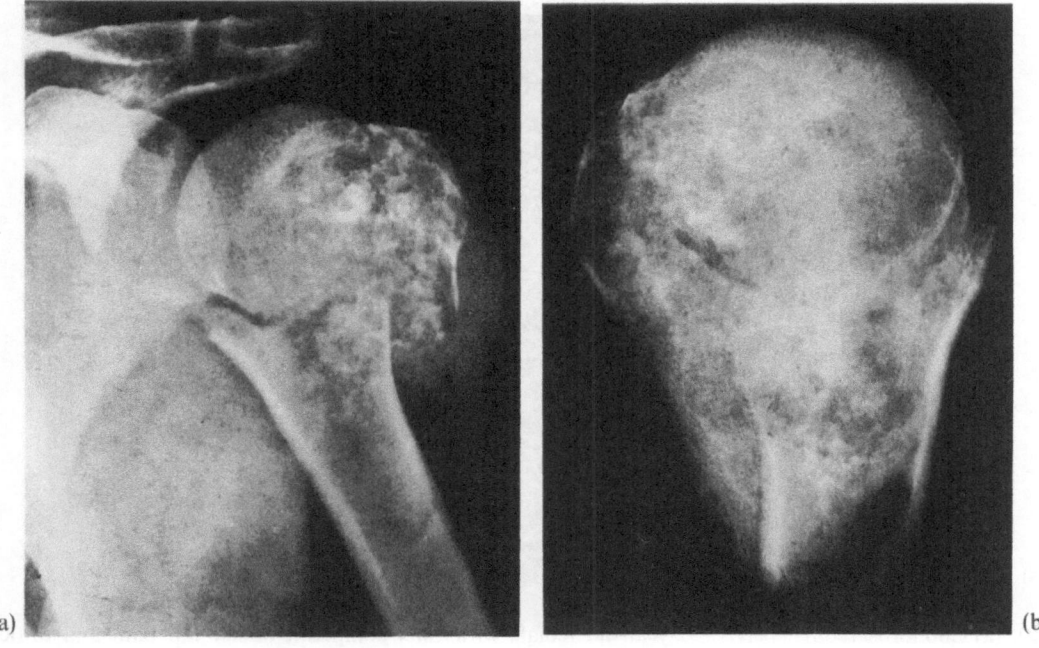

(a)   (b)

Fig. 89. (a) Chondrosarcoma, humerus: 45-year-old female with pain of 6 months' duration, which was acutely accentuated by a transverse pathologic fracture. Coarse granular "popcorn ball" calcifications are distributed throughout substance of lesion. (b) Resected specimen. Patient is alive and well 11 years post partial resection

Symptoms and physical examination are, therefore, not routinely helpful in making a diagnosis. Laboratory studies are nonspecific. Alkaline phosphatase activity is generally low. An altered carbohydrate metabolism has been reported in various neoplastic conditions. It has been shown that proliferating neoplastic tissue utilizes a greater amount of glucose (HENDERSON and LePAGE, 1959). HART and HINERMAN (1965) postulated that neoplasms may produce an anti-insulin metabolite which inactivates the peripheral utilization of glucose, thereby diverting it into the neoplastic tissue. GHOSH et al. (1973), in a qualitative and quantitative study of the pancreatic islets, obtained at autopsy from 12 control and 18 chondrosarcoma cases, noted definite hypertrophy and hyperplasia of islets in the chondrosarcoma patients. They had a greater number of cells per islet and a greater number of alpha cells as well as beta cells than the control cases. A relationship between altered carbohydrate metabolism and chondrosarcoma has also been noted clinically (MARCOVE and FRANCIS, 1963; MARCOVE et al., 1972). Oral glucose tolerance tests were abnormal in 18 of 19 patients of MARCOVE et al. (1972) with chondrosarcoma of the pelvis or upper femur. The 2 h-level was over 100 mgm/100 ml, although only 6 of the 18 patients were known diabetics. Theories involving the antigenicity (COHEN et al., 1972) and possible viral etiology of chondrosarcoma (SINKOVICS et al., 1970, 1971) will perhaps lead to other means of laboratory confirmation. In a recent study, a patient's serum reacted with cytoplasmic antigens of the autologous tumor cells in an indirect fluorescent antibody test (SINKOVICS et al., 1971).

IV. Sites

Cartilaginous tumors, both benign and malignant, may arise in any bone that is preformed in cartilage, including the base of the skull (VANDENBERG and COLEY, 1950).

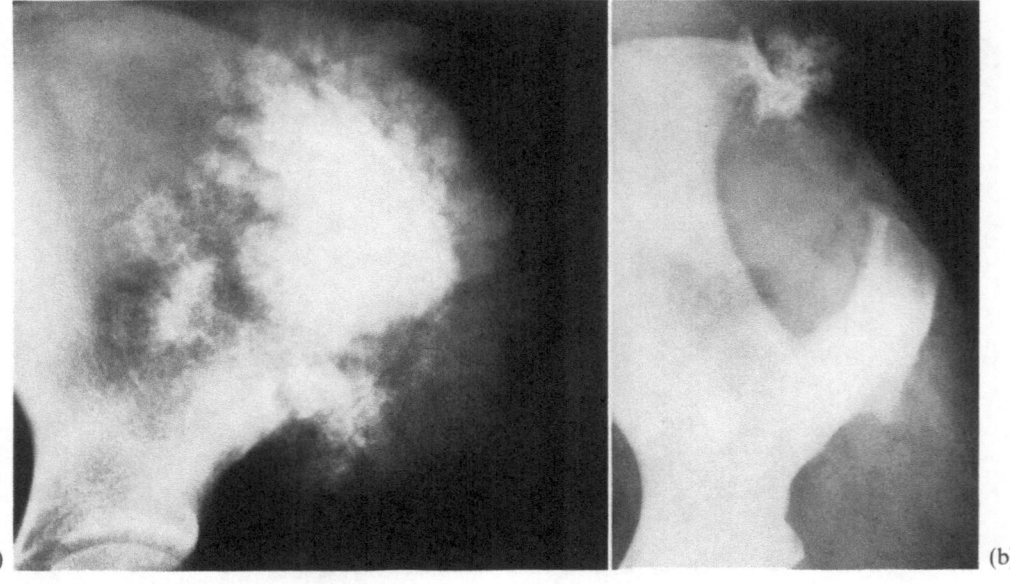

(a)   (b)

Fig. 90. (a) Chondrosarcoma, pelvis: 32-year-old female with chief complaint of left hip pain and difficulty in sitting. Lesion is heavily mineralized with marked central sclerosis suggesting bone formation. Periphery of lesion is poorly defined. Ring-shaped deposits of calcium frequently seen in association with chondrosarcoma are evident medially. (b) Recurrence 4 years post surgery. This lesion was subsequently resected. Patient is alive and well with no evidence of recurrence 18 years post second resection

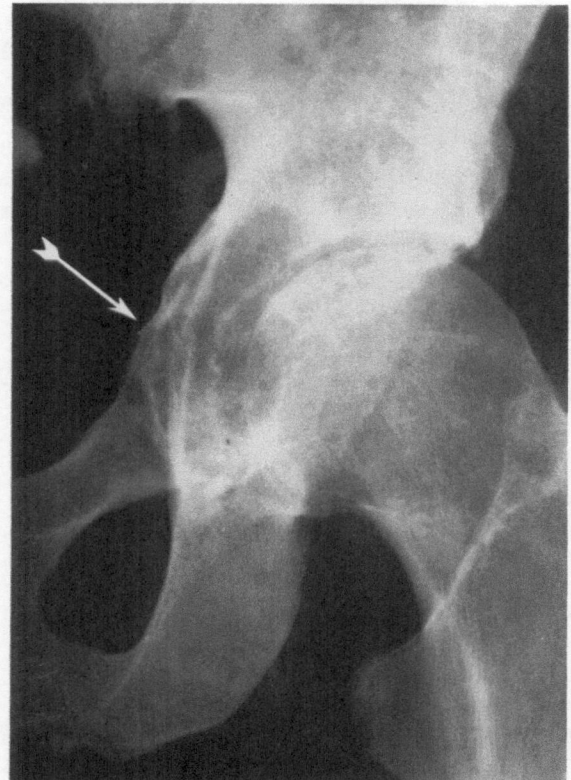 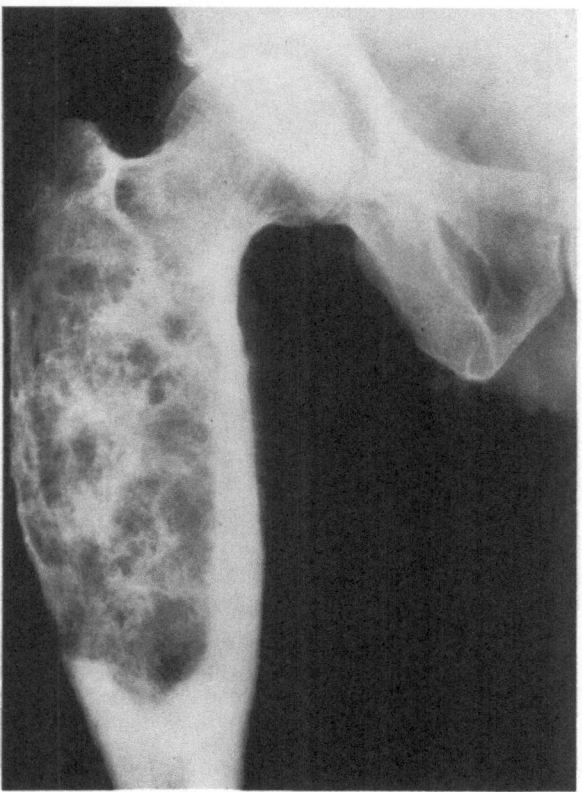

Fig. 91   Fig. 92

Fig. 91. Chondrosarcoma (lytic), pelvis: 58-year-old male with hip pain of 4 weeks duration. Note poor definition of medial acetabular cortex with completely lytic slightly expansile lesion involving acetabulum and pubic ramus (arrow). Patient is alive and well 4 years post left hemipelvectomy

Fig. 92. Chondrosarcoma, femur: Large, slowly growing, heavily mineralized tumor involves metaphysis and diaphysis. Although lesion was bordered by thickened hypertrophied cortex medially, recent periosteal reaction in form of wisps and spicules of new bone oriented perpendicularly to cortex became evident superomedially. Lateral cortex is thin and attenuated with small, localized areas of disruption. Note extension into diaphysis. Hypertrophied cortex takes on triangular or buttress-like configuration at inferior extent of lesion

The most frequent sites for both primary and secondary lesions are the pelvis (Figs. 90a, b, 91), the femoral shafts (Figs. 92, 93), and the proximal humeri (Figs. 89, 94). Other commonly involved areas are the remainder of the shoulder girdle (Figs. 95a, b) (MARCOVE and HUVOS, 1971; SCHAJOWICZ and CAMBIAGGI, 1961), the ribs, and the sternum. Uncommon skeletal sites include the vertebral column (Figs. 96a, b, c), the base of the skull, the maxilla (PADDISON and HANKS, 1971; WOLFOWITZ, 1973), and the mandible (LOVE, 1972; RICHTER et al., 1974).

In general, malignant cartilage tumors are most frequently found close to the trunk, i.e. 70% of lesions. About half of 83 chondrosarcomas reported by SINCOVICS et al. (1970) originated in the pelvis. Conversely, chondrosarcomas are rarest, with the exception of the calcaneus, in the distal extremities, which are the favorite sites for benign enchondromas. SHELLITO and DOCKERTY (1948) reported two chondrosarcomas among 40 cases of cartilaginous tumors of the hand. In a more recent review (DAHLIN and SALVADOR, 1974) of 30 chondrosarcomas of the hands and feet, 10 were found among 320 skeletal chondrosarcomas in the Mayo Clinic files. Hence, only 3% of chondrosarcomas occurred

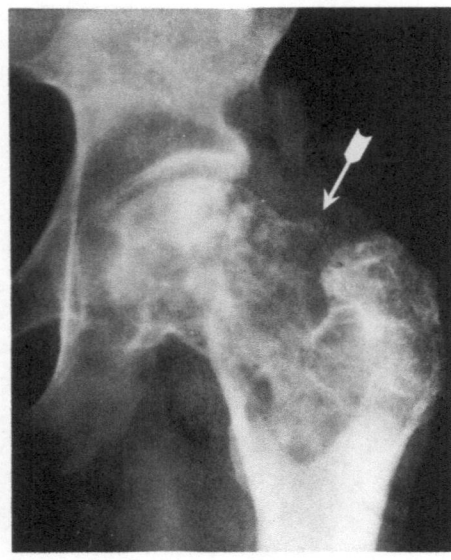
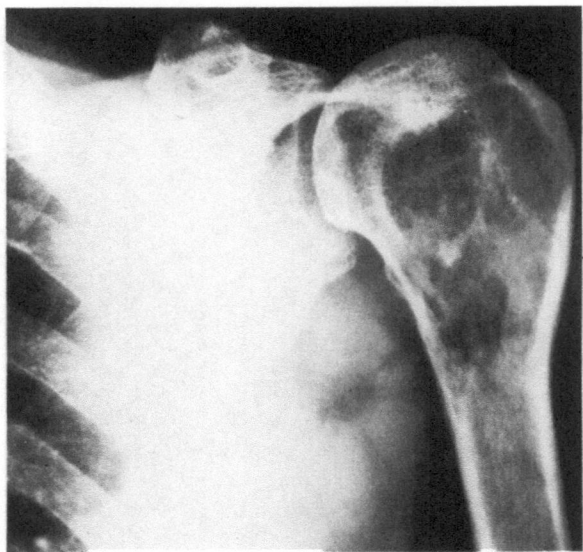

Fig. 93   Fig. 94

Fig. 93. Chondrosarcoma, femur: 61-year-old male with recurrent left hip pain. He had partial left femoral neck resection 12 years prior at another hospital where diagnosis of chondrosarcoma was made. Tumor has involved epiphyseal region, disrupted lateral cortex (arrow) and extends into soft tissues. Note sharp inferior demarcation. Patient is alive and well after insertion of proximal femoral prosthesis 19 years after initial resection and 7 years post second resection

Fig. 94. Chondrosarcoma, humerus: 53-year-old male with increasing pain and limited shoulder motion after fall 4 months prior to admission. Note central calcific deposit, thickened lateral cortex, and poor inferior demarcation of tumor which has spared end of bone

in the hands and feet. However, even this figure was felt to be high and related to the fact that the Mayo Clinic was a referral center. The incidence of chondrosarcoma of the bones of the hand alone has been estimated as representing less than 1% of chondrosarcomas that occur in man (DAHLIN and SALVADOR, 1974; HABAL et al., 1973; SHELLITO and DOCKERTY, 1948). Therefore, the site of a cartilaginous lesion is particularly significant, since it not only dictates the circumstances of its clinical discovery and symptomatology, but contributes to a clarification of the lesion's biologic behavior. This is particularly true of cartilaginous lesions.

It is of interest that enchondromas of the hands and feet frequently show histologic changes suggestive of low grade malignancy, particularly in the young, and particularly in cases of multiple enchondromatosis, while behaving in a benign manner (JAFFE, 1968). On the other hand "benign-looking" histologic sections obtained from more proximally situated lesions often belie their usually more aggressive course. A discrepancy may therefore exist between the histologic appearance and the biologic behavior of cartilaginous lesions, despite the application of classic histologic criteria as defined by LICHTEN-STEIN and JAFFE (1943). LICHTENSTEIN (1965) has also emphasized that "the rules laid down for the recognition of early chondrosarcoma apply strictly to tumors in bone, and particularly to central chondrosarcomas."

Similar histology may meet with a different interpretation, depending on whether the sample is obtained from a peripheral, central, or subperiosteal lesion and/or from a more proximally or distally situated lesion. Therefore, histologic criteria still need to be tempered by clinical circumstances such as site, in addition to symptoms and age as previously noted.

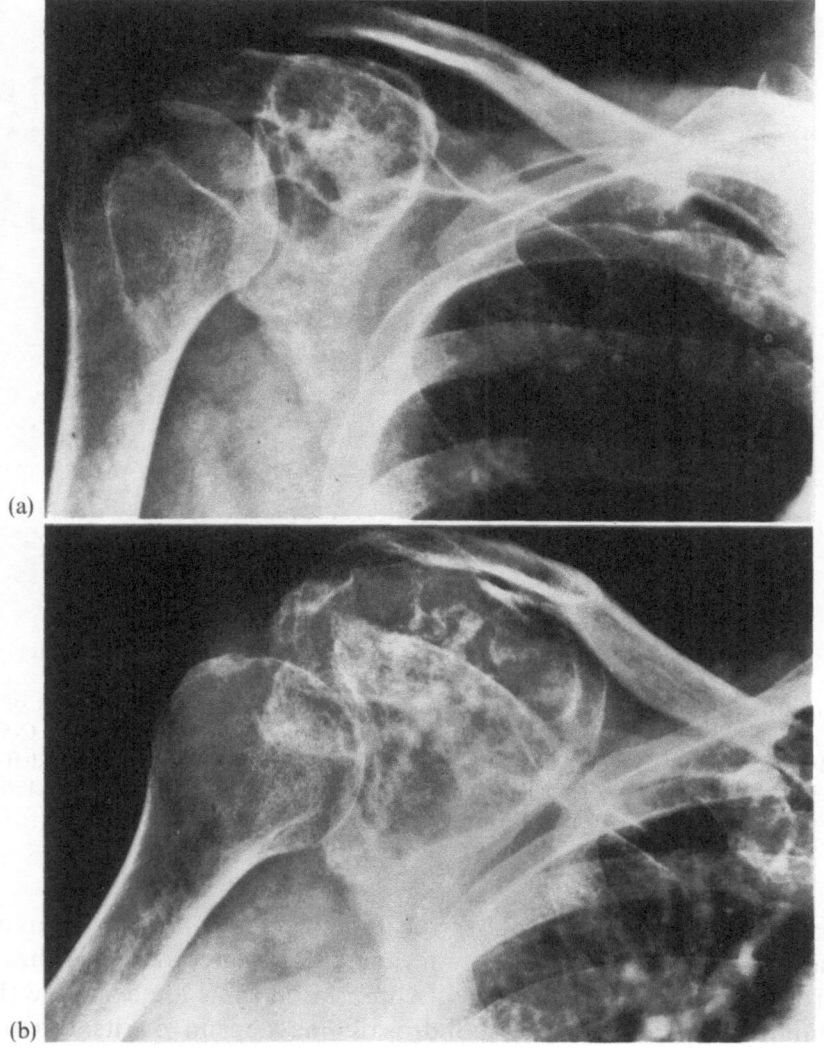

Fig. 95. (a) Chondrosarcoma, scapula: 56-year-old male complained of shoulder pain of several months' duration. Lytic expansile sharply marginated lesion with mineral within it appears to involve glenoid as well
as coracoid process of scapula on 9/5/70. (b) 1/21/74: Tumor, though still well-defined, inferomedially has
increased markedly in size. Cortex, though markedly attenuated, is still identifiable. Coarse conglomerates
of mineral are most heavily concentrated in center of lesion. (Courtesy of Dr. KENNETH JEWEL)

Histologic interpretation may additionally be modified by the size of the lesion.
The roentgenogram, therefore, in addition to helping characterize the nature of the
lesion, helps to place it in its proper perspective. The roentgenogram, therefore, together
with the histology and clinical setting, forms one of the sides of a "diagnostic isosceles"
triangle which is indispensible to the proper evaluation of cartilaginous lesions.

V. Roentgenographic Features

The roentgenogram may not only confirm the suspicion of a chondrosarcoma aroused
by the history, physical findings and pathology, but it may serve to identify the presence

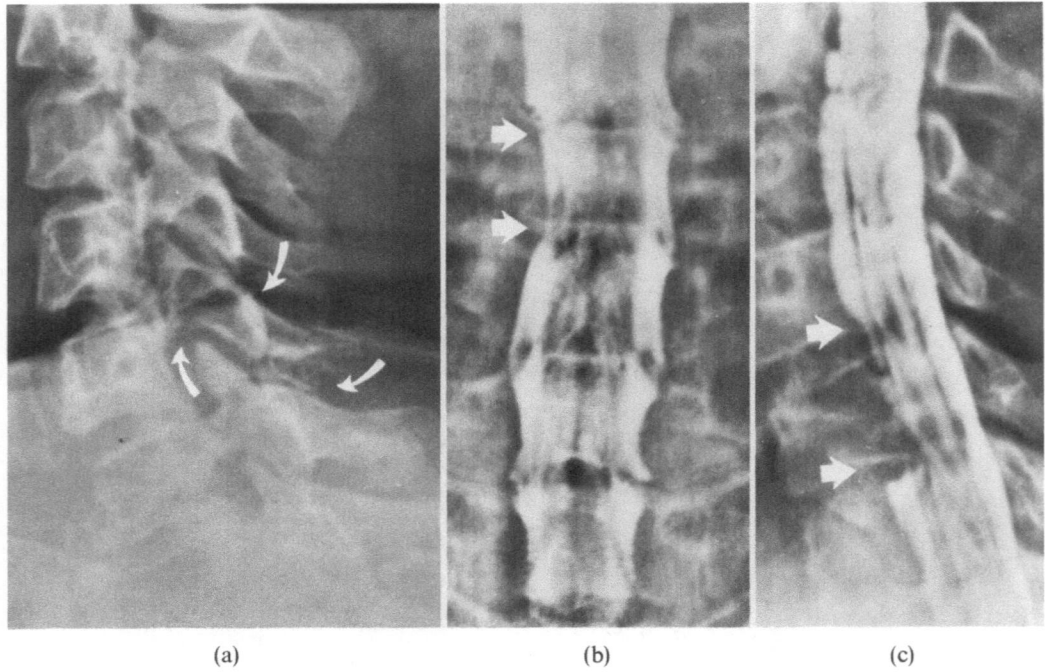

(a)   (b)   (c)

Fig. 96a–c. Chondrosarcoma, cervical spine: 58-year-old male with pain and stiffness of neck of several months'
duration. (a) Oblique view: Ill-defined radiolucent lesion involves posterior elements at C-5 level (arrows).
(b) and (c) Myelogram: PA and oblique views show that spinal cord is displaced to left and superiorly
by tumor mass which extends into spinal canal. Note persistent external pressure defect displacing spinal
cord at C-5/6 level (arrows). (Courtesy of Dr. HARVEY HECHT)

of an unsuspected lesion. It may be critical in assessing the duration of the lesion
or in evaluating its aggressive nature by means of its degree of mineralization, as well
as its size or rate of growth, particularly if comparison films are available (Figs. 95a, b).

The radiographic features of a chondrosarcoma depend on its orientation within
the bone. A central lesion in a long bone is usually situated in the metaphysis (Figs. 94,
97a, b), but may involve the diaphysis (Figs. 88, 92) and extend toward the articular
surface (Fig. 93). Impingement on the articular surface (Fig. 98), however, is less common
and rupture through articular cartilage into the joint is rarely appreciated on roentgenograms. Histologic evidence of joint invasion via articular cartilage was noted in 3 of
10 central chondrosarcomas in O'NEAL and ACKERMAN'S series (1952).

Central chondrosarcomas in long bones frequently appear as areas of hazy rarefaction
which reflect their chondroid matrix. The lesions tend to be elongated and may occasionally involve a considerable length of the medullary cavity (Fig. 88). Endosteal scalloping
and adjacent cortical expansion often result in a multilobulated appearance (GELMAN,
1974; HAMLIN et al., 1971; REITER et al., 1972).

Periosteal and endosteal reactive bone formation often produce a thickened cortex
of uniform density which is indicative of slow growth and serves as a means of identifying
the more indolent lesions (Fig. 88). Cortical thickening is often particularly prominent
at the inferior extent of the rarefied portion of the lesion, where it takes on a triangular
or "buttress-like" configuration (Figs. 92, 98). The interrupted, laminated, "onionskin"
type of periosteal new bone formation frequently noted as a hallmark of round cell
tumors is rarely observed. When associated with chondrosarcomas, an interrupted or
cyclic periosteal reaction is frequently focal with individual layers being poorly demar-

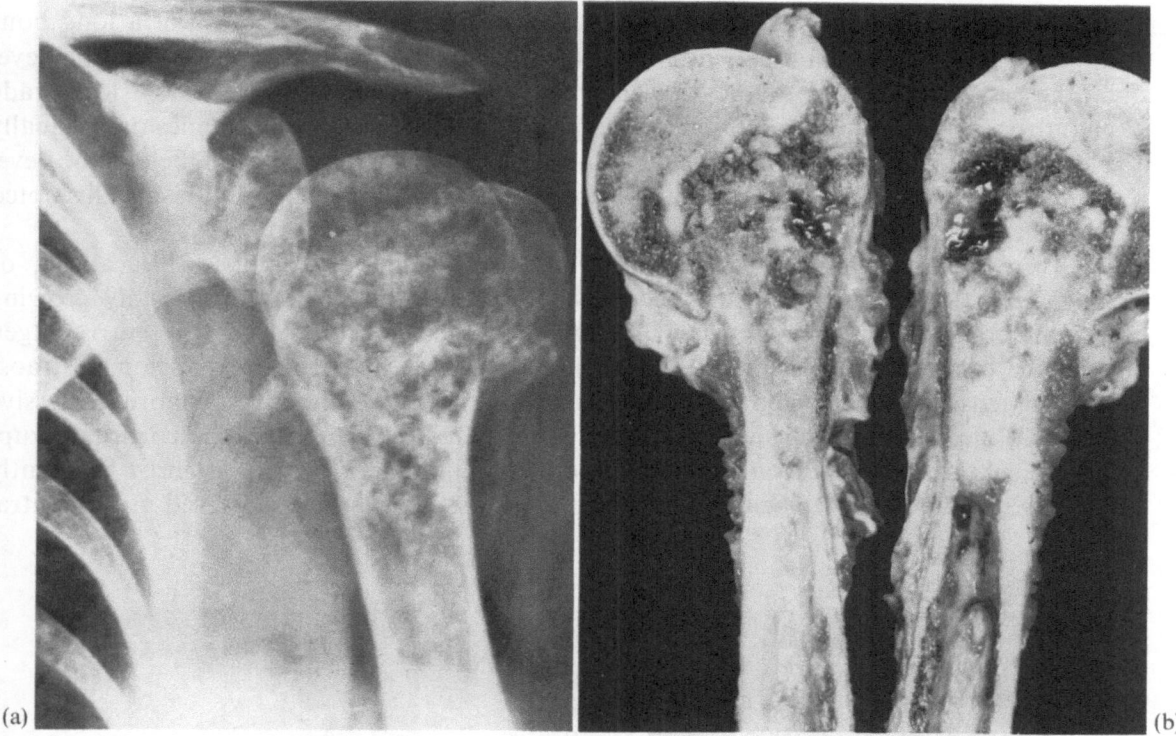

Fig. 97. (a) Chondrosarcoma, humerus. Pathologic fracture traverses central, heavily calcified portion of lesion whose superior and inferior borders are poorly defined. (b) Amputated specimen. Cut sections of proximal humerus reveal cartilaginous nature of lesion. Intramedullary calcification and focal areas of hemorrhage and necrosis are evident. Essentially metaphyseal tumor had spared epiphysis but had destroyed and penetrated cortex

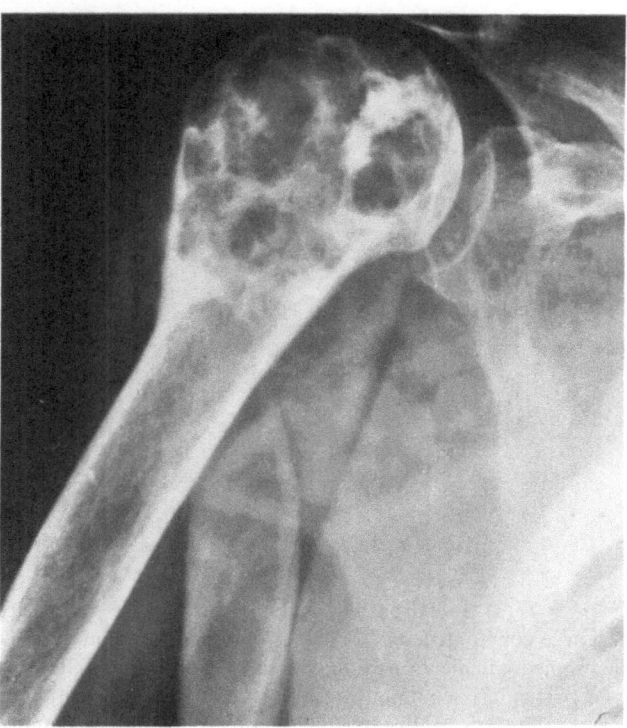

Fig. 98. Chondrosarcoma, humerus: 65-year-old male with 2 year history of shoulder pain. Large, expansile tumor abuts articular surface but respects joint space. Note proximal calcification as well as thickening and "buttressing" of inferior lateral cortex. Extremity was disarticulated

cated and indistinct. Focal periosteal reaction with new bone spicules oriented perpendicularly to the shaft are rarely noted (Fig. 92). Most commonly the cortex of a long bone appears as a single, uniform, homogeneous density of varying thickness at the level of the lesion, testifying to the slower growth characteristics of the classic low grade chondrosarcoma. A subtly ballooned or expanded shaft at the level of the lesion gradually blends with the normal diameter or contour of the bone above and below the level of the bulk of the tumor. A gradual, rather than an abrupt expansion is usually noted (REITER et al., 1972).

Even a thickened cortex may eventually be invaded by tumor and localized, or intermittent cortical interruption becomes identifiable. With the more rapidly growing lesions, cortical destruction, which is commonly focal, occurs early, with no roentgen evidence of new bone formation, remodeling, or apparent cortical expansion. Extraosseous extension as well as cortical destruction are indicative of active or more aggressive lesions. Extraosseous extension may not be appreciated, particularly when cortical disruption is subtle and the extraosseous component is unmineralized, as is most frequently the case. Extraosseous calcification within soft tissue extensions derived from central

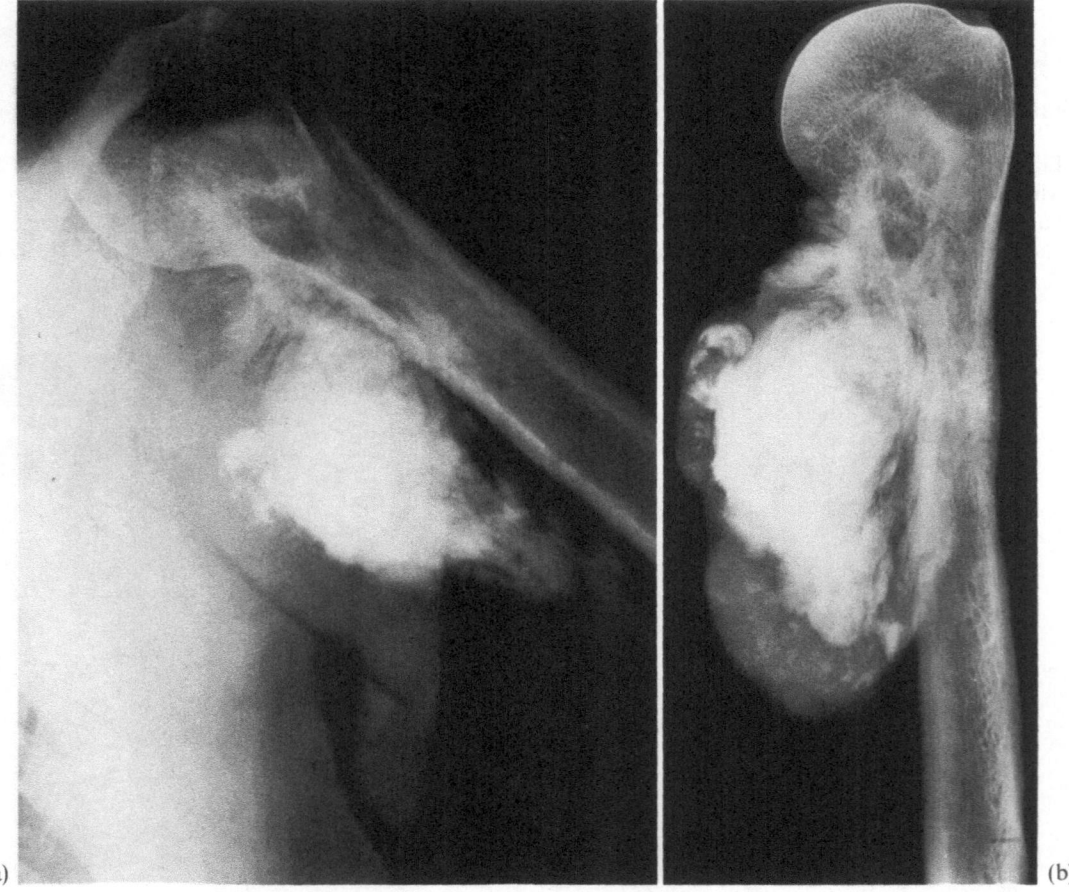

(a)   (b)

Fig. 99. (a) Chondrosarcoma, humerus: Tumor has destroyed cortex and involved surrounding soft tissues. Large conglomerate of metaplastic bone formation is seen within extrinsic mass. (b) Resected specimen. Finely stippled calcification is now discernable just peripheral to bulk of metaplastic bone (arrows). Calcification is particularly common in well-or moderately well-differentiated tumors. Foci of bone not histologically malignant, as well as myxoid zones may be noted. Tumor is reminiscent of parosteal osteogenic sarcoma

lesions is rarely discernible, either roentgenographically or histologically (O'NEAL and ACKERMAN, 1952) (Figs. 87a, b, 99a, b) as opposed to that deposited in peripheral chondrosarcomas per se. Despite the lack of mineralization, however, soft tissue extensions may appear well defined due to surrounding soft tissue structures, which tend to form a "pseudocapsule." Occasionally the tumor, by exerting pressure on neighboring muscle mass or interstitial tissue, will have its periphery etched by a thin sharp line of relatively radiolucent interstitial fat. Arteriography is often helpful in delineating the extraosseous extent of central chondrosarcomas. In addition, the fact that both the central as well as the extraosseous portions of the lesion are most commonly hypovascular in classic chondrosarcomas may offer an indirect clue as to the nature of the lesion (Figs. 100a, b, c). Xerography and roentgenograms taken with soft tissue technique may further help to define an extraosseous component (Figs. 101a, b).

The tumor in central chondrosarcoma is most commonly seen as a central, rather than eccentric, radiolucent area within the metaphyseal end of the medullary cavity. Although its medial and lateral boundaries may be bordered by a sclerotic rim of reactive new bone or a thickened cortex, the inferior and/or superior extent of the lesion is frequently poorly defined. This is in contrast to the boundaries of a benign enchondroma, which are often rounded and commonly circumferentially well-defined, frequently by a rim of bony condensation. This poor definition of superior and inferior geographic boundaries reflects the histologic appearance of the classic chondrosarcoma (Figs. 88, 94, 97). Tumor tissue is seen to subtly infiltrate among the interstices of numerous trabeculae without causing marked destruction or erosion and in this manner may commonly extend for a considerable distance throughout the medullary cavity (Fig. 102). Therefore, in chondrosarcoma, as in round cell tumors, the roentgenogram is a poor guide to the lesion's actual extent within or involvement of the medullary cavity. On the other hand, the roentgenogram is a more reliable representative of the actual size of a "classic" osteosarcoma.

The visualized area of destruction in chondrosarcoma commonly appears hazy and unclear, not only because of its chondroid matrix, but due to mineral deposition within this matrix (Fig. 88). Calcification or ossification within the lesion, either on the basis of enchondral bone formation and/or areas of degeneration (Fig. 97) further enforce the roentgen diagnosis of a cartilaginous lesion. Mineral may appear in the form of stippled or ring-like densities (LODWICK, 1965) (Fig. 89A), finely scattered throughout the lesional area or focally concentrated in large conglomerates (Figs. 94, 95, 98). The degree and distribution of mineral deposits may serve as a guide to biopsy, since a great deal of calcification is usually not present in areas of greatest activity. However, low grade chondrosarcomas may also be densely calcified by virtue of their slower growth, thereby making differentiation from a benign process, on the basis of mineral content alone, difficult. Rounder defects that are more heavily mineralized may be confused with benign enchondromas, and the more elongated mineralized lesions with bone infarcts. Size, then, becomes a pertinent factor. A previously documented calcified lesion presumed to be an enchondroma in which the calcified portion appears to "melt away" and/or which begins to enlarge, is suspect of being or having become malignant, particularly when symptomatic. Bone infarcts, in addition to being more elongated and multiple, are more heavily mineralized along the periphery (Fig. 34). They are usually silhouetted by a sharply demarcated fibro-osseous border. This is indicative of their centripetal healing pattern with attempts at bone repair being initiated from the periphery of the necrotic segment.

More highly malignant lesions may show no calcification either in the intraosseous component or within its extraosseous extension. Therefore, calcification or ossification

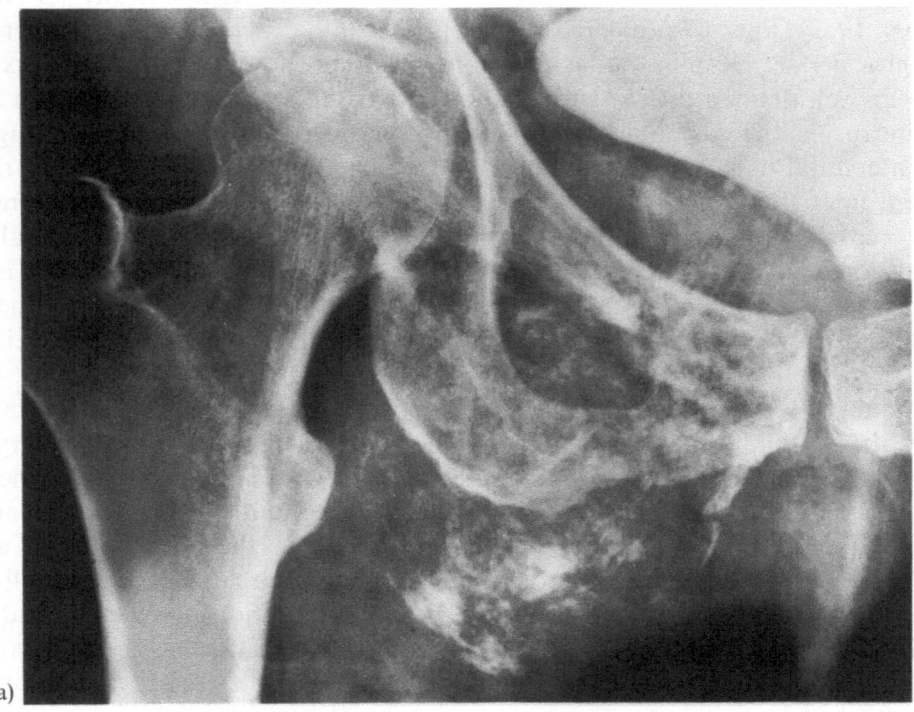

(a)

Fig. 100. (a) Chondrosarcoma, pelvis: Large, lobulated, irregularly calcified mass extends into surrounding soft tissues from ischio-pubic area of 67-year-old female. (b) Arteriogram serves to define peripheral extent of this relatively hypovascular lesion. Stretching and displacement of surrounding vessels are most marked about inferior border of tumor. (c) Subtraction film. Hypovascularity, a common finding in chondromatous tumors, is now additionally established

within the tumor may offer a clue as to its aggressiveness. Mineral is frequently not roentgenographically detectable, or may be absent in chondrosarcomas in the sacroiliac or acetabular regions (Fig. 91). These lesions may appear entirely lytic, may mimic metastases or multiple myeloma, and occur in a similar age group. The location of the lesion near the acetabulum in the region of the triradiate cartilage is a clue to the correct diagnosis (Figs. 91, 103a, b). Figure 103b shows the radiograph of a surgical specimen of an unmineralized acetabular chondrosarcoma.

When poorly mineralized, aggressive lesions involve the epiphyses of long bones, they may be radiographically indistinguishable from giant cell tumors or aneurysmal bone cysts, which have secondarily involved the end of the bone. Unicameral bone cysts, though centrally located, do not involve the epiphysis, but rather migrate towards the diaphysis with growth of the shaft.

Chondroblastomas involve the epiphyseal area but are usually smaller, well-circumscribed, rounded, or oval lesions that most commonly occur in younger patients.

Benign enchondromas are usually better defined without the degree of cortical hypertrophy and thickening so frequently associated with classic chondrosarcomas. The cortices in the vicinity of benign enchondromas, though occasionally appearing thin and expanded, are usually intact without a history of antecedent trauma. Solitary enchondromas most commonly occur in distal sites, i.e. the phalanges of the hands and feet, are usually smaller than chondrosarcomas and are asymptomatic unless fractured.

As previously emphasized, size is an important radiographic feature which may give strong support to the diagnosis of an early low grade chondrosarcoma (Fig. 88). The

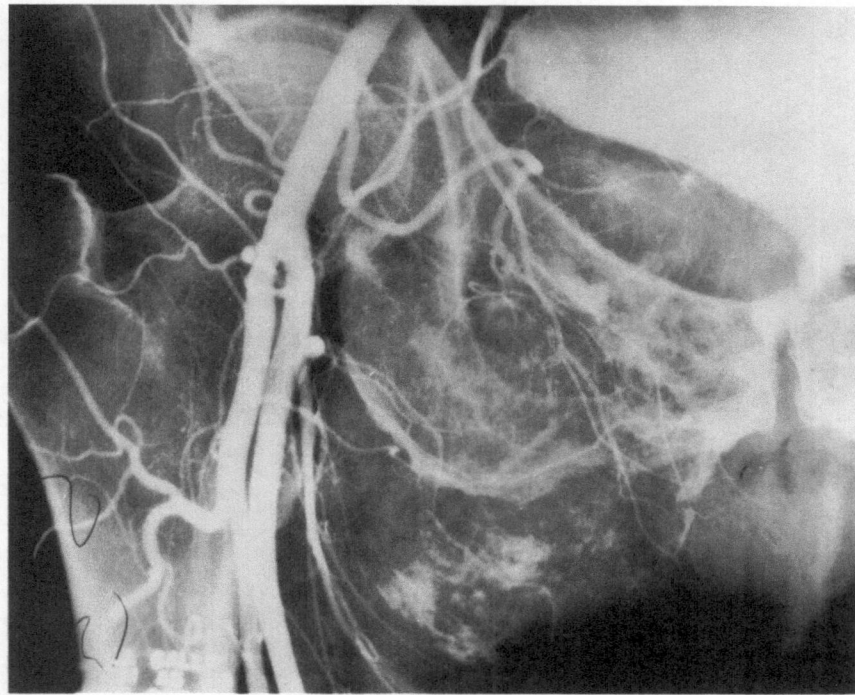

Fig. 100b

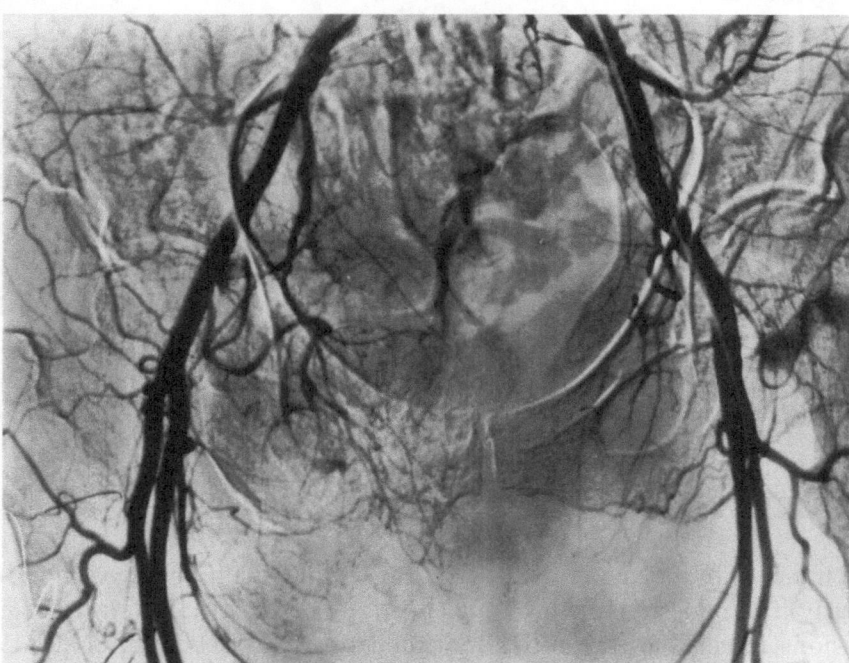

Fig. 100c

roentgenogram, despite its limitations in judging the entire extent of the lesion, is the only means, other than surgery or extirpation, of judging the volume of the lesion. Arteriography may furnish additional help in terms of defining the extent of the lesion. A centrally situated cartilaginous lesion measuring several centimeters or greater in diameter, particularly if situated proximally within the pelvis, thoracic cage, or shaft of a long bone, should arouse suspicions of malignancy (COLEY and HIGINBOTHAM, 1949; MARCOVE and HUVOS, 1971; O'NEAL and ACKERMAN, 1952; PASCUZZI et al., 1957).

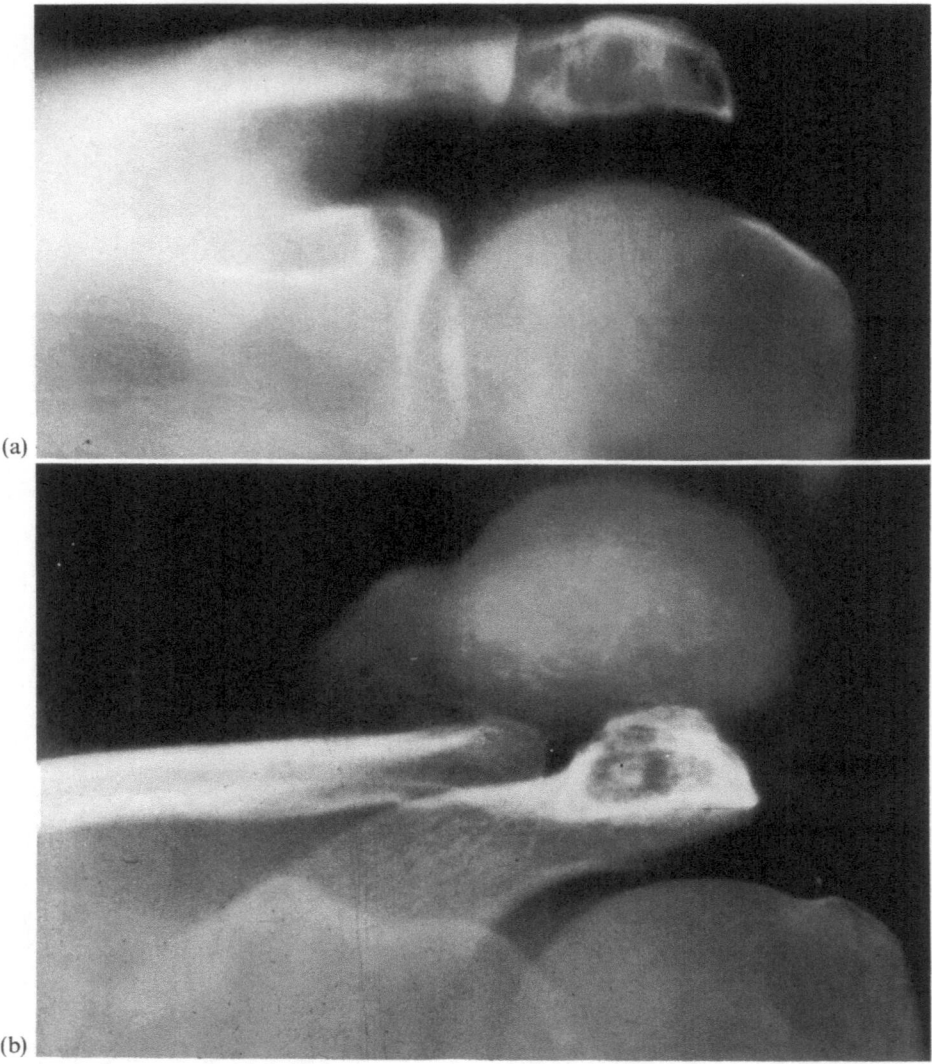

Fig. 101a and b. Chondrosarcoma, scapula: 62-year-old female with shoulder pain of 3 years duration and recent swelling. (a) Laminagrams define lytic lesion acromion with inferior cortical disruption. (b) Slight difference in technique and angulation obscures inferior cortical disruption, but defines large mass with fine stippled calcification within it. Note central acromial defect with punctate calcification within it

Some chondrosarcomas are believed to originate from benign chondromas. This is particularly true of lesions in proximal portions of the trunk and/or of more distally situated lesions in cases with multiple enchondromatosis (HAMLIN et al., 1971). It may be impossible, however, by histologic means alone, to establish the evolution of a central chondrosarcoma from a pre-existing benign endchondroma, particularly if the latter is a solitary lesion and particularly if it is situated at some distance from the trunk. The concept of malignant degeneration of solitary enchondromas has become a philosophic "bone of contention" among pathologists. Some contend that malignant degeneration of a solitary benign chondroma is a rare event and exceedingly difficult to document, either histologically or roentgenographically. Many of the lesions presumed to have undergone malignant degeneration have been diagnosed by others as examples of low grade, slow growing, primary chondrosarcoma which arose de novo. On reviewing a

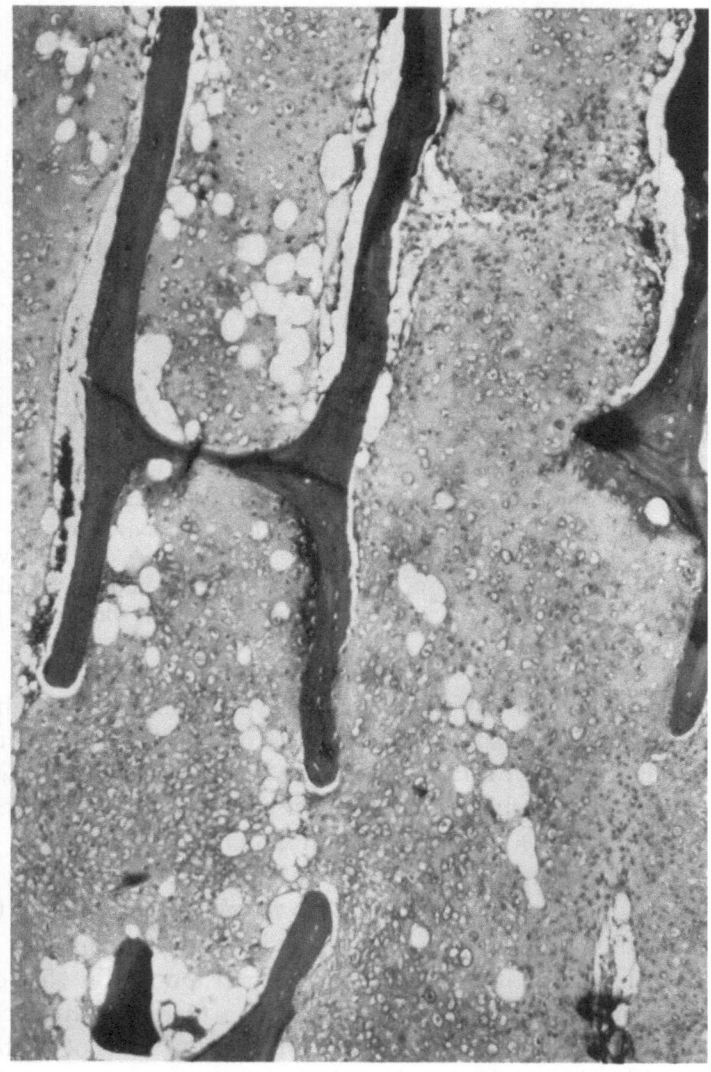

Fig. 102. Chondrosarcoma, photomicrograph (× 50): Tumor cells crowd marrow cavity interjected among trabeculae without destroying or obviously eroding them. Because of this subtle infiltration, tumor may involve considerable portion of medullary cavity and yet not be well-delineated or even appreciated roentgenographically. Roentgenogram may, therefore, be poor guide to lesions actual extent within medullary cavity

series of biopsies from chondrosarcoma said to have arisen from benign enchondromas, DAHLIN and HENDERSON (1956) describe these tumors as being low grade malignancies from the start. Some authorities claim never to have seen malignant transformation of a solitary enchondroma of the phalanges of the hands and feet (ACKERMAN and SPJUT, 1962). In DAHLIN'S series (1967) chondrosarcomatous transformation in a proved solitary benign enchondroma was not known to have occurred. He cites misinterpretation of original tissue sections, insufficient microscopic sampling of surgical material, or incomplete removal of the primary tumor as leading to underdiagnosis and the erroneous impression of malignant transformation and subsequent recurrence. In DAHLIN and SALVADOR'S (1974) recent review of 30 chondrosarcomas of the bones of the hands and feet, 26 were solitary lesions with no other known skeletal disease, while 4 arose in cases with multiple enchondromata. Multiplicity of lesions, as well as their sites, are therefore important in evaluation. Chondrosarcoma of the bones of the hands and feet was again emphasized as occurring rarely with an occasional report adding one or two cases (JAKOBSON and SPJUT, 1960; MARCOVE and CHAROSKY, 1972; PACHTER and ALPERT, 1964; SCHAJOWICZ and CAMBIAGGI, 1961). It is probable that occasional

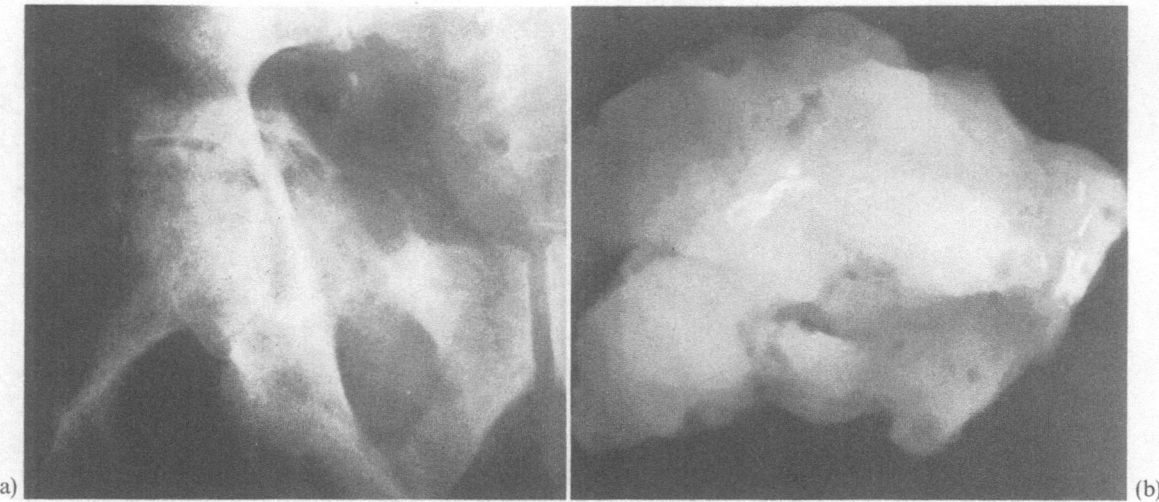

Fig. 103a and b. Chondrosarcoma, pelvis: 60-year-old male with right hip pain. (a) Lytic expansile lesion has partially destroyed acetabulum and right pubic bone. Cortex is expanded, thinned, and interrupted. Note reactive sclerosis of pubic bone. Calcification was not identified within tumor. (b) Surgical specimen. Note large soft tissue extension of tumor mass and persistent failure to delineate mineral deposition within lesion. Dense areas represent adherent bits of bone

cases reported as primary chondrosarcomas of the hands and feet, as well as those which have presumably resulted from malignant degeneration of a benign lesion, were inadequately evaluated, since criteria for differentiating these lesions from the relatively common chondromas of the bones of the hands and feet are not well delineated (DAHLIN and SALVADOR, 1974). The individual roentgenogram as well as a skeletal survey may then offer immediate additional help in determining multiplicity, as well as site and size while several roentgenograms widely spaced in time may offer a clue as to the growth potential of a particular lesion. The answers to these questions may serve as strong supporting evidence for the existence of a chondrosarcoma.

The roentgen manifestations of a classic central chondrosarcoma therefore include an indistinct area of medullary rarefaction with or without mottling, due to intralesional calcification and/or ossification; a uniformly thickened cortex which confines the lesion and/or is undergoing localized destruction and/or perforation. Such a lesion which is 2 cm or more in size, and which is situated in the proximal shaft of a long bone, the pelvis, shoulder girdle or thoracic cage, including the ribs and sternum, and particularly when associated with the onset of pain, should arouse suspicion that one is dealing with a chondrosarcoma. An associated extraosseous extension most commonly appearing as a vaguely defined, usually unmineralized, hard to delineate mass, further confirms the presence of a malignant process.

L. Peripheral Chondrosarcoma

The frequency of peripheral chondrosarcoma in general, and the development of malignant change in the cartilage cap of an osteochondroma in particular, have also been the subjects of considerable debate. The incidence of the latter complication in a solitary osteochondroma has been estimated as less than 1%. The development of condrosarcoma appears to be a rare complication of adolescent monostotic osteochondroma. In patients with hereditary multiple exostosis, however, the incidence of malignant change has ranged from 10–20% or more. This is especially true if these lesions are followed into adult life.

Again, the hazard of malignant change is more common in those lesions nearest the trunk. However, most benign osteochondromas are also situated in these areas. Of the 40 consecutive osteochondromas in O'NEAL and ACKERMAN's (1952) series, 38 (95%) involved the long bones of the extremities and chiefly arose from the upper tibia, lower femur and upper humerus.

Both roentgenographically and pathologically, the benign osteochondroma that has undergone malignant transformation may still be recognizable at its base. However, the sharp boundary at the junction between its core of cancellous bone and its cartilage cap may disappear.

In dealing with small peripheral chondrosarcomas which are associated with an exostosis, the single most important pathologic observation has been noted to be the width of the cartilage cap. If this exceeds 1 cm in an adult patient, then, according to LICHTENSTEIN (1965), the cartilage has been actively growing and as such represents a chondrosarcoma. Roentgenographic determination of the size of the cap may be roughly or inaccurately estimated on the basis of mineralization within it. However, occasionally, new calcific or ossific deposits may indicate further extension of or accretion to the lesion. Special techniques such as xerography often enhance the soft tissue or cartilaginous component of the exostosis, while an arteriogram may define its outer limits. A large thick cap persisting into adult life, or exhibiting an increase in size, whether slow or sudden, if associated with irregular mineralization at its periphery or beyond its previously established confines, is especially suspect of malignancy. Therefore, estimates of the lesion's size, and particularly of its progression as compared with previous studies, may be accomplished roentgenographically.

Another roentgen sign of peripheral chondrosarcoma or of malignant degeneration in a benign osteochondroma may be sought along the surface of a previously well-outlined cartilage cap. Its contour may become indistinct or fuzzy, with a partial or complee loss of a pre-existing thin peripheral calcific shell or of a clear zone of demarcation from the adjacent soft tissues. Unfortunately, the cartilage cap is not always well-defined at its periphery and may be irregularly mineralized within its central portion, so that roentgenograms may create a false impression of malignancy, local invasiveness, and/or inoperability. This is true both with osteochondromas and peripheral chondrosarcomas per se. The exostoses in both may attain large size. Actually, however bulky a peripheral chondrosarcoma associated with an exostosis is, at surgical exploration it is most commonly found to be a discrete circumscribed mass. It is of interest that in O'NEAL and ACKERMAN's series (1952) of exostoses, the entire projection, including the cartilage cap was encapsulated by a fibrous membrane of varying thickness that was continuous with the periosteum of the bone of origin. This was true in the benign osteochondromas as well as in the peripheral low grade chondrosarcomas treated for the first time, although the encapsulating membrane was usually thinner in the latter. The more aggressive lesions, however, often ruptured their "capsule."

Since a chondrosarcoma may destroy or obscure the pre-existing neck or pedicle of an exostosis or its origin from a large sessile cartilaginous base, the genesis of malignant from benign may then only be assumed. Again, as previously noted, this assumption is not as tenable in cases with solitary lesions as in those with multiple osteochondromatosis.

Peripheral chondrosarcomas may also arise de novo within the cortical confines of a bone and/or from the bone surface, i.e. presumably subperiosteally. However, this juxtacortical or subperiosteal location is rare. Often, at the time of diagnosis, the lesion has invaded the medullary cavity, raising the question of a central origin. Indirect evidence of its peripheral origin may lie in the fact that the bulk of the lesion is extraosseous in location, while the destruction within the medullary cavity is eccentrically situated within a large bone and of small volume in relation to the major mass of the tumor (Figs. 99, Fig. 104a, b).

The most common site of a peripheral chondrosarcoma is some part of the pelvis, and particularly the iliac part of the innominate bone (JAFFE, 1968; SINKOVICS et al., 1970) (Fig. 90a). As many as half of all peripheral chondrosarcomas involve some part of the pelvic girdle, while a large proportion of the other half develop in relation to the upper part of the femur or humerus, or to the scapula. Such lesions may be quite large, and are usually heavily mineralized centrally with streaks of calcification radiating toward the periphery. The contours of the lesion may be lobulated, ill-defined, and not calcified. The periphery is the most actively growing portion of the lesion and usually contains its most viable tissue. The pathologist most commonly relies on these well-preserved peripheral fields for accurate diagnosis rather than on those showing marked calcification or ossification. The latter are more commonly associated with areas of degeneration and/or necrobiosis.

A problem of roentgenographic differential diagnosis relates to the juxtacortical osteogenic sarcoma. However, the radiopacities of the latter lesion which extend into the

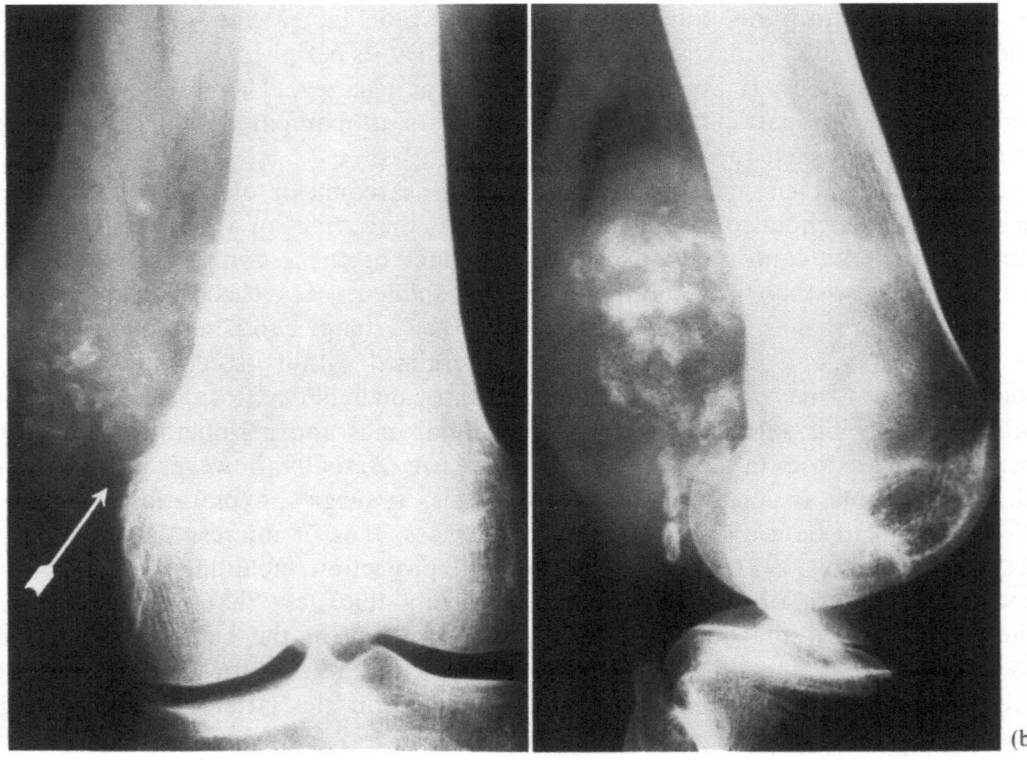

(a)

(b)

Fig. 104a and b. Chondrosarcoma, femur: 35-year-old male with pain and swelling of left knee. (a) AP view: Large, oval-shaped soft tissue mass appears cortically based with no roentgen evidence of medullary penetration. Note reactive periostitis (arrow). (b) Lateral view. Tumor mass has well-demarcated periphery with preservation of muscle and fat planes. Note heavy central mineralization

neighboring soft parts are usually fairly uniform, and just as dense as the rest of the radiopaque area, rather than spotty or fuzzy, as in chondrosarcomas. Mineral within a chondrosarcoma is also frequently deposited in the form of ring-like configurations.

What has been said about the cytologic stigmata of malignancy in connection with central chondrosarcoma applies in a general way to peripheral chondrosarcoma, although they are often not as obvious in the latter. However, no matter how subtle the histologic evidences of malignancy may be in the original lesion, they become increasingly clear-cut in any recurrences which may take place (JAFFE, 1968).

An observation made by O'NEAL and ACKERMAN (1952) in discussing the histologic criteria of peripheral chondrosarcomas may equally apply to central chondrosarcomas and may be helpful in the roentgen evaluation of both lesions. They noted that large tumors of short or long duration are usually malignant, while small tumors of long duration are usually benign.

I. Histologic Criteria

Chondrosarcoma is the most difficult of the malignant bone tumors to definitively identify. Although highly malignant lesions present no great difficulty in histologic diagnosis, considerable difficulty may be encountered in distinguishing a benign tumor from one of low grade malignancy. More than most neoplasms, cartilage tumors exhibit a large grey or middle zone which merges gradually into lesions at both ends of the spectrum. The border between the innocent tumors and the overt chondrosarcomas is often indistinct and still incompletely defined.

1. Gross

If a central tumor is examined in situ when it is still largely confined to the bone's interior, the contour of the bone is likely to appear expanded. Inspection of the outer cortical surface most commonly reveals that it is thickened, roughened, and pitted. This is the consequence on the one hand of a reactive new bone deposition by the irritated periosteum and the slow infiltrative advance of the tumor tissue along the Haversion canals of the cortex (LICHTENSTEIN, 1965).

Grossly, the tumor tissue of central chondrosarcomas, both within and external to the confines of the bone, is composed largely of faceted lobules of greyish-white to bluish cartilage. The tumor cartilage, most commonly from the bone's interior, may show gritty whitish specks, representing focal calcification and/or ossification (Fig. 97b). Large or small areas of tumor tissue particularly in bulky lesions may appear gelatinous or cystic. Such areas represent a nonspecific secondary degenerative change (Fig. 105). However, often large portions are gelatinous without degeneration (O'NEAL and ACKERMAN, 1952).

Some of the lower grade peripheral chondrosarcomas exhibit grossly well-defined bony bases and pedicles. Large degenerative cysts filled with gelatinous material are frequently noted within the cartilaginous portion of the lesion. Calcification is commonly present in almost all of the tumors of low grade malignancy and in lesser amounts in the more malignant ones. It is usually present along the active margins of the lesions.

In O'NEAL and ACKERMAN's series (1952) the tumors treated for the first time were encapsulated by a fibrous membrane continuous with the periosteum, but the more aggressive tumors had often ruptured through its confines. The encapsulating membrane of a peripheral chondrosarcoma is usually thinner than that of a benign osteochondroma and often greatly enfolded into the interstices between the nodules. The cartilage grossly

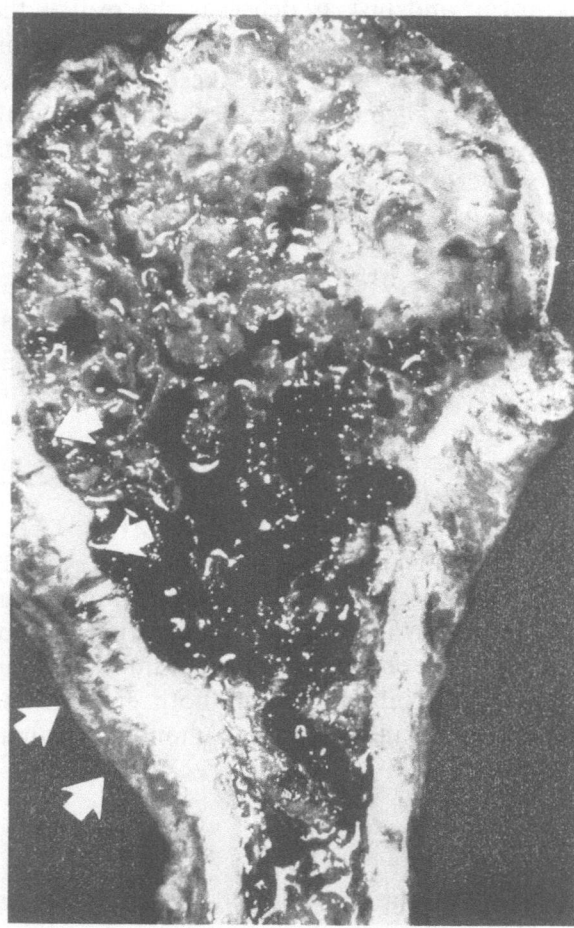

Fig. 105. Chondrosarcoma, humerus: Resected specimen. Note islands of tumor tissue superiorly intermingled with gelatinous, cystic, and hemorrhagic appearing tissue. Latter areas represent nonspecific secondary degenerative change. Thickened, hypertrophied inferior lateral cortex has triangular, buttress-like configuration. Cortical expansion and endosteal scalloping (arrows) are additional typical features

appears more finely nodular than that of an osteochondroma and the nodules separate easily. Generally, the cartilage from the central chondrosarcomas is less coherent than that from the peripheral lesions and sometimes shreds into glistening rice-sized lobules (JAFFE, 1968; LICHTENSTEIN, 1969).

2. Microscopic

Important progress in characterizing chondrosarcoma pathologically was made by LICHTENSTEIN and JAFFE in 1943 when they established the following microscopic criteria for its diagnosis: Many cells with plump nuclei, more than an occasional cell with two such nuclei, and giant cell cartilage cells with large single or multiple nuclei, which are most likely to be found in viable areas that are not heavily calcified. Nuclear hyperchromatism, nuclear and cell size variation, and mitotic figures may also be noted (Figs. 106, 107). O'NEAL and ACKERMAN (1952) further refined these histologic criteria for the identification of chondrosarcomas by adopting the grading system as represented in Table 6.

Although the incidence of abnormal nuclei is fairly uniform in some tumors, in others the distribution may be patchy with a great deal of variation from one field to another (Fig. 108). Thus, it becomes incumbent on the pathologist to make and inspect many sections. A diagnosis of chondrosarcoma may be made by finding scattered areas in which a moderate number of atypical nuclei are found, despite the fact that

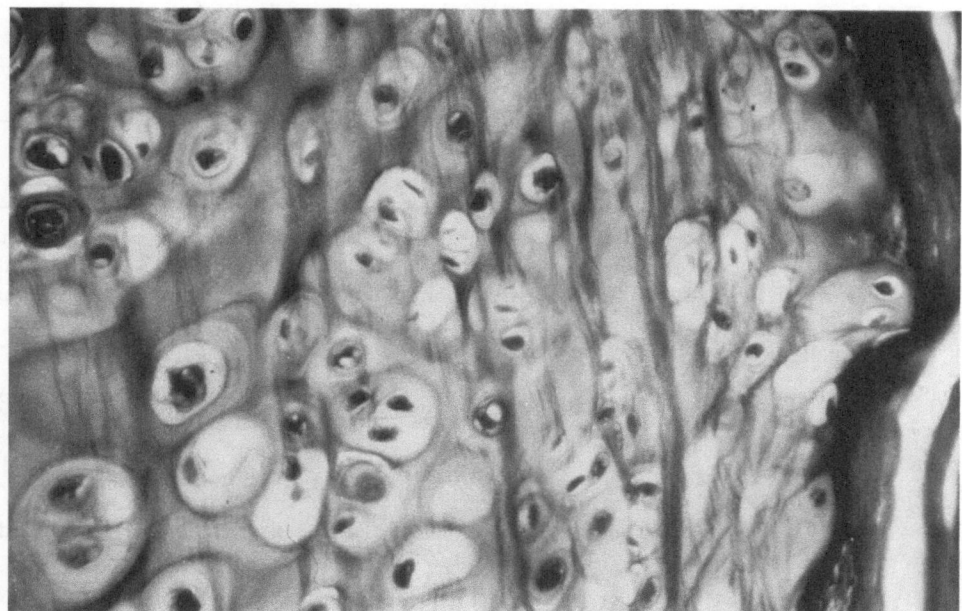

Fig. 106. Chondrosarcoma, photomicrograph (×250): Nuclear hyperchromatism, distortion, as well as nuclear and cell size variation may be noted. These are cytologic indices which contribute to diagnosis of malignancy. Generally, mitotic figures are rarely seen. (Courtesy of AUSTIN D. JOHNSTON, M.D.)

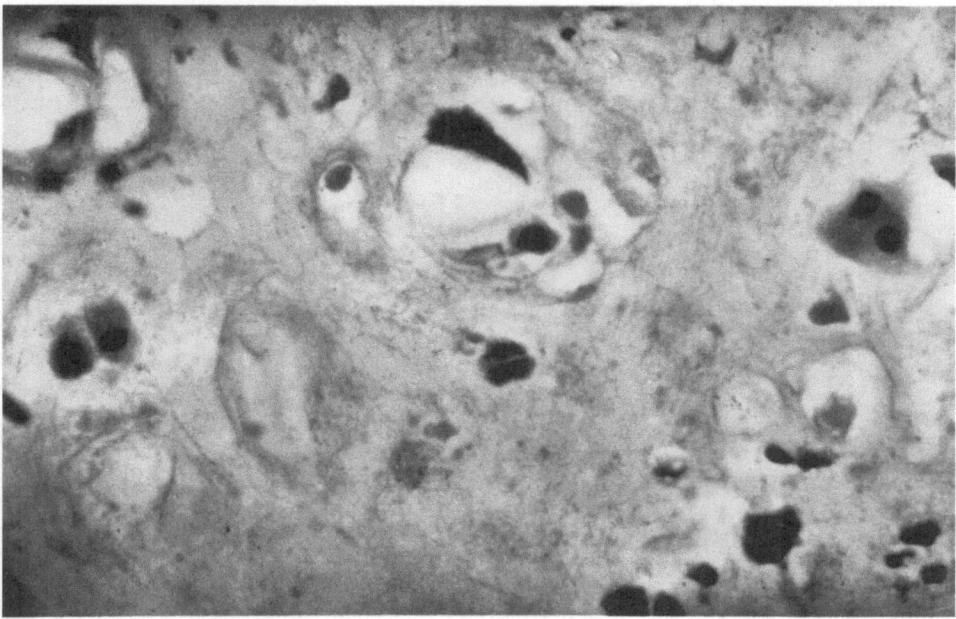

Fig. 107. Chondrosarcoma humerus, photomicrograph (×250): Bizarre giant cell, upper right, atypical cells, upper center, and questionable mitotic figure, lower right, help define chondrosarcoma histologically

the bulk of the tumor appears to be benign. It has been noted that histological malignancy generally precedes the development of clinical malignancy, sometimes by many years. O'NEAL and ACKERMAN (1952) noted in examining tissue from patients whose clinical course was known, that even quite subtle microscopic changes were indicative of a diagnosis of chondrosarcoma.

Table 6. Grading of cartilaginous tumors based on relative incidence of atypical nuclei.
(Criteria of O'NEAL and ACKERMAN, 1952)

Histologic features	Enchondroma (intramedullary chondroma)	Osteochondroma (ecchondroma)	Chondrosarcoma		
			Low-grade	Moderately malignant	Highly malignant
Variation nuclear size	Little-"0" in long bones, varies in hands and feet; small nuclei	Little-"0"; small nuclei	Occasional very plump nucleus; general plumping many nuclei	Frequent very plump nuclei; general plumping many nuclei	Great variation; large numbers very plump nuclei
Double nuclei	Rare. Not plump	Very rare	Low incidence; may be plump	Frequent plump; double nuclei	Very many
Multinucleate giant cells	0	0	0	0-rare	Occasionally-frequent
Enchondral osteogenesis[a]	0	Regular	Often regular	Bizarre, disorganized	Not found
Calcification	Frequent	Frequent	Frequent	Occasional but slight[b]	0

[a] Applies to enchondromas and peripheral chondrosarcomas. Enchondral osteogenesis occasionally seen in small areas of benign and low-grade enchondromas.
[b] In the more malignant chondrosarcomas evolving from tumors of lesser malignancy, calcification is seen only in the "older" portion of the tumor.

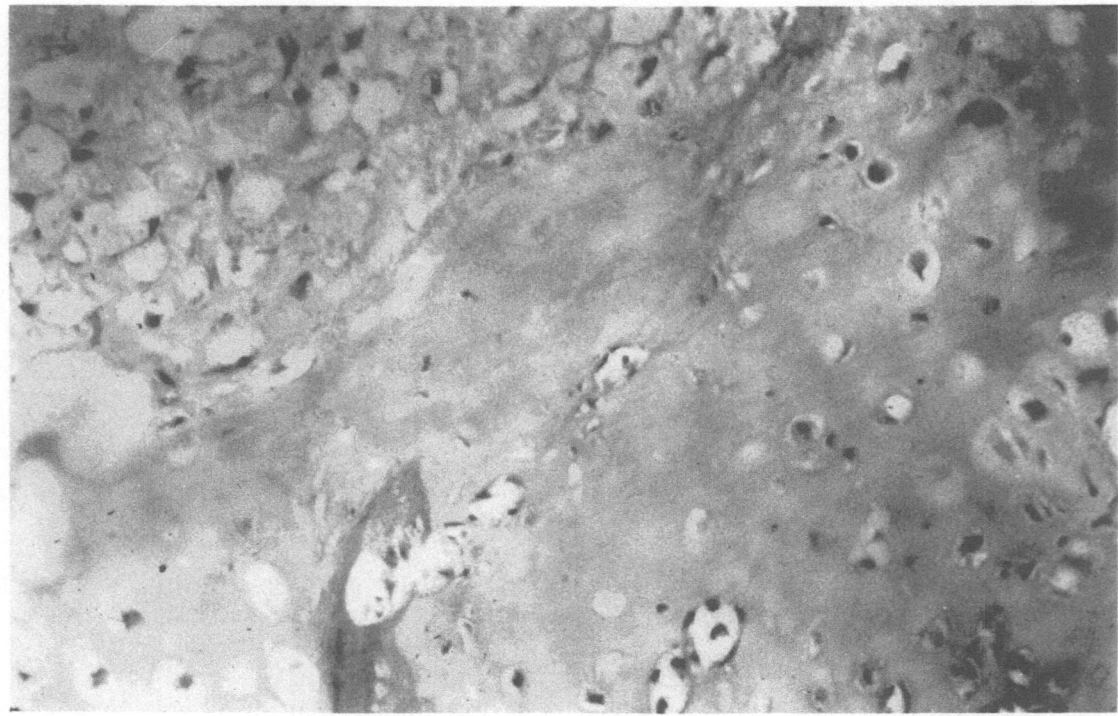

Fig. 108. Chondrosarcoma, photomicrograph ($\times 150$): Although incidence of abnormal nuclei is fairly uniform in some tumors, in others distribution may be patchy. Selected field shows two phases of chondrosarcoma. Lower part of field resembles "hyaline cartilage" of enchondroma, but has atypical enlarged cells in right mid and upper field. Left upper segment is myxomatous chondrosarcoma with definable nuclear atypism

As a rule, mitotic figures are uncommon in chondrosarcoma (Fig. 107). They are, therefore, not necessary for a diagnosis of malignancy and their absence is no guarantee of benignity. Growth in chondrosarcoma appears to be chiefly the result of amitotic division. Cellularity, too, correlates poorly with malignant potential, as emphasized by the highly cellular, but benign chondromas of the hand (JAFFE, 1968; LICHTENSTEIN and JAFFE, 1943). In addition, histologic sections from benign multiple enchondromas are more cellular than solitary enchondromas. Juxtacortical chondromas may also have an alarming histologic appearance not matched by their subsequent clinical behavior; while conversely, cartilaginous tumors of the axial skeleton and proximal limb bones often behave more aggressively then their histology would indicate. The orthopedic surgeon may then view histologic reports of benignity or malignancy with reservation when associated clinical and radiological features do not conform.

O'NEAL and ACKERMAN (1952) tried to determine whether a true capsule continuous with the periosteum was present in cases of peripheral chondrosarcoma, or whether a pseudocapsule, formed by compression of soft tissue by the advancing discrete margin of the tumor, constituted the enveloping membrane. Because of the discrete advancing border of most chondrosarcomas, true invasion of adjacent soft tissue was often difficult to differentiate pathologically from distortion by, and adherence to, an expanding noninvasive tumor. An important microscopic difference between central chondrosarcomas and benign enchondromas, however, may be found in the degree of activity of the periosteum of the overlying cortex. In central chondrosarcoma the periosteum is thickened and cellular, and is forming abundant new bone, whereas in the benign enchondroma, the periosteum usually appears more active than normal, but never as hyperplastic as that overlying a chondrosarcoma. Central chondrosarcomas that have perforated the cortex may be enveloped by periosteum for a time, but this is usually found to be ruptured in most of the larger lesions.

Another important requirement from the standpoint of accurate pathologic evaluation is the proper orientation of specimens so that the pattern of enchondral osteogenesis may be properly reflected. This varies from a regular pattern in osteochondromas (Fig. 18) to a pattern only faintly reminiscent of the normal process in the more malignant peripheral chondrosarcomas (Fig. 106). Since both recurrent and even metastatic chondrosarcomas may form bone and/or become partly calcified, these findings give no evidence that the malignant tumor has evolved from a benign one.

No single factor such as bone formation, calcification, long duration, or slow growth with increasing rate of growth has proved to be absolutely reliable in determining malignant evolution from a benign tumor. The evidence is always at best presumptive that the tumor was originally benign. In general, malignant transformation is more difficult to establish in the case of central tumors in view of the anatomically concealed nature of the initial lesion. O'NEAL and ACKERMAN (1952) note that most central and peripheral chondrosarcomas seem to be malignant from the start. They further corroborate that cartilaginous tumors of the small bones of the hands and feet cannot be judged by the microscopic criteria applicable to these lesions in other sites, since phalangeal, metacarpal, and metatarsal tumors may exhibit general plumping of nuclei, double nuclei, and occasional very large nuclei and still behave in a benign manner.

Conversely, in other areas, the histologic picture of any particular tumor does not have to be crudely and obviously sarcomatous for a diagnosis of chondrosarcoma to be made (LICHTENSTEIN, 1965). Even scattered evidence of cytologic atypism of cartilage cells should lead to recognition of the malignant character of the lesion as a whole. The tendency to underdiagnosis of an early chondrosarcoma can be overcome by observing the previously described criteria (LICHTENSTEIN and JAFFE, 1943). These histologic hallmarks will be relatively easy to find in a more fully evolved chondrosarcoma. The problem continues to revolve around defining criteria for the well-differentiated chondrosarcomas since they are most frequently erroneously diagnosed. In addition to the criteria described by Lichtenstein and Jaffe (1943), O'Neal and Ackerman (1952) have established other guidelines for grading chondrosarcomas based on the quantity of cellular alterations present, as well as the presence or absence of calcification and enchondral ossification. Diagnosis on the basis of biopsy material may be difficult or misleading, since samples are limited and, therefore, do not reveal the potential of the entire tumor; particularly one with considerable variation in pattern. A biopsy section may appear benign or equivocal while the bulk of the tumor may be unquestionably malignant. Osteosarcomas in younger individuals may exhibit extensive cartilage formation and biopsies in these cases may be interpreted as chondrosarcoma, obscuring the diagnosis of the more dangerous lesion (Dahlin and Coventry, 1967). Whether or not to perform preliminary biopsy of cartilaginous lesions is a decision that must be made by balancing the benefits to be obtained against real and possible dangers. Biopsy is expeditious and safe in accessible sites, and may be advantageous in cases in which amputation is planned, since the wound can be excised in toto. However, tumor cells may be spread by disruption of the encapsulating structures, or may be mechanically seeded into neighboring soft tissues during the procedure. This is particularly pertinent in view of the nature of the cartilage tumor cells which are prone to disseminate in soft tissues due to their exceptional capability of maintaining nutrition without a direct blood supply.

Although the ultrastructure of cartilage, and particularly articular cartilage, both normal and pathologic, has been studied, only a few papers deal with the electron microscopy of tumoral processes. Several papers dealing with the ultrastructure of chondroblastoma have included some reference to chondrosarcoma (Dahlin and Salvador, 1974; Wellman, 1969; Welsh and Meyer, 1964). One investigator described the submicroscopic and biochemical features of a single case of chondrosarcoma in the scapula of a 77-year-old woman (Anderson et al., 1963) while a more recent paper describes the ultrastructure of different grades of chondrosarcoma in 7 patients, 4 females and 3 males, ranging from 19–76 years of age (Schajowicz et al., 1974). The aim in the latter paper was to establish a correlation between the ultrastructure and the grade of histologic malignancy of these tumors. There were two cases in the femur, three in the humerus, one in the scapula and one in the sternum. Of the seven cases of graded malignancy studied, high organelle density was observed in the low grade malignancies, whereas a low organelle content and more bizarre nuclei with prominent nucleoli were seen in the tumors of a higher grade of malignancy. The more typical features of the cells included an abundant endoplasmic reticulum, which usually encircled other organelles, especially mitachondria, and which rarely presented the parallel and concentric pattern associated with the normal chondrocytes ergastoplasm. An inverse relationship between glycogen content and the histologic rate of malignancy was also noted. Endoplasmic reticulum dilatations, lipid vacuoles, and intracellular filaments were salient although nonspecific ultramorphological features of tumor cells. Although a systemic search was not made, no virus-like particles such as the A type virus-like intracysternal particles described by Morton et al. (1947, 1969) in one case of chondrosarcoma, were found.

II. Clinical Course

The natural history of chondrosarcoma varies from the rapidly fatal to the prolonged course of the low grade malignancies. Chondrosarcoma is particularly prone to massive local extension or local recurrences after unsuccessful treatment and they, rather than metastases, may be the cause of death (BARNES and CATTO, 1966). There may, additionally, be an increase in both clinical and cytologic aggressiveness after recurrence or an alteration of the basic character of the tumor with dedifferentiation to fibrosarcoma or pleomorphic sarcoma. In commenting on the former point, O'NEAL and ACKERMAN (1952) note that "though inadequate operation may increase the degree of malignancy of the low grade and equivocally malignant tumors, it should also be considered that inadequate excision is apt to leave behind the more aggressive invasive portions of the tumor." In terms of the alteration of the basic character of the lesion, DAHLIN and BEABOUT (1971) have indicated that the change or dedifferentiation may be part of the "normal" evolution of a few chondrosarcomas since 26 of their 33 cases of dedifferentiated chondrosarcomas manifested dedifferentiated zones without prior surgical intervention.

Additional factors other than nuclear morphology may play a part in the increased aggressiveness of a particular lesion after surgery. Clinical increase in malignancy following inadequate operation is often related to the disturbance of the tumor bed and to the opening up of other avenues of spread rather than to an increase in cellular malignancy in most cases. By the same virtue, primary peripheral chondrosarcomas may be encapsulated by perichondrium, while recurrent peripheral chondrosarcomas may no longer be. In addition to soft tissue extension and intramedullary spread, local involvement of regional veins and lymphatics are recorded. More advanced or aggressive chondrosarcomas have been known to break into regional venous channels and by embolization (CLARK and MALONEY, 1974; SCHWARZ et al., 1972) and/or uninterrupted intravascular growth and extension without necessarily adhering to vessel walls, have reached the heart and lungs (LICHTENSTEIN and JAFFE, 1943). The presence of severe respiratory and cardiac difficulties in a patient with chondrosarcoma may be a clinical indication that a "cord-like" intravascular growth and extension of the tumor to the heart and lungs has taken place (LICHTENSTEIN, 1965). This, however, has been rarely documented (CLARK and MALONEN, 1974; ERNST, 1900; KÓSA, 1929; SCHWARZ et al., 1972). In a case of chondrosarcoma involving the lower vertebral column, ERNST (1900) describes tumor plugs in both the renal and suprarenal veins, the left internal spermatic, the azygous veins, the inferior vena cava, the right auricle, and branches of the right and left pulmonary arteries, and still the pulmonary parenchyma was free from metastases.

Metastases, when they do occur, are most frequent in the lungs (Fig. 109c). Arterial emboli, liver, cerebral (CLARK and MALONEY, 1974), renal, and more, rarely cutaneous and bone involvement are reported. Metastases to other bones are unusual, except in cases with mesenchymal chondrosarcoma. Lymph node metastases are extremely rare. Small secondary nodules of tumor not far from the primary mass may easily be misinterpreted as representing lymph nodes that have undergone complete replacement by tumor.

An occasional chondrosarcoma may metastasize early. However, this is the exception rather than the rule. Most classic chondrosarcomas are likely to remain locally invasive for some time, even after an unsuccessful attempt at surgical removal (Figs. 109a, b, c). By the same token, inoperative or inaccessible chondrosarcoma, e.g. of a pelvis, may eventually attain tremendous size before causing the death of the patient from a variety of complications incidental to local spread and/or impingement on vital structures. However bulky a peripheral chondrosarcoma may be, it is frequently found on surgical exploration to be a discrete circumscribed mass and cure can be obtained by adequate local excision, provided that the tumor is cleared peripherally (blunt dissection should be avoided) and that the bone or pedicle at its site of attachment is resected (LICHTENSTEIN,

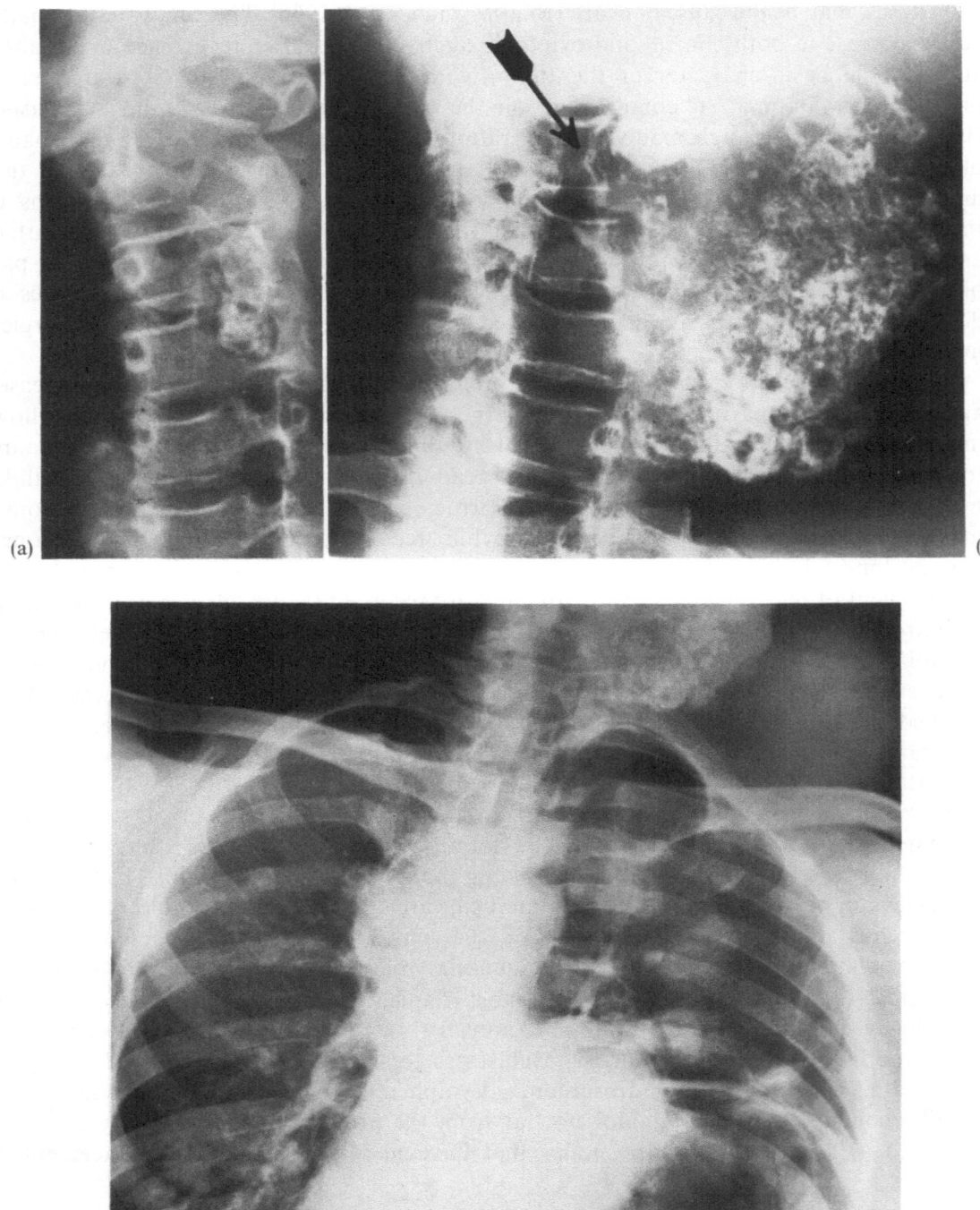

Fig. 109. (a) Chondrosarcoma, cervical spine: 58-year-old male 21 years post initial resection (1950) of left-sided cervical chondrosarcoma. Progressive motor weakness and sensory changes necessitated left hemilaminectomy in 1951, partial removal of extradural extension of tumor in 1955, and left radical neck resection followed by radiotherapy in 1960. Pulmonary metastases occurred in 1966, 16 years post initial resection. Right posterior oblique view of cervical spine (1963) 13 years post initial resection illustrates recurrent lesion with partial destruction of C-3 and C-4 pedicles, laminae and vertebral body. (b) 1971: Note marked increase in size of mass with further destruction of spine. Note bony excavation of vertebral body by tumor mass (arrows). Bony erosions are fairly well-defined. (c) PA chest film 1971. Note multiple large rounded metastatic deposits scattered throughout both lung fields. Solitary pulmonary nodule had been irradiated in 1966

1965; O'NEAL and ACKERMAN, 1950). When and if the tumor recurs, it usually does so locally. Such tumors have been known to recur repeatedly over a period of years without showing any tendency to distant metastases.

In most series no malignant tumors of the pelvis, including tumors of low grade malignancy, have been cured by local excision. Local excision may also fail in tumors considered benign. While recurrence of chondrosarcoma in the pelvis, thorax, and spine (STENER, 1971) are often incurable, even by the most radical procedures, recurrences in the extremities are more favorable and may be cured after many local recurrences. However, local resection, feasible in some selected areas and in some selected untreated low grade chondrosarcomas, is not often successful in the treatment of recurring chondrosarcomas.

Radiation therapy has been unsuccessful as a primary treatment of chondrosarcoma and generally achieves little when administered for palliation (DAHLIN and HENDERSON, 1956; LICHTENSTEIN, 1965; PADDISON and HANKS, 1971). Large series in which chemotherapy has been employed are not available (BOSTRÖM et al., 1968; GOTTSCHALK et al., 1959). Most authorities agree that obvious chondrosarcoma should be treated by appropriate radical resection or amputation on diagnosis, as outlined by several authorities (BARNES and CATTO, 1966; DAHLIN and HENDERSON, 1956; JAFFE, 1968; LICHTENSTEIN, 1965; O'NEAL and ACKERMAN, 1952). In case of doubt, preference should be given to more radical procedures in the interest of cure. Recurrent chondrosarcomas in the absence of demonstrable distant metastases may still be amenable to cure only if treated radically, and this treatment further depends on the site of the lesion.

Even metastasizing tumors may be associated with a protracted course and it is not unusual for the patient to survive for several years after the appearance of pulmonary metastases (Fig. 109c). This consideration, together with the fact that recurrences are frequent 5 years and sometimes 10 years after surgery, led DAHLIN and HENDERSON (1956) to insist that a 10 year survival without recurrence or overt metastases is mandatory before a cure is considered.

After adequate treatment, 5 year survival approaches 80% in low grade tumors and 20% in high grade tumors. In DAHLIN and HENDERSON's series (1956), however, the 10 year survival figures of 41% with adequate treatment fell to 3.7% when it was inadequate. A 10 year survival varies from 35–60% depending on the nature of the individual lesion and method of treatment. The latter is too variable for the meaningful comparison of many small series.

The prognosis in secondary chondrosarcoma associated with multiple osteochondromatosis is better than that associated with multiple enchondromatosis or with primary central chondrosarcoma.

In general, chondrosarcoma has a relatively good prognosis when compared with other bone sarcomas, and a long term survival of approximately 40% or more can be anticipated after adequate surgical treatment.

M. Mesenchymal Chondrosarcoma

This lesion was first described by LICHTENSTEIN and BERNSTEIN (1959) as one of a heterogenous group of unusual chondroid tumors. It is unique because it is composed of a paradoxical histologic combination of islands of relatively benign appearing chondroid tissue intermingled with highly cellular zones of small, anaplastic, occasionally

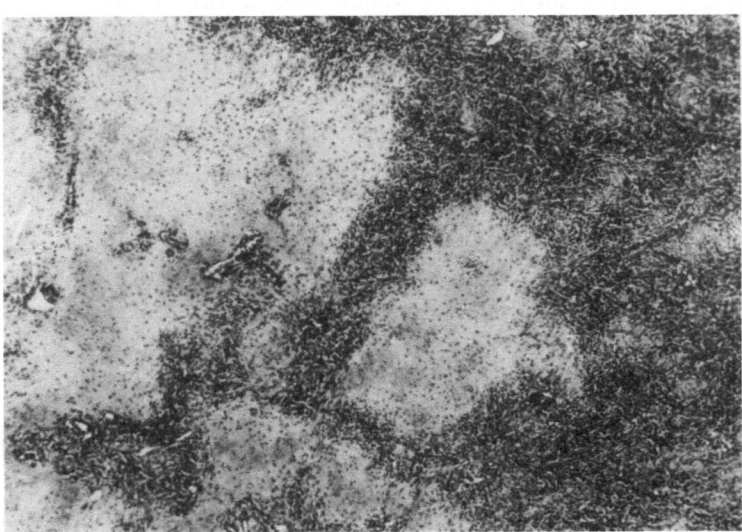

Fig. 110. Mesenchymal chondrosarcoma, photomicrograph (× 100). Typical mesenchymal chondrosarcoma with islands of well-differentiated, benign-looking cartilage and highly cellular zones composed of small undifferentiated cells. There is abrupt transition between two components. (Courtesy of A.H. SALVADOR, M.D., J.W. BEABOUT, M.D. and DAVID C. DAHLIN, M.D.)

spindle-shaped, cells (Fig. 110). In some areas either the cartilage or the stroma may dominate, and in the latter instance reticulum cell sarcoma may be simulated. The chondroid tissue contains foci of calcification and ossification. LICHTENSTEIN and BERNSTEIN (1959) believed this lesion was derived from cartilage forming mesenchyme, but that it differed from an enchondroma or the usual chondrosarcoma since it was not composed of full-fledged hyaline cartilage.

A recent electron microscopic study by STEINER et al. (1973) of a case of mesenchymal chondrosarcoma found this tumor to be composed mainly of two cell types: poorly differentiated cells, and cells showing cartilaginous differentiation (Figs. 111 a, b, 112). The matrix of the tumor consisted of thin collagenous fibrils 90–350 Å in thickness and electron dense materials. They felt that the tumor originates from primitive, cartilage forming mesenchyme with large numbers of tumor cells remaining in an early undifferentiated state, while others had undergone cartilaginous differentiation. They noted that the cartilage cells and their matrix were in an early stage of maturation, which might explain some of the morphologic similarities with young hyaline cartilage and differences from cells of ordinary chondrosarcoma (GODMAN and PORTER, 1960).

Electron micrographs of the cartilage cells of ordinary chondrosarcoma showed differences when compared with the cartilaginous areas in mesenchymal chondrosaroma. In ordinary chondrosarcoma, the cells are commonly larger and frequently show prominent dilatation of rough endoplasmic reticulum, which is seen to contain granular material (Fig. 113). These observations correlate well with those made under light microscopy in which the chondrosarcoma cells were larger and more pleomorphic than those in mesenchymal chondrosarcoma (SALVADOR et al., 1971). The matrix in ordinary chondrosarcoma as seen electron-microscopically, contains large lipid deposits and smaller amounts of collagen fibers (ANDERSON et al., 1963). In enchondroma, too, the cells are characterized by prominent indentations of the cell membrane and frequent dilatation of the rough endoplasmic reticulum (STEINER et al., 1973). Electron microscopic observations of chondroblastoma have shown a different morphology from that of mesenchymal chondrosarcoma, the cells having indented and multilobular nuclei, a small amount

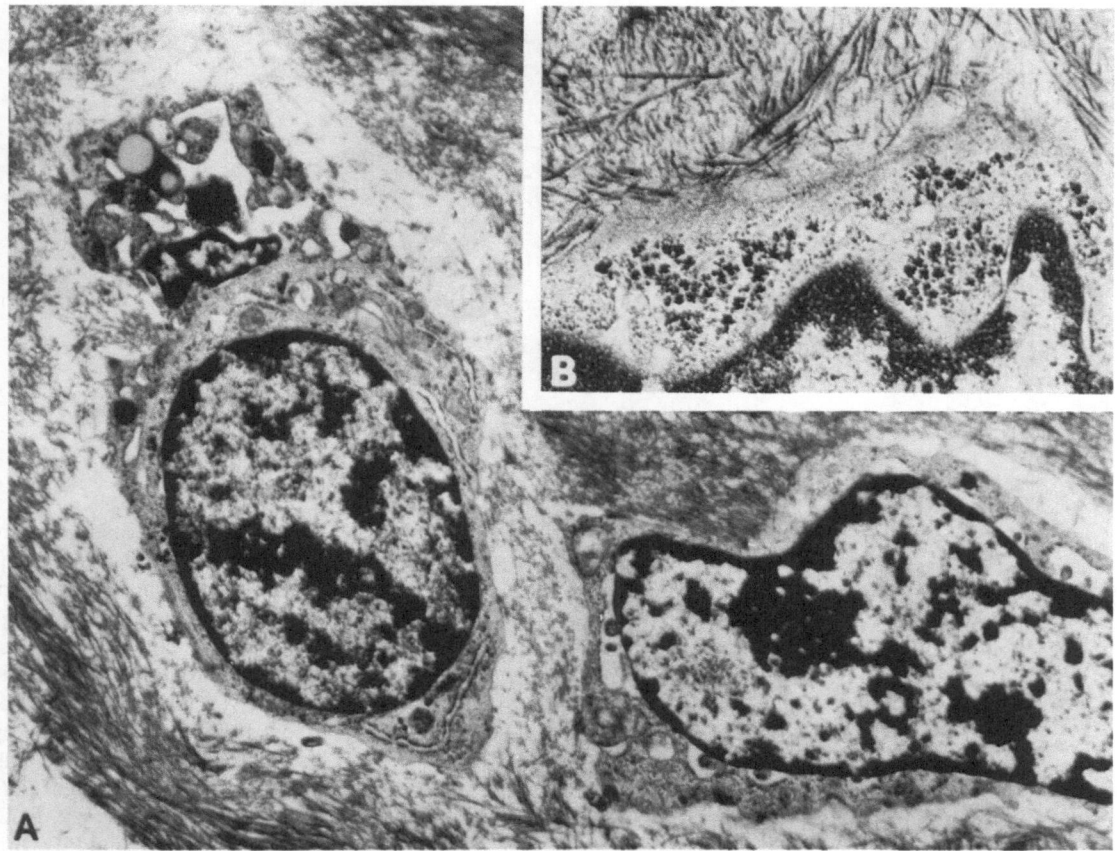

Fig. 111. (a) Mesenchymal chondrosarcoma, electron micrograph ($\times 13,400$): Electron micrograph of mesenchymal chondrosarcoma showing area of cartilaginous differentiation. Two cartilage cells and part of third cell (upper left) are surrounded by fibrillary matrix of variable density. There is moderate dilatation of rough endoplasmic reticulum in cells at right and upper left. (b) (*Inset*) $\times 34,350$. Cartilage cell cytoplasm showing dense accumulation of glycogen granules which dispose in rosettes. In addition, there are fine intracytoplasmic fibrils, and matrix adjacent to cells shows dense fibrillary pattern. (Courtesy of J.C. STEINER, M.D., J.M. MIRRA, M.D. and P.G. BULLOUGH, M.D.)

of glycogen, and the cell membrane showing microvillous processes (LEVINE and BENSCH, 1972; WELLMAN, 1969; WELSH and MEYER, 1964). In comparing the cartilage of mesenchymal chondrosarcoma with embryonal or young cartilage, similarities emerge in that the morphology of the cells in mesenchymal chondrosarcoma is consistent with that of developed chondroblasts of embryonal hyaline cartilage (GODMAN and PORTER, 1960).

HUTTER et al. (1966) published a group of malignant bone tumors under the name of primitive multipotential primary sarcoma of bone and regarded the published cases of mesenchymal chondrosarcoma as part of this entity. They felt that these tumors all had a common type of undifferentiated multipotential cell and that they all showed varying degrees of cellular and intracellular differentiation, e.g. osseous, cartilaginous, vascular. It is known that a vascular pattern resembling that seen in hemangiopericytoma is often present in mesenchymal chondrosarcoma. However, hemangiopericytoma is basically a vascular tumor that originates from capillary pericytes and should be differentiated from other tumors that may simply have a rich vascular network. It is felt by most authorities that the vascular pattern in mesenchymal chondrosarcoma as seen on light microscopy is the result of proliferation of undifferentiated cells around vascular spaces

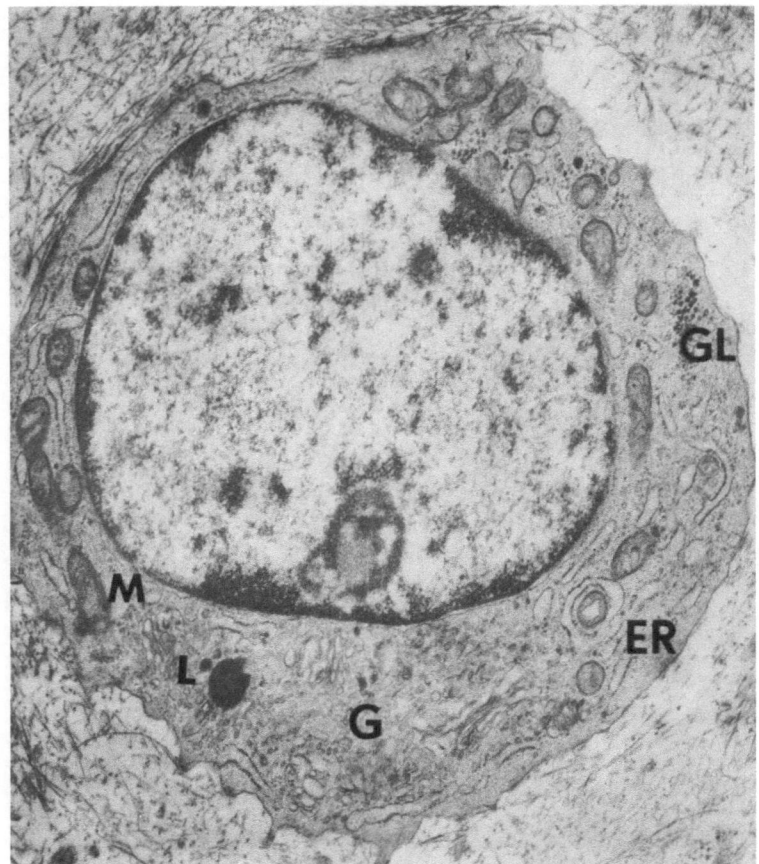

Fig. 112. Mesenchymal Chondrosarcoma, electron micrograph (×23,700) showing typical cartilage cell. Cell membrane is irregular and indented. Cytoplasm shows nonprominent rough endoplasmic reticulum (*E.R.*), well-developed Golgi apparatus (*G*), mitochondria (*M*), few lysosome-like bodies (*L*), and glycogen (*GL*). (Courtesy of J.C. STEINER, M.D., J.M. MIRRA, M.D. and P.G. BULLOUGH, M.D.)

rather than of pericytes. This has been supported by electron microscopic studies (Fig. 114). Occasionally, round and oval cells seen by means of light microscopy are suggestive of Ewing's sarcoma cells (FRIEDMAN and HANAOKA, 1971). However, glycogen, a consistent finding in cells of Ewing's sarcoma, was present in only minimal amounts or was entirely lacking as determined in the ultrastructural study of STEINER et al. (1973). There are few reports concerned with the ultrastructure of cartilaginous tumors in general, and no previous report concerning mesenchymal chondrosarcoma.

I. Clinical

Whereas males predominate in ordinary chondrosarcoma in a ratio of 5:3, females predominate in the total series of mesenchymal chondrosarcomas. The peak incidence in the latter is most commonly seen in patients between 10 and 30 years, while the peak incidence in ordinary chondrosarcoma is in the sixth decade. Differences in location are not remarkable except for the much higher percentage of mesenchymal chondrosarcomas arising in soft tissues, in addition to a large number of cases in the jaw (DAHLIN and HENDERSON, 1962; SALVADOR et al., 1971).

Patients have ranged from 5–70 years of age. More than half of the 51 Patients reported to date were in the second and third decades of life, with 29 (57%) being females.

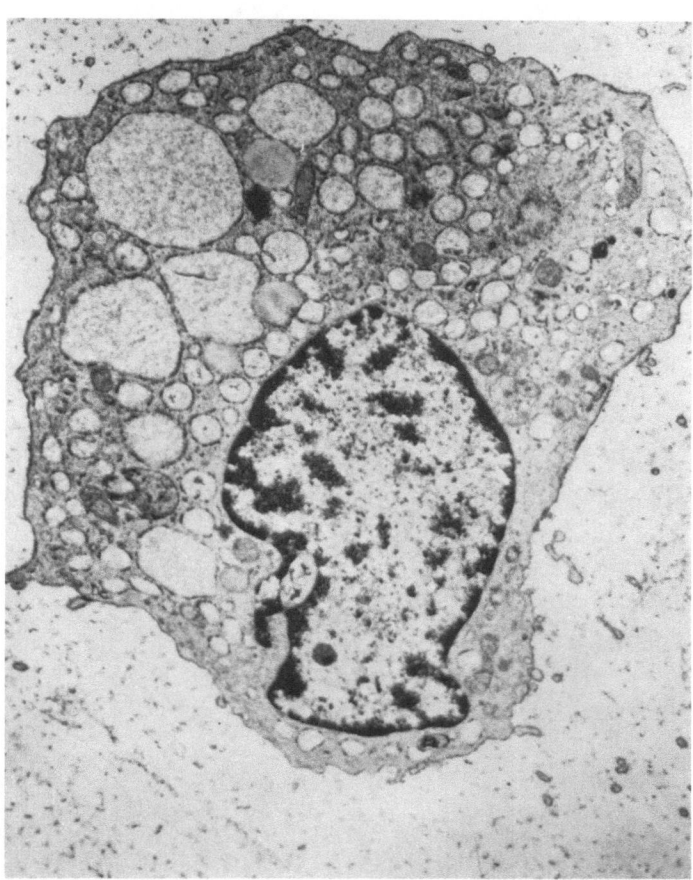

Fig. 113. Electron micrograph of cartilage cell of ordinary chondrosarcoma (×10,030). There is abundance of rough endoplasmic reticulum with dilatation containing granular material. Surrounding matrix contains sparse granular material (Courtesy of J.C. STEINER, M.D., J.M. MIRRA, M.D. and P.G. BULLOUGH, M.D.)

A total of 17 of 51 tumors (33%) arose in the soft tissues — two each in the regions of the iliac crest, paraspinal muscles, and orbits; one each in the lateral chest wall and the paramandibular area; two in the calf and two in the thigh; of the remainder, three had an intracranial location, one in the nasopharynx and one in the temporalis muscle. An additional case has been reported originating from the skull base. Of the 51 patients recently studied, 34 had tumors of skeletal origin. One of the 34 tumors of skeletal origin was multifocal when discovered (DAHLIN and HENDERSON, 1962). The sites of skeletal development of the remaining 33 included 5 tumors in major tubular bones, 1 each in the ilium, scapula, sacrum, and metatarsal, 3 in the vertebral column, 9 in the ribs, and 12 in the skull. In the latter area, 9 lesions occurred in the mandible and 3 in the calvarium. The ribs and jaws were therefore the most common sites of origin within the skeleton.

In contrast with most tumors of bone, mesenchymal chondrosarcomas rarely involve tubular bones. The ribs and jaws were most commonly involved. Skull involvement has been reported (SETH and SINGH, 1973).

II. Course

There is a great variability in the clinical course. Duration of symptoms prior to the histologic diagnosis was variable, ranging from 4 days to 4 years.

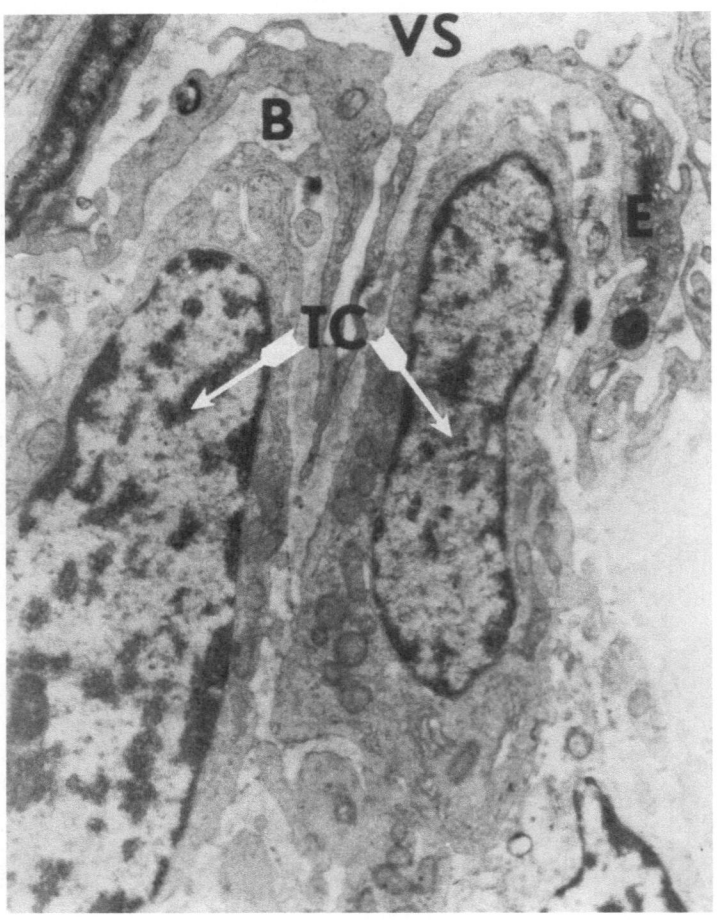

Fig. 114. Electron micrograph of mesenchymal chondrosarcoma (× 18,300) showing vascular pattern resembling hemangiopericytoma. Vascular space (*VS*), endothelial cells (*E*), and basement membrane (*B*) are seen superiorly. Poorly differentiated tumor cells (*TC*) are seen outside basement membrane. These cells appear to exert pressure on endothelial cells with protrusion into lumen. (Courtesy of J.C. Steiner, M.D., J.M. Mirra, M.D. and P.G. Bullough, M.D.)

Mean survival time is reputedly 6 years. Local recurrence is common. There is a tendency for hematogenous metastases to unusual locations, sometimes after a long delay. Metastases to other bones, lungs, liver, lymph nodes, soft tissues, kidney, pleura, and brain have been reported. Metastases may occur several years after the primary lesion has been treated. In a case with a femoral lesion (Silver et al., 1971) death occurred 10 years after diagnosis with metastases to the lung. Two patients underwent pneumonectomy for metastatic disease at intervals of 4.3 and 22 years after the initial treatment. The pulmonary lesions were histologically identical to the primary tumors. In some cases, a multicentric origin has been suggested. In addition to other bones and the lungs, metastatic sites include retroperitoneal and subcutaneous soft tissues and the breast. It is this penchant for metastases, particularly to other bones, that further justifies its distinction from other chondrosarcomas.

In commenting on their review of 51 cases, Salvador et al. (1971) noted that the series had limited value in ascertaining the results of treatment, which included excision that was defined as local removal of the tumor without an attempt to remove a wide margin of normal tissue; resection, which was defined as ablation of all tumor grossly visible, as well as surrounding tissues in which local invasion was likely to have occurred; radiation and chemotherapy, which was used as a palliative terminal measure in two cases. There was no follow-up in eight cases, six were followed for less than a year from the time of initial treatment. Three of the latter were dead and one was known to have recurrent tumor. Several patients were either alive with metastases or alive with recurrent tumor 5 years post diagnosis. The seven that died as a result of their tumors survived from 5–13.5 years. The behavior of the tumor in these protracted cases was often characterized by several local recurrences prior to generalized or pulmonary metastases and death. However, the frequency with which local recurrence preceded metastases emphasizes the importance of adequate primary radical therapy. One case was an exception since distant metastases preceded local recurrence. The protracted clinical course is further emphasized by the long survival of two patients after well-documented distant metastases had been diagnosed.

Radiotherapy was not efficacious as employed in the cases reviewed by SALVADOR et al. (1971). It failed as a primary modality in four cases and did not appear to afford significant benefit in five additional cases. A 5 year survival appears to be of limited significance since delayed death from the tumor may occur. Therefore, some current survivors will undoubtedly succumb to their tumor. One patient reported in the literature died with metastases 23 years after her first operation for the tumor (DAHLIN and HENDERSON, 1962).

Mesenchymal chondrosarcoma is a rare neoplasm, the total number of well-documented cases in the literature being approximately 55. Whereas more than 370 skeletal chondrosarcomas of the ordinary type were noted in the Mayo Clinic files, there were only 10 mesenchymal chondrosarcomas arising in bone (SALVADOR et al., 1971).

III. Histology

1. Gross

The tumors are grey to pink, firm or soft, well-defined masses, easily demarcated from surrounding tissues. Three were described as lobulated. Their maximum dimension ranged from 2–14 cm. Most tumors contained hard, mineralized material that varied in amount from scattered foci to prominent zones. Some had a cartilaginous appearance. Zones of necrosis and hemorrhage were noted in two.

With a greater number of cases to study, SALVADOR et al. (1971) reported a slightly wider spectrum than previously noted (DAHLIN and HENDERSON, 1962; DOWLING, 1964) but felt that the histology was highly characteristic. Sheets of highly undifferentiated,

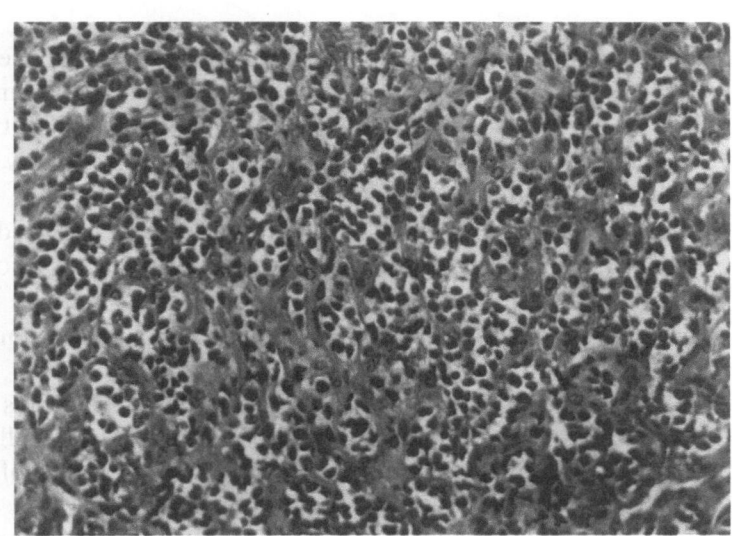

Fig. 115. Mesenchymal chondrosarcoma, photomicrograph (× 300): Ovoid and round cells predominate in this field and display definite clustering, simulating alveolar pattern seen in other types of sarcoma. (Courtesy of A.H. SALVADOR, M.D., J.W. BEABOUT, M.D. and D.C. DAHLIN, M.D.)

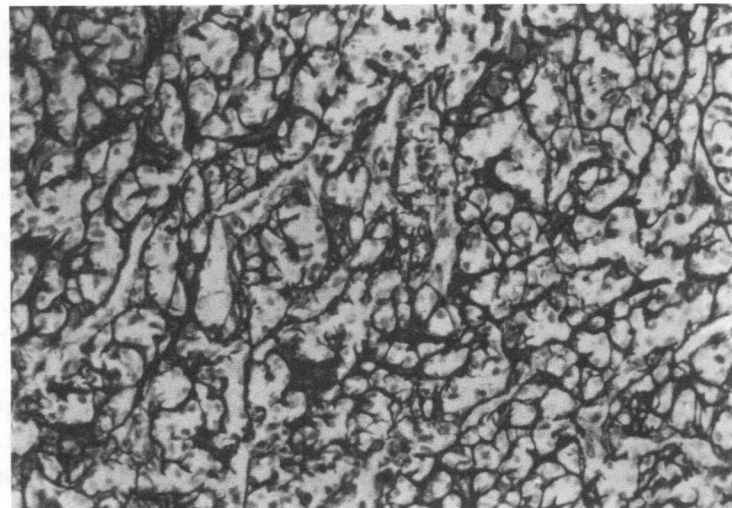

Fig. 116. Mesenchymal chondrosarcoma, photomicrograph (×290): Well-developed reticulum in cellular area. Reticulum fibers surround small clusters of neoplastic cells. (Courtesy of A.H. SALVADOR, M.D., J.W. BEABOUT, M.D. and D.C. DAHLIN, M.D.)

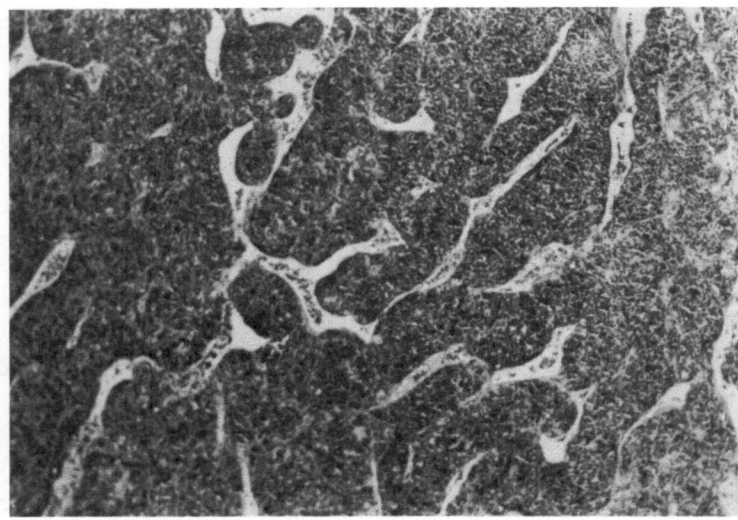

Fig. 117. Mesenchymal chondrosarcoma (×100): Another pattern of perivascular clustering not infrequently seen is shown in field. Vascular channels are well-defined and cells appear to form cords that protrude into vascular lumen. This appearance has been referred to as representing "organoid" hemangiopericytoma-like pattern. (Courtesy of A.H. SALVADOR, M.D., J.W. BEABOUT, M.D. and D.C. DAHLIN, M.D.)

small, oval, or round cells and islands of well-differentiated cartilage were noted (Fig. 110). The small cells were described as displaying a hemangiopericytoid or an alveolar pattern. Lobulation was common; and calcification and metaplastic bone formation in the chondroid islands were frequent. Occasionally the cartilaginous islands contain small but definitely malignant cells.

The cells in portions of many tumors were clustered, producing an alveolar pattern (Fig. 115) resembling the one found in reticulum cell sarcoma or in embryonal rhabdomyosarcoma. Reticulin stains showed a well-developed and usually coarse reticulin network surrounding groups of undifferentiated cells. Infrequently a fine reticulin was present around individual cells (Fig. 116).

Although foci within mesenchymal chondrosarcomas may closely simulate hemangiopericytoma, reticulum cell sarcoma, and other small cell tumors, the cartilaginous component is the differentiating feature. When the cells of this tumor are spindle-shaped or ovoid they are characteristically smaller than most of the spindle cell tumors such as fibrosarcoma. Recognition of the undifferentiated cellular element and knowledge

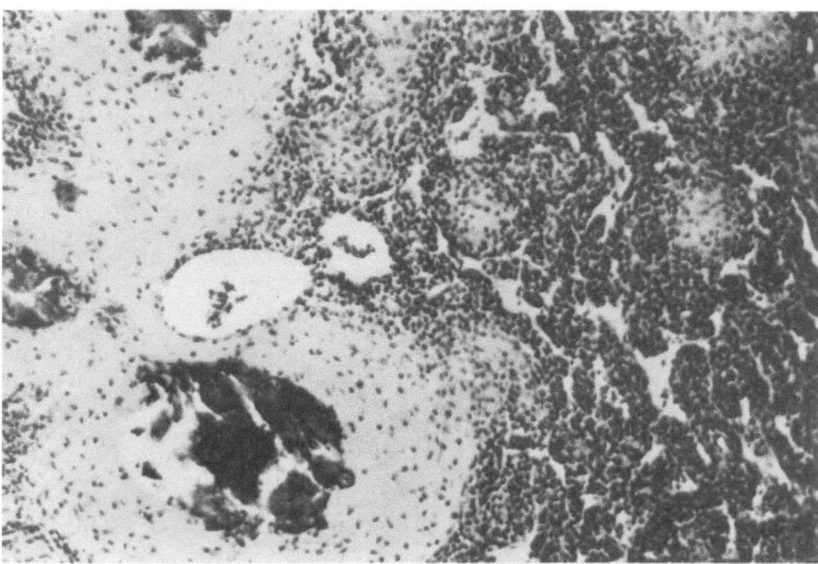

Fig. 118. Mesenchymal chondrosarcoma (×130): Another characteristic area of tumor showing chondroid islands and small undifferentiated cellular elements which here show definite hemangiopericytoid arrangement. Note small nodular-like areas of chondroid differentiation in vascular zone, and focal calcification of cartilage. (Courtesy of A.H. SALVADOR, M.D., J.W. BEABOUT, M.D. and D.C. DAHLIN, M.D.)

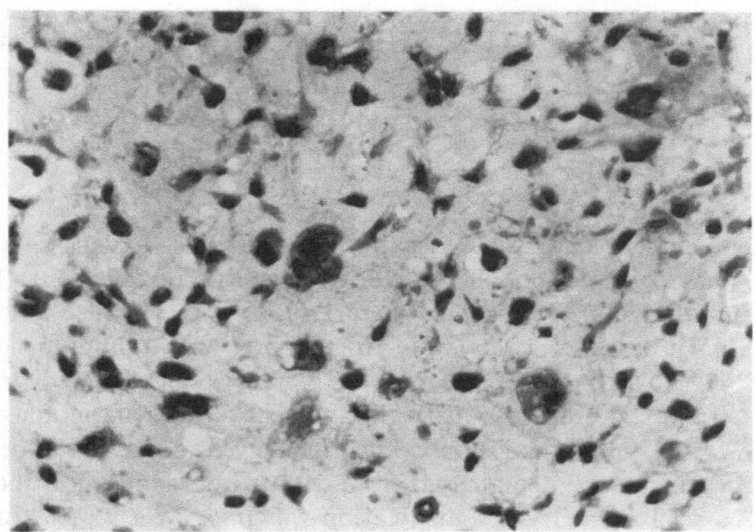

Fig. 119. Chondrosarcoma: Typical anaplastic chondrosarcoma of ordinary type. Pleomorphism and large nuclei contrast sharply with cells of mesenchymal chondrosarcoma (×250). (Courtesy of A.H. SALVADOR, M.D., J.W. BEABOUT, M.D. and D.C. DAHLIN, M.D.)

of the hemangiopericytoma-like appearance (Fig. 117) as well as the alveolar pattern (Fig. 115) are important. These elements can suggest the correct diagnosis which is proved by finding the chondroid zones (Fig. 118).

Ordinary chondrosarcomas are different from mesenchymal chondrosarcomas. When cellular zones are present in the former they merge more gradually into the chondroid islands and the cells in such zones are typically much larger than those of mesenchymal chondrosarcoma (Fig. 119). The cells in the chondroid zones of the more active chondrosarcoma usually display considerable pleomorphism, while well-differentiated chondrosarcomas (the most common type) pose no problem in differentiation because they contain no highly cellular foci.

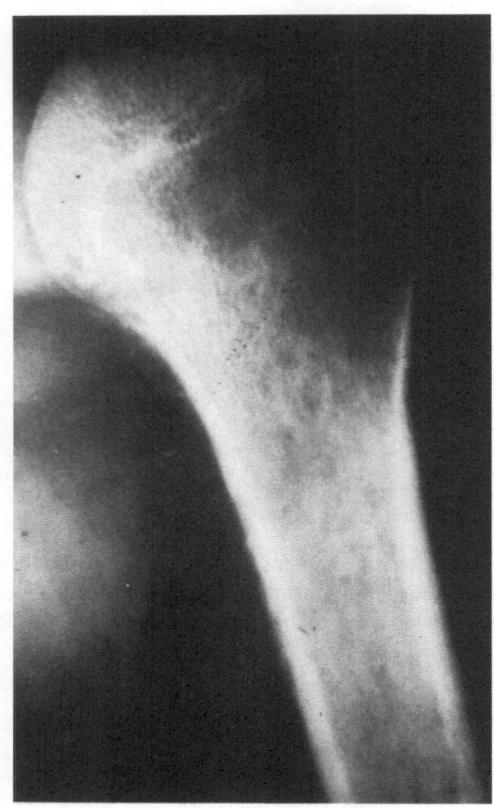

Fig. 120. Mesenchymal chondrosarcoma—humerus: 16-year-old female with 3 month history of pain and swelling of left arm and no history of trauma. Permeative destructive pattern is noted involving metaphysis with poor superior and inferior demarcation. Spicules of bone were faintly noted along lateral cortical margin. Large, soft tissue mass, not well-appreciated on this routine view was seen overlying bone. (Courtesy of AUSTIN D. JOHNSTON, M.D.)

IV. Roentgen

Roentgenograms of published cases have varying degrees of osteolysis, sclerosis, and calcification at the site of primary involvement (PAVON et al., 1971; SALVADOR et al., 1971). The skeletal metastases tend to produce lytic defects. Pulmonary metastases do not appear calcified on roentgenograms despite an identical histology (DAHLIN and HENDERSON, 1962). SALVADOR et al. (1971) reviewed 16 roentgenograms. All showed irregular stippled calcifications and 4 were of neoplasms arising in the soft tissues.

In bones, the lesions were primarily osteolytic in appearance (Fig. 120). Some defects were sharply demarcated; others faded gradually into the normal bone. None presented a sclerotic margin. Calcification was present in 9 of 12 tumors of bony origin. Although the lesions primary in bone have the appearance of a malignant neoplasm, there were no distinguishing roentgen features to differentiate them from chondrosarcoma of the ordinary type.

N. Dedifferentiation of Chondrosarcoma

Certain chondrosarcomas may, on occasion, be associated with noncartilaginous components in which areas identifiable as rhabdomyosarcoma, osteosarcoma, hemangiopericytoma, and fibrosarcoma are noted (McFARLAND and REED, 1971). It is suggested that these elements represent areas of dedifferentiation from a pre-existing well-differen-

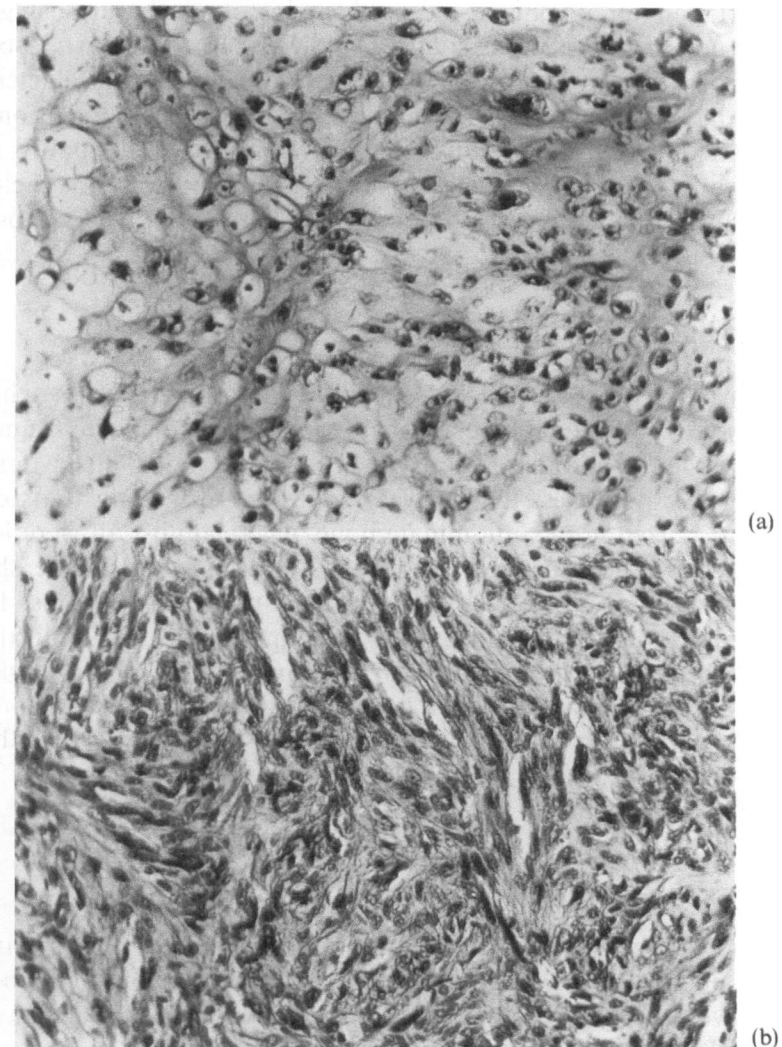

(a)

(b)

Fig. 121a and b. Dedifferentiation of low-grade chondrosarcoma: (a) *Left.* Grade I chondrosarcoma of scapula (×200). All sections studied showed this pattern. (b) *Right.* Recurrent tumor 19 months post scapulectomy was Grade III fibrosarcoma (×200). (Courtesy of D.C. DAHLIN, M.D. and J.W. BEABOUT, M.D.)

tiated chondrosarcoma, particularly in recurrent lesions (Fig. 121a, b). In a recent review, SINKOVICZ et al. (1971) in discussing a possible viral etiology of sarcoma, noted that the malignant transformation of fibroblasts in the vicinity of chondrosarcoma in vivo, resulting in the developing of fibrosarcoma may be explained by the spread of an oncogenic virus. They also noted that oncogenic viruses of the type C class were known to be able to cause neoplastic transformation of normal fibroblasts. A similar theory had been proposed by MORTON et al. (1969).

Because of the varied pattern of the non-cartilaginous component, the lesion does not appear to fit the histologic criteria of mesenchymal chondrosarcoma (SALVADOR et al., 1971; SPJUT et al., 1971). Another reason for distinguishing cartilaginous lesions with areas of dedifferentiation is that survival time has been less than 2 years after treatment, an unusually short time for either chondrosarcoma or mesenchymal chondrosarcoma. The survival time of the latter is usually longer.

In a recent study by DAHLIN and BEABOUT (1971), the pathologic requirements for inclusion was a combination of well-differentiated chondrosarcoma of the ordinary type that was usually labeled malignant with difficulty, or was "borderline" for malignancy and juxtaposed zones of anaplastic fibrosarcoma or osteogenic sarcoma. The latter zones, taken out of context, did not have histologic features suggestive of origin from a cartilaginous tumor. The cartilage usually occupied a central position and often gave evidence of being overrun and replaced by the anaplastic elements. Similar anaplastic changes have been noted without prior therapeutic intervention. The occasional higher grade chondrosarcoma, which has some spindle cell quality at the periphery of its lobule, or some zones of debatable osteosarcoma was not included in their study. It did not meet their criteria of a bimorphic combination of almost benign and highly malignant tumor.

I. Clinical

DAHLIN and BEABOUT (1971) reported 33 cases which had dedifferentiated zones of fibrosarcoma or osteogenic sarcoma. These were found among 370 well-differentiated chondrosarcomas. There were 17 women and 16 men whose ages ranged from 19–73 years. Only 1 was less than 30 years old and 16 were in the sixth decade of life. The majority occurred in the innominate bone, where almost all were located in the acetabular region. One femoral tumor was in the lower portion of the shaft, the rest of the tumors in major tubular bones affected their proximal portions. In 26 cases the dedifferentiated sarcoma was found at the first operation. The clinical characteristics including long preoperative duration of symptoms, age distribution, skeletal localization, and certain roentgen features, correlated well with the chondrosarcomatous component of these tumors. However, the rapid deterioration of most of the patients after operation was characteristic of the anaplastic portion of the tumor.

II. Pathology

Gross inspection revealed the bimorphic histologic pattern. Usually the central portion had the typically lobulated translucent quality of tumors of hyaline cartilage. The cartilage varied from firm to myxoid and often contained irregular calcific foci that were frequently detected roentgenographically. Distinct sharply limited zones were generally located peripherally. These zones appeared grossly pink or greyish-white and opaque, reflecting the histologic structure of either fibrosarcoma or osteogenic sarcoma. Occasionally these zones comprised most of the tumor, replacing the cartilaginous component.

The dedifferentiated sarcoma was usually the portion that extended into the extraosseous tissue (Fig. 122e). The original chondrosarcomas were located centrally with respect to the bone of origin in 25 cases of DAHLIN and BEABOUT (1971), 1 of which had OLLIER's enchondromatosis. Four lesions arose peripherally in a periosteal position, one in the cartilaginous cap of a pubic exostosis in a patient with multiple skeletal osteochondromatosis. Three tumors in ribs could not be classified. Generally the tumors were large, as is characteristic of chondrosarcomas.

1. Microscopic

In 22 cases reviewed by DAHLIN and BEABOUT (1971) (6% of 370 cases of well-differentiated chondrosarcoma), the dedifferentiated portion was typical of fibrosarcoma unmixed with a cartilaginous component. In 11 cases the complicating tumor was that of osteogenic sarcoma, 10 of these had zones of fibroblastic differentiation. These dedifferentiated masses usually abutted abruptly against the distinctly different cartilaginous tumor. In some tumors, however, a spindle cell component at the periphery of cartilaginous lobules shaded into the dedifferentiated sarcoma. The current tumors in three cases were fibrosarcomas throughout. Autopsy in one case revealed widespread metastatic fibrosarcoma that, without reference to the primary tumor, gave no clue to origin in a chondrosarcoma. A similar case was described by O'NEAL and ACKERMAN (1952).

III. Roentgen

All tumors had similar roentgen features, such as large size and aggressive destructive changes, indicating their malignant nature (Fig. 122). Most had calcific foci characteristic of chondrosarcoma, nearly always in a medullary location (Fig. 123). Cortical perforation and an extraosseous mass were almost always evident but the mass did not differ notably from that produced by the ordinary chondrosarcoma. It was most commonly unmineralized (Fig. 122 E). Several tumors had caused a remodeling expansion of the involved bone, indicating their initial slow growth.

The possibility of "de novo transformation" into a more malignant lesion as illustrated by DAHLIN and BEABOUT's 26 cases without prior surgical intervention, also indicates that follow-up of a possible cartilaginous tumor by use of repeated roentgenographic examinations instead of treatment may be fraught with danger.

IV. Course

Of the 28 patients treated prior to 1969, 23 are dead most with no metastatic disease; 16 livinged less than 1 year, 6 for 1–2 years and 1 for 5 years from the time of treatment for the dedifferentiated tumor. The poor prognosis contrasts with an expected 5 year survival of more than 70% for patients with adequately treated ordinary chondrosarcoma.

DAHLIN and BEABOUT's (1971) data from 33 cases indicate that about 10% of low grade chondrosarcomas can be expected to evolve into dedifferentiated sarcomas that have the features and highly malignant clinical quality of fibrosarcoma or osteogenic sarcoma. The incidence would probably be higher if the tumors in all instances of lethal recurrent and metastatic chondrosarcoma were studied. Some who have observed the clinical features of this phenomenon in recurrent tumors believe that inadequate surgical removal triggered the transformation. O'NEAL and ACKERMAN have postulated that perhaps inadequate excision is apt to leave behind the more aggressive portions of the tumor. However, DAHLIN and BEABOUT have indicated that the change is part of the "normal" evolution of a few chondrosarcomas, since 26 of 33 cases manifested dedifferentiated zones without prior surgical intervention.

These observations are of academic interest to those who study the genesis of fibrosarcomas and osteogenic sarcomas. The examination of such tumors may occasionally disclose a central cartilaginous tumor. This may be particularly cogent in cases of osteogenic sarcoma reported in older people.

However, the implication of the possibility of dedifferentiation in the course of treatment of cartilaginous tumors is of more than academic importance and emphasizes the value of adequate primary removal, so that the threat of recurrence, sometimes in the form of a highly lethal lesion, is minimized. It is, encumbent upon the pathologist to sample cartilaginous tumors thoroughly, paying special attention to zones that are grossly abnormal. This is particularly difficult in cases with limited biopsies. Surgeons

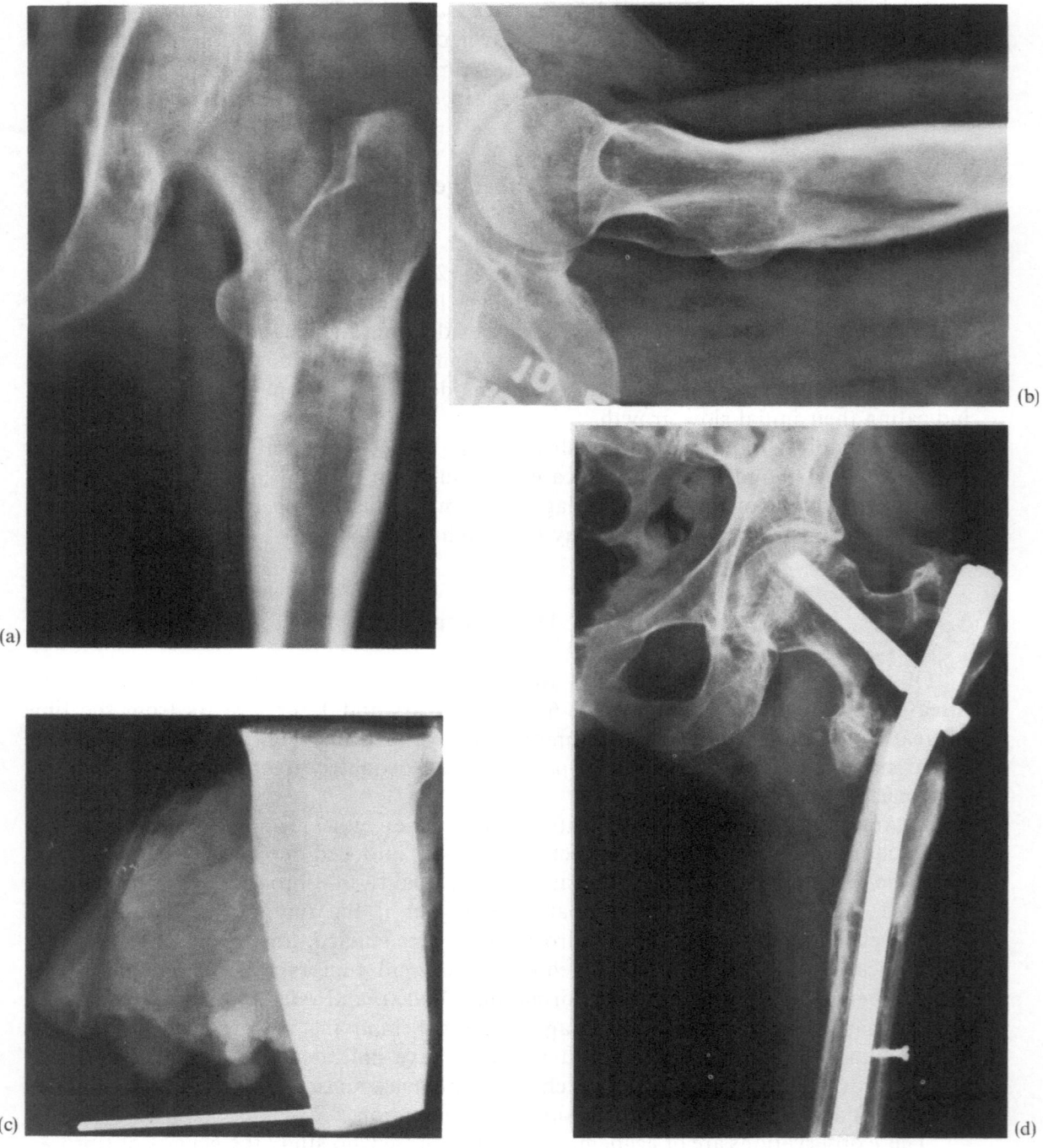

Fig. 122a–d. Dedifferentiation of low-grade chondrosarcoma: (a) Left femur, AP tomogram (10/28/67). Delineates central chondrosarcoma with atypical hazy chondroid matrix in diametaphysis. Several small calcific deposits are seen within superior substance of lesion. Note localized expansion and thickening of cortex, endosteal scalloping, and the buttress-like configuration of thickened inferior cortex. (b) Lateral view (10/28/67) again reveals centrally situated radiolucency with localized expansion of proximal femoral cortex. Note that inferior cortex appears relatively thinned. (c) Gross specimen of partially resected femur (1967). (d) AP femur (1/21/70): Bone graft placed in 1967 had successfully fused to distal femur. However, large lytic recurrent lesion is compromising proximal portion of bone graft

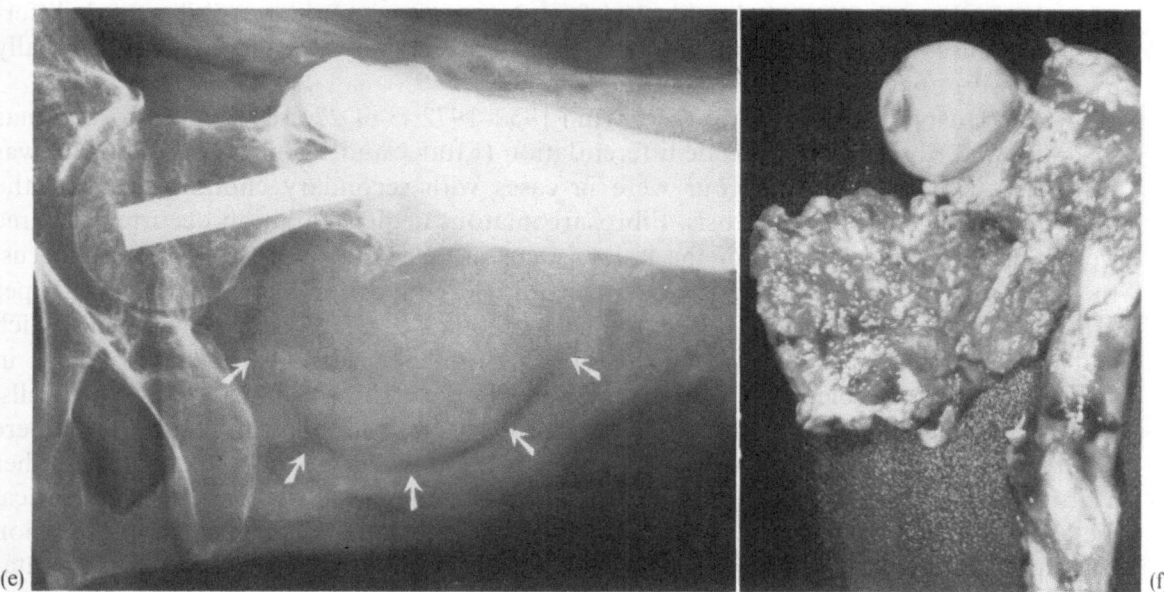

Fig. 122 e and f. Lateral view 7/21/70. Note large, rounded, soft tissue mass inferior to neck and proximal femoral shaft which represents extraosseous extension of recurrent tumor mass. Note radiolucent halo around periphery of lesion which suggests encapsulation (arrows). (f) Gross specimen of disarticulated femur: Large extraosseous extent of tumor mass is now evident. Histologically recurrent lesion proved to be fibrosarcoma

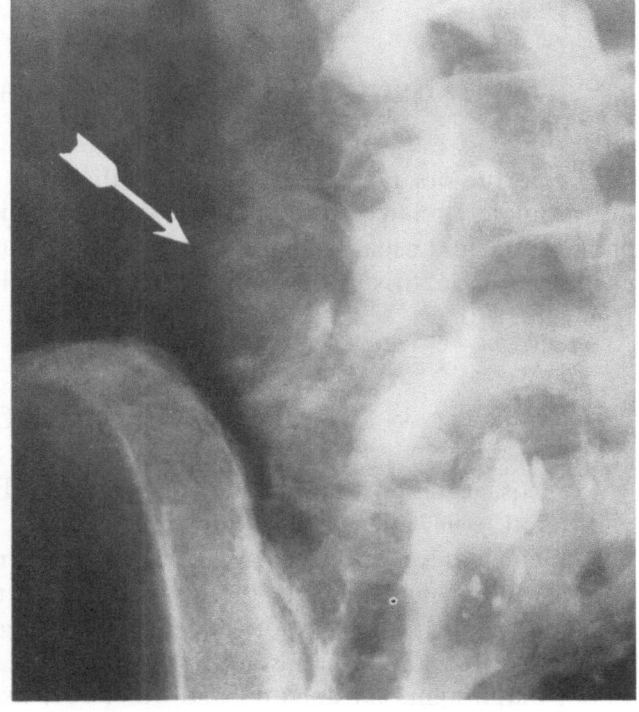

Fig. 123. Dedifferentiated chondrosarcoma: 50-year-old man with increasing pain and weakness of leg for 8 months. Note amorphous calcification in mass associated with posterior lateral aspect of lower lumbar spine (arrow). At surgery mass was found to originate from pedicles and lamina. Transverse process of L-5 was partially destroyed. Tumor had invaded posterior longitudinal ligament ventral to cauda equina and total removal could not be achieved. Histologic sections showed elements of fibroblastic dedifferentiation.
Death occurred 2 months after diagnosis

who obtain tissue for biopsy should, therefore, be cognizant of the possibility of dedifferentiated zones which are sometimes indicated both grossly and roentgenographically by aggressive appearing extension of the tumor.

At the Hospital for Special Surgery from 1952–1972, 5 of 27 (18%) chondrosarcomas seen, showed fibrosarcomatous dedifferentiation (MIRRA and MARCOVE, 1974). One was in a case with primary and four were in cases with secondary chondrosarcoma, the latter related to enchondromatosis. Fibrosarcomatous dedifferentiation occurred in three women and two men. Three of the lesions were in the femur and two in the humerus. In some areas there was a fairly sharp histologic delineation between the two types of tissue, but in others, fully differentiated malignant cartilage cells were noted which had assumed a more spindly shape, stopped producing cartilaginous matrix and in an almost imperceptible transition assumed the characteristics of fibrosarcomatous cells. The histologic evidence and the absence of primary fibrosarcoma originating elsewhere favored the concept that this association was not a collision of tumor types, but rather a fibrosarcomatous dedifferentiation of a chondrosarcoma. All five patients had clinical metastases within less than 1 year from the time of initial diagnosis. The exception was a patient with OLLIER's disease where metastases became evident 5 years after amputation. All of the patients succumbed to their disease within 1 year after the development of clinically evident metastases which were principally by vascular dissemination and involved many organ systems including the lungs, viscera, skin, muscles, and adrenals. The overall less than 20% 5 year survival rate was again emphasized.

Of additional interest was an altered carbohydrate metabolism. Either the fasting blood sugar was elevated, or the glucose tolerance test was abnormal. Altered carbohydrate metabolism had previously been noted in association with classic chondrosarcoma (MARCOVE and FRANCIS, 1963; MARCOVE et al., 1972).

O. Extraskeletal Cartilage Tumors of the Soft Tissues

These tumors may be benign or malignant. Both types are infrequeent. They are not intimately related to the periosteum of an adjacent bone, as in cases of juxtacortical chondroma, and usually do not deform or invade neighboring bone. PAGET first described cartilage tumors arising in "soft tissues completely detached from bone or normal cartilage" in 1870.

I. Malignant Soft Tissue Cartilage Tumors

Soft tissue chondrosarcomas are rare lesions (ENZINGER and SHIRAKI, 1972; GOLDENBERG et al., 1967; KAUFFMAN and STOUT, 1963; MALLORY, 1933; STOUT and VERNER, 1953) which have occurred over a wide age range, i.e. from childhood to the ninth decade, and at many sites in the body including the larynx (DE, 1972; GOETHALS et al., 1963; KURTZ, 1975; LAWSON et al., 1972), tongue (GUTMANN et al., 1974), maxillary region (JONES, 1973), kidney (GALLAGHER et al., 1974), lung (MORGAN and SALAMA, 1972), diaphragm, extrapleural and other soft tissues (ANGERVALL et al., 1973), various muscle groups, and periarticular soft tissues (REAM et al., 1973) particularly about the knee (MOORE and SHANNON, 1974). Prior to the comprehensive reports by STOUT and

VERNER (1953) and KAUFFMAN and STOUT (1963), only a few isolated cases of malignant cartilage tumors arising in extraskeletal soft tissues were published. The paucity of new reports further attests to their rarity. No extraskeletal chondrosarcomas were noted in more than 1000 cases of soft tissue tumors in 3 published series and in 3 pathology textbooks (GOLDENBERG et al., 1967). GOLDENBERG et al. (1967) recently discussed seven cases and reviewed the literature, utilizing STOUT and VERNER's criteria (1953). They excluded chondrosarcomas which arose from periosteum and normal extraskeletal cartilage, e.g. the nasal passages and the tracheal bronchial tree. Many of the reported cases of primary chondrosarcoma of lung may have originated from the latter area. Also excluded were other cartilage containing malignant tumors such as teratomas, mesenchymomas, and extraskeletal osteogenic sarcomas. Among GOLDENBERG's 26 extraskeletal chondrosarcomas, 18 were found in the gluteal region and lower extremity, 5 in the shoulder region and upper extremity, and 1 each in the tongue, thoracic wall, and urinary bladder. Of the 4 in the gluteal region, 1 arose from the ischial bursa and 2 in the gluteal muscles. Of the 5 lesions of the thigh, 3 arose in the muscle. Each of the 3 lesions about the knee was located in the popliteal space, 1 originated from the gastrocnemius muscle, 1 from the semimembraneous muscle, and 1 from the connective tissue.

In this and other series there were no distinctive clinical features. Males predominated 17:9 and the lesion had no definite age incidence since ages ranged from 2 to 73 years.

II. Pathology

Grossly the tumors may be seen to be enclosed by a tough connective tissue capsule which may be loosely attached to the surrounding tissue, or so closely adherent that complete dissection is difficult. The size of lesions in 23 cases ranged from $2 \times 1.5 \times 1.5$ cm– 20×15 cm. Large size is an ominous sign. Whitish-speckled areas of calcification may be seen grossly. However, the calcification is not always of sufficient concentration to be visible on roentgenograms. Tumors which arise in areas with little space for expansion may eventually erode adjacent bone, but in only one instance was the bone actually invaded in GOLDENBERG's series. In a few cases the exact anatomic site of origin was not determined. In others the tumor was found to arise in muscle fascia, connective tissue, or bursa.

Microscopic features are similar to those found in osseous chondrosarcomas. It may be difficult in some cases to differentiate a paraosteal or para-articular chondroma from an extraskeletal chondrosarcoma. The former tend to be small, and are usually less than 2 cm in diameter, non-movable, non-tender, and grow slowly. The paraosteal chondroma, occasionally outlined by a thin radiopaque shell, is found at the insertion of ligamentous or tendinous tissue into a bone and most frequently in the short tubular bones of the hands and feet. The para-articular chondroma arises from the fibrous coat of the capsule, or from within a joint and usually occurs in the hand. In each of these benign tumors the cartilage cells are frequently unicellular, the nuclei are neither large nor plump, and the cells show no atypism. These features serve to distinguish them from extraskeletal soft tissue chondrosarcoma. A striking histologic feature of extraskeletal chondrosarcoma is the nodular arrangement of the tumor. On occasion the nodules consist of well-formed hyaline cartilage divided by connective tissue septa. The septa are often invaded by malignant looking cells that have bizarre hyperchromatic and multiple nuclei that are irregular in size and shape.

No recorded case of malignant degeneration of a benign cartilaginous tumor of soft tissue was found by GOLDENBERG et al. (1967). There was no histologic evidence of a pre-existing benign cartilaginous tumor in any of 26 cases reviewed, although it is possible that a small focus of benign chondroma could have been rapidly overgrown and obliterated. They agree with STOUT and VERNER (1953) that extraosseous chondrosarcomas arise de novo rather than from pre-existing benign chondromas.

III. Roentgen

The majority of lesions contain scattered, rounded, or elongated areas of radiopacity (Figs. 124a, b). However, even a large lesion may show no evidence of mineralization on the roentgenogram despite the presence of calcification in the gross specimen, and the lesion may not be visualized roentgenographically. The cartilaginous nature of the lesion cannot be suspected without calcification or ossification. Conversely, many soft tissue lesions other than extraskeletal chondrosarcomas may show roentgenographic evidence of irregular calcifications, i.e. synoviomas which may calcify in 30–40% of cases. Calcified or ossified phleboliths and/or hemangiomas usually have radiolucent centers, while the calcifications of synovial chondromatosis are found within a joint, most commonly the knee and hip.

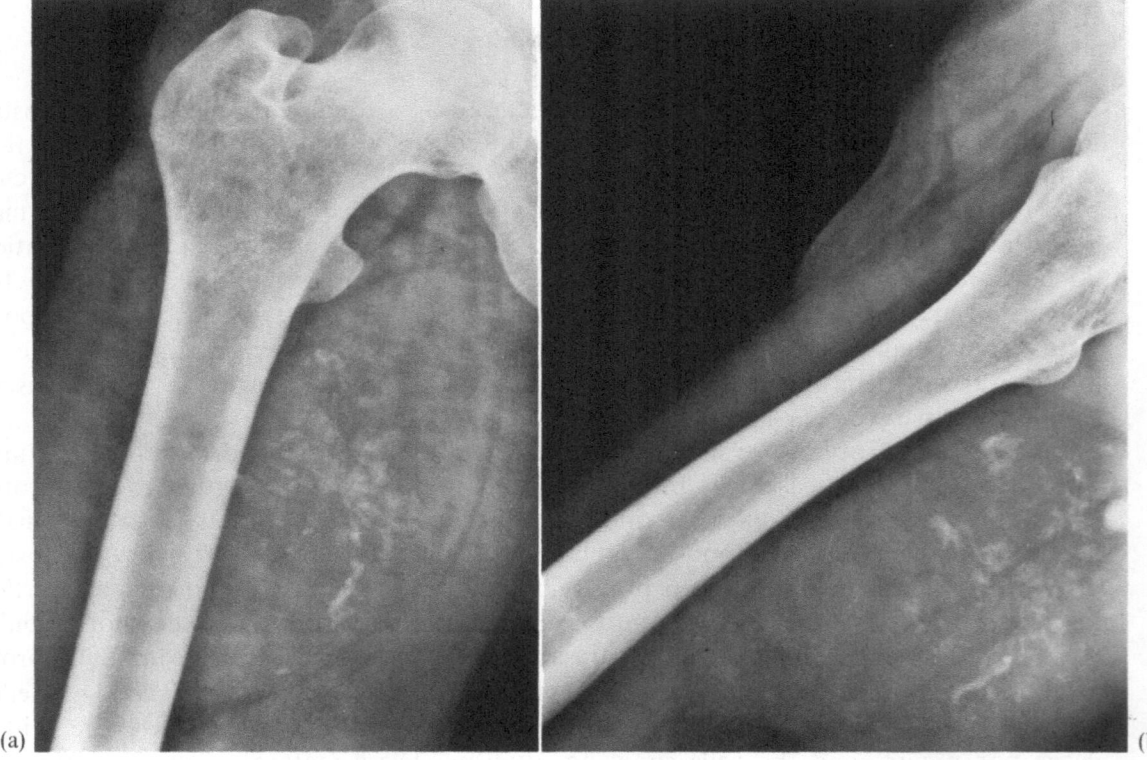

(a)		(b)

Fig. 124a and b. Extraskeletal chondrosarcoma, thigh: 29-year-old male had 9 month history of nontender proximal right thigh mass. There was no history of trauma. (a) Frontal and (b) oblique views of right proximal thigh reveal large, oval-shaped, soft tissue mass with irregular flocculent calcification within it. Note lucent halo which simulates capsule. Muscle and fat planes appear preserved. Mass was confined to soft tissues and completely divorced from bone. En bloc resection of this Grade I chondrosarcoma was performed on 3/5/75

IV. Treatment and Prognosis

Recurrence after excision is frequent and has been reported as early as 2 months and as late as 15 years after primary operation. Extraskeletal chondrosarcomas are capable of metastasizing. The exact incidence of recurrence and metastases is unknown because of inadequate follow-up. In GOLDENBERG et al.'s series (1967), 11 of the 26 tumors recurred and 4 more than once. Four metastasized. However, follow-up exceeded 5 years in only 4 cases. When the tumor recurred, or when bone had been eroded or invaded, amputation was the treatment of choice.

Complete removal of the tumor and its capsule is the only treatment which offers a prospect for cure. There are no reported cases of extraskeletal chondrosarcoma cured by radiation therapy.

V. Benign Soft Tissue Cartilage Tumors

Benign cartilage tumors in soft tissues without concomitant involvement of adjacent bone such as that displayed by juxtacortical chondromas are also rare. Benign chondromas are most common in the soft tissues of the hands and feet, but they may be seen in other areas (MAGNUSSON and ROTEMARK, 1974). They may occur within the outer fibrous coat of joint capsules and are then referred to as intracapsular chondromas, or within connective tissues in the vicinity of capsules and are then called para-articular

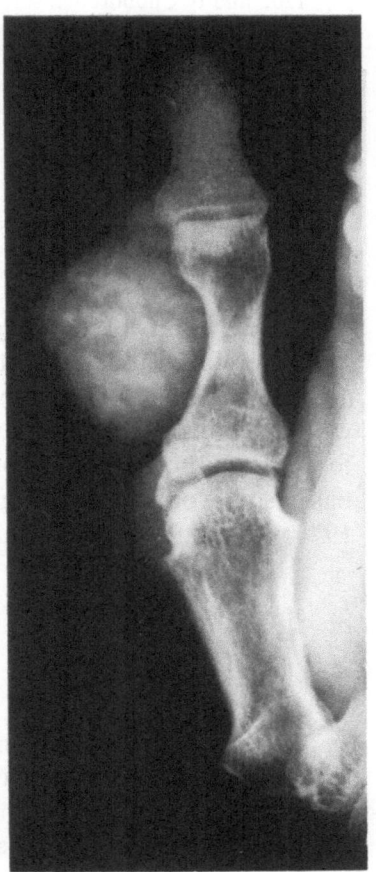

Fig. 125. Chondroma, soft tissue: 53-year-old asymptomatic female with soft tissue cartilage tumor. Large, oval, well-mineralized, well-demarcated, soft tissue mass along lateral aspect of proximal phalanx of thumb has resulted in smooth pressure erosion with sclerotic base in neighboring bone

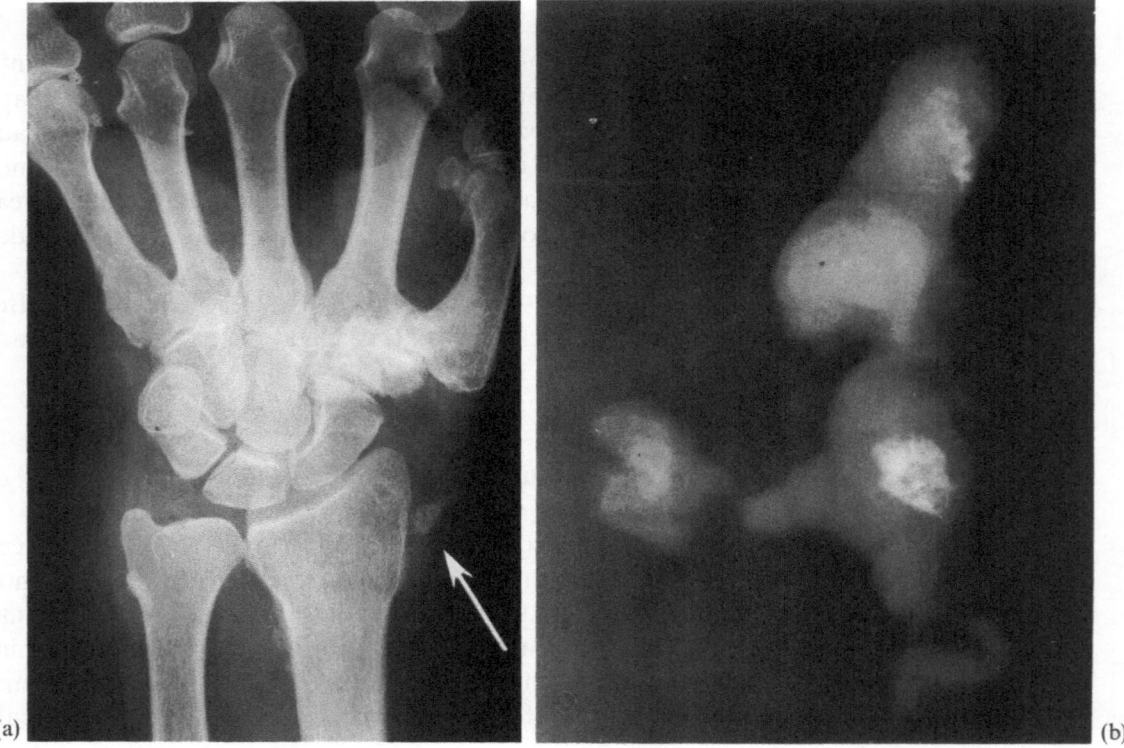

Fig. 126a and b. Chondroma, soft tissue: 58-year-old female complained of swelling about wrist. (a) Rounded, calcific deposit is seen lateral to, but separated from, distal radius (arrow) with associated prominence of neighboring soft tissues. (b) Roentgenogram of resected specimen with several calcified cartilaginous bodies which were only faintly visualized on roentgenogram and were related to the neighbouring tendon sheath

chondromas. They may also be related to the synovial surfaces of joints, bursae, or tendon sheaths (Figs. 125, 126a, b) (Jaffe, 1968; Lichtenstein, 1955; Lynn and Lee, 1972).

They exhibit a wide cytologic range as do cartilage and chondroid tumors in bone and, therefore, are frequently misdiagnosed as chondrosarcomas. Many are interpreted as being malignant since their cytologic appearance may be such that had they developed within bone they would have been so classified. This is a fallacious premise according to most authorities who point out that the appraisal of these lesions should not be based solely on their cytology, but on their natural history as well (Dahlin and Salvador, 1974; Lichtenstein and Goldman, 1964).

VI. Pathogenesis

These lesions result from extrasynovial cartilage metaplasia with subsequent cartilage proliferation occurring in the outer or fibrous coat of a joint capsule or in adjacent connective tissues most commonly in the vicinity of a joint. They should not be confused with synovial chondromatosis in which the cartilaginous metaplasia occurs in the sublining connective tissue of the synovial membrane.

VII. Clinical

There is no sex predilection. Although cases have been reported over a wide age range the vast majority of patients were over 20. They were frequently in the fourth and fifth decades in MOSHER et al.'s (1966) series, which consisted of para-articular chondromas about the knee. In this location, the presenting complaint was most commonly a mass with or without pain. Restricted motion was uncommon.

Among 70 cases of cartilaginous tumors involving the hands and feet reported by DAHLIN and SALVADOR (1974), ages ranged from 10–84 years at the time of diagnosis with a fairly even distribution from the third to the eighth decade and a peak incidence during the sixth decade. The sex distribution was nearly equal, i.e. in 35 males and 34 females. There were few symptoms related to the hands and feet. Swelling had been present from 1–50 years in 32 patients while some merely noted slowly progressive enlargement.

VIII. Site

Soft tissue hyaline cartilage tumors are common in the hands and feet. A recent compilation at the Mayo Clinic included 70 cases (DAHLIN and SALVADOR, 1974). MOSHER

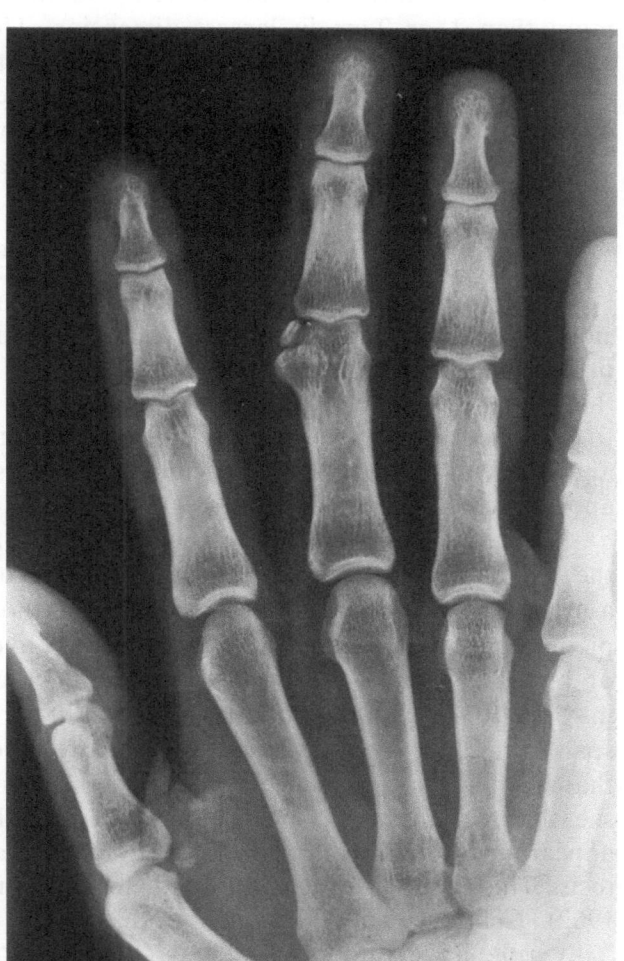

Fig. 127. Chondroma, soft tissue: Ossified chondroma lateral to proximal interphalangeal joint of 3rd finger was extracapsular in location and was situated just distal to exostosis with cartilage cap of its own. It is therefore problematic whether extracapsular chondroma arose de novo or was related to exostosis

et al. (1966) cited the knee as the most common site for para-articular chondromas and they noted that all of the reported cases in this location have been intracapsular, extrasynovial, and infrapatellar deep to the patellar tendon. SUERMONDT (1950) reported an ossified lesion in the anterior capsule of the elbow. PURSER (1956), too, reported two extraosseous osteochondral lesions in feet, one medial to the metatarsal phalangeal joint of the great toe, and the other plantar to a fourth metatarsal head. These were roentgenographically and histologically similar to the lesions about the knee. However, both lesions were extracapsular, and were separated from the adjacent joint by a bursa. It is, therefore, problematic whether these lesions represent solitary synovial chondromata in a bursa or whether the bursa formed secondary to the lesion (Fig. 127).

IX. Pathology

1. Gross

These tumors are generally small, ranging from less than 2 cm–4 cm in greatest diameter. They were 3 cm or less in 57 of DAHLIN and SALVADOR'S (1974) cases. Of these, only 6 were 5 cm or more, while the largest measured 9 cm in greatest dimension. Therefore, chondromas which develop in the vicinity of small joints are usually not more than 1 or 2 cm in largest dimension. However, those which evolve in relation to a large joint may be greater than 5 cm (CASTLEMAN, 1962). Multicentricity was demonstrated in three of DAHLIN and SALVADOR'S lesions. Two cases had separate masses and one had several masses. Their chondroid or cartilaginous quality is obvious. They are distinctly lobulated with calcific or bony flecks.

2. Microscopic

The tumors are composed of masses of hyaline cartilage, usually lobulated and occasionally partially myxoid. The cartilage may degenerate, calcify, or ossify, by means of enchondral ossification. The latter process usually follows vascular penetration of the lesion (MOSHER et al., 1966). When they have ossified, these lesions have been referred to as capsular osteomas (KAUTZ, 1945), extraskeletal osteochondromas (PURSER, 1956), and ossifying chondromas. Calcification or ossification was seen in some sections in approximately half the lesions of DAHLIN and SALVADOR (1974).

The multicentricity demonstrated in three of DAHLIN and SALVADOR'S lesions, plus the tendency for the lesion to wrap itself around bone have led to speculations of a synovial derivation for these lesions. Xanthoma-like zones dominated the histologic picture in 9 of 70 cases. Such areas have been likened to tendon sheath giant cell tumors, or benign fibrous histiocytomas, enforcing the concept that these chondroid lesions may be of synovial derivation. In fact, solitary loose bodies were seen within synovial spaces in 2 of the 70 Mayo Clinic lesions. However, this was qualified by the fact that synovial spaces might be expected to be encountered in these locations since synovial sheaths are so numerous in the hands and feet. Therefore, in some instances the histologic appearance may also resemble that seen in association with articular synovial chondromatosis. This parallelism extends to their common mimicry of sarcoma (MURPHY et al., 1962). Cells frequently have nuclei suggestive of malignancy. However, DAHLIN and SALVADOR (1974) support LICHTENSTEIN and GOLDMAN'S previous contention that these lesions are, in fact, benign and do not metastasize despite recurrence. Among the 70 tumors of DAHLIN and SALVADOR were 59 specimens sent in for consultation because of difficulty in diagnosis. Most had been considered as chondrosarcomas and many were considered "worrisome." Conversely, in their experience with 30 chondrosarcomas of the bones, of the hands, and feet, 29 began within bone. In only one case had the early roentgenogram shown no evidence of abnormality and only one lesion was considered of periosteal origin. They, therefore, had no instance of a soft tissue chondrosarcoma involving the hands or feet. No tendency to metastasize was noted among 10 cases reported by LICHTENSTEIN and GOLDMAN, who further corroborated that on pathologic examination alone they might have been inclined to overestimate the potential seriousness of a number of their tumors. They additionally noted, however, that tumors in bone of comparable cytology usually behave as insidiously invasive low grade sarcomas that are prone to recur locally and eventually require radical surgery for cure.

X. Roentgen

The roentgenogram may show an ill-defined mass which may be lobulated or oval and which may contain varying amounts of calcium and/or bone. Mineralization became visible during the course of a year in one untreated case that had originally shown roentgenographic evidence of a soft tissue mass only. Since these lesions are most commonly divorced from bone, benign and malignant hyaline cartilage tumors of bone, including those located periosteally, may be readily excluded roentgenographically. There was slight deformity or erosion of the underlying bone by the adjacent soft tissue mass in only 4 of 70 cases. Posttraumatic proliferations of bone and cartilage on a bone's surface may be difficult to differentiate, but such proliferations are rare and a history of trauma as well as previous films may be of value.

Although para-articular chondromata when they occur about the knee are most commonly situated in the infrapatellar region or in relation to the capsule, in the latter position they must occasionally be differentiated from chondrosarcoma and from synovial chondromatosis, as well as other soft tissue sarcomas (MARTIN et al., 1973). An air arthrogram is of value in substantiating an extra-articular location as opposed to the intra-articular location of synovial chondromatosis. Para-articular chondromas are often associated with single calcific or ossific densities, whereas the calcified and/or ossified intra-articular masses associated with synovial chondromatosis are usually multiple, small, and commonly of uniform size. Intra-articular loose bodies do not occur in association with para-articular chondromas. These tumors are smallest in the hands and feet, most commonly less than 3 cm in their greatest dimension, and most commonly situated in the vicinity of the small joints. They tend to be larger when they evolve in the vicinity of a large joint such as the knee and were frequently larger than 5 cm in this location. However, roentgenographic estimation of the size of unmineralized or partially mineralized lesions may be deceiving.

Recurrence was observed in 12 of 70 cases of the Mayo Clinic series. No lesion was associated with metastases. One patient with 10 recurrences had had multiple chondroid masses as large as 1 cm in diameter on the dorsal and ventral surfaces of the carpus. The lesions were cytologically active, emphasizing the ease with which these may be regarded as sarcomatous. LICHTENSTEIN and BERNSTEIN (1959) divided their 10 cases according to their degree of maturation, i.e. 4 were hyaline cartilage tumors and 6 were less differentiated chondroid tumors. None of the hyaline cartilage tumors and only 3 of the chondroid tumors recurred. The tumor cytology did not change perceptibly after recurrence.

P. Synovial Chondromatosis

Synovial chondromatosis is an uncommon, specific condition in which foci of cartilage develop, apparently through metaplasia, in the sublining connective tissue of the synovial membranes of large joints such as the hip and knee. The rarity of this condition was emphasized by MURPHY et al. (1962) who were unable to find more than 32 cases in the Mayo Clinic files over a 48-year period. The even rarer examples of chondromatosis of bursae and tendon sheaths were not included (LICHTENSTEIN, 1955; LYNN and LEE, 1972; ROBILLARD, 1941).

The literature regarding synovial chondromatosis is difficult to evaluate. The condition has often been mistakenly diagnosed in cases with intra-articular radiopaque and/or loose bodies from other causes which failed to meet JAFFE's (1968) diagnostic criteria.

I. Clinical

It occurs most frequently in young to middle-aged males. It is rare below the age of puberty. The condition is usually monoarticular. The knee joint (Fig. 128) is the favored site (MURPHY et al., 1962) while other large joints, i.e. the hip (MCIVOR and

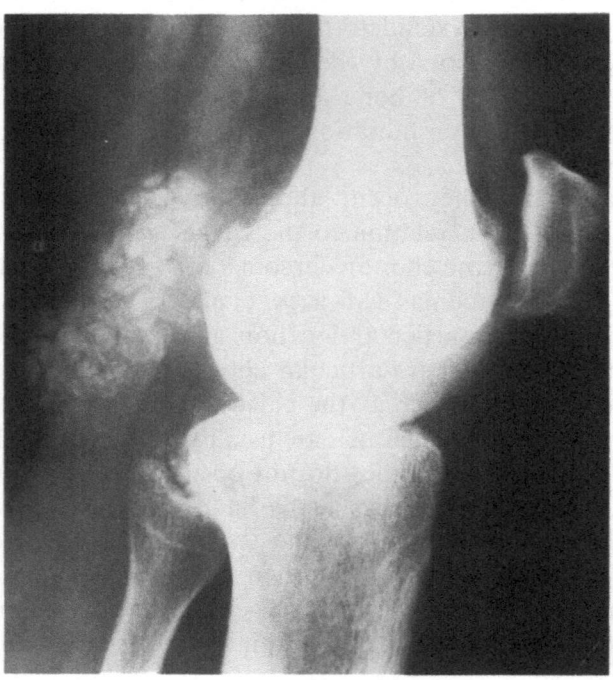 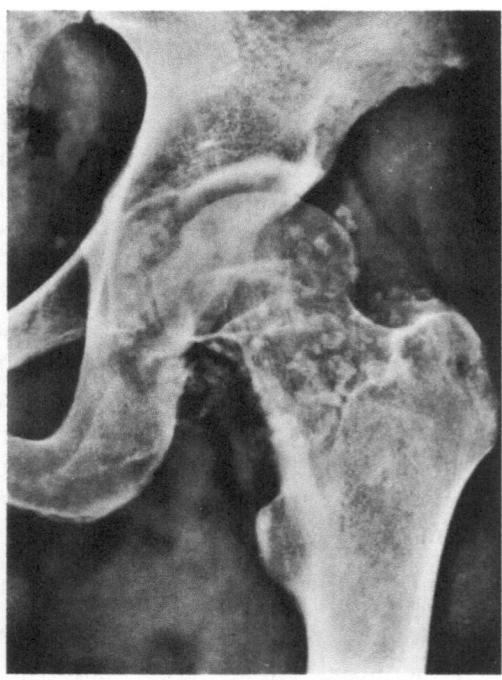

Fig. 128   Fig. 129

Fig. 128. Synovial chondromatosis, knee: 50-year-old female with 2 year history of increasing stiffness of knee. Injury sustained 4 months prior to admission had precipitated pain and swelling. Numerous discrete, fairly uniform in size, rounded, radiopaque bodies with relatively lucent centers lie posterior to knee joint. At surgery, numerous cartilaginous bodies were found within knee joint, as well as within popliteal cyst which was attached to posterior portion of joint by narrow, partially fibrosed pedicle

Fig. 129. Synovial chondromatosis, hip: Hip joint is distended with numerous radiopaque bodies which took their origin from synovial surface of articular capsule. Note smooth articular surfaces of normal hip joint with no evidence of productive or degenerative changes

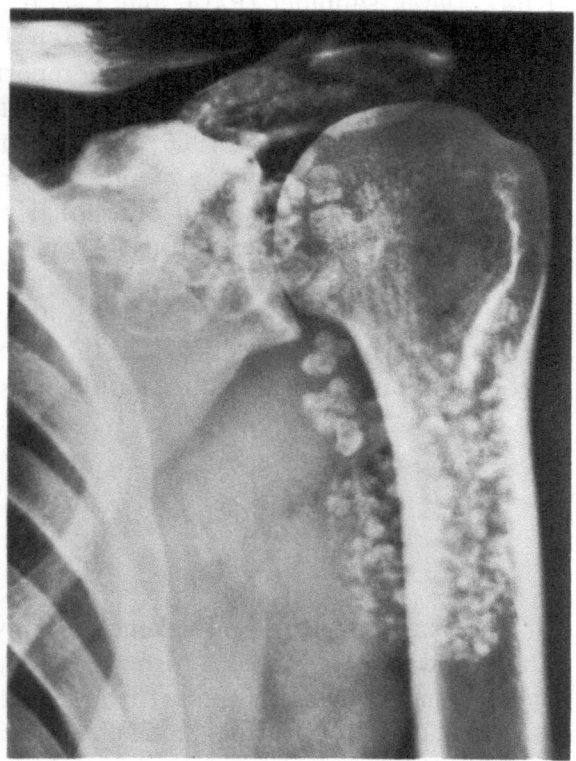

Fig. 130. Synovial chondromatosis, shoulder: Numerous cartilaginous foci are undergoing calcification. Heavy calcification of focus of cartilage is usually forerunner of ossification. Shoulder had been intermittently painful for 2 years with clicking, grating, and increasing limitation in range of motion

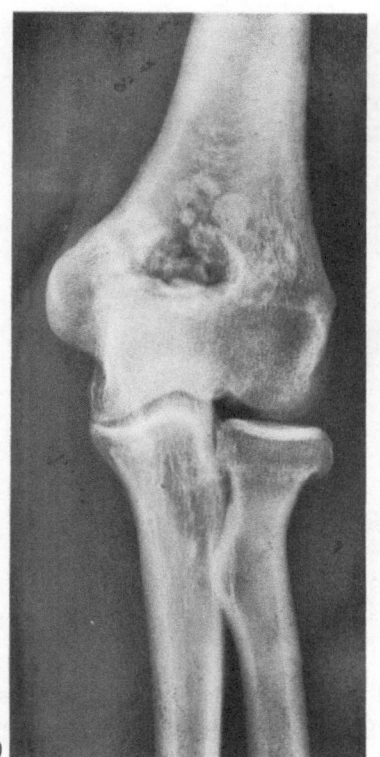

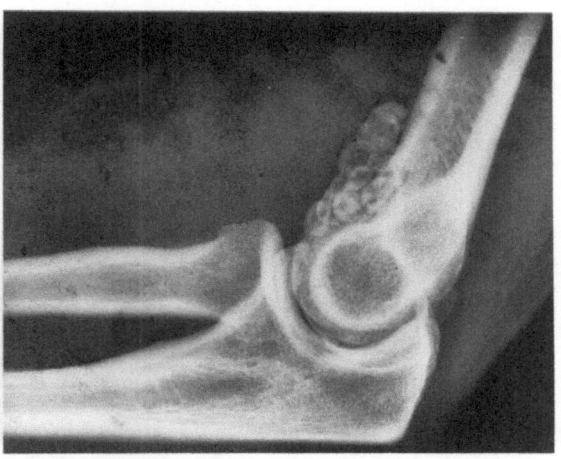

(a)

(b)

Fig. 131a and b. Synovial chondromatosis, elbow: (a) AP view. Rounded, calcified bodies are projected over olecranon fossa. (b) Numerous radiopaque bodies which were obscured on AP view are seen within joint capsule anteriorly

KING, 1962), shoulder (PAUL and LEACH, 1970), and elbow account for the majority of remaining cases (Figs. 129, 130, 131). The metacarpal-phalangeal, wrist, ankle, and tempromandibular joints are rarely reported additional sites. Therefore, the smaller diarthrodial joints are not exempt (HEIPLE and ELMER, 1972; CONSTANT et al., 1974; KETTELKAMP and DOLAN, 1966; LEWIS et al., 1974; ROBERTS, 1971; SILVER et al., 1971).

Signs and symptoms may be present for months or years and include pain, swelling, limited range of motion, and occasional grating or locking. Physical findings include limited motion, tenderness, effusion, and a local mass (EISENBERG and JOHNSTON, 1972).

The ages of 32 patients in the Mayo Clinic series (MURPHY et al., 1962) ranged from 16–67 years with an average of 40.4 years; 21 were men. The knee was affected in 22 of 32 patients, the hip in 5, the elbow in 2, and the ankle, shoulder, and wrist in 1. Symptoms ranged from 1 month to 57 years and no patient had a family history.

II. Pathology

1. Gross

The synovium may be thickened and hyperemic with numerous villous projections. Chondroid foci appear to be forming in the synovial membrane just beneath the surface. Cartilage masses vary in number from numerous to myriad and in size from microscopic to 3 cm in diameter. Cartilaginous masses may be pedunculated or may become detached. If the cartilaginous bodies have not been sequestered from their attachment to the synovium, they may stud the synovium and appear as small glistening grey-white nodules (Fig. 132). Others appear as polypoid lesions, occasionally with long stalks. The entire synovium may be involved and the nodules so numerous that they appear to form

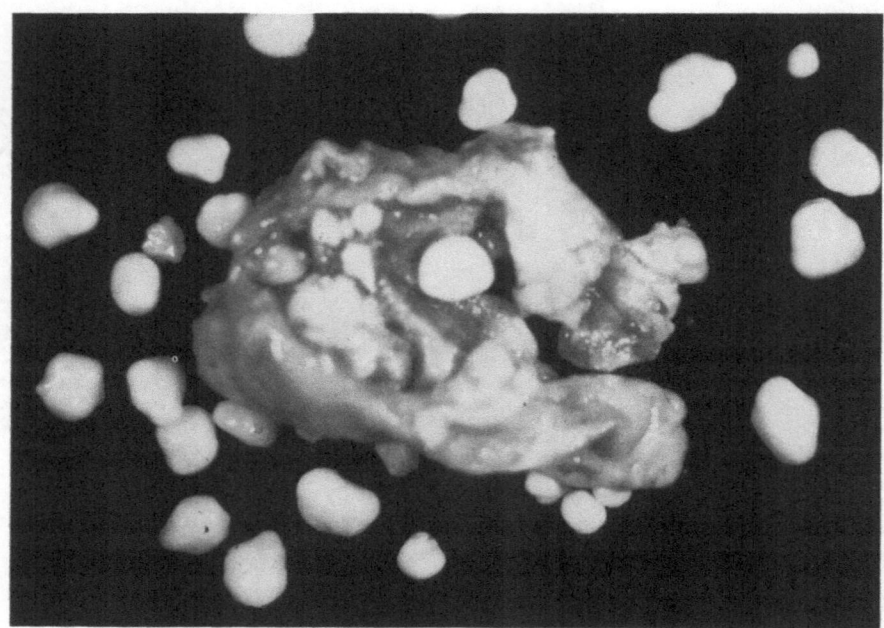

Fig. 132. Synovial chondromatosis: Gross specimen of resected synovial membrane from case illustrated in Figure 128. Affected synovium was thickened with cartilage developing immediately beneath innermost layer. Clusters of cartilage nodules of varying size protrude from surface of membrane. Many nodules had separated from synovial surface and were floating freely within joint space

a solid and/or matted mass. Cartilaginous bodies, when they become detached from the affected membrane, enter the joint cavity and increase in size, nourished slowly by synovial fluid. The loose bodies are generally white to grey-white, and most commonly oval or rounded. Infrequently they are irregular, with gross evidence of calcification and ossification. The loose bodies may be reimbedded in or attached to the synovium. Those free in the joint are histologically similar and range from masses of cartilage to bodies in which there is a mixture of cartilage that is commonly calcified and bone, which in some instances has a fatty narrow. Since many of the cartilaginous foci become calcified and/or ossified, the lesion has also been referred to as synovial osteochondromatosis.

The synovial membrane was involved in an area of at least 2 sq. cm in all 32 Mayo Clinic patients (MURPHY et al., 1962). In most, larger areas were affected and in some almost the entire synovial membrane was involved. Although in some instances synovial chondromatosis involved the peripheral attachments of the menisci, in no instance did the chondroid mass extend to the joint capsule.

2. Microscopic

Microscopically myriad cartilaginous masses were seen to be forming beneath the thin layer of cells lining the surface of the synovial membrane. Once cartilage formation is initiated at a particular synovial site, continued increase in the cartilage body results from multiplication of the cartilage cells and not from cartilage accretion by further metaplasia of the surrounding connective tissues (Figs. 133, 134).

The cartilage cells, particularly prior to mineralization, are often richly cellular, showing a fair number of cells with double and occasionally plump nuclei. This indicates

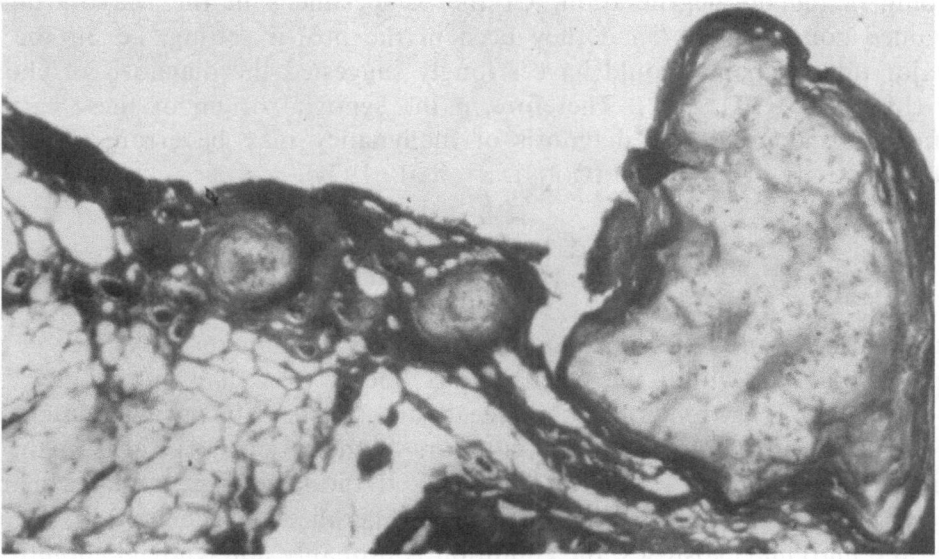

Fig. 133. Synovial chondromatosis, photomicrograph (×250): Several discrete but closely set nodules of cartilage contain varying amounts of calcium. Growing nodules of cartilage compress neighboring connective tissues so that they appear surrounded by fibrous capsule. Heavy calcification of a focus of cartilage is usually forerunner of ossification of area in question. Prerequisite of ossification appears to be invasion of calcified area by blood vessels which bring in osteoblasts on their walls. Layers of laminar bone are deposited, and bone is substituted for calcified cartilage by process of creeping replacement. One may see fatty marrow in interior of an ossific focus which has replaced a focus of calcified cartilage

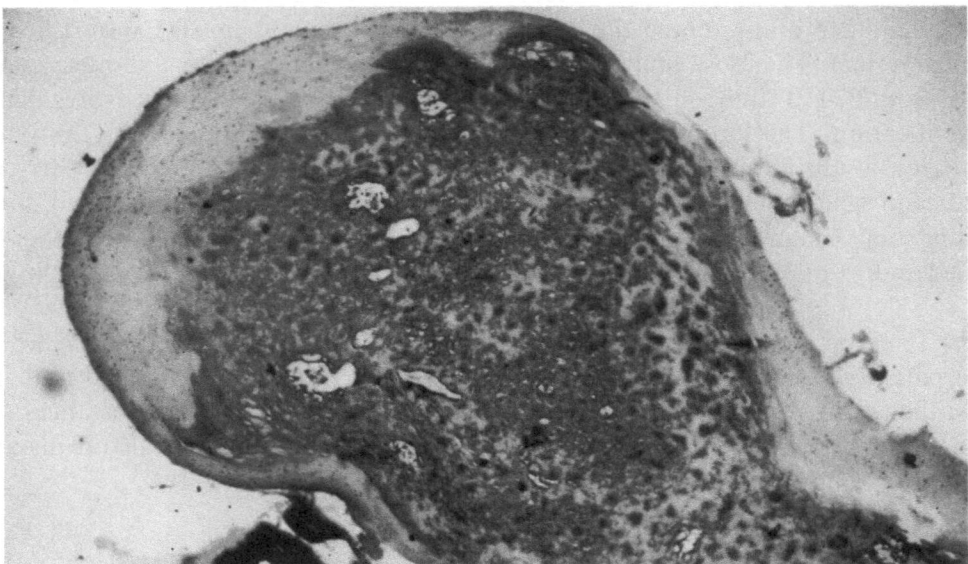

Fig. 134. Synovial chondromatosis, photomicrograph (× 250): Cartilage nodules which have not as yet become calcified or ossified are often richly cellular. Since such nodules represent actively growing foci of cartilage, fair numbers of cartilage cells with double nuclei may be present. These should not be viewed as early stigmata of chondrosarcoma, as they might be if noted in relation to a central cartilaginous lesion of bone which has undergone a spurt of growth. Cells with bizarre nuclei are usually not observed. Therefore, in connection with synovial chondromatosis, it is well to remember that presence of plumpish nuclei and more than an occasional cell with double nucleus merely indicates that cartilage area in question is actively growing

that the area in question is an actively growing cartilaginous focus rather than one undergoing malignant degeneration. Of the 32 specimens in the Mayo Clinic series, 23 contained zones which, "had they been in the proper setting, i.e. in the medulla of a major tubular bone, would have strongly suggested the diagnosis of chondrosarcoma" (Murphy et al., 1962). Therefore, if the synovial origin of these cartilaginous proliferations is ignored, the diagnosis of malignancy may be erroneously based on the cellular activity of the lesion (Constant et al., 1974).

III. Roentgen

Roentgen recognition of synovial chondromatosis depends on the degree of calcification and ossification within the cartilaginous bodies as well as upon their size and shape. Very large or extremely radiopaque bodies are usually not encountered in true synovial osteochondromatosis and the contours of the articular surfaces of the affected joint are usually unaltered (Figs. 128–131, 135). If the knee joint contains many large, extremely dense, loose bodies with associated generalized irregularity of the articular surfaces and marginal exostoses, the condition is probably not synovial chondromatosis.

Conditions which are associated with loose bodies within the joint and which may roentgenographically be confused with synovial chondromatosis are osteochondritis dissecans, osteoarthrosis, and neuropathic arthopathy. In these entities, rather than resulting from a metaplastic process, osteocartilaginous fragments are sheared or broken off from articular surfaces, may become secondarily embedded in the synovium, and/or lie free in the joint and may enlarge. Joint bodies may also form through calcification or chondri-

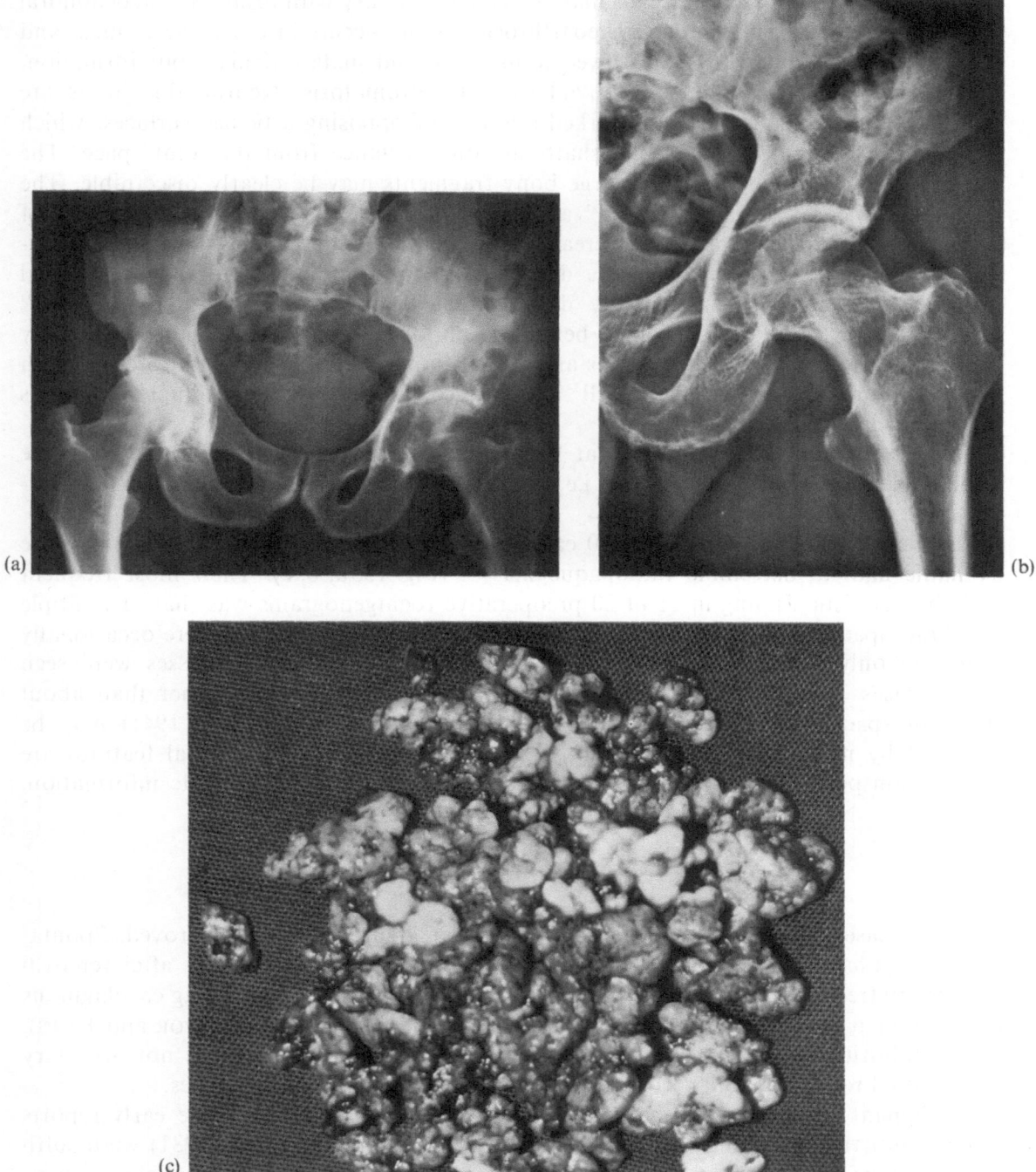

Fig. 135. (a) Synovial chondromatosis, hip: This 65-year-old male experienced repeated attacks of left hip pain with increasing limitation of motion. Other than moderate degree of osteopenia, which was attributed to disuse, no abnormality of left hip joint was noted on 11/3/73. (b) Progression in degree of osteopenia was noted in 1974. Pain had increased and extension at hip joint had become more limited. No radiopaque bodies could be identified. (c) Numerous small bodies which had not calcified sufficiently to be appreciated on roentgenogram were removed from hip joint. Partial synovectomy was done

fication of collections of fibrin that have accumulated within the joint consequent to synovitis. Osteochondritis dissecans may be related to injury with resultant osteochondral fracture or steroid arthropathy. Osteoarthrosis usually occurs in older age groups, and is usually accompanied by a narrowed joint space and juxta-articular spur formation. Neither routinely accompanies synovial osteochondromatosis. Neuropathic joints are usually lax and malaligned with marked sclerosis of opposing articular surfaces, which frequently extends down the bone shafts at some distance from the joint space. The "gouged out" donor sites of the large bony fragments may be clearly discernible. The bony and calcific "bits and pieces" associated with all these entities are usually of myriad sizes and configurations, whereas the osteocartilaginous bodies of synovial chondromatosis are usually smaller, less dense, more uniform in size, of round to oval configuration, and are occasionally described as "barley beans" or "rice bodies" (Figs. 128, 129, 130). In addition to being less uniformly dense, they may occasionally exhibit well-defined radiolucent cores and/or be stippled or peppered with calcium, with a resultant granular or "popcorn ball" appearance. They may be exceedingly numerous and ossified as well as calcified.

It is re-emphasized, however, that loose bodies, from whatever cause, can become implanted in the synovial membrane; i.e. a situation which has been duplicated experimentally (ITO, 1924).

In the Mayo Clinic series 7 of 20 cases in which preoperative roentgenograms were available had no detectable radiopaque masses (Fig. 135a, b, c). Their most frequent and characteristic finding in 11 of 20 preoperative roentgenograms was that of multiple small radiopaque masses of varying size up to 5 mm in diameter which were occasionally visible in only part of the joint area. Multiple larger radiopaque masses were seen in two cases. Proof that the radiopaque bodies are situated within rather than about the joint space, i.e. the capsule or infrapatellar fat pad (ROBILLARD, 1941) may be obtained by means of air arthrography. Therefore, although the clinical features are usually nonspecific, the roentgenogram can provide important diagnostic information.

IV. Treatment and Prognosis

All 32 cases of MURPHY et al. (1962) were treated surgically and improved. Spontaneous cures have been reported (SWAN and OWENS, 1972) as well as cures after removal of as many free bodies as possible. Spontaneous regression of the remaining cartilaginous bodies after partial or incomplete synovectomy has been described (MCIVOR and KING). Some authorities, therefore, emphasize that an extensive synovectomy is not necessary for eventual resolution and recommend simple removal of the loose bodies.

Malignant change has rarely been reported. None of the cases in the early reports of GESCHICKTER and COPELAND (1949), and REIMANN and KIENBÖCK (1931) were sufficiently documented to prove that the original condition was that of synovial chondromatosis. A case of NIXON et al. (1960) which had been reported by BRANNON and TRACEY (1957) and in which the original diagnosis was chondromatosis of the hip, had a hindquarter amputation for chondrosarcoma 1 year after onset of symptoms. This rapid progression suggests the possibility that it was a chondrosarcoma from the outset. Several other reported cases (KING et al., 1967; MULLINS et al., 1965) have also not been universally accepted as arising on a background of a previously benign lesion.

It is also noteworthy that none of 276 chondrosarcomas in the Mayo Clinic series originated in synovial chondromatosis, re-emphasizing that synovial osteochondromatosis is essentially a benign lesion. JAFFE'S (1968) experience included no case of malignant transformation. It remains difficult, if not impossible, to be certain whether malignant lesions reputedly showing areas of previously benign cartilaginous tumor took their origin from synovial osteochondromatosis.

V. Synovial Chondrosarcoma

Synovial chondrosarcoma arising de novo is also a rare malignant cartilaginous tumor arising from the synovial membrane rather than from bone. Several reported cases have not been universally accepted and include those in which a synovial origin could not be demonstrated with certainty.

A case of MULLINS et al. (1962) is referred to by SPJUT et al. (1971) as problematic. They suggested the possibility of its having been a primary chondrosarcoma of bone which secondarily invaded the neighboring soft tissues including the synovium.

Other cases have been reported by GOLDMAN and LICHTENSTEIN (1964), DUNN et al. (1974), and at the Clinicopathological Conference of the Massachusetts General Hospital in 1962 (CASTLEMAN, 1962).

GOLDMAN and LICHTENSTEIN (1964) note that, on rare occasion, chondrosarcoma may also arise from the specialized linings of tendon sheaths and possibly even bursae and make mention of a few reported instances of "ostensible tendon sheath chondrosarcomas". However, only a single case reported by ARIEL and JACOBS (1961) was known to be sufficiently well documented to be entirely convincing.

Aside from the lesion's location, synovial chondrosarcoma resembles any other chondrosarcoma. Microscopically it is similar to chondrosarcoma arising in bone, presenting with lobular masses that may invade surrounding bone as well as soft tissues. The lesion is malignant, as demonstrated by its capability of metastasizing (SPJUT et al., 1971).

Q. Summary

The family of cartilaginous lesions forms a hard-to-compartmentalize spectrum in which the distinction of an entirely benign from a frankly malignant lesion cannot always be precisely drawn. It is the separation of benign tumors from those of low grade malignancy that poses the greatest problem, and it is often a microscopic nuance that may tip the scale in terms of diagnosis. Frequently, the deciding bit of tissue may be seen solely in a small portion of these often large and bulky lesions, which are notoriously difficult to sample thoroughly and safely.

Not only a nuance of pathology, but also one of clinical or radiologic data may be important. Consequently, the proper evaluation of these lesions requires a united effort on the part of the pathologist, orthopedic surgeon, and radiologist. It is therefore advisable to have a little expertise in and appreciation of the other's discipline, as well as a basic awareness of its associated limitations, for the appropriate management of the individual case.

Interdisciplinary cooperation has proved exceptionally fruitful when dealing with this particular family of lesions since early and definitive treatment in malignant cartilaginous tumors "pays off" more than with other bone sarcomas. Therefore, though this discussion has been primarily a review of the radiologist's conventional contribution in terms of defining a set of roentgen patterns that uniquely characterize a lesion or lesions, an additional attempt was made to emphasize the clinical corrolaries associated with some of these roentgen features, and to stress the relative importance of each in a particular situation or instance.

An analysis of cartilage lesions in terms of certain key questions will help to place them in their proper perspective. The answers to these questions may additionally help to modify and refine roentgenologic impressions. Well-known biologic–pathologic paradoxes regarding discrepancies between histologic appearance and biologic behavior have been reiterated. Thus, the variation in the behavior of these lesions at certain sites is exemplified by solitary enchondromas of the hands and feet or of certain cartilaginous tumors involving the soft tissues, e.g. synovial chondromatosis. Though occasionally showing cytologic evidence of low grade malignancy, these lesions at these sites most commonly behave in a benign fashion. Benign appearing lesions of long bones, on the other hand, particularly when located in their proximal ends, more commonly behave in an aggressive manner despite an innocent histology.

Unfortunately, it is with the lesions of low grade malignancy that the greatest possibility of underdiagnosis by the pathologist exists. Despite the fact that second and perhaps third chances of salvage are possible with these generally slow growing tumors, initial underdiagnosis with resultant undertreatment may have serious repercussions. Recurrent lesions may behave in a more aggressive fashion after initial unsuccessful treatment, i.e. in 10% of recurrences, while other recurrent tumors may alter their character and assume the characteristics and more dire prognoses of other sarcomas.

Orientation at a particular site has been stressed, with the example of the juxtacortical chondroma, whose occasionally alarming histologic appearance is usually not matched by its innocuous clinical course. The multiplicity and size of the lesion or lesions, as outlined by the roentgenogram, dictates to some degree whether a cartilaginous tumor is considered benign or malignant.

A greater degree of cellularity and cellular atypism may be tolerated in the lesion of a child than in that of an adult, and a certain degree of roentgenologic change anticipated in view of continued growth in the young. Therefore, the prime importance and interplay of the position, size, site, orientation, and multiplicity of lesions in the light of age are noteworthy considerations. These questions can best be elucidated by the roentgenogram.

The roentgenologist has an additional immediate role and that is as a guide to biopsy, both in terms of localizing the lesion per se and of indicating the most fruitful and advantageous areas for sampling. The roentgenogram remains indispensible for the pathologist's proper orientation in terms of judging the lesion's milieu in view of the bits and fragments of cartilage he often receives in the way of biopsy material.

The roentgenogram furthermore has a unique long range contribution, particularly where cartilaginous lesions are concerned, since the answers may be a long while in coming. It plays an unrivaled role in recording and monitoring the progress of a lesion in time, thereby providing another graphic gauge for judging aggressiveness and prognosis. Angiography and xerography have limited application as far as cartilaginous lesions are concerned. Radiation therapy has no place in the primary treatment of chondrosarcoma and generally achieves little when administered for palliation. Chemotherapeutic agents are currently undergoing extensive trials.

The radiologist conventionally contributes importantly in the delineation and description of this interesting and challenging group of lesions. However, by additionally knowing certain salient clinical and histological facts he may further refine his interpretation, and in so doing play a more significant and occasionally a pivotal role in the successful management of these lesions.

In any event, the most rewarding approach to these lesions, i.e. the approach that yields the happiest results, heavily depends on a synthesis of biologic, clinical, pathologic, and radiologic data, any one of which may be decisive at a particular time and for a particular cartilaginous lesion.

Acknowledgments

I am indebted to Mrs. HELEN SAUER and Mrs. MARIA MACHAIN for assistance in preparation of the manuscript, and to Mr. MICHAEL CARLIN, photographer, for the excellent technical quality of the illustrations.

References

ACKERMAN, L.V., SPJUT, H.J.: Tumors of bone and cartilage. Atlas of Tumor Pathology. Sect. 2, Fasc. 4 (1962)

AEGERTER, E.: Radiol. Clin. N. Amer. 8, 215 (1970)

AEGERTER, E., KIRKPATRICK, J.A.: Orthopaedic Diseases, 3rd ed., p. 647. Philadelphia: W.B. Saunders Company 1968

ALBORES-SAAVEDRA, J., ALTAMIRANO-DIMAS, J., PENICHE, J., MARQUES-MONTER, H.: Rev. méd. Hosp. gen. (Méx.) 27, 571 (1964)

ANASTASI, G.W., WERTHEIMER, H.M., BROWN, J.R.: Arch. Surg. (Chicago) 87, 636 (1963)

ANDERSON, I.F.: S. Afr. med. J. 39, 1066–1070 (1965)

ANDERSON, C.E., LUDOWIEG, J., EYRING, E.J., HOROWITZ, B.: J. Bone Jt Surg. 45-A, 753–764 (1963)

ANDERSON, R.L., POPOWITZ, L., LI, J.K.H.: J. Bone Jt Surg. 51-A, 1199–1204 (1969)

ANDRÉN, L., DYMLING, J.F., ELNER, A., HOGEMAN, K.E.: Acta chir. scand. 126, 397 (1963)

ANGERVALL, L., ENERBÄCK, L., KNUTSON, H.: Cancer (Philad.) 32, 507–513 (1973)

ARIEL, I.M., JACOBS, P.A.: Bull. Hosp. Jt Dis. (N.Y.) 22, 129–136 (1961)

ARKIN, A.M., SIMON, N.: J. Bone Jt Surg. 32-A, 396–401 (1950)

ASSOR, D.: J. Bone Jt Surg. 55-A, 208–210 (1973)

BARNES, R., CATTO, J.: J. Bone Jt Surg. 48-B, 729 (1966)

BAUER, W.H., HARRELL, A.: J. Bone Jt Surg. 36-A, 263 (1954)

BEAN, W.B.: Arch. intern. Med. 102, 544–550 (1958)

BELL, M.S.: Brit. J. Surg. 58, 707–711 (1971)

BENEDETTI, G.B., CANEPA, G., GARCIA, M.: Arch. Putti Chir. Organi Mov. 17, 44–72 (1962)

BENSON, W.R., BASS, S., JR.: Amer. J. Clin. Path. 25, 1290–1292 (1955)

BERDON, W.E., BAKER, D.H., BOYER, J.: Amer. J. Radiol. 93, 545–556 (1965)

BERENBAUM, S.L., TZAMOURANIS, G.: Amer. J. Roentgenol. 80, 479–481 (1958)

BICK, E.M., COPEL, J.W.: J. Bone Jt Surg. 32-A, 803–814 (1950)

BLOODGOOD, J.C.: Ann. Surg. 80, 817 (1924)

Bone Tumour Committee of the Japanese Orthopaedic Association National Cancer Center Collections of the Registry of Bone Tumours in Japan, pp. 93, 99 (1966)

BOSTRÖM, H., EDGREN, B., FRIBERG, U., LARSSON, K.S., NILSONNE, U., WENGLE, B., WESTER, P.O.: Acta orthop. scand. 39, 549 (1968)

BOYER, A.: Traite des Maladies Chirurgicales 3, 594. Paris: Ve Migneret 1814

BRADDOCK, G.T.F., HADLOW, V.D.: J. Bone Jt Surg. 48-B, 145–149 (1966)

BRANNON, E.W., TRACEY, J.F.: U.S. armed Forces med. J. 8, 1517–26 (1957)

BURACZEWSKI, J., LYSAKOWSKA, J., RUDOWSKI, W.: J. Bone Jt Surg. 39-B, 705 (1957)

CAHAN, W.G., WOODARD, H.Q., HIGINBOTHAM, N.L., STEWART, F.W., COLEY, B.L.: Cancer (Philad.) I, 3–29 (1948)

CARES, H.L.: J. Neurosurg. 35, 614–618 (1971)

Case records of the Massachusetts General Hospital, Case 33–1964. New Engl. J. Med. 271, 94–100 (1964)

CASTLEMAN, B. Ed.: New Engl. J. Med. 266, 719–729 (1962)

CHIURCO, A.: Neurology 20, 275 (1970)

CLARK, J.V., MALONEY, A.F.J.: Arch. Path. (Chicago) 98, 69 (1974)

CODMAN, E.A.: Surg. Gynec. Obstet. 52, 543 (1931)

COHEN, A.M., KETCHAM, A.F., MORTON, D.L.: Surgery 72, 560–567 (1972)

COHEN, D.M., DAHLIN, D.C., MACCARTY, C.S.: Proc. Mayo Clin. 39, 509–528 (1964)

COHEN, J., CURRARINO, G., NEUHAUSER, E.B.D.: Amer. J. Roentgenol. 76, 469–475 (1956)

COHEN, J., D'ANGIO, G.J.: Amer. J. Roentgenol. 86, 502 (1961)

COLE, A.R.C., DARTE, J.M.M.: Pediatrics 32, 285 (1963)

COLEMAN, S.S.: J. Bone Jt Surg. 48-A, 1554 (1966)

COLEY, B.L., HIGINBOTHAM, N.L.: Cancer (Philad.) 2, 777 (1949)

COLEY, B.L., HIGGINBOTHAM, N.L.: Ann. Surg. **139**, 547 (1954)

COLEY, B.L., SANTORA, A.J.: Surgery **22**, 411 (1947)

CONSTANT, E., HAREBOTTLE, H., DAVIS, D.G.: Plast. reconstr. Surg. **54**, 353–358 (1974)

COPELAND, M.M., GESCHICKTER, C.F.: Ann. Surg. **129**, 724 (1949)

COWAN, W.K.: J. clin. Path. **18**, 650 (1965)

CROWELL, R.M., WEPSIC, J.G.: J. Neurosurg. **36**, 86–89 (1972)

DAHLIN, D.C.: Cancer (Philad.) **9**, 159 (1956)

DAHLIN, D.C.: Bone tumors, 2nd ed. Springfield: Charles C. Thomas 1967

DAHLIN, D.C., BEABOUT, J.W.: Cancer (Philad.) **28**, 461–466 (1971)

DAHLIN, D.C., COVENTRY, M.B.: J. Bone Jt Surg. **49-A**, 101–110 (1967)

DAHLIN, D.C., HENDERSON, E.D.: J. Bone Jt Surg. **38-A**, 1025 (1956)

DAHLIN, D.C., HENDERSON, E.D.: Cancer (Philad.) **15**, 410 (1962)

DAHLIN, D.C., IVINS, J.C.: Cancer (Philad.) **30**, 401–413 (1972)

DAHLIN, D.C., SALVADOR, A.H.: Mayo Clin. Proc. **49**, 721–726 (1974)

DAHLIN, D.C., SALVADOR, A.H.: Cancer (Philad.) **34**, 755–760 (1974)

DAHLIN, D., SWEDLOW, M.: Thirty-Fourth Seminar on Neoplasms of Bone. Chicago: American Society of Clinical Pathologists 1969

D'AMBROSIA, R., FERGUSON, A.B., JR.: Clin. Orthop. **61**, 103 (1968)

DE, P.R.: J. Laryng. **86**, 1261–1263 (1972)

DENKO, N.J., KRAUEL, L.H.: Arch. Path. (Chicago) **59**, 710–711 (1955)

DORFMAN, H.D.: Malignant transformation of benign bone lesions. Seventh National Cancer Conference Proceedings. Sep. 27–9, 1972, Los Angeles, Calif. Philadelphia: Lippincott 1973

DOWLING, E.A.: J. Bone Jt Surg. **46-A**, 747 (1964)

DREVON, P., MOURGUES, M., SANTAMARIA, F.: J. Radiol. Électrol. **31**, 80–82 (1950)

DUNN, E.J., McGAVRAN, M.H., NELSON, P., GREER, R.B., III: J. Bone Jt Surg. **56-A**, 811–813 (1974)

DUTT, A.K., DHILLON, D.S., DIN, O.: Med. J. Malaya **XXIV**, 71–73 (1969)

EDEIKEN, J., HODES, P.J.: Roentgen Diagnosis of Disease of Bone. Baltimore: Williams & Wilkins 1967

EHRENFRIED, A.: J. amer. med. Ass. **64**, 1642 (1915)

EISENBERG, K.S., JOHNSTON, J.O.: J. Bone Jt Surg. **54-A**, 176–178 (1972)

ELMORE, S.M., CANTRELL, W.C.: J. Bone Jt Surg. **58-A**, 1607–1613 (1966)

ENZINGER, F.M., SHIRAKI, M.: Hum. Path. **3**, 421–435 (1972)

ERNST, P.: Beitr. path. Anat. **28**, 255 (1900)

EWING, J.: Neoplastic Diseases. A Treatise on Tumors. 3rd ed. Philadelphia: W.B. Saunders 1928

FAIRBANK, H.A.T.: J. Bone Jt Surg. **38-B**, 237 (1956)

FANCONI, G., ILLIG, R.: Helv. paediat. Acta **14**, 425–429 (1959)

FECHNER, R.E., WILDE, H.D.: J. Bone Jt Surg. **56-A**, 413–415 (1974)

FEINTUCH, T.A.: Cancer (Philad.) **31**, 877–881 (1973)

FELDMAN, F., HECHT, H.L., JOHNSTON, A.D.: Radiology **94**, 249 (1970)

FIELDING, J.W., RATZAN, S.: J. Bone Jt Surg. **55-A**, 640–641 (1973)

FILIPPONE, J.J.: J. Amer. Pediatry Ass. **56**, 237–238 (1966)

FRANK, W.E., ROCKWOOD, C.A., JR.: Sth. med. J. (B'ham, Ala.) **62**, 1238–1253 (1969)

FRIEDMAN, B., HANAOKA, H.: J. Bone Jt Surg. **53-A**, 1118–1136 (1971)

GALLAGHER, J.C., WINSLOW, D.J., GROSSMAN, A.: Urology **III**, 473–477 (1974)

GARDNER, E.K.: Brit. J. Surg. **25**, 323–329 (1937)

GELMAN, M.I.: Rocky Mtn med. J. **71**, 38–40 (1974)

GESCHICKTER, C.F., COPELAND, M.M.: Tumors of Bone, 3rd ed. Philadelphia: J.B. Lippincott Co. 1949

GHORMLEY, R.K., MEYERDING, H.W., MUSSEY, R.D., JR., LUCKEY, C.A.: J. Bone Jt Surg. **38**, 40–48 (1946)

GHOSH, L., HUVOS, A.G., MIKÉ, V.: Amer. J. Path. **71**, 23–29 (1973)

GILMAN, W.S., JR., KILGORE, W.E., SMITH, H.E.: Clin. Orthop. **26**, 81 (1963)

GODMAN, G.C., PORTER, K.R.: J. Biophys. biochem. Cytol. **8**, 719 (1960)

GOETHALS, P.L., DAHLIN, D.C., DEVINE, K.D.: S.G.O. **117**, 77–82 (1963)

GOLDANICH, I.F.: I tumori primitivi dell'Osso, pp. 197–205. Bologna: Societa per Azione Poligrafici il Resto del Carlino 1957

GOKAY, H., BUCEY, P.C.: J. Neurosurg. **12**, 72 (1955)

GOLDEN, J.P.: Irish J. med. Sci. **140**, 118–125 (1971)

GOLDENBERG, R.R., COHEN, P., STEINLAUF, P.: J. Bone Jt Surg. **49-A**, 1487–1507 (1967)

GOLDMAN, R.L., LICHTENSTEIN, L.: Cancer (Philad.) **17**, 1233–1240 (1964)

GOORWITCH, J.: Dis. Chest **20**, 186 (1951)

GOTTSCHALK, K.F., ALPORT, L.K., ALBERT, R.E.: Cancer Res. **19**, 1070 (1959)

GRABIAS, S., MANKIN, H.J.: J. Bone Jt Surg. **56-A**, 1501–1509 (1974)

GRAVANIS, M.B., GIANSANTI, J.S.: Amer. J. clin. Path. **55**, 624–631 (1971)

GUTMANN, J., CIFUENTES, C., BALZARINI, M.A., SOBARZO, V., VICUNA, R.: Oral Surg. **37**, 75–77 (1974)

HABAL, M.B., SNYDER, H.H., JR., MURRAY, J.E.: Amer. J. Surg. **125**, 775–776 (1973)

HAMLIN, J.A., ADLER, L., GREENBAUM, E.I.: J. Canad. Ass. Radiol. **22**, 206–209 (1971)

HART, W.R., HINERMAN, D.L.: Metabolism **14**, 1158–68 (1965)

HATCHER, C.H., CAMPBELL, C.J.: Bull. Hosp. Jt Dis. (N.Y.) **12**, 411 (1951)

HEIPLE, K.G.: J. Bone Jt Surg. **43-A**, 861–864 (1961)

HEIPLE, K.G., ELMER, R.M.: J. Bone Jt Surg. **54-A**, 393–398 (1972)

HENDERSON, E.D., DAHLIN, D.C.: J. Bone Jt Surg. **45-A**, 1450 (1963)

HENDERSON, F.J., LePAGE, G.A.: Cancer Res. **19**, 887–902 (1959)

HENSINGER, R.N., COWELL, H.R., RAMSEY, P.L., LEOPOLD, R.G.: J. Bone Jt Surg. **56-A**, 1513–1516 (1974)

HERFARTH, H.: Arch. klin. Chir. **170**, 283–286 (1932)

HERNDON, N.H., COHEN, J.: J. Bone Jt Surg. **52-A**, 1241–1247 (19970)

HIGGINS, G.M., LEVY, B.M., YOLLICK, B.L.: J. Bone Jt Surg. **46-A**, 789 (1964)

HOPKINS, S.M., FREITAG, E.L.: J. Thorac. Cardiovasc. Surg. **49**, 247–249 (1965)

HUTCHISON, J., PARK, W.W.: J. Bone Jt Surg. **42-B**, 542–548 (1960)

HUTTER, R.V.P., FOOTE, F.W., JR., FRANCIS, K.C., SHERMAN, R.S.: Cancer (Philad.) **19**, 1–25 (1966)

HUVOS, A.G., HIGINBOTHAM, N.L., MILLER, T.R.: J. Bone Jt Surg. **54-A**, 1047–1056 (1972)

HUVOS, A.G., MARCOVE, R.C.: Clin. Orthop. **95**, 300–312 (1973)

HUVOS, A.G., MARCOVE, R.C., ERLANDSON, R.A., MIKÉ, V.: Cancer (Philad.) **29**, 760–771 (1972)

ILGENFRITZ, H.C.: Amer. Surg. **17**, 917–922 (1951)

ITO, L.K.: Brit. J. Surg. **12**, 31–42 (1924)

IWATA, S., COLEY, B.L.: Surg. Gynec. Obstet. **107**, 571 (1958)

JAFFE, H.L.: Arch. Path. (Chicago) **36**, 335 (1943)

JAFFE, H.L.: Bull. Hosp. Jt Dis. (N.Y.) **17**, 20 (1956)

JAFFE, H.L.: Tumors and Tumorous Conditions of the Bones and Joints. Philadelphia: Lea & Febiger 1968

JAFFE, H.L., LICHTENSTEIN, L.: Amer. J. Path. **18**, 969–991 (1942)

JAFFE, H.L., LICHTENSTEIN, L.: Arch. Surg. (Chicago) **46**, 480–492 (1943)

JAFFE, H.L., LICHTENSTEIN, L.: Arch. Path. (Chicago) **45**, 541 (1948)

JAFFE, H.L., LICHTENSTEIN, L., PORTIS, R.B.: Arch. Path. (Chicago) **30**, 993 (1940)

JAKOBSON, E., SPJUT, H.J.: Acta radiol. (Diagn.) (Stockh.) **54**, 426 (1960)

JOHNSON, L.C.: Bull. N.Y. Acad. Med. **29**, 164–171 (1953)

JONES, H.M.: J. Laryng. **87**, 135–151 (1973)

JOSEPH, W.L., FONKALSRUD, E.W.: Amer. Surg. **38**, 338–342 (1972)

KADELL, B.M., COULSON, W.F., DESILETS, D.T., FONKALSRUD, E.W.: J. pediat. Surg. **5**, 46–52 (1970)

KAHN, L.B., WOOD, F.M., ACKERMAN, L.V.: Arch. Path. (Chicago) **88**, 371 (1969)

KATZMAN, H., WAUGH, T., BERDON, W.: J. Bone Jt Surg. **51-A**, 835–843 (1969)

KAUFFMAN, S.L., STOUT, A.P.: Cancer (Philad.) **16**, 432–439 (1963)

KAUTZ, F.G.: Radiology **45**, 162–167 (1945)

KEATS, T.E.: Radiology **68**, 558 (1957)

KEITH, A.: J. Anat. **54**, 101 (1920)

KETTELKAMP, D.B., CAMPBELL, C.J., BONFIGLIO, M.: J. Bone Jt Surg. **48-A**, 746–766 (1966)

KETTELKAMP, D.B., DOLAN, J.: J. Bone Jt Surg. **48-A**, 329–332 (1966)

KING, J.W., SPJUT, H.J., FECHNER, R.E., VANDERPOOL, D.W.: J. Bone Jt Surg. **49-A**, 1389–1396 (1967)

KINGSLEY, T.C., MARKEL, S.F.: Cancer (Philad.) **27**, 203–6 (1971)

KNIGHT, J.D.S.: Brit. med. J. **I**, 1013–1015 (1960)

KOLODNY, A.: Surg. Gynec. Obstet. **44** (Suppl. 1) 1 (1927)

KÓSA, M.: Virchows Arch. path. Anat. **272**, 166 (1929)

KUHLMAN, R.E., McNAMEE, M.J.: Clin. Orthop. **69**, 264–270 (1970)

KUNKEL, M.G., DAHLIN, D.C., YOUNG, H.H.: J. Bone Jt Surg. **38-A**, 817 (1956)

KURTZ, D.M.: N.Y. St. J. Med. **85**, 86 (1975)

LAMMOT, T.R., III: J. Bone Jt Surg. **50-A**, 1230–1232 (1968)

LARSON, N.W., DODGE, H.W., RUSHTON, J.G. et al.: Proc. Mayo Clin. **32**, 728–734 (1957)

LATTES, R.: Tex. Med., **60**, 437 (1964)

LAWSON, V.G., BRYCE, D.P., BRIANT, T.D.R.: Canad. J. Otolaryng. **1**, 3 213–218 (1972)

LETTIN, A.W.F.: Proc. roy. Soc. Med. **56**, 10–12 (1963)

LEVINE, G.D., BENSCH, K.G.: Cancer (Philad.) **29**, 1546–1562 (1972)

LEVY, W.M., AEGERTER, E.E., KIRKPATRICK, J.A., JR.: Radiol. Clin. N. Amer. **2**, 327–336 (1946)

LEWIS, M.M., MARSHALL, J.L., MIRRA, J.M.: J. Bone Jt Surg. **56-A**, 180–182 (1974)

LEWIS, R.J., KETCHAM, A.S.: J. Bone Jt Surg. **55-A**, 1465–1479 (1973)

LICHTENSTEIN, L.: Cancer (Philad.) **8**, 816–830 (1955)

LICHTENSTEIN, L.: Bone Tumors, 3rd ed. St. Louis: C.V. Mosby 1965

LICHTENSTEIN, L., BERNSTEIN, D.: Cancer (Philad.) **12**, 1142 (1959)

LICHTENSTEIN, L., GOLDMAN, R.L.: Cancer (Philad.) **17**, 1203–1208 (1964)

LICHTENSTEIN, L., HALL, J.E.: J. Bone Jt Surg. **34-A**, 691–697 (1952)

LICHTENSTEIN, L., JAFFE, H.L.: Amer. J. Path. **19**, 553 (1943)

LINDBOM, A., SODERBERG, G., SPJUT, H.J.: Acta. radiol. (Diagn.) (Stockh.) **55**, 81 (1961)

LINSCHEID, R.L., DAHLIN, D.C.: J. Bone Jt Surg. **48-A**, 1359–1366 (1966)

LODWICK, G.S.: A systemic approach to roentgen diagnosis of bone tumors. Tumors of Bone and Soft Tissue. Year Book Medical Publishers. Chicago 1965

LOVE, R.T.: Mississippi St. med. Ass. J. (Journal MSMA) **13**, 465–467 (1972)

LYNN, M.D., LEE, J.: J. Bone Jt Surg. **54-A**, 650–652 (1972)

MAFFUCCI, A.: Mov. Med. Chir. Nap. **3**, 399–412 and 565–575 (1881)

MAGNUSSON, P., ROTEMARK, G.: J. Laryng. Otolaryng. **88**, 159–164 (1974)

MALLORY, T.B.: Amer. J. Path. **9**, 765 (1933)

MANGINI, U.: Bull. Hosp. Jt Dis. (N.Y.) **25**, 50–56 (1964)

MARCOVE, R.C., CHAROSKY, C.B.: Clin. Orthop. **83**, 224–31 (1972)

MARCOVE, R.C., FRANCIS, K.C.: New Engl. J. Med. **268**, 1399 (1963)

MARCOVE, R.C., HUVOS, A.G.: Cancer (Philad.) **27**, 794–801 (1971)

MARCOVE, R.C., KAMBOLIS, C., BULLOUGH, P.G., JAFFE, H.L.: Cancer (Philad.) **17**, 1209–1213 (1964)

MARCOVE, R.C., MILKÉ, V., HUTTER, R.V.P., HUVOS, A.G., SHOJI, H., MILLER, T.R., KOSLOFF, R.: J. Bone Jt Surg. **54-A**, 561–572 (1972)

MARTIN, R.F., MELNICK, P.J., WARNER, N.E., TERRY, R., BULLOCK, W.K., SCHWINN, C.P.: Amer. J. clin. Path. **59**, 623–635 (1973)

McBRYDE, A., JR., GOLDNER, N.L.: Amer. Surg. **36**, 94–108 (1970)

McFARLAND, G.B., JR., REED, R.J.: Dedifferentiation of chondrosarcoma. As quoted by SPJUT, H.J., DORFMAN, H.D., FECHNER, R.E., ACKERMAN, L.V.: Tumors of bone and cartilage. Atlas of Tumor Pathology, 2nd Series. Fasc. 5. 1971

McIVOR, R.R., KING, D.: J. Bone Jt Surg. **44-A**, 87–97 (1962)

McKENNA, R.J., SCHWINN, C.P., SOONG, K.Y., HIGINBOTHAM, N.L.: J. Bone Jt Surg. **45-A**, 1 (1966)

McLEOD, R.A., BEABOUT, J.W.: Amer. J. Roentgenol. **118**, 464–471 (1973)

MEYER, R.: Brit. J. Radiol. **31**, 106–107 (1958)

MEYERDING, H.W.: Radiology **8**, 282–288 (1927)

MIKULOWSKI, P., ÖSTBERG, G.: Acta orthop. scand. **42**, 385–390 (1971)

MILCH, R.A.: Amer. J. Surg. **87**, 134–148 (1954)

MIRRA, J.M., MARCOVE, R.C.: J. Bone Jt Surg. **56-A**, 285–296 (1974)

MOORE, J.P., SHANNON, E.: Tex. Med. **70**, 65–68 (1974)

MORGAN, A.D., SALAMA, F.D.: J. thorac. cardiovasc. Surg. **64**, 460–466 (1972)

MORTON, D.L., MOLMGREEN, R.A., HALL, W.T., SCHEDLOWSKY, G.: Surgery **66**, 152 (1969)

MORTON, J.J., MIDER, G.B.: Ann. Surg. **126**, 895 (1947)

MOSHER, J.F., KETTELKAMP, D.B., CAMPBELL, C.J.: J. Bone Jt Surg. **48-A**, 1561–1569 (1966)

MÜLLER, E.: Beitr. path. Anat. **57**, 232 (1914)

MULLINS, F., BERARD, C.W., EISENBERG, S.H.: Cancer (Philad.) **18**, 1180–1188 (1965)

MURPHY, F.D., JR., BLOUNT, W.P.: J. Bone Jt Surg. **44-A**, 662 (1962)

MURPHY, F.P., DAHLIN, D.C., SULLIVAN, C.R.: J. Bone Jt Surg. **44-A**, 77–86 (1962)

MURPHY, N.B., PRICE, C.H.G.: Clin. Radiol. **22**, 261–269 (1971)

MURRAY, R.O., JACOBSON, H.G.: The Radiology of Skeletal Disorders. Baltimore: Williams & Wilkins 1971

NAG, T.K., FALCONER, M.A.: Brit. J. Surg. **53**, 1067–1071 (1966)

NARDELL, S.G.: Brit. med. J. **2**, 555–557 (1950)

Netherlands Committee on Bone Tumors (1966) Radiological Atlas of Bone Tumours, Vol. 1. The Hague, Mouton & Co. Baltimore: The Williams & Wilkins Co. 1966

NEVIASER, R.J., WILSON, N.J.: J. Bone Jt Surg. **54-A**, 389–392 (1972)

NIXON, J.E., FRANK, G.R., CHAMBERS, G.: U.S. armed Forces med. J. **11**, 1434 (1960)

NOSANCHUK, J.S., KAUFER, H.: J. Bone Jt Surg. **51-A**, 375 (1969)

OLLIER, M.: Lyon méd. **93**, 23 (1900)

O'NEAL, L.W., ACKERMAN, L.V.: Cancer (Philad.) **5**, 551 (1952)

OPPENHEIM, J.M., BOAL, R.W.: U.S. armed Forces med. J. **6**, 279–282 (1955)

PACHTER, M.R., ALPERT, M.: J. Bone Jt Surg. **46-A**, 601–607 (1964)

PADDISON, G.M., HANKS, G.E.: Cancer (Philad.) **28**, 616–619 (1971)

PAGET, J.: Lectures on Surgical Pathology, 3rd ed. London: Longmans, Green and Co. 1870

PASCUZZI, C.A., DAHLIN, D.C., CLAGETT, O.T.: Surg. Gynec. Obstet. **104**, 390–400 (1957)

PAUL, G.R., LEACH, R.E.: Clin. Orthop. **68**, 130–135 (1970)

PAVON, S.J., BULLOUGH, P.G., MARCOVE, R.C.: N.Y. St. med. J. July, 1662–1664 (1971)

PEABODY, C.N.: J. Thorac. cardiovasc. Surg. **61**, 636–640 (1971)

PECK, J.H., JR.: J. Bone Jt Surg. **46-A**, 1379 (1964)

PEREZ, C.A., VIETTI, T., ACKERMAN, L.V., EAGLETON, M.D., POWERS, W.E.: Radiology **88**, 750 (1967)

PEROU, J.L., KOLIS, J.A., ZAESKE, E.V., BORJA, S.R.: Cancer (Philad.) **20**, 1030–1034 (1967)

PIEPGRAS, U., HIRTH, R., STÄDTLER, F., KAMMERER, V.: Neuroradiology **4**, 25–29 (1972)

PISAR, D.E.: Tex. Med. **65**, 52–55 (1969)

PLATT, H.: Proc. roy. Soc. Med. Sec. Ortho. **25**, 1 (1931)

PLUM, G.E., PUGH, D.G.: Amer. J. Roentgenol. **79**, 584 (1958)

POCHACZEVSKY, R., YEN, Y.M., SHERMAN, R.S.: Radiology **75**, 429 (1960)

PORRETTA, C.A., DAHLIN, D.C., JANES, J.M.: J. Bone Jt Surg. **39-A**, 1314–1329 (1957)

PRATT, G.D., DAHLIN, D.C., GHORMLEY, R.K.: Surg. Gynec. Obstet. **106**, 536–544 (1958)

PURSER, D.W.: J. Bone Jt Surg. **38-B**, 871–873 (1956)

RAHIMI, A., BEABOUT, J.W., IVINS, J.C., DAHLIN, D.C.: Cancer (Philad.) **30**, 726–736 (1972)

RALPH, L.L.: J. Bone Jt Surg. **44-B**, 7–24 (1962)

RAMINI, P.S.: J. Neurosurg. **40**, 107–109 (1974)

RAND, G.W.: Bull. Los Angeles neurol. Soc. **28**, 260–268 (1963)

RAVAULT, P.P., VIGNON, G., LEJEUNE, E., BOUVIEW, M., VAUZELLE, J.L., NEUNIER, P.: Rev. Rhum. **36**, 215–224 (1969)

RAY, J.J.: Lancet 1, 159 (1905)

REAM, J.R., CORSON, J.M., HOLDSWORTH, D.E., MILLENDER, L.H.: Clin. Orthop. 97, 148–152 (1973)

REICHMAN, S., THORD, L.: Acta orthop. scand. 40, 1–22 (1969)

REIMANN, H., KIENBÖCK, R.: Röntgenpraxis 3, 942–944 (1931)

REITER, F.B., ACKERMAN, L.V., STAPLE, T.W.: Radiology 105, 525–530 (1972)

RICHTER, K.J., FREEMAN, N.S., QUICK, C.A.: J. oral Surg. 32, 777–781 (1974)

ROBERTS, P.H.: Brit. J. Surg. 58, 152 (1971)

ROBILLARD, G.L.: Amer. J. Surg. 41, 442–444 (1941)

ROCKWELL, M.A., ENNEKING, W.F.: J. Bone Jt Surg. 53-A, 341–344 (1971)

ROSE, E.F., FEKETA, A.: Amer. J. clin. Path. 42, 606–609 (1964)

RUBIN, P.: Dynamic Classification of Bone Dysplasia. Chicago: Year Book Medical Publishers 1964

RUBIN, P., ANDREWS, J.R., SWARM, R., GUMP, H.: Amer. J. Roentgenol. 82, 206–216 (1959)

RYALL, R.D.H.: Brit. J. Radiol. 43, 71–72 (1970)

SACHDEVA, H.S., KASPHYAP, K.N., GREWAL, D.S., AIKAT, M.: Amer. Surg. 35, 435–438 (1969)

SALIB, P.I.: Amer. J. Orthop. 8–9, 240–242 (1966–7)

SALVADOR, A.H., BEABOUT, J.W., DAHLIN, D.C.: Cancer (Philad.) 28, 605–615 (1971)

SALZER, M., SALZER-KUNTSCHIK, M., KRETSCHMER, G.: Arch. orthop. Unfall-Chir. 64, 229–244 (1968)

SCAGLIETTI, O., STRINGA, G.: J. Bone Jt Surg. 43-A, 67–80 (1961)

SCHAJOWICZ, F., CABRINI, R.L., SIMES, R.J., KLEINSZANTO, A.J.P.: Clin. Orthop. 100, 378–386 (1974)

SCHAJOWICZ, F., CAMBIAGGI, J.E.: Bol. Soc. argent. Ortop. Traum. 25, 191–198 (1961)

SCHAJOWICZ, F., GALLARDO, H.: J. Bone Jt Surg. 52-B, 205–226 (1970)

SCHAJOWICZ, F., GALLARDO, H.: J. Bone Jt Surg. 53-B, 198–216 (1971)

SCHAUWECKER, F., WELLER, S., KLÜMPER, A., ANLAUF, B.: Bruns Beitr. klin. Chir. 217, 155–159 (1969)

SCHERER, E.: Frankfurt. Z. Path. 36, 587–605 (1928)

SCHMIDT, F.E., TRUMMER, J.J.: Ann. thorac. Surg. 13, 251–257 (1972)

SCHOENE, H.R., BERTHELSEN, S., AHN, C.: J. Bone Jt Surg. 55-A, 847–849 (1973)

SCHUTT, P.G., FROST, H.M.: Clin. Orthop. 78, 323–329 (1971)

SCHWARZ, M.I., GOLDMAN, A.L., ROYCROFT, D.W., HUNT, K.K.: Amer. Rev. respir. Dis. 106, 109–113 (1972)

SETH, H.N., RAO, B.D.P.: Indian J. Path. Bact. 7, 112–116 (1964)

SETH, H.N., SINGH, M.: Acta neuropath. (Berl.) 24, 86–89 (1973)

SHELLITO, J.G., DOCKERTY, M.B.: Surg. Gynec. Obstet. 86, 465–472 (1948)

SHERMAN, B.D., SHERMAN, R.E.: J. Amer. Ped. Ass. 61, 434–436 (1971)

SHERMAN, R.S., UZEL, A.R.: Amer. J. Roentgenol. 76, 1132–1140 (1956)

SHOJI, H., MILLER, R.M.: N.Y. St. med. J. 2786 (1971)

SIDEMAN, S., SARRAFIAN, S., TOPOUZIAN, L.K.: Northw. Univ. med. Sch. Quart. Bull. 34–35, 346–351 (1960–61)

SILVER, C.M., SIMON, S.D., LITCHMAN, H.M., DYCKMAN, J.: J. Bone Jt Surg. 53-A, 777–780 (1971)

SINKOVICS, J.G., SHIRATO, E., MARTIN, R.G., CABINESS, J.R., WHITE, E.C.: Cancer (Philad.) 27, 782–793 (1971)

SINKOVICS, J.G., SHIRATO, E., MARTIN, R.G., WHITE, E.C.: J. Med. 1, 15–25 (1970)

SIRSAT, M.V., DOCTOR, V.M.: J. Bone Jt Surg. 52-B, 741–745 (1970)

SLULITTEL, J.A., SCHAJOWICZ, F., SLULITTEL, J.: Rev. Chir. orthop. 57, 571 (1971)

SOLOMON, L.: Amer. J. hum. Genet. 16, 351 (1964)

SOLOMON, L.: S. Afr. med. J. 48, 671–676 (1974)

SPEISER, F.: Virchows Arch. path. Anat. 258, 126 (1925)

SPIESS, H.: Dtsch. med. Wschr. 35/11, 1482–1484 and 1487–1488 (1957)

SPJUT, H.J.: Cartilaginous malignant tumors arising in the skeleton. Seventh National Cancer Conference Proc. Sept. 27–29, 1972. Los Angeles, Calif.: Lippincott, Phila. 1973

SPJUT, H.J., DORFMAN, H.D., FECHNER, R.E., ACKERMAN, L.V.: Tumors of Bone and Cartilage. Atlas of Tumor Pathology, 2nd series Fasc. 5. Washington: Armed Forces Institute of Pathology 1971

SPRATT, J.S., JR.: Cancer (Philad.) 18, 14–24 (1965)

STEINER, G.C.: Cancer (Philad.) 18, 603 (1965)

STEINER, G.C., MIRRA, J.M., BULLOUGH, P.G.: Cancer (Philad.) 32, 926–939 (1973)

STENER, B.: J. Bone Jt Surg. 53-B, 288–295 (1971)

STEPHENSON, W.H.: Brit. J. Radiol. 26, 156–157 (1953)

STOUT, A.P.: Ann. Surg. 127, 706–719 (1948)

STOUT, A.P., VERNER, E.W.: Cancer (Philad.) 6, 581–590 (1953)

SUERMONDT, W.F.: Arch. chir. neerl. 2, 278–289 (1950)

SUNDARAM, T.K.S.: J. Bone Jt Surg. 48-B, 92–103 (1966)

SWAN, E.F., OWENS, W.F.: Sth. med. J. (B'ham, Ala.) 65, 1496–1500 (1972)

SWEETNAM, R., ROSS, K.: J. Bone Jt Surg. 49-B, 74 (1967)

TALERMAN, A., GOLDING, J.S.R., KIRKPATRICK, D.: J. Bone Jt Surg. 49-B, 802 (1967)

TANGHE, W., MARTENS, M.: Acta orthop. belg. 35, Fasc. 6, 996–1009 (1969)

TEITELBAUM, S.L., BESSONE, L.: J. thorac. cardiovasc. Surg. 57, 333–340 (1969)

THOMAS, M.L., ANDRESS, M.R.: Brit. J. Radiol. 44, 549–550 (1971)

TORNBERG, D.N., RICE, R.W., JOHNSTON, A.D.: Clin. Orthop. 95, 295–299 (1973)

TREVOR, D.: J. Bone Jt Surg. 32-B, 204 (1950)

TURCOTTE, B., PUGH, D.G., DAHLIN, D.C.: Amer. J. Roentgenol. **87**, 1085 (1962)

VALLS, J., OTTOLENGHI, C.E., SCHAJOWICZ, F.: J. Bone Jt Surg. **33-A**, 997 (1955)

VANDENBERG, H.J., JR., COLEY, B.L.: Surg. Gynec. Obstet. **90**, 602–612 (1950)

VARMA, B.P., GUPTA, I.M.: Clin. Orthop. **89**, 241–5 (1972)

VIRCHOW, R.: Mber. dtsch. Akad. Wiss. Berl. 760 (1875)

VIX, V.A., FAHMY, A.: Radiology **92**, 365–366 (1969)

WEIL, S.: Die angeborenen multiplen cartilaginären Exostosen. In: Handbuch der Orthopädie, HOHMANN, G., HACKENBROCH, M. and LINDEMANN, M. (Ed.), Bd. I, p. 228–232. Stuttgart: Georg Thieme 1957

WELLMAN, K.F.: Cancer (Philad.) **24**, 408 (1969)

WELSH, R.A., MEYER, A.T.: Cancer (Philad.) **17**, 578 (1964)

WILLIS, R.S.: Pathology of Tumours, 4th Edit. London: Butterworth & Co. Ltd. 1967

WISNIEWSKI, M., TOKER, C., ANDERSON, P.J., HUANG, Y.P., MALIS, L.I.: J. Neurosurg. **38**, 763–766 (1973)

WITWICKI, T., DANILUK, A., SIEDLIK, J.: Pol Tyg. lek. **24**, 1455–1457 (1969)

WITWICKI, T., DZIAK, A.: Wiad. lek. **20**, 2211–2213 (1967)

WOLFOWITZ, B.L.: J. Laryng. **87**, 409–416 (1973)

WOUTERS, H.W., SZEPESI, K., KULLMAN, L.: Arch. chir. neerl. **26**, 63–69 (1974)

WRIGHT, J.L., SHERMAN, M.S.: J. Bone Jt Surg. **46-A**, 597 (1964)

WRONSKI, J., BRYAN, S., KAMININSKI, J., et al.: J. Neurosurg. **21**, 419–421 (1964)

Giant Cell Tumor of Bone

by

Phillip A. Collins

Historically, the subject of giant cell tumor has probably provoked more controversy and confusion than any other tumor of bone. The reason for this can be found in the indiscriminate application of the diagnosis *giant cell tumor,* during the 1800's and early 1900's, to many lesions of bone, solely because they contained large multinucleated cells. Little attention was paid at that time to the stromal component. It became apparent that many lesions diagnosed as *giant cell tumors* differed from one another in their roentgenographic and histopathologic appearances, their clinical features, and their responses to therapy. Because these lesions had virtually little in common other than the presence of multinucleated giant cells as shown on histopathologic examination, the use of the terminology giant cell tumor and its *variants* developed in the earlier literature.

The unraveling of much of this confusion began when JAFFE et al. (1940) attempted histopathologically to separate true giant cell tumors from the so-called *variants.* Once the strict histopathologic criteria for the diagnosis of giant cell tumor of bone became established, the separation of the *variants* unfolded rapidly: pigmented villonodular synovitis (JAFFE et al., 1941); nonosteogenic fibroma (JAFFE and LICHTENSTEIN, 1942a); benign chondroblastoma (JAFFE and LICHTENSTEIN, 1942b); chondromyxoid fibroma (JAFFE and LICHTENSTEIN, 1948); and aneurysmal bone cyst (LICHTENSTEIN, 1950).

The separation of giant cell tumor from its variants has been of great importance, for the variants, as JAFFE (1947) stated, anatomically and clinically have little in common with true giant cell tumors. In addition to the establishment of strict histopathologic criteria for the diagnosis of giant cell tumor, the recent publication of series containing large numbers of these tumors (195 cases by DAHLIN et al., 1970; 218 cases by GOLDENBERG et al., 1970; 52 cases by McGRATH, 1972; and 53 cases by LARSSON et al., 1975) has led to a greater understanding of the clinical nature and the approach to therapy of these tumors.

A. Clinical Features

Giant cell tumor of bone is a relatively rare lesion. The overall incidence of giant cell tumor has been variously reported as 0.63 cases per million per year to 1 case per million per year by LARSSON et al. (1975) and McGRATH (1972), respectively. Giant cell tumor of bone accounted for only 4% of all bone tumors in the series of DAHLIN et al. (1970) and only 3% of all tumors in the series of McGRATH (1972). In the series of LARSSON (1975), which reported all cases recorded in the Swedish Cancer Registry for the years 1958–1968, giant cell tumor accounted for 7.8% of all primary bone tumors. Most large series indicate that approximately 75% of giant cell tumors occur in the third and fourth decades of life with the peak incidence occurring in the third decade. On the other hand, they indicate a vast range of age in which giant cell tumor of bone may occur, extending from 4 years, LARSSON et al. (1975), to 77 years, McGRATH (1972).

Most series demonstrate a large preponderance of occurrence of this tumor in females. In the series of DAHLIN et al. (1970), 59% of all the cases occurred in females, and of patients less than 20 years of age, 75% of the tumors occurred in females. In general, the other series quoted above confirm this except for LARSSON et al. (1975). In that series there were 27 females and 26 males. There were 12 patients (23%) less than 20 years old, and of this age group there were 9 males, all less than 18 years of age and 3 females, all 18 years of age or over. The finding of a large preponderance of females in any given series is attributed to the fact that females mature earlier and live longer than males. Giant cell tumor of bone is rarely encountered in patients who are skeletally immature. Whenever a tumor of bone is encountered in the presence of an unfused epiphysis, the diagnosis of giant cell tumor should be held in suspect. There have, however, been a number of reported cases where giant cell tumor of bone has occurred in skeletally immature individuals as evidenced by the report of a giant cell tumor of bone in a 4-year-old male in the series of LARSSON et al. (1975). JAFFE (1958) indicated that the occurrence of a bona fide giant cell tumor in a child of 10 years of age is not unusual, but most recent reports do not include patients this young.

The most common symptoms include pain, swelling, or both, in the region of the tumor. The pain is usually aggravated by motion and relieved by rest. When marked bony destruction is present, the pain may be constant. The tumor grows insidiously and is likely to attain a large size before manifesting symptoms. The presence of an enlarging mass and limitation of motion in the joint adjacent to the tumor are frequently encountered. Muscle atrophy from disuse is not uncommon. In the very far advanced cases, LICHTENSTEIN (1952) has reported the findings of a crackling sensation on palpation and even a pulsation. The duration of symptoms is quite variable. Some patients are asymptomatic, and the first presenting feature is pain caused by a pathologic fracture, which calls attention to the presence of a tumor. (Pathologic fracture, either as the presenting symptom or in conjunction with other symptoms, is not too uncommon a finding being reported in 19 cases of the series of DAHLIN et al., 1970, and 16 cases in the series of LARSSON et al., 1975.) Most series, however, indicate that some symptomatology has been present for at least a period of several weeks to several years. McGRATH (1972) and DAHLIN et al. (1970) indicated respectively that 33% and 50% of patients presented with symptoms that had been present for at least 6 months.

Most giant cell tumors occur at or near the end of a large tubular bone of an extremity (Fig. 1). DAHLIN et al. (1970) reported that more than 77% of these tumors are so located. Most series, with the exception of LARSSON et al. (1975), indicated that approximately 50% or more occur around the knee joint with the most frequent location being the distal femur, the proximal tibia, and the proximal fibula, respectively. In the tubular bones, excluding the knee, the distal radius and proximal humerus are the most frequent locations. In bones other than long tubular bones, the sacrum is most commonly involved (Fig. 2).

When giant cell tumors occur in the axial skeleton, they are usually located at either end of it, most frequently in the sacrum, but occasionally in the skull (usually in the sphenoid bone) (Fig. 3). Rarely are they located in the vertebral bodies above

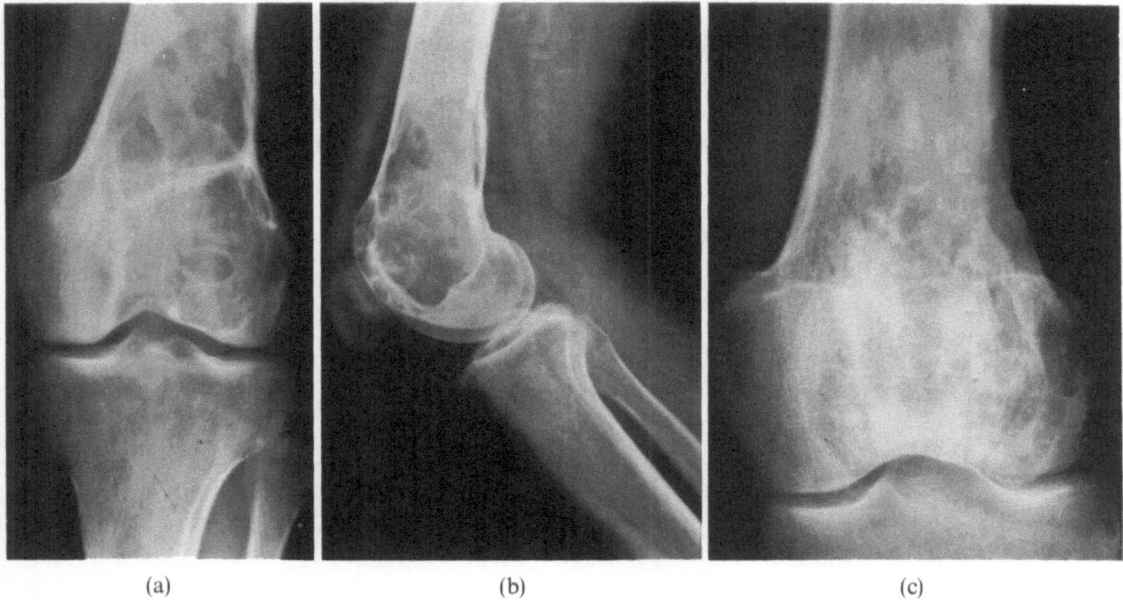

(a)   (b)   (c)

Fig. 1a–c. Giant cell tumor of distal femur. (a) and (b) Frontal and lateral views of distal right femur demonstrate a typical lytic, eccentric, expansile lesion predominantly involving lateral femoral condyle with extension into distal femoral metaphysis. Lesion erodes endosteal margin of cortex but does not break through it. (c) Demonstrates treated lesion 9 years after curettage and bone grafting

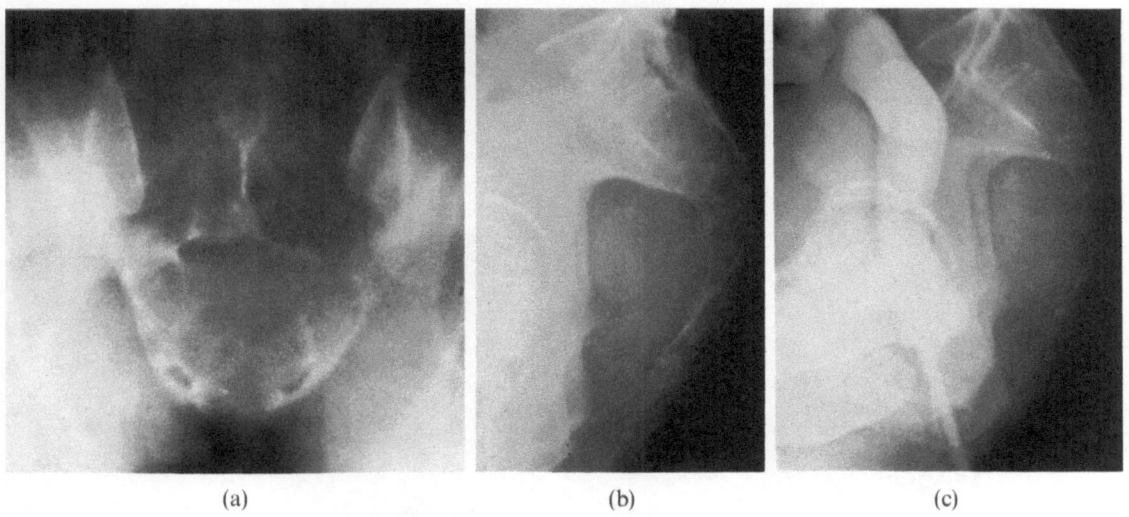

(a)   (b)   (c)

Fig. 2a–c. Giant cell tumor of sacrum. (a) Frontal body section roentgenogram of sacrum demonstrating an expansile lytic lesion in inferior portion of sacrum. (b) Lateral roentgenogram of sacrum demonstrating destruction and expansion of distal sacrum. A soft tissue mass is indistinctly seen anteriorly. (c) Lateral view of sacrum with barium in rectum more clearly demonstrating anterior expansion of the mass into the presacral space

the sacrum. Lesions suspected of being giant cell tumors and occurring in vertebral segments above the sacrum are most often finally diagnosed as aneurysmal bone cyst or osteoblastoma, and not as giant cell tumor. True giant cell tumors of the spine usually first involve the vertebral centrum, later extending into the pedicles and other posterior elements. Giant cell tumors have also been diagnosed infrequently in the iliac bone, short tubular bones of the hands and feet, the carpal and tarsal bones, the sternum, and patella and ribs. So-called *giant cell tumors* of the mandible are usually giant cell reparative granulomas and are excluded from most series of giant cell tumors.

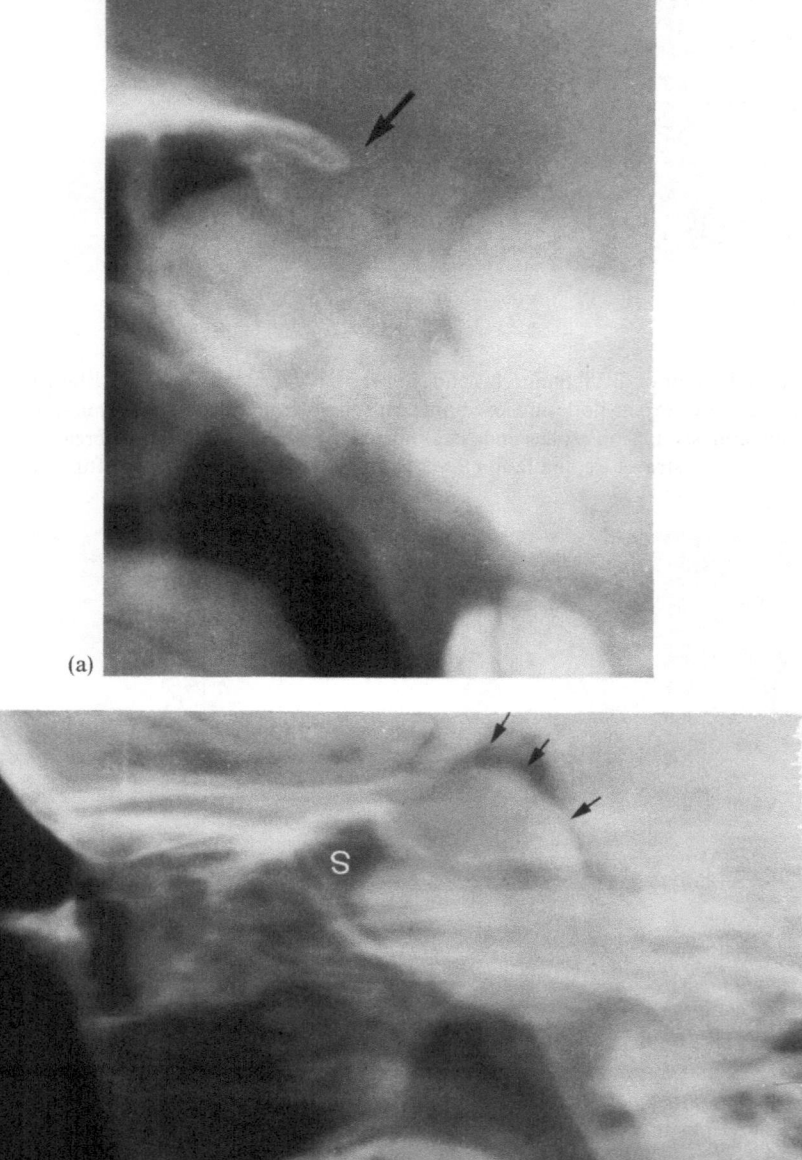

(a)

(b)

Fig. 3a and b. Giant cell tumor of clivus. (a) Lateral body section roentgenogram in region of clivus and sella turcica demonstrating a large tumor mass, which has destroyed sella turcica and invaded sphenoid sinus anteriorly and inferiorly underneath anterior clinoid process *(arrow)*. Posteriorly, extensive destruction of clivus is demonstrated. (b) Lateral body section roentgenogram taken during pneumoencephalography demonstrating intracranial extension of tumor mass *(arrows)* and invasion of sphenoid sinus *(S)*

If a suspected giant cell tumor occurs in a long tubular bone and does not involve the epiphysis, the diagnosis must be held suspect. Tumors not involving the epiphysis of long bones have been reported, but they are quite rare. DAHLIN et al. (1970) reported

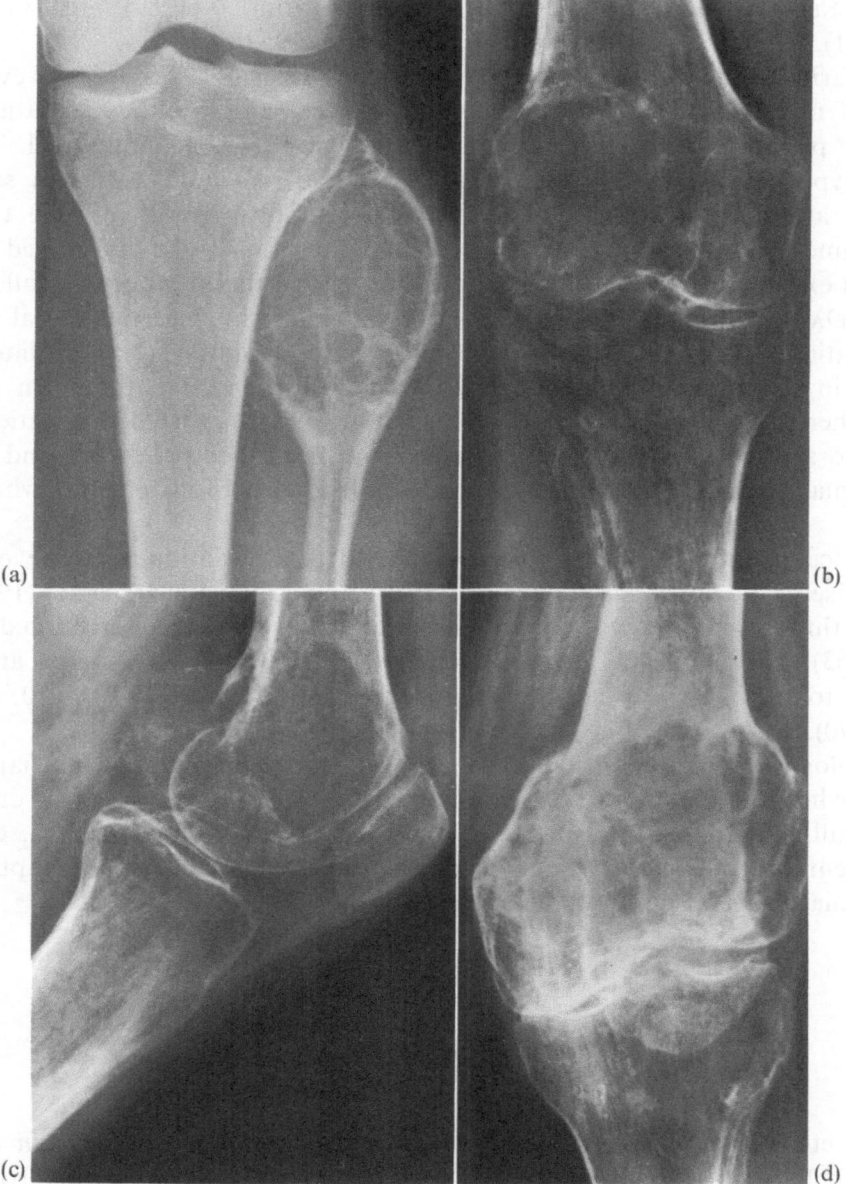

Fig. 4a–d. Multifocal giant cell tumor. (a) Demonstrates a grossly expansile lytic mass in proximal left fibula with marked thinning of endosteal surface of cortex and perforation medially. The lesion was resected, and cut section of the tumor confirmed that trabeculated appearance was due to thinning of endosteal cortical surface, which was in part penetrated by tumor. (b) and (c) Demonstrate same knee 11 years later. Patient had complained of pain in the knee for 1 year prior to this examination. An expansile lytic mass is demonstrated in distal left femur eccentrically located in lateral condyle and epicondyle and extending into metaphysis. There is marked endosteal erosion. Changes in proximal tibia are due to disuse osteoporosis. Treatment at this time consisted of curettage. Films over the next $1^1/_2$ years demonstrated a slow and partial filling in of part of the surgical defect with bone; however, the remaining surgical defect increased slightly in size. (d) A roentgenogram, taken following a fall 1 year later, demonstrated marked expansion and progression of the tumor and a pathologic fracture through lateral epicondyle. Final therapy was a midthigh amputation. There was no evidence of recurrence 20 years following that procedure

three such tumors, two which are entirely metaphyseal and one which involved the proximal humeral shaft and tuberosities. McGRATH (1972) reported a case entirely confined to a femoral shaft and another lesion involving the distal femoral metaphysis and shaft, sparing the epiphysis. Other entirely metaphyseal lesions have been reported by GOLDENBERG et al. (1970), WILKERSON and CRACCHIOLO (1969), SHERMAN and FABRICIUS (1961), JOHNSON and RILEY (1969), and JAFFE (1953).

Ordinarily giant cell tumor of bone is found as a single lesion; however, there are reports of multifocal occurrences of this tumor in a rare number of patients. Tumors which are present concurrently in the same patient are called multifocal. There is also another type of occurrence which would be considered multifocal: if a second tumor occurs in a patient who has already been successfully treated for one tumor and if enough time has elapsed so that this second tumor cannot be considered a metastasis or a local extension of the original tumor, this second tumor would be called multifocal (Fig. 4). DAHLIN et al. (1970) reported two patients who had multifocal tumors: one female patient had a tumor of the sphenoid bone and then 2 years later developed a tumor in the upper tibia; the other female patient had a tumor in the humerus and another tumor in the iliac crest. McGRATH (1972) reported one patient, who had four tumors (the distal radius, the distal ulna, a metacarpal head, and the base of the proximal phalanx). GOLDENBERG et al. (1970) reported four patients who had double lesions.

Giant cell tumor of bone has been reported in association with the occurrence of Paget's disease of bone. DAHLIN et al. (1970) and GOLDENBERG et al. (1970) reported one and three cases, respectively. Other such cases have been recorded by HUTTER et al. (1963), THOMSON and TURNER-WARWICH (1955), and SCHAJOWICZ and SLULLITEL (1966). A total of 26 cases had been reported in the literature as of 1970, GOLDENBERG et al. (1970).

Neurological symptoms occur most frequently in association with giant cell tumor of bone when these tumors are present in the sacrum, the vertebrae, or in the base of the skull, usually the basisphenoid bone. Symptoms such as sciatica, cauda equina involvement, low back pain, frontal headaches, and visual defects, or symptoms mimicking a herniated spinal disc may be encountered.

B. Pathologic Features

SPJUT et al. (1971) classified giant cell tumors as *tumors of uncertain origin*. They, along with LICHTENSTEIN (1972), felt that these tumors apparently arise from nonbone-forming mesenchymal cells of the connective tissue framework, which later differentiate into spindle-shaped or ovoid *fibroblastlike* stromal cells interspersed with multinucleated giant cells. LICHTENSTEIN (1972) stated that histologic facts favor the idea that giant cells and stromal cells have a common ancestry, and he suggested that giant cells may be derived from stromal cells by agglomeration or fusion. He pointed out that much of the confusion that existed in the past regarding the differentiation of giant cell tumor of bone from its variants resulted from undue attention having been paid to the multinucleated giant cells and not enough attention paid to the stromal cells as well as the ill-advised identification of the giant cells as osteoclasts.

Macroscopically, the giant cell tumor appears somewhat vascular and of a gelatinous, soft and friable fleshlike consistency. As stated above, it is usually eccentric and occupies the epiphyseal end of a tubular long bone extending into the metaphyseal portion of the bone and expanding and thinning its endosteal surface. It is generally red or reddish-brown in color. It may contain dark hemorrhagic areas, grayish areas of necrosis, or yellowish cystic areas following hemorrhage, necrosis, surgery, fracture, or irradiation. The tumor margin is feathery or indistinct indicating its invasiveness. Occasionally, the tumor may break through the expanded cortex and extend into the soft tissues or adjacent articular cartilage. Advanced lesions may cross a joint space either by traversing it or by extending around it through the periarticular soft tissues. Intact, unaltered, gross specimens are not often observed, because primary treatment usually consists of curettage and bone grafting or resection of the tumor in pieces. Resection *en bloc* and amputation are usually reserved for recurrent tumors or for advanced lesions, which usually demonstrate degenerative changes.

Histopathologically, most series point out that a true giant cell tumor is readily identifiable but that the cytologic details may vary considerably from one specimen to another and may also vary considerably from different parts within the same tumor. Various sections taken from the same tumor may have an appearance that runs the whole gamut from obviously *benign* to frankly *malignant*. This points out the inadequacy of punch biopsies or core biopsies and indicates the necessity of having a large amount of material from the tumor to examine and of examining numerous parts of the available specimen. The most characteristic features are best seen in areas which have not undergone any secondary changes, such as hemorrhage or necrosis.

Microscopically, the tumor tissue is a vascularized network composed of spindle-shaped or ovoid, or occasionally rounded, mononuclear stromal cells intermingled with multinucleated giant cells. The giant cells, which are usually numerous, may contain as many as 50–100 nuclei, which remarkably resemble those of the stromal cells. The stromal cells and giant cells are interspersed with a relatively meager amount of collagenous fibrils. Thin-walled blood vessels are found in various numbers in the tumor. In areas of previous hemorrhage or necrosis, large vascular sinuses lined by flattened cells may be found. Also in these areas, collagen, osteoid, and even bone may be found. This bone formation is more often identified histopathologically than roentgenographically. Approximately 35% of the tumors in the series of GOLDENBERG et al. (1970) contained microscopic evidence of osteoid or bone formation especially following fracture or unsuccessful therapy. According to them, however, the osteoid or bone appeared to be a reaction to secondary changes, such as hemorrhage, necrosis, and microfracture, and not a result of metaplasia of the stromal cells. Osteoid formation also has been reported in the periphery of lung metastases (PAN et al., 1964). Foam cells (phagocytes containing lipoid material) are infrequently encountered. SPJUT et al. (1971) also reported that the presence of osteoid was not rare. They emphasized that they had never seen cartilage in giant cell tumors.

JAFFE et al. (1940) proposed a system of a histopathologic grading of these tumors based primarily on atypism of the stromal cells. The tumors were classified into Grades I, II, and III, respectively showing insignificant, moderate, and pronounced atypism in the stromal cells. They noted that the degree of malignancy increased as the stromal cell developed a more irregular, whorled arrangement and became more abundant and densely compacted. At the same time nuclei of these stromal cells became more prominent, in that they were more variable in size, hyperchromatic, and demonstrated more frequent mitotic figures, some of which were abnormal. With increasing *malignancy* the giant cells decreased in number and contained fewer nuclei, but these showed increased abnormal mitotic activity. They stated that Grade I tumors accounted for approximately 50% of a representative series and demonstrated the least degree of aggressiveness and the most favorable prognosis. Grade II tumors followed a more aggressive course clinically with a greater tendency to recur. Grade III tumors were considered frankly malignant, possessing a sarcomatous type of stroma and a potential for metastasis, usually to the lungs. It was also felt that more often than not a malignant (i.e., Grade III) tumor is one which originally began as a Grade I or Grade II tumor but which became more aggressive, often following repeated curettage, radiation therapy, or infection. They felt that a tumor was found to be Grade III on the initial examination less frequently. In order to identify a tumor as a malignant giant cell tumor, Dahlin et al. (1970) required that histologic evidence of benign tumor must be found in sections of the lesions or in material previously removed from the same area within the lesion. They stated that if the stromal cells are malignant throughout the lesion, the lesion should probably be diagnosed as an osteogenic sarcoma or fibrosarcoma, as previously reported by Troup et al. (1960).

Lichtenstein (1972) stated that in his experience the grading of giant cell tumors still proved to be of practical value; however, Dahlin et al. (1970), Goldenberg et al. (1970), McGrath (1972), and Larsson et al. (1975) found no correlation between the histopathologic grading and recurrence rate of a given tumor or in determining which of those tumors would follow a malignant course. Cases have been reported by Jewell and Bush (1964) and Pan et al. (1964), in which histologically *benign* appearing lesions had metastasized. Spjut et al. (1971) stated that there are many recorded instances where tumor cells have invaded veins, a sign of malignancy, adjacent to giant cell tumors showing no histopathologic evidence of malignancy. Similar findings have also been reported by McGrath (1972) and Murphy and Ackerman (1956). This finding is usually not followed by the occurrence of metastasis. However, it may explain the mechanism of the development of pulmonary metastasis in the presence of apparently *benign* tumors, as reported in the literature.

C. Roentgenographic Features

The roentgenographic features of giant cell tumor of bone are, as most authors agree, not entirely specific. However, it is usually by means of the initial roentgenographic findings which, when considered with the clinical features such as age and location of the tumor, are sufficiently characteristic that the diagnosis is initially suggested. The roentgenographic features are less characteristic when the location of the tumor is somewhat unusual, such as in the sacrum, spine, or the skull. The lesion is usually radiolucent, located at the end of a tubular long bone, most frequently around the knee joint, in a skeletally mature individual (i.e., in the presence of a fused growth plate) (Fig. 1). Jaffe (1958) pointed out that the radiolucency of the giant cell tumor on the roentgenogram was due to the fact that the tumor develops rapidly causing lytic destruction, possesses little or no osteogenic capacity centrally, and causes little or no new bone formation peripherally. Therefore, on the roentgenogram, the margin of the lesion is indistinct, lacking any bony sclerosis, and, with rare exception, no stippling or calcification is seen within the tumor mass.

When the lesion occurs in a long tubular bone, it almost always involves the fused epiphysis and often extends into the adjacent metaphysis (Fig. 5). Giant cell tumors of long bones not involving the epiphysis have been mentioned elsewhere in the text, but they are exceptionally rare. More often than not, the tumor is eccentric, especially

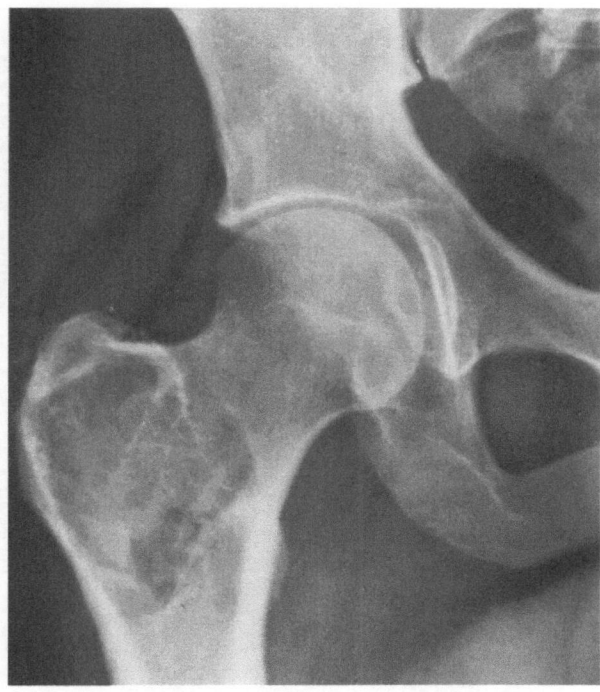

Fig. 5. Giant cell tumor of greater trochanter of femur. Roentgenogram demonstrates unusual location of giant cell tumor. Tumor arises in greater trochanter of right femur and extends into femoral neck proximally, and distally into femoral metaphysis. Lesion is lytic and expansile with considerable thinning and erosion of endosteal surface of cortex. A small cortical fracture is present in proximal portion of lesion

in a large bone; however, it may be centrally located or involve the entire width of the bone. The tumor usually abuts the articular margin of the tubular long bone. Even in a flat bone, giant cell tumors are frequently subarticular (SPJUT et al., 1971), involving the innominate bone near the sacroiliac joint and, when occurring in a rib, affecting the anterior or posterior ends. The lesion is frequently expansile with thinning of the endosteal surface of the cortex. This thinning may be irregular, forming ridges in the cortex, which results in a multicystic or multiloculated rather than a completely lucent appearance of the lesion. LICHTENSTEIN (1952) remarked that this multicystic appearance is unusual in untreated giant cell tumors and is more likely to be found in other lesions with a slower growth rate (hemangioma, nonosteogenic fibroma, fibrous dysplasia, and enchondroma). In fact, a review of many large series of giant cell tumors suggests that the opposite is true. Numerous such illustrations of well-documented, untreated giant cell tumors with visible trabeculations are found in most articles, texts, and atlases. Trabeculations developing in a previously treated lesion, which subsequently demonstrates healing, should be an alerting sign to the possibility of a recurrence of the tumor (GOLDEN-BERG et al., 1970). This is especially true if the trabeculations are coarse or thick and if the lesion has been irradiated.

The cortical margin of the lesion may contain perforations or fractures, the latter usually being of the infraction type, which do not demonstrate marked displacement of fracture fragments. Most authors describe little or no endosteal or periosteal reaction, even in the presence of a gross pathologic fracture (Fig. 6). In a small number of cases (SPJUT et al., 1971), delicate periosteal reaction has been reported in the absence of roentgenographically identifiable infractions of the cortex. In one of the larger reported series (GOLDENBERG et al., 1970), of 218 cases of giant cell tumor, approximately 25%

(a)   (b)

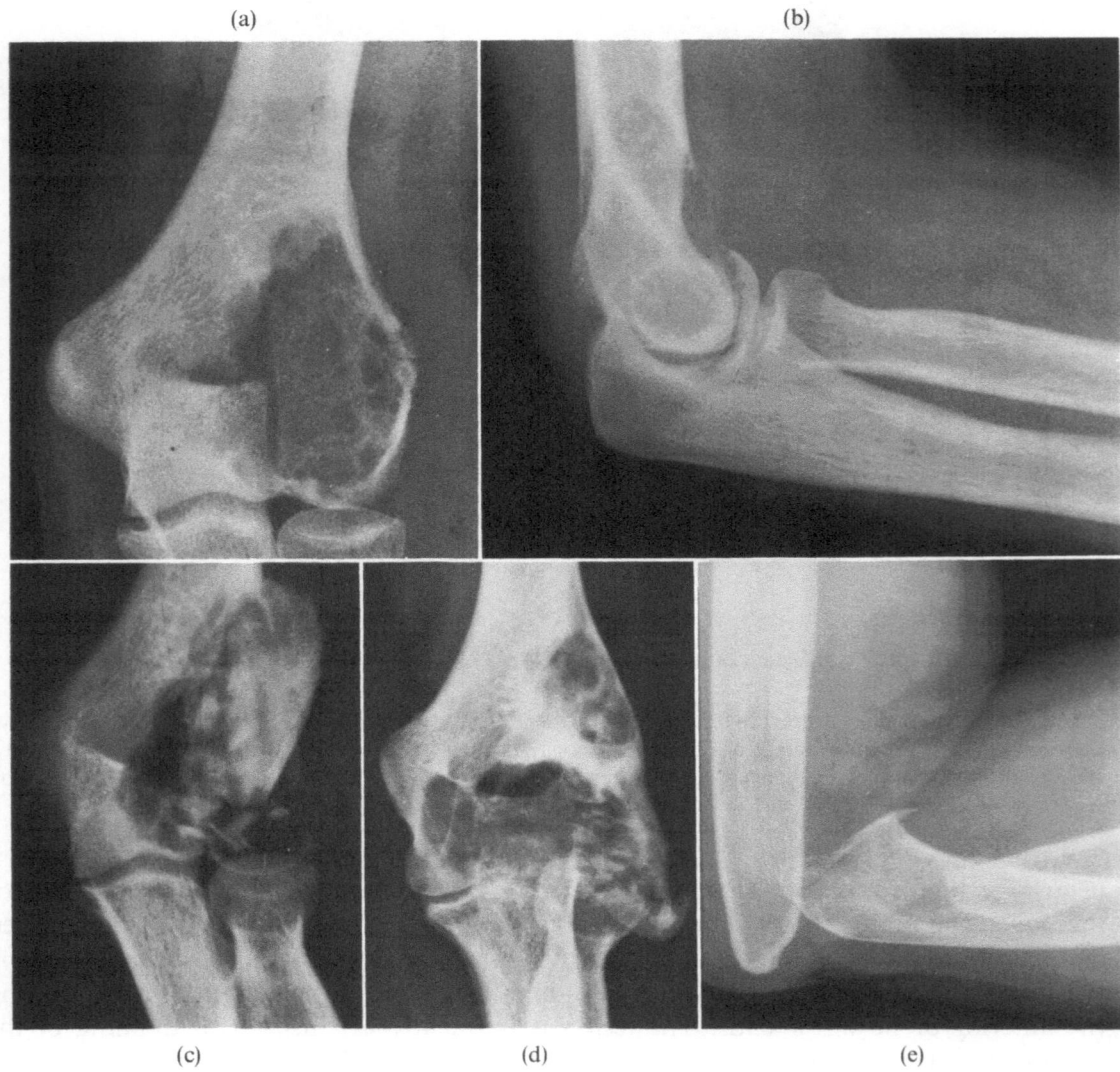

(c)   (d)   (e)

Fig. 6a–e. Giant cell tumor of distal left humerus. (a) and (b) Frontal and lateral roentgenograms demonstrating an expansile, eccentric lytic lesion arising in capitulum of left humerus. Cortex is eroded, and a pathologic fracture without evidence of periosteal reaction is present. (c) Roentgenogram following curettage and bone grafting demonstrates considerable ossification of inferior portion of surgical defect. A year following surgery a recurrence developed in capitulum. Lesion was recuretted and cavity was packed with bone chips. Following surgery patient received irradiation therapy. (d) Serial roentgenograms during following year demonstrated some initial healing, but after 2 more years follow-up, a definite recurrence was noted in lateral epicondyle along with a pathologic fracture through capitulum. (e) A biopsy of recurrence suggested sarcomatous degeneration resulting in resection *en bloc* of distal end of left humerus, elbow joint, and proximal radius and ulna. Patient was alive 26 years following initial therapy without evidence of recurrence

of the cases demonstrated cortical perforation with little or no periosteal reaction. LARSSON et al. (1975) described soft tissue extension in 21 of 53 cases in their series. This is usually more readily identifiable on examination of the gross pathologic specimen than it is on the plain roentgenogram. Special techniques such as arteriography, with or without subtraction films, may demonstrate the soft tissue component of a giant cell tumor more readily than the plain roentgenogram. Arteriography, though, is of limited value in regard to the diagnosis of giant cell tumor (Figs. 7 and 8). Some of

(a)   (b)   (c)

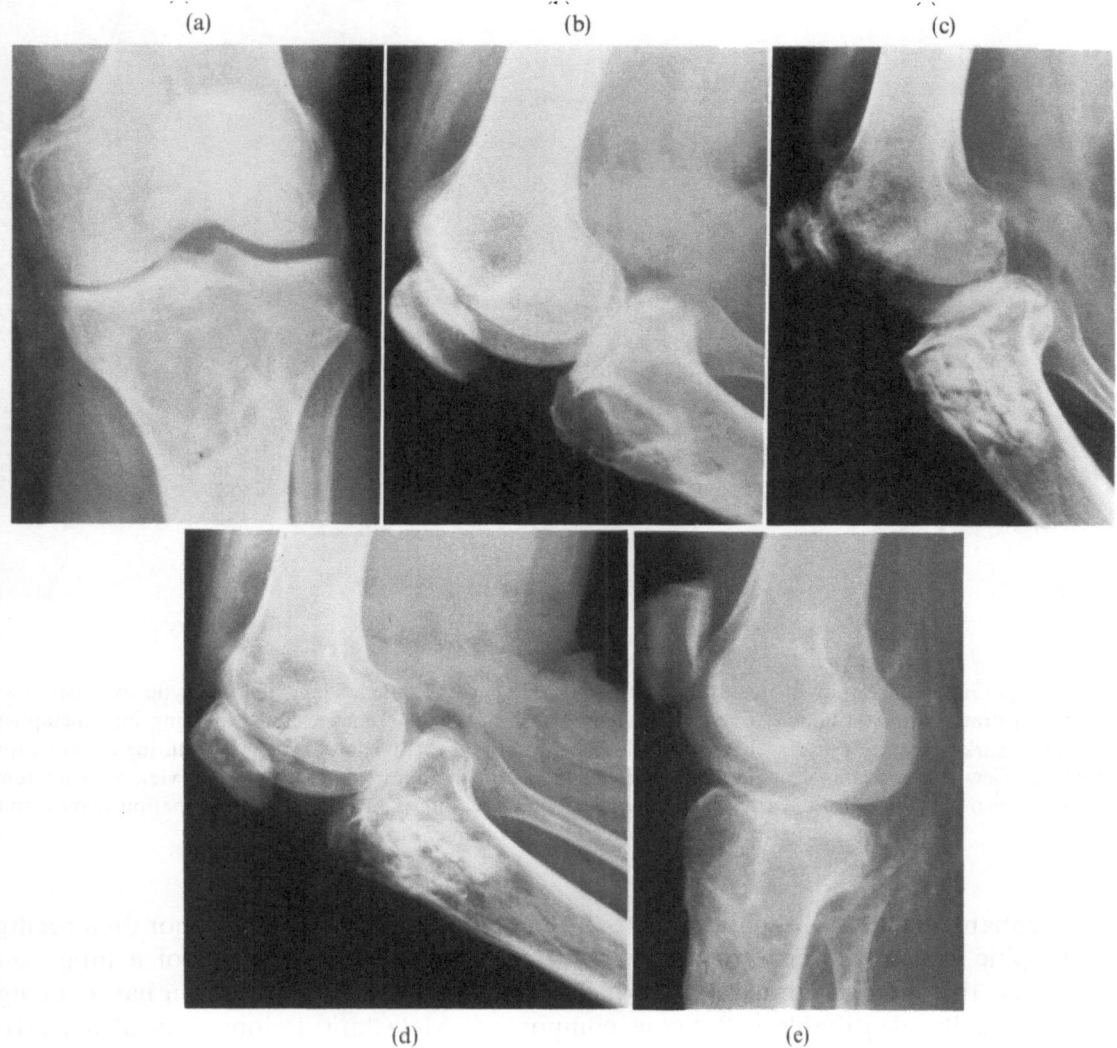

(d)   (e)

Fig. 7a–e. Giant cell tumor of proximal tibia. (a) and (b) Frontal and lateral roentgenograms of right knee demonstrating an eccentric lytic destructive lesion in proximal tibia predominantly involving epiphysis and extending into metaphysis. Minimal endosteal cortical erosion is noted along medial surface of tibial metaphysis, but considerable endosteal erosion is noted anteriorly. (c) Lateral roentgenogram of knee immediately following curettage and bone grafting. (d) Lateral roentgenogram of knee 9 months following surgery demonstrating recurrence of tumor in proximal tibia. Irregular destruction of cortex is seen, and there is partial destruction of previously dense, solid bone grafting material. (e) Lateral roentgenogram of recurrent tumor during late arterial phase of arteriography. No tumor vessels are identified, and no tumor blush or stain is seen

these tumors are vascular and some avascular. The findings are not specific. Perhaps the only value of arteriography is to demonstrate the vascular supply of the tumor and its soft tissue component prior to surgery. Xeroradiography may also prove helpful in this regard, though this is a relatively new technique and it is not mentioned in the reports of large series.

A particular problem may be encountered following irradiation of the lesion. For a period of up to 3–4 months following irradiation, there may be an apparent exacerbation of the lesion roentgenographically, and it may not be possible during this period to differentiate between lysis of tumor due to irradiation or progression of the tumor itself.

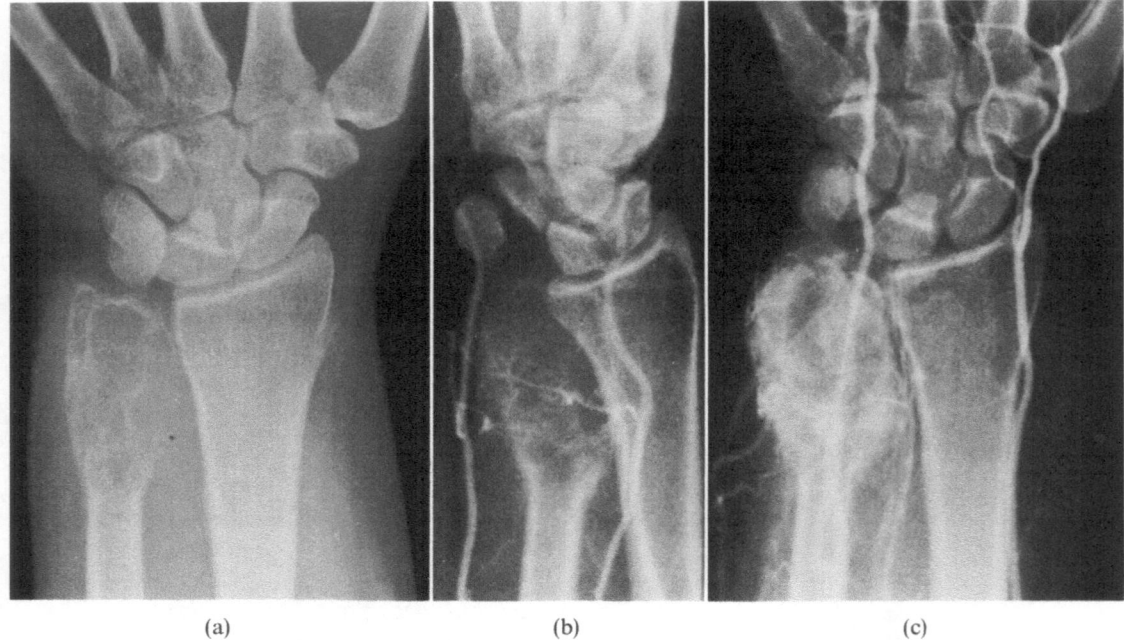

(a)   (b)   (c)

Fig. 8a–c. Giant cell tumor of distal ulna. (a) Frontal roentgenogram of left wrist. A lytic expansile lesion is demonstrated in distal ulna involving the whole width of articular margin and extending into metaphysis. There is marked cortical erosion. (b) and (c) Oblique and frontal roentgenograms of wrist during arteriography. Oblique view demonstrates irregular tumor vessels in region of tumor mass. On frontal view a dense tumor blush is seen extending around the tumor mass and encapsulating it. Microscopic examination demonstrated perforation of cortex and involvement of periosteum

Probably the most difficult lesion to differentiate from a giant cell tumor on a roentgenographic basis is a fibrosarcoma, which involves the epiphyseal end of a long bone; however, the latter lesion is more frequently metaphyseal and more often has a roentgenographically identifiable soft tissue component. Metastatic lesions may also be very difficult to differentiate from giant cell tumors on a roentgenographic basis, but they occur more frequently in an older age group. The same can be said of a central chondrosarcoma and myeloma.

Unfortunately, it is virtually impossible to distinguish a *benign* giant cell tumor from a *malignant* one on the basis of the initial roentgenographic examination, and the roentgenologist should probably eliminate these terms from his report of the appearance of the lesion. FREIBERGER et al. (1972) pointed out that the most benign appearing lesion may metastasize and cause the death of the patient. They reemphasized that the approach to the diagnosis and treatment of giant cell tumor is three-pronged, encompassing its roentgenographic, clinical, and pathologic features.

D. Treatment and Prognosis

All giant cell tumors of bone should be considered as aggressive and potentially malignant regardless of their histopathologic appearance. Much controversy has existed in the past regarding the treatment of these lesions. More recently some degree of agreement has emerged regarding management of these lesions. The poorest surgical results are obtained with curettage, with or without cautery, which results in recurrence rates as high as 68% and 85% being reported by DAHLIN et al. (1970) and GOLDENBERG et al. (1970), respectively. Recurrence in most series is defined as roentgenographic or clinical evidence of renewed activity of a tumor in a period greater than 2–3 months following primary treatment. Curettage combined with bone grafting results in a significantly fewer number of recurrences in most series, usually in the range of 25–45% of the cases. Resection *en bloc* results in even fewer recurrences, and in the series of DAHLIN et al. (1970), McGRATH (1972), and GOLDENBERG et al. (1970), amputation resulted in no recurrences. Obviously, the more radical the surgical procedure, the more likelihood there is of complete removal of the tumor. However, consideration must be given to the fact that a great number of these tumors occur about the knee or in the distal radius of young individuals. Radical surgery, such as complete resection or amputation, may not be justifiable, because it would produce considerable deformity and loss of the use of a major joint in a young individual with a long life expectancy. Curettage and grafting is not suitable for tumors that have destroyed the whole width of the ends of a long bone or have penetrated the cortex and caused soft tissue or joint space involvement. In these cases resection *en bloc* or amputation may be the only appropriate procedure.

Irradiation, either alone or in combination with surgical procedures, has been employed as a primary treatment, and cures have been reported; however, the rate of recurrence is not less than that of curettage and bone grafting, and the risk of delayed recurrence and sarcomatous degeneration (usually fibrosarcoma or occasionally osteosarcoma) is significantly higher than from surgical procedures without irradiation. Of the 195 patients in the series of DAHLIN et al. (1970), 83 patients received primary treatment at the Mayo Clinic, and an overall recurrence rate of 44.6% was observed. The recurrence rate was 47.2% for those patients who received adjunctive irradiation therapy and 42.6% for those who did not. In that same series, sarcomas were observed in 17 (8.7%) out of a total of 195 patients. Sarcomatous changes were found in 4 patients in zones of otherwise *typical* tumors at the time of initial examination. In the other 13 patients, delayed sarcomatous changes were found: sarcomatous changes developed in 2 patients whose treatment did not include irradiation and in 11 patients who were irradiated. The interval for this change to occur was 17 months to 15 years in the former group and 3.7–38 years in the latter. Most other authors concur in the concept that irradiation is a significant factor in sarcomatous transformation of giant cell tumors and advise long term follow-up of those patients whose tumors have been irradiated. Irradiation should most likely be reserved for those lesions not amenable to surgical therapy, e.g., lesions of the skull, the spine, or the sacrum.

The overall recurrence rate for all types of primary therapy is approximately 35–45%. Most recurrences are observed within the first several years following initial therapy. GOLDENBERG et al. (1970) reported that 75% of recurrences developed within 1 year and 97% within 2 years of initial diagnosis. DAHLIN et al. (1970) noted that more than 94% of recurrences developed within 3 years of primary therapy; however, as noted above, delayed recurrences, some after several decades, have been reported.

An overall malignant course of giant cell tumor resulting in the death of the patient because of the effects of the tumor itself or complications of therapy has been reported in approximately 10% of the cases (11.3% by LARSSON et al., 1975; 13.4% by McGRATH, 1972; 8.7% by DAHLIN et al., 1970; and 7.8% by GOLDENBERG et al., 1970). Most authors indicate a particularly poor prognosis for tumors of the sacrum. Total resection is seldom feasible, and they tend to have a high rate of recurrence, not uncommonly demonstrating *malignant* change. It is of interest to note that numerous series report the occurrence of metastases (usually to the lungs) but that this develops only after therapeutic intervention. Spjut et al. (1971) stated that at the time of reporting no cases were known in which metastases from giant cell tumor were present at the time the tumor was originally diagnosed. The overall incidence of metastases has been reported as high as 15% (Jaffe, 1958); however, most recent series indicate that the incidence is less. Of 218 patients (or 5.9%) in the series of Goldenberg et al. (1970), 13 developed metastases. It is of particular interest to note in that series the results of lobectomy performed for pulmonary metastasis following treatment of the original lesion. Six patients underwent thoracotomy and surgical excision for single or multiple pulmonary metastases, one patient undergoing two lobectomies. One patient died after 2 years with a mediastinal mass, but of the other five patients four were successfully treated and had not died from their tumors during a 6–18 year follow-up. One patient died 20 years later from an unrelated cause.

If a tumor recurs, a cure can usually be obtained by repetition of those procedures done initially (curettage and bone graft or resection, if the tumor is small and has not become more *malignant* histopathologically) or by more radical procedures such as resection *en bloc* or amputation. Therefore, an aggressive approach in attempting to cure giant cell tumors, even in the face of pulmonary metastases if not widely disseminated, may well be indicated. In any event, giant cell tumor of bone, as Lichtenstein (1952) has pointed out, is a formidable lesion running the whole gamut from benign to sarcomatous, and it should be managed with great respect and a full understanding that it may behave in a malignant manner in spite of a *benign* roentgenographic and histopathologic appearance.

References

Budzilovich, G.N., Truchly, G., Wilens, S.L.: Tumor giant cells in regional lymph nodes of a case of recurrent giant cell tumor of bone. Clin. Orthop. **30**, 182–187 (1963)

Dahlin, D.C.: Bone tumors. 2nd ed. Springfield, Ill.: Charles C Thomas 1967

Dahlin, D.C., Cupps, R.E., Johnson, E.W.: Giant cell tumor: a study of 195 cases. Cancer (Philad.) **25**, 1061–1070 (1970)

Freiberger, R.H., Keats, T.E., Norman, A., Pritzker, H.A., Theros, E.G.: Bone disease syllabus (disorders of the skeleton, Set 2). Chicago, Ill.: Amer. Coll. Radiol. 1972

Goldenberg, R.R., Campbell, C.J., Bonfiglio, M.: Giant cell tumor of bone: an analysis of two hundred and eighteen cases. J. Bone Jt Surg. **52-A, No. 4,** 619–664 (1970)

Hutter, R.V.P., Foote, F.W., Frazell, E.L., Francis, K.C.: Giant cell tumors complicating Paget's disease of bone. Cancer (Philad.) **16,** 1044–1056 (1963)

Jaffe, H.L.: Tumors of the skeletal system; pathological aspects. Bull. N. Y. Acad. Med. **23**, 497–511 (1947)

Jaffe, H.L.: Giant-cell tumour (osteoclastoma) of bone; its pathologic delimitation and the inherent clinical implications. Ann. Roy. Coll. Surg. Engl. **13**, 343–355 (1953)

Jaffe, H.L.: Tumors and tumorous conditions of the bones and joints. Philadelphia, Penn.: Lea & Febiger 1958

Jaffe, H.L., Lichtenstein, L.: Non-osteogenic fibroma of bone. Amer. J. Path. **18**, 205–221 (1942a)

Jaffe, H.L., Lichtenstein, L.: Benign chondroblastoma of bone. Amer. J. Path. **18**, 969–991 (1942b)

Jaffe, H.L., Lichtenstein, L.: Chondromyxoid fibroma of bone; a distinctive benign tumour likely to be mistaken especially for chondrosarcoma. Arch. Path. (Chicago) **45**, 541–551 (1948)

Jaffe, H.L., Lichtenstein, L., Portis, R.B.: Giant cell tumour of bone. Its pathological appearance, grading, supposed variants and treatment. Arch. Path. (Chicago) **30**, 993–1031 (1940)

Jaffe, H.L., Lichtenstein, L., Sutro, C.J.: Pigmented villonodular synovitis, bursitis and tenosynovitis. Arch. Path. (Chicago) **31**, 731–765 (1941)

Jewell, J.H., Bush, L.F.: *Benign* giant-cell tumor of bone with a solitary pulmonary metastasis. A case report. J. Bone Jt Surg. **46-A**, 848–852 (1964)

Johnson, K.A., Riley, L.H.: Giant cell tumor of bone.

An evaluation of 24 cases treated at The Johns Hopkins Hospital between 1925 and 1955. Clin. Orthop. **62**, 187–191 (1969)

LARSSON, S., LORENTZON, R., BOQUIST, L.: Giant-cell tumor of bone: a demographic, clinical, and histopathological study of all cases recorded in the Swedish Cancer Registry for the years 1958 through 1968. J. Bone Jt Surg. **57-A(2)**, 167–173 (1975)

LICHTENSTEIN, L.: Aneurysmal bone cyst, a pathological entity commonly mistaken for giant cell tumour and occasionally for hemangioma and osteogenic sarcoma. Cancer (Philad.) **3**, 279–289 (1950)

LICHTENSTEIN, L.: Bone tumors. 1st ed. St. Louis, Mo.: C. V. Mosby Co. 1952

LICHTENSTEIN, L.: Bone tumors. 4th ed. St. Louis, Mo.: C. V. Mosby Co. 1972

MCGRATH, P.J.: Giant-cell tumour of bone: an analysis of fifty-two cases. J. Bone Jt Surg. **54-B(2)**, 216–229 (1972)

MURPHY, W.R., ACKERMAN, L.V.: Benign and malignant giant-cell tumors of bone: a clinical-pathological evaluation of thirty-one cases. Cancer (Philad.) **9**, 317–339 (1956)

Netherlands committee on bone tumours: Radiological atlas of bone tumours. Vol. I. Baltimore, Md.: Williams and Williams Co. 1966

PAN, P., DAHLIN, D.C., LIPSCOMB, P.R., BERNATZ, P.E.: *Benign* giant cell tumor of the radius with pulmonary metastasis. Proc. Mayo Clin. **39**, 344–349 (1964)

SCHAJOWICZ, F., SLULLITEL, I.: Giant-cell tumor associated with Paget's disease of bone. A case report. J. Bone Jt Surg. **48-A**, 1340–1349 (1966)

SHERMAN, M., FABRICIUS, R.: Giant-cell tumor in the metaphysis of a child. Report of an unusual case. J. Bone Jt Surg. **43-A**, 1225–1229 (1961)

SPJUT, H.J., DORFMAN, H.D., FECHNER, R.E., ACKERMAN, L.V.: Tumors of bone and cartilage: atlas of tumor pathology. Series 2, Fasc. 5. Washington, D.C.: Armed Forces Institute of Pathology 1971

THOMSON, A.D., TURNER-WARWICK, R.T.: Skeletal sarcomata and giant-cell tumour. J. Bone Jt Surg. **37-B**, 266–303 (1955)

TROUP, J.B., DAHLIN, D.C., COVENTRY, M.B.: The significance of giant cells in osteogenic sarcoma: do they indicate a relationship between osteogenic sarcoma and giant cell tumor of bone? Proc. Mayo Clin. **35**, 179–186 (1960)

WILKERSON, J.A., CRACCHIOLO, A.: Giant-cell tumor of the tibial diaphysis. J. Bone Jt Surg. **51-A**, 1205–1209 (1969)

Marrow Tumors

by

Harry J. Griffiths

The term "marrow tumors" suggests different tumors to the histologist and to the radiologist. For the purposes of this volume, tumors of the bone marrow include not only the plasma cell or round cell tumors (i.e., Ewing's sarcoma, reticulum cell sarcoma, and multiple myeloma), but also Hodgkin's disease and lymphosarcoma. However, this is not too surprising because there is enormous overlap in the radiologic appearances of metastatic reticulum cell sarcoma and lymphoma of bone, as well as in the clinical presentation, course, and radiologic features of Ewing's sarcoma and reticulum cell sarcoma.

Each of these tumors is dealt with separately, and consideration of the presentation, clinical and pathologic features, treatment, and prognosis is given; based not only on the author's experience, but also on the literature. Due weight is given to the radiologic features, and a discussion of the common roentgenologic findings is given with mention of some of the more rare appearances—particularly in multiple myeloma where there are illustrations of "shaggy dog" myeloma, as well as the exceptionally rare osteosclerotic type of myeloma. Solitary plasmacytoma and soft-tissue myeloma are also considered in this section.

A. Ewing's Sarcoma

I. Introduction

Ewing's sarcoma was first described in 1921 by JAMES EWING as a diffuse tumor arising from the endothelial cells of the bone marrow. However, it has recently been shown (FRIEDMAN and GOLD, 1968) that it arises in fact from either the immature reticulum cells or from the primitive mesenchyme of the medullary cavity and thus at least histologically could be considered to be one of the primary lymphomas of bone. In view of the fact that clinically and therapeutically Ewing's sarcoma differs from this group of tumors, it will be considered here as a separate entity.

II. Incidence

In the Mayo Clinic series, Ewing's sarcoma represented 7% of malignant bone tumors and 5% of all bone tumors (DAHLIN, 1967). However, ACKERMAN (1968) found that

Ewing's sarcoma represented 4% of all bone tumors seen in Washington. Other authors give its incidence ranging from 0.5% to 10% of all malignant bone tumors.

III. Age

Ewing's sarcoma is a malignant tumor of childhood and adolescence with an age range of 5 months to 83 years. The mean age incidence lies somewhere between 16 and 19 and about two-thirds of cases of Ewing's sarcoma present before age 20, and 90% before age 30.

IV. Sex Incidence

In most series there is a predominance of males, generally with a 2:1 ratio, although JENKIN (1966) reports a slight preponderance of female patients in his group of 45 cases.

V. Bones Involved

Ewing's sarcoma has been described involving nearly every bone in the body, although it is very rare in the spine and fairly uncommon in the small bones of the hands and feet. Most authors have found that the majority of cases involve the long tubular bones of the arms and legs, but both the pelvis and shoulder girdle are frequently involved (Table 1). Although Ewing's sarcoma is said to classically involve the midshaft of long bones, in the reported series only 22% of cases are purely diaphyseal. They are almost invariably placed centrally within the medullary cavity.

Table 1. Bones involved in Ewing's sarcoma

Leg	503	44%
Pelvis	224	20%
Axial skeleton (includes ribs and skull)	173	16%
Arm	152	13%
Shoulder	80	7%
	1,132	

After BHANSALI and DESAI (1963), SPJUT et al. (1971), JENKINS (1966), and PRITCHARD et al. (1975)

Some 60% of cases appear to arise from the metaphysis and spread into the diaphysis secondarily. These tumors involve the junction of the upper and middle thirds of the long bones as frequently as the junction of the lower and middle thirds, and are usually eccentric in position. Epiphyseal involvement is extremely rare. It is of interest that the site of the tumor is directly related to the survival of the patient in that there is a 5-year survival rate of 22% in patients with involvement of the long bones, whereas the 5-year survival rate for involvement of the skull and scapula is 0%.

VI. Clinical Presentation

There is a history of trauma in a few patients (7–20%), although the majority of patients present with pain and swelling, usually of 9–12 months duration. The pain is often intermittent initially and then increases in severity until there may be limited range of motion in adjacent joints. A palpable mass is present in most patients which is often tender and has dilated blood vessels in the overlying skin. A localized elevation in temperature occurs in 33% of patients with Ewing's sarcoma.

Fever, weight loss, and cachexia occur in 25% of patients and are a poor prognostic sign since they imply generalized disease. Pathologic fractures occur in from 2 to 5% of patients and are more frequent in metaphyseal lesions. Occasionally increasing weakness in association with general debility and paresthesia has been described in Ewing's sarcoma and in a few patients this may progress onto frank paraplegia.

VII. Laboratory Data

Unlike, reticulum cell sarcoma, generalized symptoms are common in Ewing's sarcoma. The tumor is associated with anemia in 25% of cases and a leukocytosis in the majority of patients. There is an elevated erythrocyte sedimentation rate in 90% of patients, and the more elevated this becomes, the worse the prognosis.

VIII. Radiologic Features

1. Periosteal Reaction

a) Onion-Skin Pattern of Subperiosteal Bone Formation

This is a characteristic but not specific feature since it also occurs in such conditions as syphilitic osteitis. Onion-skin lamellation occurs in 36% of patients with Ewing's sarcoma overall, although it was present in 100% of patients with central diaphyseal lesions of long bones in SHERMAN and SOONG's (1956) series (Figs. 1, 2). Onion-skin lamellation is due to reactive new bone formation which occurs secondary to penetration of the periosteum by the tumor and is rarer in metaphyseal tumors, which often show one of the other types of periosteal reaction.

b) Right-Angled Spiculation (Sunray Appearance)

This represents perpendicular periosteal new bone formation and occurs in about 30% of cases of Ewing's sarcoma involving the metaphysis and in 12% of all types of Ewing's sarcoma (Fig. 3). The sunray appearance may make the radiologic differential diagnosis from osteosarcoma difficult. It is caused by rapid growth of the tumor in the soft tissues, carrying with it periosteal cells so that the new bone is laid down perpendicular to the cortex rather than in lamellations parallel to the bone, which is inclined to occur in more slowly growing tumors.

c) Codman's triangle

This will also occur rarely in a very rapidly growing Ewing's sarcoma, particularly those involving the metaphysis (see Fig. 9).

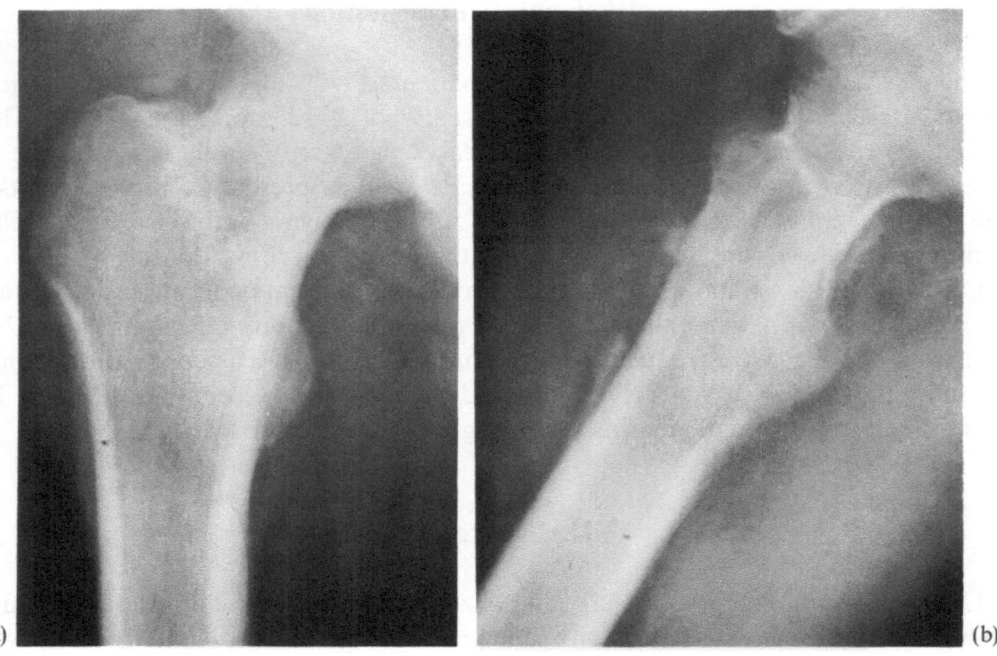

(a)   (b)

Fig. 1. (a) Ewing's sarcoma of upper femur: 22-year-old male patient complaining of pain in hip. Note laminated "onion skin" perosteal reaction (AP view). (b) Frog leg view: note poorly defined osteolytic lesion with overlying periosteal reaction

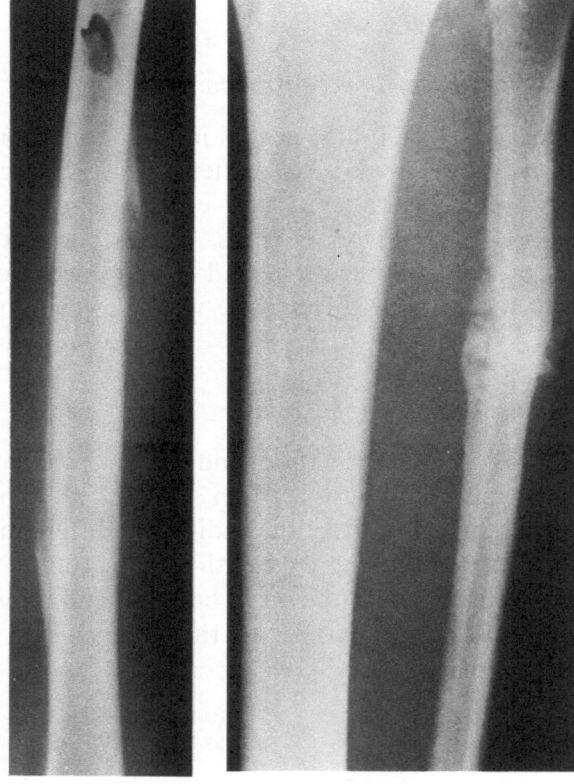

Fig. 2. Ewing's sarcoma—humerus: Lamellated periosteal reaction is present in this Ewing's sarcoma without obvious underlying bone destruction. Note Codman's triangles

Fig. 3. Ewing's sarcoma—fibula: Right-angled periosteal spiculation is present in this 18-year-old patient with Ewing's sarcoma of fibula

Fig. 2   Fig. 3

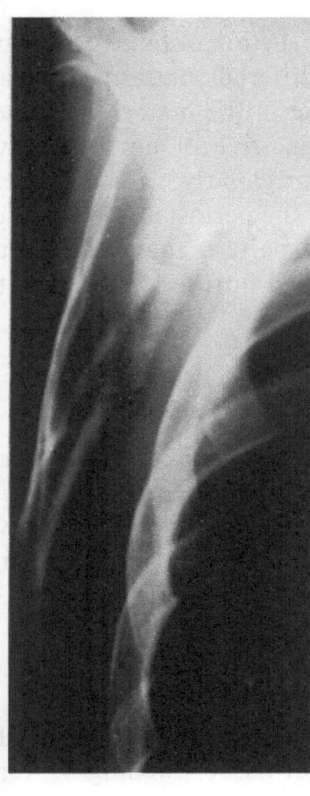

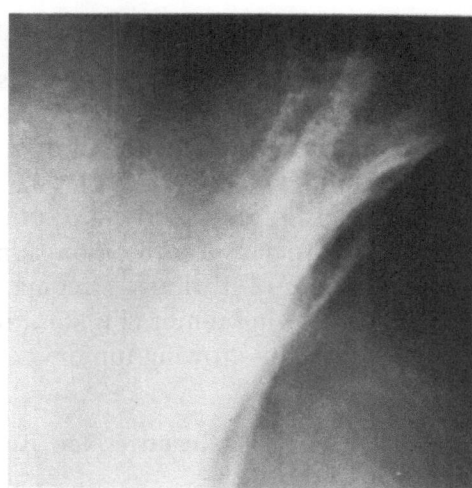

Fig. 5

Fig. 4. Ewing's sarcoma—scapula: This was a rapidly growing destructive tumor producing cortical destruction and periosteal reaction

Fig. 5. Ewing's sarcoma—anterior superior iliac spine: The irregular mottled appearance of this bone is typical of Ewing's sarcoma in a flat bone. Note also loss of cortex and periosteal reaction

Fig. 4

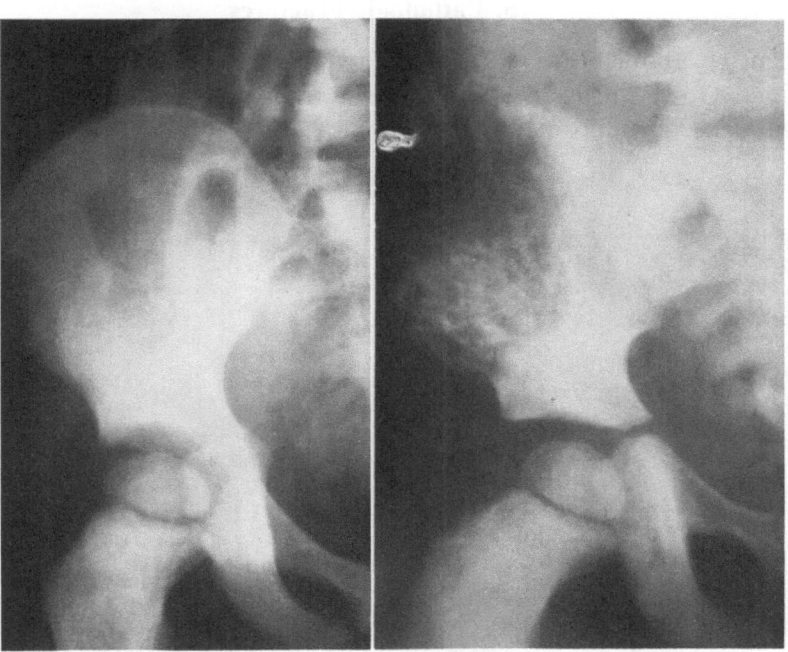

Fig. 6. Ewing's sarcoma—iliac bone: This child complained of pain in the right hip, and initial radiograph appeared normal. 8 months later there was marked destruction of iliac bone with a honeycomb pattern

2. Destruction of Bone

Another characteristic appearance of Ewing's sarcoma is destruction of bone occurring mainly in the intramedullary canal. There are a number of different patterns with an irregular mottled appearance with cortical destruction occurring in the majority of cases (39% in BHANSALI and DESAI's series, 1963), and this is suggestive of an infiltrative permeative lesion (Figs. 4, 5). Superficial cortical erosions—particularly with endosteal bone destruction—in association with onion-skin lamellation of the periosteum is another characteristic appearance of Ewing's sarcoma. A honeycomb pattern may also occur due to a more slowly growing tumor (Fig. 6). Finally a widespread diffuse loss of density may occur in a very rapidly growing tumor.

3. Reactive New Bone Formation

Usually there is little or no reactive new bone formation in the intramedullary canal of long bones, but there are sporadic case reports of purely sclerotic types of Ewing's sarcoma. However, a tumor with mixed, mottled, destructive areas, and patchy reactive new bone is fairly common in flat bones (PRITCHARD et al., 1975). It gives a "moth-eaten" appearance, which may be difficult to distinguish from widespread metastases (Figs. 7, 8).

4. Soft-tissue Swelling

This is invariably present and is usually obvious not only clinically but radiologically (Fig. 9). In about 50% of cases of Ewing's sarcoma, the soft-tissue swelling is very large and will distort and destroy the soft-tissue planes. There is often some reactive new bone formation within the mass—either periosteal onion-skin lamellation or perpendicular streaks giving a sunray appearance.

5. Pathologic Fractures

These occur in about 10% of cases of Ewing's sarcoma and are often one of the presenting signs. However, not every pathologic fracture is painful and a certain number of tumors will cause asymptomatic fractures.

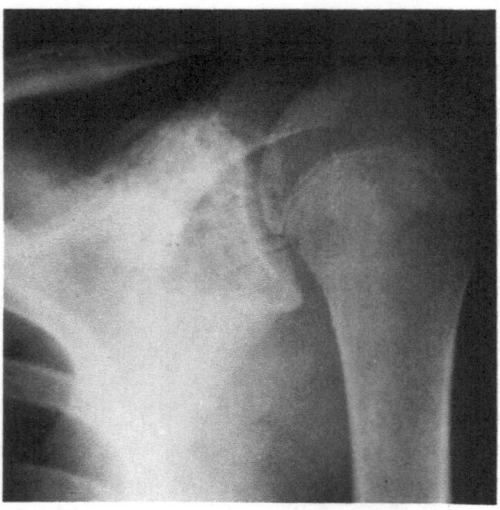

Fig. 7. Ewing's sarcoma—scapula: Glenoid has a mixed sclerotic and lytic appearance ("moth-eaten") which is typical of Ewing's sarcoma of flat bones

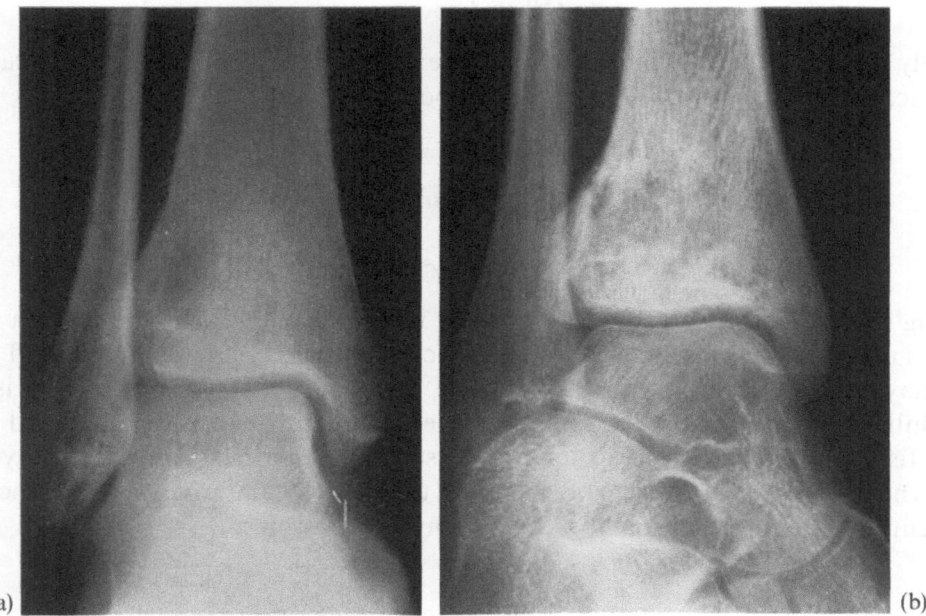

Fig. 8. (a) Ewing's sarcoma—distal tibia: This 20-year-old woman was complaining of pain in her ankle, and a poorly defined lytic area was seen in metaphysis of lower tibia. (b) Ewing's sarcoma—distal tibia: A mottled sclerotic and lytic lesion appeared 6 months later, which on biopsy was found to be Ewing's sarcoma

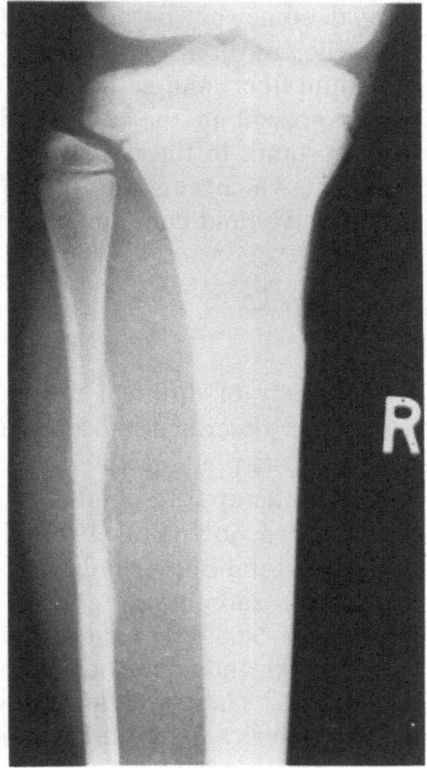

Fig. 9. Ewing's sarcoma-fibula: Note marked soft-tissue swelling with loss of normal soft-tissue planes and lengthy periosteal reaction, with Codman's triangle

6. Other Appearances

Rarely there will be cavitation within the lesion in the bone giving a radiologic appearance similar to that of an aneurysmal bone cyst.

IX. Pathology

1. Gross

Ewing's sarcoma is a soft, semisolid tumor which glistens when cut. It has a grayish-white or gray-pink appearance and commonly contains areas of hemorrhage and necrosis which may be so extensive that they replace most of the tumor. Its origin is within the medullary cavity, but Ewing's sarcoma permeates through the cortex and invades the soft tissues rapidly. The periosteum at first resists the invasion so that layer upon layer of new bone is laid down parallel to the periosteum (onion-skin lamellation). The extent of the tumor is usually greater than that seen on x-rays.

2. Microscopic

The histologic appearance of Ewing's sarcoma is similar to some other tumors, particularly neuroblastoma, reticulum cell sarcoma, and metastatic undifferentiated carcinoma. The tumor consists of distinctive, small, rounded, closely packed, uniform cells which are highly anaplastic and are about two to three times the size of lymphocytes. These cells form dense sheets or nests which often congregate around blood vessels to impart a rosettelike pattern. Nests of tumor cells with intervening fibrous septa are characteristic but not often seen.

The cell membranes are indistinct with scanty cytoplasm and the nuclei are round to oval, somewhat basophilic with few nucleoli and clear-cut nuclear membranes. There is rarely any bone or cartilage formation within the tumor. There is also a lack of reticulum fibers and with periodic acid-Schiff stain (PAS), a PAS-positive staining glycogen is present in the cells of Ewing's sarcoma. These are two histologic differences of importance in the differential diagnosis between Ewing's sarcoma and reticulum cell sarcoma, which contains plentiful reticulum fibers and no glycogen within the cells, but do have lipid containing vacuoles (SPJUT et al., 1971).

X. Treatment

A variety of different modes of therapy has been used for Ewing's sarcoma since it was first described and these include local resection, amputation, the use of Coley's toxins, (COLEY et al., 1948), the use of radioactive phosphorus (^{32}P), chemotherapy, and radiotherapy. A combination of radiotherapy with surgery and/or chemotherapy is advocated now (PHILLIPS and HIGINBOTHAM, 1967), although some authors suggest the use of total body irradiation (MILLBURN et al., 1968; and JENKIN, 1966).

Ewing's sarcoma is a fairly radiosensitive tumor and suggested dose rates range from 3,000–6,000 R over the course of 5–6 weeks. JENKIN (1966) suggests 4,500–5,000 R in 3–5 weeks and advocates radiotherapy to the whole bone as well as to the surrounding soft tissues. There is almost invariably a dramatic response with a reduction in the pain as well as a marked shrinkage in the size of the tumor. However, when the sarcoma recurs, the response to a second dose of radiotherapy is poor. Radiotherapy is also used for metastatic spread of the tumor — either as treatment for solitary bone metastases, or for generalized disease including intrapulmonary metastases. A suggested dose is 2,000 R and this will palliate pain and often reduce the metastases in size.

Of the many forms of chemotherapy that have been used to treat Ewing's sarcoma, cyclophosphamide, vincristine, and cytoxan appear to be in most common use today. In the past, nitrogen mustard, methotrexate, leukeran, 6 mercaptopurine, and melphalan have all been tried. The suggested therapeutic regimen of cyclophosphamide begins with two intravenous doses of 100–150 mg followed by 100–150 mg by mouth daily until some response is seen (either palliation of pain or decrease in the size of the primary tumor or its metastases). Once this has occurred, a maintenance dose of 50 mg orally daily is suggested (JENKIN, 1966).

XI. Prognosis

The 5-year survival rate in the literature appears to vary from 0–30%. However, a number of early studies undoubtedly contained tumors other than Ewing's sarcoma and thus caution is advised in the interpretation of these early survival rates. Most recently, PRITCHARD et al. (1975) found an overall 5-year survival rate of 16%, which decreases to 14% at 10 years and $11^1/_2$% at 20 years. Nearly one-half of the patients die in the first year and the 5-year survival rate with known metastases was found to be nil, whereas the 5-year survival rate without known metastases was 19%. In Pritchard et al.'s group of patients, the 5-year survival rate in patients with the tumor in an extremity treated by surgery without metastases was 45% compared to 13% in other groups of patients. Another valuable prognostic sign is the lack of generalized signs and symptoms, e.g., no fever, normal erythrocyte sedimentation rate, and no anemia. BHANSALI and DESAI (1963) collected from the literature a total of 646 patients on whom the overall 5-year survival rate was 9%. But 251 of these patients were treated by radiotherapy alone with a 5-year survival rate of 10%, and a further 100 patients only received surgical therapy with a 20% 5-year survival rate.

POMEROY and JOHNSON (1975) reported on 66 patients who received local irradiation and chemotherapy with alternating high doses of adriomycin and cyclophospha-mide/vincristine. There was a 56% 2-year survival rate and 35% 5-year survival rate in this group. But more impressive is the group of 43 patients without metastases who had a 64% 2-year survival rate and a 52% 5-year survival rate on this regimen.

In most patients there is a rapid progression of the tumor with only about one-quarter of the patients having metastases at the start of the treatment, whereas 85% are dead in 2 years. Metastases may go anywhere, but are most common in other bones (particularly the skull), the lungs, and lymph nodes (local as well as distant). At autopsy, between 50 and 75% of patients have evidence of metastases to the skeleton, whereas POTDAR (1971) found radiologic evidence of bony metastases in only 15% of his patients.

XII. Differential Diagnosis

There are two distinct groups of conditions from which Ewing's sarcoma has to be differentiated — and one group depends on radiographic grounds while the other depends on histologic factors (see Table 2). The most important radiologic differential diagnosis is between Ewing's sarcoma and osteomyelitis, but usually the rapid history of the latter plus the clinical findings make the diagnosis of osteomyelitis relatively

Table 2. Differential Diagnosis of Ewing's sarcoma

Radiological	Benign	Osteomyelitis
		Eosinophilic granuloma
	Malignant	Osteosarcoma
		Central chondrosarcoma
		Multiple myeloma (older people)
		Lymphoma
		Reticulum cell sarcoma
Histological	Benign	Eosinophilic granuloma
	Malignant	Reticulum cell sarcoma
		Neuroblastoma
		Metastatic undifferentiated carcinoma

simple. Other malignant tumors, such as osteosarcoma and chondrosarcoma have different radiologic and clinical appearances and histologically are easily differentiated from Ewing's sarcoma. One problem may be in the differentiation of Ewing's sarcoma from reticulum cell sarcoma and other lymphomas in younger patients, and from multiple myeloma in older patients, but often the histologic picture is specific enough for an exact diagnosis to be made.

B. Reticulum Cell Sarcoma of Bone

I. Introduction

Primary reticulum cell sarcoma of bone is histologically indistinguishable from the sarcoma which involves the reticuloendothelial system elsewhere in the body. Moreover, there appear to be two separate and distinct types of reticulum cell sarcoma involving bone. One is a primary condition of the skeleton, in which usually only a solitary bone is involved and presents classically as an infiltrative lesion in the shaft of one of the long bones. The other is a sarcoma of the reticuloendothelial system (involving particularly the lymph nodes of the thorax) which eventually metastasizes to bone, and then its appearance is similar to that of lymphoma involving bone. The two conditions have distinctive presentations, differing radiologic appearances, and follow separate clinical courses. Whereas generalized reticulum cell sarcoma (which is a true malignant lymphoma involving the spleen and lymph nodes) occurs in middle to old age, primary reticulum cell sarcoma of bone is a disease of young people and carries a better prognosis. A further problem in the diagnosis of primary reticulum cell sarcoma of bone is that it is sometimes difficult to differentiate both radiologically and histologically from Ewing's sarcoma, and this is particularly true in adolescent patients.

II. History

The first case of a sarcoma arising from the reticuloendothelial cells of bone was described by OBERLING in 1928. Sporadic cases of this tumor were described up to 1939 when PARKER and JACKSON reviewed the clinical and radiologic findings of primary reticulum cell sarcoma of bone. Since that time several review articles have appeared — notably SHERMAN and SNYDER (1947), McCORMACK et al. (1952), IVINS and DAHLIN (1953), and WILSON and PUGH (1955).

III. Incidence

Primary reticulum cell sarcoma of bone represents 2.7% of all tumors of bone or 3.4% of primary malignant tumors of bone in a recent Mayo Clinic review (DAHLIN, 1967). But ACKERMAN (1968) puts the incidence at 6% of all bone tumors. In my own experience, reticulum cell sarcoma represents about 4% of all true primary bone tumors — both benign and malignant.

IV. Age

Primary reticulum cell sarcoma appears to be rare under 10 years of age. It occurs more commonly over 30 and WANG and FLEISCHLI (1968), in a series of 21 patients, found that 50% occurred in the third and fourth decades (range 11–75). FRANCIS et al. (1954), in a series of 44 cases, described an age range of 11–67 (mean 34), while WILSON and PUGH (1955), in a series of 33 patients, showed an age range of 9–67 (mean 39). This is in contradistinction to Ewing's sarcoma which occurs in the first two decades and the generalized form of reticulum cell sarcoma which occurs in the sixth decade.

V. Sex Incidence

Males appear to be involved more frequently with primary reticulum cell sarcoma of bone than females with a 2:1 or 3:1 ratio, although WANG and FLEISCHLI (1968) found a 1:1 male to female ratio in a group of 21 patients.

VI. Bones Involved

Primary reticulum cell sarcoma of bone may involve almost any bone in the body, but it appears to involve primarily the long tubular bones of the upper arm and about the knee (Table 3). 67% of most series of reticulum cell sarcoma involve the long bones, whereas the tumor is rare in the radius and small bones of the hands and feet. In one series (IVINS and DAHLIN, 1953) 15% occurred in the mandible and, although three cases of primary reticulum cell sarcoma involving the skull were described by STRANGE

Table 3. Bones involved in primary reticulum cell sarcoma in a series of 99 patients

Femur	31	Vertebrae	5
Tibia	15	Rib	4
Humerus	13	Mandible	4
Pelvis	9	Fibula	3
Scapula	6	Foot	2
Ulna	5	Sternum	2

Based on WANG and FLEISCHLI (1968), FRANCIS et al. (1954), and WILSON and PUGH (1955)

(1954), it is probable that this represented metastatic generalized reticulum cell sarcoma rather than true primary reticulum cell sarcoma of bone, because no cases of involvement of the skull have been reported since. Other bones which may be involved include the clavicle and patella.

VII. Clinically

There is a remarkable contrast between the well-being of the patient with primary reticulum cell sarcoma of bone and the size and severity of the lesion. This is in marked distinction to the generalized form of reticulum cell sarcoma, which is invariably accompanied by chronic low grade fever, fatiguability, and loss of weight.

Reticulum cell sarcoma of bone presents with pain and swelling of the involved bone which have been frequently present for 1–2 years. Pain is present in 100% of patients with this tumor, and varies from being intermittent and dull or occasionally sharp, to a constant nagging pain unrelieved by rest and often most distressing at night. Swelling is present in 85% of cases of reticulum cell sarcoma and this may be associated with localized heat overlying the swelling (24%) or local tenderness (58%).

If the tumor occurs in the metaphysis, reticulum cell sarcoma may progress toward the joint causing inflammation of the synovium with an associated joint effusion; but extension into the joint space itself is rare. Generalized fever is also rare in reticulum cell sarcoma and this is a helpful method of distinguishing the lesion from Ewing's sarcoma in young people in whom fever is common.

Pathologic fractures are fairly common—in PARKER and JACKSON's (1939) series they occurred in 18% and in BETHGE's (1955) series of patients, pathologic fractures occurred in 21%. In many patients with reticulum cell sarcoma this is often the presenting sign and although there is an old theory that previous trauma led to the occurrence of the reticulum cell sarcoma, there is no proof that this may be true.

VIII. Laboratory Data

The biochemical tests in reticulum cell sarcoma of bone are usually not helpful; the serum calcium and phosphate, as well as the alkaline phosphatase are normal. Occasionally there may be a secondary anemia with a leukocytosis.

IX. Radiologic Features

Classically the first change is patchy infiltration with bone destruction arising in the medullary cavity of the diaphysis of a long bone. The lucencies have poorly defined margins which represent direct infiltration and destruction of bone by malignant cells. This patchy infiltration will eventually spread until it reaches the cortex, at which stage the first symptoms occur. Once reticulum cell sarcoma has involved the cortex then a periosteal reaction is common. The appearance in the cortex is essentially the same as in the medullary cavity initially, with patchy lucencies which eventually become confluent.

WILSON and PUGH (1955), in a classical radiologic paper divide the radiologic features under a number of separate subgroupings and this classification will be followed here.

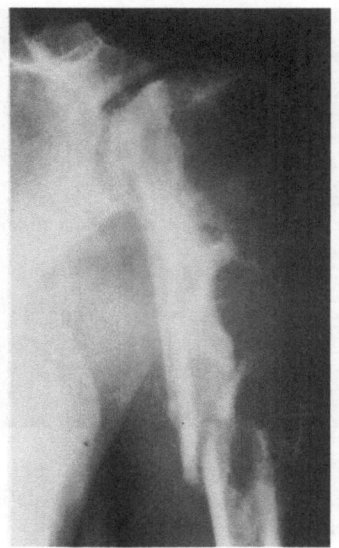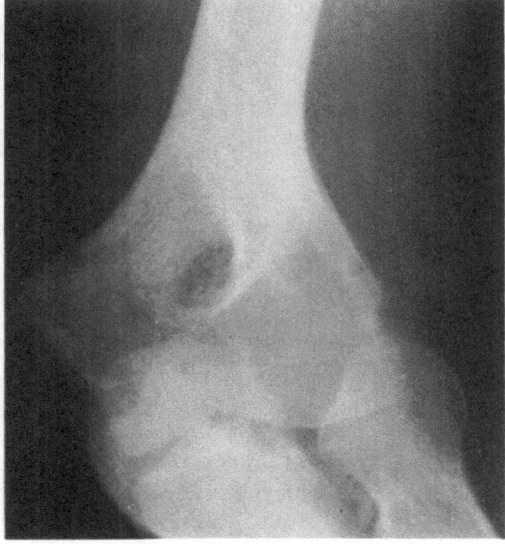

Fig. 10   Fig. 11

Fig. 10. Reticulum cell sarcoma—proximal humerus: This 20-year-old man had generalized reticulum cell sarcoma, and following minor trauma developed pathologic fracture through this large destructive lesion in proximal humerus. Note periosteal reaction

Fig. 11. Reticulum cell sarcoma—distal humerus: This young male patient had multiple lytic lesions in skeleton, and generalized reticulum cell sarcoma involving mediastinal and abdominal nodes. On turning over in bed he heard his elbow crack and developed a pathologic fracture through this secondary area of reticulum cell sarcoma

1. Location of Tumor in Bone

In Wilson and Pugh's series, 27% of reticulum cell sarcoma of bone involved the proximal end and 27% the distal end of the long tubular bones, while 45% involved the diaphysis. Usually between one-quarter and one-half of the involved bone is affected, but in some cases the entire bone may be involved. If reticulum cell sarcoma occurs in bones like the clavicle, scapula, or ribs, it may be metaphyseal or diaphyseal and frequently spreads to involve both. Should reticulum cell sarcoma involve the pelvis, then it may be a generalized permeative lesion throughout the rami or the iliac bone.

The metastatic form of reticulum cell sarcoma involves the metaphysis rather than the diaphysis, and this may have led to confusion between the two lesions in the past (Figs. 10, 11). In the leg, there is a prepondency for this tumor to involve the bones around the knee whereas in the arm, reticulum cell sarcoma seems to have a predilection for involvement of the upper humerus near the shoulder.

2. Destruction of Cancellous Bone

This is a constant feature and is the predominant radiologic finding (Figs. 12, 13, 14). Reticulum cell sarcoma is a patchy, mottled, infiltrative lesion which blends imperceptibly with normal bone. The destruction of bone is normally marked, occurring in 50% of patients; and these lucencies frequently coalesce.

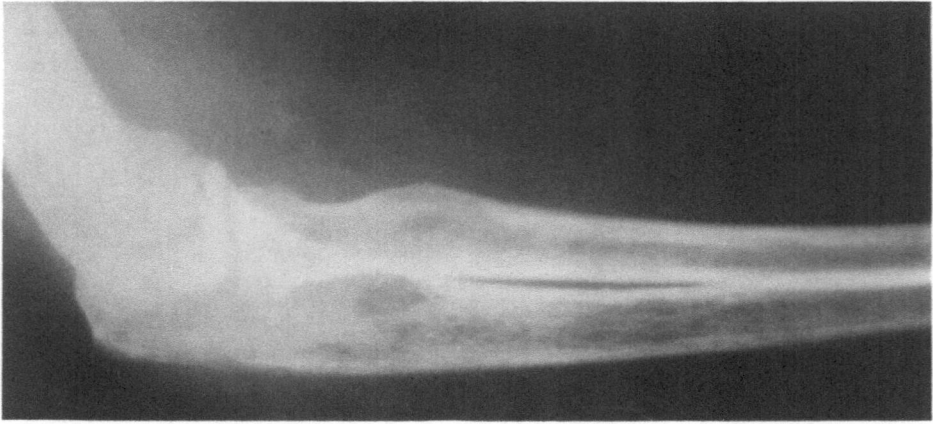

Fig. 12. Reticulum cell sarcoma—ulna: This permeative lesion in metaphyseal/diaphyseal part of this ulna is classical appearance of reticulum cell sarcoma of a long bone. There are multiple, poorly defined lucencies with a soft-tissue mass, and there is a faint periosteal reaction

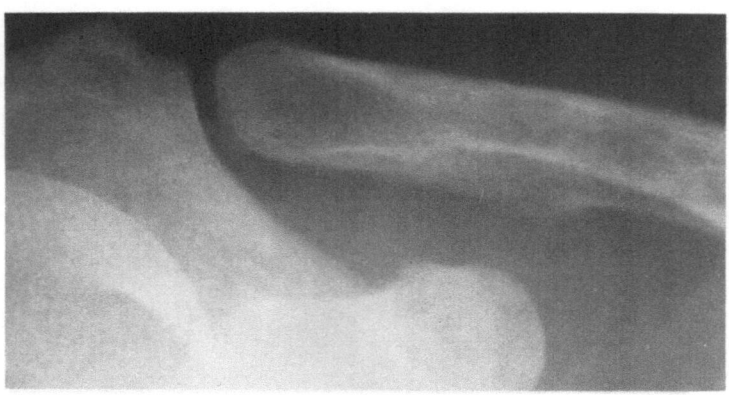

Fig. 13. Reticulum cell sarcoma— clavicle: This young male patient complaining of shoulder pain had this lesion picked up on a routine chest x-ray. On biopsy it proved to be a reticulum cell sarcoma of clavicle. Following total excision (1965) the patient has had no recurrence

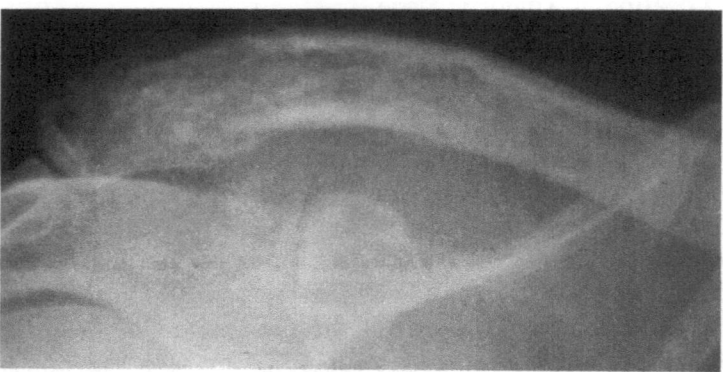

Fig. 14. Reticulum cell sarcoma— clavicle: This young male physician was complaining of shoulder pain and a reticulum cell sarcoma of clavicle was demonstrated (this is a separate case from Fig. 13). Ill-defined lucencies can be seen involving diaphysis of clavicle and spreading into distal end, and there is some periosteal reaction

3. Destruction of Cortical Bone

This occurs in some 90% of patients with reticulum cell sarcoma of bone and will vary from small irregular areas of infiltration to complete destruction of the cortex (Fig. 15). This total destruction usually only occurs if the medullary cavity is severely involved and is invariably associated with a large soft-tissue mass. Mild to moderate cortical bone destruction occurs in one-third of cases, whereas total dissolution of the cortex occurs in approximately 20% (Fig. 16, 17).

Fig. 15. Reticulum cell sarcoma—diaphysis of humerus: This young female patient was complaining of pain in the arm. Radiograph showed destructive diaphyseal lesion with multiple ill-defined lucencies involving cancellous and cortical bone. On biopsy this proved to be a reticulum cell sarcoma which responded well to radiotherapy

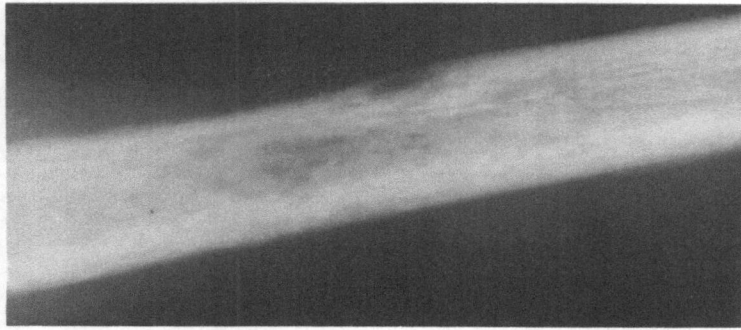

Fig. 16. Reticulum cell sarcoma—clavicle: (This is a different case from both Figs. 13 and 14). There is a rapidly growing destructive lesion involving distal clavicle with an obvious periosteal reaction superiorly

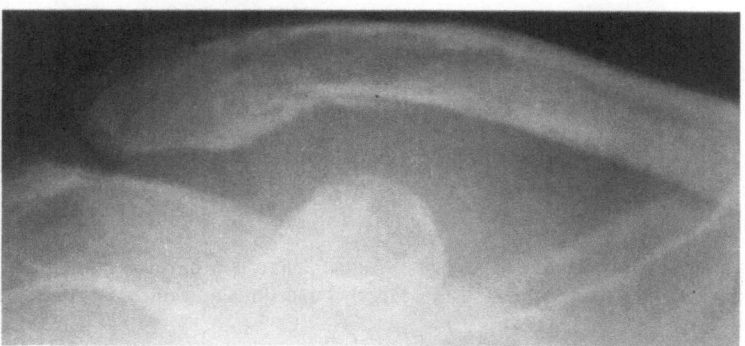

Fig. 17. Reticulum cell sarcoma—clavicle: This tumor was markedly destructive and spread rapidly. Patient died 6 months later

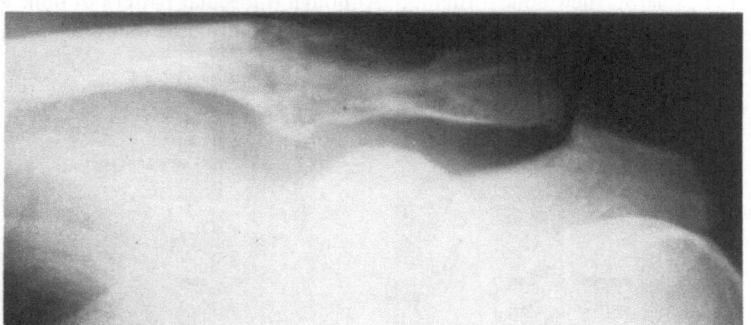

4. Reactive Proliferation of Bone

Occasionally foci of new bone may be seen radiographically and these represent reactive proliferation of bone. It occurs because the reticulum cell sarcoma tumor cells stimulate the normal cells to produce new bone. This occurs in 40% of cases to a minimal or moderate degree and is often seen histologically rather than roentgenologically (Figs. 18, 19). It is rare for reactive proliferation of bone to be a predominant feature of reticulum cell sarcoma, but in 15% of WILSON and PUGH'S (1955) patients, new bone formation was more evident than destruction of bone.

5. Cortical Thickening

In almost every situation where there is a reactive process occurring in the medullary cavity, endosteal new bone formation may be stimulated and this will lead to apparent

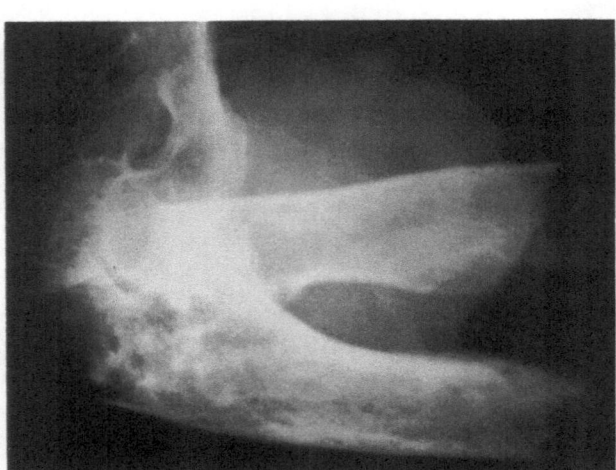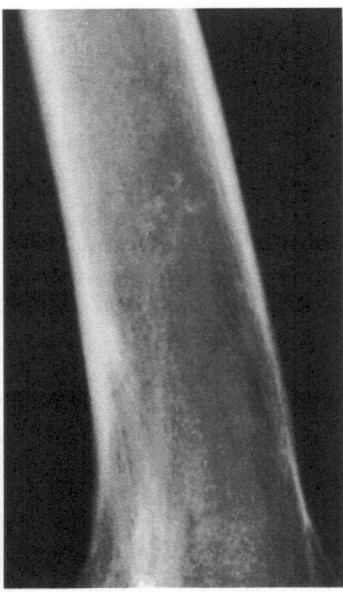

Fig. 18   Fig. 19

Fig. 18. Reticulum cell sarcoma—ulna: There is a mottled lytic and sclerotic lesion involving proximal ulna. Tumor appears to be largely cancellous and on biopsy was a typical reticulum cell sarcoma

Fig. 19. Reticulum cell sarcoma—distal femur: This middle-aged patient was complaining of increasing pain in the knee. This radiograph demonstrates some poorly defined areas of sclerosis, which on biopsy proved to be sclerotic new bone formation. Although trabecular pattern of bone appears relatively normal roentgenologicylly, on biopsy the bone marrow had been totally replaced by reticulum cell sarcoma

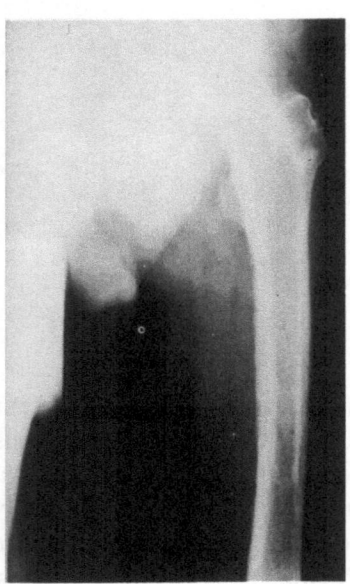

Fig. 20. Reticulum cell sarcoma—femur: This 80-year-old male patient had pain in the left hip and leg. Roentgenologically a "bone within a bone" can be clearly seen. At autopsy this was found to be due to reticulum cell sarcoma

cortical thickening, although radiologically the "bone within a bone" appearance is classical (Fig. 20). This endosteal reaction, although rare in primary reticulum cell sarcoma of bone, does occur in about one-quarter of cases—and in this author's experience is more common in older patients.

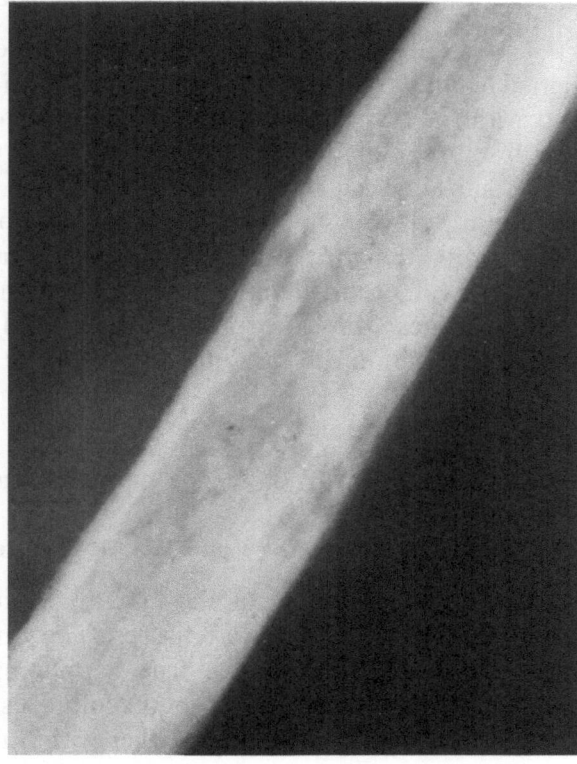

Fig. 21. Reticulum cell sarcoma—midshaft humerus: (Same case as Fig. 15) This radiograph taken at a slightly later stage shows lamellated periosteal reaction over multiple areas of destruction

6. Periosteal Reaction

This is a controversial subject because some authors say that periosteal reaction occurs commonly in reticulum cell sarcoma whereas others find it rare. In WILSON and PUGH's (1955) series, periosteal reaction occurred in 45% of their patients. It was minimal in 24%, moderate in 18% and marked in only one patient, with onion-skin lamellation, which appeared radiologically similar to a classical Ewing's sarcoma; but at histology, it appeared to be a reticulum cell sarcoma of bone. It is probable that periosteal reaction occurs in two situations—one is when the cortex is broached and there is an attempt of the skeleton to wall off the tumor (Figs. 16, 21). The other cause of periosteal reaction is when there is reactive new bone formation in the soft-tissue mass which is frequently associated with reticulum cell sarcoma of bone.

7. Soft-Tissue Involvement

Three-quarters of the patients with reticulum cell sarcoma of bone will have a soft-tissue mass. In 50% it is marked and often one of the major presenting signs. This mass undergoes calcification in 15% of cases—either as a result of direct stimulation of the cells to calcify or as a result of dystrophic calcification. Once the tumor has invaded the soft tissues, it will both push the soft-tissue structures away and also infiltrate them, and this is a useful sign in the radiologic differential diagnosis between reticulum cell sarcoma and chronic osteomyelitis.

8. Pathologic Fracture

This occurs in 20–30% of patients with reticulum cell sarcoma and is often a presenting sign. The underlying destruction and infiltration is usually obvious roentgenographically and with the classical x-ray appearances as well as a history of minimal trauma leading to a fracture, a diagnosis of underlying bone tumor is easy to make.

Perhaps one final word should be said on the radiologic differences between primary reticulum cell sarcoma and the generalized form of the disease. In metastatic reticulum cell sarcoma the appearances are those of a large lytic destructive lesion, which is often asymmetrical, occurring in the region of the metaphysis (Fig. 11). They occur particularly commonly near the elbow and the knee, and are often impossible to differentiate from primary reticulum cell sarcoma on radiologic grounds alone.

X. Pathology

1. Gross

There is involvement of the marrow cavity with extension into the cortex and frequently beyond into the soft tissues. The tumor often contains areas of necrosis and hemorrhage and resembles a true lymphoma in that it is fleshy, homogeneous, soft, and friable. It has a grayish-pink color, usually with ill-defined margins, and often containing reactive new bone—either within the tumor itself or subperiosteally.

2. Microscopic

Histologically it is impossible to differentiate reticulum cell sarcoma of bone from reticulum cell sarcoma of lymph nodes—they both are highly cellular tumors with a loose stroma of collagenous bundles and reticulum fibers. The reticulum cells are fairly uniform in size and have indistinct boundaries. The cells have a faintly acidophilic or basophilic cytoplasm and their nuclei are lobular with distinct indentation. There is a marked fibrous stroma which can be visualized using special reticulum stains and these are areas of necrosis as well as foci of extravasated blood.

Although occasionally cells similar to Reed-Sternberg cells may be seen, most cases of reticulum cell sarcoma of bone have a somewhat mixed cell population, often with a lymphocytic component. IVINS and DAHLIN (1953) claim that because of these appearances, reticulum cell sarcoma represents a true malignant lymphoma.

XI. Treatment

As our understanding of primary reticulum cell sarcoma of bone has evolved, so the various forms of therapy have altered. Initially radical surgery or amputation was the treatment of choice. This era was followed by the use of Coley's toxins and more recently by chemotherapy. However, radiotherapy has now become the treatment of choice. The tumor is moderately radiosensitive and the use of supervoltage therapy has markedly increased the 5-year survival rate. WANG and FLEISCHLI (1968) use 4,500–5,000 R over the course of 4–5 weeks and irradiate the entire bone. If it is feasible to do easily, some authorities suggest removal of the bone (e.g., a clavicle or rib) and then advocate the use of radiotherapy subsequently.

XII. 5-Year Survival Rate

This varies from 22–50% in the literature, although the most recent figures from WANG and FLEISCHLI (1968) suggest a 5-year survival rate of 50%. FRANCIS et al. (1954) found a 48% 5-year survival rate but a 30% 10-year survival rate, which suggests that patients with primary reticulum cell sarcoma of bone should have a lengthy follow-up period.

XIII. Metastases

Metastases are present between 40 and 50% of cases, and they spread via lymphatics, mainly to regional lymph nxdes (22%), other bones, and the lung.

XIV. Differential Diagnosis

Only one nonmalignant condition could be mistaken for primary reticulum cell sarcoma of bone and that is chronic osteomyelitis. The skeletal changes may be identical, although typically osteomyelitis involves the junction of the diaphysis and the metaphysis where the blood supply is poorest. Osteomyelitis is asymmetrical and involves the periosteum more rapidly than does reticulum cell sarcoma. If osteomyelitis involves the central part of the shaft of a long bone, then an awareness of the soft-tissue changes is essential for the differential diagnosis. In osteomyelitis the soft-tissue planes are removed and the fat lines are lost, whereas in reticulum cell sarcoma the soft-tissue planes are distorted but not destroyed. Also in chronic osteomyelitis there are more systemic signs of chronic illness and frequently the two may be differentiated on the clinical picture alone.

With regard to the differential diagnosis from other malignant tumors, the overlap between Ewing's sarcoma and primary reticulum cell sarcoma in young people may be so great that the clinical and radiologic features are identical, although the histologic appearances are usually different.

Eosinophilic granuloma of bone usually has a number of separate foci and rather than being permeative, it appears as one or more separate lucencies particularly involving the skull and pelvis. Once again the histologic pattern is distinctive, as it is in both osteosarcoma and metastatic neuroblastoma.

However, the differentiation between primary reticulum cell sarcoma of bone and the more generalized form of reticulum cell sarcoma may be impossible, and is probably of little clinical importance. A normal chest x-ray should exclude mediastinal and hilar lymph nodes and the clinical differences between the two conditions have already been emphasized (see Table 4).

Table 4. Differential diagnosis of reticulum cell sarcoma of bone

Benign	Chronic osteomyelitis
	Eosinophilic granuloma
Malignant	Osteosarcoma
	Ewing's sarcoma
	Metastatic neuroblastoma

C. Multiple Myeloma and Solitary Plasmacytoma

Although the radiologic appearances of multiple myeloma are well known, some understanding of the different types of plasma cell dyscrasias is necessary to perceive how these various conditions may overlap, not only radiologically but also clinically and histologically (see Table 5). This is a relatively new field and the interested radiologist is referred to a recent article by Renner and Smith (1974).

Table 5. Plasma cell dyscrasias

A. *Major pathologic varieties of importance*
   I.   Solitary plasmacytoma
   II. Multiple myeloma
   III. Primary macroglobulinemia (Waldenström)
   IV. Amyloidosis

B. *Secondary nonpathologic varieties*
   I.   Chronic inflammatory processes
      1. Liver disease: hepatitis and cirrhosis
      2. Chronic tuberculosis
      3. Subacute bacterial endocarditis
      4. Systemic lupus erythematodes
   II. Neoplasia
      1. Lymphoma
      2. Leukemia
      3. Carcinoma: pancreas and prostate
   III. Drug reactions
      1. Penicillin

C. *Idiopathic*
   Precursor to myeloma in later years

After Abramson and Shattil, 1973

The so-called solitary osseous myeloma is probably rather different in origin to the extramedullary plasmacytoma, although both will almost invariably progress onto disseminated myelomatosis eventually. These entities will be considered under the title Solitary plasmacytoma and their appearances will be discussed in this article, as well as both the classical appearances and the rarer roentgenologic aspects of multiple myeloma. Mention will also be made of some of the nonosseous changes which may occur in this common form of primary bone neoplasia. Currently a controversy is raging over a rare condition called plasma cell leukemia in which the patient will present with hepatosplenomegaly, leukocytosis, and a large number of plasma cells in the peripheral blood. There appears to be no evidence that it is directly related to multiple myeloma, although it is presumably related to the plasma cell dyscrasias. But since it has no specific radiologic appearances, plasma cell leukemia will not be considered further in this chapter.

I. Incidence and Pathogenesis

Although multiple myeloma is the commonest primary malignant tumor of bone (accounting for over 40% in the Mayo Clinic series—Spjut et al., 1971), and it is the cause of 1.7 deaths per 100,000 population per year (JAFFE, 1958), the pathogenesis is completely unknown. Attempts have been made to relate myeloma to chronic myeloproliferative disorders, trauma, virus infections, and chronic irritation. However, it is essentially a disease of the elderly, and although a number of familial cases have become apparent and there are even a few reports of spouses developing myeloma, it is probable that multiple myeloma represents a primary neoplasm of the primitive reticulum cell.

II. Age

Myelomatosis is classically a disease of the elderly, with three-quarters of cases occurring between the ages of 50 and 70 (mean age 64). It is rare before 40, but some young patients under 20 years of age have been found to have the condition. Solitary plasmacytoma has an age range of 12–72 with most patients presenting in the sixth and seventh decades.

III. Sex

There is an overall sex incidence of about 2:1 male to female, but in the rare sclerotic type of myelomatosis, this increases to 4:1, male to female, which is a similar sex incidence as that mentioned by TODD (1965) for solitary plasmacytoma.

IV. Bones Involved

Both solitary myeloma and multiple myelomatosis occur predominantly in marrow (plasma) bones, whereas extramedullary plasmacytomas occur in the soft tissues predominantly of the head and neck. The vertebrae, ribs, and skull are the bones most frequently involved, but the pelvis and hip girdle as well as the shoulder girdle are also often involved (Table 6). Myelomatosis only rarely involves the periphery and then almost invariably only after the central skeleton is extensively involved.

Solitary myeloma is usually metaphyseal in origin when it occurs in long bones, but 20% occur in the vertebrae and 20% in the pelvis. Rarely there may be a series of recurrent individual solitary myeloma deposits in the same patient spread over many years before the almost inevitable progression on to the disseminated type of myelomatosis. On the other hand, extramedullary plasmacytoma usually occurs in the soft tissues

Table 6. Bone involvement in 78 patients with multiple myeloma

	% of total	% of cases with pathologic fracture
Vertebrae	66	62
Rib	44	23
Skull	41	—
Shoulder girdle	38	7
Pelvis	28	5
Femur	24	11

After CARSON et al. (1955) and SPJUT et al. (1971)

of the sinuses or upper respiratory tract (nasopharynx, soft palate, and nasal fossa). This accounts for 50% of cases in TODD's series (1965) and the remainder may occur anywhere in the soft tissues—pleura, tonsils, skin, ovary, breast, and lymph nodes (HELL-WIG, 1943).

V. Clinical and Laboratory Data

The majority of patients present with bone pain—frequently backache related to the vertebral micro-fractures or the true compression fractures which are a common feature of multiple myeloma. In fact, 92% of SNAPPER and KAHN's (1964) series had bone pain. Neurologic signs are also frequent and are usually associated with vertebral compression fractures: 66% of patients with vertebral lesions had compression fractures in another series (CARSON et al., 1955). Another classical method for myelomatosis to present is unexplained osteoporosis in a middle-aged patient—often a man. Under these circumstances it is *always* essential to exclude myeloma.

Generalized signs and symptoms such as weight loss, cachexia, and weakness are common. There is often a progressive normocytic anemia associated with a decrease in the platelet count, elevation of the ESR, and rouleaux formation of red cells. The leukocyte count may be normal or there may be a slight leukocytosis. Hyperuricemia, as a result of the increased turnover of nucleoproteins is common, and hypercalcemia occurs in 33% of patients with myeloma. Azotemia is not infrequent, and renal failure occurs in about 20% of patients with myelomatosis. Hepatosplenomegaly is fairly common. Hemorrhage may occur and there appears to be an association between polycythemia and the sclerotic form of myeloma (HIMMELFARB et al., 1974).

VI. Diagnosis and Classification

The diagnosis is usually made on electrophoresis of either the blood or the urine. A total of 90% of patients with multiple myeloma have abnormal plasma protein electrophoresis—a wide M band paraprotein. Over 60% of patients with myelomatosis have Bence-Jones proteinuria (a light chain immunoglobulin) and this may be the only detectable abnormality for many years. To demonstrate Bence-Jones protein requires the urine to be heated and the abnormal protein will come out of solution to form a white precipitate at about 50°C, which will disappear if the urine is further heated. Then Bence-Jones protein will reprecipitate out on cooling, and although it is a very simple method for detecting myeloma, it must be remembered that Bence-Jones protein does not occur exclusively in that disease as it may also occur in small amounts in patients with primary amyloid, leukemia, and lymphoma.

Other methods of diagnosis include biopsy or bone marrow aspiration, both of which will demonstrate a plasmacytosis.

Various methods of classification of the types of abnormal protein have been used in an attempt to understand the disease better. Older classifications used to divide myeloma into four types are:

1. raised gammaglobulin
2. raised "M" globulin (beta or in between beta and gamma)
3. normal electrophoretic patterns (less than 5% of patients with multiple myeloma)
4. other abnormalities (alterations of albumin, etc.).

More recently a classification based on the specific type of protein has been used (BERGSAGEL et al., 1967):

1. G myeloma globulin 55%
2. light chain protein 25%
3. A myeloma globulin 20%.

VII. Radiologic Features

The appearance of solitary plasmacytoma will depend on whether it is in bone or in the soft tissues. In the soft tissues extramedullary plasmacytoma will present as a soft-tissue mass without calcification or ossification, although it will erode through adjacent bone structures—particularly in the nose and sinuses.

Solitary myeloma of bone will usually have a multicystic soap bubble appearance and occur in the metaphyseal region of a long bone or above the acetabulum in the pelvis (Figs. 22, 23, 24). It is destructive but will contain thick trabeculae and often balloon out the cortex, similar to a giant cell tumor. A periosteal reaction is rare and characteristically solitary myeloma of bone looks benign. However, it will often send off disseminated lesions within 2 or 3 years, although a number of patients with long-term follow-up (over 20–35 years) of a solitary lesion have been reported (WRIGHT, 1961).

The classical radiologic appearance of multiple myeloma is of multiple, sharply-defined lucencies to which the term "punched out" is accurately applied. But there are many other forms of myeloma in bone ranging from a rather moth-eaten appearance to a pure osteoblastic sclerotic reaction. Thus, an attempt will be made to categorize these differing appearances.

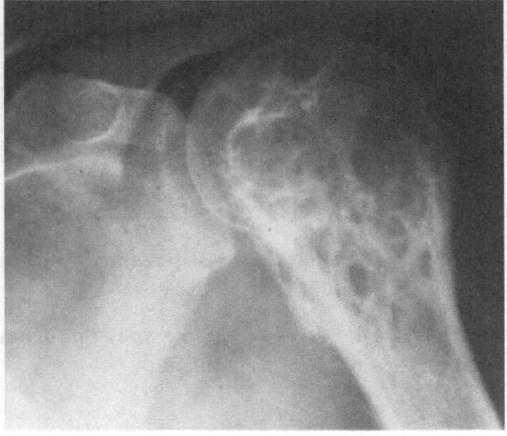

Fig. 22

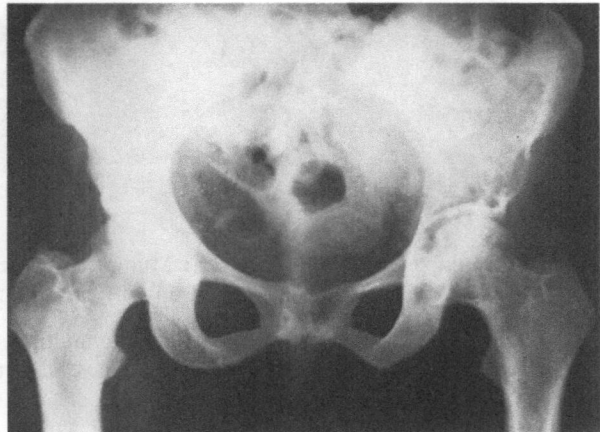

Fig. 23

Fig. 22. Solitary plasmacytoma—upper humerus: This large expansatile tumor of metaphysis of the upper humerus resembles a giant cell tumor or aneurysmal bone cyst. It appears benign with clear-cut margins and some periosteal reaction. However, on biopsy it was found to be a solitary plasmacytoma

Fig. 23. Solitary plasmacytoma—acetabular roof: This large multicystic lesion over othe roof of the left acetabulum has produced expansion of bone. Its appearances are those of a benign tumor (resembling giant cell tumor), however, on biopsy it was found to be a solitary plasmacytoma

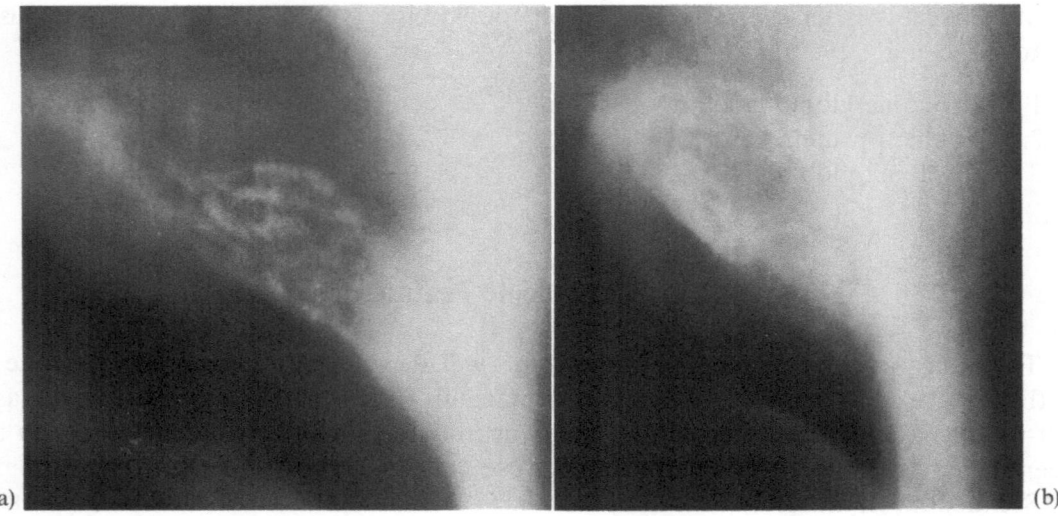

Fig. 24a and b. Solitary plasmacytoma—rib: Tomographic views show soft-tissue mass surrounding this expansatile lesion of the left sixth rib. Exaggerated honeycomb trabecular pattern of this solitary lesion is typical of plasmacytoma

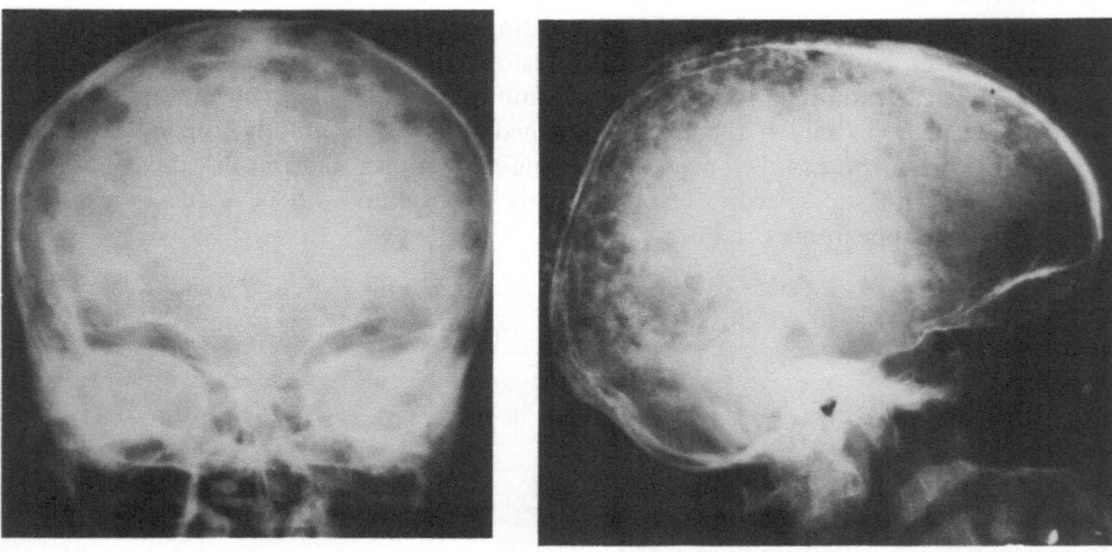

Fig. 25   Fig. 26

Fig. 25. Multiple myeloma—AP skull: Multiple, well-defined, punched-out lucencies are present throughout vault of the skull in this 70-year-old male patient with multiple myeloma

Fig. 26. Multiple myeloma—lateral skull: Note multiple, punched-out, lytic areas of varying sizes throughout skull, some of which appear to have sclerotic margins as a result of chemotherapy

1. Destructive Osteoclastic Lesions

This is by far the most common radiologic appearance seen in multiple myeloma.

a) Sharply Defined "Punched Out" Lesions

These may be small or large and are often varied in size. They occur most frequently in the skull, clavicles, ribs, and pelvis (Figs. 25, 26, 27, 28).

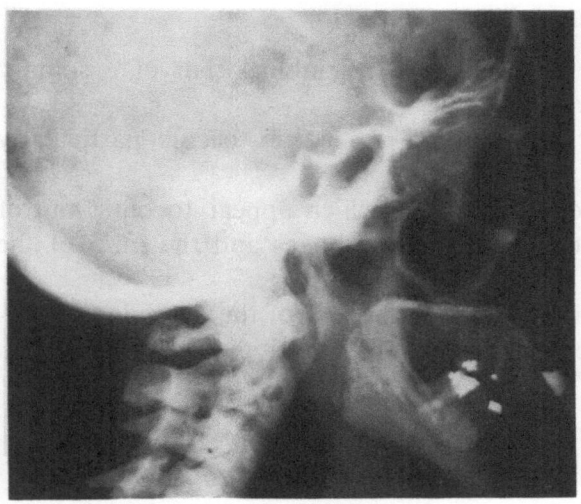 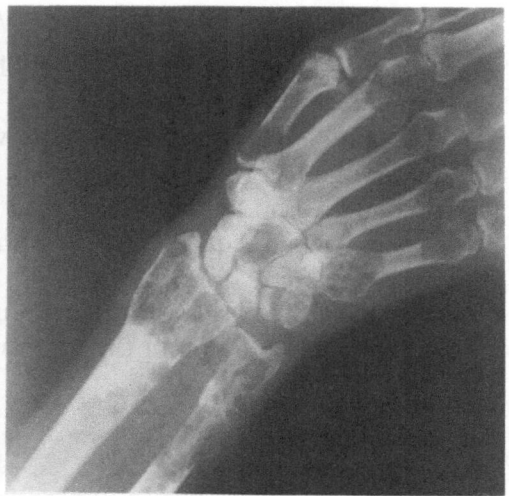

Fig. 27   Fig. 28

Fig. 27. Multiple myeloma involving skull and mandible: Note multiple, punched-out lesions in calvarium and involving mandible. Mandibular involvement is rare in metastatic lesions

Fig. 28. Multiple myeloma involving distal arm: Note multiple, punched-out lesions distorting normal architecture of all visualized bones

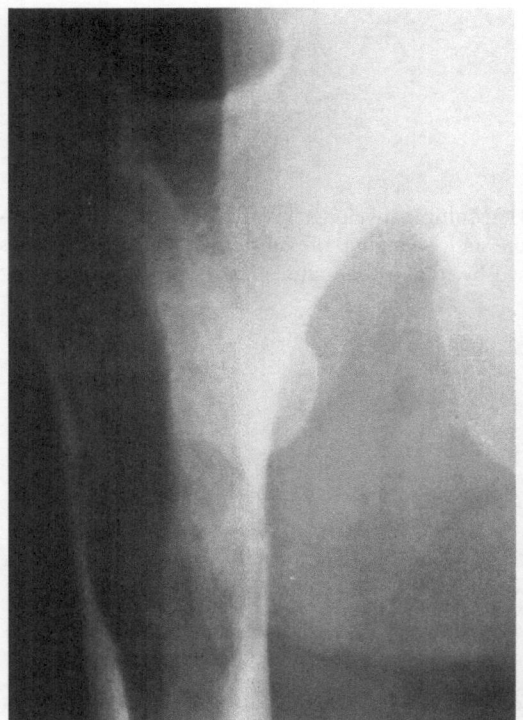 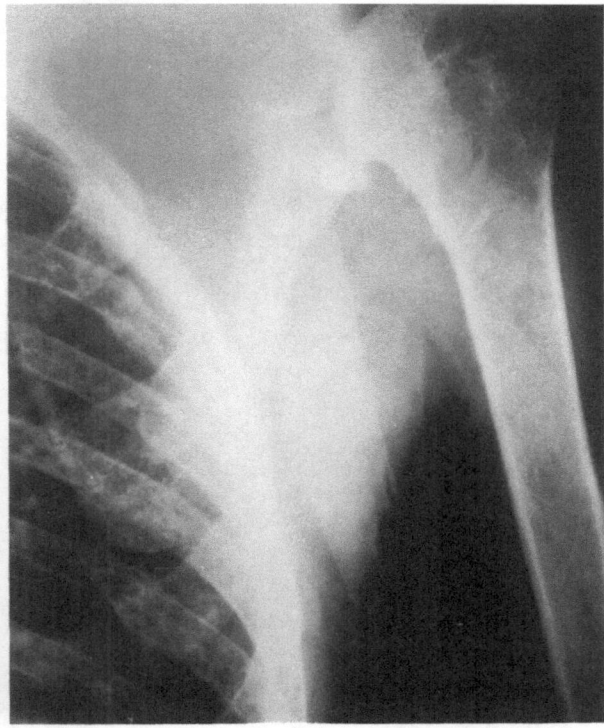

Fig. 29   Fig. 30

Fig. 29. Multiple myeloma of upper femur: This large, centrally placed, lytic lesion with cortical destruction resembles solitary myeloma — except this male patient had multiple, punched-out lesions elsewhere in the skeleton

Fig. 30. Multiple myeloma of ribs and upper humerus: Note honeycomb pattern of rib with multiple, odl pathologic fractures and expansion of a number of ribs

b) Expansile Lytic Areas

1. Single multilocular soap bubble or cystic pattern resembling that of a solitary myeloma (Fig. 29).

2. Multiple honeycomb pattern with expansion of the cortex occurs particularly in the ribs and sternum (Figs. 30, 31).

3. Purely destructive lesions with ill-defined margins which appear to burst out of the bone—most frequently seen in the metaphysis of long bones and the rami of the pelvis (Fig. 32).

4. Endosteal erosions with clear-cut margins and destruction of the overlying cortex. These are very common in the disseminated form of multiple myeloma (Fig. 33).

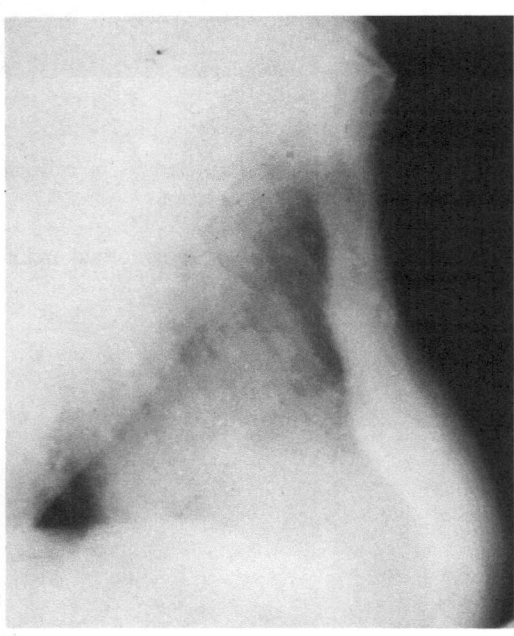

Fig. 31. Multiple myeloma involving sternum: Note expansion and widening of substernal soft-tissue planes caused by total myelomatous involvement of sternum

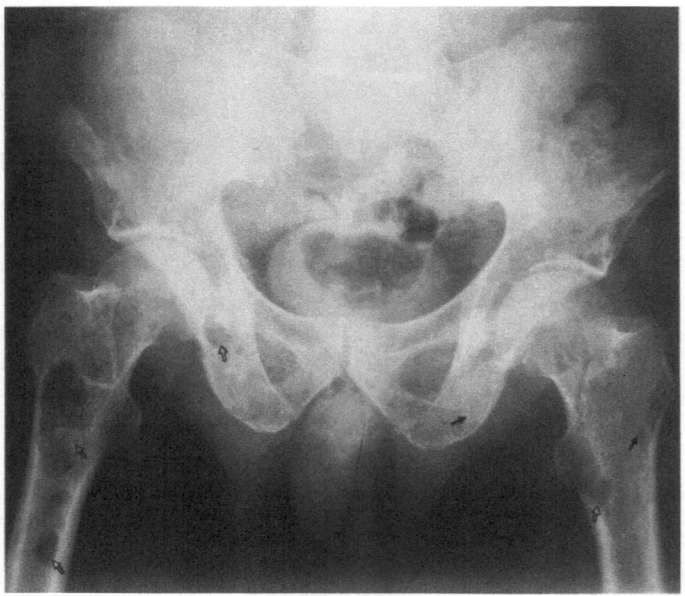

Fig. 32. Multiple myeloma: Widespread involvement of all visualized bones with destruction and expansion of both cancellous and cortical bones (*arrows*)

c) Generalized Osteoporosis

This occurs particularly in the young male patient and is caused by a generalized increase in osteoclastic activity with the patient frequently presenting with back pain. Radiologically this type of osteoporosis is usually visible earliest in the lumbar region of the spine where there may be associated compression fractures of the vertebral bodies (Fig. 34).

d) Pathologic Fractures

Some 50% of patients with multiple myeloma have pathologic fractures—most frequently of the vertebral bodies (Fig. 35). But they do occur in long bones, although there is rarely any evidence of callus formation and the fracture rarely heals spontaneously. However, following local radiotherapy, there may be regression of the tumor with healing and eventual callus formation.

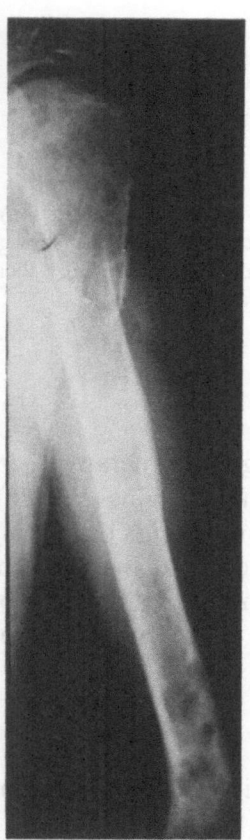

Fig. 33. Multiple myeloma: Widespread lytic areas with pathologic fracture of upper humerus. Note apparent expansion and destruction of normal cortex produced by many of the lesions

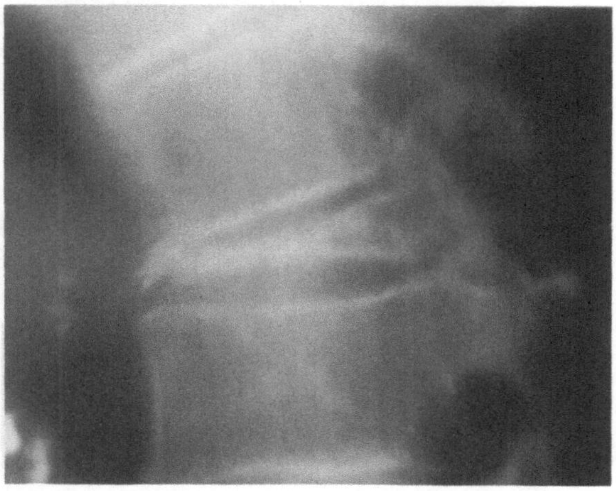

Fig. 34. Multiple myeloma—osteoporosis: This man of 45 was followed for 3 years by a nutritionist before this vertebra collapsed and patient developed Bence-Jones proteinuria

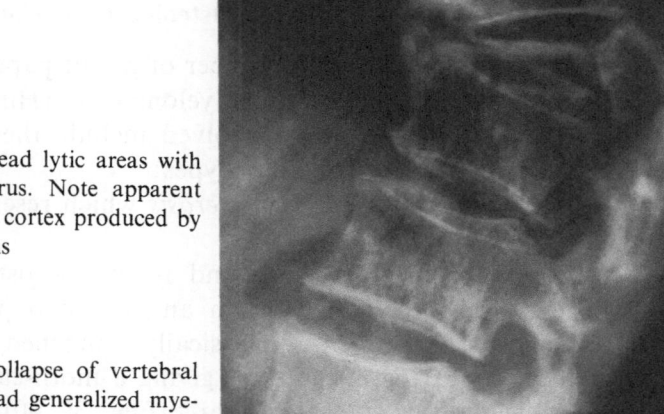

Fig. 35. Multiple myeloma—total collapse of vertebral body: This man of 65 with widespread generalized myeloma complained of pain in his back. Total collapse of anterior part of vertebral body with maintenance of posterior part (and pedicles) is typical of myeloma

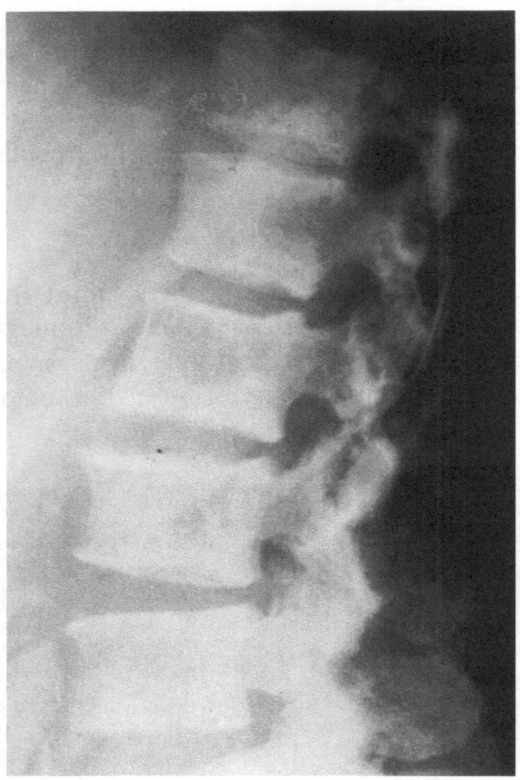

Fig. 36. Multiple myeloma—effects of radiotherapy: Spine in this patient with widespread myeloma showed patchy increase in bone density following local radiotherapy

2. Mixed Osteolytic and Osteoblastic Lesions

These are very rare in untreated myeloma, although following radiotherapy there is often some attempt at healing and lucent areas may develop sclerotic margins (Fig. 36). Rarely a moth-eaten or mottled appearance may be seen in the skull in patients presenting with myeloma without treatment. Presumably this reflects the widespread involvement of the calvarium with surrounding osteoblastic activity. Another mixed lesion may be due to a periosteal reaction and this occurs very rarely and will be discussed in the next group of lesions.

3. Purely Osteoblastic Lesions

These are also rare, although a number of recent papers have highlighted the occurrence of primary sclerotic lesions in myelomatosis (HIMMELFARB et al., 1974; PETCH, 1971; LOWBEER, 1969). The bones involved include the ribs, vertebrae, sternum, and pelvis. There are a number of different types:

Diffuse, generalized, uniform osteosclerosis which resembles myelosclerosis or hemolytic anemia (Fig. 37).

Diffuse patchy sclerosis also rare and resembles osteoblastic metastases (Fig. 38).

Diffuse sclerosis with lucent areas in an untreated patient. This is more common and the lucencies may be large and classically "punched out" lesions, or may be small areas particularly occurring in the skull giving a moth-eaten appearance. However, this situation is exaggerated by fluoride therapy (Figs. 39, 40).

Localized sclerotic lesions are excessively rare and impossible to differentiate from a solitary metastasis.

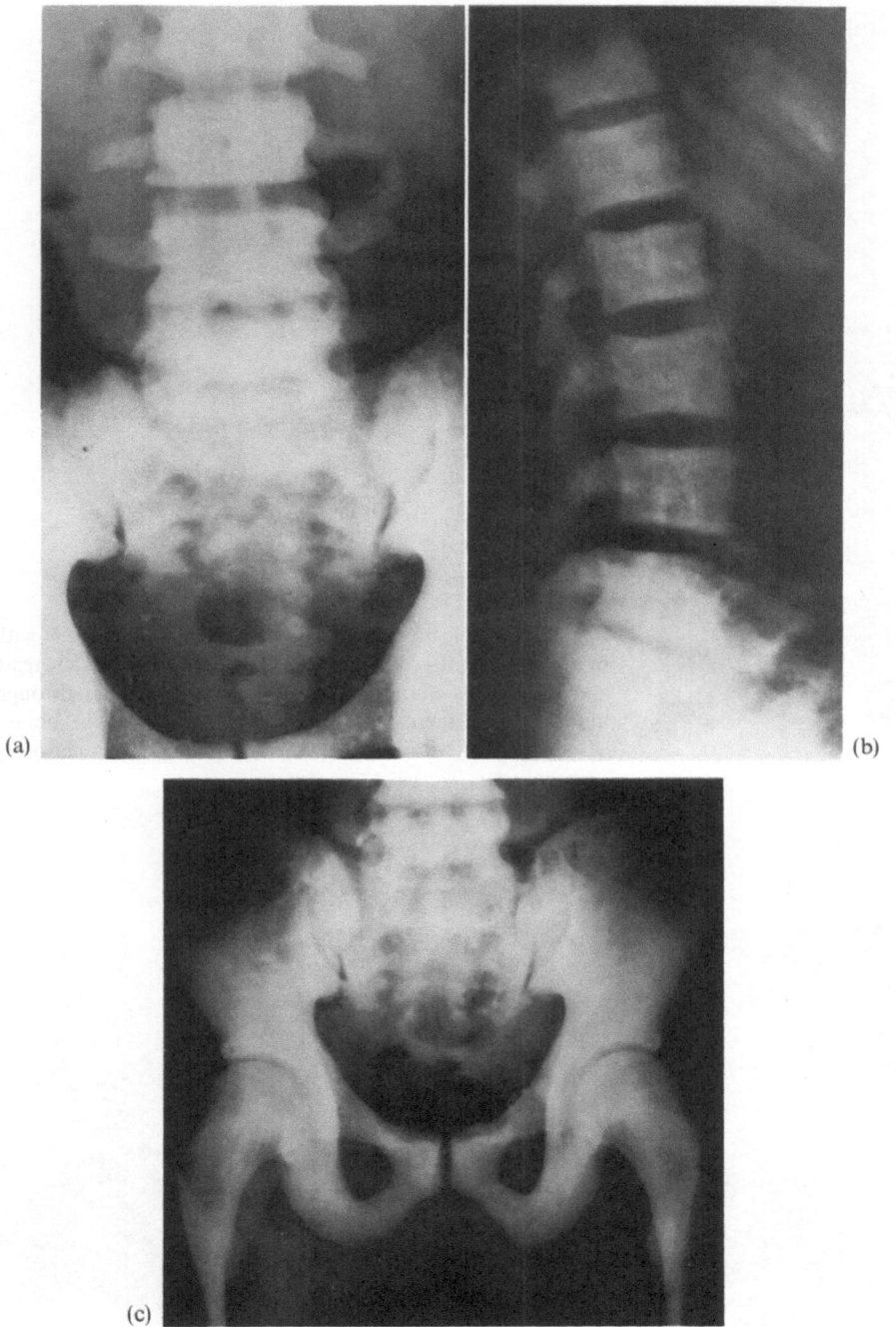

Fig. 37. Multiple myeloma—widespread osteoblastic response without therapy: this 71-year-old black man developed generalized increased density in all visualized bones (a) lumbar spine—AP view, (b) lumbar spine— lateral film, (c) pelvis

Periosteal new bone formation may occur in solitary myeloma, but is otherwise very rare in multiple myeloma.

"Shaggy dog" myeloma is a curiosity and also excessively rare. It represents an intense periosteal reaction occurring perpendicularly to the long axis of the bone, and has only been described in very widespread bone disease in myelomatosis (Fig. 41).

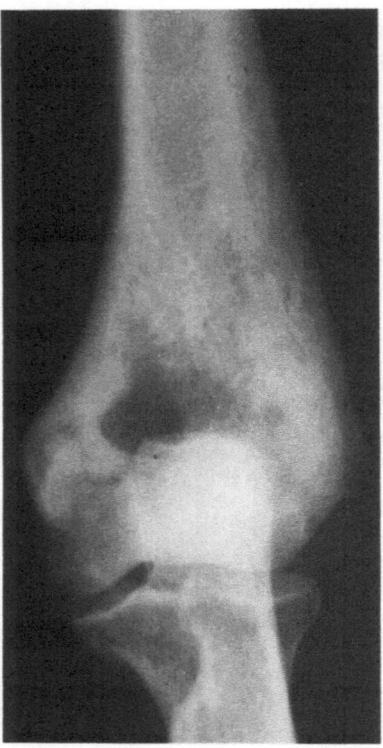

Fig. 38. Multiple myeloma—patchy osteoblastic response without therapy: This 50-year-old patient developed rapidly widespread myeloma and pain in his elbow. There are discrete lucencies throughout lower humerus, and there is a diffuse patchy increase in bone density in same area. At autopsy these were found to be due to myeloma

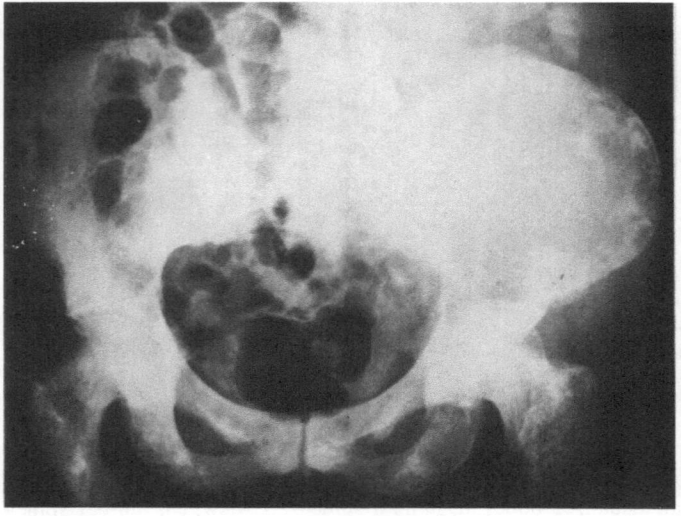

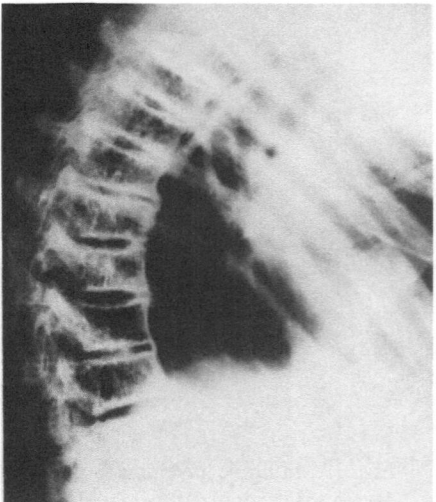

Fig. 39   Fig. 40

Fig. 39. Multiple myeloma—effects of fluoride therapy: This patient with severe myeloma was on high doses of fluoride for 2 years which enhanced density of normal bone. However, the disease progressed rapidly and multiple, small, punched-out lucencies can be seen, as well as a large destructive area in the left iliac bone

Fig. 40. Multiple myeloma—effects of fluoride therapy: This elderly female patient received fluoride therapy for many years. Note enhancement of remaining trabeculae, as well as punched-out lucencies throughout spine

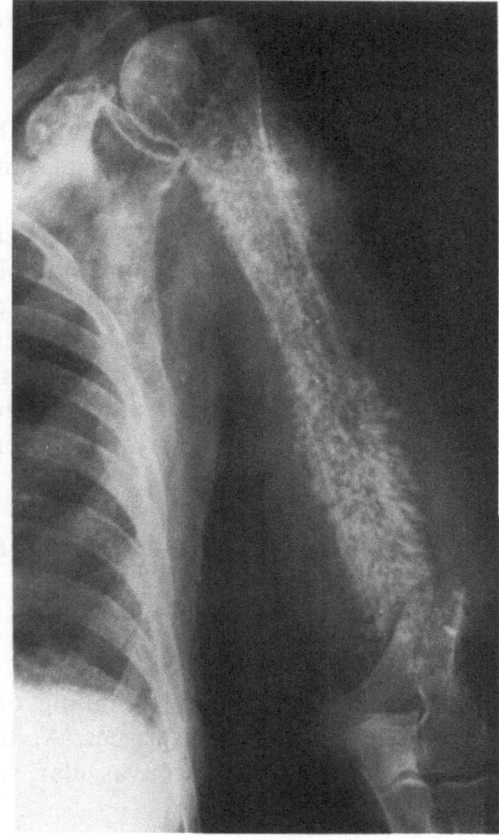

41

Fig. 41. "Shaggy Dog" myeloma: This elderly patient with widespread myeloma developed this intense, right-angled spiculated periosteal reaction, and finally a pathologic fracture occurred through lower humerus. This appearance is result of intense periosteal osteoblastic response to underlying tumor

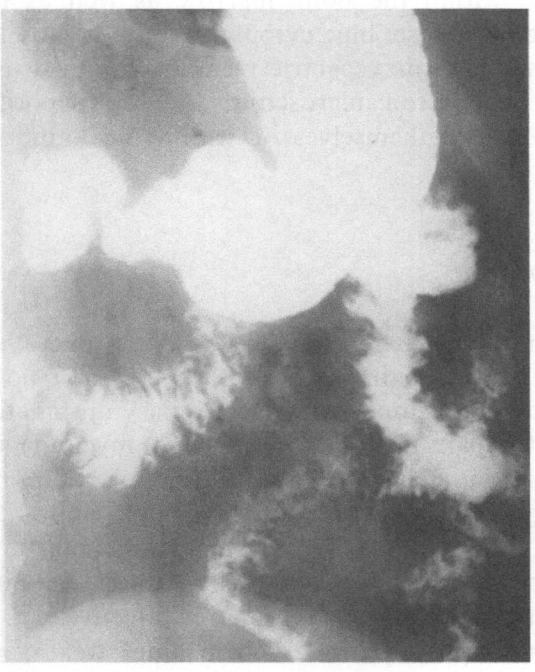

Fig. 42

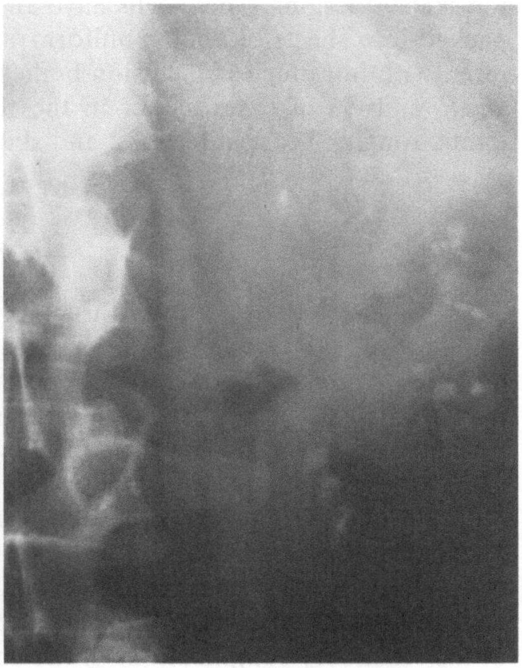

Fig. 43

Fig. 42. Amyloid of intestine: This 60-year-old male patient with longstanding myeloma developed malabsorption syndrome and these intestinal changes. Note irregularity of jejunal mucosa, which is nonspecific. On autopsy patient was found to have widespread amyloid deposits in lungs, kidneys, heart, and intestine

Fig. 43. Amyloid of kidney: Note generalized enlargement as well as nephrocalcinosis in kidney of this 77-year-old male patient with longstanding myeloma

4. Other Radiologic Features

Other radiologic features include the presence of a soft-tissue mass, either adjacent to a long bone lesion or occurring as an increase in the paraspinal shadows. The presence of a soft-tissue mass adjacent to a long bone lesion is more common in multiple myeloma than in metastases and may be used as a method of differentiation between the two.

The lungs are involved in about half the patients with myelomatosis—often with recurrent pneumonias or with diffuse plasma cell infiltrates which are usually terminal. The liver is enlarged in 40% of patients and there is splenomegaly in one-quarter of patients with myeloma. Amyloidosis may involve the heart causing cardiomegaly, the intestine (Fig. 42), giving rise to malabsorption syndromes and characteristic radiologic appearances, and the kidneys where renal failure often ensues (see Fig. 43).

VIII. Pathology

1. Gross

Multiple myeloma is a malignant reticulosis with focal neoplastic proliferation of plasma cells which causes thinning of bone with eventual erosion of the cortex and spread into adjacent soft tissues. At this stage, pathologic fractures are common. The tumor is reddish-gray, nonvascular, soft, and very cellular. It resembles lymphoma.

2. Microscopic

There are abnormal cells (myeloma cells) within the bone marrow as well as in the skeletal lesions. These cells have an abundant, dense, blue cytoplasm and are closely packed into sheets of almost uniform size. They have an eccentric pleomorphic nucleus, often with intranuclear inclusion bodies seen on electron microscopy. Amyloid deposits occur in 10% of cases, either in the tumor masses themselves or within the kidneys, joints, tongue, heart, intestines, and skin.

IX. Treatment

As in most bone tumors, the therapy for multiple myeloma has evolved over the last 50 years and whereas surgery used to be the main form of therapy, it is now only rarely used—and then only to excise a solitary lesion in an otherwise asymptomatic patient. Radiotherapy is particularly useful for painful bone lesions since myeloma is very radiosensitive, and recently Bergsagel (1971) has advocated total body irradiation.

However, the treatment of choice currently is chemotherapy, and although a number of agents has been tried over the years, a combination of 1 phenylalanine mustard (Melphalan), prednisone, and procarbazine produces a 59% response rate (Alexanian et al., 1972). Long-term cyclophosphamide also appears to be reasonably effective.

The current therapy for a patient with multiple myeloma also includes treatment of the secondary complications of the condition such as anemia, renal failure, infections, and fractures. Treatment of the various metabolic disturbances is also important, and hisodium hydrogen phosphate (10 g/day) is advocated for the hypercalcemia of myelomatosis. Of patients with multiple myeloma, 4% develop a hyperviscosity syndrome (decreasing vision, coma, congestive cardiac failure, renal failure, and hemorrhage) which is relieved by plasmaphoresis.

A discussion of the treatment for multiple myeloma would not be complete without mention of the use of fluoride (COHEN, 1966). Apart from the generalized increase in bone density because of the morphologic alterations in the hydroxyapatite crystal which fluoride produces, fluoride is probably more dangerous than useful (CARBONE et al., 1968; HARLEY et al., 1971). Some authorities still advocate small doses of fluoride plus vitamin D and calcium for bone pain. Its efficacy is unproven.

X. Prognosis

Multiple myeloma has a varied prognosis which depends on the rate of tumor growth and its spread (MALPAS, 1974). There is some evidence to suggest that the prognosis depends on the differentiation within the lesion itself — and that of patients with poorly differentiated lesions, 75% were dead in 2 years whereas those tumors that are well differentiated have a better prognosis — with $3^1/_2$ years being the average survival rate (NORDENSON, 1966). However, this is very controversial and some authorities disagree (COHEN et al., 1964). The presence of Bence-Jones proteinuria in association with renal failure gives a poor prognosis, as does a poor response to therapy as shown by immunoglobulin levels (JOHANSSON, 1971). A better prognosis is suggested when the initial presenting feature of multiple myeloma is generalized osteoporosis.

However, the overall 5-year survival rate is about 20%. The cause of death in 48 patients being infections (particularly pneumonia) (31%), cardiopulmonary complications 17%, uremia 2%, myeloma 6%, and hemorrhage 8% (WINTROBE, 1967).

The 5-year survival rate of solitary plasmacytoma is much higher — in the region of 60%. However, it must be remembered that these solitary lesions inevitably become multiple and disseminated with a concomitantly poor 5-year survival rate.

Two complications of myeloma will be mentioned separately, (1) renal disease, and (2) amyloid.

1. Renal Disease in Multiple Myeloma

The patient with renal involvement in myelomatosis presents with an intense proteinuria (15–20 g/day). This usually signifies the presence of recurrent renal infections in association with collections of actual myeloma cells in the renal parenchyma. Amyloidosis of the kidney also occurs in 5–15% of patients with myelomatosis. Renal failure will frequently supervene, mainly due to renal casts obstructing the tubules (often the loops of Henle), but also due to precipitation of proteins and tubular atrophy. Calcium deposition may occur in both the tubules and in the casts themselves. It is obvious that matters will get considerably worse on dehydration and a patient in incipient renal failure due to sludging in the tubules, may be pushed over the brink into total failure by withholding fluids. Thus when intravenous pyelography required dehydration, a number of patients inadvertently died because of the deposition of this abnormal protein in the renal tubules. If intravenous pyelography is considered essential today, a patient with multiple myeloma may safely undergo this radiologic procedure on condition they receive adequate hydration — even to the extent of giving extra fluids (Fig. 43).

2. Amyloid

Some 10–15% of patients with myeloma develop amyloidosis, and it is a well-known but poorly understood complication of myeloma. The distribution of amyloid deposits in myeloma resembles that of primary amyloidosis, hence the differential diagnosis be-

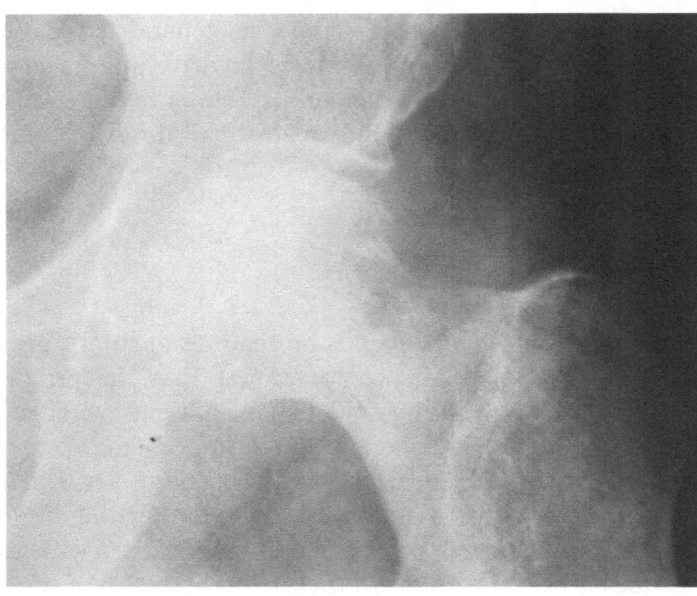

Fig. 44. Amyloid of hips: This elderly patient developed multiple myeloma 5 months before she had pain in her left hip. Large destructive lesion with poorly defined margins on superior surface of femoral neck is typical of amyloid of bone

tween primary amyloid and secondary amyloid in myeloma is often impossible (HIMMEL-FARB et al., 1974). Apart from cardiomegaly, hepatosplenomegaly and amyloid deposits adjacent to the intestine, amyloid may be deposited in the bone. Its characteristic appearance is that of a destructive lesion in the metaphyseal region of a long bone—particularly in the upper femur (Fig. 44). The amyloid substance is probably excreted by the reticuloendothelial cells and cases of amyloid may demonstrate elevated IgG, IgA, and IgM levels as well as Bence-Jones proteinuria. Thus, there appears to be considerable overlap between amyloidósis and myeloma.

XI. Differential Diagnosis

The differential diagnosis between multiple myeloma and metastases (particularly from breast and thyroid) may be difficult, although there are some helpful pointers:

1. myeloma involves intervertebral discs and metastases usually do not,
2. myeloma often has a soft-tissue mass associated with it,
3. myeloma is rare in the pedicles of the vertebrae, whereas metastases commonly involve this area,
4. myeloma is common in the mandible but metastases are rare (Fig. 27).

The more benign-appearing myeloma deposits may resemble lesions of sarcoid or eosinophilic granuloma, and the sclerotic type of myeloma may resemble lymphoma, fluorosis, myelosclerosis, mastocytosis, and osteoblastic metastases (e.g., prostate).

Histologically myeloma may have to be differentiated from an inflammatory process but the latter will have fibrosis and vascularization will be present, whereas myeloma will not demonstrate either of these features.

The differential diagnosis of solitary plasmacytoma is the same as above apart from the benign-appearing metaphyseal expansile lesion which may look identical to a giant cell tumor, an aneurysmal bone cyst, or a brown tumor of hyperparathyroidism.

D. Lymphoma of Bone

I. Introduction

Both lymphosarcoma and Hodgkin's disease are primary neoplasms of the lymphatic and hematopoetic systems. Involvement of the skeleton occurs secondarily and may either be by direct extension or due to hematogenous dissemination. There seems to be a likelihood that Hodgkin's disease is either virus-induced or represents a true immunologic disorder. It has been postulated that the body's normal T cells (immunocompetent thymus derived lymphocytes) react against other T cells which have been altered by an infection to produce a neoplastic histiocyte (Reed-Sternberg cell). It is of interest that there is a relationship between high doses of corticosteroids and an increased risk of lymphoma – particularly post renal transplantation where the risk is 200 times normal.

Although the first description of Hodgkin's disease involving bone was made in 1911 by ZIEGLER, there is little agreement as to the incidence of osseous involvement in lymphoma. In Hodgkin's disease the incidence of radiologically visible skeletal lesions appears to vary from 34% (UHLINGER, 1933) to 10% (GRANGER and WHITAKER, 1967) with a mean value of about 15% (DRESSER and SPENCER, 1936; FUCILLA and HAMANN, 1961; VIETA et al., 1942; and GOLDING, 1959). But EWING (1940), in his classic work on the subject points out that at autopsy most patients with longstanding Hodgkin's disease will have osseous lesions. Hodgkin's disease involves the skeleton at a late stage of the condition, whereas bone lesions in lymphosarcoma may appear early in the clinical course of the disease.

Although the current method of staging Hodgkin's disease lies outside the scope of this book, a simplified system is given by AISENBERG (1973).

Stage I — Hodgkin's disease only involves a single lymph node region or organ
Stage II — means that two or more organs and/or node regions are involved on the same side of the diaphragm
Stage III — signifies that the disease has spread to involve both sides of the diaphragm
Stage IV — refers to diffuse or disseminated involvement of extralymphatic organs; for example, bones.

II. Incidence

Table 7 outlines the incidence of involvement of the skeleton in Hodgkin's disease according to a number of authors. COLES and SCHULZ (1948) give an incidence of 21% of bone involvement in systemic reticulum cell sarcoma, 13% in Hodgkin's disease,

Table 7. Incidence of osseous involvement in Hodgkin's disease

1. UEHLINGER (1933)	34% of	50 patients
2. STUHLBARG and ELLIS (1965)	19% of	158 patients
3. CRAVER and COPELAND (1934)	16% of	172 patients
4. VIETA et al. (1942)	15% of	257 patients
5. GOLDING (1959)	14% of	1,525 patients
6. HORAN (1969)	14% of	201 patients
7. FUCILLA and HAMANN (1961)	12% of	94 patients
8. DRESSER and SPENCER (1936)	11% of	172 patients
9. GRANGER and WHITAKER (1967)	10% of	951 patients

and 12% in lymphosarcoma; whereas Vieta et al. (1942) found that x-ray changes of Hodgkin's disease were present in 15% of their patients and in 7% of patients with lymphosarcoma.

The two forms of spread are related to the prognosis of the diseases as well as to the radiologic features. Those cases in which the skeleton has direct extension from contiguous lymph nodes have a better prognosis (Pear, 1974). But those patients with hematogenous spread (mainly from the para-aortic lymph nodes via the spleen into the blood and thence into the bone marrow) may have few radiologic features because bone marrow involvement may be all that has occurred, although widespread marrow involvement will suggest a worse prognosis.

III. Age

There appear to be two distinct peak ages at which lymphoma occurs, but the age range is from 14 to 70 years. Lymphosarcoma occurs in generally older patients (peak 52–56, mean 48), but those with skeletal involvement are somewhat younger (peak 32–36, mean 37); whereas Hodgkin's disease with or without skeletal lesions has a peak incidence in the midtwenties (20–24) with a mean of 34 years.

IV. Sex

The sex incidence of lymphoma is equal for both Hodgkin's disease and lymphosarcoma, although in Granger's (1967) group of over 900 patients, the ratio was male to female 2:1.

V. Bones Involved

Lymphoma of bone will involve the marrow-containing bones predominantly — namely vertebrae, pelvis, ribs, sternum, shoulder girdles, and upper femurs. Of patients with Hodgkin's disease, 91% have involvement of the lymph nodes. Lymphosarcoma is inclined to have a more generalized distribution with less involvement of lymph nodes

Table 8. Involvement of various parts of the skeleton in Hodgkin's disease and lymphosarcoma

	Hodgkin's disease[a] in %	Lymphosarcoma[b] in %
Spine	47	23
Pelvis	14	8
Long bones	10	31
Ribs/sternum	23	27
Clavicle	2	3
Scapula	2	3
Skull	2	5
Multiple sites	65	60
Lymph nodes	91	60

[a] Taken from 810 patients reported in the literature in which the site is given
[b] Taken from Vieta et al. (1942).

(60% of cases), but a higher proportion of cases have involvement of the GI tract (21%) than in Hodgkin's disease.

Table 8 is a summary of the bones involved in lymphoma of the skeleton. Of patients with skeletal involvement in Hodgkin's disease, 65% have lesions in multiple bones, as opposed to 60% of patients with lymphosarcoma.

VI. Clinical Presentation

Often the clinical signs and symptoms of lymphoma involving the osseous system precede the radiologic features by many months, but it may take years before the characteristic lytic areas of destruction can be seen in the skeleton. The most usual clinical presentation is of localized pain which may be intermittent or persistent. This is often accompanied by tenderness on pressure and there is usually either local swelling or a palpable mass present. If the lymphoma involves the spine, then neurologic deficits may also occur. There are also usually generalized constitutional changes, such as fever, sweats, and chills which are accompanied by the appropriate laboratory changes.

VII. Laboratory Data

Most patients with lymphoma have a leukocytosis which will turn into a leukopenia following therapy. There is often also a secondary anemia. However, the only laboratory investigation of interest in skeletal involvement by lymphoma is the alkaline phosphatase level. VIETA et al. (1942) found that 73% of patients with radiologically visible skeletal lesions in Hodgkin's disease had an elevated alkaline phosphatase, as opposed to elevation in 58% of cases without osseous involvement. Similarly, in lymphosarcoma 62% had an elevated alkaline phosphatase with involvement of the skeleton in comparison to 33% without any bone lesions. The serum alkaline phosphatase is related to osteoblastic activity, so that elevation of the level above normal does occur in a large number of conditions other than malignancy (WOODARD and CRAVER, 1940).

VIII. Radiologic Features

The radiologic features of lymphoma will vary depending on whether the skeletal involvement is from direct extension or from dissemination into the blood stream. Since there are also differences between lymphosarcoma and Hodgkin's disease, these will be considered separately.

1. Lymphosarcoma

The skeletal lesions in lymphosarcoma are generally due to dissemination and are more often purely destructive.

Destructive osteolytic lesions occur in 85% of cases of lymphsarcoma involving the skeleton. The lesions are frequently multiple and often more extensive and invasive than lytic lesions in Hodgkin's disease. They may be large and geographic or highly aggressive, permeative, "moth-eaten" lesions (Figs. 45, 46, 47).

Mixed osteolytic and osteoblastic lesions are rare, in 10% (Fig. 48).

Pure osteoblastic lesions are extremely uncommon, only 5% and may not occur in pure lymphosarcoma.

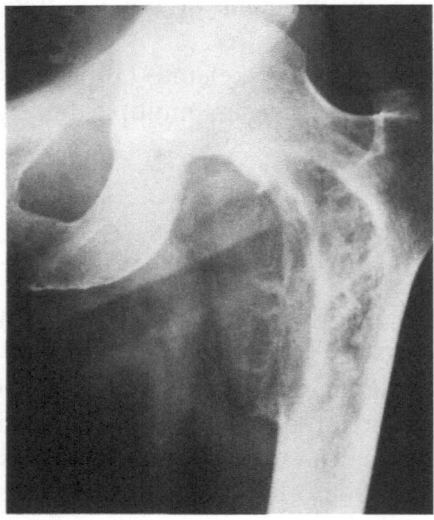
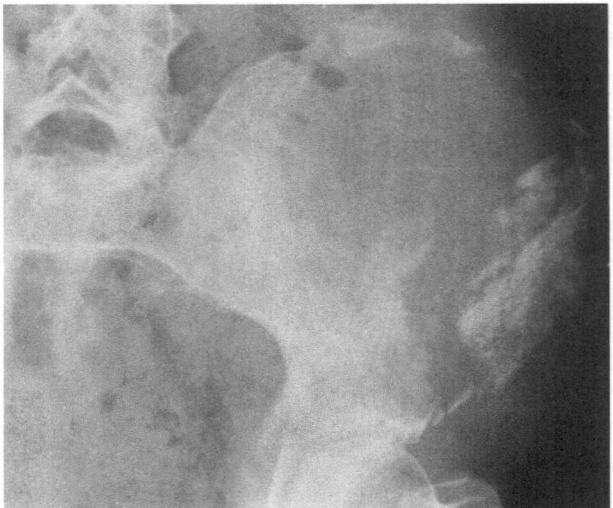

Fig. 45   Fig. 46

Fig. 45. Lymphosarcoma—femur: Solitary osteolytic destructive lesion invading soft-tissue in region of lesser trochanter. On biopsy this proved to be lymphosarcoma

Fig. 46. Lymphosarcoma—pelvis: Osteolytic destructive lesion causing dissolution and expansion of the left iliac wing in this 45-year-old female patient with widespread lymphosarcoma

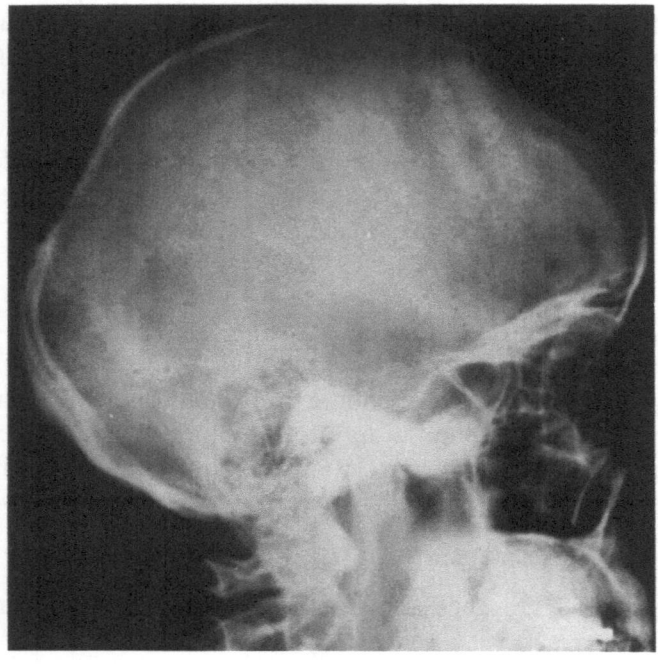

Fig. 47. Lymphosarcoma—skull: Osteolytic destructive lesion on posterior aspect of vault of the skull in this 46-year-old male with widespread lymphosarcoma

Pathologic fractures are more common than in Hodgkin's disease, particularly in the spine. Vertebral lesions—compression fractures of the vertebrae—are more common and complete than those which occur in Hodgkin's disease (Fig. 49).

Periosteal reaction is rare, but may occur in lymphosarcoma involving long bones (see Fig. 45).

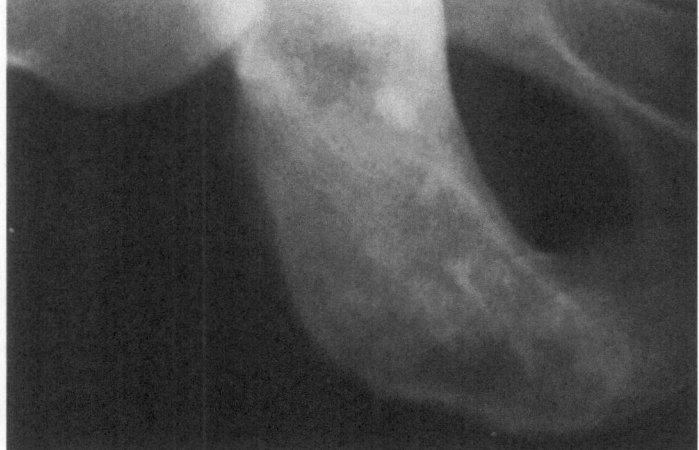

Fig. 48. Lymphosarcoma—mixed osteolytic and osteoblastic lesions in ischial ramus: This young male patient presented with pain in buttock. On biopsy this was found to be lymphosarcoma

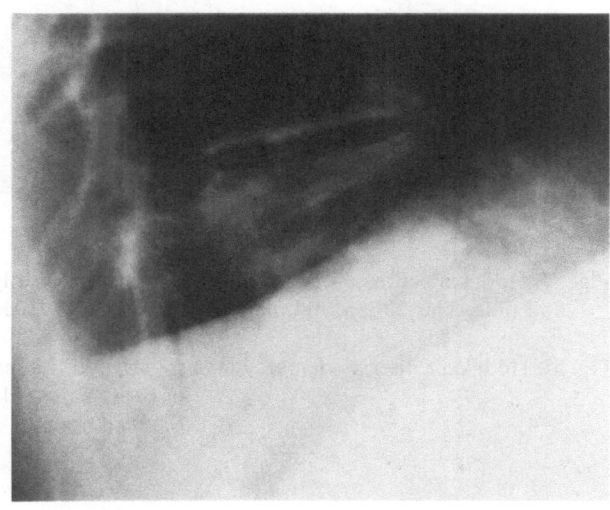

Fig. 49. Lymphosarcoma—vertebra: Note the almost total collapse of vertebral body in this severely osteopenic spine. At autopsy, all vertebral bodies were found to be invaded by lymphosarcoma

2. Hodgkin's Disease

Multiple osseous lesions occur in about two-thirds of cases of Hodgkin's disease and pure lytic lesions are considerably rarer than in lymphosarcoma; whereas pure sclerotic lesions, particularly those involving the vertebral bodies (ivory vertebra), are far more common than in lymphosarcoma.

Destructive osteolytic lesions are more predominant in the pelvis where they are less sharply circumscribed and often diffuse. In addition, there may be expansion of the bone, particularly occurring in the ribs and sternum. Purely lytic lesions accounted for 28% of cases in VIETA's et al. (1942) series (Figs. 50, 51).

In the pelvis, Hodgkin's disease produces multiple lytic geographic areas with marginal sclerosis particularly occurring in the region of the sacroiliac joints, possibly as a result of contiguous spread from the para-aortic nodes (Fig. 52). In the ribs and sternum, Hodgkin's disease produces destructive expansatile lesions which often have some form of periosteal reaction and in fact more than 90% of Hodgkin's disease lesions in the ribs are purely lytic (GRANGER and WHITAKER, 1967).

Mixed osteolytic and osteoblastic lesions are the most common lesions seen in Hodgkin's disease involving the skeleton (60% in VIETA's et al. series, 1942). These lesions

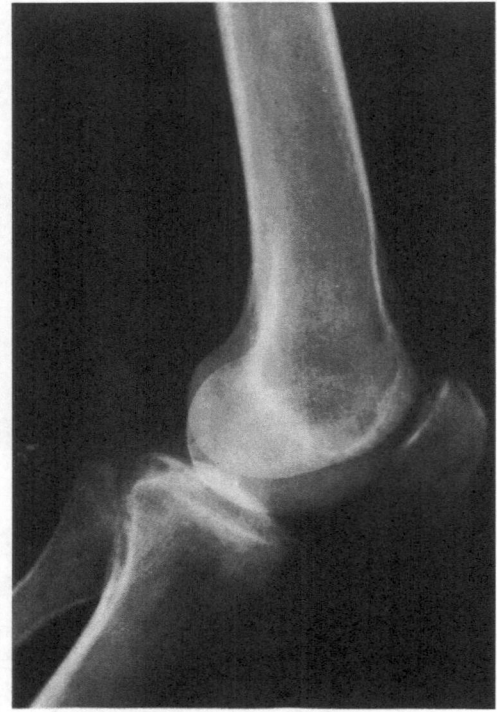 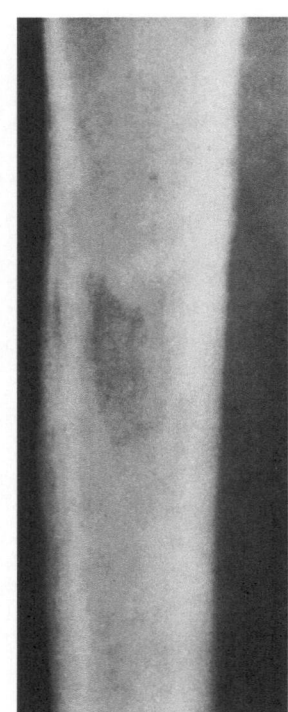

Fig. 50   Fig. 51

Fig. 50. Hodgkin's disease—knee: Multiple poorly defined lytic areas can be seen, particularly in upper fibula and tibia. This 28-year-old male patient had Stage III Hodgkin's disease until he developed knee pain

Fig. 51. Hodgkin's disease—femur: Large solitary lytic lesion in diaphysis of a long bone. There is a suggestion of early periosteal reaction

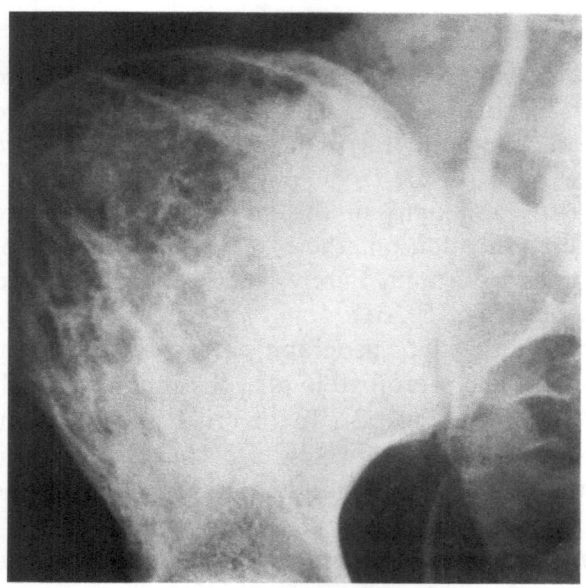

Fig. 52. Hodgkin's disease—pelvis: Patchy osteolytic areas are present in iliac crest in this young male patient. Note surrounding osteoblastic reaction, particularly in region of right sacroiliac joint

are irregular in outline, often with poorly demarcated margins with gradual transition into normal bone (Figs. 53, 54). In long bones, these lesions may have sharp demarcation but there is no involvement of either cartilaginous surfaces or intervertebral discs. Although the classical lesion in the spine is the "ivory vertebra," mixed osteolytic osteoblastic lesions of the vertebral column are in fact more common. But it is important to note that collapse of involved vertebrae in Hodgkin's disease is considerably more rare

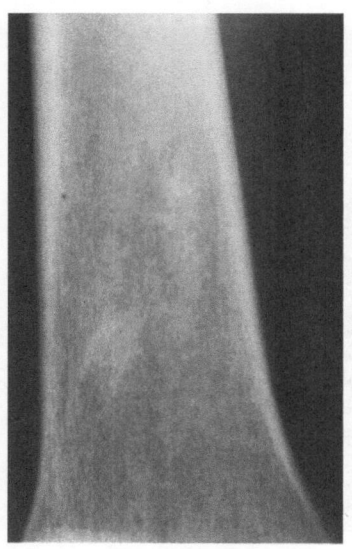 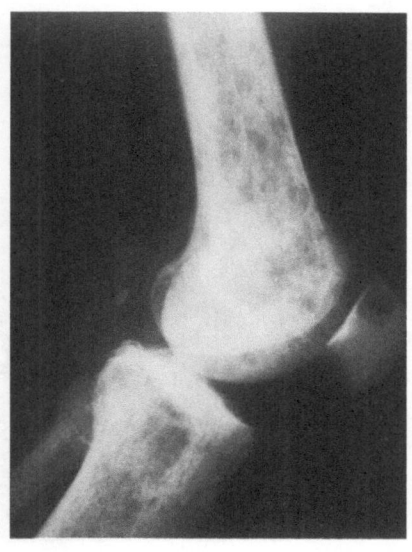

Fig. 53   Fig. 54

Fig. 53. Hodgkin's disease—lower femur: Small, poorly defined lytic and blastic lesion in metaphysis of left femur was only radiologic evidence of skeletal involvement in this 36-year-old male patient with mediastinal node involvement

Fig. 54. Hodgkin's disease—knee: Mixed osteolytic and osteoblastic lesions in lower femur and upper tibia were caused by widespread involvement of skeleton in this young patient with Hodgkin's disease

Fig. 55. Hodgkin's disease—vertebral bodies: This female patient of 45 developed pain in the back and this anterior scalloping of L4 and L5. There was a fluffy periosteal reaction and sclerosis of remaining vertebral bodies, and on biopsy this lesion was found to be due to Hodgkin's disease with widespread para-aortic node involvement in this region

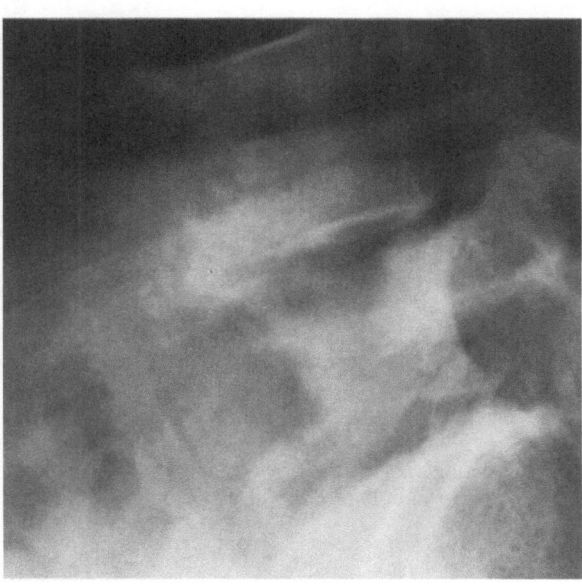

than in lymphosarcoma or in metastatic disease and this fact may help in the differential diagnosis of a lesion in the spine.

A characteristic, but rare vertebral lesion described by both GRANGER and WHITAKER (1967), and PEAR (1974) is scalloping of the anterior margin of the vertebral body with a fluffy periosteal reaction and this is due to contiguous spread via the para-aortic nodes. It occurs in Hodgkin's disease, lymphosarcoma and leukemia, but is never seen in metastases (Fig. 55).

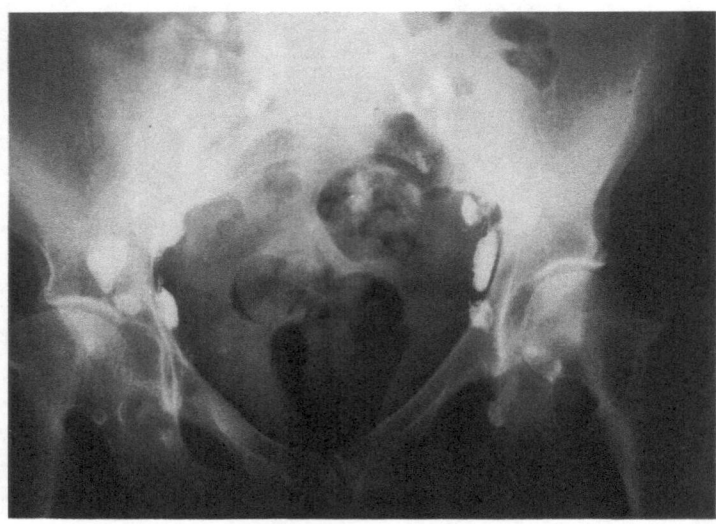

Fig. 56. Hodgkin's disease—lymph nodes and pubic ramus: Large foamy nodes are present in pelvis and para-aortic region. Solitary sclerotic area in right pubic ramus was biopsied and found to be due to Hodgkin's disease

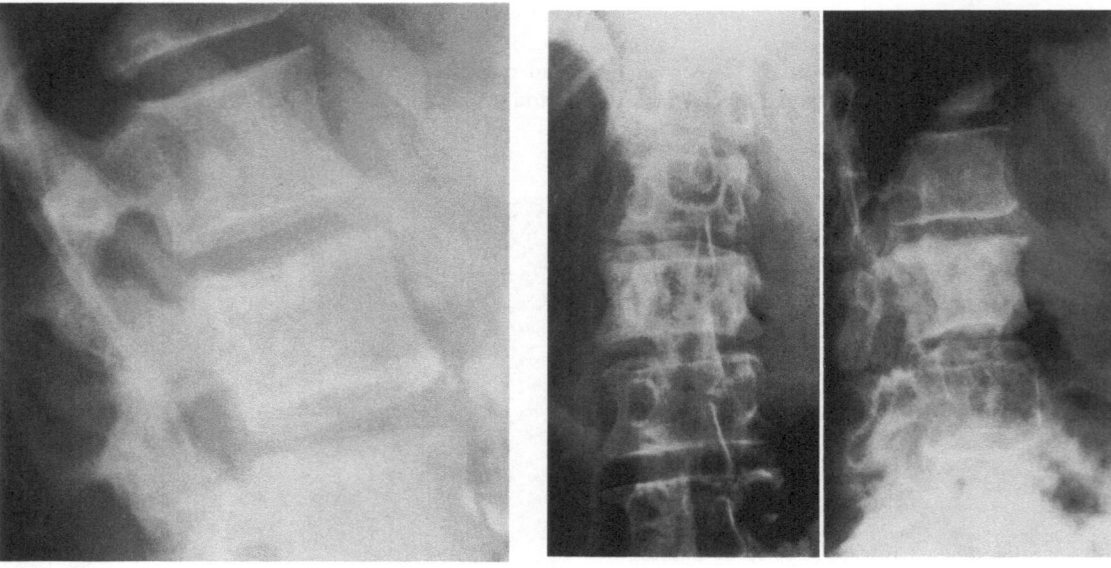

Fig. 57   Fig. 58

Fig. 57. Hodgkin's disease—sclerotic lesions in vertebral bodies: There are a number of poorly defined sclerotic areas in lumbar vertebral bodies which developed in a patient with widespread Hodgkin's disease

Fig. 58. Hodgkin's disease—ivory vertebra: Note overall increase in density of body of L2 (AP+lateral view)

Pure osteoblastic lesions are rare outside the vertebral column in Hodgkin's disease. However, sclerotic lesions are seen in 15% of cases of Hodgkin's disease overall (Fig. 56). In the vertebral body there is a coarse increase in the size and density of the trabeculae, often beginning anteriorly until the whole vertebral body is involved ("ivory vertebra") (Figs. 57, 58). This is often associated with a paraspinal mass (Fig. 59). When sclerotic lesions occur outside the spine, histologically there appear to be nests of neoplastic cells within narrowed marrow spaces and new bone surrounding them. It has been postulated that this reaction is mediated by a hormone (prostaglandin?) (see Table 9).

Pathologic fractures may occur in the ribs in Hodgkin's disease but are very rare in most series. The variety of pathologic compression fractures in the spine has already been discussed.

Periosteal reaction may occur in long bones, but is never lamellated, unlike Ewing's sarcoma, and only rarely spiculated (differential diagnosis—osteogenic sarcoma). Some

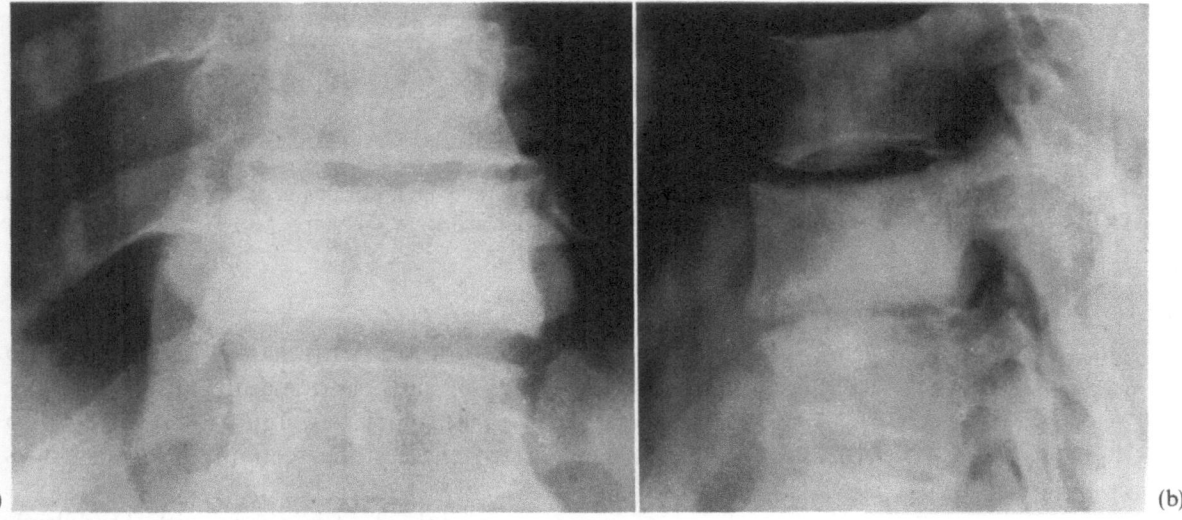

(a)   (b)

Fig. 59. Hodgkin's disease—ivory vertebra with paraspinal soft-tissue mass: Note dense sclerosis involving posterior part of T11 and widening of paraspinal lines. (a) AP film, (b) lateral film

Table 9. Differential diagnosis of an ivory vertebra

I. Paget's disease

There should be enlargement of the bone with particular disorganization of the internal structure (picture-frame vertebra).

II. Blastic metastases

Particularly from prostate in males, and treated breast carcinoma in females (usually with clinical evidence of the primary neoplasm and widespread bone lesions).

III. Hodgkin's disease

Usually associated with periosteal reaction and/or a paravertebral soft-tissue mass. Also often mediastinal and/or paratracheal nodal enlargement.

IV. Hemangioma of vertebra

Vertical linear streaking of widened primary trabeculae, characteristically in an asymptomatic patient.

V. Rare infections

Brucella and salmonella infections are both indolent conditions with exceptionally rare bone involvement and some constitutional signs and symptoms of infection which may produce an ivory vertebra.

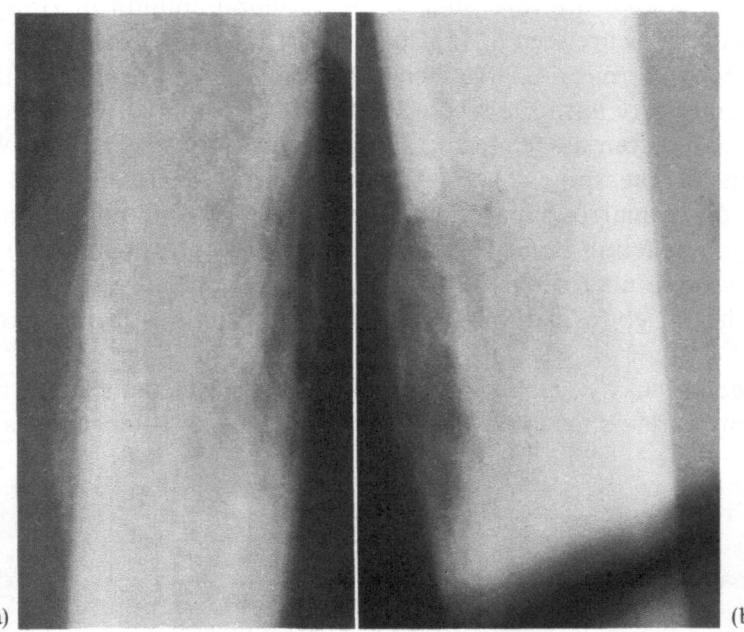

Fig. 60. Hodgkin's disease—upper femur: This infiltrative lesion in upper femur with cortical destruction and posterial reaction was found to be a focus of Hodgkin's disease on biopsy. (a) AP film, (b) oblique film

authors claim that it is very rare, but GRANGER and WHITAKER (1967) found it to be present in 30% of their patients at a total of 43 sites, and mainly at the anterior aspect of the vertebral bodies in association with an ivory vertebra (25%). They also described periosteal reaction in more than half of the lesions seen in the long bones (Fig. 60).

Paravertebral masses may be seen in nearly one-third of patients with Hodgkin's disease involving the spine (particularly in the lower thoracic region) (Fig. 59).

Ligamentous calcification of the anterior longitudinal ligaments of the spine has been reported in two patients by DUNCAN (1973). Some other cases of ligamentous calcification occurring *de novo* have been mentioned in the literature, but most cases of soft-tissue or ligamentous calcification occur after a course of radiotherapy; presumably as a result of dystrophic calcification—a similar process to that producing calcification in lymph nodes after radiotherapy. Both patients had ivory vertebrae and the two may be connected in some way, but it is more likely that this form of ligamentous calcification represents an intense periosteal reaction.

Hypertrophic osteoarthropathy has been reported in association with mediastinal Hodgkin's disease (PEAR, 1974).

IX. Pathologic Features

1. Gross

The lesions in lymphoma vary from microscopic foci to large gray-white or yellow-white nodules occurring in the bone marrow. They may be of a nodular type which is associated with a better prognosis (53% 5-year survival rate).

2. Microscopic

There is a large range of cellular types with varying proportions of endothelial cells, giant cells, lymphocytes (both small and large), plasma cells, and eosinophils. The characteristic feature of Hodgkin's disease is the Reed-Sternberg cell which is from 12 to 40 μ in diameter, with a double mirror-image nucleus, dense chromatin, and large nucleoli.

In lymphosarcoma the characteristic appearance is of sheets of uniform lymphocytes which are often fairly small. The poorly differentiated types of cell in both conditions are associated with a poor prognosis (3% 5-year survival rate).

X. Treatment

The standard treatment for the various forms of lymphoma is radiotherapy with a dose of 3,500–4,000 R over the course of $3^1/_2$–4 weeks, although there is some evidence that total nodal irradiation gives a better 5-year survival rate. However, lymphomatous involvement of bone is largely radio-resistant so that radiotherapy is given mainly for the palliation of pain. An adjunct therapy being used increasingly is chemotherapy—either using a drug such as vinblastine, procarbazine, bleomycin, or prednisone separately, or using them in some combination such as MOPP—nitrogen *M*ustard, *O*ncovin (vincristine), *P*rednisone and *P*rocarbazine—which produces a 100% response rate (AISENBERG, 1973).

XI. Prognosis

The prognosis is related to the cell type and the more poorly differentiated the tumor cell type, the worse the prognosis. The overall 5-year survival rate for lymphosarcoma is between 10 and 15% and there appears to be little difference if the skeleton is involved or not. The overall 5-year survival rate for all forms of Hodgkin's disease in 1950 was 21% male and 29% female, and in 1974 it was 52% male and 56% for women, showing that at least some forms of cancer appear to be manageable (SILVERBERG, 1975).

With regard to Hodgkin's disease, the relationship to cell type and ultimate prognosis has been more clearly worked out (BUTLER, 1971) with the *lymphocytic predominant variety* having the highest 5-year survival rate (73%) down to the *lymphocytic depleted variety* having the poorest prognosis (13%). In Hodgkin's disease it appears that those patients with skeletal involvement have a rather better prognosis, although a number of authors disagree (COLES and SCHULZ, 1948, and PEAR, 1974). STUHLBARG and ELLIS (1965) found a 1-year survival rate of 93% with bone involvement (66% without) and a 5-year survival rate of 57% with osseous involvement and 16% (5-year survival rate without any bony changes. This was confirmed by VIETA et al. (1942).

XII. Differential Diagnosis

The differential diagnosis of lymphomas involving the skeleton depend on whether the lesions are single or multiple and if they are lytic or blastic. The differential diagnosis of an ivory vertebra has already been discussed (Table 9) and the remainder is outlined in Table 10.

Table 10. Differential diagnosis of lymphomas

Single lytic lesion
    Osteomyelitis
    Tuberculosis (particularly in spine)
    Ewing's sarcoma
    Reticulum cell sarcoma
    Osteogenic sarcoma

Single blastic lesion
    Paget's disease (particularly in pelvis)
    Ivory vertebra (Table 9)
    Solitary metastasis (prostate)

Multiple lytic lesion
    Metastases (breast)
    Multiple myeloma

Multiple blastic lesion
    Metastases (prostate)

Acknowledgments

I thank Mary Margaret Franclemont for her secretarial assistance, and the Visual Education Department of Children's Hospital Medical Center, Boston for the majority of the illustrations. Also my thanks are due to Dr. Ellen Philips for Figures 8, 10, and 24; Dr. Robert Wilkinson for Figures 1, 2, and 6, and Dr. Elliot Himmelfarb of the University of Tennessee College of Medicine for Figure 37.

References

Ewing's Sarcoma

ACKERMANN, L.V.: Bone and joint, pp. 799–878. In: Surgical pathology, 4th ed., St. Louis: The C.V. Mosby Company 1968

BHANSALI, S.K., DESAI, P.B.: Ewing's sarcoma: observations on 107 cases. J. Bone Jt. Surg. **45A**, 541–553 (1963)

COLEY, B.L., HIGINBOTHAM, N.L., BOWDEN, L.: Endothelioma of bone (Ewing's sarcoma). Ann. Surg. **128**, 533–560 (1948)

DAHLIN, D.C.: Ewing's tumor, pp. 186–195. In: Bone tumors, 2d ed., Springfield, Ill.: Charles C Thomas, 1967

EWING, J.: Diffuse endothelioma of bone. Proc. N.Y. path. Soc. **21**, 17–24 (1921)

FRIEDMAN, B., GOLD, H.: Ultrastructure of Ewing's sarcoma of bone. Cancer (Philad.) **22**, 307–322 (1968)

JENKIN, R.D.T.: Ewing's sarcoma: a study of treatment methods. Clin. Radiol. **17**, 97–106 (1966)

MILLBURN, L.F., O'GRADY, L., HENDRICKSON, F.R.: Radical radiation therapy and total body irradiation in the treatment of Ewing's sarcoma. Cancer (Philad.) **22**, 919–925 (1968)

PHILLIPS, R.F., HIGINBOTHAM, N.L.: The curability of Ewing's endothelioma of bone in children. J. Pediat. **70**, 391–397 (1967)

POMEROY, T.C., JOHNSON, R.E.: Combined modality therapy of Ewing's sarcoma. Cancer (Philad.) **35**, 36–47 (1975)

POTDAR, G.G.: Ewing's tumour. Clin. Radiol. **22**, 528–533 (1971)

PRITCHARD, D.J., DAHLIN, D.C., DAUPHINE, R.T., TAYLOR, W.F., BEABOUT, J.W.: Ewing's sarcoma: a clinicopathological and statistical analysis of patients surviving five years or longer. J. Bone Jt. Surg. **57a**, 10–16 (1975)

SHERMAN, R.S., SOONG, K.Y.: Ewing's sarcoma: its roentgen classification and diagnosis. Radiology **66**, 529–539 (1956)

SPJUT, H.J., DORFMAN, H.D., FECHNER, R.E., ACKERMAN, L.V.: Tumors of bone and cartilage. Washington, D.C.: Armed Forces Institute of Pathology, 1971

Reticulum Cell Sarcoma

ACKERMAN, L.V.: Table 40, p. 817. In: Surg. Path., 4th ed., St. Louis: The C.V. Mosby Company 1968

BETHGE, J.F.J.: Die Ewingtumoren oder Omoblastome des Knochens. Differentialdiagnostische und kritische Erörterungen. Ergebn. Chir. Orthop. **38**, 327–425 (1955)

DAHLIN, D.C.: Malignant lymphoma of bone (reticulum cell sarcoma), pp. 126–137. In: Bone tumors, 2d ed. Springfield, Ill.: Charles C Thomas, 1967

FRANCIS, K.C., HIGINBOTHAM, N.L., COLEY, B.L.: Primary reticulum cell sarcoma of bone. Report of 44 cases. Surg. Gynec. Obstet. **99**, 142–146 (1954)

IVINS, J.C., DAHLIN, D.C.: Malignant lymphoma (reticulum cell sarcoma) of bone. Mayo Clin. Proc. **38**, 375–385 (1953)

McCORMACK, M.L.J., DOCKERTY, M.B., GHORMLEY, R.K.: Ewing's sarcoma. Cancer **5**, 85–99 (1952)

McCORMACK, L.J., IVINS, J.C., DAHLIN, D.C., JOHNSON, E.W.: Primary reticulum cell sarcoma of bone. Cancer (Philad.) **5**, 1182–1192 (1952)

OBERLING, C.: Les réticulosarcomes et les réticuloendothéliosarcomes de la moelle osseuse (sarcomes d'Ewing). Bull. Ass. franç. Cancer **17**, 259–296 (1928)

OBERLING, C., RAILENAU, C.: Nouvelles recherches sur les réticulosarcomes de la moelle osseuse (sarcomes d'Ewing). Bull. Ass. Franç. Cancer **21**, 333–347 (1932)

PARKER, F., JR., JACKSON, H., JR.: Primary reticulum cell sarcoma of bone. Surg. Gynec. Obstet. **68**, 45–53 (1939)

SHERMAN, R.S., SNYDER, R.E.: The roentgen appearances of primary reticulum cell sarcoma of bone. Amer. J. Roentgenol. **58**, 291–306 (1947)

STRANGE, V.M.: Reticulum cell sarcoma primary in the skull. Amer. J. Roentgenol. **71**, 40–50 (1954)

WANG, C.C., FLEISCHLI, D.J.: Primary reticulum cell sarcoma of bone: with emphasis on radiation therapy. Cancer (Philad.) **22**, 994–998 (1968)

WILSON, T.W., PUGH, D.G.: Primary reticulum cell sarcoma of bone, with emphasis on roentgen aspects. Radiology **65**, 343–351 (1955)

Multiple Myeloma

ABRAMSON, N., SHATTIL, S.J.: M-components. J. Amer. med. Ass. **223**, 156–159 (1973)

ALEXANIAN, R., BONNET, J., GEHAN, E., HAUT, A., HEWLETT, J., LANE, M., MONTO, R., WILSON, H.: Combination chemotherapy for multiple myeloma. Cancer (Philad.) **30**, 382–389 (1972)

BERGSAGEL, D.E.: Total body irradiation for myelomatosis. Myeloma Workshop. Brit. med. J. **2**, 325 (1971)

BERGSAGEL, D.E., GRIFFITH, K.M., HAUT, A., STUCKEY, W.S.: The treatment of plasma cell myeloma. Advanc. Cancer Res. **10**, 311–359 (1967)

CARBONE, P.P., ZIPKIN, I., SOKOLOFF, L., FRAZIER, P., COOK, P., MULLINS, F.: Fluoride effect on bone in plasma cell myeloma. Arch. intern. Med. **121**, 130–140 (1968)

CARSON, C.P., ACKERMAN, L.V., MALTBY, J.D.: Plasma cell myeloma: a clinical, pathologic and roentgenologic review of 90 cases. Amer. J. clin. Path. **25**, 849–888 (1955)

COHEN, D.M., SVIEN, H.J., DAHLIN, D.C.: Long-term survival of patients with myeloma of the vertebral column. J. Amer. med. Ass. **187**, 914–917 (1964)

COHEN, P.: Fluoride and calcium therapy for myeloma bone lesions. J. Amer. med. Ass. **198**, 115–118 (1966)

HARLEY, J.B., SCHILLING, A., GLIDEWELL, O.: Ineffectiveness of fluoride therapy in multiple myeloma. New Engl. J. Med. **286**, 1283–1288 (1971)

HELLWIG, C.A.: Extramedullary plasma cell tumors as observed in various locations. Arch. Path. (Chicago) **36**, 95–111 (1943)

HIMMELFARB, E., SEBES, J., RABINOWITZ, J.: Unusual roentgenographic presentations of multiple myeloma: report of three cases. J. Bone Jt. Surg. **56 A**, 1723–1728 (1974)

JAFFE, H.L.: Tumors and tumorous conditions of bones and joints (Chap. 23). Philadelphia: Lea and Febiger 1958

JOHANNSSON, B.: Prognostic factors in myelomatosis. Section of Myeloma Workshop. Brit. med. J. **2**, 319–328 (1971)

LOWBEER, L.: Occurrence of osteosclerosis in multiple myeloma. Lab. Med. 396–397 (1969)

MALPAS, J.S.: Blood and neoplastic diseases: myelomatosis. Brit. med. J. **4**, 520–522 (1974)

NORDENSON, N.G.: Myelomatosis: a clinical review of 310 cases. Acta med. scand., Suppl. 445, **179**, 178–183 (1966)

PETCH, M.C.: Opaque bones. Proc. roy. Soc. Med. **64**, 393 (1971)

RENNER, R.R., SMITH, J.R.: Plasma cell dyscrasias (except myeloma), Semin. Roentgenol. **9**, 209–218 (1974)

SNAPPER, I., KAHN, A.I.: Multiple myeloma. In: Multiple myeloma, MIESCHER, P.A. (ed.). New York: Grune and Stratton 1964

SPJUT, H.J., DORFMAN, H.D., FECHNER, R.E., ACKERMAN, L.V.: Tumors of bone and cartilage. Washington, D.C.: Armed Forces Institute of Pathology 1971

TODD, I.D.H.: Treatment of solitary plasmacytoma. Clin. Radiol. **16**, 395–399 (1965)

WINTROBE, M.M.: Multiple myeloma, pp. 1188–1201. In: Clinical hematology, 6th ed. Philadelphia: Lea and Febiger 1967

WRIGHT, C.J.E.: Long survival in solitary plasmacytoma of bone. J. Bone Jt. Surg. **43 B**, 767–771 (1961)

Lymphoma

AISENBERG, A.C.: Malignant lymphoma. New Engl. J. Med. **288**, 883–890, 935–941 (1973)

BUSY, J., LOTE, J., PALLARDY, G.: Etude radiologique des localisations osseuses de la maladie de Hodgkin. J. Rad. Electrol. **39**, 239–247 (1958)

BUTLER, J.J.: Relationship of histological findings to survival in Hodgkin's disease. Cancer Res. **31**, 1770–1775 (1971)

COLES, W.C., SCHULZ, M.D.: Bone involvement in malignant lymphoma. Radiology **50**, 458–462 (1948)

CRAVER, L.F., COPELAND, D.: Changes in bone in Hodgkin's granuloma. Arch. Surg. (Chicago) **28**, 1062–1086 (1934)

DRESSER, R., SPENCER, J.: Hodgkin's disease and allied conditions of bone. Amer. J. Roentgenol. **36**, 809–815 (1936)

DUNCAN, A.W.: Calcification of the anterior longitudinal vertebral ligaments in Hodgkin's disease. Clin. Radiol. **24**, 394–395 (1973)

EWING, J.: Neoplastic diseases: a treatise on tumors, 4th ed. Philadelphia: W.B. Saunders Company 1940

FUCILLA, I.S., HAMANN, A.: Hodgkin's disease in bone. Radiology **77**, 53–60 (1961)

GOLDING, F.C.: Textbook of x-ray diagnosis, 3rd ed. London: Lewis 1959

GRANGER, W., WHITAKER, R.: Hodgkin's disease in bone, with special reference to periosteal reaction. Brit. J. Radiol. **40**, 939–948 (1967)

HARDER, J.: Über Knochenlymphogranulomatose. Fortschr. Röntgenstr. **93**, 445–455 (1960)

HORAN, F.T.: Bone involvement in Hodgkin's disease. Brit. J. Surg. **56**, 277–281 (1969)

PEAR, B.L.: Skeletal manifestations of the lymphomas and leukemias. Semin. Roentgenol. **9**, 229–240 (1974)

SILBERBERG, E.: Major trends in cancer: 25 year survey. CA: Cancer J. Clin. **25**, 1 (1975)

STUHLBARG, J., ELLIS, F.W.: Hodgkin's disease of bone: favorable prognostic significance? Amer. J. Roentgenol. **93**, 568–572 (1965)

UEHLINGER, E.: Über Knochen-Lymphogranulomatose. Virchows Arch. path. Anat. **288**, 36–118 (1933)

VIETA, J.O., FRIEDELL, H.L., CRAVER, L.F.: A survey of Hodgkin's disease and lymphosarcoma in bone. Radiology **39**, 1–15 (1942)

WOODARD, H.Q., CRAVER, L.F.: Serum phosphatase in lymphomatoid diseases. J. clin. Invest. **19**, 1–7 (1940)

ZIEGLER, K.: Hodgkin's disease. Gustav Fischer J. Jena (1911)

Vascular Tumors of Bone

by

Michael C. Beachley

A. Hemangiomas

Hemangiomas (angiomas, benign hemangioendotheliomas) are primary vascular tumors which may occasionally originate in bone. The qualifying terms "cavernous" and "capillary" are used to describe the histologic form of hemangioma under discussion.

The capillary hemangioma is less common in bone, although it represents the most common tumor of infancy and childhood. In this age group it is almost entirely limited to the skin, and is usually of congenital origin. Capillary hemangiomas of bone are soft, dark bloody areas which may be traversed with dense, sclerotic trabeculae. Histologically, the tumor is formed by fine capillary loops, often radiating in a sunburst fashion, lined by small cells.

The more common hemangioma of bone is the cavernous type. The blood vessels are much more dilated than in the capillary type, and they are felt by some authors to represent a capillary hemangioma in which there has been expansion of the connection between the general circulation and the vascular channels, so that the capillaries become distended and form pools or sinuses. Consequently, the entering vessels are larger than in the capillary hemangioma (PACK and MILLER, 1950). These widely dilated spaces or sinuses are usually filled with blood and are lined by a single layer of flattened endothelial cells. This is the typical type of hemangioma found in the skull and in the vertebrae, and, incidentally, is also the type typically found in the liver and gastrointestinal tract.

Hemangiomas are uncommon bone tumors reported to represent 0.6–1.0% of all primary bone tumors (DAHLIN, 1967). These tumors are found in patients of all ages, but most commonly in the middle decades of life. The only location in which they occur with any frequency is the spine, where they are usually asymptomatic. SCHMORL (1927), in a study of 3,829 vertebral columns, found hemangiomata in 10.7%. TÖPFER (1928), in a study of over 2,000 vertebral columns, found hemangiomas in 12%.

Spinal hemangiomas are usually single lesions, but occasionally two or more vertebral bodies are involved. They are most often confined to the vertebral body, but occasionally may extend into the posterior elements and transverse processes.

The skull is the second most frequent area of involvement; more than half of all hemangiomas of bone occur in either the skull or spine (SHERMAN and WILNER, 1961). They are also occasionally seen in ribs, facial bones, other flat bones, and long bones. SHERMAN and WILNER (1961) have indicated that the capillary type of hemangioma is more common in the flat bones and metaphyses of long bones, whereas the vertebrae and skull are more frequently involved with cavernous hemangiomas.

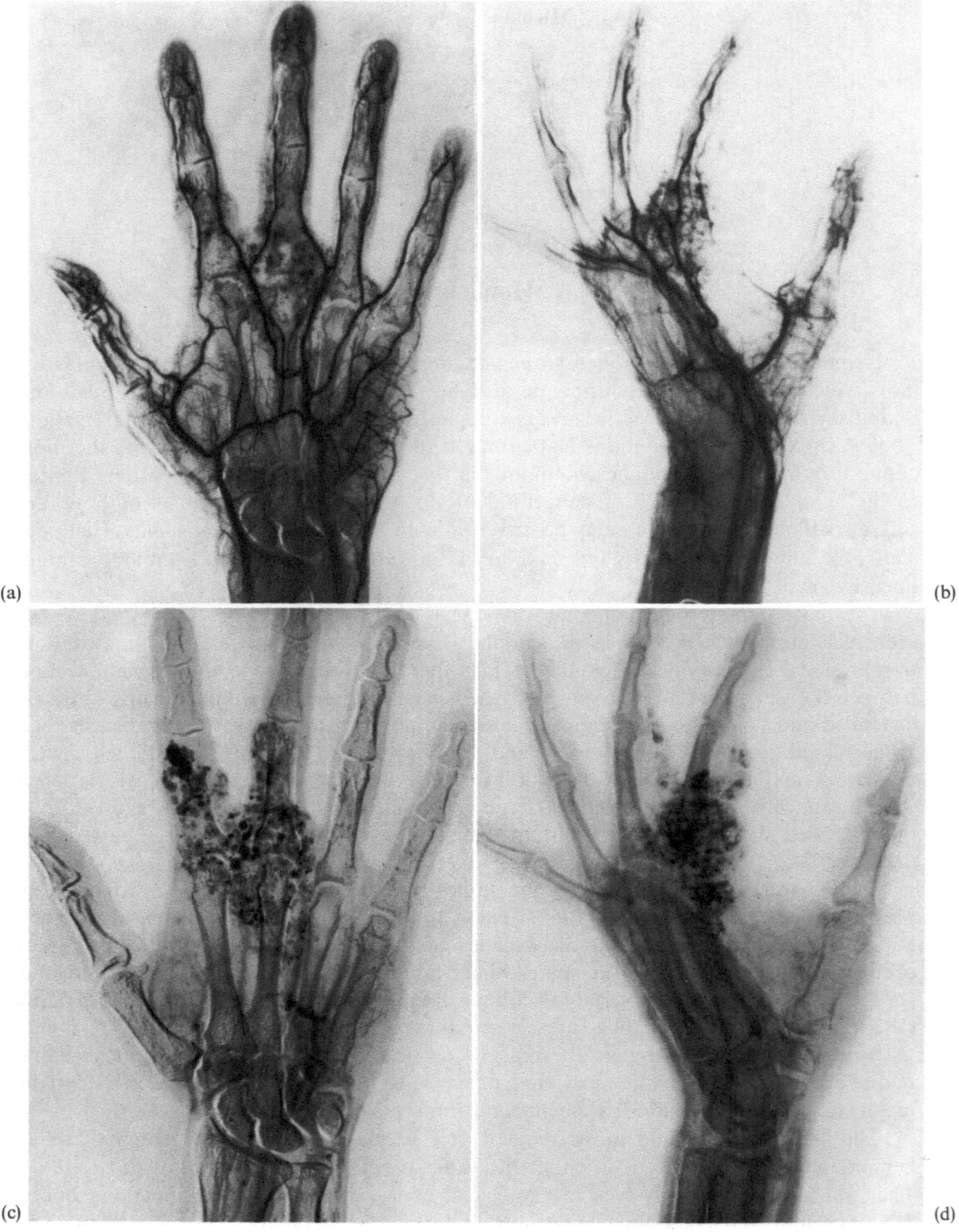

Figs. 1a–d. Arteriogram of hand in anteroposterior (a, c), and oblique (b, d) views. The soft tissue hemangioma is opacified early in arterial phase. Blood supply is derived mainly from common digital arteries. During late venous phase (c, d), there is retention of contrast medium in tumor, with exact demarcation of involved tissue areas. (Ben-Menachem, Y., and Epstein, M.J.: 1974, with permission)

The etiology of hemangiomata is not known, but many consider these to be congenital lesions which usually remain asymptomatic and are discovered incidentally. The congenital hemangiomas probably begin as capillary types and then progress to a cavernous type as described above.

Numerous reports are included in the literature which suggest a close association with trauma. Although it is true with many bone tumors that trauma to the area first draws the patient's attention to a pre-existing lesion, some of the reports have indicated that the soft tissue swelling or bony mass produced by trauma did not regress, and was subsequently proven to be a hemangioma. There is greater evidence with hemangiomas than with other bone tumors that trauma may indeed be a primary or contributory cause in their development. A case in point is described by ROSENBAUM et al. (1969), in which a patient was hit on the head with a metal pipe, and within 3 months developed a gradual mass and soreness over the area. Roentgenograms revealed a zone of rarefaction with a scalloped, sclerotic rim with a radial arrangement of bone trabeculae. The plain films were typical of a hemangioma, and selective external carotid arteriography demonstrated the hemangioma fed by the superficial temporal artery and middle meningeal arteries. The resected specimen showed a typical cavernous hemangioma. The authors also refer to six other articles in which local trauma was related to calvarial hemangiomas, and one article in which a nasal hemangioma was related to a fracture.

A similar type of case has been reported by BEN-MENACHEM and EPSTEIN (1974). A crush injury to the hand resulted within 2 months in the development of a tender mass which was subsequently proven to be a capillary hemangioma of soft tissue (Figs. 1a–d).

Primary hemangiomas of bone are usually slow-growing and asymptomatic, and many such tumors exist throughout life undetected. They are frequently discovered coincidentally at the time of radiographic examination for some other problem. Symptomatic hemangiomas are usually noticed by the patient because of swelling, pain, or occasionally a pathologic fracture. Vertebral lesions may produce a vague intermittent type of pain, or may result in collapse of a vertebra with resulting pain and neurologic signs and symptoms. This may be in the form of spasm and rigidity of the muscles of the lumbar region, or result in signs of cord compression with spastic paraplegia and peripheral sensory loss.

Roentgenographic Appearance

The roentgenographic appearance of hemangiomata of vertebrae is usually characteristic and diagnostic. The diagnosis is also usually readily made in skull lesions, but in other flat bones and particularly in long bones, a variety of roentgen descriptions have been reported, and differential diagnostic considerations are necessary.

The typical roentgen appearance in vertebrae is a demineralization of the vertebral body, with the presence of parallel vertical linear streaks resembling corduroy cloth. Ordinarily this is best seen in the lateral projection, and in the frontal projection usually resembles a demineralized vertebra with honeycomb appearance (Figs. 2a and b). The cortex is usually intact, although ill-defined in some areas. The lesion may be confined to the vertebral body, or occassionally may extend into the pedicles, posterior elements, and transverse processes of the vertebrae, which also show a honeycomb texture with coarse trabeculae and demineralization. Body-section radiography can be very helpful to demonstrate the typical roentgen appearance in cases in which the plain roentgenograms are not diagnostic. In those cases with a compression fracture, the characteristic changes may be completely lost, and the etiology of the compression cannot be determined unless characteristic changes of the posterior elements of the vertebrae are seen.

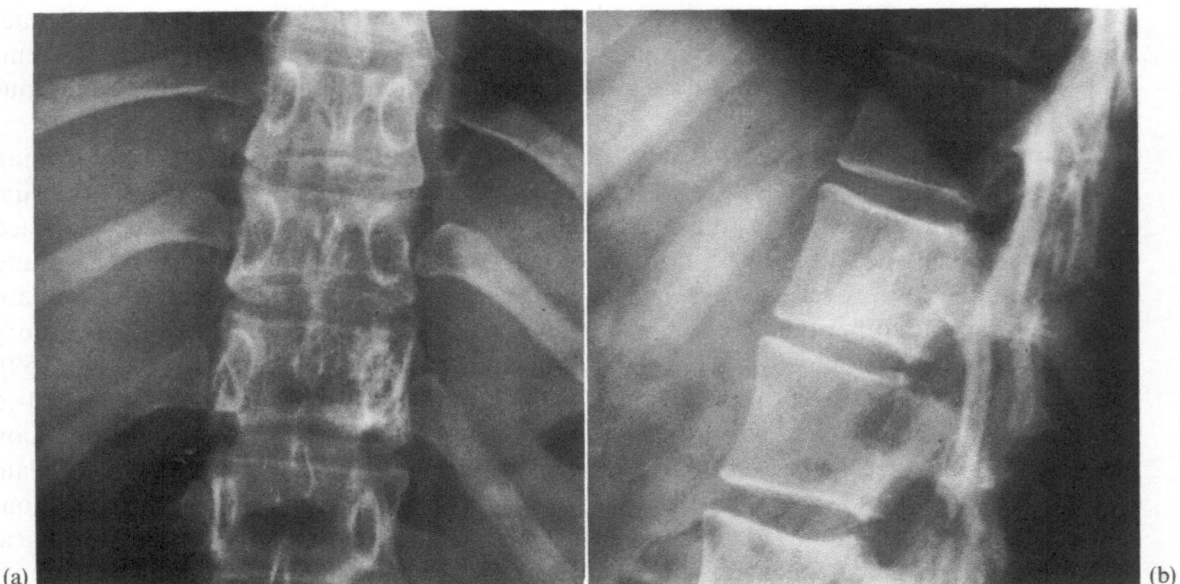

Fig. 2a and b. Anteroposterior roentgenogram (a) shows typical vertebral hemangioma involving primarily the left side of D12 vertebral body. The lesion has reticulated honeycombed appearance of coarsened trabeculae. Lateral view (b) shows vertical striations caused by remaining large trabeculae, characteristic of vertebral hemangiomas

In the differential diagnosis, hemangiomata of the vertebrae must occasionally be distinguished from Paget's disease, although the latter is usually more dense, with an increased density of the end plates and margins of the vertebrae resembling a picture frame. Occasionally, multiple myeloma, metastatic carcinoma, or lymphomas must be considered in the differential diagnosis. In most cases, however, vertebral hemangiomas are so characteristic as to be diagnostic.

Hemangiomata of the skull also have a typical roentgenographic appearance in most cases, being a solitary area of rarefaction varying from 1.0 to 7.0 cm in diameter. The central portion is characterized by a honeycomb or grossly granular appearance when seen en face, surrounded by a well-defined margin (Fig. 3). The smallest lesions may be entirely lytic with no visible internal structure, and a few large hemangiomata of the skull have been demonstrated which are entirely lytic. The most characteristic roentgen finding, however, is seen in the tangential view of the lesion. The lesion typically involves the diploë and outer table of the skull with an intact inner table, although rarely the inner table may bulge inward. A sunburst pattern of radiating striations resembling a "hair-on-end" appearance within the lesion is seen. When the lesions extend into the facial bones, they are typically honeycombed in appearance, and the parallel striations may not be seen.

In the differential diagnosis, meningiomas may at times closely resemble hemangiomas, but are intracranial and typically involve the inner table of the skull. Purely lytic hemangiomas closely resemble epidermoids, although the epidermoids are usually more serpiginous in outline with a dense peripheral margin. Metastatic tumors and multiple myeloma are also occasional differential considerations.

A spectrum of roentgen appearances is exhibited by hemangiomas in the flat bones. In the mandible, hemangiomas are usually coarsely trabeculated, multiloculated, expanding lesions, with the trabeculae radiating from the central portion of the tumor. The cortex may be quite thin, but remains intact and no soft tissue component is seen.

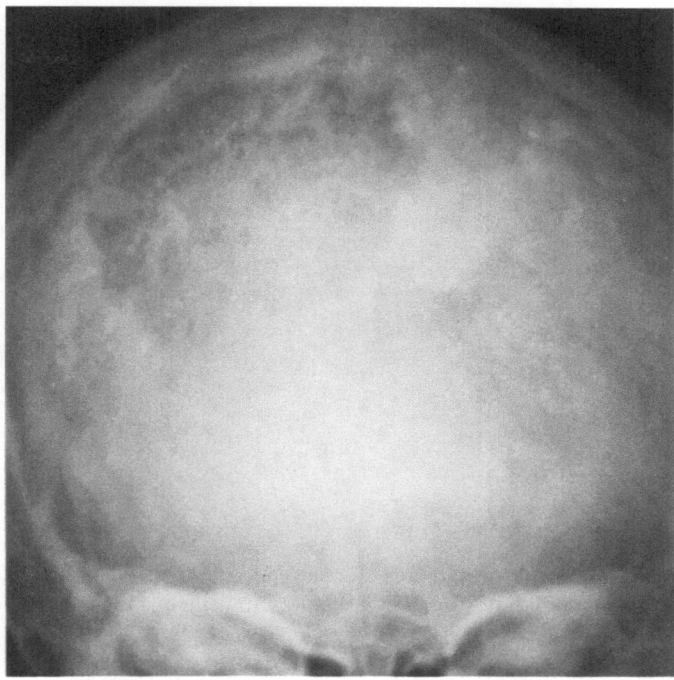

Fig. 3. Posteroanterior roentgenogram of skull shows lacelike osteolytic hemangioma of right frontal bone with scalloped margins

The multiloculated, reticulated, or honeycomb pattern is typical of hemangiomata of flat bones, but unfortunately is not always present.

In ribs, the lesions may be entirely lytic and expansile, maintaining a faint cortical rim and a sharp demarcation with normal bone. It may then be confused with many expansile, purely lytic lesions of ribs including giant cell tumors, fibrous dysplasia, or chondroma. A typical vacuolated appearance may be seen with irregular, thinned cortex, which suggests a hemangioma, but a soft tissue mass may also be present. Confusion with osteogenic sarcoma is possible in these cases. Occasionally, the cortical margins in ribs may be so thinned and distorted that they appear to be destroyed, particularly along the inferior margins. When a honeycomb lesion of rib is seen, the diagnosis of hemangioma is not difficult, but it is important to realize that hemangiomas in ribs may be completely lytic, may appear to destroy cortex, and may rarely be accompanied by a soft tissue mass.

In the long bones, a hemangioma normally has loculations interspersed with a fine fibrillary network (Figs. 4a and b). The oval or round locules of the lytic lesion involve the cortex up to the level of the periosteum. These lesions may closely resemble giant cell tumors, fibrous dysplasia, or eosinophilic granuloma.

Hemangiomata of soft tissue may occasionally involve adjacent bone (Figs. 5a–c). In many cases, the hemangiomata of the soft parts will have multiple calcified phleboliths, which is not a finding in primary hemangiomata of bone (Figs. 6a–c).

The simplest type of secondary change is a smooth indentation or cortical erosion of the bone, secondary to the constant pressure, sometimes pulsatile, of the nearby hemangioma. The margins of the bone may be irregular and show combined bone destruction and attempts at regeneration.

Occasionally an exostosis or osteoma may develop at the site of a soft tissue hemangioma. The cause of the development of the exostosis is not known. There may be a more generalized overgrowth or hypertrophy of bone with an expansion of the diameter,

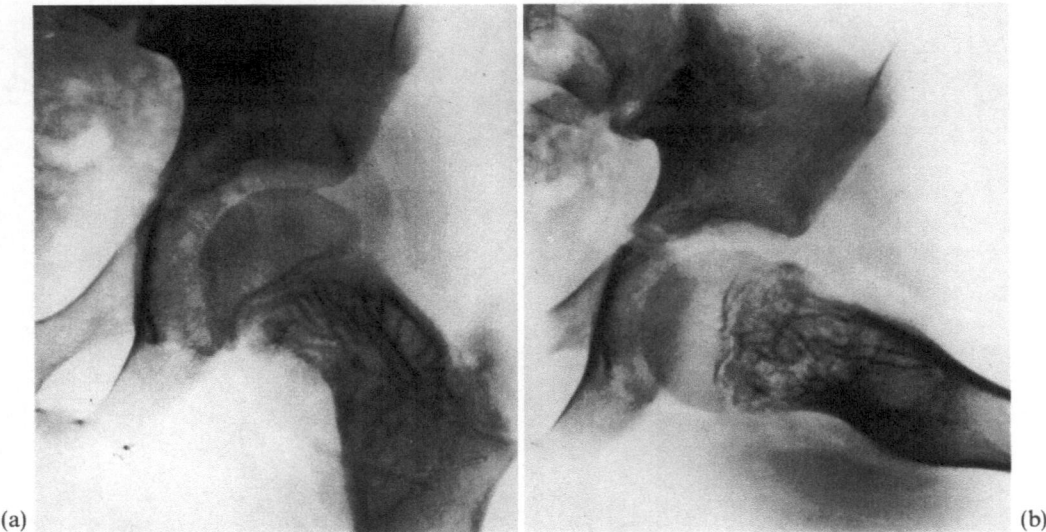

Fig. 4a and b. Anteroposterior (a) and lateral (b) roentgenogram of proximal femur showing typical lacelike pattern of osteolysis secondary to hemangioma of metaphysis. (Horvath, 1970, with permission)

and thickening and hypertrophy of the cortex. The bony trabecular structure is frequently coarsened, and in places, the cortex may be thin. In addition to enlargement in the width of the bone, elongation of the long bones of an extremity may occur, particularly in the presence of a hemangioma involving an entire extremity. This is probably due to the altered circulation of bone with venous stasis and more direct arteriovenous communications than through the usual capillary network (Pack and Miller, 1950).

To summarize the plain roentgen appearance of hemangiomata of bone, the most typical appearance is a honeycomb and coarsely trabeculated demineralized region in bone. Vertical striations resembling corduroy cloth is the typical appearance in the vertebrae. In the skull, vertical striations involving the diploë and outer table as seen on the tangential view is the classic appearance. A variable roentgen appearance may be seen in flat bones and long bones where lesions may be either lytic or loculated. A variety of bone changes may be seen secondary to soft tissue hemangiomata, but typically these have calcified phleboliths in the soft tissue, which is not seen in primary hemangiomata of bone.

Arteriography may be of value in demonstrating hemangiomas of bone (Forrest and Staple, 1971, and McNeill et al., 1974). Multiple examples of the angiographic demonstration of deep hemangiomas of the extremities have been recorded, including some cases with secondary bone involvement (Fig. 5c). However, several reports have described the angiographic findings in primary bone hemangiomata involving vertebrae and skull.

Hacker and Alonso (1969) described a typical hemangioma of the cervical spine, in which the arteriogram initially would probably be called normal, but subtraction technique demonstrated a recognizable stain in the capillary phase. They felt that angiography was of help in demonstrating the extent of the lesion, and in demonstrating the feeding vessels and draining vains. Manelfe and Djindjian (1972) demonstrated the value of lateral subtraction angiography in determining the posterior extent of vertebral hemangiomata. In a normal vertebra, a unilateral intercostal or lumbar injection

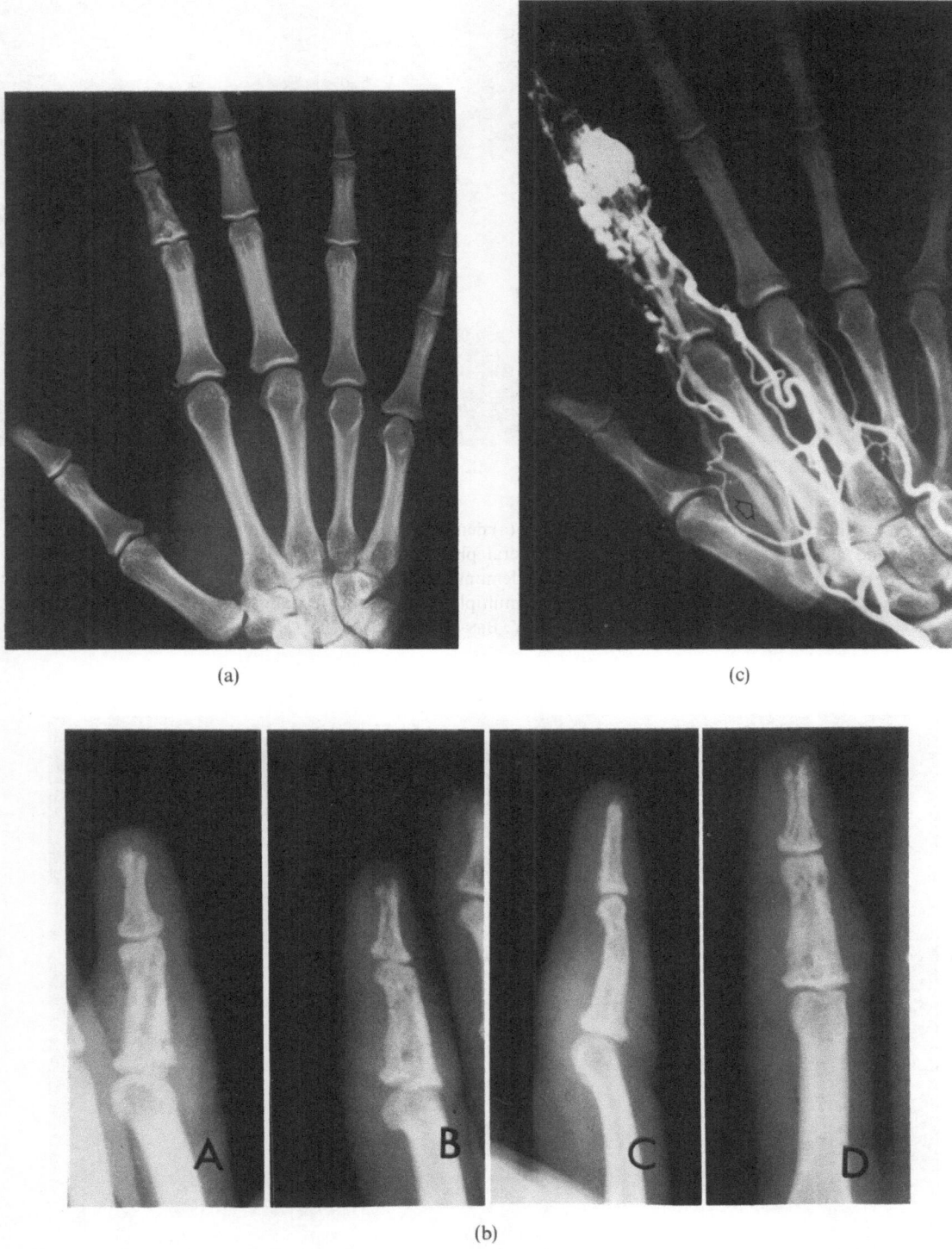

Fig. 5a–c. Anteroposterior roentgenogram (a) of hand shows osteolytic lesion of middle phalanx of index finger. Close-up views (b) *A, B, C, D* demonstrate vacuolated osteolytic appearance in more detail. Arteriogram (c) demonstrates lesion to be highly vascular, involving both bone and soft tissue, and early venous drainage is apparent (*open arrow*). (Courtesy of J.J. BROSNAN, M.D., Chicago)

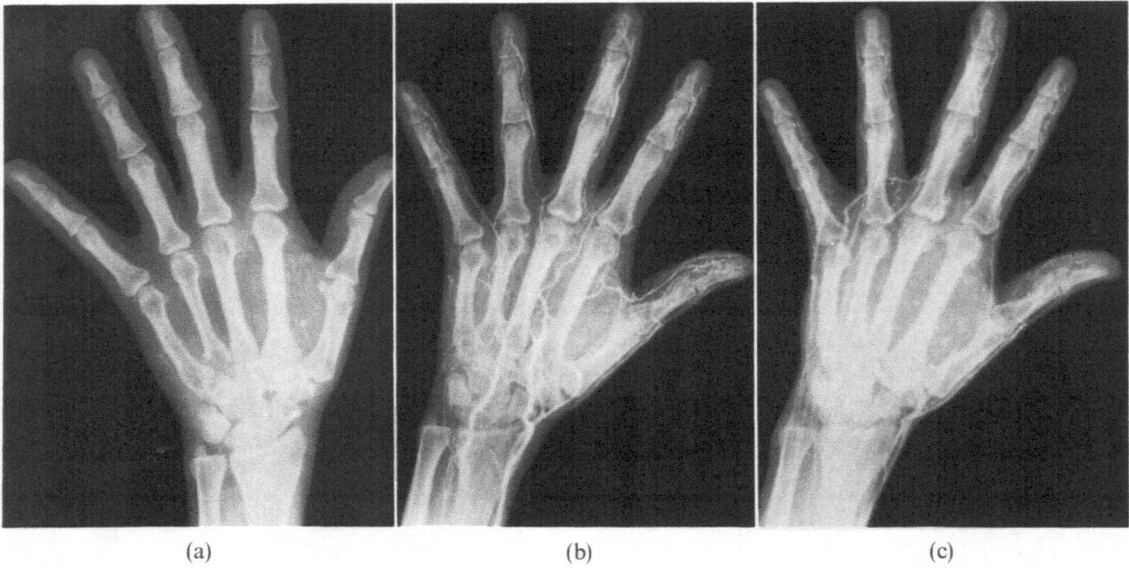

(a)   (b)   (c)

Fig. 6a–c. Anteroposterior roentgenogram of hand (a) demonstrates undulating, solid periosteal reaction involving second and third metacarpal bones, and several phleboliths along radial aspect of second metacarpal. The arterial phase of arteriogram (b) does not demonstrate rapid filling of lesion, but late venous phase (c) shows late retention of contrast medium in multiple lakes within hemangioma between first and third metacarpal bones. (Courtesy of Y. Ben-Menachem, M.D., Houston, Texas)

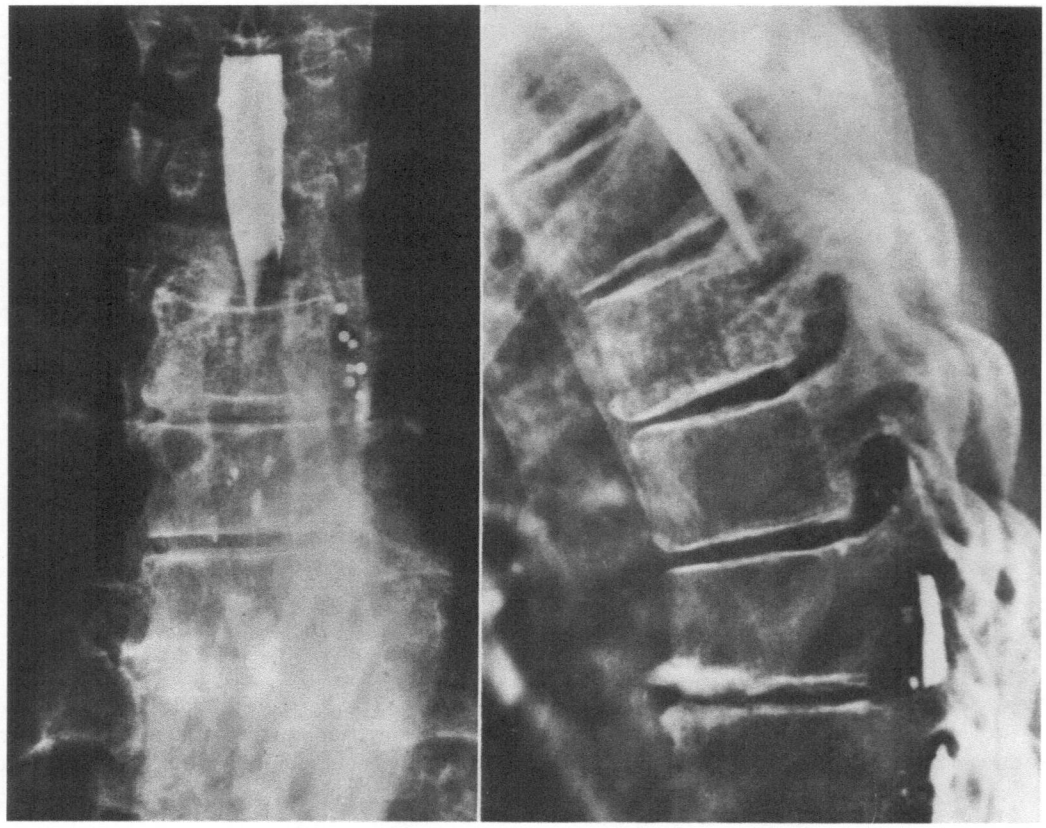

Fig. 7a   Fig. 7b

will fill only the hemivertebra on the side injected. In the presence of a hemangioma, both sides of the vertebra are opacified. Dorsal extension of the tumor into the epidural space with possible cord compression can be nicely demonstrated by these techniques.

THIEMANN (1970) used the venous approach in the differential diagnosis of aneurysmal bone cysts from hemangiomata of the cervical spine. By injection of contrast material into the spinous process, he was able to demonstrate spinal hemangiomata.

ROSENBAUM et al. (1969) described the angiographic findings in a calvarial hemangioma. They demonstrated that a considerable quantity of contrast media (15 cc. of

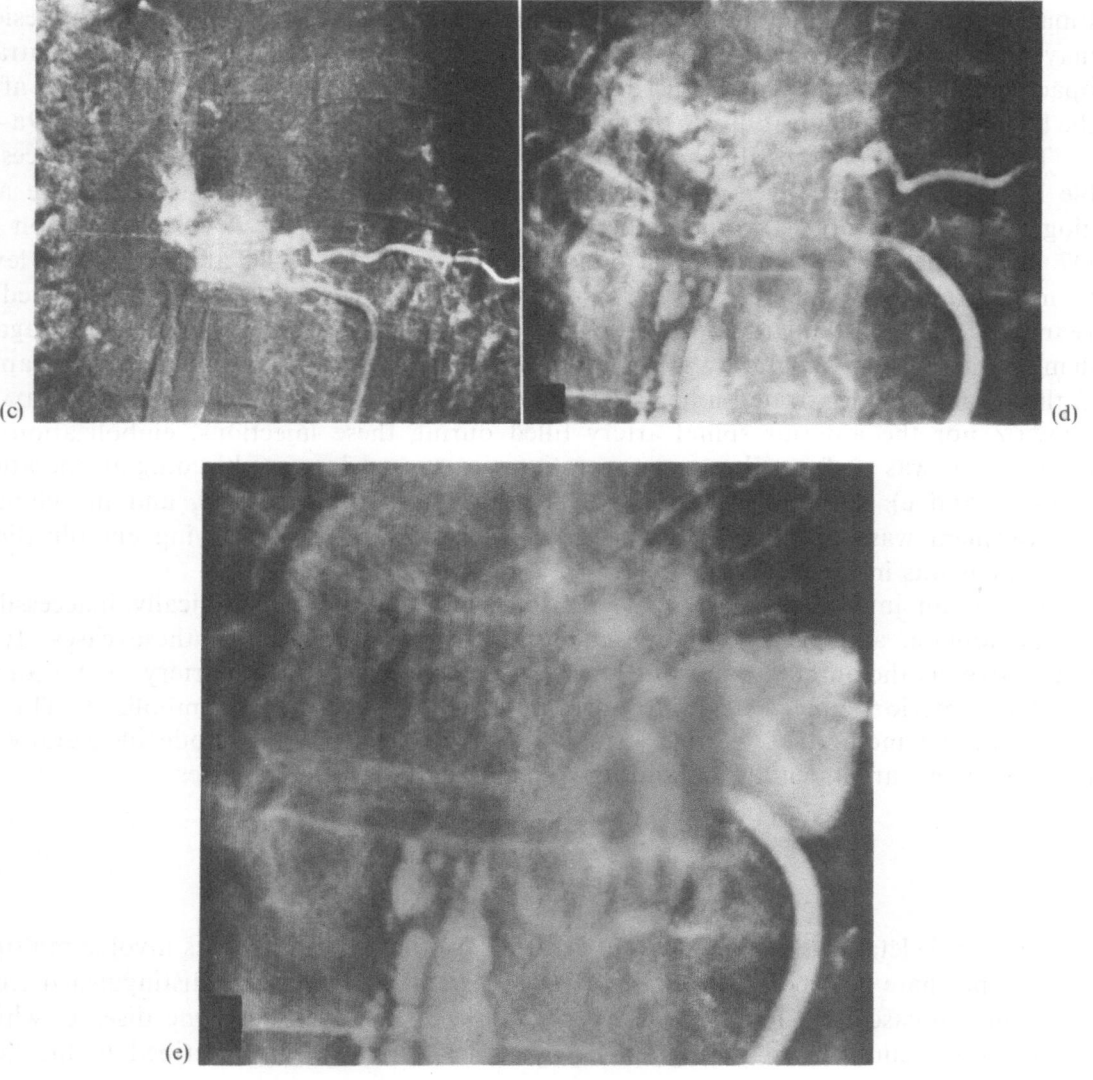

Fig. 7a–e. Anteroposterior (a) and lateral (b) roentgenograms demonstrate typical plain film findings of hemangioma of D7 dorsal vertebra. Suboccipitally introduced positive contrast medium discloses complete block due to extradural process. The anteroposterior subtraction selective angiogram (c) of left seventh intercostal artery demonstrates the blush of hemangioma in dorsal vertebra. The hemangioma extended posteriorly, corresponding to area of complete subarachnoid blockage at D7 level. Repeat anteroposterior arteriogram of D7 vertebral body just prior to embolization (d), and following introduction of emboli (e), demonstrates complete obliteration of flow to D7 hemangioma. (HEKSTER et al. 1972, with permission)

60% Renografin) must be injected selectively into the external carotid artery to demon-strate some of these lesions. Despite the fact that the hemangioma was 6.0 cm in diameter, only a single 3 mm zone of the tumor opacified with contrast media. At surgery, on the other hand, the lesion was shown to be highly vascular. This difficulty in opacifying the hemangioma was accounted for by the effect of hemodilution of the opaque material in the large pool of blood within the hemangioma. The contrast media coming through this small feeding vessel becomes immediately diluted and no longer visible on the radiographs. Only in large hemangiomas are the sunburst blood-filled channels opacified, and in lesions in which the plain film morphology is not of the sunburst configuration, opacification with contrast may occur as coarse dots or "colonies" of contrast media. Finally, an abrupt termination of an afferent vessel in close juxtaposition to the lesion may be seen as the opaque column discharges into the large blood pool. Contrast opacification of the lesion may be quite prolonged, extending greater than 10 sec after the beginning of opacification. A similar case is illustrated by YAGHMAI in Figures 19a–d.

The treatment of accessible hemangiomas is normally by surgical resection; inaccessi-ble lesions are treated by x-ray therapy. HEKSTER et al. (1972) have described the an-giographic therapy of a symptomatic spinal hemangioma. This involved a lesion of D7 in a patient with a neurologic deficit and a complete block at the D7–D8 level at myelography. A laminectomy was successful, but recurrent symptoms occurred 2 years later and spastic paraparesis developed 3 years later. A complete block was again demonstrated by myelography (Figs. 7a and b), and selective intercostal angiography at the D7 level demonstrated a hemangioma (Fig. 7c). Since neither the artery of ADAM-KIEWICZ nor the anterior spinal artery filled during these injections, embolization of these vessels was performed as a preoperative measure to decrease bleeding at operation (Figs 7d and e). The patient also had 3,000 R of radiation therapy, and the clinical improvement was such that surgery was cancelled; 7 months following embolization, the patient was in excellent condition.

This is an intriguing method of treating symptomatic and surgically inaccessible hemangiomata, and possibly radiation therapy is not necessary in these cases. It is imperative, as the authors point out, that critical vessels such as the artery of ADAMKIE-WICZ or anterior spinal artery are not fed from the vessel to be embolized. This is not a routine method of treating hemangiomata, but is another mode of therapy in the physicians' armamentarium, and may be applicable in selected cases.

I. Diffuse Skeletal Hemangiomatosis

Diffuse skeletal hemangiomatosis is a disease in which hemangiomas involve multiple bones, and there may be associated visceral involvement. It must be distinguished from Gorham's disease, also termed massive osteolysis or disappearing bone disease, which has a unique clinical and radiographic appearance, and will be described in the next section.

Diffuse skeletal hemangiomas are usually of blood vessel origin, but they may be partly or predominantly lymphatic. This syndrome may be seen at any age, and there is an approximately equal sex incidence.

The most common sites of involvement are the skull, pelvis, ribs, scapula, humerus, tibia, and femur. Of 26 cases reviewed by WALLIS et al. (1964), 9 cases did not have visceral involvement and 17 had involvement of viscera. Of the latter 17 cases, 13 were benign and 4 were malignant. The spleen was involved in 8, the liver in 9, the lymph nodes in 6, the mediastinum and pleura in 7, the lungs in 6, the kidney in 4, the thymus in 3, muscle in 2, the brain in 1, and the adrenals in 1. In the nonvisceral group, the only extraosseous structures involved were subcutaneous tissues, lymphatics, and lymph nodes.

The gross appearance of these lesions demonstrates numerous irregularly rounded, dark red and tan cystic areas surrounded by dense sclerotic bone, somewhat accentuating the trabecular pattern (SPJUT et al., 1971). Histologically, the lesions of diffuse skeletal hemangiomatosis are no different than localized hemangiomas, although often representing a combination of cavernous and capillary formation. The lesions are at times entirely lymphangiomatous in origin, but histologically this is identical to hemangiomas except that erythrocytes are not seen in the vascular spaces. It is of interest that needle biopsies of these lesions are frequently inadequate, and only serve to delay the diagnosis. In addition, pulmonary involvement has been described in a diffuse miliary nodular pattern in which the biopsy reveals small capillary spaces lined by single endothelial cells scattered irregularly in the stroma of dense fibrous tissue. The vascular spaces, filled with erythrocytes and leukocytes, serve to classify this as hemangiomatosis (WALLIS et al., 1964). Other visceral involvement, including the liver, may also show the histologic picture of a mixed capillary and cavernous hemangioma.

The clinical presentation of most patients was bone pain and fractures, particularly compression fractures of the back. WALLIS et al. (1964) found that back pain without evidence of fracture carried a more serious prognosis since most of these patients had visceral involvement, either benign or malignant. It was also evident from this series that pulmonary involvement carried a very poor prognosis and that those cases with visceral involvement did far worse than those without visceral involvement. The group of patients without visceral involvement were younger, and they had a benign course with slow progression and eventual stabilization. In the group with benign visceral involvement, 8 of the 12 patients who were followed were dead within 1–12 years; all 4 patients with malignant visceral involvement were dead within 3–7 months after the initial study.

Roentgenographic Appearance

Diffuse skeletal hemangiomas are roentgenographically similar to hemangioma of bone, except that they are in multiple locations and may be primarily sclerotic. The multiplicity of the tumors immediately suggests the possibility of hyperparathyroidism, metastatic carcinoma, multiple myeloma, or histiocytosis. Although lytic components were seen in all patients with hemangiomatosis, sclerotic lesions were also seen in 50% of the patients, suggesting a differential diagnosis including agnogenic myeloid metaplasia, lymphoma, multiple myeloma, osteopoikilosis, Paget's disease, urticaria pigmentosa, and osteopetrosis (WALDRON and ZELLER, 1969).

Although the mixed pattern may be characteristic, some lesions may be purely osteoblastic and be indistinguishable from osteoblastic metastases (Figs. 8a–c). Compression fractures of vertebrae are reasonably common, and pathologic fractures are seen in other bones. Lytic lesions may expand bone, yet have a rather indolent appearance.

The differential diagnosis of mixed lytic and blastic lesions of bone as described above is a process of exclusion. Failure to discover a primary lesion will help exclude metastases. The typical distribution and roentgen characteristics of some lesions in the differential diagnosis, and the clinical findings in others, serve to direct the differential considerations toward the correct diagnosis.

In cases with visceral involvement, angiography may be of considerable help (Fig. 8d). Celiac angiography with demonstration of hemangiomas of the liver or spleen is of

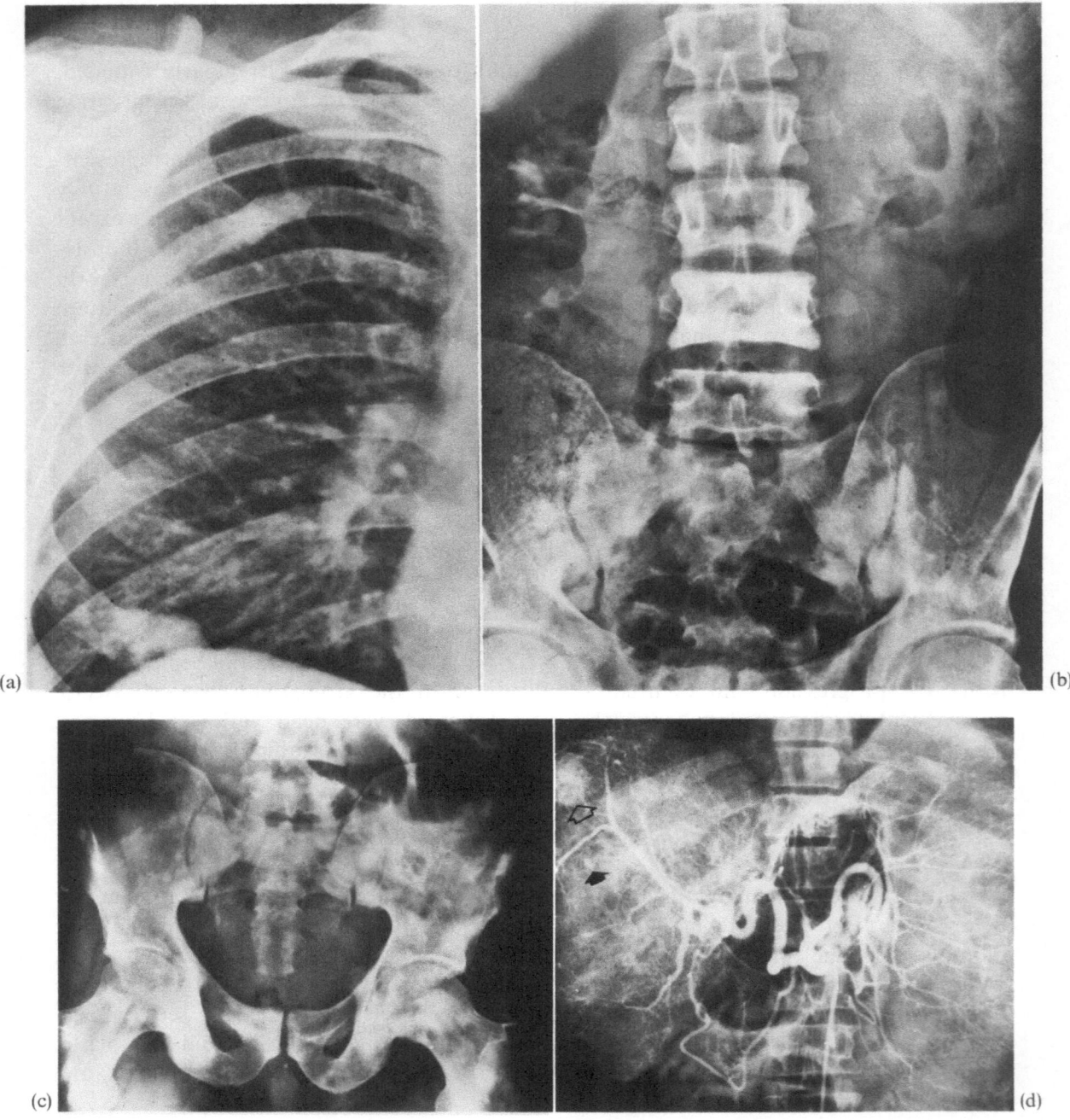

Fig. 8a–d. Anteroposterior roentgenogram of right side of chest (a) demonstrates osteosclerotic lesions of right posterior fifth rib and anterior sixth rib. Biopsy of right sixth rib was interpreted as multifocal sinusoidal telangiectasis, and subsequently determined to be diffuse skeletal hemangiomatosis. Anteroposterior view of lumbar spine (b) shows L4 to be "ivory vertebra," and there is also increased density in right infrapedicular portion of L2 and left suprapedicular portion of L5. Anteroposterior view of pelvis (c) shows mixed sclerotic and lytic process in both innominate bones, sacrum, and both femora. These lesions were reported to have shown no significant change during a 16-year follow-up period. Selective celiac arteriogram (d) demonstrates massive splenomegaly and distorted, reticulated arterial vascularity within liver. Small collection of contrast material in right hepatic lobe (*solid arrow*) was considered to be suspicious for hemangioma in view of patient's known disease elsewhere. *Open arrow* points to expanded, sclerotic right anterior sixth rib. (WALDRON, R.L., and ZELLER, J.A., 1969, with permission)

great prognostic significance, as described above (WALDRON and ZELLER, 1969; SCHIMMEL et al., 1974). Chest radiography for the evaluation of possible pulmonary, pleural, or mediastinal involvement will also be of great importance from a prognostic point of view.

If the tumors are localized, surgical excision of either bone or visceral lesions can be performed. Roentgen therapy has also been given to involved bones, generally with a favorable result. In the group without visceral involvement, there is usually eventual stabilization and the patient enjoys reasonably good health. It is important to detect those with associated visceral involvement, especially thoracic involvement, since this will predict the clinical prognosis of diffuse skeletal hemangiomatosis.

To summarize, diffuse skeletal hemangiomatosis is a syndrome of hemangiomas in multiple bones, frequently with associated visceral involvement. The histologic appearance is that of a hemangioma, and the roentgenographic appearance is frequently typical of hemangioma, but occurring in multiple bones. It does, however, have a higher incidence of sclerotic lesions, and the typical appearance is mixed lytic and sclerotic lesions of bone. The presence and extent of visceral involvement, and particularly thoracic involvement, will determine the clinical outcome. Those patients without visceral involvement in general have a self-limited course with stabilization, whereas those with visceral involvement, whether benign or malignant, will usually have a fatal outcome.

II. Massive Osteolysis

This is a rare syndrome of bone, first recognized as an entity by GORHAM et al., in 1954. This has also been called Gorham's disease, disappearing bone disease, or phantom bone disease.

There is no sex predisposition, and the majority of patients with this syndrome have been under the age of 30, the youngest being an 18-month-old boy. There have been no hereditary, endocrine, or metabolic disorders implicated as a causative factor in this disease.

It is characterized pathologically by benign angiomatosis, which may be either hemangioma, lymphangioma, or a combination of both. The walls of these sinusoid-like spaces cannot be differentiated histologically into lymphangioma and hemangioma, and both blood and lymph may gain entrance into the sinusoids. It is the material contained within the sinusoids which leads to the histologic classification.

The clinical course is characterized by an insidious focal onset which may be accompanied by a pathologic fracture, with a slowly progressive destruction of the bone, without skipped areas. The lesions are almost always unilateral, and soft tissue involvement is usually confined to the areas near the bone lesions. The disease readily crosses joint boundaries so that both the involved and adjacent bones may completely disappear.

Roentgenographic Appearance

The roentgen appearance is initially seen as a focal bone destruction with a relatively rapid progression to complete osteolysis over a period of months (Figs. 9a–c, 10a and b). The edge of the lesion is usually a tapered-down, conelike spicule of bone (Figs. 11a and b), apparently due to intraosseous involvement removing the medullary support, and extraosseous involvement that presses on the bone externally (HALLIDAY et al., 1964). The disease is self-limited and the progression will eventually cease, following an unpre-

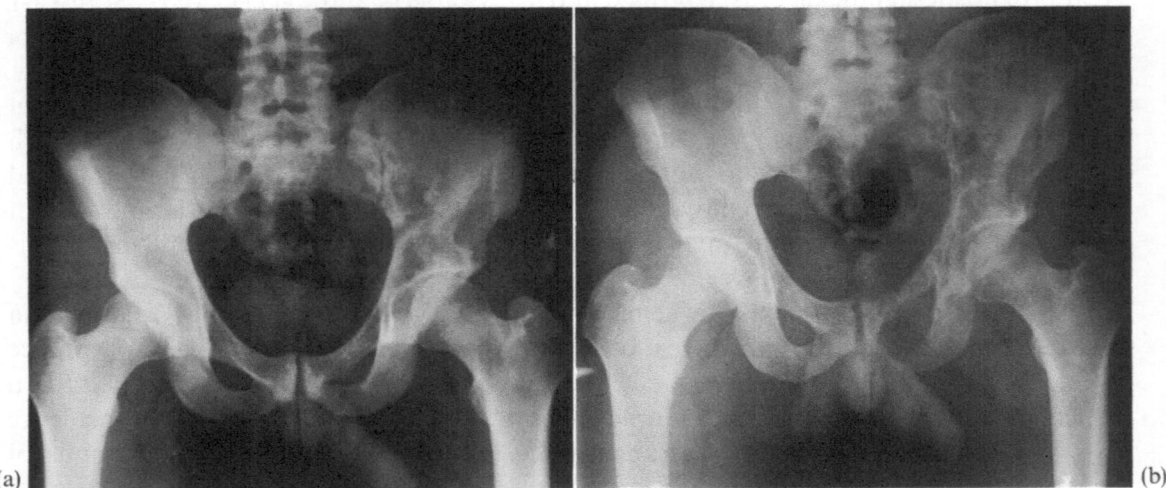

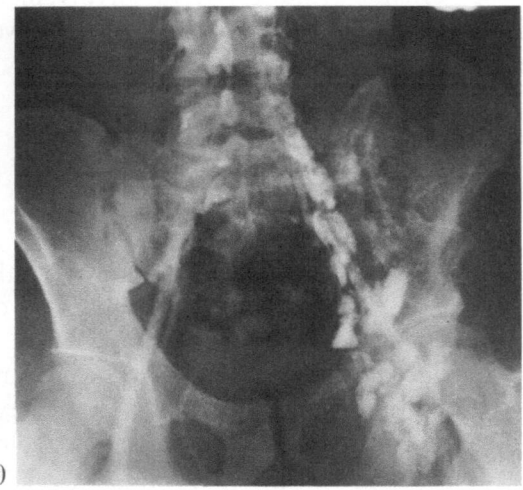

Fig. 9a–c. Anteroposterior roentgenogram (a) demonstrates widespread demineralization of medial half of left ilium and several areas of localized destruction. Left half of sacrum is affected, with lower segments apparently completely destroyed, and wing of sacrum showing mottled destruction. A repeat roentgenogram 17 months later (b) shows much more extensive destruction of left innominate bone and left half of sacrum. Rami of left pubis are badly damaged with pathologic fractures. Aortogram and residual contrast medium from lymphangiogram (c), both performed before operation, disclosed no abnormality or communication between osseous lesions and arterial or lymphatic circulation. (HALLIDAY et al., 1964, with permission)

dictable amount of destruction and deformity. There is no evidence of reossification, and the patient is left with the deformity resulting when the active osteolysis is arrested.

The progression of this disease is quite characteristic and cannot be easily confused with any other disease. The roentgen description above differs markedly from diffuse skeletal hemangiomatosis in that it is of focal nature and progresses in a single extremity or the vertebral column. It tends to be unilateral, and no blastic activity is seen.

There is no known treatment for this disease, with the possible exception of radiation therapy, but the unpredictable activity of this syndrome makes it difficult to evaluate the results of therapy. Reconstructive orthopedic procedures may help correct some of the deformity remaining after the phase of active osteolysis. Deaths have been reported from this disease, either due to hemorrhage from the hemangiomas, or due to severe involvement of the thoracic cage or vertebrae, with respiratory embarrassment.

To summarize, massive osteolysis is a rare syndrome in which focal hemangiomas, lymphangiomas, or a combination of both progresses without regard to joint spaces, resulting in a complete disappearance of bone in a progressive fashion. It is self-limited, and there is no evidence of restoration of bone once osteolysis has occurred. Although histologically benign, the degree of deformity may be severe, and occasionally fatal. The roentgenographic appearance is typical and is the basis for making this diagnosis.

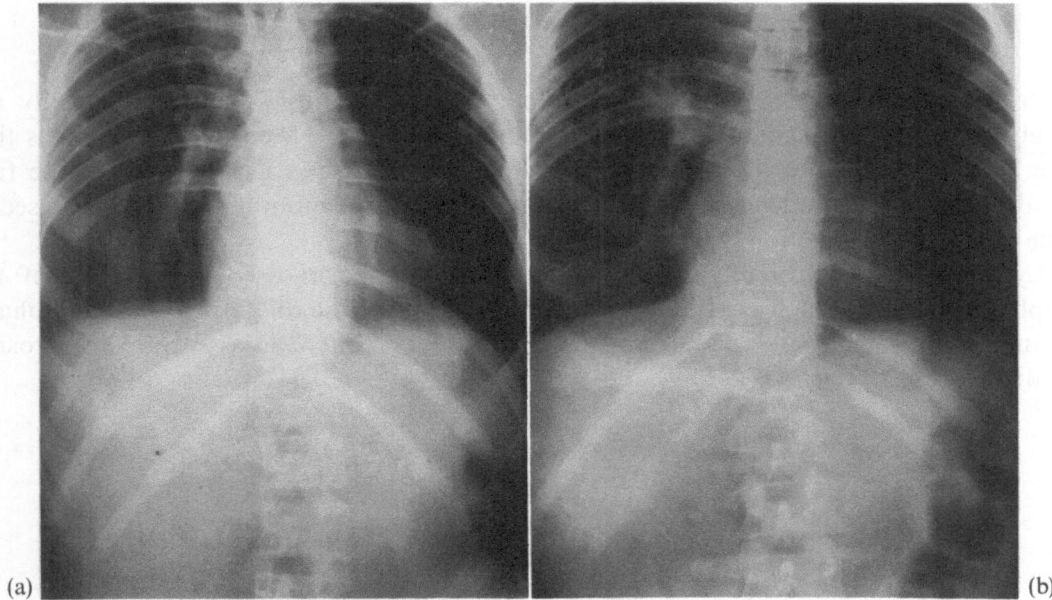

Fig. 10a and b. Anteroposterior chest roentgenogram (a) demonstrates partial disappearance of right eighth, ninth, and tenth ribs. A repeat roentgenogram 7 months later (b) demonstrates loss of all of right ribs previously involved, and beginning of dissolution of right eleventh rib. (HALLIDAY et al., 1964, with permission)

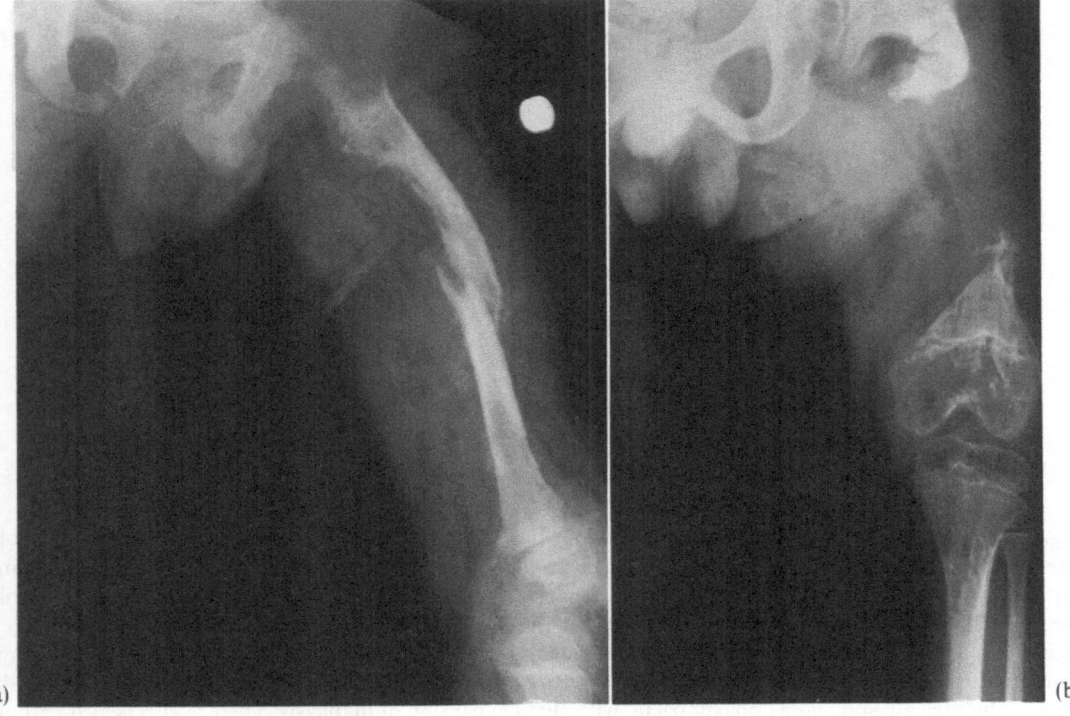

Fig. 11a and b. Anteroposterior roentgenogram of left femur (a) shows pathologic fracture in mid shaft. Progressive resorption of femur, which has not been limited to site of fracture, is noted. A roentgenogram 5½ years later (b), after several operative procedures with grafting, shows complete resorption of entire mid shaft of femur. (HALLIDAY et al., 1964, with permission)

B. Lymphangioma

Primary lymphangiomas of bone may be single or multiple, and histologically are closely related to hemangiomas or hemangiomatosis of bone. Most lymphangiomas that have been reported have been in multiple sites. The disease is usually seen in the first two decades of life, and has been seen in one patient at 3 months of age. There seems to be no sex predisposition.

Lymphangiomas probably originate from abnormal intraosseous dilatation of the lymphatic channels which exist in the periosteum of bone. The dilatation of the lymphatic channels results in cystic spaces, and as these enlarge, there is a progressive erosion of adjacent bone.

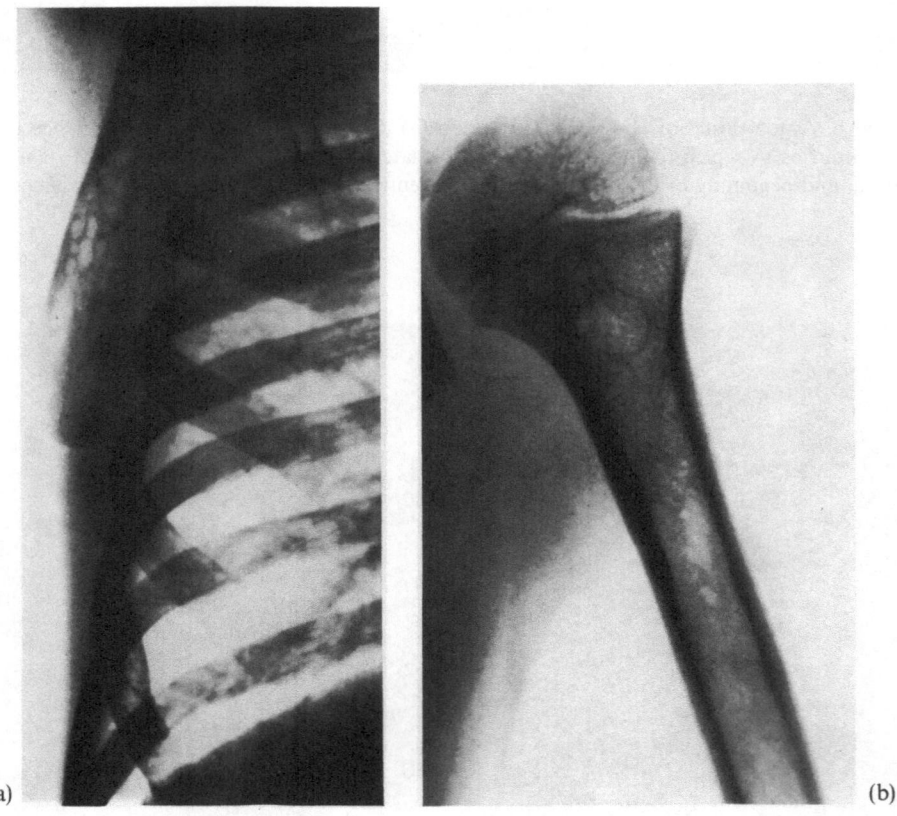

(a)   (b)

Fig. 12a–i. Anteroposterior roentgenogram of right side of chest (a) shows honeycomb lucent process involving lateral aspect of wing of scapula. Rib involvement is also present, with expansion of one of ribs. Left humerus (b) shows well-defined cystic lucency in left humeral metaphysis, and less well-defined changes involving proximal diaphysis. Left pelvis and proximal femur (c), taken in February, 1971, demonstrates multiple cystic lucencies in bones. Rapidity of osteolytic process is demonstrated in film taken 6 months later (d), demonstrating marked progression of process, particularly in intertrochanteric region, but also in pelvis. Left thigh (e) shows multiple lucencies in spongiosa and compacta, with slight expansion of diaphysis. There is also healed pathologic fracture. Lymphangiogram of extremity shows normal lymphatic channels. Film of lumbar spine and pelvis (f) during parenchymal phase of lymphangiogram shows multiple cystic lucencies in pelvis, and no filling of para-aortic lymph nodes. There is contrast media in bodies of L2 and L3. Lateral view of lumbar spine (g) confirms presence of contrast media in cystic cavities in body and lamina of L2 and L3. Tomograms (h and i) demonstrate well contrast medium within vertebral body. (KOHOUTEK, 1973, with permission)

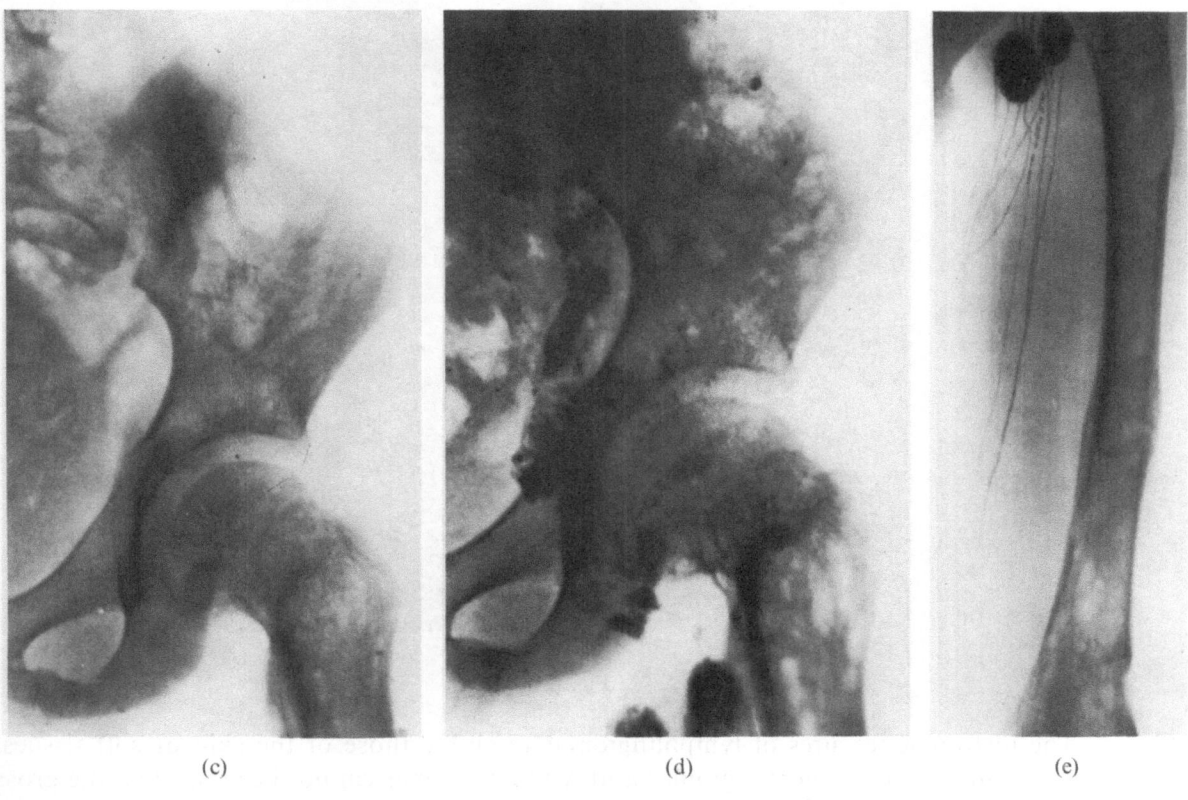

(c) (d) (e)

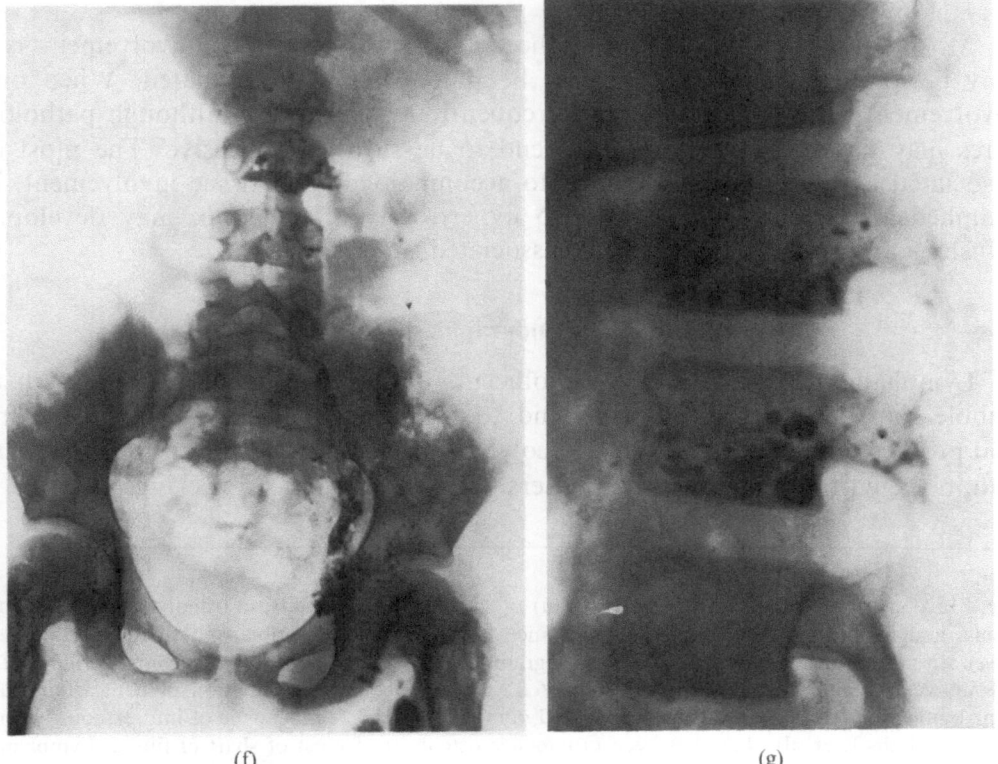

(f) (g)

Fig. 12c–g

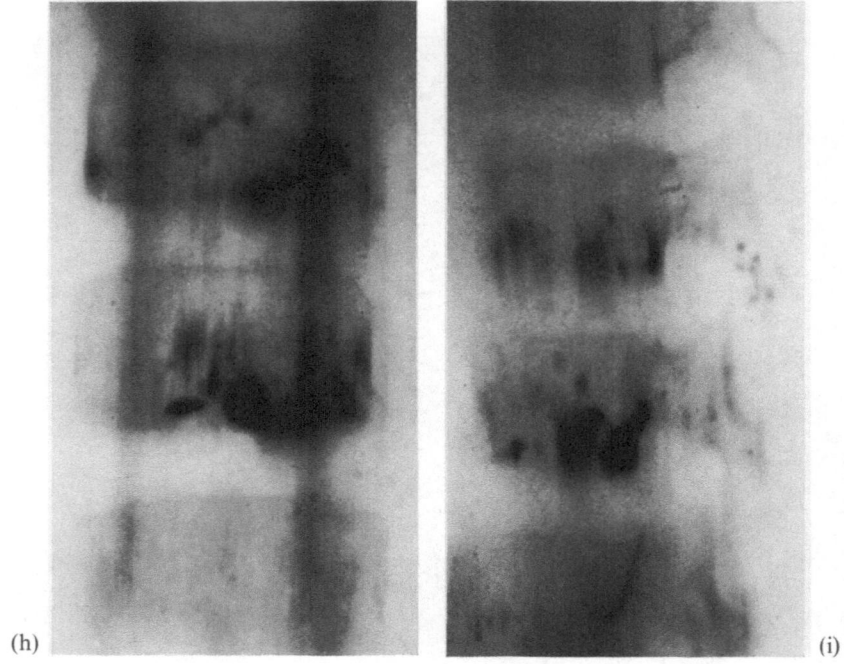

(h)   (i)

Fig. 12h–i

The histologic features of lymphangiomas resemble those of the skin or soft tissues. Although histologically hemangiomas and lymphangiomas cannot be separated, the gross appearance at operation with milky fluid exuding from the cysts, in association with the radiographic appearance, is thought to be diagnostic of a lymphangioma (STEINER et al., 1969).

Most lymphangiomas occur in the soft tissues, and bone involvement is rare. It may be limited to a single bone or be more widely disseminated. When only bone involvement is present, patients are frequently asymptomatic, although pathologic fractures may occur. The bone lesions tend to be slowly progressive. The most common associated abnormalities are related to accompanying soft tissue involvement, in which lymphedema, occasionally leading to hypertrophy of the limb, may develop. Pleural effusions and splenomegaly may be associated findings.

Roentgenographic Appearance

Lymphangiomas are usually radiolucent, well-outlined lesions, often with a "soap bubble" appearance. The lesions tend to be purely lytic in nature, well-demarcated, and progression is unpredictable. Osteolytic defects are seen both in the medullary cavity and in the cortex. Fine sclerotic borders surround the lytic areas (Figs. 12a–d).

Fig. 13a–d. Anteroposterior roentgenogram (a) of lower legs shows diffuse osteolytic process of right tibia, fibula, and femur. A "soap bubble" appearance is evident in lower tibia and fibula. Soft tissues of right lower leg are markedly enlarged. Lymphangiogram of right leg (b) demonstrates contrast filling of dysplastic subcutaneous lymphatics 1 h after injection. 6 days later (c), there is retention of contrast media in cystic bone lesions of tibia, fibula, calcaneous, cuboid, and patella. This is diagnostic of intraosseous lymphangiomatosis. 6 months later (d), there has been progressive osteolysis of most of shaft of fibula. Lymphangiographic contrast material is still retained in dilated lymphatics of bone and soft tissues. (HAFNER et al., 1972, with permission)

(a) (b)

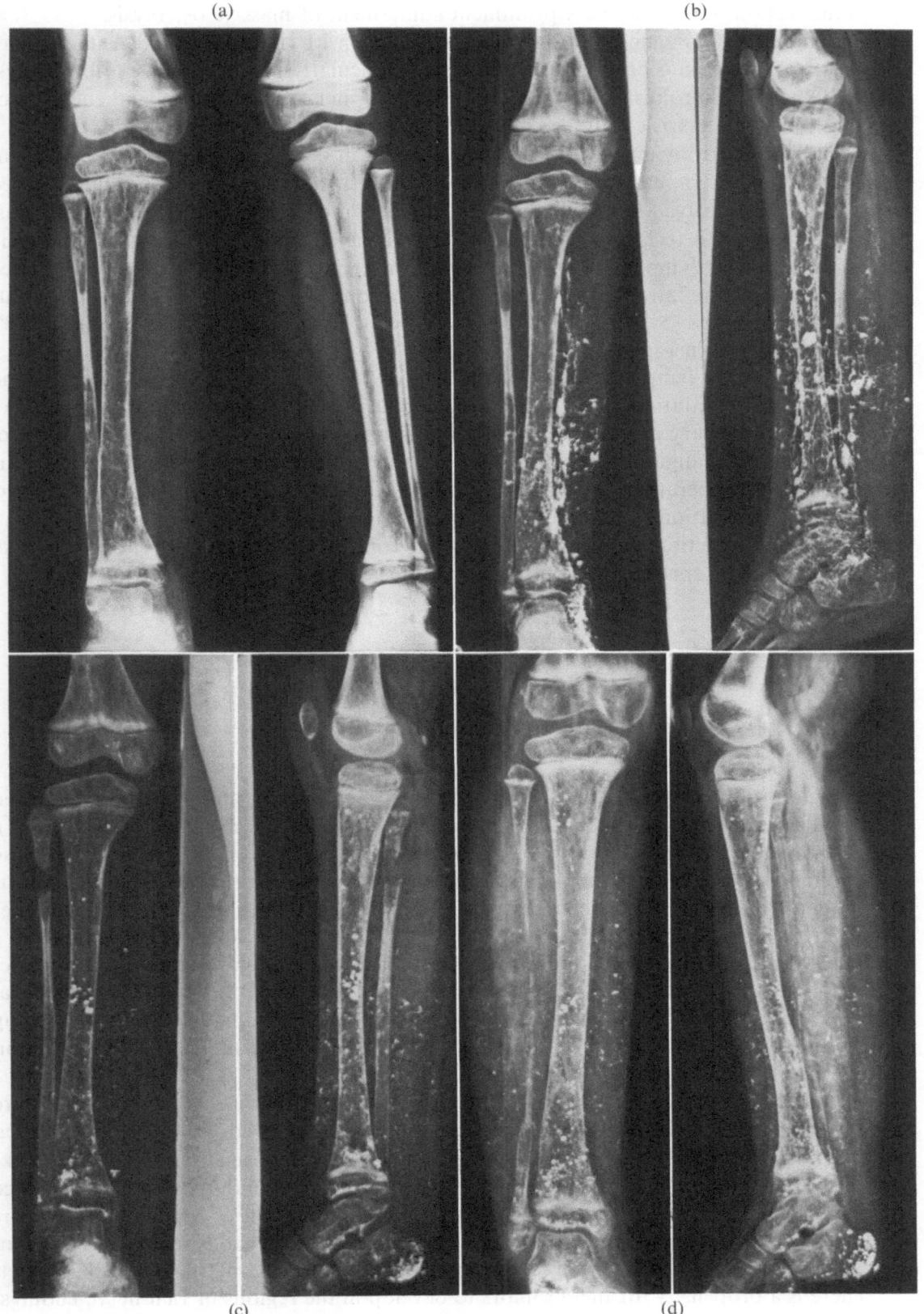

(c) (d)

Fig. 13a–d

Rarely, the lymphangiomas may be much more aggressive. As mentioned in the previous section, these may be a prominent component of massive osteolysis.

The differential diagnosis in the young age group with multiple lytic defects includes neoplastic, storage, and proliferative disorders, particularly histiocytosis X. Fibrous dysplasia, hyperparathyroidism, congenital fibromatosis, neurofibromatosis, and enchondromatosis must also occasionally be considered in the differential diagnosis.

Lymphangiography may be of considerable help in demonstrating primary lymphangiomas of bone. Lymphangiographic changes which have been described include dilated lymphatics with delayed drainage and a paucity of lymph nodes in the involved regions. The most important technical point is to obtain delayed films at 24 and 48 h following the injection of the lymphangiographic contrast material, since these are the films which will demonstrate the intraosseous lymphatic dilatation. Good examples of this technique have been described by Nixon (1970), Hafner et al. (1972), and Kohoutek (1973), and are illustrated in Figures12e–i, and 13a–d.

To summarize, lymphangiomas of bone are closely related to hemangiomas and represent cystic dilatation of intraosseous lymphatics, resulting in pressure erosion of cortical and medullary portions of bone. Lymphangiomas cannot be distinguished histologically from hemangiomas except for the presence or absence of red cells within the sinusoids, but at operation, the presence of milky fluid in the cystic spaces is diagnostic. Preoperative evaluation should include lymphangiography, which, by using delayed films 48 h after the injection of lymphangiographic contrast material, may show filling of intraosseous cystic spaces, pathognomonic for this disease.

C. Glomus Tumor

The glomus tumor has been referred to as an angioneuroma, and was first recognized as an enlarged caricature of the normal neuromyoarterial glomus by Masson (1924). He initially felt that these tumors could occur only in the fingers and toes because this is the location of the normal anatomical structures giving rise to the glomus tumor. Subsequently, both he and other authors have reported this tumor occurring in other locations.

The normal glomus acts as a regulatory mechanism diverting flow through arteriovenous communications or through a capillary bed. This serves to regulate interstitial pressure, control and regulate capillary flow, and act as a thermoregulator by controlling heat dissipation. These normally measure 1 mm in diameter, and are most common in the fingertips and ends of the toes.

The glomus tumor is felt to simply be hypertrophy of the normal glomus structure rather than a true neoplasm. Murray and Stout (1942) first discovered that the so-called epithelioid cells in glomus tumors were cells which had initially been described by Zimmermann (1923). By using a silver technique, Zimmermann found these on the surface of capillaries and called them pericytes. Murray felt that these epitheloid cells were pericytes which occurred in capillaries in all portions of the body, and furnished an explanation for the development of glomus tumors away from the hands and feet.

There is a propensity for these tumors to develop in the regions of rich nerve endings, and they have been reported following trauma. They may be very sensitive to touch, and may be quite painful when exposed to cold, with relief when exposed to warm water (MERCIER et al., 1970, and NATALI et al., 1966). The single most common location for glomus tumors is in the subungual region of the fingers.

Histologically, these have the same appearance as the normal glomus, with the exception that the capillaries have thicker walls and the caliber of the spaces may be larger. In addition, there may be an increase in their neural plexus. It is an organoid and highly differentiated lesion.

The glomus tumor is rare in bone, and most cases with bone involvement actually are secondary involvement due to soft tissue glomus tumors. The plain films may show a localized external cortical erosion of the bone adjacent to the lesion (Fig. 14 a), or may show a "punched-out" osteolytic lesion (Fig. 15). The local affect on bone appears to be entirely a pressure phenomenon from the adjacent tumor. The tumor itself does not contain calcification or other roentgenographically distinctive findings.

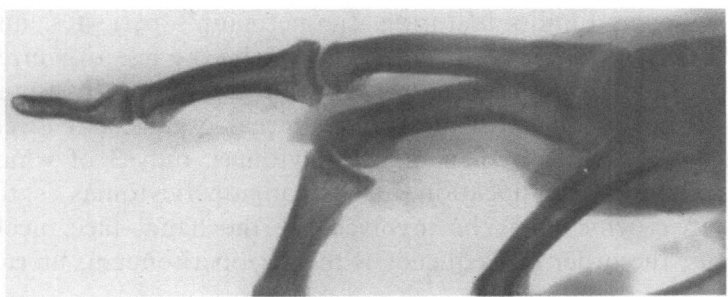

Fig. 14a

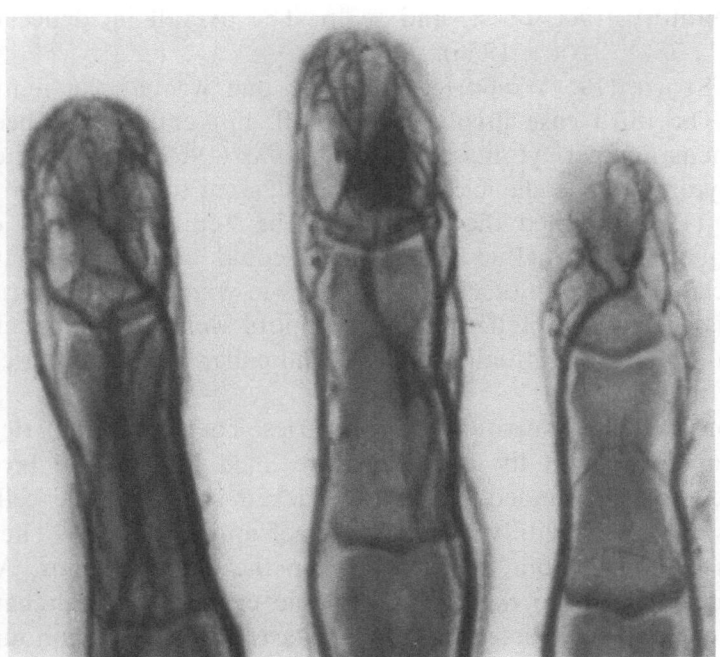

Fig. 14b

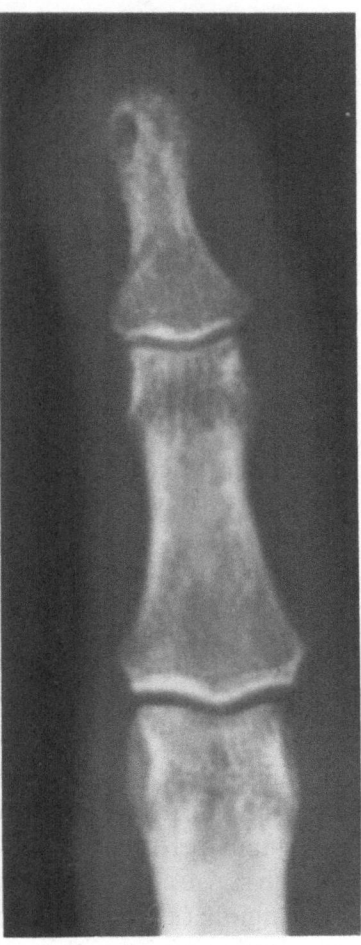

Fig. 15

Fig. 14a and b. Lateral roentgenogram of finger (a) demonstrates smooth external cortical pressure defect on dorsal aspect of distal phalanx. Digital arteriogram (b) outlines subungual glomus tumor by vascular blush. (LORD, G., and DUPONT, J.Y., 1974, with permission)

Fig. 15. Small "punched-out" lesion of distal phalanx was a proven glomus tumor

Angiography is helpful to define the lesion, make a specific diagnosis, and to define the presence of other asymptomatic lesions. The angiographic findings are characterized by enlarged feeding vessels with a hypervascular appearance composed of vascular lakes and a late blush. Rapid circulation and early venous filling is seen in some cases, but not in others (Natali et al., 1966, and Mercier et al., 1970). The vascular abnormality is usually confined precisely to the painful subungual tumefaction or discoloration (Fig. 14b), but occasionally other areas of involvement may be seen.

These tumors are treated by surgical excision. Incomplete removal, however, may result in a recurrence.

D. Hemangiopericytoma

Hemangiopericytomas are vascular tumors featuring Zimmermann's pericytes, and were first described by Stout and Murray in 1942. This is felt to be the less organized and more malignant counterpart of the glomus tumor. This tumor is usually found as a painless mass in the soft tissues of the extremities and internal organs, but rarely in bone. In 1956, Stout collected 197 cases of hemangiopericytomas, only 3 of which were primary in bone. The most common location for hemangiopericytomas is the thigh. Other extra-abdominal areas which may be involved are the hand, face, neck, and chest. Of the internal organs, the order of frequency is the retroperitoneum, uterus, and oral cavity and pharynx.

Of the tumors which metastasize, the most frequent primary site is the lower extremity, particularly the thigh, followed by the retroperitoneum, mediastinum, and occasionally the gastrointestinal tract, respiratory tract, chest, and scalp. The overall incidence of metastases is 23 of 197 cases (11.7%) (Stout, 1956).

Of the three cases which Stout (1956) reported in bone, one was in the femur and the other in the fibula. The third case involved the skull, but could have been an extension of a meningeal hemangiopericytoma. Marcial-Rojas (1960) has reported a primary lytic hemangiopericytoma of the clavicle which metastasized to lung.

After Murray and Stout (1942) defined the pericyte as the "epitheloid" cell of glomus tumors, the authors questioned whether this pericyte could be the malignant component of a previously unclassified group of vascular tumors in which the capillaries were lined by normal epithelial cells. They felt that these tumors were the malignant counterpart of the glomus tumor, and were initially reported and called hemangiopericytomas by Stout and Murray in 1942.

The pericyte is a normal contractile cell surrounding capillaries. The hemangiopericytoma is made up of many capillaries, but the capillaries are lined by a single layer of endothelial cells. Capillaries are surrounded by closely packed small spindle cells, sometimes arranged in clusters or whorls, with varying degrees of mitotic activity. These malignant pericytes do not have the organoid structure seen in the glomus tumor. Although Stout (1956) has made attempts to establish histologic criteria for malignant hemangiopericytomas, he found that the predictability of metastasis based on the amount of mitotic activity within the primary tumor was impossible. Hence, all hemangiopericytomas must be considered malignant.

Roentgenographic Appearance

Hemangiopericytomas in bone are rare tumors with only a few descriptions recorded in the literature. Most commonly, bone involvement is by external pressure erosion from adjacent soft tissue hemangiopericytomas. They may rarely contain calcification, which may be whorled in appearance (MUJAHED et al., 1959), or be in the form of spicules within the tumor mass (KENT, 1957).

The primary tumors of bone have been lytic lesions which may expand the bone, perforate the cortex, or completely destroy the involved portion of bone (Figs. 16a and b). This is clearly not a unique roentgen description, and the rarity of this tumor places it very low on any list of lytic expansile lesions of bone. Bone involvement by a partially calcified soft tissue tumor, however, particularly in the lower extremity, should suggest the diagnosis of hemangiopericytoma.

A review of the angiographic findings of hemangiopericytomas indicates that these usually are quite vascular with a tumor blush and enlarged venous drainage (DEVILLIERS et al., 1967). These descriptions, however, relate to soft tissue tumors and there is no description of the angiographic findings in a primary hemangiopericytoma of bone. There is no criteria by which the soft tissue hemangiopericytomas could be differentiated from other highly vascular lesions of soft tissue, and, presumably, this also applies to primary tumors of bone.

In summary, the hemangiopericytoma is the malignant counterpart of the glomus tumor, characterized by many capillaries lined by a single layer of endothelial cells, with a nonorganoid stroma of malignant pericytes. The histologic criteria does not allow a prediction of metastatic potential; therefore, all hemangiopericytomas must be treated aggressively. The roentgen appearance is a nonspecific, aggressive osteolytic lesion of bone. When associated with a partially calcified soft tissue tumor, particularly in the lower extremities, the diagnosis of a hemangiopericytoma should be suggested. Surgery is the primary mode of therapy, and many advocate follow-up radiation therapy to the resected site because of the high local recurrence rate and possibility of metastases.

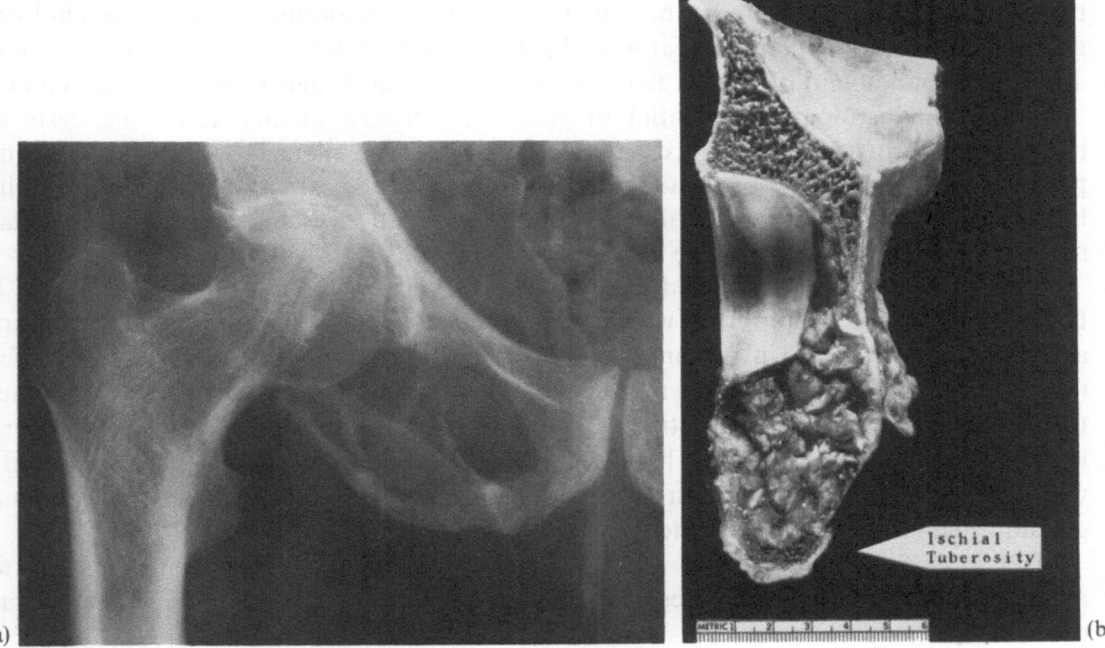

Fig. 16a and b. Anteroposterior roentgenogram (a) of right ischium demonstrating slightly expansile and destructive hemangiopericytoma of ischium. This gross specimen (b) demonstrates that lesion is well-circumscribed. (UNNI et al., 1971, with permission)

E. Hemangioendothelioma (Angiosarcoma)

Hemangioendotheliomas have been placed in the intermediate category of aggressiveness. There has been confusion in the classification of this group of tumors, but most pathologists presently equate hemangioendothelioma with angiosarcoma, and consider all to be malignant (UNNI et al., 1971). Various names have been given to this tumor, including malignant hemangioendothelioma, malignant hemangioma, malignant metastasizing angioma, granulation tissue sarcoma, angioblastoma, angioendothelioma, hemangiosarcoma, angiomyosarcoma, and even lymphangiosarcoma when the quantity of red blood cells within the tumor makes it impossible to distinguish primary lymphangiomatous from hemangiomatous tissue.

Hemangioendotheliomas of bone are considerably less common than hemangiomas of bone, but somewhat more common than hemangiopericytomas. In a group of 69 cases of bone tumors of vascular origin reported from the Mayo Clinic, 9 were angiosarcomas (UNNI et al., 1971). This tumor occurs in patients 3–78 years of age, and has a predominance in males with a 2:1 ratio.

Hemangioendotheliomas are also more common in soft parts than in bone. There is a predilection for involvement of the femur and vertebral column, but approximately one third of the patients will have multifocal involvement. This may be manifested by the diffuse involvement of one bone or multiple bones.

Grossly, these lesions are usually fairly well-circumscribed, dark red, friable lesions. There is little sclerotic reaction at the margins of the lesions, and the tumor may penetrate the cortex and secondarily involve the surrounding soft tissues.

Microscopically, the basic pattern in hemangioendotheliomas is neoplastic new blood vessel formation. The proliferating malignant endothelial cell is the hallmark of this tumor, with formation of atypical endothelial cells in greater numbers than are required to line the vessels with a simple endothelial membrane, and the formation of vascular tubes with a delicate framework of reticulin fibers and a tendency for their lumens to anastomose. In many areas, there will appear to be budding of the endothelial cells, giving the tumor a papillary appearance. There are no histologic criteria for the differentiation of hemangioendothelioma from angiosarcoma, and, hence, the two are equated.

The main histologic differential diagnosis is between aneurysmal bone cysts and hemangioendotheliomas, and occasionally differentiating metastatic carcinoma from a primary vascular tumor. Metastatic hypernephromas are particularly prone to mimic hemangioendotheliomas, especially if it is an unusually vascular tumor and contains foci with spindling, sarcoma like cells (UNNI et al., 1971).

The etiology of hemangioendotheliomas is unknown in the majority of cases, but two factors have been reported which may be contributory. Trauma has been reported as an antecedent factor in the onset of hemangioendothelioma in at least five patients (SPJUT et al., 1971). It is possible that hemangioendotheliomas develop from the granulation tissue capillaries of traumatized areas. The second factor which has been reported is radiation therapy to benign hemangiomas. Three examples have been reported in which patients have had radiation therapy to benign hemangiomas, and developed hemangioendotheliomas following a latent period of 4–15 years (SPJUT et al., 1971).

Hemangioendotheliomas are usually clinically manifested by pain and swelling, and in an extremity, by a limp. These tumors are usually very aggressive, and metastases occur early.

Roentgenographic Appearance

Hemangioendotheliomas are destructive and often expansile "soap bubble" lesions (Fig. 17). The roentgenographic appearance frequently will closely parallel the histologic grade of the neoplasm. In low-grade tumors, scattered trabeculae may be seen within the tumor, and the margins are fairly well-demarcated. In high-grade tumors, however, the margins are indistinct and irregular, and no trabeculae remain within the lesion (Fig. 18). Periosteal reactive new bone formation is not seen except in the most advanced lesions. The lesion may extend over a considerable length of the involved bone, and have a "Swiss cheese" type of appearance (Figs. 19a and b).

Soft tissue hemangioendotheliomas are characterized angiographically by numerous irregular and tortuous vessels with vascular lakes, arteriovenous shunting, and early venous filling. Presumably primary bone hemangioendotheliomas have a similar appearance. Because of mesenchymal origin of this tumor, venography and lymphangiography should also be performed to detect involvement of these other vascular systems (COLLARD et al., 1966).

Treatment for hemangioendotheliomas is surgery followed by radiation therapy, but prognosis is very poor. One-third of patients will live 3 years, and the 5-year cure rate is 9% (MCCARTHY and PACK, 1950). Hemangioendotheliomas metastasize widely to lung, brain, pleura, liver, and occasionally to lymph nodes.

In summary, angiosarcomas and hemangioendotheliomas are equated histologically. This is an extremely malignant tumor which may be seen at any age, characterized by malignant proliferation of endothelial cells forming a highly vascular tumor. It is purely osteolytic and may expand bone, but is not characterized by periosteal reactive new bone formation. This is a highly malignant tumor which metastasizes early, and carries a 5-year cure rate of only 9%.

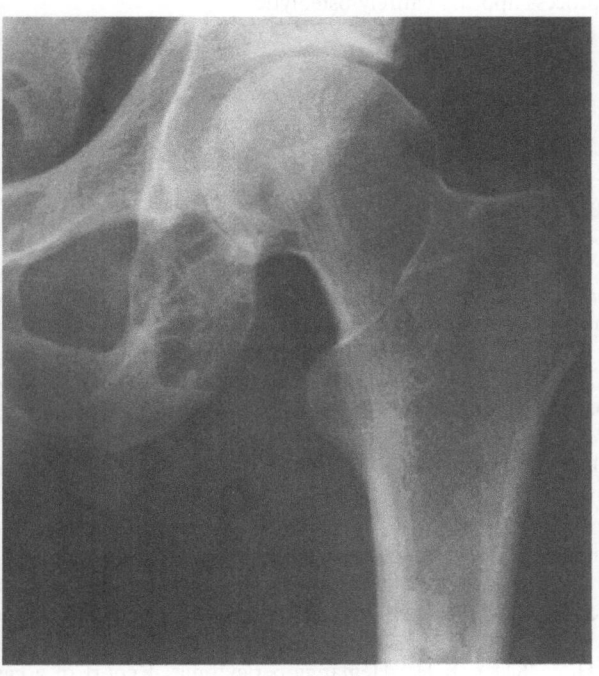
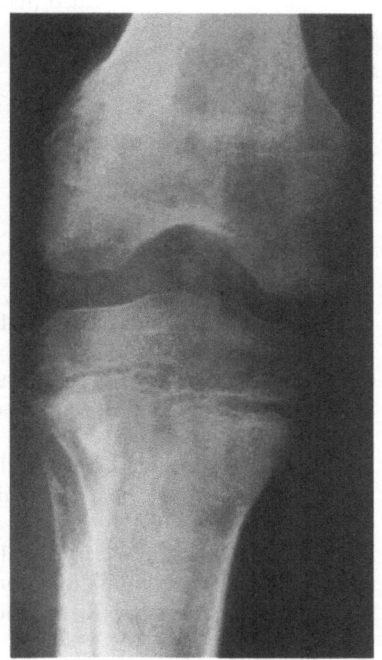

Fig. 17   Fig. 18

Fig. 17. Roentgenogram of left ischium shows well-defined, slightly expansile, bubbly lesion of bone which was hemangioendothelioma, Grade I. (DAHLIN et al., 1967, with permission)

Fig. 18. Anteroposterior roentgenogram of knee shows osteolytic lesion of proximal fibula, with indistinct and irregular margins, representing hemangioendothelioma, Grade III. (DAHLIN, 1967, with permission)

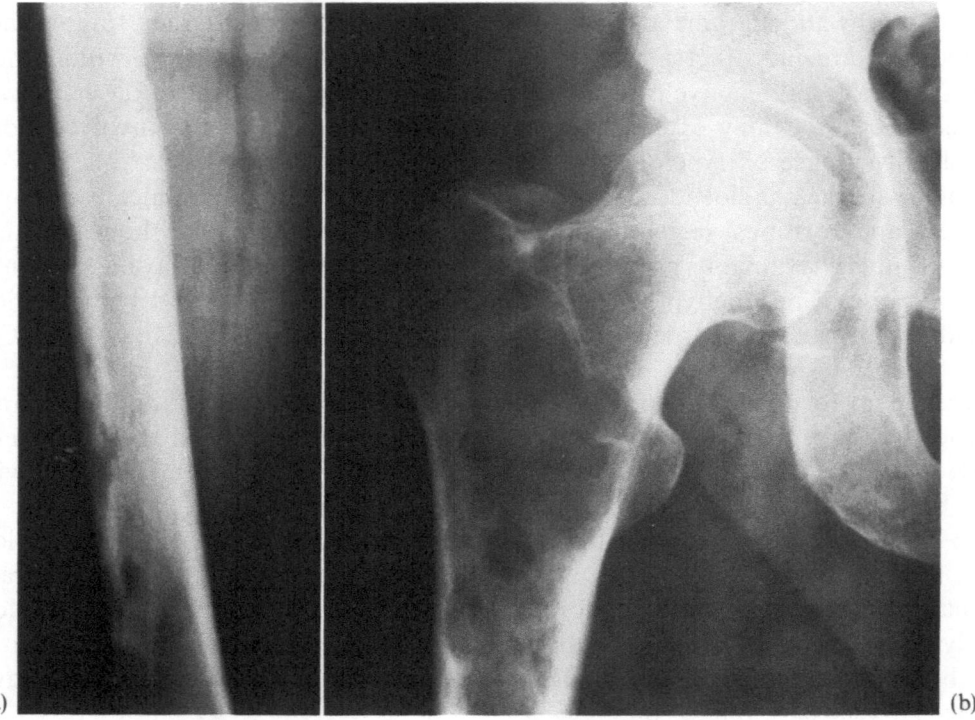

(a)   (b)

Fig. 19a and b. Anteroposterior roentgenograms of femoral shaft (a) and femoral neck (b) show extensive and multifocal osteolytic hemangioendothelioma involving entire femur. Some lesions are much better demarcated than others, but process appears entirely osteolytic

References

Ben-Menachem, Y., Epstein, M.J.: Post-traumatic capillary hemangioma of the hand. J. Bone J. Surg. **56A**, 1741–1743 (1974)

Collard, M., Collette, J.M., Mayall, R.C.: L'Etude angiographique des angiosarcomes. J. belg. Radiol. **49**, 126–133 (1966)

Dahlin, D.C.: Bone tumors: General aspects and data on 3987 cases 2nd Ed., Springfiled, Ill.: Charles C Thomas 1967

Forrest, J., Staple, T.W.: Synovial hemangioma of the knee: Demonstration by arthrography and arteriography. Amer. J. Roentgenol. **112**, 512–516 (1971)

Gorham, L.W., Wright, A.W., Shultz, H.H., Maxon, F.C., Jr.: Disappearing bones: A rare form of massive osteolysis: Report of two cases, one with autopsy findings. Amer. J. Med. **17**, 674–682 (1954)

Hacker, H., Alonso, A.: Die angiographische Darstellung eines Wirbelkörperhämangioms. Fortschr. Röntgenstr. **111**, 581–583 (1969)

Hafner, E., Fuchs, W.A., Kuffer, F.: Lymphangiography in Lymphangiomatosis of bone. Lymphology **5**, 129–131 (1972)

Halliday, D.R., Dahlin, D.C., Pugh, D.G., Young, H.H.: Massive osteolysis and angiomatosis. Radiology **82**, 637–644 (1964)

Hekster, R.E.M., Luyendijk, W., Tan, T.I.: Spinal-cord compression caused by vertebral hemangioma relieved by percutaneous catheter embolization. Neuroradiology **3**, 160–164 (1972)

Horvath, M.F.: Quelques aspects du diagnostic radiologique des angiomes osseux. J. Radiol. Électrol. **51**, 139–148 (1970)

Kent, K.H.: Hemangiopericytoma; Report of a case with special reference to roentgen therapy. Amer. J. Roentgenol. **77**, 347–356 (1957)

Kohoutek, V.: Zur lymphographischen Diagnose der multiplen Knochenlymphangiomatose. Fortschr. Röntgenstr. **118**, 559–565 (1973)

Lord, G., Dupont, J.Y.: Tumeurs glomiques sous-unguéales. Nouv. Presse méd. **3**, 445–446 (1974)

MANELFE, C., DJINDJIAN, R.: Exploration angiographique des angiomes vertébraux. Acta radiol. [Diagn.] (Stockh.) 13, 818–828 (1972)

MARCIAL-ROJAS, R.A.: Primary hemangiopericytoma of bone. Cancer (Philad.) 13, 308–311 (1960)

MASSON, P.: Le glomus neuro-myo-arteriel des regions tactiles et ses tumeurs. Lyon chir. 21, 257–280 (1924)

MCCARTHY, W.D., PACK, G.T.: Malignant blood vessel tumors. Surg. Gynec. Obstet. 91, 465–482 (1950)

MCNEILL, T.W., CHAN, G.E., CAPEK, V., RAY, R.D.: The value of angiography in the surgical management of deep hemangiomas. Clin. Orthop. 101, 176–181 (1974)

MERCIER, R., BRESSON, P., VIALLET, J.F., VANNEUVILLE, G.: Intérêt de l'artériographie dans les tumeurs glomiques sous-unguéales. J. Radiol. Électrol. 51, 303–304 (1970)

MURRAY, M.R., STOUT, A.P.: The glomus tumor: Investigation of its distribution and behaviour, and the identity of its "epithelioid" cell. Amer. J. Path. 18, 183–203 (1942)

MUJAHED, Z., VASILAS, A., EVANS, J.A.: Hemangiopericytoma; Report of four cases with a review of the literature. Amer. J. Roentgenol. 82, 658–666 (1959)

NATALI, J., ECARLAT, B., VINARDI, G., BATISSE, F.: Artériographie d'une tumeur glomique. J. Chir. (Paris) 92, 481–484 (1966)

NIXON, G.W.: Lymphangiomatosis of bone demonstrated by lymphangiography. Amer. J. Roentgenol. 110, 582–586 (1970)

PACK, G.T., MILLER, T.R.: Hemangiomas: Classification, diagnosis, and treatment. Angiology 1, 405–426 (1950)

ROSENBAUM, A.E., ROSSI, P., SCHECHTER, M.M., SHEEHAN, J.P.: Angiography of haemangiomata of the calvarium. Brit. J. Radiol. 42, 682–687 (1969)

SCHIMMEL, D.H., MOSS, A.A., KOROBKIN, M.: Use of abdominal arteriography in assessing diffuse skeletal haemangiomatosis. Brit. J. Radiol. 47, 142–144 (1974)

SCHMORL, G.: Die pathologische Anatomie der Wirbelsäule. Verh. Dtsch. orthop. Ges. 21, 3–41 (1927)

SHERMAN, R.S., WILNER, D.: The roentgen diagnosis of hemangioma of bone. Amer. J. Roentgenol. 86, 1146–1159 (1961)

SPJUT, H.J., DORFMAN, H.D., FECHNER, R.E., ACKERMAN, L.V.: Tumors of bone and cartilage. Atlas of Tumor Pathology, Second Series, Fascicle 5. Armed Forces Inst. Path. Washington, D.C., pp. 325–340 (1971)

STEINER, G.M., FARMAN, J., LAWSON, J.P.: Lymphangiomatosis of bone. Radiology 93, 1093–1098 (1969)

STOUT, A.P.: Tumors featuring pericytes: Glomus tumor and hemangiopericytoma. Lab. Invest. 5, 217–223 (1956)

STOUT, A.P., MURRAY, M.R.: Hemangiopericytoma: A vascular tumor featuring Zimmermann's pericytes. Ann. Surg. 116, 26–33 (1942)

THIEMANN, K.J.: Zur Differentialdiagnose der aneurysmatischen Knochenzyste und des Hämangioms in der Halswirbelsäule. Fortschr. Röntgenstr. 112, 641–645 (1970)

TÖPFER, D.: Über ein infiltrierend wachsendes Hämangiom der Haut und multiple Kapillarektasien der Haut und inneren Organe; Zur Kenntnis der Wirbelangiome. Frankfurt. Z. Path. 36, 337–345 (1928)

UNNI, K.K., IVINS, J.C., BEABOUT, J.W., DAHLIN, D.C.: Hemangioma, hemangiopericytoma, and hemangioendothelioma (angiosarcoma) of bone. Cancer (Philad.) 27, 1403–1414 (1971)

VILLIERS, DE, D.R., FARMAN, J., CAMPBELL, J.A.H.: Pelvic haemangiopericytoma: Preoperative arteriographic demonstration. Clin. Radiol. 18, 318–323 (1967)

WALDRON, R.L., ZELLER, J.A.: Diffuse skeletal hemangiomatosis with visceral involvement. J. Canad. Ass. Radiol. 20, 119–123 (1969)

WALLIS, L.A., ASCH, T., MAISEL, B.W.: Diffuse skeletal hemangiomatosis. Amer. J. Med. 37, 545–563 (1964)

ZIMMERMANN, K.W.: Der feinere Bau der Blutcapillaren. Z.: Anat. Entwickl. Gesch. 68, 29–109 (1923)

Connective Tissue Tumors of Bone

by

Paul H. Pevsner

The major conditions of interest are those of the chondrogenic series which include chondromyxoid fibroma and its malignant counterpart, chondromyxoid sarcoma, infantile fibrochondroma, and infantile periosteal chondroma; and the fibrogenic series which includes calcifying fibroma, nonossifying fibroma, and the malignant counterpart fibrosarcoma. The nonhematopoietic series of intramedullary lesions that arise from fat which include lipomas and their malignant counterparts liposarcoma will also be discussed.

A. Chondrogenic Series

Chondromyxoid fibroma is generally accepted as a distinctive tumor of cartilaginous derivation, however, many authors disagree on its clinical behavior (AEGERTER and KIRKPATRICK, 1963; LICHTENSTEIN, 1965b). Several authors have remarked on the benign quality of this tumor in spite of frequent and often early recurrences. DAHLIN (1957a), JAFFE and LICHTENSTEIN (1948), SCHAJOWICZ and GALLARDO (1971), and SPJUT et al. (1971) and others have commented on malignant transformation. AEGERTER and KIRKPATRICK (1963) have suggested that chondromyxoid fibroma is a slowly progressive malignant tumor which is usually cured by conservative resection but which may, over many years, become locally invasive and even metastasize. A more aggressive course has been noted in younger individuals (RALPH, 1962).

Numerous descriptions of chondromyxoid fibroma as well as individual case reports have appeared since the original paper by JAFFE and LICHTENSTEIN (1948), including those by FELDMAN et al. (1970), FRANK and ROCKWOOD (1969), MARCOVE et al. (1964), SACHDEVA et al. (1969), SETH and RAO (1964), and WRENN and SMITH (1954).

However, accurate evaluation of the total number is difficult because there is much histologic overlapping in the various series. SCHAJOWICZ and GALLARDO (1971) reported 32 cases from 10 Latin American countries and fewer than 100 well-documented cases in the literature. The two largest series referred to in their paper were the 11 cases reported by the Netherlands Committee on Bone Tumors and the 41 cases in the collection of the Bone Tumor Committee of the Japanese Orthopedic Association National Cancer Center. SALZER and SALZER-KUNTSCHIK (1965) had collected 117 cases and FELDMAN et al. (1970) reported 207 cases from the literature. FRANK and ROCKWOOD (1969) reported 4 cases and gathered more detailed information on 90 cases in the literature. RAHIMI et al. (1972) documented 20 of 24 cases from the Mayo Clinic. At that time approximately 250 cases of chondromyxoid fibroma had been reported. The incidence of the tumor appears to be less than 1% of all tumoral and tumorlike lesions of bone.

There is no obvious sex distribution, the incidence of chondromyxoid fibroma is equal in both males and females. The age incidence is predominately in the second and third decades but cases have been reported ranging from age 6 to age 79, and in all series 60% occur in patients under 30 years of age.

It appears that chondromyxoid fibroma may occur in any age at which a group of chondroblasts left behind in the metaphysis by the advancing epiphyseal frontier, develops the ability to proliferate. Thus, the common metaphyseal location may also explain the age incidence.

Symptoms that are most prominent include pain and swelling. The duration of pain in various series ranges from 2 weeks to 32 months with an average of approximately 22 months. Often a pathologic fracture is responsible for the pain, though often only swelling and induration of the extremity involved is demonstrated clinically. The duration of the swelling ranges from 2 to 72 months with an average of 10 months.

In the long bones, the chondromyxoid fibroma has always been reported in the metaphysis. In the short cylindrical bones of the hands and feet it may begin in the metaphysis, but ultimately involves the entire shaft. The lesion is usually small, averaging 2–3 cm in diameter, but lesions of greater than 10 cm have been reported. In the metaphysis of long bones it is usually eccentric, slowly growing, producing a thin line of reactive sclerotic bone along the margin in contact with the cancellous bone tissues. Occasionally there is erosion of the cortex without reactive bone formation, producing lifting of the cortex without invading or penetrating it. The cortex may be thin to the point of fracture. The resulting callus formation following the fracture mixed in with the expanding cartilaginous tumors presents a confusing picture. The epiphyseal line and the distal pole of the lesion are usually separated by at least 1 cm or more of normal bone. However, occasionally the lesion may about directly upon the epiphysis, which makes the differentiation between chondromyxoid fibroma and chondroblastoma extremely diffcult. Aegerter and Kirkpatrick (1963) point out that the differentation between the two lesions may not be justifiable because the histologic elements are so similar, but rather that they represent the same lesion with peculiar features secondary to the environmental differences of location, the one in the epiphysis and the other in the shaft.

The radiologic features of the chondromyxoid fibroma vary, depending on the site of the lesion. In the tubular bones, the lesion typically appears as a well-demarcated, eccentrically located, metaphyseal lesion. It is round or oval, and has its long axis paralleling that of the bone. Feldman et al. (1970) reported that the average size of the tumor in long bones was $3 \times 2 \times 2$ cm, with a range of about 1–10 cm in its greatest dimension, which concurs with the findings of Rahimi et al. (1972). The tumor typically has a scalloped border with a rim of sclerosis. In some cases, specifically those of Vix and Fahmy (1969) this sclerosis was so pronounced as to simulate that of osteomyelitis. The tumor itself is radiolucent and appears as a defect with a trabecular pattern. The trabeculae do not represent complete bony septa, they are pseudotrabeculations from reflections of corrugation and scalloping of the bone at the edge of the tumor. The smaller tumors appear as smooth, punched out cystic defects. The tumor usually spares the epiphyseal cartilaginous plate. The lobulated masses of cartilage that characterize the chondromyxoid fibroma have the density of soft tissue, resulting in the appearance of a radiolucent lesion in contrast with the surrounding bone. Uncommonly, spotty calcification is present reflecting calcifying chondroid. In the long bones this neoplasm arises eccentrically and thins and expands the overlying cortex as it grows, but rarely involves the epiphyseal line. In the flat bones, the lesion is usually evident as a radiolucent defect with sclerotic, scalloped borders which often contains many trabeculations.

Occasionally there is marked soft tissue invasion by the tumor when it has eroded through the cortical margin. The peripheral edge of the tumor abutting soft tissue may show remnants of the cortex pushed away from the bone, but though periosteal reaction has been reported, this is only occasionally seen as a Codman's triangle. Pathologic fracture is a frequent finding of the lesion in both the long bones and metatarsals. The spotty calcification, though seen only occasionally radiographically, is seen in as high as one-third of the cases microscopically (RAHIMI et al., 1972). The tumor size tends to be very much larger when it occurs in flat bones.

The gross pathologic features of the tumor are that of a fibrous semi-translucent, rubbery mass with a smooth, bosselated outer surface. They are usually of a bluish hue, and areas of yellow, gray, or brown discoloration are often seen. The tumors are usually well-demarcated from the surrounding tissues, and myxoid foci, small cysts, or hemorrhagic zones can be seen. The cysts can sometimes be filled with a significant amount (up to 5 or 10 cc) of clear fluid. Microscopically the tumor is characterized by lobules with extensive fusion with neighboring lobules. Between the lobules of tumor and adjacent bone a narrow space occupied by a loose, highly vascularized, non-neoplastic, connecutive tissue is often demonstrated. This connective tissue can be seen within the tumoral mass incompletely filling the spaces between the lobules. Bony septa do not usually divide the tumor and the lobules are invariably connected. The central part of the lobules usually appears myxoid and blends into a more cellular periphery where spindle-shaped fibroblastic cells are noted. Occasionally mitotic figures are seen in these cellular zones and resemble those of fibrosarcoma. In some tumors parts of lobules are more fibrous and hypocellular, and microcysts containing a mucinous or hyaline material are seen. SALZER and SALZER-KUNSCHIK (1965) relate collagenization of central myxoid parts of the lobules to aging of the lesion. Cells with large and multiple nuclei are seen in more than one-third of the lesions. The presence of such multinucleated cells imparts an ominous appearance, and introduces the possibility of mistaking these tumors for chondrosarcomas. Necrotic foci are often seen within the lobules in as high as 10% of the cases. Polygonal or round, closely packed, peripheral cells are sometimes seen in the lobules. These cells resemble those of benign chondroblastoma, and may be intermingled with fibroblasts and multinucleated benign giant cells. Osteoid or fine bony trabeculae, as described by BENEDETTI et al. (1962), are found in many of the tumors. When minimal, the trabeculae appear as faint osteoid in the peripheral parts of the tumor lobules. When it is more prominent the trabeculae show mineralization and extend into interlobular connective tissue.

Mucinous lesions, or those with a highly myxoid quality recur more frequently. In addition, these more mucinous lesions tend to occur in younger individuals. Therefore, a combination of mucinous lesions with large or atypical nuclei in young individuals should suggest a high probability of recurrence following curettage. RAHIMI et al. (1972) reported postirradiation sarcomatous change with development of a fibrosarcoma 6 years following irradiation at the site of the initial lesion. That patient died with evidence of metastasis 1 year later, despite amputation for the sarcoma.

The prognosis for this lesion is somewhat mixed considering that in one-third of the cases reported, malignant degeneration with features of chondrosarcoma have been described (AEGERTER and KIRKPATRICK, 1963).

Benign giant cells have been described as a constant finding in chondromyxoid fibroma (JAFFE and LICHTENSTEIN, 1948). However, other authors find the presence of such cells in less than half of the tumors in their series (RAHIMI et al., 1972; FELDMAN et al., 1970).

The differential diagnosis of chondromyxoid fibroma includes, most importantly, chondrosarcoma. The problem is exaggerated by the large nuclei present in about one-third of the chondromyxoid fibromas. Paradoxically, because of the fear of unnecessary radical treatment for benign tumors, pathologists have often considered or made the diagnosis of chondromyxoid fibroma when the lesion in question was actually a chondro-sarcoma; disastrously inadequate treatment results. Even though the chondrosarcoma may have prominent myxoid areas, this tumor has a more distinct hyaline cartilage quality and it lacks the characteristic admixture of fibromatous elements. Further, it lacks the abrupt boundary of chondromyxoid fibroma, and this aggressive quality is reflected in a radiographic appearance which contrasts with the benign appearance of the chondromyxoid fibroma.

Malignant degeneration of chondromyxoid fibroma is somewhat controversial in the literature. RAHIMI et al. (1972) reported one case of malignant change and that was in a patient irradiated as part of the primary treatment of the original lesion. In all other cases which they reviewed, elements of histologic changes characteristic of chondrosarcoma could be found in the original biopsy material. Therefore, they suggest that since the risk of malignant transformation of true chondromyxoid fibroma is so low, unnecessary radical treatment should not be employed. However, this does not exclude complete removal of chondromyxoid fibroma by resection. Resection should include the tumor bed to prevent the relatively high rate of occurrence seen after curettage alone. The efficiency of more complete resection has been documented by SCHAJOWICZ and GALLARDO (1971) and is indicated by the success with such treatment of recurrent tumors in the series of RAHIMI et al. (1972) (Figs. 1–5).

A very rare lesion that is only seen in children, and has a similar appearance to chondromyxoid fibroma is infantile chondroma or periosteal fibrochondroma of child-hood. These lesions are generally periosteal in origin as determined from radiographs

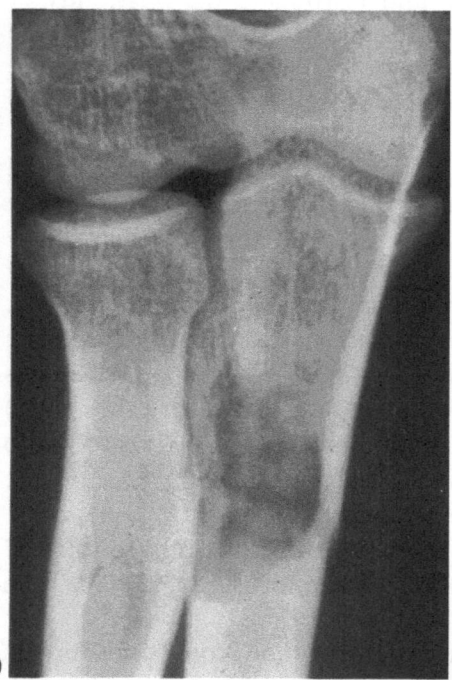

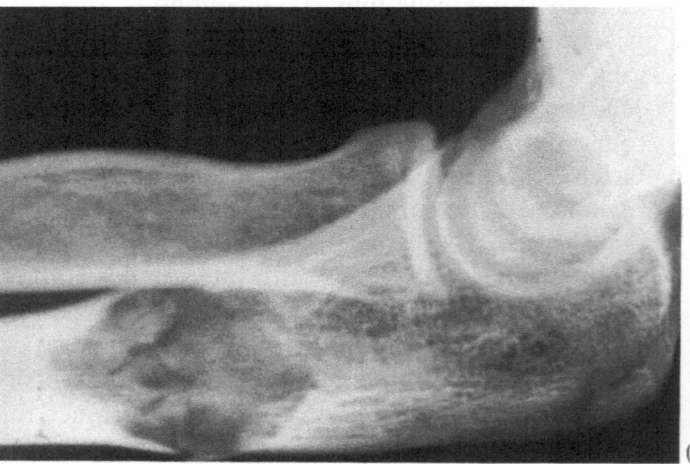

(a)   Fig. 1a and b. Chondromyxoid fibroma of proximal ulna
                                      with pathologic fracture through fracture site

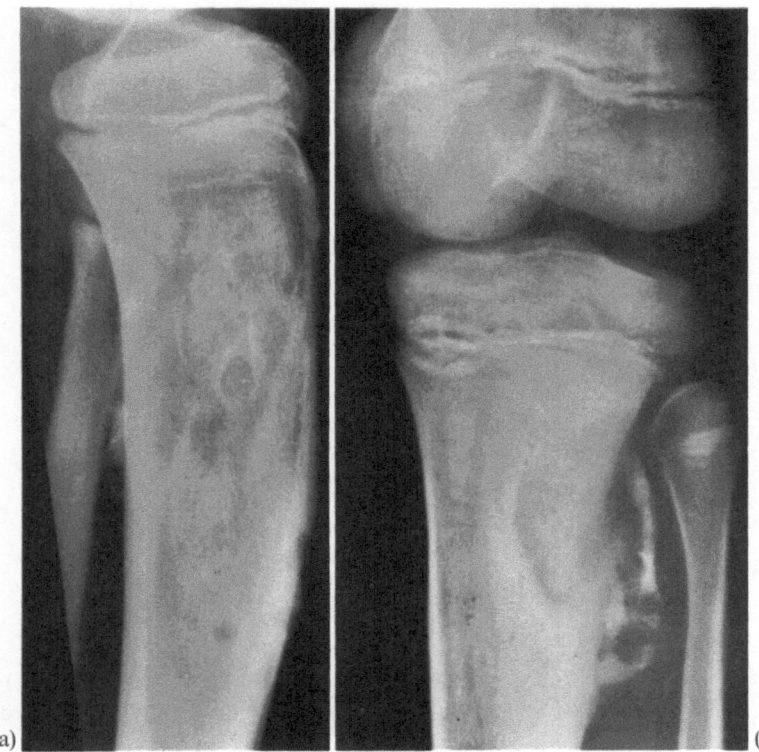

(a)   (b)

Fig. 2a and b. Chondromyxoid fibroma of proximal tibia with extra cortical expansion and periosteal elevation

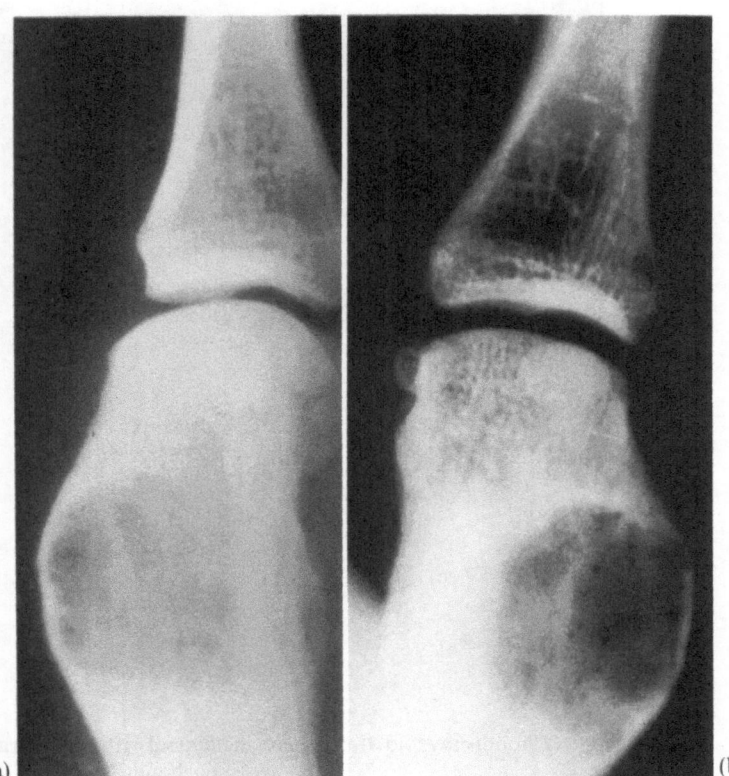

Fig. 3a and b. Chondromyxoid fibroma of proximal metacarpal of the thumb

(a)   (b)

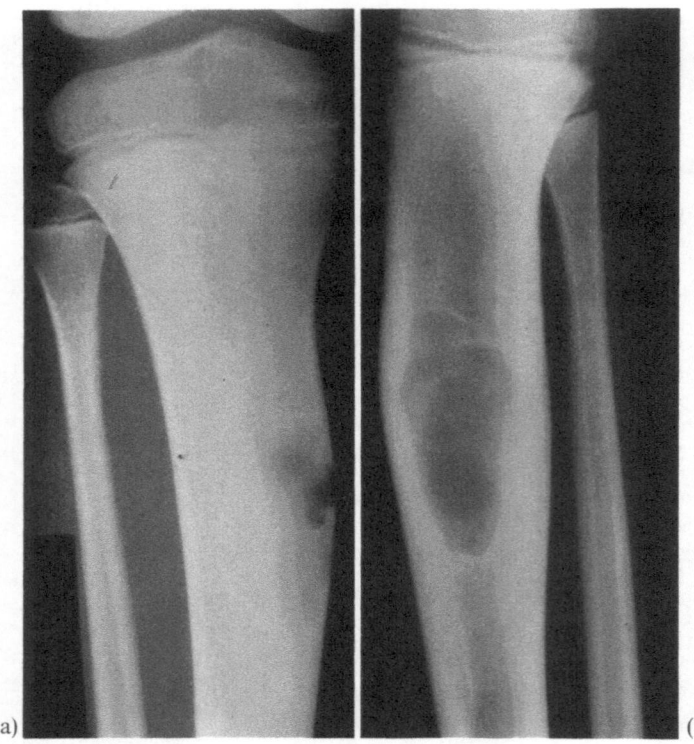

Fig. 4a and b. Chondromyxoid fibroma of proximal tibia showing marked, scalloped margination

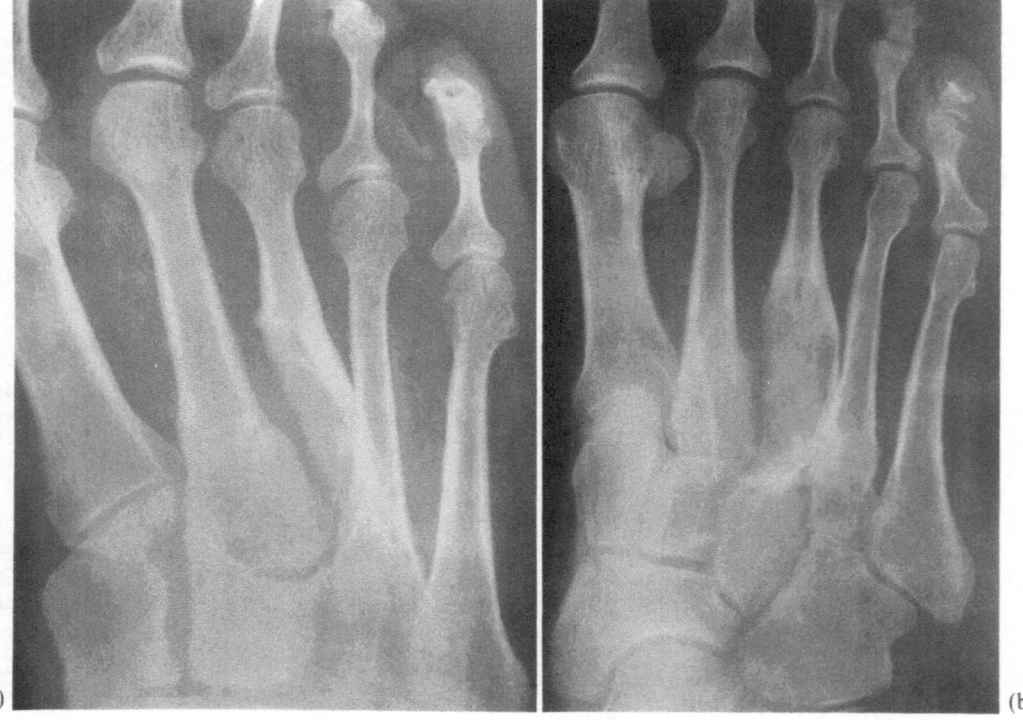

Fig. 5a and b. Chondromyxoid fibroma of metatarsal with radiographic appearance very similar to that of enchondroma

and microscopic sections. A fine diffuse calcification on the radiographs is matched by spotty areas of calcification in the microscopic section. These lesions produce cartilage, but many of the cells fail to develop hyaline cartilage and instead produce fibrocartilage with spotty calcification. These lesions have a benign appearance radiographically and are not known to metastasize (Figs. 6–8).

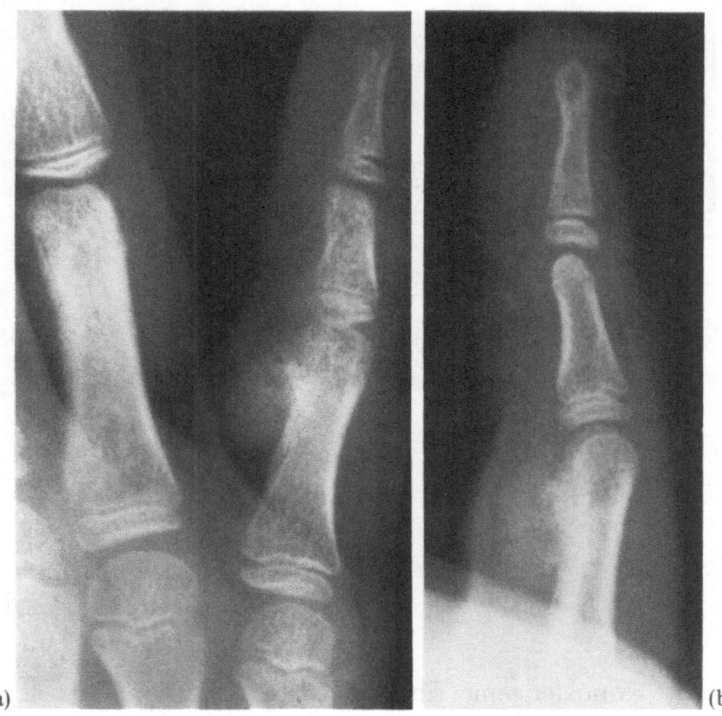

Fig. 6a and b. Periosteal fibro-chondroma of proximal phalanx of a child

(a)   (b)

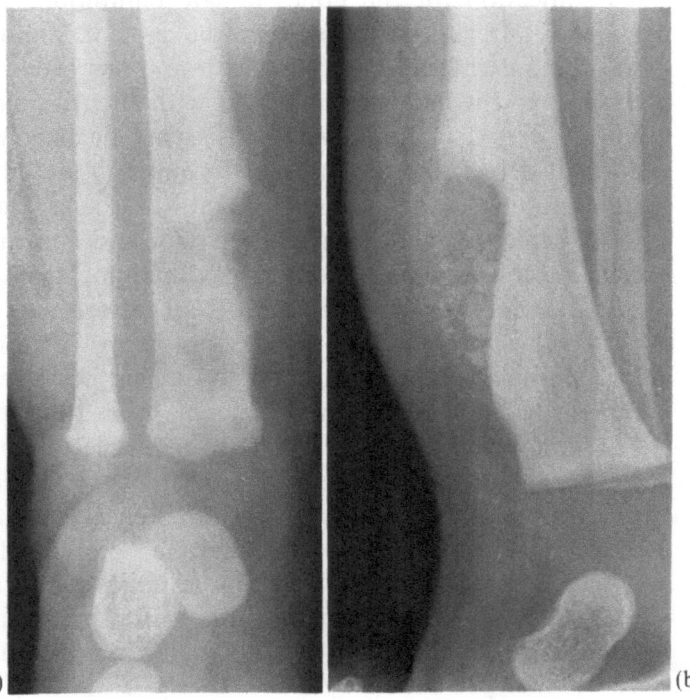

Fig. 7a and b. Juvenile periosteal fibro-chondroma of distal tibia

(a)   (b)

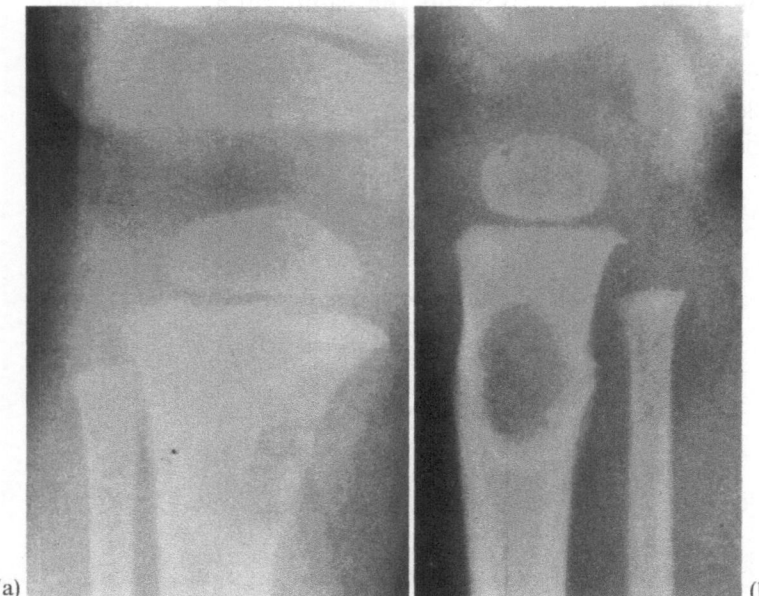

(a)   (b)   Fig. 8a and b. Infantile chondroma
                                                              of proximal tibia

B. Fibrogenic Series

Nonosteogenic fibroma is a rather common degenerative and proliferative lesion of the medullary and cortical tissues of bone. It occurs most commonly near the ends of the diaphyses of the large long bones, particularly of the lower extremities. It has a predilection for the bones of late childhood, adolescence, and early adult life. The majority of cases occur between the ages of 5 and 15 years. Very often multiple lesions are demonstrated. In the past the lesion has been referred to as a xanthoma or fibroxanthoma, and it has been confused with such lesions as a solitary cyst, giant cell tumor, fibrous dysplasia, lipid histiocytosis, chronic osteomyelitis, bone infarct, and subperiosteal cortical defect. Nonosteogenic fibroma is a definite clinical entity with specific clinical, radiographic, and microscopic features. JAFFE and LICHTENSTEIN (1942) were the first to recognize the characteristic behavior and appearance which enables one to distinguish this lesion from a large number of others mentioned. The lesion is entirely nonneoplastic and therefore the word fibroma is an unfortunate term because it has placed the lesion within the classification of bone tumors in which it does not really belong.

One-half of the lesions diagnosed as nonosteogenic fibroma has given rise to no symptoms and is discovered incidentally in routine radiographs made for other reasons. For this reason the true incidence of the lesion is unknown and difficult to determine. Trauma, as an antecedent historical event, occurs just as often as it does not and probably bears no relationship to the development of these lesions. Pain is the common complaint and it may be of weeks or months duration, suggesting that it is usually not of a very severe nature. The lesions usually appear near the end of the diaphysis of long bones and the pain is often interpreted as arthritic in character. If a slender bone such as the fibula, or the ulna is involved and there is expansion, the mass may be the first presenting sign.

The majority of these lesions occur in the first two decades, but occasionally an older individual has been seen to have a nonosteogenic fibroma. The lesions are seen in the flat bones as well as the long bones; and lesions of the ilium and bilateral lesions have been described. The radiographic appearance is that of a confluent area of deossification, the whole having a bosselated outer surface which involves both cancellous and compact bone and appears to begin just deep to the cortical laminae and destroys bone tissue in both directions. It is often within a centimeter of the unclosed epiphyseal line. The average size at the time of discovery is usually 3–5 cm. The lesion is usually eccentric, but gradually extends across the entire diameter of the bone and becomes sealed off from the normal medullary tissue above and below by a margin of sclerotic bone and laterally it is usually covered by a fusiform bulging shell of cortex. If the patient is followed long enough, the lesion will appear to "drift" toward the mid-diaphysis as enchondral bone growth pushes the epiphysis away from it. It usually does not extend beyond the midpoint of the shaft of the long bones. Eventually new bone grows in from the periphery and obliterates the entire area of the lesion. The complete healing of a few cases reported in the literature has been over a period from 2 to 5 years. A curetted lesion may appear to heal only to re-occur later, further toward the mid-diaphysis, at a point corresponding to the original site in the younger bone (HATCHER, 1945).

Frequently a fracture of the cortical shell can occur through the lesion, and the callus induced following the fracture makes both the radiographic and microscopic picture more complex. Usually pain becomes extremely severe. If the biopsy is not chosen carefully, the microscopic picture is that of reparative fracture rather than a nonosteogenic fibroma. The microscopic picture is that of an area of cancellous and overlying cortical deossification and replacement by fibroblastic proliferation. Whether a true ischemic degenerative process precedes the fibrous hyperplasia or whether a primary uncontrolled fibrous hyperplasia causes the bone erosion to accommodate its bulk is unclear. The expansion of the cortex over many of these lesions suggests the latter explanation. The

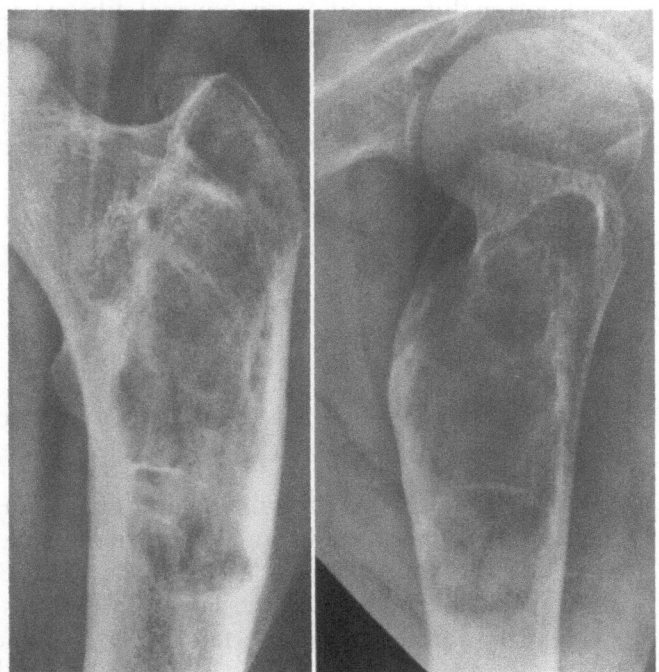

Fig. 9a and b. Nonosteogenic fibroma   (a)   (b)
    of proximal femur

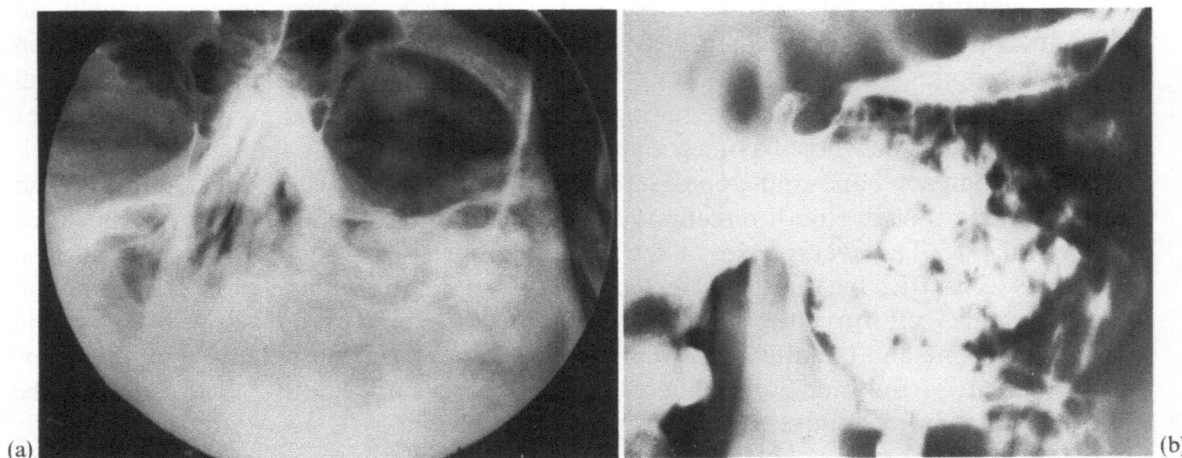

Fig. 10a and b. Calcifying fibroma of the left maxilla

cause for this overgrowth is unknown. Focal ischemia secondary to vascular occlusion following trauma or embolism has been suggested as the initiating agent, however, this does not stand up to careful examination. In most lesions at least a few xanthoid cells, large, pale polyhedral cells with abundant finely granular cytoplasm can be found. Often these cells are arranged in aggregates or cell islands and occasionally they dominate the microscopic field. These cells are macrophages, or phagocytizing fibroblasts, if a distinction can be made, that have taken up lipid material, largely cholesterol. Prussian blue reaction identifies this material as hemosiderin. This is considered by some to be further evidence that these lesions have their origin in bone infarcts (Fig. 9a and b).

From the evidence currently available, a nonosteogenic fibroma should disappear in 2–5 years from the time it is diagnosed. If it is unusually large and thereby jeopardizes the strength of the bone, or if a fracture occurs and causes pain or disability, conservative surgical management may be necessary with curettage.

Occasionally one finds an unusual fibrous lesion in the jaw and maxillary region which, on microscopic examination, is a mass of collagen without any evidence of atypical tissue, or neoplastic elements. It is usually very acellular, but has a rather disturbing picture on radiographs. These lesions are often calcified and are not known to be malignant other than locally deformative of surrounding tissue. Such lesions are fibromas and the term calcifying fibroma accurately describes both the radiographic and microscopic picture. These lesions are very similar to the microscopic appearance of fibrous dysplasia, but are far less cellular microscopically (Fig. 10a and b).

C. Fibrosarcoma

Fibrosarcoma is a rare malignant neoplasm of bone that is reported to be less than 4% of primary malignant bone tumors (Dahlin, 1967b; Eyre-Brook and Price, 1969; Jaffe, 1947c, 1958; Lichtenstein, 1965a; Stout, 1948). One-half of these tumors occur in the long bones of the lower extremities with 40% in the region of the knee. This distribution has been reported by Dahlin and Ivins (1969), Eyre-Brook and Price (1969), Gilmer and MacEwen (1958), and Cunningham and Arlen (1968). Other sites include the mandible, humerus, radius, ulna, calvarium, maxilla, rib, scapula, clavicle, sacrum, vertebrae, and ilium as well as the more common locations in the femur and tibia. Most of the lesions in the long bones are metaphyseal, although in a few instances they have occurred in the shaft of a femur, humerus, or tibia.

Symptomatology and signs are entirely nonspecific. The patient may complain of pain or mass in the region of the tumor and symptoms vary from a few weeks to as long as 2 or more years. Of 50 patients reported by EYRE-BROOK and PRICE (1969), 7 presented with a fracture through the tumor site. Other authors have described pulmonary metastases as the primary presentation. Multiple lesions are rare, but diffuse involvement has been reported by STEINER (1944) and by NIELSEN and POULSEN (1962). There is a high rate of local recurrence especially if incomplete excision has been performed (JAFFE, 1958c).

The most common age of occurrence is in the second, third, and fourth decades but ranges from 6 to 88 years. If one includes lesions that have arisen in pre-existing conditions such as Paget's disease, treated giant cell tumors, and in irradiation osteitis, the mean age is somewhat higher, in fact, the occurrence of this lesion at a later age than osteosarcoma is a factor that implies the presence of a primary lesion and not a variant of osteosarcoma. Females appear to show a slight predominance over males in terms of occurrence.

The radiographic appearance shows such marked destructiveness by the tumor that it is sometimes difficult to distinguish fibrosarcoma from an osteolytic osteosarcoma. The osteolytic characteristic of this tumor very often produces marked erosion to cortical bone with a major portion of the tumor appearing in the contiguous soft tissues. Periosteal bone reaction is not uncommon. There may be slight sclerosis at the margins of the tumor which is more distinct in well-differentiated lesions. The permeative appearance giving a mottled radiolucency on radiographs like Ewing's sarcoma is another characteristic of this lesion.

Most authors believe fibrosarcoma arises de novo in bone, however, STOUT (1948) and GESCHICKTER (1932) denied the existence of a primary fibrosarcoma of bone. These authors believe that a careful study of the lesion microscopically will reveal osteoid or cartilage, or that the lesion began as a sarcoma of the periosteum or adjacent soft tissues with secondary invasion of the underlying bone. This, however, is not the general view (JAFFE, 1947, 1958b; LICHTENSTEIN, 1965a; DAHLIN and IVINS, 1969; GILMER and MACEWEN, 1958; EYRE-BROOK and PRICE, 1969). It is the opinion of these authors that the fibrosarcoma arises directly from the supportive connective tissues of bone marrow and only rarely arises from the periosteum. The tumor is made up of entirely fibrous elements and nowhere in a careful histologic examination will neoplastic osteoid or cartilage formation be identified as a component of the tumor.

Secondary fibrosarcoma is a term applied to sarcoma occurring in preexisting lesions such as Paget's disease. Sarcoma that occurs following radiation to either diseased or normal bone sometimes take the form of fibrosarcoma. Rarely, fibrous dysplasia has been complicated by fibrosarcoma. Secondary fibrosarcoma has been reported to have occurred in osteomylitis sinus tracts (MORRIS and LUCAS, 1964; DORFMAN et al., 1966). In the series of DAHLIN and IVINS (1969), 30% of the fibrosarcomas arose in precursor lesions, which included treated and untreated giant cell tumors.

The gross appearance of these lesions is rather distinct. Pseudoencapsulation may occur in some areas permitting the tumor to be "shelled out" with relative ease. Zones of cystic degeneration, necrosis, and hemorrhage may be identified. The tumors have an irregular shape dependent on the visible areas of bony destruction and extraosseous extensions of the tumor can occasionally break through an adjacent joint surface. The

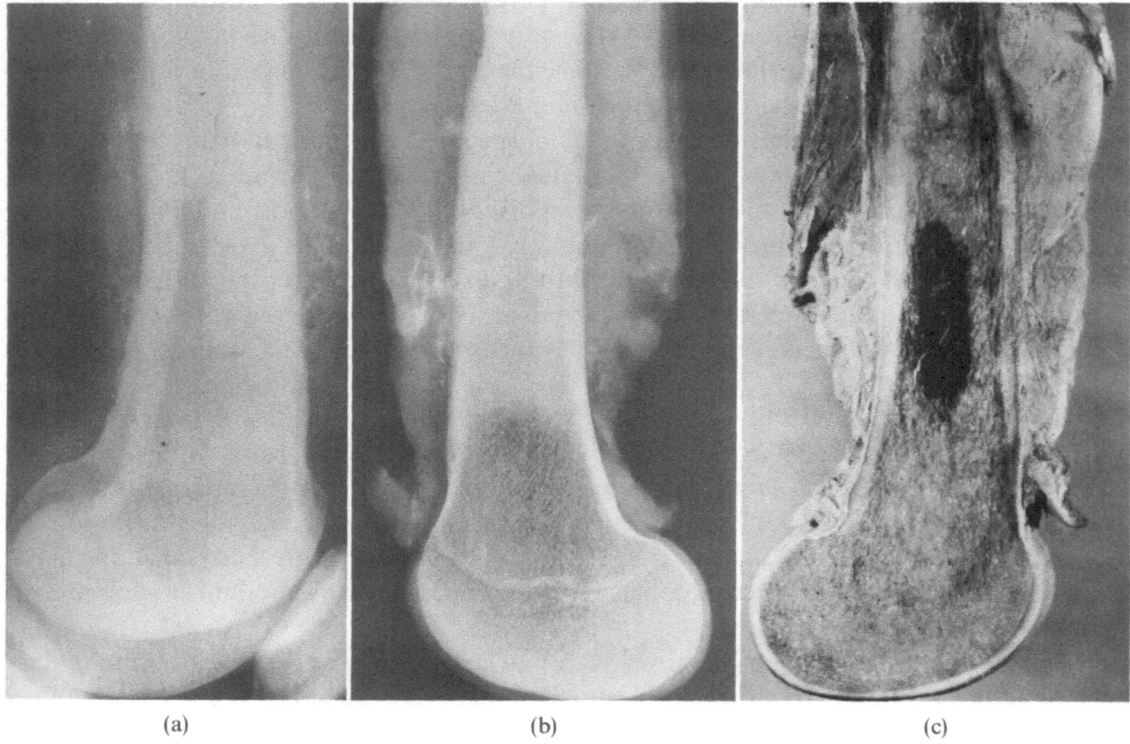

(a)   (b)   (c)

Fig. 11 a–c. Periosteal fibrosarcoma of distal femur with specimen radiograph and gross specimen. This tumor arose in periosteum and then enveloped and invaded the cortex and medullary cavity of the bone

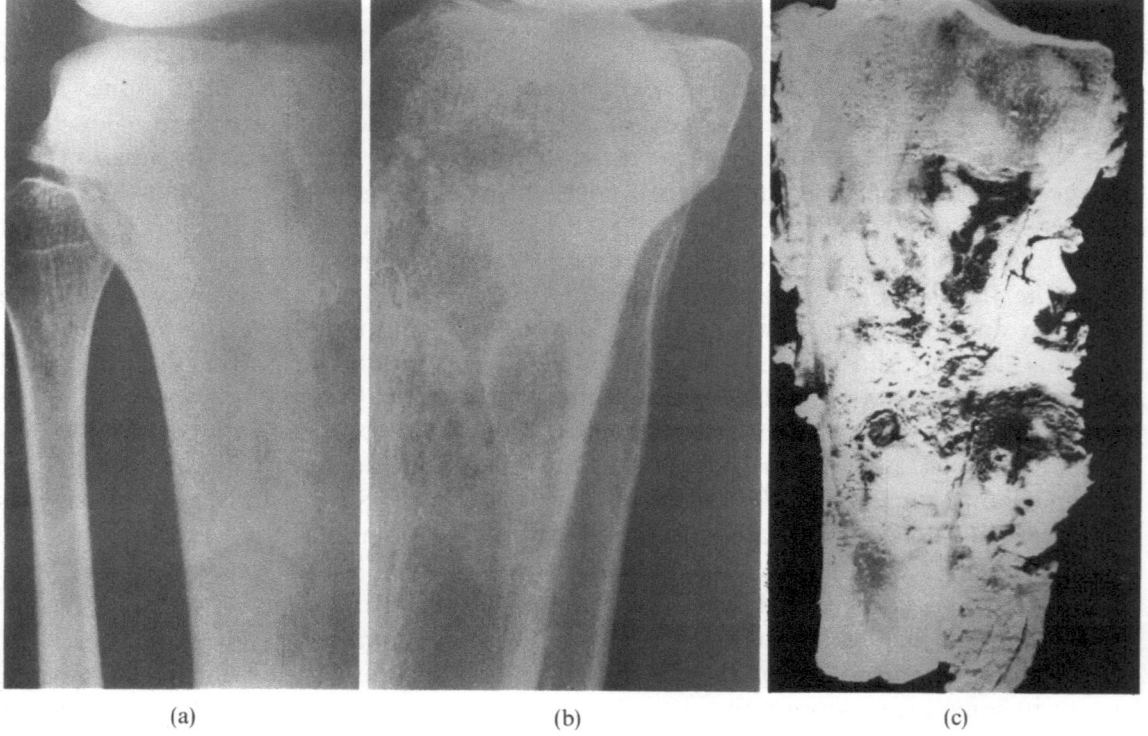

(a)   (b)   (c)

Fig. 12a–c. Fibrosarcoma of proximal tibia with erosion through the bone into the soft tissues as demonstrated on the gross specimen

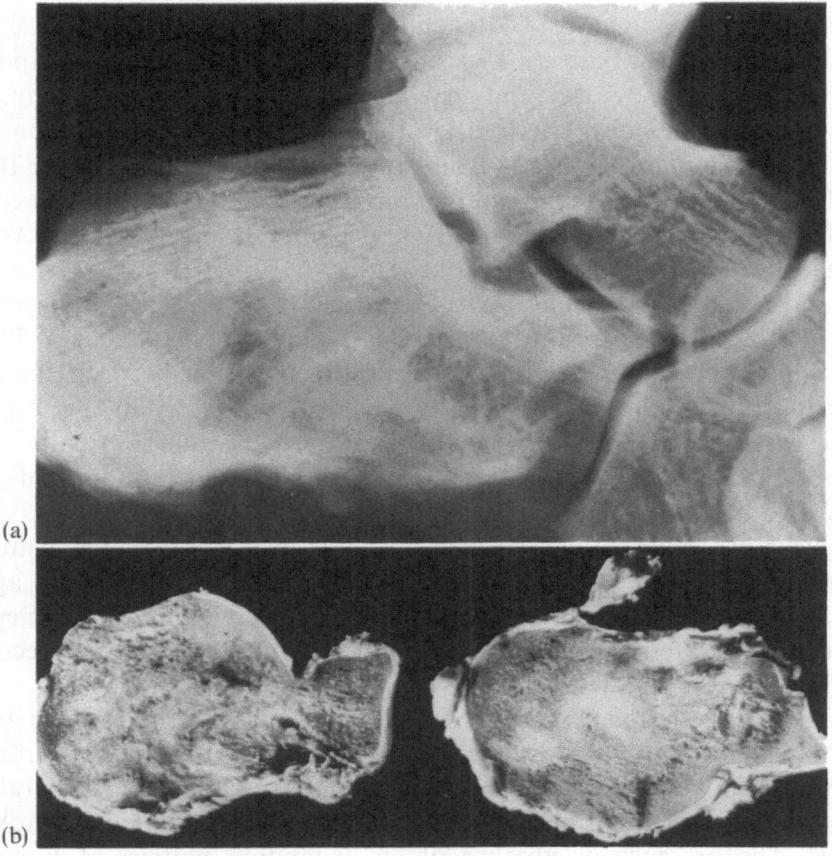

Fig. 13a and b. Fibrosarcoma of calcaneus. The surgical specimen demonstrating diffuse permeative destruction of both medullary cavity and cortex

tumor size varies from 1 to 20 cm in diameter. The periosteal form of fibrosarcoma is rather rare, and these lesions may be limited to the surface bone or may erode the cortex and involve the medullary cavity secondarily. They also tend to be of low histologic grade for malignancy. The histologic pattern of this tumor is very similar to that of the fibrosarcoma seen in soft tissues. Broder's classification has been used by several authors to classify their cases of fibrosarcoma. This is true of the series of GILMER and MacEWEN (1958), and DAHLIN and IVINS (1969). Most of the lesions are poorly differentiated with very few being well-differentiated. The nuclei are frequently fairly uniform in outline even though multinucleated forms and bizzare forms may be seen (Figs. 11–13).

D. Lipoma

Intraosseous lipomata are among the rarest of all bone tumors. JAFFE (1958a) and LICHTENSTEIN (1965b) stated that they personally had not seen a case. In 1967(a) DAHLIN quoted an incidence of 1/1000 of all bone tumors seen at the Mayo Clinic. Most authors quote less than 10 cases in the literature but a recent search has revealed 28 cases reported over a 100-year period (HART, 1973). Osseous lipomata are of two basic types:

the periosteal lipomata, which arise from the subperiosteal tissue and may deform bone by pressure or induce a periosteal reaction (BARTLETT, 1930; FLEMING et al., 1962; KURLAND and KENNARD, 1965; SCHWEITZER, 1970), and intraosseous lipomata, which arise from the medullary cavity and may expand the bone from within. Both forms of osseous lipomata are characterized by the presence of mature adipose tissue and are indistinguishable microscopically from soft-tissue lipomata except for their location. Periosteal lipomata are more common than intraosseous lipomata (FLEMING et al., 1962). The small fatty inclusions described in vertebral bodies at autopsy (MAKRYCOSTAS, 1927) are not regarded as true lipomas (LICHTENSTEIN, 1965b).

The average age of presentation is 38.5 years. There is no predilection for any age group. The ages range from $5^1/_2$ years old (WEHRSIG, 1910) to age 70 (ACKERMAN and SPJUT, 1962). There appears to be an equal distribution between the sexes (HART, 1973). The location of the intraosseous lipomata are primarily in the long bones with 60% of the cases occurring in the tibia and fibula. The tumor usually occurs in the metaphyses of the affected bones. The skull, ribs, and small bones of the feet and hands have also been described as sites of lipomata.

The clinical presentation can be extremely varied, from an incidental finding to frank pain and swelling at the site of the lesion, which is occasionally aggravated by activity. The spectrum can include some or all of these patterns to varying degrees. In the cases in the literature the duration of symptoms was rarely recorded, it has been reported as short as 5 weeks and as long as 30 years (HART, 1973).

Radiologically the lesions appear as cystic cavities within the affected bones. Trabeculae are present in many of the lesions and produce a loculated appearance. Sclerosis in a cyst wall can be seen but is not a prominent feature and generally periosteal reaction is not demonstrated. Bone expansion has been reported in more than 50% of the cases. The presence or absence of an expanding pattern of bone depends to a large extent on the particular bone affected. The fibular lesions and those found in the ribs are invariably expanded on radiographs, however, lesions in the larger long bones usually do not show evidence of expansion. Frequently there is marked cortical thinning without expansion of the outer margins of the bone. The absence of specific features, wide age range, and the multiple sites of occurrence make the radiologic diagnosis of intraosseous lipoma extremely difficult.

The gross pathology of the tumors is that of a bright yellow, lobulated, somewhat glistening mass. They closely resemble a mass of adipose tissue within the bone. The size of the lesions reported in the literature vary from 2 to 13 cm in the greatest dimension. The size of the tumor has not been shown to be related to the bone in which it was located nor to the duration of symptoms. The tumors are usually clearly demarcated from the surrounding bone.

The histologic features of the lipomata are interesting in that bony trabeculae are likely to be constant features of this tumor. The tumors are composed of lobules of mature adipose tissue (CARUOLO and DAHLIN, 1953; NEWMAN, 1957; THEVENOUT et al., 1965; WEHRSIG, 1910; ORINGER, 1948; ACKERMAN and SPJUT, 1962; KAGANSKI, 1963; DAHLIN, 1967).

Intraosseous lipomata may not be as rare as has been previously believed because of the high incidence of asymptomatic lesions found on routine examinations of chest films or extremities for other reasons. The relatively high incidence in the ribs may be explained just by the greater number of routine radiographs of the chest. The case described by COWDELL (1954) illustrates this point. Trauma may be a factor in the pathogenesis as suggested by MUELLER and ROBBINS (1960), who described a patient that sustained a fracture of the tibia 2-years prior to the diagnosis of an intraosseous lipoma at the fracture site. At the time of the fracture there was no evidence of cystic lesion in the bone. A history of antecedent injury has been described in three other patients (SMITH and FIENBERG, 1957; SKINNER and FRASER, 1957; BAGNOUD et al., 1967). In the first two patients the injury preceded the definitive radiograph by only 1 week and in the last the injury occurred over many years to the affected lower limb of a sportsman. This patient had an injury at the site of the lesion from which time her symptoms began. It is difficult, however, to establish a definite causal relationship over such a long period, particularly when radiologic evidence of the tumor did not appear until 15 years following the original injury. Previous injury was denied by 10 patients and it must be concluded that injury has not been shown to be a significant part of the history and therefore fracture is an unlikely etiology. BAGNOUD and his colleagues (1967) noted evidence of infarction in the inner cortical bone overlying the lesion in the tibia; also the trabeculae within the lesion were atrophic. They felt that the wedge shape of the tumor suggested bone infarction and concluded, therefore, that intraosseus lipoma was an expression of chronic infarction of bone and pointed to the high frequency of intraosseous lipomata in the metaphyses of long bones which corresponded closely with the distribution of chronic infarcts in the same bones. One of DAHLIN's (1967a) cases is of interest because there was some doubt expressed as to whether the lesion was a bone infarct or true intraosseous lipoma. SMITH and FIENBERG (1957) and AZIZI (1968) noted no evidence of a vascular bone either within or surrounding the lesion. However, the presence of expanded bone in over 50% of the cases and the lack of radiographic sclerosis of the margin does not support the theory of chronic bone infarction.

Many of the features of localized osteoporosis resemble those seen in intraosseous lipomata and the suggestion has been made that the presence of thin trabeculae, a relative increase in the amount of intertrabecular tissue, the absence of any osteoblastic

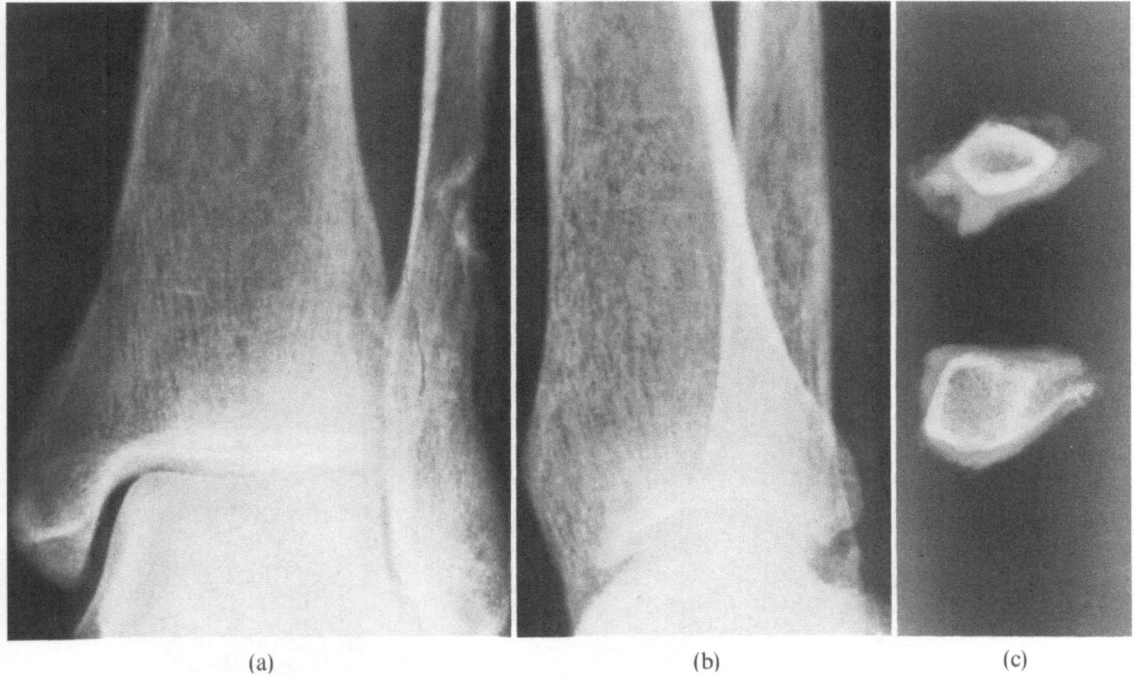

(a)   (b)   (c)

Fig. 14a–c. Lipoma of distal fibula showing destruction of cortex in both clinical and surgical specimen radiographs. There was microscopic evidence of early sarcomatous change

or osteoclastic activity, and the cortical thinning are all histologic features of osteoporosis as well as of the lipomata reported in the literature (COLLINS, 1966). However, COLLINS described bony trabeculae with osteocytes in the lacunae of osteoporotic bone, whereas the lacunae in intraosseous lipomata are usually acellular. This and the finding of bone expansion makes localized osteoporosis very likely.

Both the microscopic appearance of the lesion as a discrete mass within the bone as well as the frequent occurrence of bone expansion combined with the fact that no report of an intraosseous lipoma ever metastasizing or becoming malignant suggest that it is truly a benign tumor (Figs. 14–16).

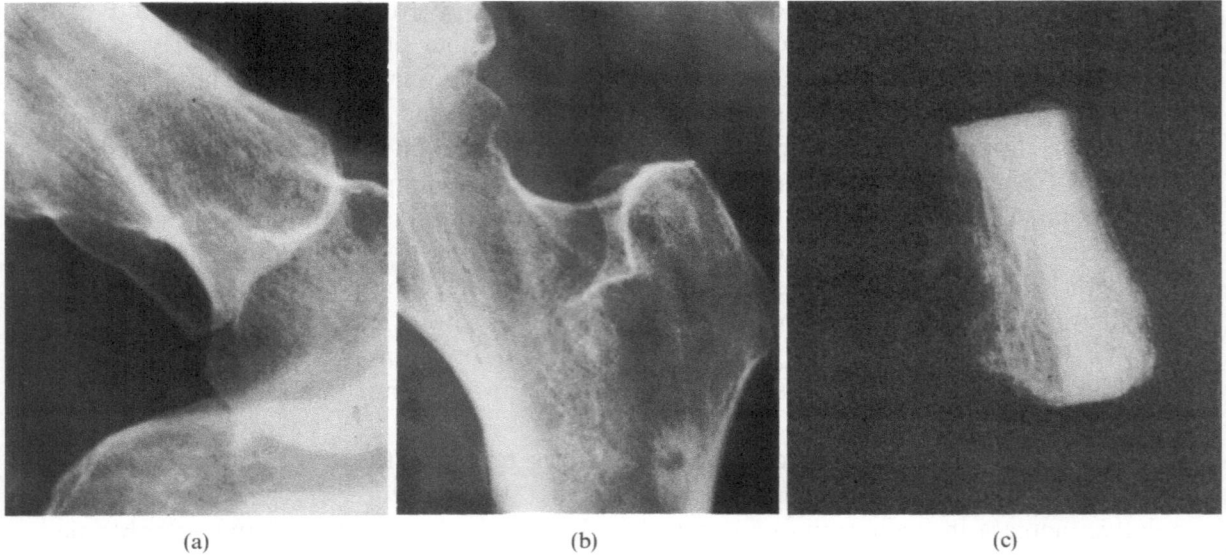

(a)   (b)   (c)

Fig. 15a–c. Lipoma of proximal femur with a sclerotic margin abutting cortex demonstrated on both clinical and specimen radiographs

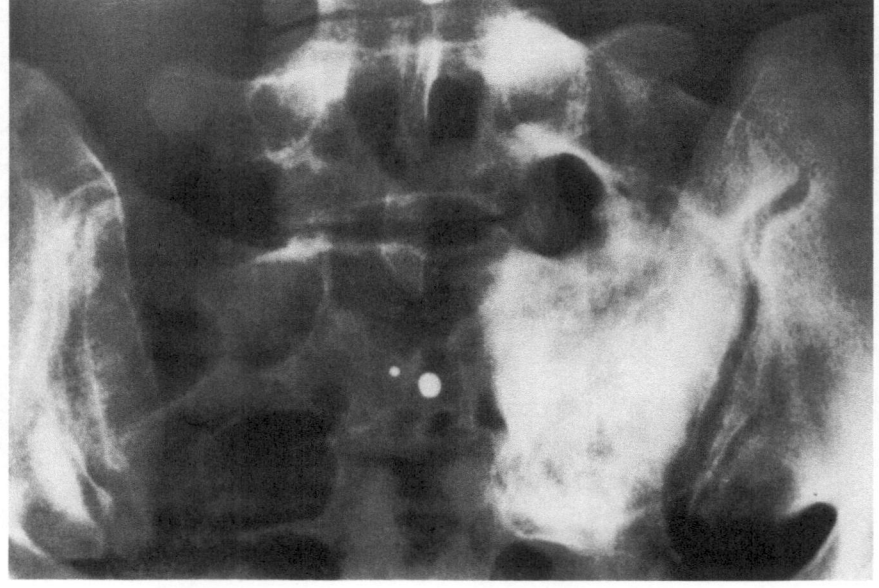

Fig. 16. Ossifying lipoma of sacrum

E. Liposarcoma

Liposarcoma is the second most common of the malignant soft tissue tumors. However, despite the fact that adipose tissue is an important constituent of bone marrow, liposarcomas arising in bone are extremely uncommon (JAFFE, 1958c). Liposarcoma arising in the soft tissue adjacent to bone rarely infiltrates the bone, and when bone invasion occurs, deep penetration into the cortex is unusual. STEWART (1931), one of the first to report liposarcoma of bone, described three cases. Subsequent cases were reported by BARNARD (1934), DUFFY and STEWART (1938), DAWSON (1955), MASTRAGOSTINO (1965), FIALHO and BARCELLOS (1958), COSTE et al. (1959), RETZ (1961), JOHNSON et al. (1962), CATTO and STEVENS (1963), GOLDMAN (1964), and ROSS and HADFIELD (1968). Two criteria must be met before a tumor of bone can be classified as a primary liposarcoma of bone. First, one must prove that the tumor has characteristic gross and microscopic features. Second, one must prove that the tumor arose within the bone rather than from the periosteal soft tissues or as a metastases. Part of the difficulty in diagnosing liposarcoma lies in the extremely varied histologic appearance which this tumor presents. This has been well documented by STOUT (1944) and ENTERLINE et al. (1960) in tumors arising in soft tissues. STOUT describes four histologic types while ENTERLINE and associates described five histologic types. STOUT's classification of cell types is as follows:

1. Well-differentiated myxoid with small adult lipocytes and embryonal stellate or spindle-shaped fat cells.

2. Poorly differentiated myxoid, similar to the well-differentiated type with bizarre monstrous lipoblasts, decreased lipoid materials, occasional signet ring forms, and rare fibrosarcomatous areas.

3. Round cell or adenoid type, with lipoblasts that have central nuclei and voluminous foamy cytoplasm containing lipoid with some extremely large cells measuring 120 μ in length with hyperchromatic nuclei.

4. The mixed group composed of two or more elements of the preceding groups. The most common cell type reported in the literature has been of the mixed variety. There does not appear to be any prognostic significance related to the cell type.

The mean age of occurrence has been 31.5 years with a four to one male to female ratio in the cases reported in the literature. The youngest age in which the tumor has been described has been in a 15-year-old male and the oldest age has been that of a 53-year-old male. Over 60% of the tumors have appeared in the lower extremity, and the tibia was the most frequently involved bone (29%). Survival ranged from 11 days to 6 years with the mean about 2 years.

In both cases reported by JOHNSON et al. (1962), the tumor arose in a bone cyst while in one other case, that reported by RETZ (1961), the tumor arose in a nonossifying fibroma.

The histologic picture in most cases was of the mixed type with areas of spindle-shaped fibroblastic cells, lipoblasts, and matured fat cells in the well-differentiated tumors and giant cells and atypical mitotic figures in poorly differentiated tumors. Special stains for fat such as Sudan IV or Sudan black revealed positive cytoplasmic droplets.

Although extremely rare, primary liposarcoma of bone is a well-defined entity. The variability of cell type should not be interpreted as militating against this diagnosis, since this same variability has been well documented in liposarcomas arising in the soft tissues.

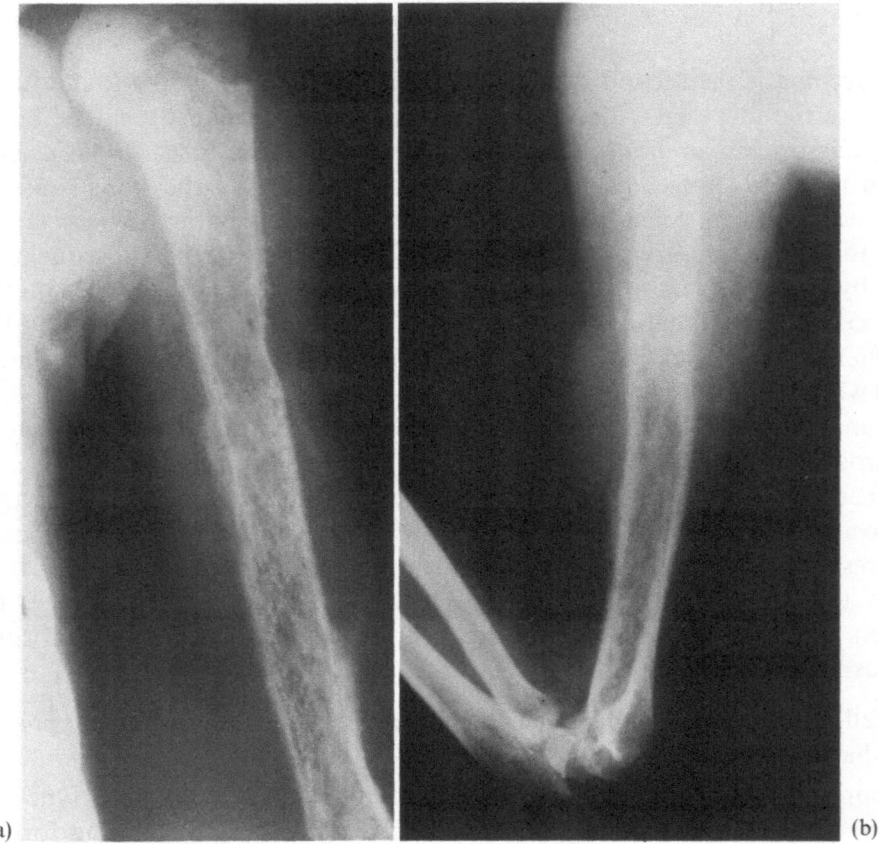

Fig. 17a and b. Liposarcoma of humerus

The radiographic picture of intraosseous liposarcoma is quite variable from a benign appearance (Fig. 14) to one of severe bone distruction with a permeative appearance and marked soft tissue extension similar to that of fibrosarcoma (Fig. 17a and b).

This is to acknowledge the excellent efforts of David C. Dillard, R.T., Mrs. Alice Smith, reference librarian, and Mrs. Judy Lee, secretary.

References

Ackerman, L.V., Spjut, H.J.: Tumors of bone and cartilage. Atlas of tumor pathology, Section 2, fascicle 4. Washington, D.C.: Armed Forces Institute of Pathology 1962

Aegerter, E., Kirkpatrick, J.A., Jr.: Orthopedic diseases: Physiology, pathology, radiology, 2nd. ed. Philadelphia: W.B. Saunders Company, pp. 580–587, 1963

Azizi, D.: Le lipome intra-osseux. J. Chir. 96, 557 (1968)

Bagnoud, F., Thevoz, F., Taillard, W.: Le lipome intra-osseux, expression d'un infarctus chronique. J. Chir. 94, 165 (1967)

Barnard, L.: Primary liposarcoma of bone. Arch. Surg. (Chicago) 29, 560–565 (1934)

Bartlett, E.I.: Periosteal lipoma. Arch. Surg. (Chicago) 21, 1015 (1930)

Benedetti, G.B., Canepa, G., Garcia, M.: Il fibroma condromixoide dell'osso; revisione critica delle letteratura ed indagini istologiche ed istochimiche su

8 casi. Arch. Putti Chir. Organi Mov. **17**, 44–72 (1962)

Caruolo, J.E., Dahlin, D.C.: Lipoma involving bone and simulating malignant bone tumor. Proc. Mayo Clin. **28**, 361 (1953)

Catto, M., Stevens, J.: Liposarcoma of bone, J. Path. **86**, 248–253 (1963)

Collins, D.H.: Pathology of bone. London: Butterworths 1966

Coste, F., Lapresle, J., Basset, F.: Un cas de liposarcome à départ vraisemblablement osseux et ayant intéressé secondairement la moelle épiniére. Presse méd. **67**, 834–837 (1959)

Cowdell, R.H.: Intra-osseous lipoma of rib. Brit. J. Surg. **41**, 664 (1954)

Cunningham, M.P., Arlen, M.: Medullary fibrosarcoma of bone. Cancer (Philad.) **21**, 31–37 (1968)

Dahlin, D.C.: Fibrosarcoma, pp. 212–221. In: Bone tumors, 2nd ed. Springfield, Ill.: Charles C Thomas 1967b

Dahlin, D.C.: Bone tumors, pp. 238, 2nd ed., Springfield, Ill.: Charles C Thomas 1967a

Dahlin, C.C.: Bone tumors: General aspects and data on 3,987 cases, 2nd ed. Springfield, Ill.: Charles C Thomas, pp. 48–57, 1967c

Dahlin, D.C., Ivins, J.C.: Fibrosarcoma of bone. A study of 114 cases. Cancer (Philad.) **23**, 35–41 (1969)

Dawson, E.K.: Liposarcoma of bone. J. Path. Bact. **70**, 513–520 (1955)

Dorfman, H.D., Norman, A., Wolff, H.: Fibrosarcoma complicating bone infarction in a caisson worker. A case report. J. Bone Jt Surg. **48A**, 528–532 (1966)

Duffy, J., Stewart, F.W.: Primary liposarcoma of bone. Report of a case. Amer. J. Path. **14**, 621–626 (1938)

Enterline, H.T., Culberson, J.D., Rochlin, D.B., Brady, L.W.: Liposarcoma. A clinical and pathological study of 53 cases. Cancer (Philad.) **13**, 933–950 (1960)

Eyre-Brook, A.L., Price, C.H.G.: Fibrosarcoma of bone. Review of fifty consecutive cases from the Bristol Bone Tumour Registry. J. Bone Jt Surg. **51B**, 20–37 (1969)

Feldman, F., Hecht, H.L., Johnston, A.D.: Chondromyxoid fibroma of bone. Radiology **94**, 249–260 (1970)

Fialho, F., Barcellos, J.M.P.: Liposarcoma do sacro. Rev. bras. Cir. **35**, 419–422 (1958)

Fleming, R.J., Alpert, M., Garcia, A.: Parosteal lipoma. Amer. J. Roentgenol. **87**, 1075 (1962)

Frank, W.E., Rockwood, C.A., Jr.: Chondromyxoid fibroma: review of the literature and report of four cases. Sth. med. J. (Bgham, Ala.) **62**, 1248–1253 (1969)

Geschickter, C.F.: So-called fibrosarcoma of bone. Bone involvement by sarcoma of the neighboring soft parts. Arch. Surg. (Chicago) **24**, 231–291 (1932)

Gilmer, W.S., Jr., MacEwen, G.D.: Central (medullary) fibrosarcoma of bone. J. Bone Jt Surg. **40A**, 121–141 (1958)

Goldman, R.L.: Primary liposarcoma of bone. Report of a case. Amer. J. clin. Path. **42**, 503–508 (1964)

Hart, J.A.L.: Intraosseous lipoma. J. Bone Jt Surg. **55B**, 624–632 (1973)

Hatcher, L.H.: The pathogenesis of localized fibrous lesions in the metaphyses of long bones. Ann. Surg. **122**, 1016 (1945)

Jaffe, H.L.: Tumors of the skeletal system: Pathological aspects. Bull. N.Y. Acad. Med. **23**, 497–511 (1947)

Jaffe, H.L.: Tumors and tumorous conditions of the bones and joints. London: Henry Kimpton 1958a

Jaffe, H.L.: Tumors and tumorous conditions of the bones and joints, p. 507. Philadelphia: Lea and Febiger 1958b

Jaffe, H.L.: Desmoplastic fibroma and fibrosarcoma, pp. 298–313. In: Tumors and tumorous conditions of the bones and joints. Philadelphia: Lea and Febiger 1958c

Jaffe, H.L., Lichtenstein, L.: Amer. J. Pathol. **18**, 969 (1942)

Jaffe, H.L., Lichtenstein, L.: Chondromyxoid fibroma of bone: an distinctive benign tumor likely to be mistaken especially for chondrosarcoma. Arch. Path. (Chicago) **45**, 541–551 (1948)

Johnson, L.C., Vetter, H., Putschar, W.J.G.: Sarcomas arising in bone cysts. Virchows Arch. path. Anat. **335**, 428–451 (1962)

Kaganski, V.E.: Lipoma kosti. Vop. Onkol. **9**, 97 (1963)

Kurland, K.Z., Kennard, J.W.: Parosteal lipoma arising from the proximal radius: A case report. Clin. Orthop. **41**, 140 (1965)

Lichtenstein, L.: Fibrosarcoma of bone, pp. 229–240. In: Bone tumors, 3rd ed. St. Louis: C.V. Mosby Company 1965a

Lichtenstein, L.: Bone tumors, 3rd ed. St. Louis: C.V. Mosby Company, pp. 58–70, 1965b

Makrycostas, L.: Über das Wirbelangiom, -lipom und -osteom. Virchows Arch. path. Anat. **265**, 259 (1927)

Marcove, R.C., Kambolis, C., Bullough, P.G., Jaffe, H.L.: Fibromyxoma of bone: a report of 3 cases. Cancer (Philad.) **17**, 1209–1213 (1964)

Mastragostino, S.: Tumor lipoblastici primitivi dello scheletro. Chir. Organi Mov. **44**, 18–36 (1965)

Morris, J.M., Lucas, D.B.: Fibrosarcoma within a sinus tract of chronic draining osteomyelitis. Case report and review of literature. J. Bone Jt Surg. **46A**, 853–857 (1964)

Mueller, M.C., Robbins, J.L.: Intramedullary lipoma of bone. J. Bone Jt Surg. **42A**, 517 (1960)

Newman, C.W.: Fibrolipoma of the mandible. J. oral Surg. **15**, 251 (1957)

Nielsen, A.R., Poulsen, H.: Multiple diffuse fibrosarcomata of the bones. Acta path. microbiol. scand. **55**, 265–272 (1962)

Oringer, M.J.: Lipoma of the mandible. Oral Surg. 1, 1134 (1948)

Pound, E., Pickrell, K., Huger, W., Barnes, W.: Fibrous dysplasia (ossifying fibroma) of the maxilla: Analysis of fourteen cases. Ann. Surg. 161, 406–410 (1965)

Rahimi, A., Beabout, J.W., Ivins, J.C., Dahlin, D.C.: Chondromyxoid fibroma: A clinicopathologic study of 76 cases. Cancer (Philad.) 30, 726–736 (1972)

Ralph, L.L.: Chondromyxoid fibroma of bone. J. Bone Jt Surg. 44, 7–24 (1962)

Retz, L.D., Jr.: Primary liposarcoma of bone. Report of a case and review of the literature. J. Bone Jt Surg. 43A, 123–129 (1961)

Ross, C.F., Hadfield, G.: Primary osteo-liposarcoma of bone. (Malignant mesenchymoma.) J. Bone Jt Surg. 50B, 639–643 (1968)

Sachdeva, H.S., Kasphyap, K.N., Grewal, D.S., Aikat, M.: Chondromyxoid fibroma of bone. Amer. Surg. 35, 435–438 (1969)

Salzer, M., Salzer-Kuntschik, M.: Das Chondromyxoidfibrom. Langenbecks Arch. klin. Chir. 312, 216–231 (1965)

Schajowicz, F., Gallardo, H.: Chondromyxoid fibroma (fibromyxoid chondroma) of bone: a clinico-pathological study of thirty-two cases. J. Bone Jt Surg. 53, 198–216 (1971)

Schweitzer, G.: Parosteal lipoma of the radius. S. Afr. med. J. 44, 648 (1970)

Seth, H.N., Rao, B.D.: Chondromyxoid fibroma of bone: report on three cases. Indian J. Path. Bact. 7, 112–116 (1964)

Shapiro, R., Francisco, J., Finkelman, A.: Ossifying fibroma of the maxilla. J. oral Surg. 23, 539–543 (1965)

Skinner, G.B., Fraser, R.G.: Medullary lipoma of bone. J. Canad. Ass. Radiol. 8, 19 (1957)

Smith, A.G., Zavateta, A.: Osteoma, ossifying fibroma, and fibrous dysplasia of facial and cranial bones, Amer. med. Ass. Arch. Path. 54, 501–727 (1952).

Smith, J.F.: Fibrous dysplasia of jaws. Arch. Otolaryng. (Chicago) 87, 592–603 (1965)

Smith, W.E., Fienberg, R.: Intraosseous lipoma of bone. Cancer (Philad.) 10, 1151 (1957)

Spjut, H.J., Dorfman, H.D., Fechner, R.E., Ackerman, L.V.: Tumors of bone and cartilage. In: Atlas of tumor pathology, 2nd series, fasc. 5. Washington, D.C.: Armed Forces Institute of Pathology, pp. 50–59, 1971

Steiner, P.E.: Multiple diffuse fibrosarcoma of bone. Amer. J. Path. 20, 877–893 (1944)

Stewart, F.W.: Primary liposarcoma of bone. Amer. J. Path. 7, 87–93 (1931)

Stout, A.P.: Liposarcoma — malignant tumor of lipoblasts. Ann. Surg. 119, 86–107 (1944)

Stout, A.P.: Fibrosarcoma. The malignant tumor of fibroblasts. Cancer (Philad.) 1, 30–63 (1948)

Thevenot, P., Peloux, Y., Michelin, C.: Le lipome intramédullaire osseux. Méd. trop. 25, 745 (1965)

Thoma, K.H.: Differential diagnosis of fibrous dysplasia and fibro-osseous neoplastic lesions of the jaw and their treatment. J. oral Surg. 14, 185–194 (1965)

Thomas, K.H., Goldman, H.: Oral pathology, 5th ed., St. Louis, Mo.: C.V. Mosby Co. 1960

Vix, V.A., Fahmy, A.: Unusual appearance of a chondromyxoid fibroma. Radiology 92, 365–366 (1969)

Wehrsig, G.: Lipom des Knochenmarks. Zbl. allg. Path. path. Anat. 21, 243 (1910)

Wrenn, R.N., Smith, A.G.: Chondromyxoid fibroma. Sth. med. J. (B'gham, Ala.) 47, 848–854 (1954)

Chordoma

by

Hossein Firooznia and Richard S. Pinto

A. Introduction

Chordoma is a rare malignancy which arises from the remnants of notochord (chorda dorsalis). The tumor bears distinct histologic resemblance to this primitive embryologic structure. It occurs along the midline in the axial skeleton. It arises most commonly from the distal and proximal ends of the axial skeleton, i.e., the spheno-occipital and the sacrococcygeal regions. These two locations account for 85–90% of all the reported instances of chordoma. The remaining 10–15% occur along the course of the spine, the commonest sites of involvement, in descending order of frequency, being cervical spine, particularly C1–C2 region, lumbar spine, and thoracic spine. Chordomas are locally invasive, growing slowly and destroying the adjacent bone and soft tissue structures. Bone destruction, formation of a soft-tissue mass containing calcification and/or fragments of bone in more than half the patients, associated with gradual but relentless compression and invasion of the surrounding structures are the cardinal manifestations of this neoplasm and account for its varied clinical manifestations.

These tumors, particularly the intracranial cases, are seldom totally resectable surgically, or curable by irradiation, and local recurrence, therefore, is very common. More than half the chordomas are very slow growing and the tumor may recur, several years later, following its initial treatment. Chordomas do not metastasize readily although occasional instances of distant secondary deposits, particularly to the lungs, liver, lymph nodes, and brain, have been reported mainly from the sacrococcygeal and vertebral tumors.

B. Embryology

I. General Considerations

The pathologic characteristics, the histologic peculiarities, and the unique anatomic localization of chordomas cannot be appreciated without some conception of the evolution of chorda dorsalis (MULLER, 1858; WILLIAMS, 1908; HASS, 1934; HOROWITZ, 1941; SENSENIG, 1949, 1956).

In the animal kingdom the highest phylum in the evolutionary ladder are the chordata. The major characteristics of these animals is an axial cylindrical-shaped structure, which serves as the main back-support of the animal and is called chorda dorsalis or notochord. The notochord has received considerable attention from the comparative morphologist because of its phylogenetic significance and from the pathologist who is concerned with tumors that may have origin in its tissues.

The highest group of the chordata is the vertebrata. In the vertebrates, among mammals, a notochordal rod serves as a transient axial support during the early embryonic life, but it soon undergoes regression and only traces of it remain in the adult.

II. Formation of Notochord

In the developing embryo, intimately associated with the formation of the primitive streak, is the origin of an axially located cylindrical mass of cells which give rise to the notochord. These cells arise from the cephalic end of the primitive streak and soon appear as a midsagittal rod of cells lying ventral to the neural tube, with which its dorsal surface is in contact, and forming the roof of the archenteron in the midline. In embryos of 2–3 mm, the cellular mass located in front of the anterior end of the primitive streak has already differentiated sufficiently to form the chordal anlage. Thus, a groove with a ventral concavity is formed at first. It then closes off ventrally to form an elongated cylinder but it temporarily retains its contact with the neural tube and gut. As the cells of the developing notochord close in to form a cylindrical rod, a mass of mesodermal tissues surround them. Thus, simultaneously with this stage of development of notochord, a mass of mesodermal cells begin to form the primordia of the axial skeleton, which form surrounding the notochord. By 20 days ovulation age the notochord begins to separate from both the neural tube and gut, and by STREETER'S (1945) age group 28–30 days (ovulation age), the separation is complete throughout the cervical and thoracic segments (SENSENIG, 1949). At this time in human embryos the notochord forms a longitudinal, nonsegmented rod of cells which extends from the region of Rathke's pouch (future sphenoidal region) to the most caudal segment. It is a midaxial structure around which the occipital and vertebral segments are formed. At this stage the notochord is located as a rod in the center of the developing vertebral bodies. In the animals with a cartilagenous spine, ringlike cartilagenous vertebrae are formed about the notochord. Although somewhat compressed where the vertebrae encircle it, the notochord persists in these animals as a well-defined, continuous structure extending throughout the length of the vertebral column. As the cartilagenous vertebrae are replaced by the more highly developed bony vertebrae in the higher animals, the notochord is still more compressed. But even in the higher animals a minute canal in the centra of the vertebrae still remains to mark its existence. In man, as condensation of the mesenchymal anlage of the vertebral bodies progresses, the cells of the notochord are gradually extruded into the intervertebral regions. During this period vacuolation and mucoid degeneration of the notochordal cells appear. By the time the vertebral bodies have assumed the morphology of cartilage, the notochordal cells, as a rule, are confined entirely to the central portions of the intervertebral discs. The notochordal cells gradually undergo adaptive changes, and aid in forming the nucleus pulposus. The original tract of the chorda in the vertebrae is marked by a streak of mucoid material, but cells may persist here (although less frequently than in the nucleus pulposus) well into adult life (HASS, 1934).

At the cephalic and caudal extremities of the axial skeleton, i.e., the occipitosphenoidal and sacrococcygeal regions, the development and regression of notochordal cells varies from the typical course already described. At the occipitosphenoidal region the developing notochord extends as far forward as the buccopharyngeal membrane, and temporarily remains attached to its caudal wall as the hypophyseal pocket forms.

Detailed studies of the occipitosphenoidal region reveal the cephalic tip of the notochord to be lying in contact with the infundibular process. Toward the end of the 4th week of embryonic life, the infundibular process invaginates, to constitute the pars neuralis of the adult hypophysis. Regression of the notochord starts at this stage, and by the 6th week the regression is more evident, so that sagittal sections give the impression of its pulling away from the infundibular process and also losing its own continuity. The primary fusion of the cephalic tip of the notochord to the infundibular process is very important from a pathologic and clinical point of view. The notochordal cells, which originally are in contact with the infundibulum, may invaginate into the sella turcica with the pars neuralis. They may be carried similarly to the suprasella region. These remnants, following neoplastic transformation, will present as intrasellar, suprasellar, or parasellar mass lesions without a concomitant destructive lesion of the sellar structures or the basisphenoid, which is usually encountered with chordomas of this region.

In the caudal region the notochord undergoes a marked variation in its development through its regression within the last four terminal segments. Far more variation is encountered here than in the occipital region. In some cases the notochord shifts to a more dorsal position in the future sacral and caudal segments and may even lie dorsal to the anlage of the vertebral bodies within the vertebral canal. In other embryos both dorsal and ventral extensions of the notochord project beyond the limits of the vertebral rudiments. With the reduction and assimilation of the more distal caudal vertebral rudiments the notochordal tissues fail to undergo equal reduction and form masses of cells within and about the 4th coccygeal segment. Similar massing of cells is also seen, occasionally, at various levels in the future sacral and coccygeal segments. Finally, there is the rare occurrence of a duplication of the notochord in the more caudal segments (SENSENIG, 1956).

III. Origin of Notochord

Three phases in the development of the chorda dorsalis have been defined (ALEZAIS and PEYRON, 1914, 1920, 1922). At an early stage it is a hollow tube lined by cells of entodermal origin. Then the tube is transformed to a solid cord of closely approximated, polyhedral epithelial cells. Finally, as the structure is adapted to a supporting role, the cells become vacuolated, and presumably elaborate a mucinous material which escapes into the intercellular spaces. As differentiation progresses, the cells undergo variable morphologic changes, and become widely dispersed in a voluminous mucinous matrix. HASS (1934), in a review of 56 cases of chordoma of the cranium and the cervical portion of the spine, compared the three stages described by ALEZAIS and PEYRON (1922) with the variable histology of the chordomas. In only one tumor was there an architecture which resembled the primitive tubal structure of the chorda (HASS, 1934). A reduplication of the second stage was more common. In these instances the chordoma was composed almost exclusively of a mosaic of lightly acidophilic nonvacuolated, round, or polyhedral epithelial cells separated by a small amount of homogenous intercellular material, mucin. The majority of the tumors exhibited the sequences of evolution through the second and third stages. In these neoplams there were columns and clusters of epithelial cells which seemed to serve as germinal centers about which there were less cellular fields in which progressive differentiation to an adult type of chordal tissue had taken place. These germinal centers usually were near the periphery of the lobulations, while centrally a mucinous matrix comprised almost the whole of the structure.

IV. Chordal Ectopia and Chordal Remnants

By a series of comparative anatomical studies MULLER, in 1858, showed that vestiges of notochordal tissue could be demonstrated in the basilar cartilage of man and animals, and that in the fetus the notochord in fact reaches quite up to the sella turcica. In the spheno-occipital synchondrosis it remains as a small, soft mass exactly analogous to the nucleus pulposus of the other intervertebral discs; this tissue can still be found here after birth, when it has disappeared from the neighboring bone and cartilage. MULLER first showed that in the very region of the future spheno-occipital synchondrosis the notochord has a decided tendency to approach the superior surface of the basilar cartilage. He further found in human embryos, along the track of the notochord through the basilar cartilage, a number of little cavities or canals filled with notochordlike tissues.

MULLER'S work was not accepted as final and the nature of this malformation was disputed until 1894–1895. In 1894 MULLER'S views received confirmation at the hands of RIBBERT (1894), who reviewed the whole question and based his opinion on a series of five cases studied in STEINER'S laboratory. He adduced the following reasons for accepting the notochordal origin of these clival excrescences. (1) They all arise along the midline from the clivus. (2) In no case has transition from cartilage to tumor tissue been demonstrated. (3) The tumor and the cartilage merely coexist side by side—a persistence of intracartilagenous notochordal vestiges. (4) In a cartilage tumor, undergoing gelatinous softening, the cells do not present the typical physaliphorous appearance, and there is no gelatinous intersubstance between the cell groups. There is, on the other hand, a close resemblance between the tissue of these jellylike masses and that of the notochordal vestiges in the intervertebral discs. RIBBERT applied the name *chordoma* to these lesions in 1894.

NEBELTHAU (1897) published three cases of spheno-occipital ecchondrosis, and found sufficient reason for accepting their notochordal origin in their histological structure, and specially in the character of their cells. He discarded the concept of cartilagenous origin of ecchondrosis, and pointed out the fact that chondromas undergoing mucoid degeneration, unlike clival excrescences, are not composed of young cells and show no evidence of cellular proliferation.

1. Ecchordosis Physaliphora

STEWART and MORIN (1926) suggested the more appropriate name ecchordosis physaliphora, instead of ecchondrosis physaliphora, for these lesions. This designation is helpful because it acknowledges the notochordal origin of these clival remnants, puts to rest the notion of their cartilagenous origin, and segregates these innocuous notochordal remnants from the true neoplasms or chordoma. It should be recalled that the term "chordoma" was originally applied to these clival excrescenses by RIBBERT in 1894. Currently, the term chordoma is used for true neoplasms of notochordal origin. As already discussed, small, proliferated rests of heterotopic notochordal tissue are occasionally found along the path of the original notochord, from the pituitary fossa to the tip of the coccyx. The term "benign chordoma" is occasionally used by some authors to refer to these small proliferated notochordal rests, irrespective of their site. However, since the term "chordoma" has acquired the connotation of a malignant tumor, the term benign chordoma should perhaps be avoided in any connection (JAFFE, 1958).

Ecchordosis represents a proliferated mass of ectopic notochordal tissue occurring at the base of the skull, in the region of the clivus. It is a gelatinous nodule, and has a translucent whitish appearance. The lesion usually measures no more than a few millimeters in diameter. It usually has a fragile, slender stalk which passes through an aperture in the dura and attaches the nodule usually to the middle of the dorsum sellae. The lesion may also be loosely adherent to the pia arachnoid, over the pons. The lesion can easily be differentiated from a lipoma both by its translucent whitish appearance and its attachment to the underlying bone. Microscopically, the nodule shows few cells, and those present are highly vacuolated and contain mucin. These notochordal remnants are poorly nourished and often show advanced degeneration microscopically. In different microscopic fields one sees larger intercellular collections of homogenous material which in places gives the staining reaction of mucin (JAFFE, 1958; RUSSELL and RUBINSTEIN, 1963).

An ecchordosis does not tend to produce pressure or tissue destruction at the site of its growth and hence does not produce clinical complaints. It is discovered at autopsy incidentally, and often only when a special search is made for it. In a series of 500 autopsies, RIBBERT (1904) found 10 instances (2%) of clival ecchondrosis. STEWART and MORIN (1926) reported 4 instances in 350 necropsies.

2. Other Notochordal Remnants

Notochordal remnants normally persist in the adult in the apical ligament of the odontoid process and in the nucleus pulposus of the intervertebral discs. As was discussed previously, notochordal remnants are also occasionally found elsewhere along the path of the original notochord from the region of the pituitary fossa to the tip of the coccyx.

Ecchordosis physaliphora, a small jellylike nodule of proliferated notochordal remnants arising from the middle of dorsum sellae, has already been considered (see IV 1).

Other reported notochordal vestiges are as follows:

Spheno-occipital region. As was discussed in embryology of the cephalic tip of the notochord, it is evident that notochordal tissues may be carried with the evolving infundibulum and pars neuralis of the pituitary gland to the intrasellar or suprasellar regions (MATHEWS and WILSON, 1974). Notochordal vestiges have been found imbedded in the dorsum sellae in 4–5% of normal adults (WILLIS, 1967). These remnants are also found in the substance of bone close to the floor of sella turcica; adjacent to the cranial surface of the clivus just caudal to the sella; in the substance of bone at spheno-occipital synchondrosis; and on the cranial surface of the clivus just anterior to the foramen magnum.

Vertebral column (C_1 to L_5). Notochordal vestiges have been found on the pharyngeal surface of the base of the skull along the midline and in the soft tissues of the nasopharynx from the region of the sphenoid sinus to the upper cervical spine.

In 1889, KIRSCHBERG and MARCHAND described the occurrence of persisting notochordal vestiges in the substance of the vertebrae in a rachitic subject. LINCK and WARSTAT (1922) reported four cases of small protrusions of chordal tissue on the anterior and posterior surfaces of the vertebral bodies in the lumbar region of the human fetus (40–50 mm). These authors found throughout the vertebral bodies connecting bands between these foci and the main notochordal strand. They postulated that these ectopic collections of chordal tissue had been squeezed out of the vertebrae by the pressure of the developing cartilage.

SCHMORL (1928) demonstrated spinal chordal remnants in nine adult cadavers in dissections of over 3000 human vertebral columns. He found notochordal vestiges to

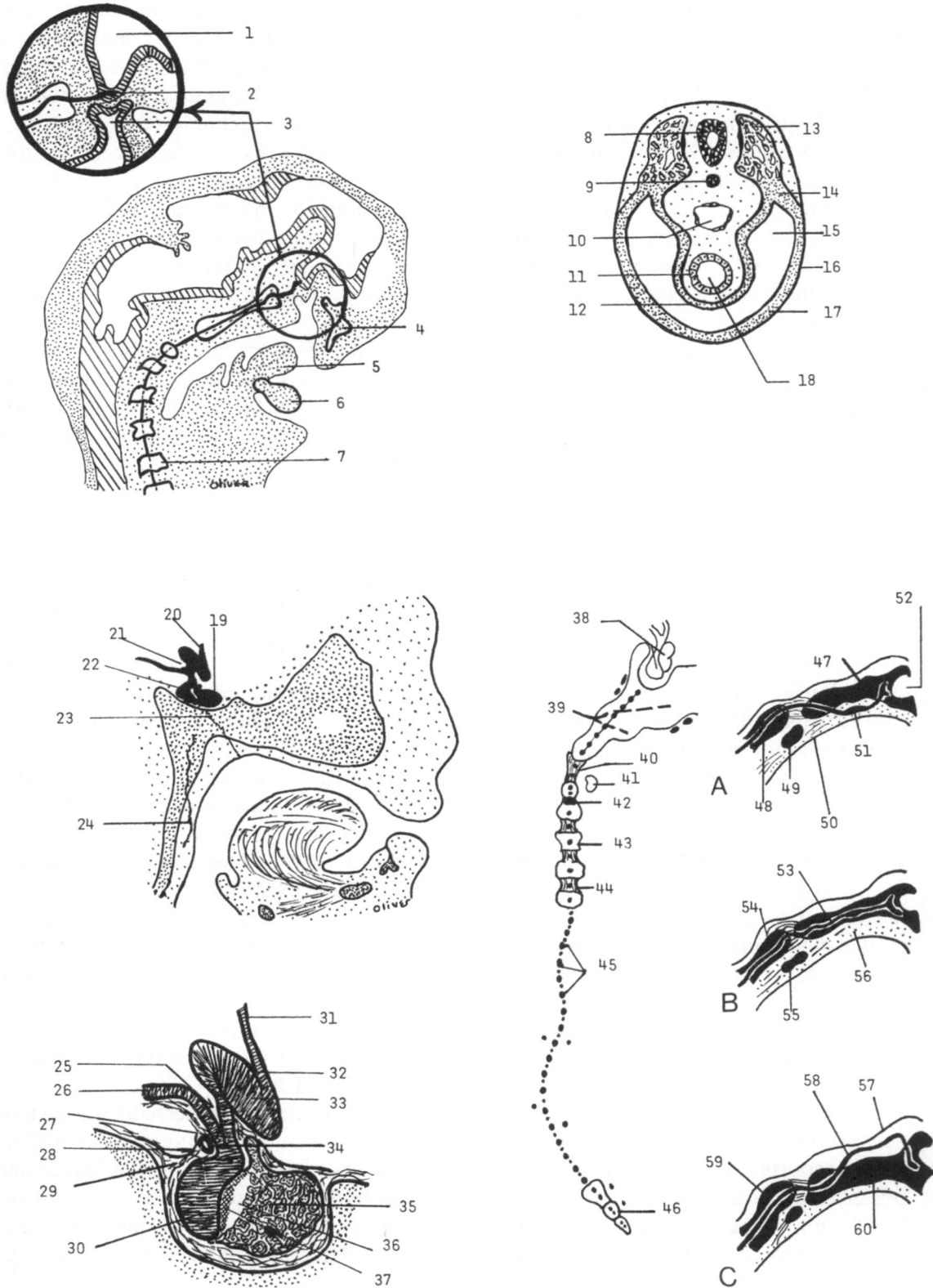

Fig. I

be located posteriorly in the vertebral bodies in six cases, centrally in two, and laterally in one instance.

CAPPELL (1928) found, in transverse sections of the lumbar region of a 21 mm embryo, small strands of chordal tissue extending from the central chordal mass into the surrounding mesenchyme, and also, small islets of notochordal cells on the anterior surface of the developing cartilage.

Sacrococcygeal region. BERARD et al. (1922), in a study of 50 human embryos and fetuses, found developmental displacements of chordal tissues in this region. The notochordal rests were located beneath the perichondrium of the developing bones and in the surrounding mesenchyme on the anterior and posterior surfaces.

SCHWABE (1933) demonstrated nests of well-preserved chordal cells within the disc zones of the sacrum in every decade of life up to the fifth decade, and, in a degenerated stage, even thereafter. These strands of cells were observed to extend to the surface of the sacrum and to the margins of the spinal canal. Since the sacral segments become fused together, the notochordal remnants within the disc zones of the sacrum are in reality intraosseous, a position resembling that of chordal vestiges within the vertebral bodies of the specimens described by SCHMORL.

3. Relationship of Notochordal Remnants to Chordoma

The notochordal remnants in the nucleus pulposus of the intervertebral discs and in the apical ligament of the dens are designated as normally placed chordal vestiges. The notochordal remnants encountered elsewhere, i.e., in the spheno-occipital region (including clival ecchordosis); in the posterior wall of the nasopharynx; in the substance of bone in the vertebral bodies, or in the tissues surrounding them, are designated as abnormal or ectopic remnants, because they are located where notochord should have regressed (centra of the vertebral bodies) or in locations where they are truly ectopic (i.e., remnants eccentrically placed in the vertebrae and particularly vestiges located in the extraosseous tissues).

Fig. I. Embryology of the notochord. Numbers *1–7*, schematic diagram of a 4-week-old embryo. Inset demonstrates relationship between cephalic tip of notochord and infundibulum: *1* infundibulum, *2* cephalic tip of notochord, *3* Rathke's pouch, *4* nasal bone, *5* tongue, *6* mandible, *7* vertebral body.

Numbers *8–18*, schematic transverse section of a vertebrate embryo: *8* neural tube (nervous system), *9* notochord, *10* aorta, *11* entoderm, *12* splanchnic mesoderm, *13* somite (skeleton, muscles), *14* nephrotome (urogenital system), *15* coelom, *16* ectoderm, *17* somatic mesoderm, *18* gut (digestive and respiratory systems).

Numbers *19–24*, diagram showing sagittal section of hypophyseal region: *19* pars distalis, *20* lamina terminalis, *21* infundibular recess, *22* pars neuralis, *23* location of regressed stalk of Rathke's pouch, *24* notochord.

Numbers *25–37*, details of adult pituitary: *25* infundibular recess, *26* tuber cinerum, *27* infundibular stalk, *28* diaphragma sellae, *29* sella turcica, *30* pars neuralis, *31* lamina terminalis, *32* pars distalis, *36* residual lumen, *37* pars intermedia.

Numbers *38–46*, relationship of notochord to neuraxis. Sites where notochordal remnants may persist are indicated by black dots. Note intraosseous (skull base and vertebrae) as well as extraosseous remnants at base of the skull, discs, and extravertebral tissues: *38* pituitary gland, *39* basisphenoid and basioccipital, *40* apical ligament of the odontoid process, *41* anterior arch of atlas, *42* notochordal remnant at the juncture of the odontoid process and the body of axis, *43* third cervical vertebra, *44* intervertebral disc, *45* notochordal remnants at centers of intervertebral discs, *46* sacrococcygeal region.

Numbers *47–60* depict relationship between notochord and skull base, in a sagittal section of this region in the embryo. A is the most common arrangement and C is the least common. *47* and *60* Cartilage of basal plate of the skull, *48, 54, 59* axis, *49* and *55* anterior arch of atlas, *50* pharyngeal wall, *51* notochord in roof of pharynx, *52* hypophyseal fossa, *53* notochord in substance of the basal plate, *56* mesoderm in base of the skull, *57* dura, *58* notochord on cranial side of basal plate beneath dura mater

Some investigators believe most of the chordomas evolve out of proliferated vestiges of these ectopic notochordal tissues (Stewart and Morin, 1926; Horowitz, 1941; Jaffe, 1958; Epstein, 1969). This concept is supported by the striking similarity in the topographic distribution of the chordomas on the one hand, and ectopic notochordal remnants on the other. The majority of chordomas, as will be considered later, occur at either end of the axial skeleton, i.e., spheno-occipital and sacrococcygeal regions, precisely where the notochordal aberrations commonly occur and ectopic notochordal remnants are found; and not in the rest of the axial skeleton, where the normally placed remnants of the notochord are most abundant (i.e., within the nucleus pulposus). In the case of vertebral chordomas, it is noteworthy that most investigators believe the tumor invariably arises within the vertebral body, i.e., from the ectopic remnants, and not from the nucleus pulposus of the intervertebral discs (Stewart, 1922; Jaffe, 1958; Epstein, 1969). Although the indirect evidence for this malignant transformation is fairly convincing, nevertheless, this evolution cannot be proved, since, unless they undergo malignant transformation, these ectopic rests are innocuous and clinically silent. On the other hand, it is possible that some chordomas arise from notochordal tissues within the nucleus pulposus. Only a small number of authors, however, accept this possibility (Hansson, 1941; Lichtenstein, 1972; Dahlin, 1967).

We believe this possibility, although probably very rare, nevertheless exists. In some cases of vertebral chordoma, when two or more adjacent vertebrae are affected, and as is usually the case, the corresponding discs spaces are destroyed, the lesion appears primarily as a lesion of the disc with invasion and erosion of the adjacent vertebrae, and not vice versa. Primary malignancies of the vertebrae do not ordinarily invade and cross the intervertebral discs; and do not as a rule, invade the adjacent vertebrae, via this route. Vertebral chordomas, as will be discussed later, not uncommonly occur in two or more adjacent vertebral bodies and the intervening discs are seen to be destroyed. Although the slow but relentless growth behavior of chordoma may explain this prominent characteristic (namely a primary vertebral tumor growing slowly and successively destroying the vertebra and then the adjacent disc and eventually crossing into the next vertebra).

Nevertheless, the possibility of a primary tumor of the disc cannot be ruled out. Certainly, this possibility appears very appealing in patients who have a destroyed disc and destructive lesions of the adjacent vertebrae of more or less equal magnitude. Similarly, some patients with vertebral chordoma affecting two or more vertebrae, may indeed have multicentric chordomas of the corresponding discs with secondary invasion and destruction of the adjacent vertebrae, rather than a primary intravertebral chordoma producing these findings.

C. Pathology

I. Gross Pathology

1. General Considerations

Chordoma is a relatively soft tumor with a somewhat lobulated or bossed surface. The tumor is usually invested with a fibrous capsule, except in the region of bone invasion, where the boundaries of the tumor are indistinct. It may have a grayish color in some areas, while other areas are likely to be glistening and semitranslucent, on account of their mucin content. The gross tumor may resemble chondrosarcoma or mucous adenocarcinoma. The cut surface of the tumor presents a lobular pattern in which the lobules are delimited by septae of fibrous tissue. More importantly, the cut surface is likely to present a distinctly mucinous or gelatinous character, although this feature may be more pronounced in some specimens than in others. Areas of discoloration of varying sizes secondary to recent or old hemorrhage are also usually noted. The smaller tumors may appear relatively firm and present as a solid mass. The bulkier tumors, on the other hand, tend to be more lobulated and usually contain areas of cystic softening, as well as foci of hemorrhage and necrosis. Occasionally, some large tumors, despite significant amount of mucin, appear firm and tense because of the thickness and firmness of their interlobular septa and capsule (LEWIS, 1921; STEWART, 1922; STEWART and MORIN, 1926; ROBBINS, 1945; JAFFE, 1958; LICHTENSTEIN, 1972; DAHLIN, 1967).

STEWART (1922) relates the degree of malignancy of the tumor to its macroscopic characteristics, stating that with increasing malignancy the tumor becomes more and more solid and opaque, the formation of mucin being in inverse ratio to the rate of cellular multiplication. HASS (1934), following a comprehensive review of the literature, expressed a similar opinion.

Some chordomas may contain areas of calcification and/or ossification. Calcification in the tumor may be microscopic or very extensive; it may be associated with areas of necrosis or hemorrhage. The areas of ossification likewise range from microscopic foci to fragments of bone measuring few or several centimeters in size. As the tumor invades and destroys the adjacent bony structures it commonly expands the invaded bone. Fragments of bone may become completely surrounded by the tumor and become sequestered and displaced from the donor site with the enlarging tumor. Thus, areas of calcification and ossification in chordomas may be an integral part of the tumor, or the result of invasion of the adjacent osseous structures.

Some chordomas may become extremely gelatinous, and contain significant amount of mucin, sometimes as much as 50% of their volume or even more. ROBBINS (1945) described a large lumbar chordoma in which, on section through its more solid portions, an almost pure white, glassy surface, covered with a tenacious glairy mucus was seen. This mucus pulled out into long, filamentous strands, so copious in amount that they layered the instruments, hands, and dissecting table.

A remarkable characteristic of chordomas is its ability to invade and destroy bone. The bone destruction may be very extensive. For example, a large segment of the base of the skull, or practically the entire sacrum may be destroyed. Interestingly, despite this prominent local destructiveness, widespread soft tissue destruction and invasion by chordomas is uncommon. Invasion of the veins by chordoma has been described in occasional instances (HASS, 1934; JAFFE, 1958).

2. Classification of Chordoma

Chordoma occurs with predictable regularity in the midline in the axial skeleton along the path of the primitive notochord. It is encountered most frequently at the sites were notochordal vestiges (particularly ectopic vestiges) are found. These sites are: dorsum sellae, floor of the sella, spheno-occipital synchondrosis, cranial surface of the clivus just caudal to the dorsum and just anterior to the foramen magnum, pharyngeal surface of the base of the skull from the sphenoid sinus region to the C_2 vertebra, and sacrococcygeal region. Chordomas are also infrequently found in the rest of cervical spine, thoracic spine, and lumbar spine. Very few documented chordomas have been reported occurring in atypical locations. These latter tumors presumably arise from notochordal tissues which have been displaced for unusual distances by growing cartilage or other nearby structures.

COENEN (1925), after a review of the clinical aspects of chordomas and consideration of their embryology, proposed the first classification for this tumor. Following his report other investigators employed this classification with minor modifications. We prefer the following classification because it is complete, as well as helpful, for clinical and pathologic purposes.

Classification of Chordoma

I.   Intracranial
     1. Sellar and perisellar regions
     2. Clivus
     3. Foramen magnum region
II. Nasopharyngeal
     1. Epipharynx
     2. Atlantoaxial region
III. Vertebral
     1. Cervical spine
     2. Thoracic spine
     3. Dorsal spine
IV. Sacrococcygeal including presacral and retrosacral
V.   Atypical locations
     1. Maxillary sinuses and bones
     2. Frontal sinuses
     3. Occipital bone (other than basiocciput)
     4. Visceral
     5. Other

Some investigators (KAMRIN et al., 1964) believe separation of intracranial chordomas into those arising from the clivus and those arising elsewhere in the cranium does not serve a useful purpose because of great overlapping of the symptoms. This is true in advanced cases. In early cases, however, a precise knowledge of the tumor's site of origin is very important. In these cases, the tumor may present as a sellar mass lesion or a lesion of the clivus. Although association of chordoma and clivus is well known, chordomas are usually not thought of as sellar lesions. As will be discussed later, approximately one-half of all intracranial chordomas present as masses in the sellar or perisellar regions. Although this fact has been pointed out by several authors in the past (BAILEY and BAGDASAR, 1929; HASS, 1934; WOOD and HIMADI, 1950; POPPEN and KING, 1952; KAMRIN et al., 1964; SCHECHTER et al., 1974), chordomas are not usually included in the differential diagnosis of the lesions of this region. Therefore, we feel it is important to emphasize the sellar origin of intracranial chordomas as well as their clival origin.

Another problem in this regard is the relationship between nasopharyngeal and intracranial chordomas. Some intracranial chordomas, at least in the beginning, are strictly confined to the intracranial space, and have no extracranial component. On the other hand, chordomas may arise in the nasopharynx without having any intracranial component. However, sometimes when a chordoma is initially discovered, it is noted that the tumor has intracranial as well as extracranial components. For example, the tumor may have destroyed the sellar region and the sphenoid sinus, and produced a mass in the sellar region as well as in the nasopharynx, or, a tumor that appears retropharyngeal may be noted to have a large intracranial component as well. In these instances, it is difficult, if not impossible, to classify these tumors.

3. Topographic Distribution of Chordoma

As was discussed previously, chordomas occur mainly in the cranial and sacrococcygeal regions. Due to the rarity of this tumor, very few large series have been reported in the literature. Following description of clival "ecchondrosis" by VIRCHOW (1857), and particularly after subsequent demonstration of their notochordal origin by MULLER (1858) and RIBBERT (1894 and 1895), a considerable number of cases were reported. COENEN (1925), in a comprehensive study, collected not only most of the published cases of chordoma but also most of the cases of clival notochordal heterotopia which were reported up to 1925.

It must be recalled that the term "chordoma" was first applied by RIBBERT (1895) to the innocuous experimental notochordal masses which were produced following needle puncture of the intervertebral discs of young rabbits. Following RIBBERT's experiments, the term chordoma was applied to clival notochordal vestiges as well as true neoplasms of the notochord. STEWART (1922) reported a sacrococcygeal chordoma and collected 26 cases of true notochordal neoplasms reported in the literature up to that time. STEWART (1922) reported his case as "malignant sacrococcygeal chordoma" and stated that malignant neoplasms of the notochord, which are symptomatic, should be considered separately; and pointed out the fact that clival chordal vestiges, which were reported by several authors as chordoma, are merely innocuous benign asymptomatic nodules, which are not true neoplasms. In 1926 STEWART and MORIN published an excellent comprehensive review of chordoma, reported a new sacrococcygeal case, and collected another 28 cases of chordoma from the literature. These authors also suggested the more appropriate name "ecchordosis physaliphora" for the clival heterotopic notochordal remnants. Other large series of cases were reported by MABREY (1935), 150 cases; FAUST et al. (1944), 248 cases; HERZOG (1944), 138 cases; TONELLI (1950), 317 cases; and DAHLIN (1967), 122 cases. It must be realized, however, that some of these reported series include cases included in other series, and therefore there is a great overlap in these computations. HOROWITZ (1941) collected 245 cases and FORTI and VENTURINI in 1960 collected 548 cases of chordoma from the world literature. There are, however, few large series in the recent literature which have been reported from a single institution: CONGDON (1952), 22 cases; WINDEYER (1959), 29 cases; DAHLIN (1967), 122 cases; and HIGHINBOTHAM et al. (1967), 46 cases.

For the purpose of evaluation of topographic distribution of this tumor, the series reported by HOROWITZ (1941), 245 cases; the series by TONELLI (1950), 317 cases; and the series by DAHLIN (1967), 122 cases, were selected and compiled. In these 684 patients, the anatomic localization of the tumors is as follows: 239 cranial (35%), 91 vertebral (13%), and 354 sacrococcygeal (52%). The formula suggested for ease of remembering of this numerical distribution is one-half sacrococcygeal, one-third intracranial, and one-sixth vertebral (see Fig. II).

For a more detailed evaluation of the intracranial chordomas, a search of the literature was made and 63 cases of intracranial chordomas were compiled from our own material and the following reports (WOOD and HIMADI, 1950; UTNE and PUGH, 1955; PLAUT and BLATT, 1967; FALCONER et al., 1968; SCHECHTER et al., 1974). To achieve some measure of statistical accuracy, single case reports were not included. Furthermore,

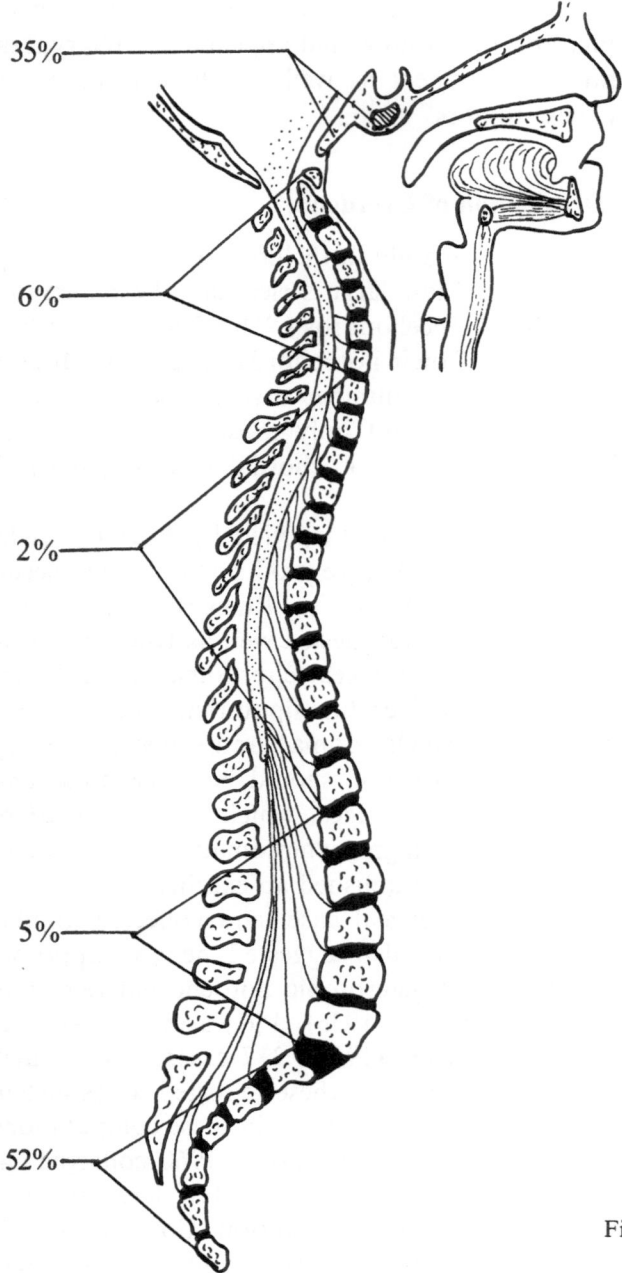

Fig. II. Percentage frequency distribution of chordoma along the axial skeleton

only reports describing a series of chordoma with sufficient detail to ascertain the precise intracranial location of the lesion were selected.

In 63 intracranial chordomas compiled in this fashion, 31, or 49%, presented as a sellar or perisellar mass lesion without concomittant destruction of the clivus. There was 1 case presenting as a perisellar mass without any bony destruction. In 30 patients various degrees of destruction of the sella turcica and sphenoid sinus were present. There were 32 patients who had a mass arising along the course of the clivus, with various degrees of erosion and destruction of the adjacent osseous structures. It is of considerable interest to note that the clivus was intact in 49% of these intracranial tumors.

Regarding vertebral chordomas, the distribution in descending order of frequency is as follows: cervical spine, lumbar spine, and thoracic spine. In the cervical spine, the atlantoaxial region is a frequent site. An interesting feature of vertebral chordomas is the fact that they commonly involve more than one vertebra. In these cases the lesion, which is thought to be a single primary tumor, is seen to extend along the course of the spine into two or more vertebrae with involvement of the corresponding intervertebral discs. An interesting entity is multicentric chordoma of the spine reported by BELLET et al. (1970). These authors reported chordoma of the second lumbar vertebra and third and fourth thoracic vertebrae in a 69-year-old patient, and found three similar cases in the literature.

4. Gross Pathology of the Intracranial Chordomas

In this region the tumor rarely attains a comparatively large size. The tumor is usually covered by the dura. However, in advanced cases, the dura is penetrated and in some cases destroyed, and the tumor may be found adherent to the brain or actually invading it. It typically occurs in the posterior part of the sella and dorsum, or further inferiorly along the clivus, particularly the region of spheno-occipital synchondrosis. Thus, the bulk of the tumor is initially in the midline. However, later in the course of the disease, the tumor may be found to be situated mostly, or even entirely, on the side of the midline.

At surgery the tumor may be seen as several lobules connected by small bridges of tumor tissue, rather than a single large mass. In advanced cases, the tumor is seen as a sheet of cells covering the surface of the base of the skull with many large lobules arising from this sheet.

The intracranial chordomas usually invade the underlying bone with ease and compress and displace the nearby soft-tissue structures. From its point of origin the tumor extends in several typical directions. Thus, the tumor may extend anteriorly and superiorly into and over the hypophyseal fossa, laterally into the floor of the middle fossa, into the cerebellopontine angles in the posterior fossa, posteriorly and inferiorly along the clivus and into the spinal canal, inferiorly into the sphenoid sinuses and nasopharynx, and superiorly and posteriorly into the base of the brain.

The sellar lesions are usually found to have destroyed the sellar floor, dorsum sellae, and posterior clinoids. The invasion may be very extensive and all the sellar components, including the anterior clinoids, may be destroyed. The sphenoid sinuses are commonly invaded and the tumor tissue is found filling the sinuses. In some cases the walls of the sphenoid sinuses are largely destroyed and the tumor tissue is found extending into the nasopharynx. Contrary to expectations, the volume or extent of the nasopharyngeal growth does not parallel the size of the intracranial neoplasms in the majority of the cases (HASS, 1934). The involvement of the nasopharynx may become very extensive, and the tumor may be found extending through the posterior choanae into the nose and even into the maxillary antra.

Anteriorly the tumor may extend into and over the sella turcica, producing various degrees of sellar destruction and displacement or invasion. The tumor may be found as far anteriorly as the olfactory groove (TAVERAS and WOOD, 1964). Occasionally, invasion of the ethmoids and the osseous walls of the orbital cavities are encountered (HASS, 1934). Suprasellar and parasellar extension commonly occurs in the chordomas of the sellar region. These tumors compress, displace, and, occasionally, even invade the suprasellar and parasellar structures. Thus the optic chiasm may be compressed, and the floor of the third ventricle and its recesses may be distorted and displaced superiorly. The compression of the optic pathways by these chordomas frequently causes visual defects similar to the defects produced by the pituitary tumors. Lateral parasellar extension of the tumor leads to the invasion of the cavernous sinus and displacement and eventually encasement of the carotid artery and cranial nerves.

Purely intrasellar chordomas without significant bony erosions are very uncommon. Belza (1966) reported an intrasellar chordoma that had eroded the sellar floor, leaving the dorsum sellae intact. Mathews and Wilson (1974) reported a 41-year-old American Indian in whom a purely intrasellar chordoma was found. The sella was ballooned, but it was intact otherwise. Mathews and Wilson (1974) made an extensive search of the literature and found no other instance of a chordoma entirely confined within an intact sella.

Occasionally, the tumor is mainly suprasellar or parasellar without having any other significant component. In these instances the tumor is usually attached with a stalk to the dorsum sellae or clinoid processes (Plaut and Blatt, 1967; Falconer et al., 1968).

Sellar chordomas often extend posteriorly as well as inferiorly along the course of the clivus. Although this downward extension is occasionally very extensive in sellar chordomas, this feature is particularly seen in clival chordomas, especially in chordomas arising just anterior to the foramen magnum. In these cases the tumor may pass anteriorly beneath the basilar process of the occipital bone into the retropharyngeal tissues or laterally into the paravertebral tissues. The tumor may even grow into the spinal canal, usually ventral to the cord and outside the dura (Hass, 1934).

Chordomas of the clivus typically cause erosion of the clivus, and extend in the direction of the nasopharynx as well as posteriorly. These tumors, as well as the sellar chordomas, depending on their location, may compress the interpeduncular and/or pre-pontine cisterns, displace cerebral peduncles, aqueduct, pons, and the fourth ventricle posteriorly. Thus hydrocephalus may be produced as the result of aqueductal compression, as well as collapsing of the basilar absorbing surfaces. Clival chordomas are less prone to produce nasopharyngeal extension than are the sellar chordomas (Gardner and Turner, 1941). Clival chordomas may extend laterally over the floor of the posterior cranial fossa, producing various degrees of erosion and destruction of the petrous bones.

5. Gross Pathology of Nasopharyngeal Chordomas

The tumors presenting in the nasopharynx may have their origin in the nasopharyngeal mucosa, base of the skull, atlanto-occipital membrane, or atlantoaxial region. They may also be the result of upward extension of the high cervical chordomas or tumors of the lower end of the clivus just anterior to the foramen magnum, or downward extension from intracranial, particularly sellar chordomas. The former group, i.e., true nasopharyngeal chordomas, are very rare tumors and comprise about 3% of all chordomas. This includes chordomas of the atlantoaxial region. On the other hand, most nasopharyngeal chordomas belong to the latter group. Approximately one-third of all intracranial chordomas have a nasopharyngeal mass sometime during their course (Hass, 1934; Dahlin and MacCarty, 1952; Ormerod, 1960; Batsakis, 1963; Kamrin et al., 1964; Wright, 1967).

A nasopharyngeal chordoma originating from the mucosa of the nasopharynx or atlantoaxial membrane may be, at least at the outset, confined to the nasopharynx without having any intracranial component, or attachment to the base of the skull or cervical spine. These instances are rare, however. Wright (1967) reported two cases of chordoma of the nasopharynx without any associated osseous destructive lesions or attachment to the cervical spine. Similar cases have been reported by others (Hass, 1934; Livingstone, 1935; Handousa-Bey, 1949; Windeyer, 1959; Ormerod, 1960).

On the other hand, more commonly the tumor may be attached to the cervical vertebrae, with or without bony destruction; or it may be associated with, or cause, erosion of the base of the skull and eventually produce an intracranial mass.

Some nasopharyngeal tumors may produce extensive destructive lesions of the base of the skull, nasopharynx, paranasal sinuses, orbits, maxillary bone, and face. The tumor may extend into the soft tissues of the face, retropharyngeal or parapharyngeal region, or neck. A large intraspinal extension, producing an epidural mass and cord compression is often found. The dura is not usually invaded. As elsewhere, despite extensive osseous destruction, the soft tissues are rarely destroyed by this tumor. The tumor usually presents as a round, smooth, firm mass in the epipharynx or the retropharyngeal region, displacing the pharyngeal wall, the soft palate, or other structures. It may bulge into the oropharynx and displace and distort the tonsils and peritonsilar structures or it may extend into the nose and cause nasal obstruction. The tumor is usually in the midline, although occasionally it grows predominantly to one side. Although the tumor is usually found attached to spine or the base of the skull, the nasopharyngeal mucous membrane is usually not invaded nor attached to the tumor. The tumor usually has a wide base, although in rare instances it may be pedunculated.

Some nasopharyngeal chordomas develop during the course of an intracranial chordoma, particularly, tumors of the region of the sella turcica and the lower end of the clivus just anterior to the foramen magnum. In most of these patients the nasopharyngeal mass is clinically silent, at least at the outset, and it is incidentally discovered on the roentgenograms of the skull (HASS, 1934; LIVINGSTONE, 1935; GARDNER and TURNER, 1941; TAMPLIN, 1949; HANDOUSA-BEY, 1949; DAHLIN and McCARTY, 1952; ORTON, 1953; WINDEYER, 1959; ORMEROD, 1960; KAMRIN et al., 1964; WRIGHT, 1967; SCHECHTER et al., 1974).

6. Gross Pathology of Vertebral Chordomas

In the spine the tumor occurs most commonly in the cervical spine (particularly upper cervical spine), followed by lumbar spine, and thoracic spine. Tumors of the upper cervical spine and skull base may produce a large retropharyngeal mass, and, when first seen, they may appear to be restricted to the nasopharynx. The tumor, however, when traced posteriorly will be seen to arise from the base of the skull or the cervical vertebrae. At necropsy, an intracranial or intraspinal extension of the tumor is almost always noted. These tumors have been considered in discussion of nasopharyngeal chordomas.

It is of interest that very few instances of vertebral chordoma were reported in the literature following recognition of chordoma as a distinct pathologic entity. In all likelihood, this was due to lack of familiarity with this entity, particularly as a spinal tumor. Considering the difficulty of histologic diagnosis of this tumor, it is probable that some vertebral chordomas are still not correctly identified. The true incidence of vertebral chordomas, therefore, is probably higher than 13% reported in the literature.

Chordomas of the thoracic spine are very rare. HUTTON and YOUNG (1929) described a case of chordoma of the thoracic spine that affected the fourth, fifth, and sixth thoracic vertebrae, associated with epidural extension and compression of the spinal cord. Other cases of chordoma in this region have been reported by other authors (CAPPELL, 1928; HANSSON, 1941; DAHLIN and MacCARTY, 1952; HUSAIN, 1960; EPSTEIN, 1969).

Chordomas of the lumbar spine have been described by several authors (POPPEN and KING, 1952; ROBBINS, 1945; MORRIS and RABINOVITCH, 1947; WOOD and HIMADI, 1950; DAHLIN and MacCARTY, 1952; CONGDON, 1952; BAKER and COLEY, 1953; ALLEN,

1955; Windeyer, 1959; Jones, 1960; McCormack, 1960; Kamrin et al., 1964; Leman et al., 1965; Hartofilaikidis-Garofalidis et al., 1968; Epstein, 1969).

Chordoma of the spine presumably arises from the notochordal remnants in the vertebral body. The tumor commonly affects two or more vertebrae, causing gradual destruction of the body at first, followed by destruction of the arch and eventual collapse of the vertebrae. The intervertebral discs, usually spared by other malignancies, are commonly found to be invaded by the tumor and substantially or completely destroyed. Thus the tumor, originating in the body of one vertebra, crosses the intervening discs and destroys the nearby vertebrae. The involvement of several adjacent vertebrae was thought by Dyke (1941) to be more frequent with chordoma than any other type of malignant disease. This view is now shared by most investigators. A vertebral chordoma may have affected only one vertebra when initially discovered, however, clinical follow-up of the patient, and eventually necropsy, commonly reveal evidence of involvement of multiple adjacent vertebrae and corresponding intervening discs. On the other hand, a review of the literature reveals that when diagnosis of vertebral chordoma is established, approximately one-half of all patients have two or more vertebrae involved (Syme and Cappell, 1926; Dyke, 1941; Wood and Himadi, 1950; Dahlin and MacCarty, 1952; Poppen and King, 1952; Utne and Pugh, 1955; Jaffe, 1958; Epstein, 1969).

We have had personal experience with nine vertebral chordomas. Involvement of two or more vertebral bodies and intervening discs was present in eight patients. In two of these patients invasion and destruction of the intervertebral discs was verified by surgical and pathologic examination.

As was discussed previously, most investigators believe vertebral chordomas arise from the ectopic notochordal remnants within the vertebral bodies, and not from the normally placed remnants in the intervertebral discs. However, in rare instances pathologic examination of the tumor suggests this possibility. For example, Hansson (1941) described a 45-year-old man with neurologic findings pointing to the sixth and seventh thoracic segments. Radiographic examination revealed erosion of the inferior surface of the seventh and superior surface of the eighth thoracic vertebrae, as well as destruction of the corresponding neural arches. Surgical exploration revealed that the disc between the seventh and eighth thoracic vertebrae had been transformed into a blush tumor mass which penetrated into the adjacent vertebral bodies. Epstein (1969) described a 52-year-old woman with low back pain radiating along the sciatic nerve distribution suggestive of a herniated disc. Plain radiographs were negative. Myelography revealed an epidural defect at the fourth lumbar interspace. At surgery an epidural tumor was discovered. This was a soft, gelatinous, friable mass which involved the body of the third lumbar vertebra inferiorly and the fourth lumbar vertebra superiorly as well as the intervertebral disc.

Vertebral chordomas replace the vertebral body partially or substantially with tumor tissue and extend into the perispinal soft tissues. In the neck the tumor commonly produces a retropharyngeal or retroesophageal mass. Occasionally a tumor mass is found laterally in the neck. A similar pattern of anterior or lateral extension occurs in the thoracic and lumbar regions. Thus the tumor may grow in the retropleural or retroperitoneal spaces, producing a mass in front or the side of the spine. At surgery the mass is found to be attached to the spine at one or more levels. The tumor often breaks out of the body of the vertebra posteriorly and infiltrates beneath the posterior longitudinal ligament. The intervertebral discs are often found to be invaded and destroyed by the tumor. With further posterior extension the tumor enters the epidural space and produces spinal cord compression. In advanced cases, at necropsy, the tumor is seen surrounding the dura and extending up and down in the spinal canal. The dura is usually not penetrated, although local spinal nerves are usually found surrounded by, or imbedded in, the tumor tissue.

Invasion of the dura, intradural extension, and invasion of the spinal cord is rare in spinal chordomas and very few documented cases have been reported. POPPEN and KING (1952) reported six cases of spinal chordomas, three lumbar, and three sacral in location. In all these patients the tumor was extensive, and the spinal cord, the cauda equina and the nerve roots were compressed by extradural masses. At times the dura was penetrated, with marked intradural extension. FOX et al. (1968) reported a 58-year-old woman with a sacrococcygeal chordoma that was treated surgically by partial resection of the sacrum and coccyx. The patient was treated by irradiation in the following 16 years for pelvic recurrence. At necropsy, there was extensive replacement of the remainder of the sacrum and adjacent pelvis by a nodular mucoid neoplasm. The spinal canal, up to the level of the sixth thoracic vertebra, was filled with neoplasm and the spinal cord and cauda equina from this level distally were difficult to recognize.

We have had experience with nine vertebral chordomas in three of whom an intradural extension of the tumor was demonstrated at myelography and subsequently at surgery. The first patient was a 33-year-old woman when originally seen with chordoma of the second cervical vertebra. She was followed for 39 years and underwent decompression laminectomy and local resection of the tumor several times. The tumor gradually involved the cervical vertebrae and discs from the level of the axis to the fifth cervical spine. Epidural extension of the tumor was noted all along, and at last surgical exploration, invasion of the dura and intradural extension was noted. The second patient was a 24-year-old woman with chordoma affecting the second, third, and fourth cervical vertebrae. At surgery, dural invasion and intradural extension was noted. The third patient, a 47-year-old man had chordoma of the ninth and tenth thoracic vertebrae. The patient died 4 years following the diagnosis. At necropsy, invasion of the dura was present. Extensive seeding of the leptomeninges at the base of the brain, as well as the cervical and thoracic spinal cord, was noted.

Some vertebral chordomas may attain a very large size. ROBBINS (1945) described a 41-year-old man who was admitted to the hospital with a large abdominal mass. At surgery the peritoneal cavity contained 5 l of a serosanguinous fluid, removal of which revealed a slippery mucinous material covering most of the serosal surfaces. The region of the transverse mesocolon was filled with solid tumor tissue, which was fused to the stomach, pancreas, transverse colon, and left kidney. The mass extended posteriorly and completely enveloped the aorta and vena cava. The patient died 9 days after his entry into the hospital. At postmortem the tumor was found to be densely adherent to the prevertebral fascia in the region of the second and third lumbar vertebrae. No bony erosion or destruction of the vertebrae of intervertebral discs were demonstrable.

Vertebral chordomas, despite their remarkable ability to invade and destroy bone, do not ordinarily invade and destroy the soft-tissue structures in their path of growth. This characteristic is seen even with large tumors and in tumors with prominent cellular anaplasia. The large abdominal chordoma described by ROBBINS (1945), was found to have enveloped the pancreas, adrenal gland, spleen, kidney, ascending colon, and part of the stomach. However, investigation of these organs showed that the tumor tissue extended up to the external limits of these structures without actual invasion of any of them. The mucosa of the entire gastrointestinal tract was intact. We found no documented cases of ulceration of the gastrointestinal mucosa secondary to invasion by vertebral chordoma, a fact which has been pointed out by ACKERMAN and DEL REGATO (1962).

7. Gross Pathology of Sacrococcygeal Chordomas

In this region, the tumor usually originates in the substance of bone in the sacrum or coccyx. In these cases, destructive lesions of the sacrum and/or coccyx are an integral part of the tumor. On the other hand, some chordomas in this region apparently arise from the notochordal remnants in front or behind the sacrum. In these patients, the tumor may, at least at the outset, appear as a pelvic or a retrosacral mass without evidence of a estructive lesion of the sacrum or coccyx (WILLIS, 1930; HSIEH and HSIEH, 1936; DAHLIN and MacCARTY, 1952). WILLIS (1967) reported a 36-year-old woman with a pelvic chordoma which, over a period of 4.5 years, occupied most of the pelvic cavity and extended into the soft tissues of the proximal thigh. The tumor was adherent to the sacrum, but no destructive lesion of the sacrum was present. DAHLIN and MacCARTY (1952) studied 32 sacrococcygeal chordomas. No lesion of the sacrum or coccyx was present in 3 of these patients. We have had experience with nine sacrococcygeal chordomas. Eight patients had a destructive lesion of the sacrum and/or coccyx. One patient, however, had a small retrosacral chordoma without evidence of osseous destruction.

Chordomas of this region usually produce a smooth, somewhat lobulated, presacral, extrarectal mass attached to the anterior surface of the sacrum and/or coccyx. The tumor may be almost liquid in consistency and is rarely very firm. It has a definite elastic feeling to it. Mucus-producing adenocarcinomas and soft chondromas or chondrosarcomas may simulate a pelvic chordoma grossly.

In approximately one-third of the cases, a retrosacral mass, firmly attached to the posterior aspect of the sacrum and/or coccyx, is present. The tumor is usually in the midline, but it may gradually occupy most of the dorsal surface of the lower back. Occasionally a retrosacral chordoma may have a prominent lateral extension into the soft tissues of the buttocks or the proximal thigh (DAHLIN and MacCARTY, 1952). Almost all patients with retrosacral chordoma have a presacral extension as well.

Pelvic chordomas may grow upward into the lumbar region. Extension of the tumor inside the pelvis displaces the rectum and pelvic colon anteriorly, or to one side. As in the rest of the neuraxis, chordoma of the sacrococcygeal region does not invade the soft-tissue structures of the pelvis. The tumor may encircle and encase the rectum, uterus, or bladder, but actual invasion of the wall of these viscera is rare, and ulceration of their mucosa practically never occurs (DAHLIN and MacCARTY, 1952; WINDEYER, 1959; ACKERMAN and DEL REGATO, 1962).

Extension into the spinal canal in the epidural space is very common. An epidural mass causing compression of the dural sac is often found. The epidural mass ordinarily is on the ventral aspect of the canal, but occasionally is mainly on one side. The mass usually extends up and down the epidural space for a short distance, however, not uncommonly, a large epidural mass extending along several levels in the lumbosacral region is found. Vertebrosacral chordomas usually cause destruction of the body of the vertebrae. However, occasional cases of invasion and destruction of the vertebral elements (transverse process, pedicle, lamina, spinous process) have been recorded. In some cases, long-standing and persistent compression may cause erosion and thinning of the neural arches without actual osseous invasion and destruction (POPPEN and KING, 1952, WINDEYER, 1959). POPPEN and KING reported a 36-year-old woman who had had partial resection of the coccyx 7 years previously for "coccygodynia." The complaints did not subside and the patient developed progressively worsening signs and symptoms of compression of the sacral and lower lumbar nerves. At surgery, destructive lesions of the bodies of the vertebrae from the second lumbar to the fourth sacral were found. A huge extradural tumor was present. The spinous processes and laminae of these vertebrae were eroded and paper thin. Histologically, the tumor was a typical chordoma.

Dural invasion and intradural extension of the tumor is very rare. DAHLIN and MacCARTY did not report a case of dural invasion in their 44 vertebral and sacrococcygeal cases (see Sect. I-6, Gross Pathology of Vertebral Chordoma)

8. Histology of Chordoma

a) Histogenesis

As was previously discussed, because of its close relationship during the embryonic life with ectoderm, endoderm, and mesoderm, much controversy exists as to which blastodermic layer the notochord should be ascribed. PATTEN (1968) considers the notochord as belonging with the mesoderm. Some authorities, including GESCHICKTER and COPELAND (1949), consider the notochord as an endodermal structure. LICHTENSTEIN (1965) considers it to be a derivative of both mesoderm and ectoderm. STEWART and MORIN (1926) and ROBBINS (1945) consider the notochord to be a tissue of ectodermal origin, in which its cellular structure assumes a mesenchymal characteristic because of notochord's purely mechanical function. These authors consider this dual "origin" to be significantly reflected in the cellular composition of the chordomas. The presence of predominantly epithelial-like structures in some chordomas and cells resembling spindle-cell sarcoma in others, or in the same tumor, are thought to be reflections of this fact.

b) Cytology

As stated by EVANS (1966), the microscopic picture of chordoma is characteristically pleomorphic and a wide range of structural variations is ordinarily noted in different tumors and in various segments of the same tumor. The salient features include the almost constant arrangement of the tumor cells into lobules or alveoli, the tendency of the cells to grow in cords, and be transformed into syncytial masses, the production of an abundant mucinous matrix, and the presence of large physaliphorous cells. A framework of fibrous trabeculae, most prominent at the periphery of the tumor and disappearing centrally, is seen dividing the tumor into lobules. The blood supply of the tumor comes from thin-walled blood vessels which are carried inside the tumor by these fibrous septae.

The number of the cells and their morphology varies with the size and the age of the lobule, and in different segments of the tumor. The younger and smaller nodules, especially those at the invasive border of the tumor, are composed of well-formed cells associated with minimal amounts of intercellular mucin, whereas the older and larger lobules may show much cellular disintegration accompanied by abundant mucin production. In the very young nodules, polygonal or prismatic cells are seen in close juxtaposition resembling epithelial cells. In the larger lobules the cells may be arranged in columns extending toward the central zone in a radial fashion. In between the columns of cells the amount of mucin increases toward the central regions, where it is usually abundant and may form large irregular pools. The amount of mucin usually increases with the size and the age of the lobule; some lobules appear to be composed almost entirely of mucinous lakes, in which a few isolated cells are scattered.

Intracellular cytoplasmic vacuoles are a prominent feature of chordoma. Vacuolation is a continuous process and its various stages can be followed from cell to cell. In smaller cells single or multiple vacuoles develop. They get larger and more numerous until the characteristic physaliphorous cells are produced. In physaliphorous cells, large vacuoles surround a central or eccentrically placed nucleus. As the process of vacuolation proceeds, the cell outlines become increasingly more difficult to define, until a highly vacuolated syncytium is produced.

A striking feature of chordoma is the formation of varying amounts of extracellular mucin. This may be very abundant and, at times, large segments of the tumor are composed of scattered disintegrated cells, and a syncytium lying in a sea of mucus.

UTNE and PUGH (1955) reviewed 72 instances of chordoma and reported intracellular cytoplasmic vacuoles in some portion of the tumor in all their patients. The physaliphorous cells were prominent in one-half of the cases. Extracellular mucin, of varying amounts, was found in every case.

An occasional confusing problem can be the differentiation of a sacrococcygeal chordoma from an unusual example of mucin-producing adenocarcinoma of the rectosigmoid with insignificant mucosal ulceration. Some of the earlier case reports of pelvic tumors, reported as chordoma, causing colonic obstruction and mucosal ulceration, in all likelihood, are instances of mucin-producing adenocarcinoma of the colon (e.g., LEWIS, 1921).

Occasionally, another diagnostic problem is the differentiation of chordoma from chondroma and chondrosarcoma. FALCONER et al. (1968) reported four cases of tumors of the skull base which had been originally diagnosed as chordoma and subsequently proved to be chondromas with a benign course. HERNDON and COHEN (1970) reported a lumbar chondroma resembling a chordoma. DAHLIN and MACCARTY (1952) state that chondromas and chondrosarcomas ordinarily offer no problem in the differential diagnosis, because their cells lie in lacunae and lack intracellular vacuoles. However, two tumors had to be discarded by these authors from a group of 63 cases originally designated as chordoma, because the differentiation from chondrosarcoma could not be made with certainty. DAHLIN (1967), in a review of 122 cases of chordoma, noted 3 instances of sacrococcygeal chordoma which contained discrete foci of chondrosarcoma. One of these also contained islands of osteogenic and fibrosarcoma.

Histologic separation of chordomas into benign and malignant (CONGDON, 1952) has not gained wide usage. In the majority of the cases, the tumor manifests an indolent and progressive course, often over a period of years. The degrees of cellular differentiation, anaplasia, and mitotic activity, do not accurately portend the biological behavior of the neoplasm and are unrelated to the clinical course and the length of survival in the majority of the cases (ROBBINS, 1945; DAHLIN and MACCARTY, 1952; POPPEN and KING, 1952; CRAWFORD, 1958; JAFFE, 1958; DAHLIN, 1967; FOX et al., 1968).

9. Metastasis

The overall incidence of metastasis in chordoma is not very high. DAHLIN and MAC-CARTY reported a series of 59 cases of chordoma, but did not observe a biopsy-proved instance of metastasis, although the clinical findings were suggestive of this possibility in 2 patients. The incidence often cited in the literature is 10%. In sharp contrast is the overall 43% incidence of distant metastasis reported by HIGHINBOTHAM and associates (1967) in a report on 46 cases of chordoma encountered during a 35-year study. We observed 2 instances of pathologically verified distant metastasis in 24 cases of chordoma.

There is strong circumstantial evidence, as suggested by KAMRIN et al. (1964) and FOX et al. (1968), that long clinical duration, repeated recurrences, and even radiation therapy play a role in the determination of the capability to metastasize. The series of HIGHINBOTHAM et al. (1967) and the course of the patient reported by FOX et al. (1968) seem to support this assumption. FOX and associates (1968) collected 48 cases of chordoma associated with metastasis from the literature. An analysis of a total of

52 cases, including 4 instances from our material and 2 other cases found in the literature (see References), reveals the following observations. The sacrococcygeal chordomas associated with distant metastasis accounted for 33 cases and were the leading group, an observation which has been made by several other authors in the past. Vertebral chordomas made up 15 cases of the total, and intracranial tumors were responsible for only 3 instances of metastasis. An instance of a primary chordoma of the scapula with pulmonary metastasis has been reported (HIGHINBOTHAM et al., 1967). Metastasis is usually by the hematogenous route (DAHLIN, 1967). Metastatic deposits have been reported in practically every organ of the body and in unusual locations, including the skin. Recurrence usually produces multiple nodules in the region of previous surgical excision. The most frequent sites of secondary deposits, in descending order of frequency, include the lungs (31 cases), liver (13), regional and remote lymph nodes (11), bones (10), brain (5), skin (5), and peritoneum (3). In most of these patients metastasis is not widely disseminated; there were only 11 instances with widespread metastases (Fig. 1).

10. Chordoma in Unusual Locations

There are only a few instances of chordoma reported in the literature occurring in locations not adjacent to the path of the primitive notochord. These include two tumors, one of the upper and one of the lower jaw (KORITSKI, 1914), and a tumor each of left superior occipital bone (ALEZAIS and PEYRON, 1914b), frontal sinus (ADAMS, 1948), maxillary antrum and nares (PASTORE et al., 1949), in the ethmoid and maxillary sinuses (BERDAL and MYHRE, 1964), and scapula (HIGHINBOTHAM et al., 1967). These tumors presumably arise from notochordal tissues which have been displaced for unusual distances by growing cartilage or other nearby structures.

D. Clinical Findings

I. General Considerations

The presenting complaints and physical findings vary according to the location and direction of spread, but in all cases the findings are due to the presence of a slowly expanding tumor mass causing destruction of the nearby bony structures of the base of the skull or the vertebral axis, as well as compression of the adjacent brain, spinal cord and/or the nerves issuing from them.

1. Age and Sex

Intracranial chordomas occur predominantly in the third, fourth, and fifth decades of life, with a mean age of onset of 35 years. These tumors, however, occur in all age groups including old age and childhood. STEWART and MORIN (1922, 1926) collected 55 chordomas from the literature. The mean age in cranial chordomas in this group was 35 years. The average age of onset in 56 cases of cranial and cervical spine chordomas compiled by HASS (1934) was 36. MABREY (1935) found the cranial chordomas to be more frequent during the fourth and fifth decades of life (49 patients). Similar figures have been reported by other investigators.

Cranial chordomas are distinctly uncommon in childhood, although several cases have been reported. Hennig (1900) reported a case as early as the 7th month of fetal life. Koritski (1914) and Rubaschow (1929) reported a tumor in a 1.5-month-old, and 1-day-old babies respectively, but these tumors were in unusual locations (mandible). Whether these cases represent true chordomas is open to question. Arauz and Podesta (1923) quoted a patient in whom symptoms began at 5 years of age. Highinbotham et al. (1967) reported a 2.5-year-old patient. The youngest patient in Schechter et al.'s (1974) 30 patients was 8 years old.

Vertebral chordomas occur most frequently in the third, fourth, and fifth decades of life. A review of the literature indicates that the mean age of onset in these patients is very similar to the cranial chordomas (35 years).

Sacrococcygeal chordomas occur usually a decade or so later than cranial chordoma. The mean age of onset in these tumors is about 50 years. In Stewart and Morin's (1922), 1926) compilations, the mean age was 50 years (28 patients). Mabrey (1935) found these tumors to be more frequent during the fifth and sixth decades of life (87 patients). In 40 patients compiled by Utne and Pugh (1955), the mean age was 50 years. Similar figures have been reported by other investigators (Jaffe, 1958; Dahlin, 1967; Epstein, 1969). Sacrococcygeal chordomas are distinctly uncommon prior to the third decade of life. However, the tumor has been reported in patients as young as 2 years (Montgomery and Woltman, 1933). In Mabrey's (1935) collected series of 85 sacroccygeal chordomas, 4 patients were below the age of 9 years.

Cranial chordomas occur somewhat more frequently in males than in females. When the series of Stewart and Morin (1922, 1926), Utne and Pugh (1955), and Dahlin (1967) are compiled, the male to female ratio is 43:37. Vertebral chordomas do not have any significant predilection for either of the sexes. Sacrococcygeal chordoma, on the other hand, affect males approximately three times as commonly as females. When the series of Stewart and Morin (1922, 1926), Utne and Pugh (1955), and Dahlin (1967) are compiled, the male to female ratio is 100:31.

2. Symptomatology

In the majority of the cases, the onset of chordoma is very insidious. Cranial chordomas, by virtue of their location, produce symptoms early during their course, while vertebral and particularly sacrococcygeal tumors may exist for a relatively long period of time without causing any significant symptoms or signs. There is also usually a delay between the onset of symptoms and the discovery of the true nature of the disease. In intracranial chordomas this delay is usually in order of a few months, while in sacrococcygeal lesions this interval may be significantly longer.

a) Clinical Findings in Intracranial Chordomas

The findings in these patients result from the slow, but relentless growth of the tumor at the base of the brain, usually originating near the midline. This space occupying mass causes increased intracranial pressure as well as findings related to the invasion of the base of the skull and compression of the nearby structures. The tumor's originating in the region of the sella turcica cause destruction of the pituitary gland and compression of the first seven cranial nerves. The lesions occurring further posteriorly and inferiorly along the course of the clivus, by virtue of their position, present mainly as a posterior fossa space-occupying mass, and produce findings related to the compression of the pons, cerebellum, and the lower cranial nerves. The lesions occurring further inferiorly may produce findings of compression at the foramen magnum region.

These considerations are applicable only when these lesions are discovered fairly early during their course. As is known, sellar lesions may extend infratentorially along the clivus causing extensive bony destruction and compression of the posterior fossa structures. Similarly, lesions of the clivus may extend into, and over, the sella turcica with extensive destruction and compression of the nearby structures. As it is seen, therefore, a marked overlapping of the clinical finding may be noted in these lesions.

The clinical findings, on the whole, do not present in a well-ordered sequence. However, findings caused by increased intracranial pressure are usually the first disturbances noted by the patient. Thus, headache and visual disturbances (subjective complaints of diplopia or blurred vision and objective ocular disturbances of choked disk or optic atrophy), and constitutional findings (fatigue, weakness, lethargy, forgetfulness, depression, and emotional instability) are experienced by the patient initially. These findings are gradual in onset. There may be unexplained periods of remission lasting for a few months. These temporary remissions may be complete, i.e., the findings may disappear completely. However, the disturbances will recur and will get progressively worse. It is not unusual to note patients who develop headache and ocular findings (diplopia, blurred vision), lasting for a few weeks then subsiding totally or substantially, only to recur with greater severity and extent in a few months. The second group of findings which usually follow, but may occur concurrently with, the manifestations of increased intracranial pressure are those caused by invasion of, and pressure upon, the structures which are adjacent to the mass. This group consists of pain in the head and neck region, pituitary insufficiency, and paralysis of the cranial nerves.

Table 1. Predominant presenting findings of intracranial chordoma (152 patients)

	No.	%
Headache	112	73
Diplopia	93	60
Blurred vision	65	42
Visual field defect	38	25
Dysphagia	36	23
Endocrine dysfunction	20	13
Anosmia	10	6
Ptosis	37	24
Decreased hearing	29	19

A summary of the predominant clinical findings in 152 patients compiled from the literature (KAMRIN et al., 1964; UTNE and PUGH, 1955) is presented in Table 1. The most frequent symptom at the onset is headache. It is usually referred to either the frontal or the occipital region. The headaches are usually of increasing severity with temporary periods of relief lasting up to a few months. There may be pain felt deep within, or in the back of the neck. The most common visual disturbance is diplopia. Blurred vision and decreased visual acuity are also seen fairly frequently. Although it is rare for a patient to report visual field defects, this finding is found in approximately one-fourth of all patients on testing. Papilledema and optic atrophy are seen with equal frequency, being present in 20% of the patients (HASS, 1934; GIVNER, 1945; UTNE and PUGH, 1955). In predominantly sellar lesions the visual disturbances generally are the result of compression of the optic chiasm and/or the sixth nerve. In the former instance, reduction of visual acuity and bitemporal hemianopsia are the most important findings, which almost without exception prompt the diagnosis of a primary tumor of the hypophysis or its anlage. In some instances the sixth nerve is the only structure affected initially. This is responsible for the not infrequent occurrence of diplopia or blurring of vision as the first presenting disturbance, preceding the onset of headache by a few weeks. In later stages, depending on the extent and direction of growth of the neoplasm, various defects in the visual fields, including asymmetrical and unilateral defects, and total blindness may be noted. Other occular manifestations include internal strabismus, altered pupillary reactions, dilatation of the pupils, and anisocoria. The tumor may also compress or stretch various cranial nerves in this region. Although the typical tumor is in midline, there is a pronounced tendency for involvement of the cranial nerves to be unilateral. In these patients, the findings are similar to those produced by other sellar, suprasellar, or parasellar lesions, such as pituitary tumors, meningioma, craniopharyngioma, and aneurysm. When the impairment is bilateral, it is almost always more complete and more widespread on one side than on the other (Hass, 1934). The olfactory nerve is only occasionally involved, because the tumor rarely extends into the anterior cranial fossa. The ocular nerves, aside from the optic nerve which has already been considered, are frequently affected as the mass involves the cavernous sinus. Paresis of the abducens nerve (6th) is most frequent, and it usually precedes the onset of paralysis of the other ocular nerves. Paralysis of the third and fourth nerves occurs in one-third of the patients. These disturbances are most commonly unilateral, although in late stages of the disease, bilateral paralysis is encountered. Involvement of the fifth nerve is less common, being seen in only 12% of the patients. Impairment of the motor function of this nerve is rare, while various sensory disturbances, as frequently bilateral as unilateral, are noted. In almost every instance in which the function of the facial nerve is disturbed (14%) the sixth nerve and, less commonly, the fifth nerve are also involved (Hass, 1934).

Disturbances of endocrine function on the basis of pituitary insufficiency include amenorrhea, sterility, loss of libido, and marked gain of weight. These findings are only occasionally noted at the onset. Most often these disturbances present insidiously a year or so after the onset of the disease.

Nasopharyngeal symptoms, secondary to invasion of the nasopharynx, although they accompany or follow the onset of headaches and visual disturbances, occasionally are the first manifestation of the disease. Occasionally, nasopharyngeal manifestations precede the onset of intracranial symptoms for many years, the longest duration having been 12 years (Arauz and Podesta, 1923). On the other hand, a relatively silent, and occasionally large, retropharyngeal mass, starting at the base of the skull and extending in front of C_1–C_2 region, is often found in these patients. Occasionally, such a nasopharyngeal mass may be the only finding.

In the predominantly clivus chordoma, presenting symptoms are those of a tumor of the posterior fossa, with compression of the pons and cerebellum and involvement of the lower cranial nerves. Commonly, because of extradural extension of the tumor, disturbances secondary to the compression of the upper cervical cord are also noted. Thus, paralysis of various cranial nerves, from trigeminal to hypoglossal, disturbances of gait, various sensory and motor findings involving the neck, shoulders, and extremities are usually seen. Pain deep within, or in the back of the neck, although usually late in onset, may occasionally be the first complaint (4%). The tumor may produce predominantly unilateral findings. In one-sixth of all patients with intracranial chordoma, symptoms of a cerebellopontine-angle tumor are present. Other findings in these patients include decreased hearing, dysphagia, tongue deviation, and nasopharyngeal obstruction.

In two-thirds of all patients with lower cranial nerve involvement, a nasopharyngeal mass is also present. This is a valuable clinical finding and should always be searched for in the presence of lower cranial nerve dysfunction. If a mass can be seen, persistent attempts at biopsy will usually result in a positive tissue diagnosis. Several attempts at biopsy are often necessary as the tumor does not invade the mucosa but is deep in the pharyngeal wall, pushing normal structures before it as it grows out from the cervical spine (KAMRIN et al., 1964).

Tumors of the clivus often extend superiorly and anteriorly into and over the sellar region. In later stages, manifestations of involvement of the hypophysis and compression of the perisellar cranial nerves are often present.

Occasionally, manifestations which are caused by compression of the brain stem, or pressure against the spinal cord in the region of the foramen magnum, are noted as the initial presenting disturbances. More often, these abnormalities develop during the course of the disease as the tumor gradually expands. The resulting manifestations are varied, but they are, as a rule, secondary to involvement of the pyramidal or sensory tracts. Hemiparesis, the most important of these, is seen in 9% of the patients. More commonly, weakness of the shoulder and/or the upper extremity is present. This is usually associated with pain in the neck, shoulder, and arm. These findings are often unilateral, although on occasion they may be noted to affect one upper extremity alternately or concurrently with the other. Among these findings, neck pain has been emphasized by several authors. The pain is accentuated by motion of the head and occasionally is so severe that the patient is obliged to hold his head rigidly in a fixed position. Paraparesis, hyperactive reflexes, muscular atrophy, colonic convulsions, incontinence, hypalgesia, hemianesthesia, hypesthesia, ataxia, and loss of deep reflexes are other infrequent manifestations (HASS, 1934).

Involvement of the upper cervical vertebrae is seen in 15% of these patients. A nasopharyngeal mass is almost always present in this latter group. These lesions have been classified as tumors of the dens epistrophei by some authors. As was discussed previously (see pathology), a nasopharyngeal mass may be present when the patient is initially seen (35%), it may be the predominant (15%), or the sole initial presentation, or it may develop during the course of the disease when the tumor extends into the nasopharynx (STEWART, 1922; STEWART and MORIN, 1926; HASS, 1934; ADSON et al., 1935, MABREY, 1935; HARVEY and DAWSON, 1941; FAUST et al., 1944; GIVNER, 1945; DAHLIN and MACCARTY, 1952; POPPEN and KING, 1952; UTNE and PUGH, 1955; JAFFE, 1958; WINDEYER, 1959; KAMRIN et al., 1964; HIGHINBOTHAM et al., 1967; DAHLIN, 1967).

b) Clinical Findings in Nasopharyngeal Chordoma

Nasopharyngeal chordomas may have no extension outside this region and be primarily nasopharyngeal tumors (WRIGHT, 1967), but these are uncommon. It is more likely they are a downward extension from an intracranial tumor (BATSAKIS and KITTLESON, 1963), or an upward extension of a high cervical growth (see Gross Pathology). These lesions are indistinguishable from other tumors arising in this region such as craniopharyngioma or nasopharyngeal carcinoma until a correct histologic diagnosis is made.

Nasopharyngeal symptoms may be the predominant presenting complaints in patients with intracranial tumors (UTNE and PUGH, 1955). These disturbances include obstructed breathing, which usually is of short duration averaging less than 6 months, nasal obstruction, conductive deafness, anosmia, and rhinolalia clausa. Secondary infection leads to purulent nasal discharge and sometimes to epistaxis.

Unilateral or bilateral paresis of the vocal cords is seen in some patients. This is, however, secondary to the involvement of the vagus nerve and is seen primarily with the tumors of the clivus. In these patients, disturbances of taste (glossopharyngeal), as well as involvement of the 11th, and often the 12th, cranial nerves are also present (SYME and CAPPELL, 1926; HASS, 1934; RIDPATH, 1938; ADAMS, 1948; PASTORE et al., 1949; ORTON, 1953; UTNE and PUGH, 1955; WINDEYER, 1959; ORMEROD, 1960; KAMRIN et al., 1964; WRIGHT, 1967).

c) Clinical Findings in Vertebral Chordoma

The clinical manifestations of these lesions is the result of (1) a slowly growing tumor mass causing destruction of the vertebrae, (2) compression of the spinal cord and/or the spinal nerves, and (3) compression of the nearby extraspinal structures. Vertebral chordoma often involves two or more vertebrae, and produces a para- or prespinal mass in almost all cases.

Chordomas of the cervical spine, depending on their location, may produce a retropharyngeal, retroesophageal, or a predominantly lateral mass in the neck. Prespinal extension of the mass may cause dysphagia, and less commonly, difficulty of breathing. The presence of a tumor in the neck was noted by 6 patients in a group of 14 vertebral chordomas reported by UTNE and PUGH (1955). KAMRIN et al. (1964) reported four patients with cervical chordoma in whom three had a palpable mass. In nine patients with cervical chordoma (DAHLIN and MACCARTY, 1952; UTNE and PUGH, 1955), four patients presented with initial symptoms of compression of the spinal cord or nerve roots; three had prespinal masses, causing dysphagia; and two patients presented with masses in the lateral surface of the neck. WINDEYER (1959) reported three cervical chordomas. One patient's first complaint was swelling of the neck, and slight discomfort on swallowing associated with right arm pain and pins and needles in the fingers. A second patient developed a lump in the right side of the neck, approximately 1.5 years following onset of persistent neck pain, and 1 year prior to the admission for treatment. These masses are usually firm, most often measure between 5–10 cm, and on the average are discovered 1 year prior to the time the definitive diagnosis is established.

In the thoracic and lumbar spine, extraspinal extension of the neoplasm usually does not cause significant symptoms related to the pressure by the tumor. Occasionally, a feeling of "tightness" or "heaviness" in the chest is experienced by the patient. Abdominal masses may attain a very large size, and produce various manifestations of a large intraabdominal or retroperitoneal neoplasm (ROBBINS, 1945; HARTOFILAIKIDIS-GAROFALIDIS, 1968).

Neoplastic invasion of the vertebrae results in focal pain, which may have a constant dull aching characteristic at first, but usually gets progressively worse. Compression of the cord and spinal nerves leads to various neurologic disturbances depending on the level and extent of the involvement. The earliest complaints in most of the patients, consist of sensory disturbances, such as numbness and paresthesia followed by pain, affecting the neck, arms, or legs on one or both sides. These symptoms may be of intermittent nature at first, although they invariably get progressively worse and more extensive at each recurrence and soon become constant. The sensory disturbances may be present for 6 months to 3 years before significant motor deficit develops and the diagnosis is established. Periods of remission, lasting one to several months were seen in six of our nine patients with vertebral chordoma, and have been observed by other authors. As the tumor enlarges, other disturbances of cord or spinal nerve compression, such as long tract signs, pathologic reflexes, paralysis of various groups of muscles in the upper and/or lower extremities, and urinary and fecal sphincter disturbances will be noted. Motor deficit is rarely the sole initial presenting disturbance although the constellation of motor deficit (such as weakness of arms or legs), pain and paresthesia is the most common presenting complaint. Paresthesia, pain, and motor deficit (mild paresis to complete paralysis of one extremity) lasting a few months to a few years prior to the discovery of the true nature of the disease, has been observed in 25% of the patients with vertebral chordoma. In patients with lumbar chordoma, back pain and radicular pain in the distribution of the sciatic nerve, mimicking a herniated intervertebral disk, are commonly noted. Back pain may be present for 3–6 years before the definitive diagnosis is established. Occasionally the presenting complaint is urinary or fecal incontinence (HUTTON and YOUNG, 1929; HASS, 1934; ADSON et al., 1935; POPPEN and KING, 1952; ROBBINS, 1945; MORRIS and RABINOVITCH, 1947; POPPEN and KING, 1952; SENNETT, 1953; BAKER and COLEY, 1953; ALLEN, 1955; WINDEYER, 1959; ROSENQUIST and SALTZMAN, 1959; KAMRIN et al., 1964; EPSTEIN, 1969).

d) Clinical Findings in Sacrococcygeal Chordoma

Sacral chordomas as a rule produce destructive lesions of the sacrum and/or coccyx, compress the cauda equina and pelvic nerves, and produce a presacral or retrosacral mass. The most common presenting complaint is pain (95%). Only rarely a silent perisacral mass or lytic lesion of sacrum is found accidentally. We encountered a patient in whom a silent sacral destructive lesion (later found to be chordoma) was discovered on a pelvic film taken for intravenous pyelography. The pain is usually felt in the sacrococcygeal region or in the rectum. It is usually mild, but often with progression of the disease it becomes intractable with radiation along the sciatic nerves. The pain is usually present for 2–5 years before the definitive diagnosis is made. Occasionally, this interval is much longer. UTNE and PUGH (1955) reported two patients (5%) in whom pain of gradually increasing severity had been present for 18 years. Also, a diagnosis of hemorrhoids treated surgically without relief was part of the history in 14 patients (35%) reported by these authors.

Sensory disturbances, other than pain, are less prominent in these patients, although saddle numbness and anesthesia is seen in 20% of the patients, usually occurring long after the onset of the pain. A mass is usually present in these patients. On rectal examination it is usually firm, smooth, or lobulated, fixed to the sacrum, and clearly extraluminal. Occasionally, a retrosacral mass is also present (see Pathology). The mass may become very large and fill most of the pelvic cavity, displacing and compressing rectum, bladder, and other pelvic structures. Although the tumor may actually surround and encase the pelvic structures, it usually does not cause mucosal invasion and destruction. However, rectal bleeding, secondary to venous stasis and engorgement, may occasionally be seen (5–10%).

Constipation is a common feature. Of 40 patients, 29 had constipation in the series of UTNE and PUGH (1955). Fecal incontinence is usually seen as a late complication. Disturbances related to the lower urinary tract, such as difficulty in starting urination, dysuria, frequency, and urgency are encountered less commonly (10–15%), and are not usually severe at the onset. However, late in the course of the disease, disturbances of the bladder function often become very troublesome. This may be due to a neurogenic bladder, or the result of severe encasement of the bladder by the tumor. Other neurologic disturbances, such as paresthesia and muscle paralysis, are usually far less prevalent (5%) in sacrococcygeal chordomas than in any other region (STEWART and MORIN, 1926; MABREY, 1935; FAUST, 1944; GENTIL and COLEY, 1948; DAHLIN and MACCARTY, 1952; LITTMAN, 1953; UTNE and PUGH, 1955; KAMRIN et al., 1964; EPSTEIN, 1969).

E. Roentgenologic Findings

I. Intracranial Chordomas

1. Plain Film Findings (Including Body-Section Radiography)

Although intracranial chordoma may present with clinical signs of an intracranial mass without plain films change, a high percentage of cases will have evidence of bone involvement at the time of admission to the hospital. UTNE and PUGH (1955) demonstrated bone involvement in 80% of their cases. WOOD and HIMADI (1950) recorded that all seven of their intracranial chordomas showed destruction of the clivus, dorsum sellae, posterior clinoids, sellar floor, or invasion into the sphenoid sinus. SCHECHTER et al. (1974) reported that 87% of their patients showed destruction of bone either from direct pressure by tumor growth or demineralization of the dorsum sellae and posterior clinoids secondary to raised intracranial pressure (Fig. 2). The tumor usually originates in the midline and, the dorsum sellae, clinoids, medial tips of the petrous bones, and clivus are the predominant intracranial structures which are affected (Figs. 2, 3, 4). The degree of destruction of the sella may be variable. UTNE and PUGH (1955) reported some portion of the sella to be involved in 69% of their cases. It was involved in all seven of Wood and Himadi's reported intracranial cases. The dorsum sellae is usually destroyed before the posterior clinoids (Fig. 2). The erosion and undercutting of the anterior clinoids to total destruction of both clinoids may occur, but this is usually a feature of very large tumors (WOOD, 1950; SCHECHTER et al., 1974; Figs. 5, 6, 7). UTNE and PUGH (1955), in their review of intracranial chordomas from the literature, stated 69% of cases to have showed dorsum sellae destruction. The sella is rarely bal-

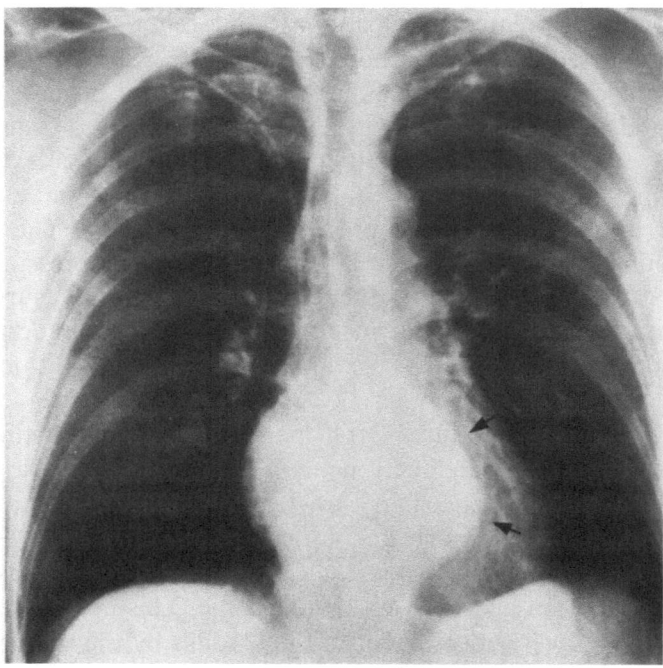

Fig. 1. PA chest film, thoracic chordoma: Well-defined paravertebral mass is seen in lower thoracic region with multiple parenchymal densities within both lung fields which, at postmortem examination, proved to be metastatic chordoma (*arrows*)

looned as with pituitary tumors, though BELZA (1966) and MATHEWS and WILSON (1974) each recorded an intrasellar chordoma which eroded the sellar floor and left the dorsum sellae intact, thereby having the appearance of an intrasellar pituitary adenoma. Since a high percentage of cases have been reported with only destruction of

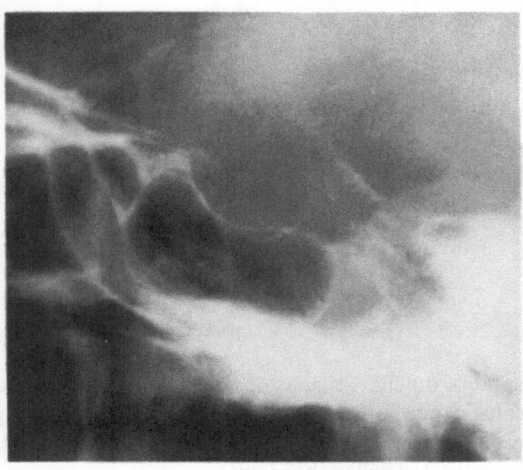 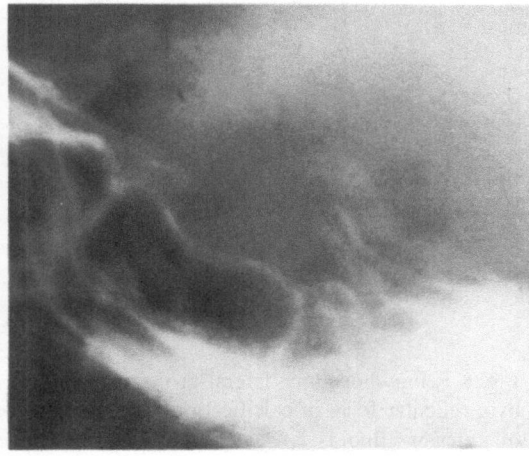

Fig. 2   Fig. 3

Fig. 2. Sellar chordoma, coned down view, lateral projection: There is deossification of the dorsum sellae with incomplete visualization of lamina dura of the pituitary fossa. There is no definite demonstration of suprasellar calcification. Sella is not enlarged. No intrasphenoidal soft-tissue mass density is seen. Anterior clinoids are intact. These findings are not unlike those in chronic increased intracranial pressure

Fig. 3. Sellar chordoma coned down view, lateral projection, sella turcica: This is the same patient as in Figure 2 at 1-year interval from previous radiologic examination. There is further destruction of dorsum sellae with involvement of clivus at the junction of clivus and dorsum sellae. No appearance of retrosellar or suprasellar calcifications has occurred in the year interval. Unlike pituitary adenomas, intracranial chordomas destroy bone in a slow and relentless process instead of eroding and expanding pituitary fossa

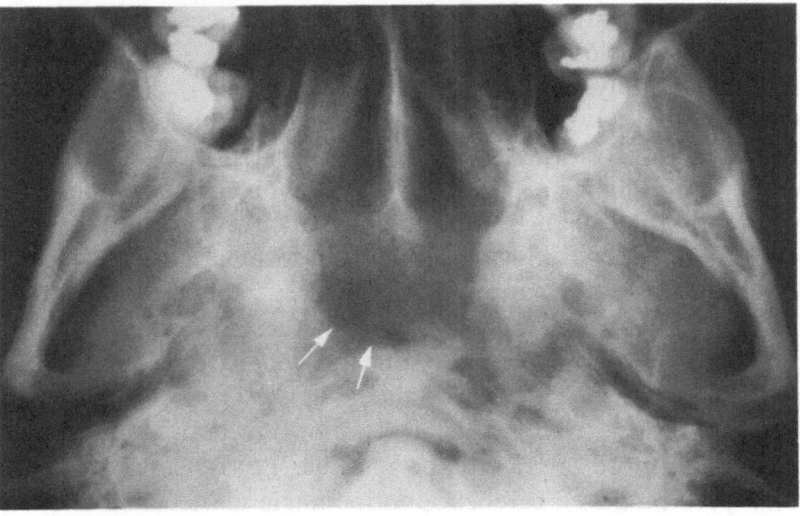

Fig. 4. Clival chordoma, submentovertex view: This projection is helpful since it shows destruction of clivus without aid of tomography. Further information may be gotten from the base view in that a definite soft-tissue density is seen encroaching upon the air shadow of posterior nasopharynx (arrows). Destruction of medial petrous tip on the left is not clearly seen on this reproduction

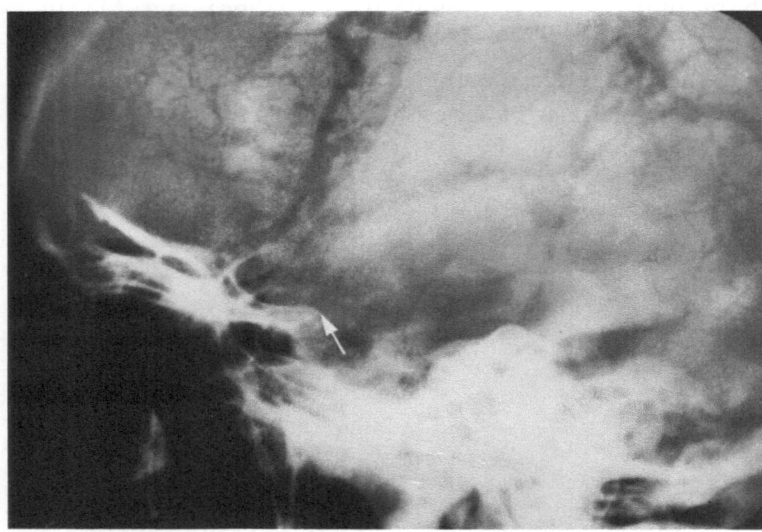

Fig. 5. Sellar chordoma, lateral projection of skull: Destruction of dorsum sellae is observed, which is replaced by a reticular form of calcification and scattered flecks of calcification noted in suprasellar area. Undercutting of anterior clinoids is demonstrated (*arrow*). The mixture of different types of calcifications in the sella, parasellar, and suprasellar area is not unusual in sellar chordomas

the dorsum sellae without involvement of the clivus, it is acceptable to classify these cases as sellar or hypophyseal in origin. This opinion is held by UTNE and PUGH (1955) in which they subdivide their intracranial cases as hypophyseal, spheno-occipital, and nasopharyngeal in location. FALCONER et al. (1968) also group their intracranial chordomas into anatomic locations consisting of sellar, parasellar, and clival. This is helpful in that a different gamut of differentiation from other intracranial neoplasms will be utilized when chordoma originates primarily in the sellar region than when it originates in the spheno-occipital or clival area.

The spheno-occipital synchondrosis is the commonest site of origin of chordomas. UTNE and PUGH (1955) state that destruction of the clivus was seen in 62% of their reported intracranial chordomas. They recommended the submentovertex view as best to demonstrate the osteolysis involving the clivus (Fig. 4). DI CHIRO and ANDERSON (1965) stated that body-section radiography is indispensable for evaluation of the clivus since the dense structures of the mastoids on lateral projection are superimposed on the main body of the clivus. As with primary involvement of the sella, osteolysis is the prominent radiographic change associated with a clival chordoma (Fig. 8). SCHECHTER et al. (1974), in their report of 30 intracranial chordomas, stated that no case showed evidence of reactive bone formation in the area of the neoplasm. UTNE and PUGH (1955) stated that 15% of their cases showed increased density in the location of the tumor. In our experience we have seen one proven case of a clival chordoma with osteosclerosis of the clivus and dorsum sellae (Fig. 9). Osteosclerosis involving the base of the skull is felt to be an extremely rare feature of intracranial chordoma. Infrequently, chordomas may arise more lateral to the midline. POPPEN and KING (1952) described two cases which presented as a cerebellopontine angle mass. IRACI et al. (1973) reported a case with Vernet's syndrome, that is, involvement of the 9th, 10th and 11th cranial nerves with cerebellar dysfunction. In their case, destruction of the anteroinferior aspect of the petrous pyramid was demonstrated in the area of the jugular fossa. Other areas of bone destruction that have been reported associated with chordomas are enlargement

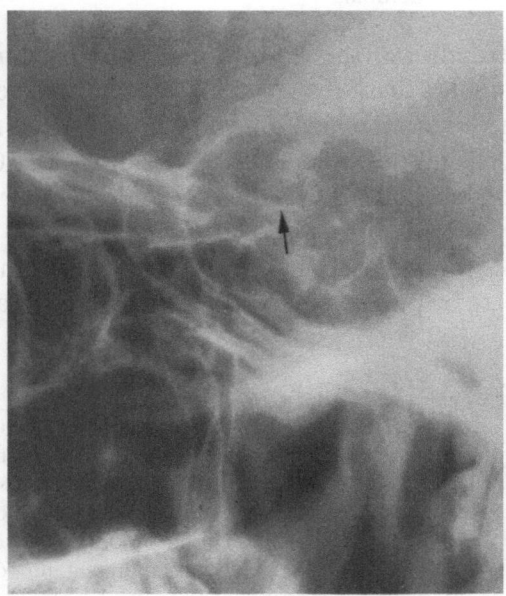
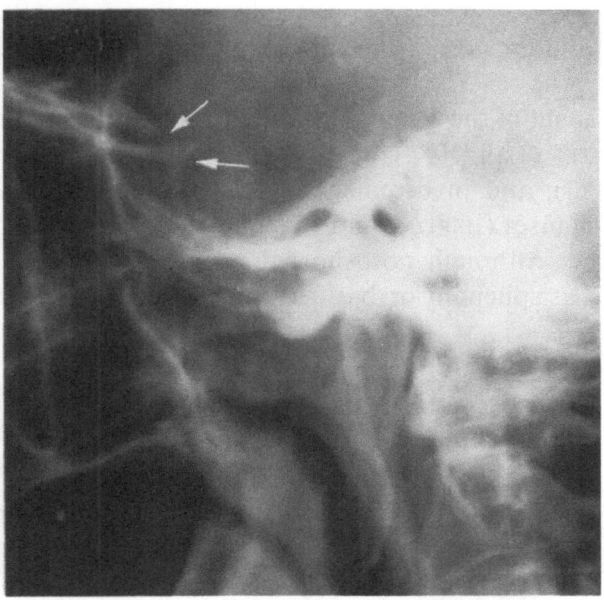

Fig. 6   Fig. 7

Fig. 6. Sellar chordoma, lateral projection of skull: Dense nodular and amorphous types of calcifications are seen in suprasellar and intrasellar areas. Destruction of posterior clinoids are observed and undercutting of anterior clinoids is present (*arrow*). Dense calcification of sellar chordoma is also present within sphenoid sinus. The lamina dura of posteroinferior portion of pituitary fossa is intact. This type of calcification is not unusual for a sellar chordoma nor is involvement of sphenoid sinus or undercutting of clinoids a differentiating point between a pituitary adenoma and a sellar chordoma. The lack of expansion of pituitary fossa as well as presence of calcification should lead one to consider a sellar chordoma instead of a pituitary adenoma. Differentiation from a craniopharyngioma would be extremely difficult in this case

Fig. 7. Sellar chordoma, lateral projection of skull: There is complete erosion of floor of the pituitary fossa and sphenoid sinus. Dorsum sellae has been completely destroyed. Destruction of one anterior clinoid is seen (*upper arrow*) and undercutting of other anterior clinoid is present (*lower arrow*). No calcifications are observed in sella or suprasellar region. Note is made of soft-tissue mass within nasopharynx indicative of extension of intracranial chordoma into superior portion of nasopharynx. This feature of chordomas is not uncommon. A nasopharyngeal mass which has been histologically diagnosed as a chordoma should lead one to evaluate for origin of chordoma either intracranially or from upper cervical spine

Fig. 8. Sellar chordoma, midline complex motion tomogram: There is osteolysis of basisphenoid inferior to dorsum sellae. The floor of pituitary fossa and dorsum sellae are eroded. Destruction of nasopharyngeal surface of basisphenoid is also seen. A soft-tissue density is present within superior aspect of nasopharynx, indicative of extension of chordoma into this region (*arrows*). No calcifications within region of osteolysis is observed in this case. Tomography is invaluable in clearly demonstrating osteolysis and destruction of bony structure of the base of the skull and may aid in localizing an area for surgical biopsy

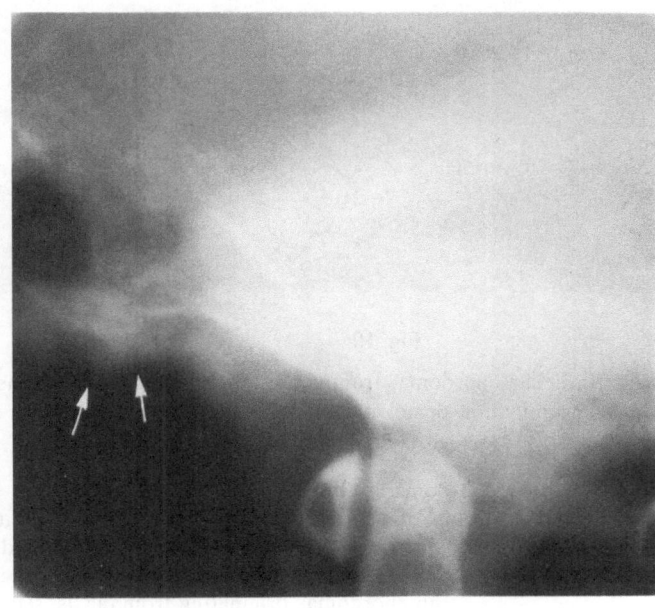

and erosion of the superior orbital fissures, destruction of the medial tips of the petrous bones (SCHECHTER et al., 1974), erosion of the jugular fossa (IRACI et al., 1973), involvement of the sphenoid sinus and enlargement of the foramen ovali (WRIGHT, 1967; SCHECHTER et al., 1974), destruction of the ethmoid air cells (WOOD and HIMADI, 1950) (Figs. 10, 11), and involvement of the frontal sinus (ADAMS, 1948) and ethmoid and maxillary sinuses (BERDAL and MYHRE, 1964; PASTORE et al., 1949).

Although notochordal rests may be isolated to the nasopharyngeal surface of the basisphenoid or basiocciput, and may give rise to a purely nasopharyngeal chordoma,

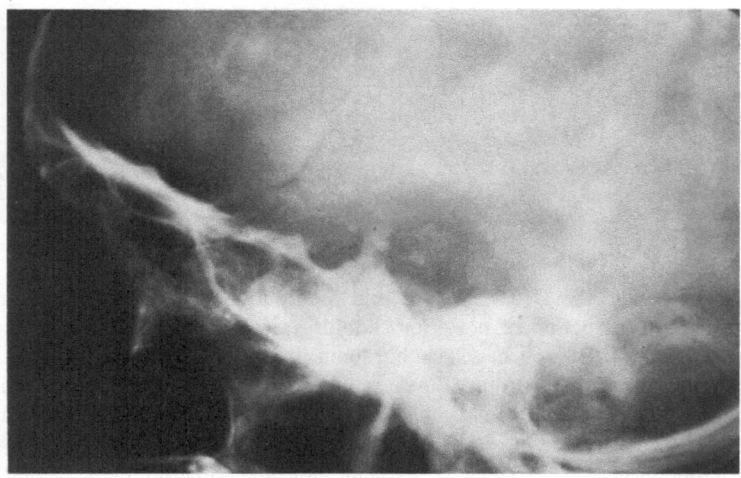

Fig. 9. Clival chordoma, lateral projection of skull: There is increased bony production of basisphenoid and basiocciput which forms clivus and dorsum sellae. This is an unusual presentation of clival chordoma and osteosclerosis of clivus would lead one to consider a clival meningioma rather than a clival chordoma. Numerous scattered flecks of calcification in retrosellar region are not atypical of a clival chordoma. There is destruction of posterior clinoids and a dense intrasphenoidal mass is present

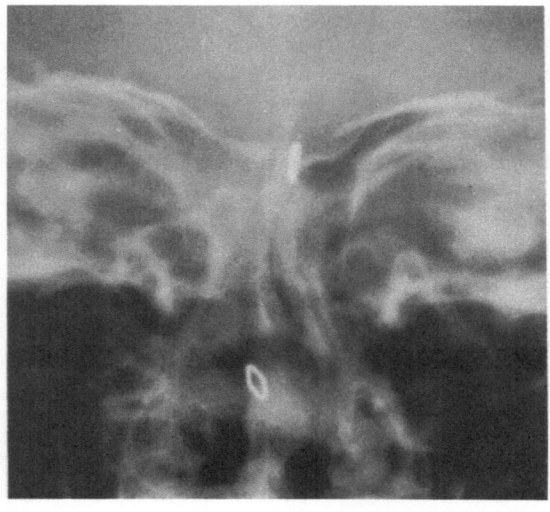

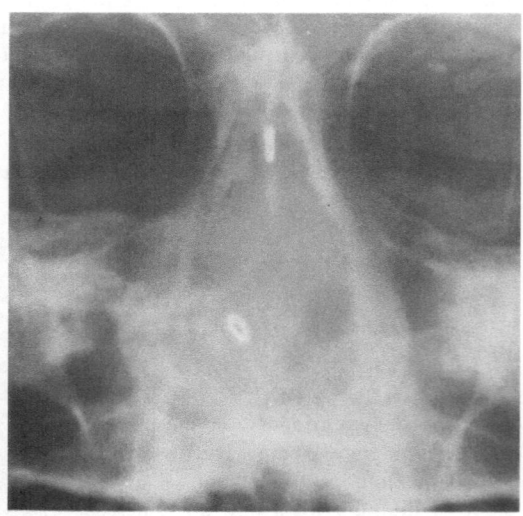

Fig. 10   Fig. 11

Fig. 10. Sellar chordoma, frontal projection of paranasal sinuses: A sellar chordoma proven 3 years prior to this examination demonstrates clouding of ethmoid air cells due to extension of chordoma from posterior nasopharynx

Fig. 11. Sellar chordoma, Caldwell projection: Same patient as in Figure 10, 1 year later, shows further growth and extension of chordoma, now involving nasal cavity with destruction of perpendicular plate of ethmoid and all turbinates. Extension anteriorly into ethmoid air cells and nasal cavity is uncommon in chordomas but may, at times, be observed. Extension to these areas occurs from posterior nasopharynx in chordomas originating from clivus, sella, or upper cervical spine

most nasopharyngeal chordomas are extensions from intracranial neoplasms (WOOD and HIMADI, 1950; UTNE and PUGH, 1955). KAMRIN et al. (1964) and SCHECHTER et al. (1974) reported that a soft-tissue mass was observed in a third of their intracranial chordomas. Extension of this nasopharyngeal mass into the nasal cavity may occur. Nasopharyngeal chordoma extending from the nasal cavity into the maxillary antrum has been described (PASTORE et al., 1949). No calcification within the nasopharyngeal soft-tissue mass has been described.

2. Calcifications

Roentgenographic demonstration of calcifications on plain skull films have been reported to be associated with intracranial chordomas. KAMRIN et al. (1964) described suprasellar calcifications in 30% of their intracranial chordomas. WOOD and HIMADI (1950) were the first authors to emphasize that intracranial chordomas are associated with calcification. Of the chordomas reported by SCHECHTER et al., 50% showed calcification on plain film examination. Analyzing the calcification of suprasellar tumors, LINDGREN and DI CHIRO (1951) divided the calcifications into five types: (1) reticular (Fig. 5), (2) a solid nodular mass, (3) scattered flecks of calcifications measuring 1–2 mm, (4) a cystic type of calcification, and (5) a mixed type, that is, a combination of the nodular and cystic calcification (Fig. 6). Of their four chordomas, the appearance of the calcifications were mixed in three, and nodular in one. SCHECHTER et al. (1974) showed that intracranial chordomas may also demonstrate a reticular form of calcification as well as demonstrating a purely cystic type of calcification. SCHECHTER et al. (1974) stated that three of their cases had a reticular form of calcification with seven showing a nodular mass and four demonstrating scattered flecks of calcification. One of their cases showed a purely cystic type of calcification. The location of the calcification demonstrate the predominately midline location of intracranial chordomas. SCHECHTER et al. (1974) reported one-third of their cases having calcifications localized to the midline behind the clivus and dorsum sellae. In less than 10% of their cases was the calcification in the parasellar region. In 20% of their cases scattered flecks of calcification were localized in the retrosellar area or in the intrasellar area. MATHEWS and WILSON (1974) demonstrated nodular calcifications purely within the hypophyseal fossa. DI CHIRO and ANDERSON (1965) demonstrated dense retrosellar calcification in seven of nine cases of clival chordomas and state that when this is associated with bony destruction of the clivus, dorsum sellae, and petrous bones, it is almost pathognomonic of a clival chordoma. Therefore, calcification, that is, midline or paramedian to the sella, or in the retrosellar area, coupled with bony destruction of either the clivus or the dorsum sellae, would be highly suggestive of intracranial chordoma.

Pathologically, the calcifications within intracranial chordomas originate primarily via two mechanisms: (1) calcification has been shown to be secondary to areas of tissue necrosis and cystic degeneration within the tumor (WOOD, 1950) and (2) the calcification may represent sequestered bone which has been advanced within the expanding tumor (SCHECHTER et al., 1974).

3. Angiography

a) Carotid Angiography

Current investigation of intracranial masses begins with carotid angiography. The angiographic changes in chordomas depend on the location of the main tumor mass,

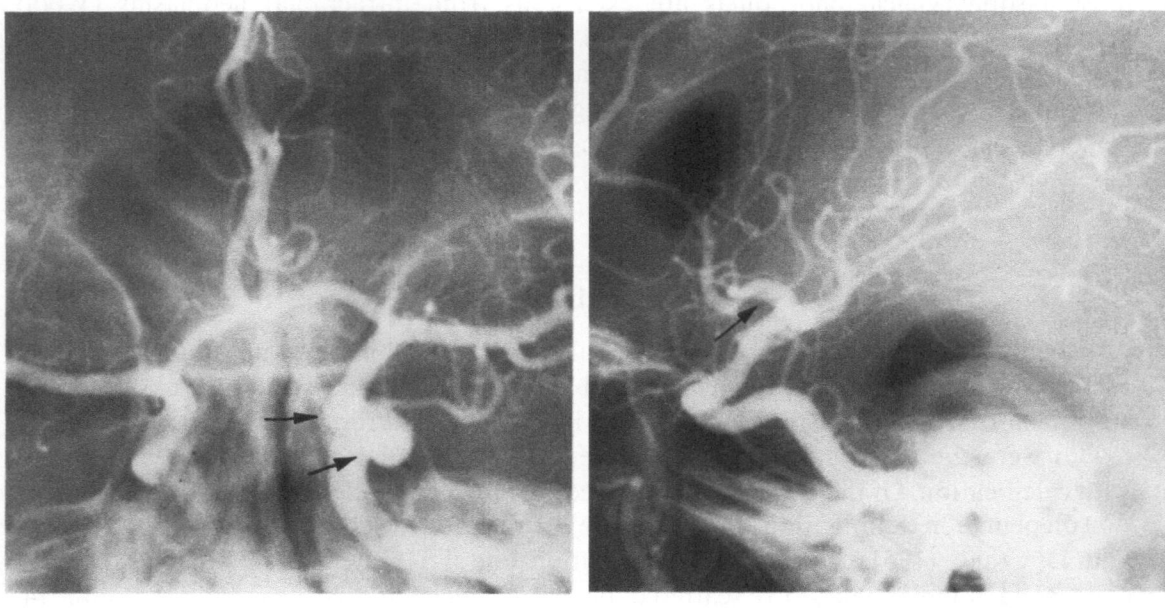

Fig. 12   Fig. 13

Fig. 12. Sellar chordoma: Selective left internal carotid angiogram in Caldwell projection demonstrates intrasellar lesion which has extended to anterior suprasellar area. There is lateral displacement of cavernous sinus on left which is demonstrated by displacement of posterior portion of intracavernous carotid artery laterally (*lower arrow*) when compared to anterior portion of intracavernous portion of internal carotid artery (*upper arrow*). Horizontal portions of the left and the right anterior cerebral arteries are bowed upward. Lateral deviation of supraclinoid segment of the left internal carotid artery is seen

Fig. 13. Sellar chordoma: Lateral projection of a left common carotid angiogram (same patient as in Fig. 12) reveals closing of siphon as has been described in anterior suprasellar masses with superior deviation of anterior cerebral arteries (*arrows*). No abnormal vasculature or tumor blush is observed

its size, and, of course, its direction of growth. CHASE and TAVERAS (1961) have described the vascular displacements of the intracranial vasculature in suprasellar tumors. Carotid angiography may show no vascular abnormalities in small tumors (HILAL, 1971). With larger tumors we will see lateral displacement of the intracavernous portion of the internal carotid artery when the tumor is mainly intrasellar in location and impinging on the medial aspect of the cavernous sinus (Fig. 12). The supraclinoid segment of the internal carotid artery will be closed with an anteriorly located mass (Fig. 13), or open when the mass is directly above the sella or in the retrosellar area. Elevation and upward bowing of the horizontal segment of the anterior cerebral artery will be seen with anteriorly situated masses, as well as masses which are directly suprasellar (Figs. 12, 13). With larger masses which have an infratemporal parasellar extension, elevation of the horizontal segment of the middle cerebral artery will be seen (Figs. 14, 15). If obstruction of the ventricular system is seen either at the foramen of Monroe or at the aqueduct, lateral displacement of the ascending frontal branches will be observed, which is secondary to ventricular dilatation. Supralateral displacement of the posterior communicating arteries will be observed with more posterior masses (Figs. 16, 17). The anterior choroidal artery may be superiorly or laterally displaced or flattened with the more posteriorly situated chordomas which encroach upon the lateral borders of the suprachiasmatic cistern. Massive tumors in the suprasellar area which may be associated with obstruction at the foramen of Monroe will show elevation of the septal vein and

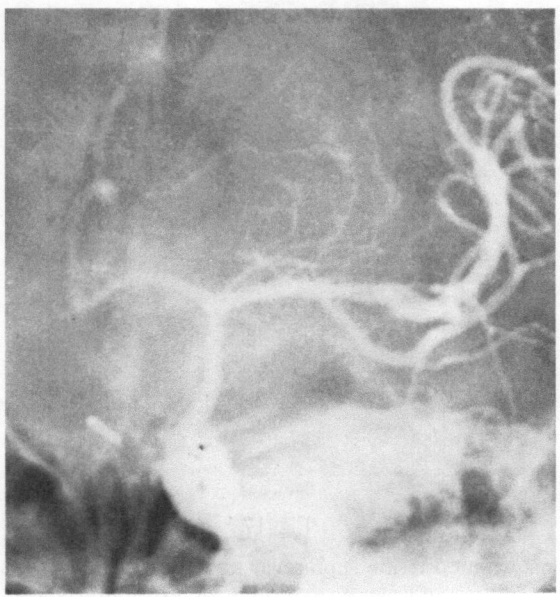 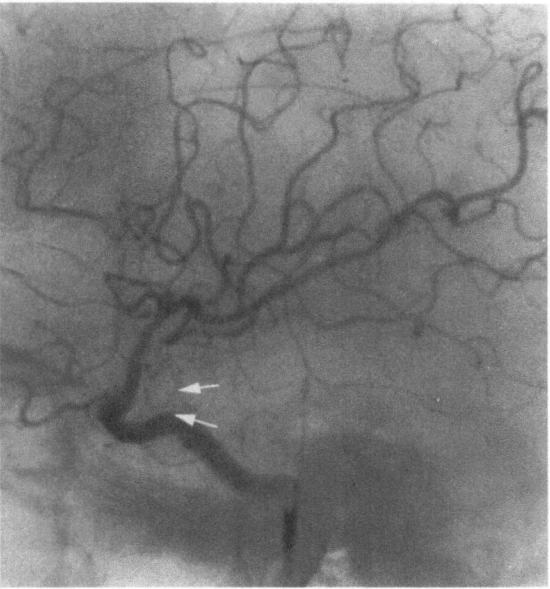

Fig. 14   Fig. 15

Fig. 14. Sellar chordoma: frontal projection of internal carotid angiogram in same patient as in Figures 12 and 13 1 year after a subtotal removal of a sellar chordoma reveals a marked increase in size of suprasellar component which has involved not only the anterior suprasellar region but also the straight suprasellar area and has extended parasellarly elevating horizontal portion of left middle cerebral artery. Supraclinoid segment of internal carotid artery is straightened and narrowed by circumferential growth of tumor. Early recurrence of sellar chordomas is not an unusual feature nor is parasellar growth with perivascular infiltration of vital arteries

Fig. 15. Sellar chordoma: Lateral projection of selective internal carotid artery corresponding to Figure 14 shows supraclinoid artery to be displaced upward with marked narrowing indicative of circumferential growth of tumor with encasement of this artery. Hypertrophy of inferior cavernous artery originating from intracavernous portion of internal carotid artery is seen. It supplies bulk of intrasellar and suprasellar portion of the tumor (*arrows*). A definite tumor blush on delayed serial filming was not appreciated

the anterior portion of the internal carotid artery may be displaced laterally, medially, or superiorly (CHASE and TAVERAS, 1963). FALCONER et al. (1968) reported one case of a sellar and suprasellar chordoma which demonstrated an uniform tumor blush above the sella during the venous phase of the angiogram. No other instance of a tumor stain in an intracranial chordoma has been recorded.

b) Vertebral Angiography

Vertebral angiography is indispensible for the evaluation of a spheno-occipital or clival chordoma. When the tumor is originating from the clivus and extends posteriorly in the midline, the lateral projection will show displacement of the basilar artery in an arcuate configuration away from the base of the skull (Fig. 18). With tumors which are growing asymmetrically and extending to one side of the midline there may be displacement of the basilar artery to the contralateral side. With further lateral asymmetrical growth of chordomas, particularly with extension into the cerebellopontine (CP) angle, angiographic signs of a CP angle mass may be observed, which include superior displacement of the ipsilateral posterior cerebral and superior cerebellar arteries and posterior displacement of the ipsilateral anterior inferior and posterior inferior cerebellar

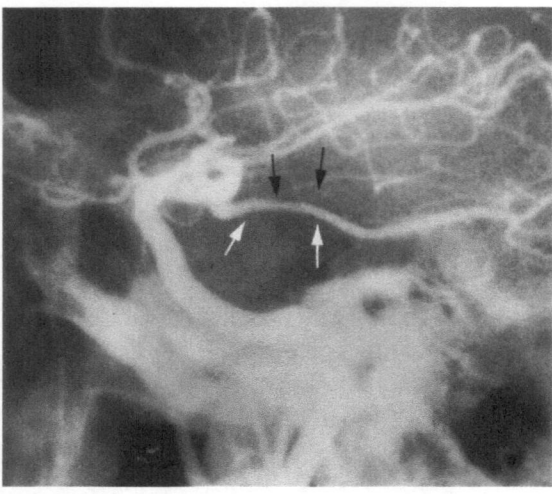 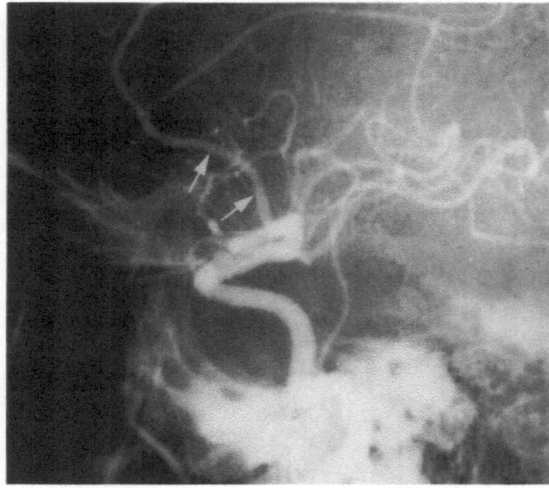

Fig. 16   Fig. 17

Fig. 16. Common carotid angiogram of sellar chordoma with posterior suprasellar extension demonstrates anteroinferior displacement of cavernous portion of internal carotid artery indicative of extradural spread of tumor. Posterior suprasellar extension of tumor is observed by superior elevation of posterior cerebral artery (*lower arrows*) and superior elevation of anterior chorodial artery (*upper arrow*)

Fig. 17. Sellar chordoma with extradural parasellar and anterior suprasellar extension: Lateral projection of common carotid angiogram reveals intracavernous portion of internal carotid artery elevated superiorly due to extradural extension of chordoma. Carotid siphon is closed due to anterior suprasellar extension by chordoma which is also bowing anterior cerebral artery superiorly (*arrows*)

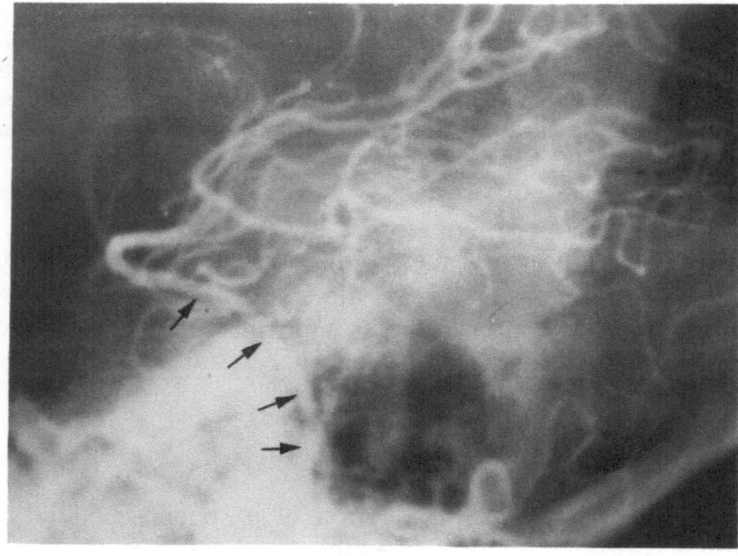

Fig. 18. Selective left vertebral angiogram, arterial phase, demonstrates bowing of basilar artery away from clivus indicative of extra-axial mass within prepontine cistern (*arrows*). This configuration is typical for clival chordoma

arteries. The venous phase of the vertebral angiogram will demonstrate posterior displacement of the anterior pontomesencephalic vein and the precentral cerebellar vein with a midline mass (Fig. 19), and with extension of the tumor into the CP angle, the petrosal vein may be pushed laterally (Schechter et al., 1974). No pathophysiologic abnormalities have been described in clival chordomas, that is, abnormal tumor vascularity, tumor stain, early venous opacification, or vascular encasement.

Fig. 19. Lateral projection of the
left vertebral angiogram, venous
phase, in same patient as Figure 18 reveals posterior displacement of anterior pontome-
sencephalic vein in convec configuration away from clivus (arrows). Superior foramen ceacum,
formed by interpeduncular vein
joining with anterior pontomesencephalic vein, is displaced posteriorly indicative of extension of tumor into interpeduncular fossa
(crossed arrow). Precentral cerebellar vein is displaced posteriorly
(double crossed arrows). Arterial
and venous portions of the left
vertebral angiogram definitely
places lesion in prepontine cistern
and interpeduncular fossa and ex-
cludes intra-axial pontine mass

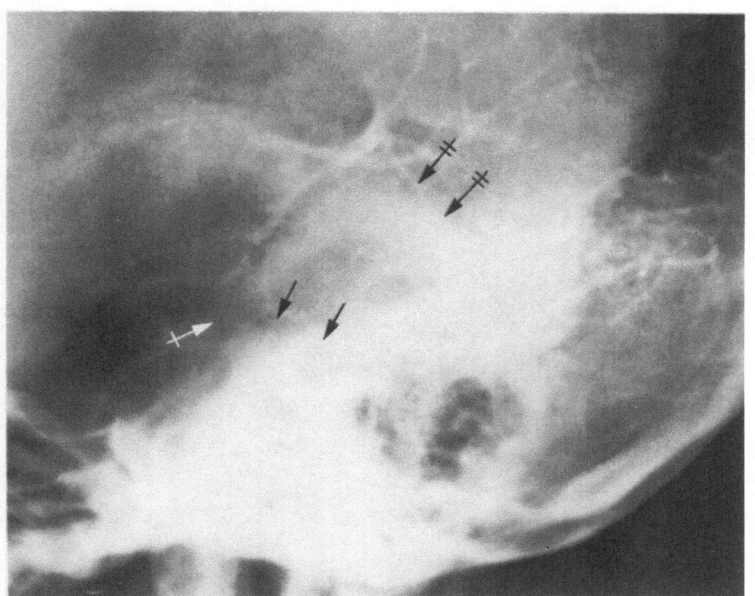

Fig. 20. Lateral projection of PEG
in clival chordoma demonstrates
posterior displacement of fourth ventricle with superoposterior displacement of aqueduct of Sylvius. Note
enlargement of prepontine cistern
which differentiates extra-axial prepontine lesion from intra-axial pontine mass

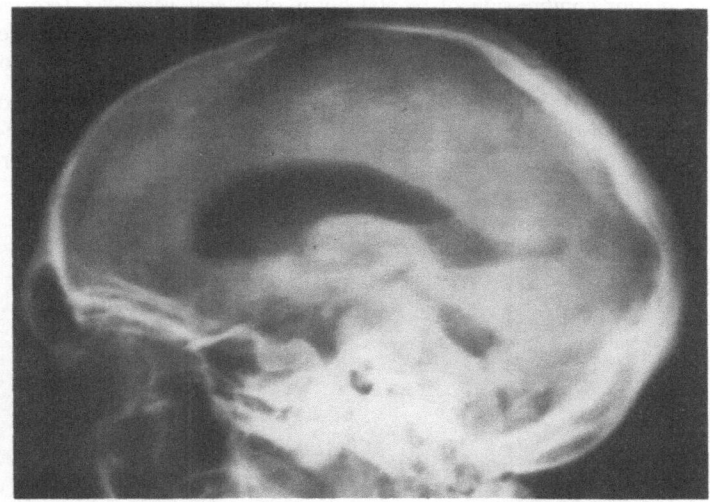

4. Pneumoencephalography

WOOD and HIMADI (1950) and SCHECHTER et al. (1974) have given excellent descriptions of the ventricular displacements by intracranial chordomas as demonstrated on
air studies. WOOD and HIMADI have described obstruction of the aqueduct in two patients
at the posterior end of the third ventricle in the retrosellar area. In four of their patients
a filling defect in the prepontine cistern was demonstrated. Demonstration of the prepontine cistern is most important in spheno-occipital or clival chordomas since this will
distinguish an extra-axial prepontine lesion from an intra-axial pontine mass (Fig. 20).
The fourth ventricle is displaced posteriorly as well as superiorly in clival chordomas.
The aqueduct will also be displaced posteriorly with prepontine masses. WOOD and
HIMADI (1950) (seven patients) demonstrated the dome of the mass to be retrosellar
in four cases. In SCHECHTER et al.'s series of 30 intracranial chordomas (1974), the
radiographic findings in clival chordomas are that of a prepontine mass with displacement

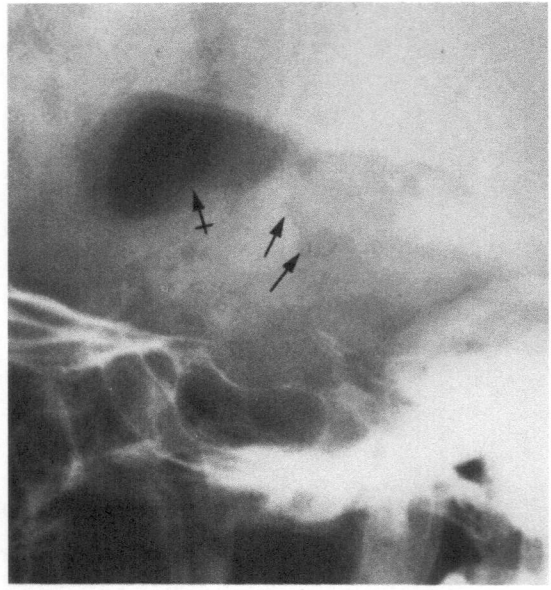 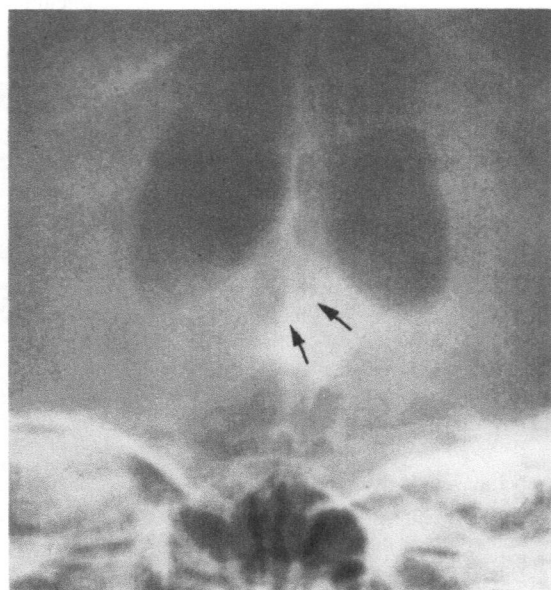

Fig. 21   Fig. 22

Fig. 21. Lateral projection from PEG in sellar chordoma (same patient as Fig. 2) demonstrates anterior suprasellar extension of mass which has obliterated anterior recesses of third ventricle (*arrows*) and has produced inferior compression of frontal horns of lateral ventricles (*crossed arrow*). For lesions in suprasellar region only, a small amount of ventricular air is used so as not to obscure anterior recesses of third ventricle by superimposed subarachnoid air

Fig. 22. AP projection in brow-up position of PEG corresponding to Figure 21 reveals compression and elevation of anterior third ventricle (*arrows*) which shows oblique cutoff of air within anterior third ventricle indicative of eccentric midline suprasellar mass

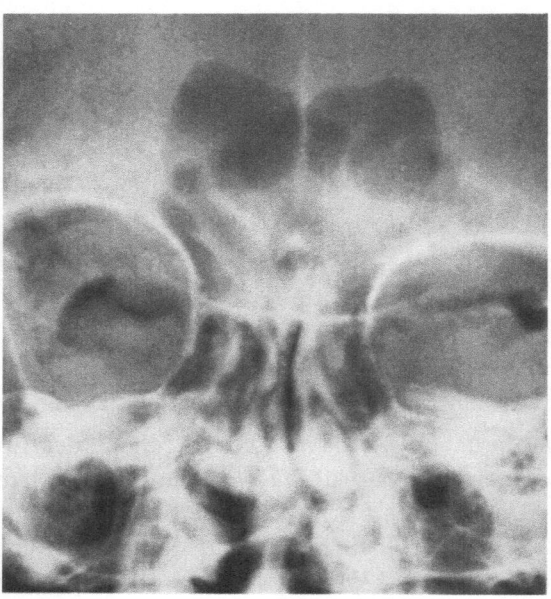 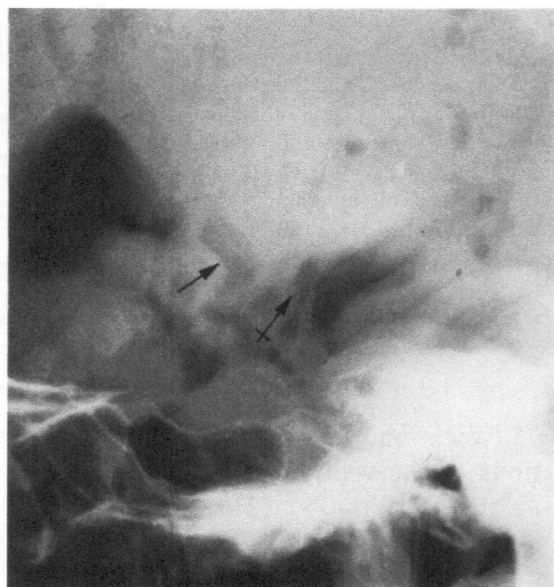

Fig. 23   Fig. 24

Fig. 23. Caldwell projection from PEG reveals parasellar extension of sellar chordoma which has produced superior and lateral displacement of the left temporal horn (compare the left air-filled temporal horn with that of normal right temporal horn)

Fig. 24. Lateral projection from PEG in brow-up position (same patient as in Fig. 23) reveals compression of anterior third ventricle by suprasellar extension of sellar chordoma (*arrow*) with superior displacement of the left temporal horn by parasellar extension of tumor (*crossed arrow*)

of the pontine cistern and fourth ventricle posteriorly, as well as posterior displacement of the aqueduct of Sylvius.

With primarily sellar and parasellar tumors, superior displacement of the third ventricle at pneumoencephalography is the predominent feature. Elevation and splaying of the anterior recess of the third ventricle, not unlike a pituitary tumor, is commonly seen (Figs. 21, 22). With larger tumors, as well as tumors which extend anteriorly, a filling defect in the floor of the anterior end of the lateral ventricles may be observed (Fig. 21). Marked hydrocephalus is not a feature of chordomas, therefore, obstruction of the foramen of Monroe usually will not be demonstrated. With parasellar extension of the tumor, lateral, superior, and posterior displacement of the temporal horn on the ipsilateral side will be observed (Figs. 23, 24). With filling of the suprachiasmatic cistern, marked obliteration may be observed and the subarachnoid air may cap the dome of the tumor.

5. Brain Scan (Technetium 99m pertechnetate)

Few reports are in the literature concerning the brain scan in cases of intracranial chordomas. SCHECHTER et al. (1974) reported one case with a well-defined area of isotopic uptake in the parasellar region. We have observed one case where brain scan demonstrated an area of increased isotopic uptake in the suprasellar region in a patient with a sellar and suprasellar chordoma (Figs. 25, 26).

6. Computerized Tomographic (CT) Scan

No instance of chordoma demonstrated on CT scan has yet been reported in the literature. We have observed one case of a proven intracranial chordoma in the retrosellar

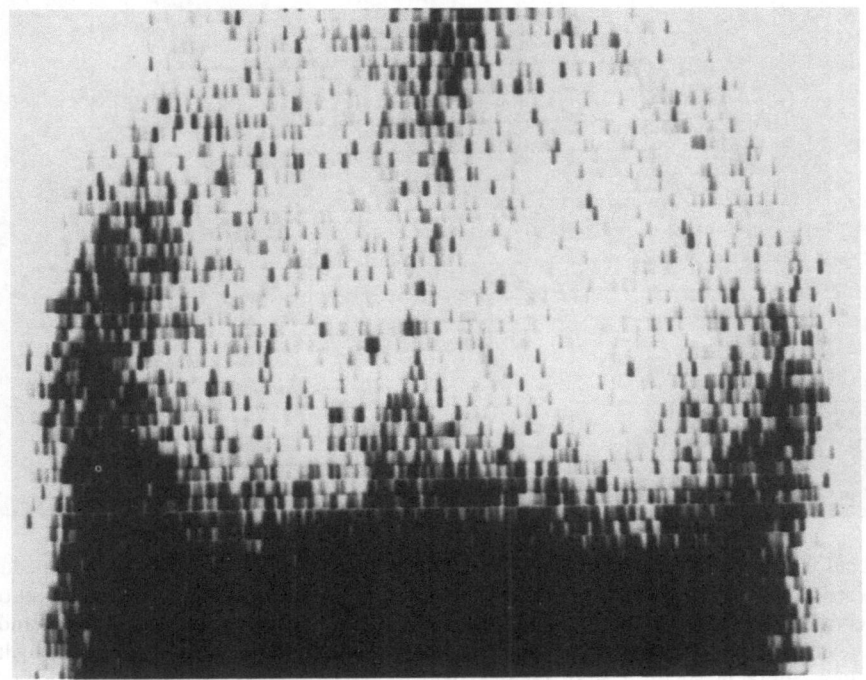

Fig. 25. Brain scan: Anterior projection after administration of 99m technetium pertechnetate demonstrates increased uptake in midline and to the left of midline

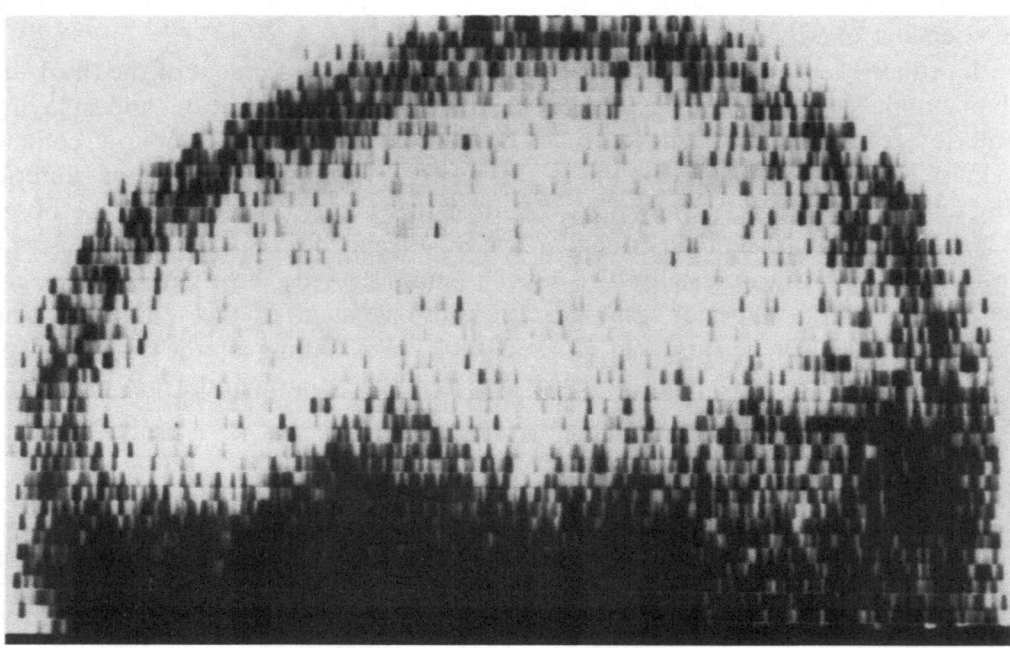

Fig. 26. Brain scan: Left lateral projection of same patient as in Fig. 25 reveals increased uptake in region of sella turcica by a proven sellar chordoma

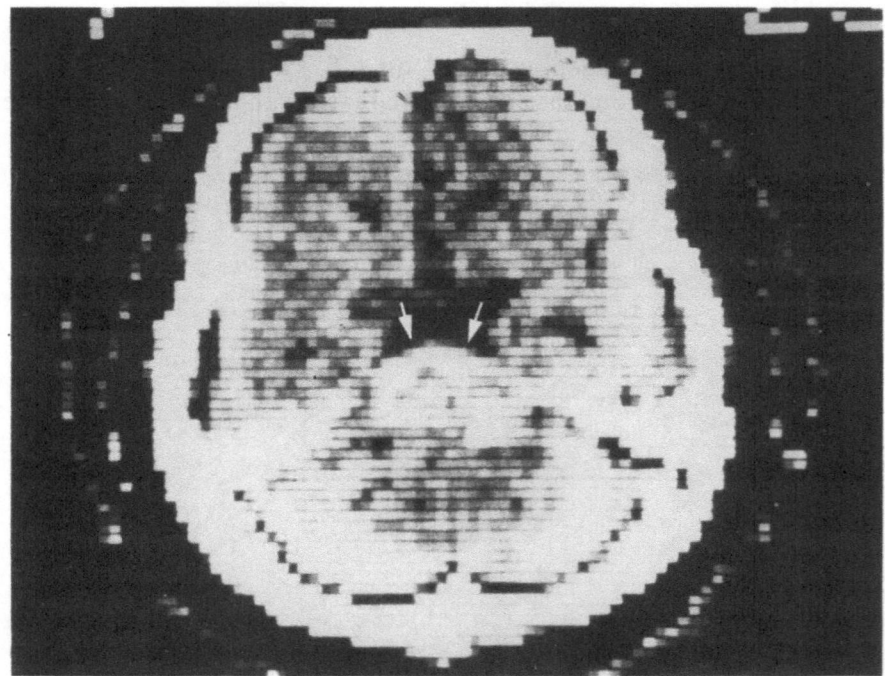

Fig. 27. Basal cut utilizing computerized axial tomography demonstrates obliteration of interpeduncular fossa and circum-mesencephalic cisterns by a large retrosellar lesion. Impingement upon posterior aspect of suprasellar cistern is observed (*arrow*). Areas of increased densities in region of interpeduncular fossa and prepontine cistern indicate calcification within tumor. Retrosellar location with obliteration of interpeduncular fossa and impingement upon suprachiasmatic cistern coupled with presence of scattered areas of calcification should include chordoma in differential diagnosis. Absorption coefficient of mass which is similar to normal brain tissue should exclude clival cholesteatoma, which typically has lower absorption coefficients. A craniopharyngioma or a clival meningioma would be difficult to exclude

area which, on the basal cuts of the CT scan, demonstrated destruction of the dorsum sellae with obliteration of the interpeduncular fossa and the circummesencephalic cistern (Fig. 27). The tumor mass had a measure (absorption coefficient) similar to that of brain tissue, though, interspaced within the tumor mass small flecks of calcification were observed. A contrast enhancement scan was not done on this patient. Again location of the mass in the retrosellar or prepontine cistern with evidence of calcification and destruction of the dorsum sellae supports the provisional diagnosis of an intracranial chordoma on CT scanning.

II. Nasopharyngeal Chordomas

Most reported cases in the literature of chordomas which involve the nasopharynx have their origin either intracranially (BATSAKIS, 1963) or arise from the upper cervical vertebrae (WRIGHT, 1967). Though ectopic remnants have been observed in the soft tissues of the nasopharynx, it is impossible to exclude a tumor originating from ectopic remnants within the skull base (sellar or clival) when osseous destruction is associated with the nasopharyngeal mass. Two of four nasopharyngeal chordomas reported by WRIGHT (1967) did not show any destruction or bony involvement of the base of the skull or the upper cervical vertebrae. WOOD and HIMADI (1950) reported one nasopharyngeal chordoma without evidence of osseous destruction. The presence of a nasopharyngeal mass histologically diagnosed as chordoma should lead to a search for either an intracranial chordoma, which has grown into the nasopharynx, or a tumor of the upper cervical vertebrae. If radiologic, as well as clinical and surgical evaluation fail to demonstrate any evidence of osseous involvement, then, it may be concluded that the nasopharyngeal chordoma has originated from ectopic remnants within the nasopharyngeal soft tissues. It must be emphasized, however, that true nasopharyngeal chordomas for the most part, eventually invade and destroy the base of the skull during their course.

III. Vertebral Chordomas

Vertebral chordomas comprise 13% of reported chordomas in the literature (Fig. II). UTNE and PUGH (1955) reported 88% of vertebral chordomas to have bone involvement and 75% of their patients had osteolysis, which began in the vertebral bodies. Half of their cases showed extension of the tumor to involve three or more adjacent vertebral bodies. Vertebral chordomas have a predilection for the cervical region with the lesion reported more often involving the upper cervical region (MURRAY and JACOBSON, 1971) (Figs. 28, 29). A compilation of several series of vertebral chordoma reported in the literature (Table 2) reveals the cervical spine to be involved in 44% of the cases, followed by lumbar spine (41%), and thoracic spine (14.5%).

1. Plain Film Findings

The most commonly reported plain film findings in vertebral chordomas are destruction and infiltration of bone. UTNE and PUGH (1955) showed destruction of vertebral bodies in 75% of their patients and in half of these patients there was involvement of three or more adjacent vertebral bodies. Furthermore, when invasion of the posterior elements, as well as the vertebral body was considered, 88% of the patients had evidence of involvement. WOOD and HIMADI (1950) described bone destruction to occur in each

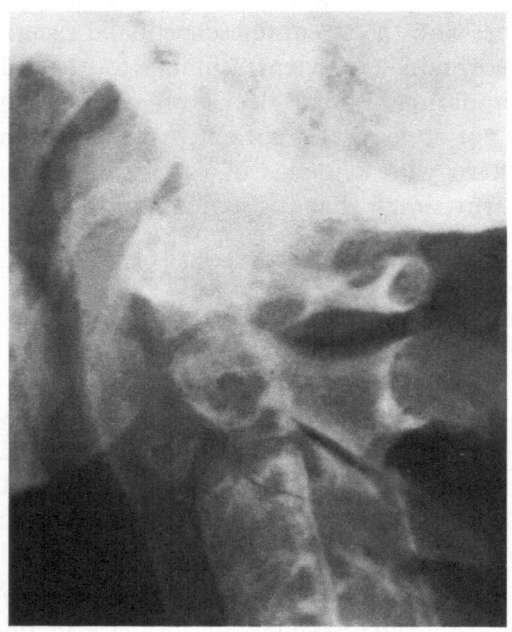 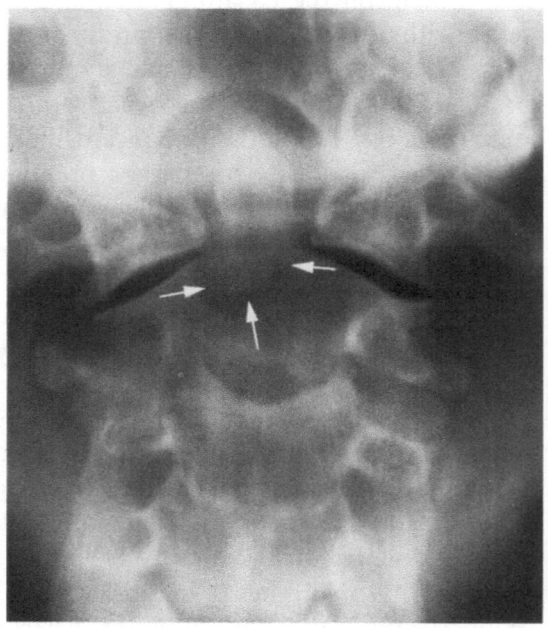

Fig. 28   Fig. 29

Fig. 28. Cervical chordoma, C2: Lateral projection of upper cervical spine reveals destructive lesion involving body of C2 with localized soft-tissue mass impinging upon air laryngogram. Intervertebral space between C2 and C3 is narrowed. Incidentally, congenital fusion of bodies and lateral masses of C3 and C4 is noted

Fig. 29. Same patient as in Figure 28: Frontal tomogram further demonstrates destruction of body of C2 with pathologic fracture of odontoid process (*arrows*). There is destruction of right lateral mass and pedicle of C3. Inferior vertebral plate of C2 is totally destroyed and involvement of right superior articulation facet and superior vertebral plate of C3 is seen with irregularity as main radiographic sign. Chordoma typically involves multiple vertebral bodies, including intervening intervertebral disc space. No definite osteosclerosis is observed. Localized soft-tissue density in precervical region is frequently observed with chordomas

Table 2. Distribution of vertebral chordomas

	Cervical	Thoracic	Lumbar
STEWART and MORIN (1926)	1	–	–
MABREY (1935)	7	2	5
ADSON et al. (1935)	1	–	–
WOOD (1950)	1	1	3
POPPEN and KING (1952)	3	–	1
SENNETT (1955)	–	–	1
ALLEN (1955)	–	–	1
UTNE and PUGH (1955)	37	12	32
ROSENQUIST and SALTZMAN (1959)	–	1	2
WINDEYER (1959)	5	1	2
HARTOFILAIKIDIS-GAROFALIDIS et al. (1968)	–	–	2
RAO BALAPARAMESWARA and DINAKAR (1970)	–	2	3
Total	58	19	54
Incidence	44%	14.5%	41%

of their five cases of vertebral chordomas and all had involvement of two or more adjacent vertebral bodies. KAMRIN et al. (1964), reporting on nine vertebral chordomas, showed bone destruction to occur in a majority of their patients with little evidence of collapse of the involved vertebral body, reporting vertebral compression in two patients, one with involvement of the second cervical vertebrae and a second patient with compression of a lumbar vertebral body. POPPEN and KING (1955) again emphasized the multiple vertebral body destruction, which is highly characteristic of the reported cases of vertebral chordomas in the literature. They also reported an osteoblastic reaction occurring along with the bone destruction that was observed in one cervical and in one lumbar case of chordoma. WOOD and HIMADI (1950) had demonstrated associated osteoblastic reaction in two of their five cases. UTNE and PUGH (1955) reported an osteoblastic reaction occurring in 50% of their cases but they stated this was associated with compression of bone rather than osteosclerosis due to new bone formation. An "ivory" vertebra secondary to infiltration by chordoma has been reported (RAO BALAPARAMESWARA and DINAKAR, 1970). The most significant radiographic feature in our series of nine vertebral chordomas is the demonstration of multiple contiguous vertebral body destruction. In our series only one case had evidence of osseous involvement of a single vertebral body (Figs. 30, 31). Osteosclerosis, secondary to the slow progressive growth of chordoma in the bone, was present in half of our vertebral chordomas. At no time was the presence of increased bone density associated with a significant compression fracture or collapse of a vertebral body. We feel osteosclerosis is a valid radiographic finding, even though a difference of opinion exists within the literature. Osteosclerosis, coupled with osseous destruction, forms an important differentiating feature of vertebral chordomas.

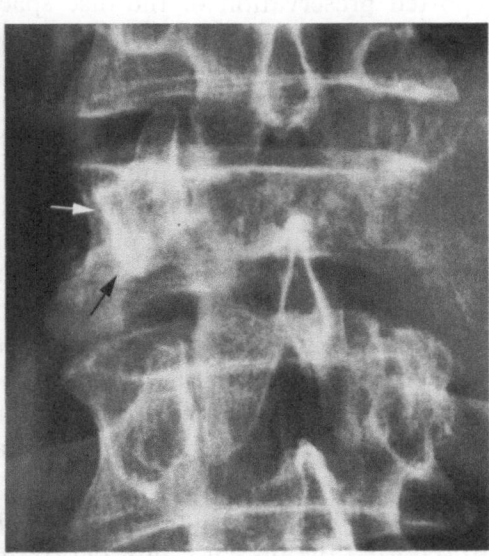
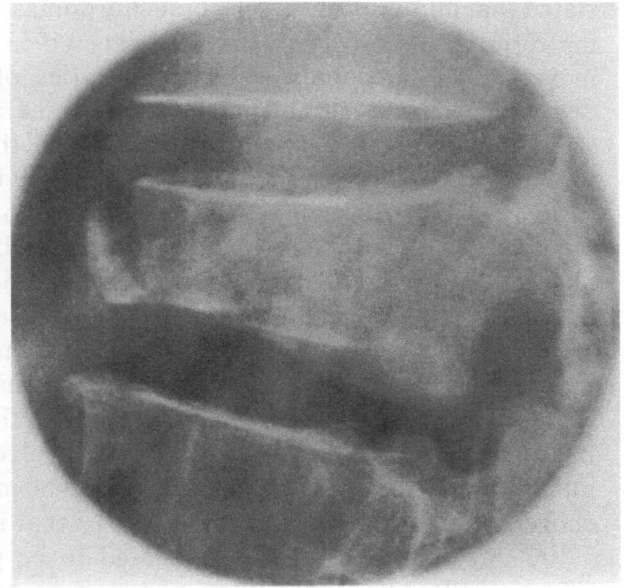

Fig. 30   Fig. 31

Fig. 30. Lumbar chordoma: AP projection of L2 demonstrates destruction of the left lateral aspect of body and pedicle of L2 with a well-defined paravertebral mass containing scattered flecks of calcification. Osteosclerosis of the right pedicle of L2 is observed (*arrows*). The combination of osteolysis with osteosclerosis and a soft-tissue mass containing scattered flecks of calcification virtually eliminates other malignancies such as metastases or myeloma, and with preservation of intervertebral disc spaces tuberculosis can be excluded

Fig. 31. Lumbar chordoma: Lateral projection of same patient as in Figure 30 reveals compression of second lumbar vertebra with adjacent intact vertebral disc spaces

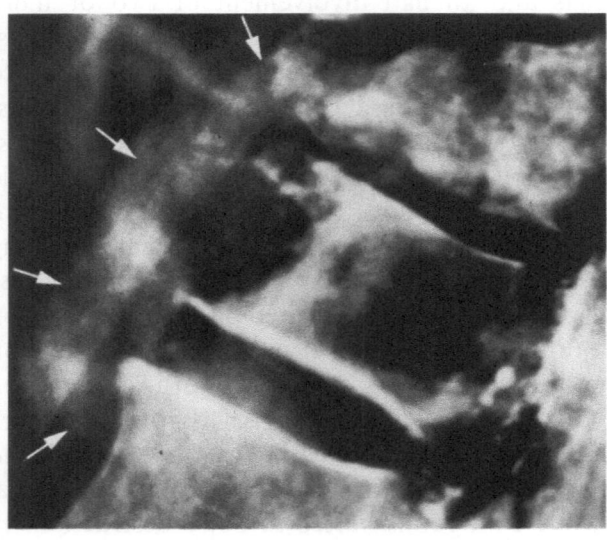

Fig. 32. Thoracic chordoma: Lateral projection of lower thoracic spine in a patient with chordoma reveals lytic and destructive lesions of T9 and T10 with involvement of intervertebral disc spaces between T8 and T9 and T10. Paravertebral soft-tissue mass is observed containing numerous flecks of calcification (*arrows*). Involvement of intervertebral disc spaces is a prominent feature of vertebral chordomas

KAMRIN et al. (1964) stated that the disc interspaces are preserved in vertebral chordomas. Currently, most investigators believe that vertebral chordomas originate from the notochordal rests within the vertebral bodies. Whether or not primary chordomas may originate from notochordal remnants, which make up the nucleus pulposus, is an interesting hypothesis, but has not gained acceptance within the literature as the prime mechanism of development of vertebral chordomas. WOOD and HIMADI (1950) stated that all five of their vertebral chordomas demonstrated involvement of the intervening discs. MABREY (1935) and SENNETT (1953) reported preservation of the disc space in vertebral chordomas. We, in our series of nine vertebral chordomas, have noted disc space narrowing and irregularity of the adjacent opposing vertebral endplates in six patients (Figs. 29, 32). Involvement of the intervening vertebral disc was shown pathologically at postmortem examination to be secondary to tumor infiltration in two cases (Fig. 32). Though we do not have pathologic proof of disc-space infiltration in our cases, radiographic evidence of intervertebral disc space narrowing and irregularity may indeed represent tumor infiltration and destruction of the intervening nucleus pulposus. An alternate explanation is possibly related to altered stress patterns which occur secondary to vertebral body destruction. This may produce degeneration of the intervening disc which is followed by spondylotic changes of the opposing vertebral margins, thereby creating a radiographic pattern which may be similar to tumor invasion. No matter which mechanism of disc-space involvement is in effect, an abnormality of the intervertebral disc space is a useful adjunct in the differentiating complex of vertebral chordomas from other malignant lesions that involve the axial skeleton.

A soft-tissue mass has been stated to be present in 100% of vertebral chordomas (UTNE and PUGH, 1955). WOOD and HIMADI (1950) reported the presence of a paravertebral soft-tissue mass in two of their five reported vertebral chordomas. ALLEN (1955) stated that soft-tissue swelling may be seen in the absence of bone invasion with spinal chordomas (Fig. 33). In our series of nine vertebral chordomas, a precervical or paravertebral mass was seen in five patients. Flecks of calcifications were present in the soft-tissue mass in two patients (Figs. 30, 31, 32). As with calcification within the intracranial chordomas, the two mechanisms offered as explanation for these calcifications are cystic degeneration within the tumor mass with subsequent calcification, and sequestered bone fragments which have been caught within the expanding tumor mass. In one

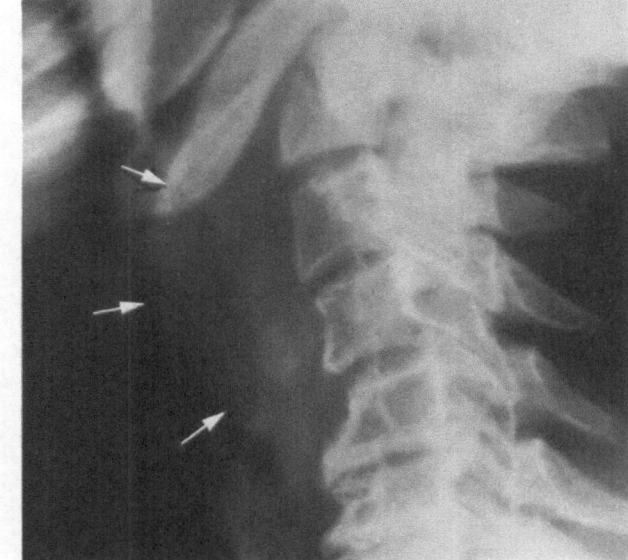

Fig. 33. Cervical chordoma: Lateral projection of upper cervical spine demonstrates large, localized soft-tissue mass displacing larynx anteriorly (*arrows*) without evidence of vertebral body involvement. This is an unusual presentation of cervical chordoma. Calcification is present within inferior aspect of mass

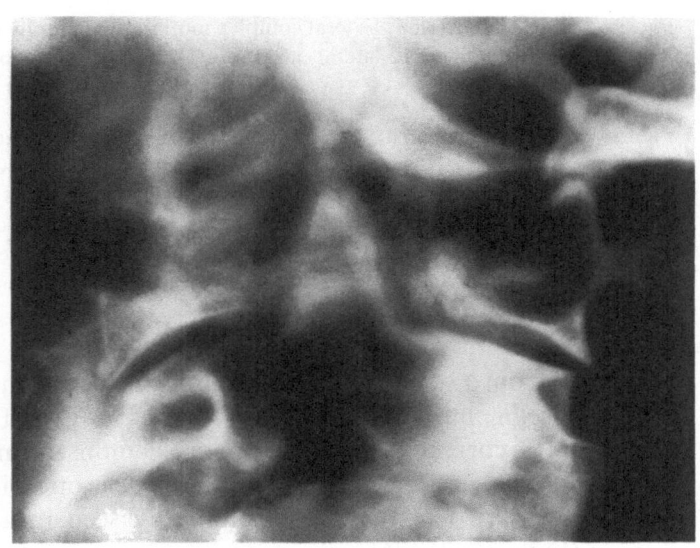

Fig. 34. Cervical chordoma: Frontal complex motion tomography reveals lytic lesion of body of C2 and expansile lytic lesion of the left lateral mass of C1. The right lateral mass of C1 also shows destructive process

vertebral chordoma in our series the calcification was found to be within areas of necrosis within the tumor (Fig. 32). Although the presence of a paravertebral mass does not in any way aid in the differentiation of a chordoma from other malignant or inflammatory lesions of the axial skeleton, the presence of calcifications within the soft-tissue mass will lessen the diagnostic possibilities. It virtually eliminates myeloma and metastasis of the involved vertebral bodies. It is very unlikely that an acute pyogenic inflammatory mass secondary to vertebral osteomyelitis will demonstrate soft-tissue calcifications. It, however, does not rule out tuberculous osteomyelitis involving the axial skeleton, which also involves the precervical or paravertebral soft-tissues. Calcifications within the soft-tissue mass may be observed in this disease entity (MURRAY and JACOBSON, 1971).

Bone expansion in vertebral chordomas is rarely encountered (WOOD and HIMADI, 1950). At times it may be extremely difficult to differentiate a chordoma with bone

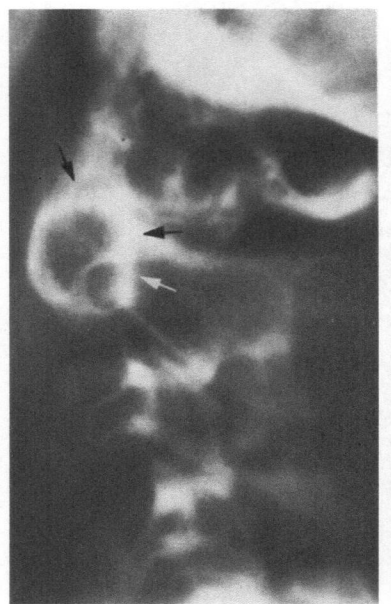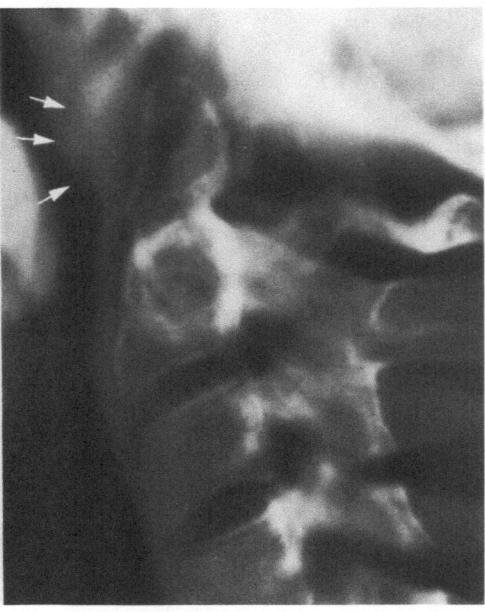

Fig. 35   Fig. 36

Fig. 35. Cervical Chordoma: Lateral complex motion tomography in same patient as Figure 34 reveals expansile lytic lesions involving left lateral mass of C1 and anterior portion of body of C2 which has a ense sclerotic rim (*arrows*)

Fig. 36. Cervical chordoma: Lateral projection, midline cut, utilizing complex motion tomography (same patient as in Figs. 34, 35) demonstrates lytic lesion of body of C2 to be surrounded by thick sclerotic rim. Note involvement of odontoid process by an osteolytic process and total destruction of anterior mass of C1. There is soft-tissue density (*arrows*) which is impinging upon posterior aspect of oropharynx. Though an expansile lytic process is unusual for vertebral chordoma, the presence of multiple vertebral body involvement coupled with peripheral sclerosis and precervical soft-tissue mass should make chordoma the prime diagnosis

expansion from a benign giant cell tumor or aneurysmal bone cyst expanding the involved vertebral segment. Some differentiating features of vertebral chordomas may aid in arriving at a correct diagnosis, such as demonstrating multiple vertebral body involvement, and the presence of a thick osteosclerotic rim surrounding the expanded area of osteolysis; two features not commonly seen in aneurysmal bone cysts or giant cell tumors (Figs. 34, 35, 36).

In summary, vertebral chordomas may be diagnosed preoperatively if a definitive differentiating complex is present. This complex includes multiple asymmetrical adjacent vertebral body destructions with evidence of involvement of the disc interspace coupled with a paravertebral or prevertebral soft-tissue mass, which may contain scattered flecks of calcification. The presence of osteosclerosis at the margins of the osteolysis is an important feature in the differentiation from a tuberculous osteomyelitis, particularly with involvement of the cervical vertebrae in which tuberculous osteomyelitis uncommonly produces proliferation of new bone (MURRAY and JACOBSON, 1971).

2. Myelography

Most vertebral chordomas will show posterior extension into the spinal canal, which is best evaluated with a lumbar myelogram. WOOD and HIMADI (1950) demonstrated posterior epidural extension in two of three cases of vertebral chordomas which underwent myelographic examination. Two of Sennett's reported vertebral chordomas at myelo-

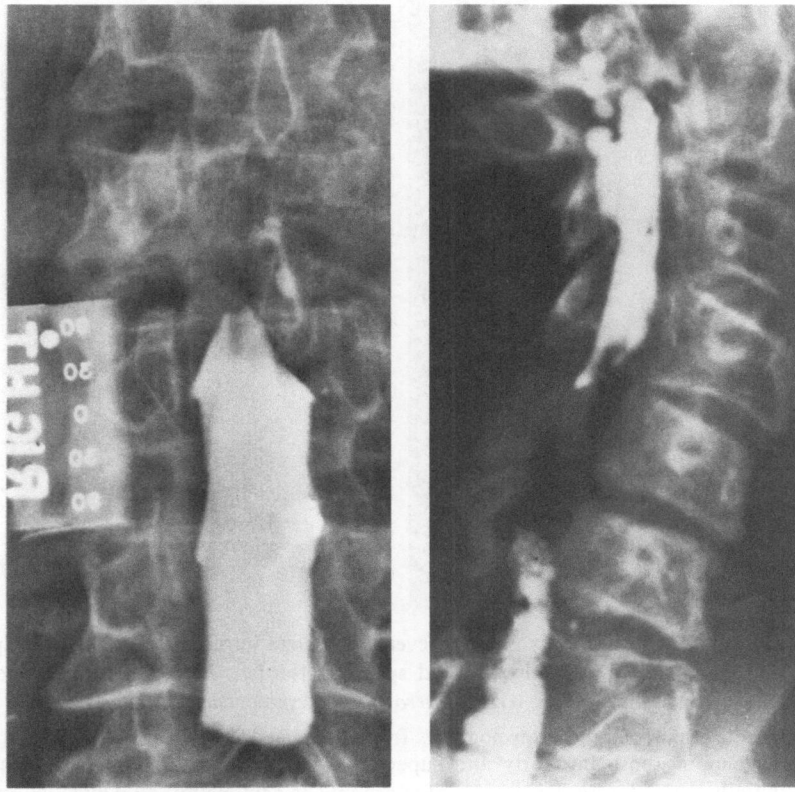

Fig. 37   Fig. 38

Fig. 37. Lumbar chordoma: A lumbar myelogram demonstrates a complete epidural block at L2/3 disc interspace secondary to intraspinal extension of a lumbar chordoma (same patient as in Figs. 30, 31, and 42)

Fig. 38. Cervical chordoma: Prone cervical myelogram, lateral projection, reveals imcomplete epidural defect with displacement of subarachnoid space posteriorly. Epidural defect is confined to area of vertebral body involvement. Note sclerosis of body of C6

graphy showed a complete epidural block. In our series eight patients underwent myelographic examination, and all eight patients manifested intraspinal extension of the tumor. Six patients demonstrated an epidural defect localized to the destroyed vertebral bodies with two showing a complete epidural block (Figs. 37, 38). In two cases an intradural block was observed (Figs. 39, 40). Both cases of complete intradural block showed a small epidural component as well. In one of these patients an oblique cervical spine film revealed widening of multiple intervertebral foramina and a preoperative diagnosis of multiple neurofibromas was made (Fig. 41). At surgery intradural extension of the tumor was found in these two patients. The intradural extension of chordomas has received little stress within the literature (HSIEH and HSIEH, 1936; POPPEN and KING, 1952; SENNETT, 1953), but vertebral chordomas, particularly cervical lesions, have been mistaken for a cervical neurofibroma at both plain film examination and at myelography (Figs. 39, 41). The clue in differentiation of chordoma from neurofibroma at myelography rests in the demonstration of osseous changes typical of chordoma at the area of the myelographic intradural block; which does not rule out a dumbbell neurofibroma, but would direct one to consider other possibilities for this myelographic configuration.

The presence of an epidural defect or complete epidural block does not differentiate chordoma from other malignant lesions involving the axial skeleton. Diagnosis of chordomas rests primarily on the osseous changes of the involved bodies.

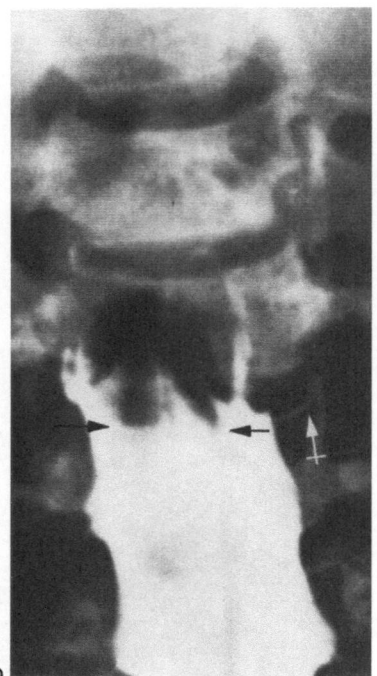 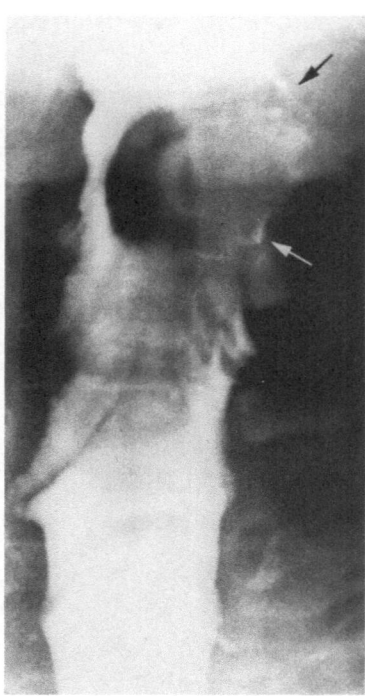

Fig. 39

Fig. 40

Fig. 39. Cervical chordoma: Cervical myelogram reveals complete intradural block with displacement of cord to the right (*arrows*) and cupping of subarachnoid space on the left. Note epidural component to complete intradural block (*crossed arrow*). Same patient as in Figure 41

Fig. 40. Cervical chordoma: Cervical myelogram, frontal projection, reveals well-defined intradural lesion with subarachnoid cupping both inferiorly and superiorly (*arrows*) in patient with cervical chordoma from C3–C6. Patient initially had extradural extension of chordoma as demonstrated on myelogram 1 year previously (Fig. 38). Patient underwent a surgical decompression procedure which showed intradural extension of chordoma. Demonstration of intradural lesion at myelographic examination is indicative of dural invasion by chordoma

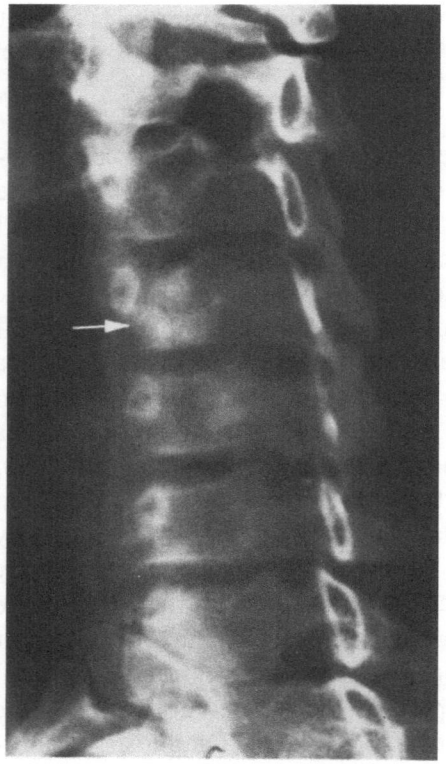

Fig. 41. Cervical chordoma: Left oblique projection of cervical spine reveals widened intervertebral foramina at C3/4 and C4/5. Osteosclerosis of body of C4 is observed (*arrow*). Cervical myelogram in this patient demonstrated a complete intradural block and neurofibroma was preoperative diagnosis. Intradural extension of vertebral chordomas are an infrequent occurrence and frequently are misdiagnosed as neurofibroma

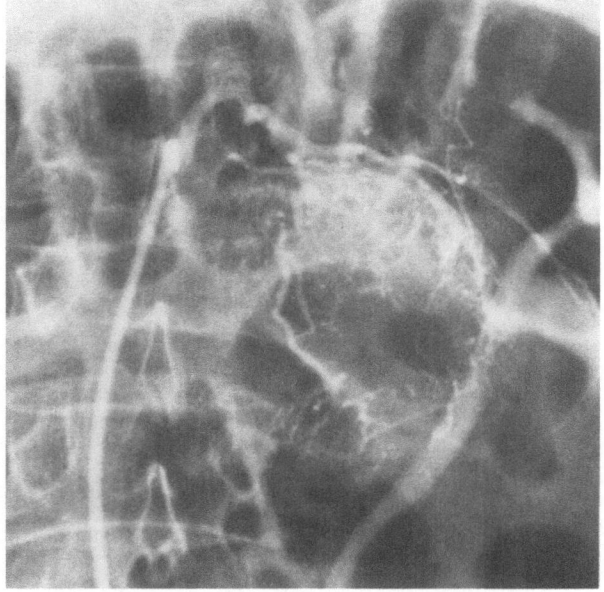

Fig. 42. Lumbar chordoma: Selective lumbar arteriogram demonstrates vascular paravertebral soft-tissue mass with pathologic vessels (vessels which are disorganized, ragged, and exhibit no diminution in caliber as they proceed from their origin) which aids one to suggest malignant lesion. Coupled with plain film findings (Figs. 30 and 31) one can, with a high degree of assurance, conclude that this is a malignant vertebral chordoma

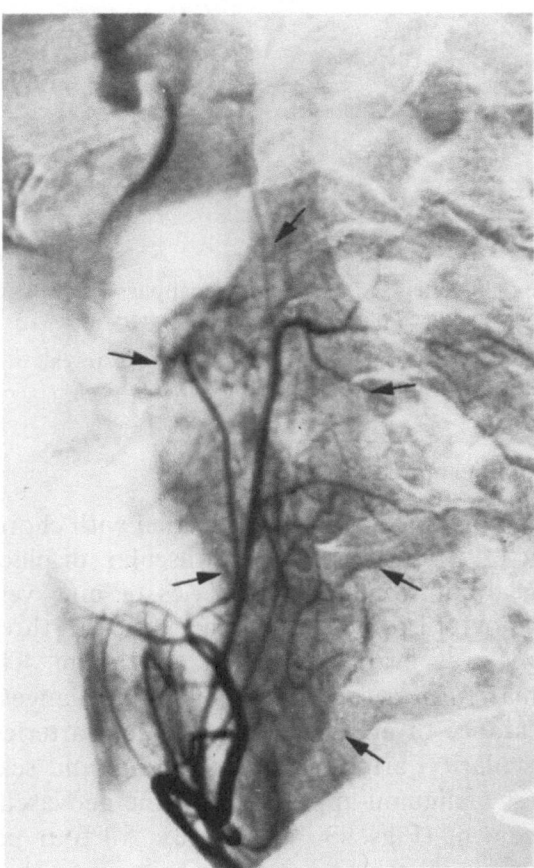

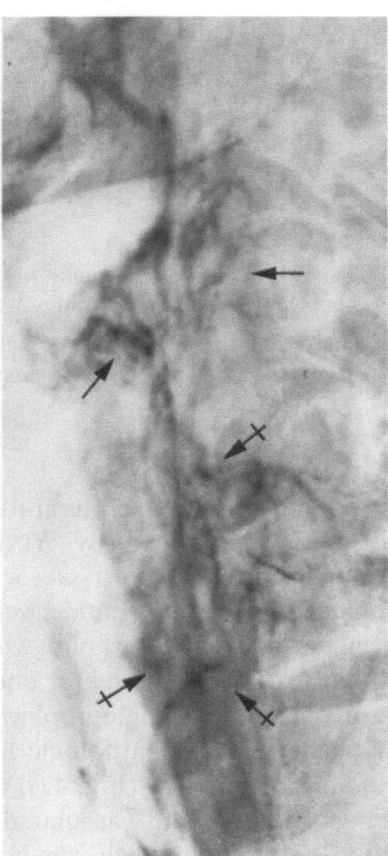

Fig. 43

Fig. 44

Fig. 43. Cervical chordoma: Selective injection of the right thyrocervical trunk, arterial phase, lateral projection, reveals increased neovascularity with tumor blush extending from C4–C6 (*arrows*)

Fig. 44. Same patient as Figure 43, intermediate phase, reveals arteriovenous shunts along superior aspect of soft-tissue tumor (*arrows*) and areas of contrast pooling within bulk of tumor (*crossed arrows*)

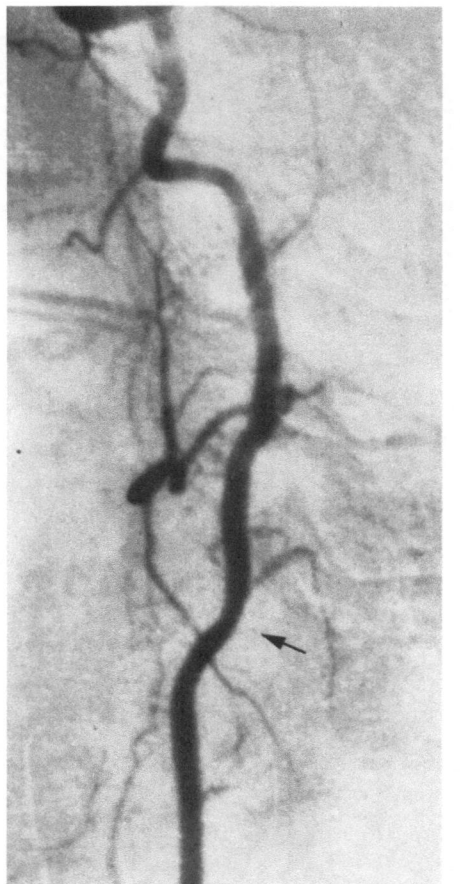
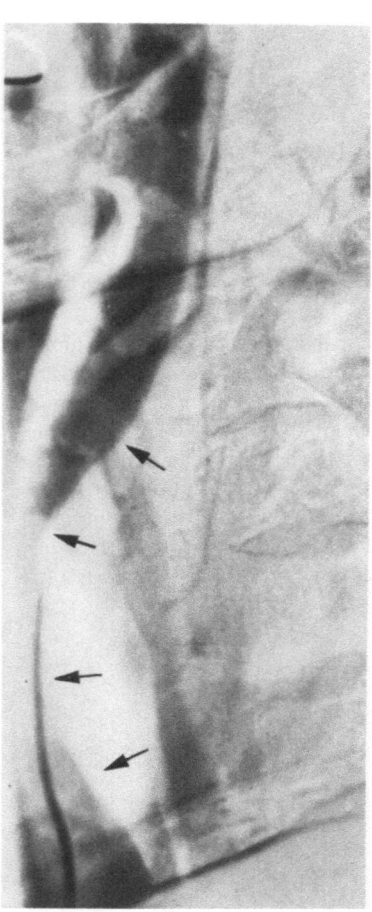

Fig. 45   Fig. 46

Fig. 45. Same patient as Figures 43 and 44, selective right vertebral angiogram, arterial phase, reveals surgically proven perivascular infiltration which narrows lumen of the right vertebral artery (*arrow*)

Fig. 46. Same patient as Figures 43–45, right common carotid angiogram, venous phase, reveals soft-tissue mass displacing jugular vein anterolaterally without evidence of invasion (*arrow*)

3. Angiography

The only mention in the literature of angiographic changes associated with chordomas outside of the cranium is by WINDEYER (1959) who described vascular displacement of the iliac vessels due to a sacrococcygeal chordoma. In our series of nine vertebral chordomas, four patients underwent angiography. Of these four patients, three had subselective spinal angiography while one was evaluated by an aortogram. The angiographic features of vertebral chordomas form a spectrum of variant changes from a blatantly malignant angiographic appearance of enlargement of feeding arteries with large ragged, irregular pathologic neovascularity, arteriovenous shunting, and scattered areas of contrast pooling (Fig. 42); to a less malignant appearance of fine neovascularity, vascular narrowing, and vascular displacement (Figs. 43, 44, 45, 46). All four patients showed a tumor stain which was homogenous in two and nonhomogenous in the other two patients. Though a great degree of overlap has been reported in the angiographic features of benign and malignant lesions of the axial skeleton, angiography may delineate the total extent of the mass and aid in localization of a biopsy site for a definitive tissue diagnosis (COCKSHOTT, 1964; DOS SANTOS, 1950; HALPERN and FREIBERGER, 1965; LAGERGREN et al., 1958; STAPEL et al., 1968; STRICKLAND, 1959; YAGHMAI et al., 1971).

Two angiographic signs which have been reported to give a high degree of assurance that one is dealing with a malignant lesion of bone and/or soft tissues are: (1) demonstration of pathologic vessels, which have been described as an irregular network of new vessels, demonstrating disordered branching and showing no progressive diminution in caliber, and (2) encasement of vessels (COCKSHOTT, 1964; DOS SANTOS, 1950; HALPERN and FREIBERGER, 1965; STAPEL et al., 1968; STRICKLAND, 1959; YAGHMAI et al., 1971).

Chronic inflammatory masses generally produce no angiographic features other than vascular displacement, though hypertrophy of feeding arteries, a hyperemic pattern of vascularity with blush, arteriovenous shunting, and contrast pooling have been reported with inflammatory lesions (COCKSHOTT, 1964; LAGERGREN et al., 1958; STAPEL et al., 1968; YAGHMAI et al., 1971). A malignant lesion, in addition to the above angiographic signs described in chronic inflammatory lesions, may demonstrate pathologic vessels and/or perivascular infiltration (encasement) of otherwise normal vessels. In our four angiographic cases, the morphologic appearance of pathologic vessels was seen in two cases corroborating the radiographic impression of a malignant lesion made on the plain film findings. Vascular encasement was present in one case, which is indicative of perivascular infiltration by a malignant tumor. In our other two cases, hypervascularity with tumor blush, arteriovenous shunting, and contrast pooling were considered nonspecific in differentiating an inflammatory lesion from a malignant one. In no way did arteriography give a histologic diagnosis, though it was helpful in determining the malignant nature of the lesion in half of our angiographic cases as well as having aided the operating surgeon by defining the total extent of the mass, and was definitely of help in demonstrating areas of encasement of important arteries.

IV. Sacrococcygeal Chordoma

The sacrococcygeal region is the most frequent location of chordomas (Fig. II). The incidence of involvement of the sacrum by chordomas, as reported in the large series in the literature, is 52%. The roentgenographic examination of the pelvis will show bone involvement in a high percentage of cases (UTNE and PUGH, 1955). Bone destruction is the most consistent feature of chordoma involving the sacrococcygeal area (HSIEH and HSIEH, 1936; GENTIL and COLEY, 1948; FLETCHER et al., 1935; CAMP and GOOD, 1938; WINDEYER, 1959).

UTNE and PUGH (1955) stated that 75% of sacrococcygeal chordomas will show bone involvement, primarily bone destruction on radiographic examination. A lytic lesion expanding the sacrum, with irregular scalloped margins, was noted by these authors to be a frequent finding. There was calcification within the tumor in 50% of their patients.

KAMRIN et al. (1964) reported that 80% of sacral chordomas in their series had erosion of bone, primarily of the sacrum, without evidence of osteoblastic reaction. The osseous lesion may have an extraosseous component which will displace the bladder and rectum. POPPEN and KING (1952) reported evidence of osteosclerotic reaction adjacent to the osteolysis in two cases. SENNETT (1953) described four lesions, all of which were situated in the midline and showed irregular destruction and expansion of the sacrum. Two of his reported cases showed bone reaction and small spicules of "bone" within the tumor mass. The radiographic findings of sacrococcygeal chordomas were first described by HSIEH and HSIEH (1936), in which patients with sacrococcygeal chordomas showed destruction of bone to be invariably present with an appearance of multiple-lobulated radiolucent areas of osteolysis. Expansion of the sacrum was noted by them

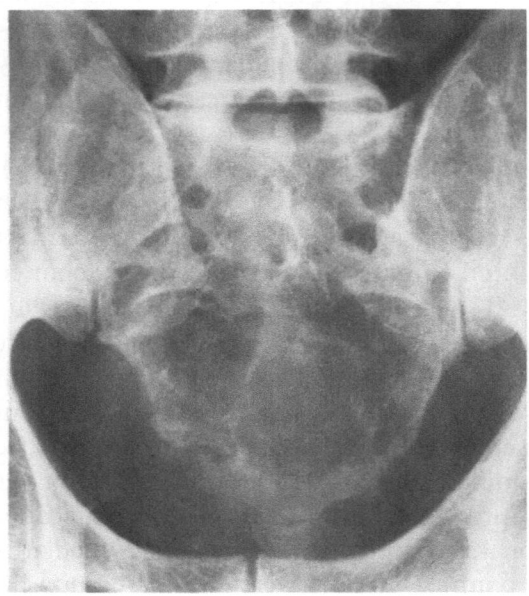 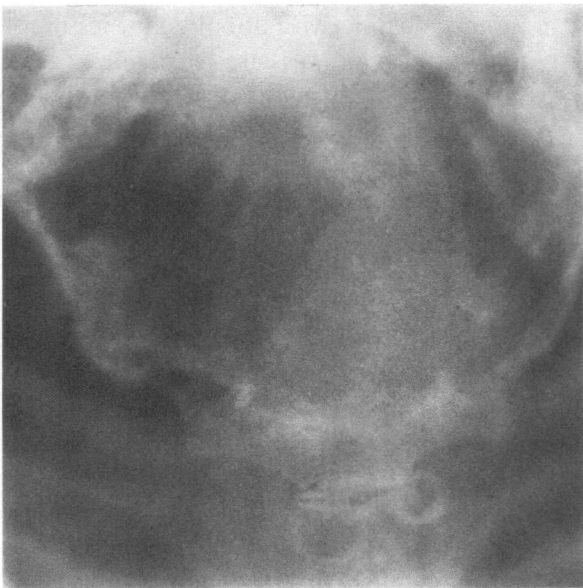

Fig. 47   Fig. 48

Fig. 47. Sacrococcygeal chordoma: Typical plain film changes of sacrococcygeal chordoma are present. Destruction of multiple sacral segments with scalloped, ill-defined border is seen with numerous linear and nodular calcifications within lesion. Destructions of sacrum in sacrococcygeal chordomas are primarily located in midline, though they may be eccentric. Relatively wide zone of transition between normal architecture of sacrococcygeus and osteolysis points to malignant lesion. Calcifications within lytic lesion tends to exclude other malignancies of sacrococcygeus such as plasmocytoma or metastases. Differentiation from primary chondrosarcoma of sacrum is difficult

Fig. 48. Sacrococcygeal chordoma: Frontal tomography of sacrum in same patient as Figure 47 demonstrates scalloped peripheral margins of osteolysis and slight expansion of sacrum by this tumor. Numerous nodular calcifications are seen throughout osteolysis. Tomography is important in evaluation of patients when overlying gas and feces obscure bony architecture of sacrum

and felt to be due to the expanding growth of the tumor mass. Calcification was also seen within the tumor mass which they described to be either due to reactive bone formation or deposits of calcification in the tumor as a result of degeneration and necrosis. As in other regions, a fragment of bone may be engulfed by and displaced within the tumor (WOOD, 1950; ALLEN, 1955).

According to UTNE and PUGH (1955), 85% of reported sacrococcygeal chordomas present with a pelvic mass which produces displacement of the rectum and bladder as well as medial displacement of the pelvic ureters secondary to the presacral growth of the tumor. Not all authors list the primary direction of growth of the tumor. Many large series such as MABREY (1935) and STEWART and MORIN (1926) show that presacral growth of the sacrococcygeal chordomas occurred in 46% and 44% respectively, whereas retrosacral growth was seen 33% of the time in Mabrey's series and 30% of the time in Stewart's and Morin's series. The rest of their sacrococcygeal chordomas showed an equal distribution of the soft-tissue mass both retrosacrally and antesacrally. Though there have been several instances in the literature which have shown a negative pelvic roentgenogram with proven chordomas, this may be due to superimposition of the pelvic soft tissues, as well as gas and fecal contents of the pelvic colon on the sacrum. It is therefore recommended, particularly in patients who complain of persistent localized sacral pain and/or discovered to have a fixed presacral mass on digital examination

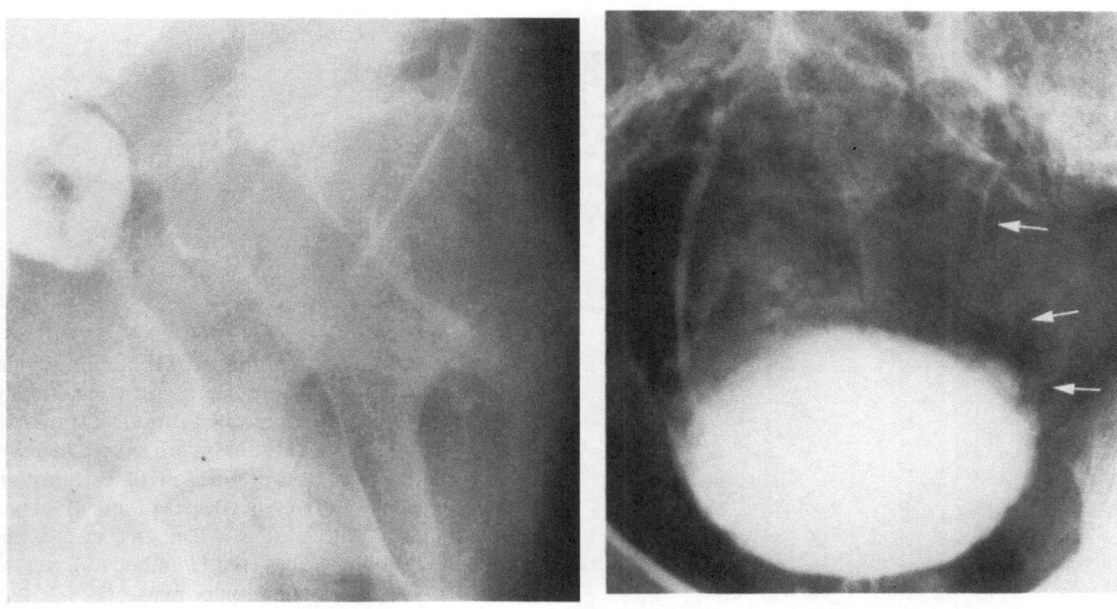

Fig. 49   Fig. 50

Fig. 49. Sacrococcygeal chordoma: Lateral projection from air contrast barium enema, reveals increase in presacral space which commonly occurs with presacral growth of sacrococcygeal chordoma. Sacrococcygeal chordomas on digital examination present as presacral mass

Fig. 50. Sacrococcygeal chordoma, intravenous pyelogram: Medial displacement of distal ureters is observed with presacral growth of sacrococcygeal chordomas (*arrows*). Not uncommonly sacrococcygeal tumors present as large bulky pelvic mass

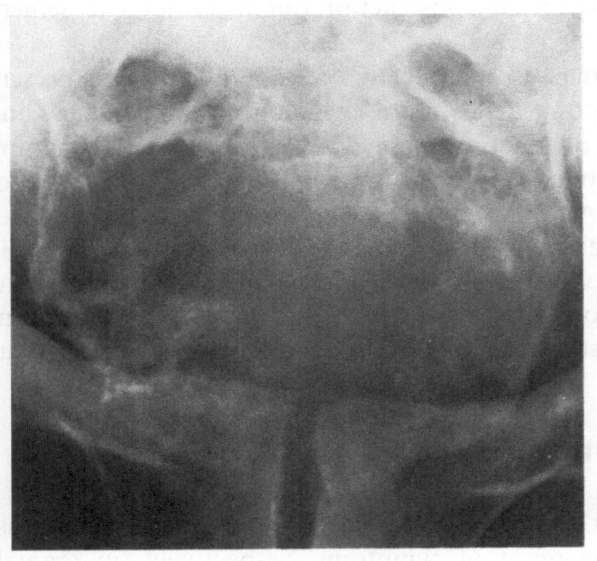
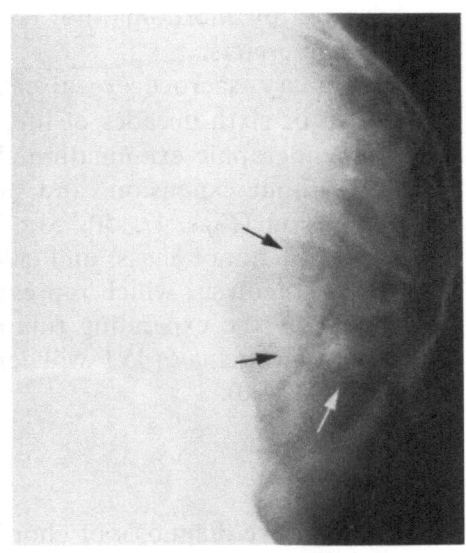

Fig. 51   Fig. 52

Fig. 51. Sacrococcygeal chordoma: Osteolysis of body of the sacrum which is eccentric in location with dense calcification within tumor. Note relatively wide zone of transition between normal sacrum and osteolysis

Fig. 52. Sacrococcygeal chordoma: Same patient as Figure 51, lateral projection. There is destruction of multiple sacral segments with amorphous calcification in presacral space (*arrows*). Calcifications tend to exclude many malignancies which involve sacrum, such as myeloma and metastases, though it would be difficult to differentiate from sacral chondrosarcoma

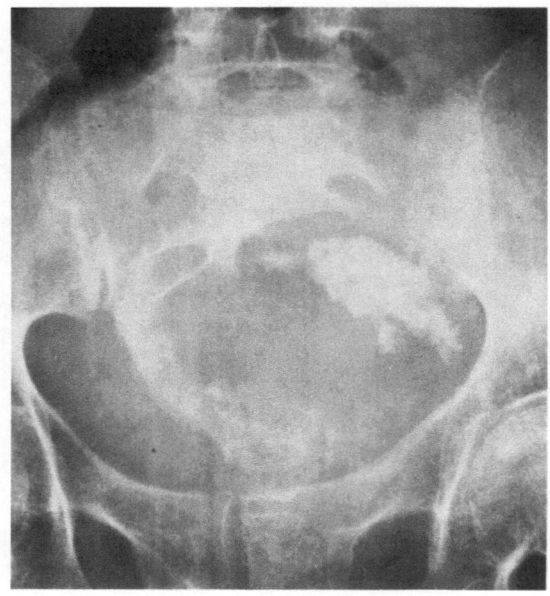

Fig. 53. Sacrococcygeal chordoma: Frontal projection of sacrum reveals multiple sacral segments totally destroyed with dense area of calcification and multiple nodular densities within area of lysis. Two mechanisms have been described for production of calcification within chordomas: (1) cystic degeneration of tumor with subsequent calcification, which this case exemplifies, and (2) bone sequestered from body of sacrum by expanding tumor mass

of the rectum, that body-section radiography of the sacrum both in AP and lateral projections be performed to demonstrate more clearly areas of osteolysis within the sacral segments (Figs. 47, 48). Barium enema and intravenous pyelography (IVP) may show displacement of the rectum and ureters indicative of the antesacral location of the expanding soft-tissue mass of the sacrococcygeal chordoma (Figs. 49, 50); however, no accepted report in the literature has shown either ulceration of the rectal or rectosigmoid mucosa by chordoma, nor complete urinary obstruction due to tumor encasement of the pelvic ureters.

In summary, sacrococcygeal chordomas are characterized as tumors which present in the fifth or sixth decades of life, affecting males more commonly than females, and on roentgenographic examination show destruction of several segments of the sacrum, with or without expansion, and occasionally with scalloped margins to the edge of the lytic lesion (Figs. 47, 50, 51, 52). A thick sclerotic rim may be associated with the expanding tumor mass, and calcification of fragments of bone may be seen within the area of osteolysis, which represents either cystic degeneration of the tumor or bone sequestered by the expanding tumor growth (Figs. 42, 51, 53). Ancillary examinations such as barium enema or IVP will demonstrate the antesacral component of the soft-tissue mass (Figs. 49, 50).

V. Diagnosis

The definitive diagnosis of chordoma is often delayed for an average of 18 months, 27 months, and 3–5 years following the onset of symptoms, respectively, in cranial, vertebral, and sacrococcygeal chordomas.

A clinical diagnosis of intracranial chordoma should be suspected whenever there is clinical evidence for a predominantly midline mass lesion of the base of the skull. The clinical findings may be indistinguishable from pituitary adenoma, craniopharyngioma, intrasellar or retrosellar meningioma, or other mass lesions of this region. A nasopharyngeal and particularly, a retropharyngeal, mass lesion, is a very valuable finding. Except for craniopharyngioma and carcinoma of the nasopharynx, other intracranial tumors, such as pituitary adenoma and meningioma, do not ordinarily cause a nasopharyngeal mass. Very large pituitary tumors may completely replace the sphenoid sinus and produce a nasopharyngeal mass. However, a retropharyngeal mass is unlikely in these patients. A nasopharyngeal mass is seen in one-third of all intracranial chordomas. Furthermore, posterior and downward extension of the lesion along the clivus toward the foramen magnum region, as is the case with sellar chordomas, is most uncommon in pituitary adenoma. Epidural extension of the lesion into the spinal canal, seen in chordomas, is very unlikely in other intracranial lesions. Differentiation of chordoma from an unusual instance of sellar or clival osteochondroma may be impossible (FALCONER et al., 1968). Nasopharyngeal carcinoma (either primary or metastatic) may produce extensive destruction of the base of the skull and a soft-tissue tumor mass in the nasopharynx. In these patients, lymphadenopathy is often found in the neck, a finding which is most unusual in nasopharyngeal chordoma (PASTORE et al., 1949).

Diagnosis of chordoma can rarely be made on clinical ground alone. By combining the clinical findings with roentgenologic features, however, the diagnosis may be strongly suspected (KAMRIN et al., 1964).

The demonstration of a midline suprasellar space-occupying lesion which destroys the dorsum sellae, though highly suggestive of a chordoma, would make it most difficult to exclude a pituitary adenoma or craniopharyngioma. The presence of calcification within the tumor mass would be less likely in a pituitary adenoma (LINDGREN and DI CHIRO, 1951). The lack of a "tumor blush" on carotid angiography would also make a pituitary adenoma unlikely (BAKER, 1972). The absence of prominent tumor vascularity on carotid angiography would tend to exclude a tuberculum or tentorial meningioma.

When a prepontine calcified lesion is demonstrated in the absence of osteosclerosis of the clivus, a clival meningioma is less likely. Again, differentiation from a craniopharyngioma which has extended into the prepontine cistern or from an intracranial cholesteatoma, will be extremely difficult on plain film examination or by angiography. The presence of calcification will, of course, make an intracranial cholesteatoma unlikely. Angiography will also differentiate a clival chordoma from a clival meningioma in that no tumor stain or neovascularity has been reported with a clival chordoma (SCHECHTER et al., 1974). With the advent of computerized tomography more specific diagnostic features may be observed to differentiate histologic groups which involve the same intracranial areas, an example being a cholesteatoma that has an absorption coefficient in the minus (fat density) range (PAXTON and AMBROSE, 1974). What effect contrast enhancement with CT scanning will have in differentiating a clival meningioma from a chordoma will require further work with this very important and new modality before any definite conclusions can be reached.

Vertebral. The findings of multiple adjacent vertebral body and disc destruction with presence of osteosclerosis and a soft-tissue mass containing calcification virtually eliminates consideration of any other malignant lesion of the axial skeleton such as myeloma or metastases. The prime difficulty one encounters with chordoma is in the differentiation from a chronic osteomyelitis, primarily of the granulomatous type (tuberculosis). MURRAY and JACOBSON (1971) have stated that tuberculosis of the cervical spine uncommonly produces osteosclerosis, and since chordomas most often involve the cervical spine, the presence of osteosclerosis may in fact be a feature which would place chordoma as the prime provisional diagnosis in this area. In our opinion this is not a hard and fast rule and difficulty will arise in differentiating chordoma from a chronic inflammatory mass, not only in the cervical spine, but also in the rest of the axial skeleton.

Angiography may not be helpful in differentiating a chordoma from a chronic inflammatory mass unless definite pathologic vessels are seen within the soft-tissue component of the mass, or the presence of perivascular infiltration (encasement) is demonstrated (involving arteries). The demonstration of neovascularity and tumor blush, arteriovenous shunting, and contrast pooling are nonspecific and will not allow one to differentiate a chronic inflammatory lesion from a vertebral chordoma. Myelographic examination, though important in demonstrating posterior intraspinal extension of the tumor, is also unable to differentiate a primary malignant lesion of the axial skeleton from metastases, myeloma, or an inflammatory lesion. When vertebral chordomas have an expansile appearance, differentiation from a giant cell tumor or aneurysmal bone cyst of the axial skeleton may be readily made in that chordomas involve multiple vertebral bodies and may show evidence of osteosclerosis. A further differentiating feature is the presence of a thick sclerotic rim which may be associated with chordomas.

Sacrococcygeal. Metastases to the sacrum with pure osteolysis is the most frequent lesion destroying this structure that one sees in the every day practice of radiology. The absence of a thick sclerotic rim may aid to differentiate metastases from a sacrococcygeal chordoma. A chondrosarcoma involving the sacrum may present difficulty in differentiation from chordoma. A plasmocytoma of the sacrum again may present difficulty in differentiation from a chordoma, but the presence of calcification within the tumor mass will favor the latter diagnosis. Sacromeningoceles will show intraspinal origin of the erosive process as well as widening of the sacral foramina, and are easily differentiated from the destructive changes that are seen with chordomas. Sacromeningoceles also do not show calcifications, a wide zone of transition between involved and noninvolved segments of the sacrum, or evidence of a thick sclerotic rim at the periphery of the erosive defect. Sacrococcygeal teratomas seen in infants and children, may show characteristic dental remnants, and therefore, may be easily differentiated from a sacrococcygeal chordoma.

To establish the histologic diagnosis the simplest biopsy method available should be utilized, such as pharyngeal and sphenoidal biopsy, which, if repeated a few times, usually yield diagnostic results. However, if the diagnosis is not established, an exploratory operative procedure becomes indicated.

VI. Treatment

At the present time complete surgical resection can only be accomplished in sacrococcygeal chordomas via a radical excision with total sacrectomy (Kamrin et al., 1964; MacCarty et al., 1961). MacCarty et al., in their series of 18 patients treated by radical sacrectomy, reported 12 of 18 patients surviving an average of 6 years after operation. Total evaluation of their therapy is complicated by the fact that 13 patients received postoperative radiotherapy. For vertebral chordomas surgical resection may result in long-term survival in addition to relieving acute spinal cord compression. Dahlin and MacCarty (1952) reported a patient where resection of a cervical chordoma, which had destroyed the bodies of three cervical vertebrae, has remained free of disease for 15 years after removal of the tumor. Kamrin et al. (1964) state that for vertebral chordomas the only indication for surgical intervention, other than for biopsy, is for impending paraplegia.

Surgical treatment for intracranial chordomas is performed primarily for decompression of vital structures (Kamrin et al., 1964). Kamrin et al. further state that, except for emergency situations demanding surgical decompression for the preservation of life or vital structures, surgical treatment of nonsacrococcygeal chordomas has little to offer. FALCONER et al. (1968) reported a series of cases which showed sufficient improvement after surgical intervention to return to normal functioning, but they agree that surgery is mainly for palliation.

It is generally stated that chordomas are relatively radioresistent except when they occur in children where they exhibit a higher degree of radiosensitivity than those chordomas which occur in adults (WOOD, 1950; ORMEROD, 1960; WINDEYER, 1959). There have been reports in the literature of long-term survival following a course of supervoltage radiation. WINDEYER (1959), in his series of 19 chordomas, had 8 patients with sacrococcygeal chordomas who were treated with supervoltage radiation, 6 being without symptoms or signs of disease for 4 years. Though he himself considered radiotherapy as palliative treatment he did report that 1 patient has remained well for 18 years after 13,500 R were given in three separate treatments. ORMEROD (1960) reported a case of a nasopharyngeal chordoma which received a total of 10,000 R, and has not recurred after a 4-year follow-up. He further stated that the impression of radio-resistance of chordomas may be related to the fact that 6,000 R, the usual therapy for chordomas, may be insufficient to destroy the tumor and that higher doses may be required to reach a curative dose. The case reported by ORMEROD in 1960 was further reported by WRIGHT in 1967, in which the patient received an additional 3,175 R for a local recurrence, and is at present free from evidence of disease 13 years after initial presentation. Most authors agree that radiotherapy has some value in the treatment of chordomas in that it may prolong survival and be of help in relieving pain. Complicating evaluation of high-dose radiotherapy is the opinion of KAMRIN et al. (1964), that distant metastases are related to longer survival and massive radiation to the tumor site.

In an evaluation of different methods of therapy of a series of patients which were treated at one institution, DAHLIN and MacCARTY (1952) concluded that a combination of surgery and radiotherapy offered the best chance of prolonging survival. WRIGHT (1967) concluded that higher doses may be required in the treatment of chordomas, a trend which appears to be followed by many other radiotherapists.

References

ACKERMAN, L.V., DEL REGATO, J.A.: Cancer: Diagnosis, treatment and prognosis, 3rd ed. St. Louis: E.V. Mosby Co. pp. 380, 678 (1962)

ADAMS, W.S.: Chordoma of the right frontal sinus. J. Laryng. **62**, 93–95 (1948)

ADSON, A.W., KERNOHAN, J.W., WOLTMAN, H.W.: Cranial and cervical chordomas. A clinical and histologic study. Arch. Neurol. Psychiat. (Chicago) **33**, 247–261 (1935)

ALLEN, A.L.: Detection of chordoma: Report of four new cases. Clin. Orthop. **6**, 158–165 (1955)

ANDERSON, W.B., MEYERS, H.L.: Multicentric chordoma. Report of a case. Cancer (Philad.) **21**, 126–128 (1968)

BAKER, H.L.: The angiographic delineation of sellar and parasellar masses. Radiology **104**, 67–78 (1972)

BATSAKIS, J.G., KITTLESON, A.C.: Chordomas – Otorhinolaryngologic presentation and diagnosis. Archives Otolaryng. **78**, 168–175 (1963)

BELZA, J.: Double midline intracranial tumors of vestigial origin: contiguous intrasellar chordoma and suprasellar craniopharyngioma. Case report. J. Neurosurg. **25**, 199–204 (1966)

BERDAL, P., MYHRE, E.: Cranial chordomas involving the paranasal sinuses. J. Laryng. **78**, 906–919 (1964)

CAMP, J.D., GOOD, C.A.: The roentgenologic diagnosis of tumors involving the sacrum. Radiology **3**, 398–403 (1938)

CHALMERS, J., HEAD, B.E.: A metastasing chordoma. J. Bone Jt Surg. **54B**, 526–529 (1972)

CHASE, N.E., TAVERAS, J.M.: Cerebral angiography in the diagnosis of suprasellar tumors. Amer. J. Roentgenol. **86**, I, 154–165 (1961)

CHASE, N.E., TAVERAS, J.M.: Carotid angiography in

the diagnosis of extradural parasellar tumors. Acta radiol. (Stockh.) 1, 214–244 (1963)

Cockshott, W.P.: The place of soft tissue arteriography. Brit. J. Radiol. 37, 367–375 (1964)

Congdon, C.C.: Benign and malignant chordomas. A clinico-anatomic study of twenty-two cases. Amer. J. Path. 28, 793–821 (1952)

Dahlin, D.C.: Bone tumors: General aspects and data on 3,987 cases, 2nd ed. Springfield, Ill.: Charles C Thomas, pp. 222–233 1967

Dahlin, D.C., Mac Carty, C.S.: Chordoma: A study of fifty-nine cases. Cancer (Philad.) 5, 1170–1178 (1952)

Di Chiro, G., Anderson, W.B.: Clivus. Clin. Radiol. 16, 211–223 (1965)

Dos Santos, R.: Arteriography in bone tumors. J. Bone Jt Surg. 32B, 17–29 (1950)

Falconer, M.A., Bailery, I.C., Duchen, L.W.: Surgical treatment of chordoma and chondroma of the skull base. J. Neurosurg. 29, 261–275 (1968)

Faust, D.B., Gilmore, H.R., Mudgett, C.S.: Chordomata: A review of the literature with report of a sacrococcygeal case. Ann. intern. Med. 21, 678–698 (1944)

Fletcher, E.M., Woltman, H.W., Adson, A.W.: Sacrococcygeal chordomas: A clinical and pathologic study. Arch. Neurol. Psychiat. (Chicago) 33, 283–299 (1935)

Fox, J.E., Batsakis, J.G., Owano, L.R.: Unusual manifestations of chordoma. A report of two cases. J. Bone Jt Surg. 50A, 1618–1628 (1968)

Gardner, W.J., Turner, O.: Cranial chordomas. A clinical and pathologic study. Arch. Surg. (Chicago) 411–425 (1941)

Gentil, F., Coley, B.L.: Sacrococcygeal chordoma. Ann. Surg., 127, 432–455 (1948)

Halpern, M., Freiberger, R.H.: Arteriography in orthopedics. Amer. J. Roentgenol. 94, 194–206 (1965)

Hartofilaikidis-Garofalidis, G., Papathanassiou, B.T., Kambouroglou, G.: Chordoma of the lumbar spine. Int. Surg. 5D, 566–570 (1968)

Harvey, W.F., Dawson, E.K.: Chordoma. Edinb. med. J. 48, 713–730 (1941)

Herndon, J.H., Cohen, J.: Chondroma of a lumbar vertebral body resembling a chordoma. J. Bone Jt Surg. 52A, 1241–1247 (1970)

Hilal, S.K.: Angiography of juxtasellar masses. Semin. Roentgenol. 6, 75–88 (1971)

Hsieh, C.K., Hsieh, H.H.: Roentgenologic study of sacrococcygeal chordoma. Radiology 27, 101–109 (1936)

Iraci, G., Gerosa, M., Pardatscher, K.: Isolated Vernet's syndrome: An unusual manifestation of intracranial chordoma. Surg. Neurol. 1, 295–298 (1973)

Jaffe, H.L.: Tumors and tumorous conditions of the bones and joints. Philadelphia: Lea & Febiger, 451–462 1958

Joy, H.H., Ecker, A., Riemenschneider, P.A.: Role of cerebral angiography in ophthalmology. Amer. J. Ophthal. 37, 55–68 (1954)

Kamrin, R.P., Potanos, J.N., Pool, J.L.: An evaluation of the diagnosis and treatment of chordoma. J. Neurol. Neurosurg. Psychiat. 27, 157–165 (1964)

Lagergren, C., Lindbom, A., Soderberg, G.: Hypervascularization in chronic inflammation demonstrated by angiography. Angiographic, histopathologic and microangiographic studies. Acta radiol. (Stockh.) 49, 441–452 (1958)

Lichtenstein, L.: Bone tumors, 4th ed. St. Louis: C.V. Mosby, pp. 335–342 (1972)

Lindgren, E., Di Chiro, G.: Suprasellar tumours with calcification. Acta radiol. (Stockh.) 36, 173–195 (1951)

Mabrey, R.E.: Chordoma: A study of 150 cases. Cancer (Philad.) 25, 501–517 (1935)

Mac Carty, C.S., Waugh, J.M., Conventry, M.B., O'Sullivan, D.C.: Sacrococcygeal chordomas. Surg. Gynec. Obstet. 113, 551–554 (1961)

Mathews, W., Wilson, C.B.: Ectopic intrasellar chordoma. Case report. J. Neurosurg. 39, 260–263 (1974)

Money, R.A., Vanderfield, G.K.: Angiography in management of intrasuprasellar tumors. J. Neurosurg. 12, 203–215 (1955)

Murray, R.O., Jacobson, H.G.: The radiology of skeletal disorders: Exercises in diagnosis. Baltimore: Williams & Wilkins, 1971

Ormerod, R.: A case of chordoma presenting in the nasopharynx. J. Laryng. 74, 245–254 (1960)

Pastore, P.N., Sahyoun, P.F., Mandeville, F.B.: Chordoma of the maxillary antrum and nares. Arch. Otolaryng. (Chicago) 50, 647–658 (1949)

Paxton, R., Ambrose, J.: The EMI scanner. A brief review of the first 650 patients. Brit. J. Radiol. 47, 530–565 (1974)

Pendergrass, E.P., Schaeffer, J.P., Hodes, P.J.: The head and neck in roentgen diagnosis, Vol. II. Springfield, Ill.: Charles C. Thomas 989–997, 1956

Pinto, R.S., Lin, J.P., Firooznia, H., Lefleur, R.S.: The osseous and angiographic features of vertebral chordoma. Neuroradiology 9, 231–241 (1975)

Plaut, H.F., Blatt, E.S.: Chordoma of the clivus: A report of four cases. Amer. J. Roentgenol. 100, 639–648 (1967)

Poppen, J.L., King, A.B.: Chordoma: Experience with thirteen cases. J. Neurosurg. 9, 139–163 (1952)

Rao Balaparameswara, S., Dinakar, I.: Vertebral chordomas. Neurol. India. 19, 112–115 (1971)

Rao Balaparameswara, S., Dinakar, I.: Ivory vertebra associated with chordoma. Indian. J. Radiol. 24, 182–184 (1970)

Ridpath, R.F.: Chordoma with report of two cases. Ann. Otol. Rhin. Laryng. 47, 649 (1938)

Robbins, S.L.: Lumbar vertebral chordoma. Arch. Path. (Chicago) 40, 128–132 (1945)

ROSENQUIST, H., SALTZMAN, G.F.: Sacrococcygeal and vertebral chordomas and their treatment. Acta radiol. (Stockh.) **52**, 177–193 (1959)

SASSIN, J.F., CHUTORIAN, A.M.: Intracranial chordoma in children. Arch. Neurol. **17**, 89–93 (1967)

SCHECHTER, M.M., LIEBESKIND, A.L., AZAR-KIA, B.: Intracranial chordomas. Neuroradiology **8**, 67–82 (1974)

SENNETT, E.J.: Chordoma: Its roentgen diagnostic aspects and its response to roentgen therapy. Amer. J. Roentgenol. **69**, 613–622 (1953)

STAPEL, T.W., EVENS, R.G., STEIN, A.H.: Arteriography in orthopedics. Arch. Surg. (Chicago) **97**, 682–690 (1968)

STEWART, M.J.: Malignant sacrococcygeal chordoma. J. Path. Bact. **25**, 40–63 (1922)

STEWART, M.J., MORIN, J.E.: Chordoma: A review with report of a new sacrococcygeal case. J. Path. Bact. **29**, 41–60 (1926)

STRICKLAND, B.: The value of arteriography in the diagnosis of bone tumours. Brit. J. Radiol. **32**, 705–713 (1959)

TAMPLIN, E.C.: The last ten years, some experiences and reflections. J. Laryng. Otol. **63**, 314–319 (1949)

TAVERAS, J.M., WOOD, E.: Diagnostic neuroradiology. Baltimore: Williams and Wilkins Company, 151, 152, 437, 438, 443, 926; 1964

TOOLE, H., IOANNOVICH, D.: Cervical chordoma: Diagnosis and operation: Discussion with a report of a case. Arch. Otolaryng. (Chicago) **72**, 219–226 (1960)

UTNE, J.R., PUGH, D.G.: The roentgenological aspects of chordoma. Amer. J. Roentgenol. **74**, 593–608 (1955)

WANG, C.C., JAMES, A.E.: Chordoma with a brief review of the literature and report of a case and widespread metastases. Cancer (Philad.) **22**, 162–167 (1968)

WILLIS, R.A.: Sacral chordoma with widespread metastases. J. Path. **33**, 1035–1043 (1930)

WINDEYER, B.W.: Chordoma. Proc. roy. Soc. Med. **52**, 1088–1100 (1959)

WOOD, E.: The roentgenologic diagnosis and treatment of chordoma. Trans. Amer. neurol. Ass. 17–23 (1950)

WOOD, E.H., HIMADI, G.M.: Chordomas: A roentgenologic study of sixteen cases previously unreported. Radiology **54**, 706–716 (1950)

WRIGHT, D.: Nasopharyngeal and cervical chordoma — Some aspects of their development and treatment. J. Laryng. **81**, 1337–1355 (1967)

YAGHMAI, I., SHAMSA, A.Z., SHARIAT, S., AFSHARI, R.: Value of arteriography in the diagnosis of benign and malignant bone lesions. Cancer (Philad.) **27**, 1134–1147 (1971)

ZINGESSER, L.H., SCHECHTER, M.M.: Radiology of masses lying within and adjacent to the tentorial hiatus. Brit. J. Radiol. **37**, 486–510 (1964)

Historical Review and Embryology of Chordoma

ALEZAIS, M., PEYRON, A.: Contribution a l'etude des chordomes; chordomes de la region occipitale. Bull. Ass. franç. Cancer, Paris: **7**, 194 (1914a)

ALEZAIS, M., PEYRON, A.: Sur une tendence évolutive remarquable de certains chordomes — Passage de l'épitheliome au sarcome polymorphe. Bull. Ass. franç. Cancer, Paris: **7**, 437 (1914b)

ALEZAIS, M., PEYRON, A.: Sur l'évolution cellulaire du tissu notochordal dans les tumeurs. C.R. Soc. Biol. (Paris) **83**, 368 (1920)

ANDRÉ-THOMAS, H., JUMENTIE, J.: Chordome de la region sphéno-basilaire. Rev. neurol. **30**, 300–304 (1923)

ARAUZ, S.L., PODESTA, R.: Cordomas malignos del cavum. Pren. méd. argent. **24**, 461–471 (1923)

AREY, L.B.: Developmental anatomy. A textbook and laboratory manual of embryology. Philadelphia: W.B. Saunders 1965

BAILEY, P., BAGDASAR, D.: Intracranial chordoblastoma. Amer. J. Path. **5**, 439–440 (1929)

BELLET, M., LE TREUT, A., AZALOUX, H., REBOUL, J.: Chordome vertébral à double localisation. Chaire Carcinol., Hôp. St. André, Bordeaux méd. **3**, 12, 2987–2998 (1970)

BERARD, L., DUNET, C.L., PEYRON, A.: Les chordomes de la region sacro-coccygienne et leur histogenèse. Bull. Ass. franç. Cancer, **2**, 28 (1922)

CAPPELL, D.F.: Chordoma of the vertebral column, with three new cases. J. Path. Bact. **31**, 797 (1928)

COENEN, H.: Das Chordom. Brun's Beitr. z. klin. Chir. **133**, 1 (1925)

FISCHER, B., STEINER: Über ein malignes Chordom der Schädel-Rückgratshöhle. Ziegler's Beitr., Jena **40**, 109 (1907)

FRORIEP, A.: Kopftheil der chorda dorsalis bei menschlichen Embryonen. Beitr. Anat. Embryol. als Festschr. f. F. G. J. Henle, pp. 26–40 (1882)

GAGE, S.P.: The notochord of the head in human embryos of the third to the twelfth week, and comparisons with other vertebrates. Science **24**, 295–296 (1906)

GRAHL, O.: Eine Ecchondrosis physalifora spheno-occipitalis ungewöhnlichen Umfangs (Inaug. Diss., Göttingen) 1903

HANSSON, C.J.: Chordoma in a thoracic vertebra. Acta radiol. (Stockh.) **22**, 598 (1941)

HASS, G.M.: Chordomas of cranium and cervical portion of the spine: Review of the literature with report of case. Arch. Neurol. Psychiat. (Chicago) **32**, 300–327 (1934)

HASSE: Ein neuer Fall von Schleimgeschwulst am Clivus. Virchows Arch. path. Anat. vol. **11**, 395 (1857)

HELLMANN, K.: Ein malignes Chordom des Nasenrachenraumes. Verh. dtsch. Ges. Hals-, Nas.- u. Ohrenärzte, p. 111 (1921)

Hennig, L.: Über congenitale echte Sacraltumoren. Beitr. path. Anat. **23**, 593–619 (1900)

Hirsch, C.: Zur Frage des malignen Chordoms. Z. Hals-, Nas.- u. Ohrenheilk. **28**, 140–146 (1931)

Horowitz, T.: Chordal ectopia and its possible relation to chordoma. Arch. Path. (Chicago) **31**, 354–362 (1941)

Huber, G.C.: On the relation of the chorda dorsalis to the anlage of the pharyngeal bursa of median pharyngeal recess. Anat. Rec., **6**, 373–404 (1912)

Hutton, A.J., Young, A.: Chordoma, report of two cases. A malignant sacrococcygeal chordoma and chordoma of the dorsal spine. Surg., Gynec. Obstet. **48**, 333–344 (1929)

Jaffe, H.L.: Tumors and tumorous conditions of bones and joints. Philadelphia: Lea & Febiger, 1958

Killian, G.: Über die Bursa and Tonsilla pharyngea. Eine entwicklungsgeschichtliche und vergleichende anatomische Studie. Morph. Jb. **14**, 618–711 (1888)

Kirschberg, A., Marchand, F.: Über die sogenannte fötale Rachitis (Micromelia Chondromalacia). Beitr. path. Anat. **5**, 183 (1889)

Klebs, E.: Ein Fall von Ecchondrosis spheno-occipitalis amylacea. Virchows Archiv, path. Anat. **31**, 396 (1864)

Klebs, E.: Die allgemeine Pathologie. Jena, **2**, 693 (1889)

Koritski, G.E.: Histogenesis and Localisation of Chordomata, Charkowsky med. J., **17**, 62 (1914)

Kunitoma, K.: The development and reduction of the tail and of the caudal end of the spinal cord. Contr. Embryol. Carneg. Inst. **8**, 163–197 (1918)

Lewis, N.D.C.: A contribution to the study of tumors from the primitive notochord. Arch. intern. Med., **28**, 434 (1921)

Lichtenstein, L.: Bone tumors, 4th ed.. St. Louis: C.V. Mosby Co. 1972

Linck, A.: Chordoma malignum, ein Beitrag zur Kenntnis der Geschwülste an der Schädelbasis. Zieglers Beitr., Jena **46**, 573 (1922a)

Linck, A.: Beitrag zur Kenntnis der menschlichen Chorda dorsalis im Hals und Kopfskelet. Anat. Hefte, **42**, 605–736 (1911)

Linck, A.: Über die Chorda dorsalis beim Menschen und die malignen Chordome an der Schädelbasis. Z. Hals-, Nas.- u. Ohrenheilk. **3**, 487–496 (1922b)

Linck, A., Warstat, H.: Zur Kenntnis der malignen Chordome in der Sacrococcygealgegend. Beitr. klin. Chir., **127**, 612–626 (1922)

Luschka, H.: Die Altersveränderungen der Zwischenwirbelknorpel. Virchows Arch. path. Anat. **9**, 311 (1856)

Luschka, H.: Über gallertartige Auswüchse am Clivus Blumenbachii. Virchows Arch. path. Anat. **11**, 8 (1857)

Miller, J.: Relationship of the notochord to the carti-

lage of the skull and its correlation with the location and frequencies of chordomata. Anat. Rec. **112**, 362 (1952)

Minot, C.S.: Segmental flexures of the notochord. Anat. Rec. **1**, 42–50 (1907)

Muller, H.: Über das Vorkommen von Resten der Chorda dorsalis bei Menschen nach der Geburt und über ihr Verhältnis zu den Gallertgeschwülsten am Clivus. Z. rationelle Med. **2**, 202 (1858)

Nebelthau, L.A.: Über die Gallertgeschwülste am Clivus Blumenbachii, Diss., Marburg, 1897

Orts Llorca, F., Sternberg, H.: Über regelwidrige Verbindungen der Chorda dorsalis mit dem Medullarrohre bei jungen menschlichen Embryonen. Anat. Anz. **78**, 335–341 (1934)

Patten, B.M.: Fusion of the notochord to neural tube in a human embryo of the sixth week. Anat. Rec. **95** (3), 307–309 (1946)

Patten, B.M.: Human embryology. New York: McGraw-Hill, 3rd ed. 1968

Peyron, A.: Tumeurs de la notochord. Atlas du cancer. Ass. franç. Cancer II 1923

Piraud, G.: La notochorde. Embryologie générale et experimentale. Vestiges et tumeurs. Paris: LeFrançois, 1933

Pototschnig, G.: Ein Fall von malignem Chordom mit Metastasen, Ziegler's Beitr., Jena, **65**, 356 (1919)

Ribbert, H.: Über die Ecchondrosis physalifora spheno-occipitalis. Centralb. allg. Path., Jena, **5**, 457 (1894)

Ribbert, H.: Über die experimentelle Erzeugung einer Ecchondrosis physalifora. Verh. d. Congr. inn. Med. Wiesbaden, **13**, 455 (1895)

Ribbert, H.: Geschwulstlehre, Bonn, p. 149, 1904

Rubaschow, S.: Zur onkologischen Kasuistik: Chordom mit ungewöhnlichem Sitz. Zbl. Chir. **56**, 137–138 (1929)

Russell, D.S., Rubinstein, L.J.: Pathology of tumours of the nervous system. Baltimore: Williams & Wilkins, 2nd ed. 1963

Schmorl, G.: Über Chordareste in den Wirbelkörpern. Zbl. Chir. **55**, 2305 (1928)

Schwabe, R.: Notochordal remnants in sacrum. Virchow's Arch. path. Anat. **287**, 651 (1933)

Sensenig, E.C.: The early development of the human vertebral column. Pub 583, Contr. Embryol, Carneg. Inst. **33**, 23–42 (1949)

Sensenig, E.C.: Adhesions of notochordal and neural tube tissues in the formation of chordomas. Anat. Rec. **112**, 388 (1952)

Sensenig, E.C.: Adhesions of notochord and neural tube in the formation of chordomas. Amer. J. Anat. **98**, 357 (1956)

Snook, T.: The later development of the bursa pharyngea: Homo. Anat. Rec. **58**, 303–320 (1934)

Stewart, M.J., Le F. Burrow, J.: Ecchondrosis physaliphora spheno-occipitalis. J. Neurol. Psychopath. **4**, 218–220 (1923)

Streeter, G.L.: Developmental horizons in human

embryos. Publ. 541, Contr. Embryol, Carneg. In-
stu. **30**, 211–245 (1942)

STREETER, G.L.: Developmental horizons in human
embryos. Publ. 557, Contr. Embryol. Carneg. Inst.
31, 27–63 (1945)

STREETER, G.L.: Developmental horizons in human
embryos. Publ. 575, Contr. Embryol. Carneg. Inst.
32, 133–203 (1948)

STREETER, G.L.: Developmental horizons in human
embryos. Prepared for publication by C.H. HENSER
and G.W. CORNER. Pub. 592, Contr. Embryol. Carneg. Inst. **34**, 165–196 (1951)

VIRCHOW, R.: Untersuchungen über die Entwicklung
des Schädelgrundes im gesunden und krankhaften
Zustand und über den Einfluß derselben auf Schä-
delform, Gesichtsbildung und Gehirn. Berlin: Reimer, 1857

WADDINGTON, E.M.: Principles of embryology, 2nd
ed. New York: Mac Millan Company, 1960

WILLIAMS, L.W.: The later development of the notochord in mammals. Amer. J. Anat. **8**, 251 (1908)

WILLIS, R.A.: Pathology of tumors, 2nd ed. London:
Butterworth 1967

ZENKER, F.A.: Über die Gallertgeschwülste des Clivus
Blumenbachii (Ecchondrosis prolifera, Virchow).
Virchows Arch. path. Anat. **12**, 108 (1857)

Pathology and Clinical Manifestations of Chordoma

Intracranial

DANZINGER, J., LEWER, A.K., BLOCH, S.: Intracranial
chordomas. Clin. Radiol. **25**, 309–316 (1974)

FORTI, E., VENTURINI, G.: Contributo alla conoscenza
delle neoplasie notocordali. Riv. Anat. pat. **17**,
317–396 (1960)

GIVNER, I.: Ophthalmologic features of intracranial
chordoma and allied tumors of the clivus. Arch.
Ophthal. N.Y., 2nd series **33**, 397–403 (1945)

GODTFREDSEN, E.: Eye and nerve symptoms in connection with cranial chordomas. Acta ophthal. (Kbh.)
21, 224–236 (1943)

HERZOG, G.: Chordome. HENKE, F., LUBERSCH, O.
(eds.). Handb. d. spez. path. Anat. u. Histol., Berlin, part 5, 9: 380–389, 451–454, 1944

LEWER-ALLEN, K., KERR, W.A.: Chordomas of the
clivus and the cervical spine. S. Afr. med. J. **42**,
1165–1174 (1968)

TONELLI, L.: I tumori della notocorda; clinica delle
diverse localizzazioni, studio istologico e proposta
di un nuovo schema ordinativo. Arch. Vecchi Anat.
pat. Med. clin. **15**, 471–607 (1950)

Nasopharyngeal

BATSAKIS, J.G.: Chordomas: Otorhinolaryngologic
presentation and diagnosis. Arch. Otolaryng. (Chicago) **78**, 168–175 (1963)

BOYLE, T.M.: The management of nasopharyngeal
chordoma by repeated irradiation. J. Laryng. **80**,
533–535 (1960)

CRIKELAIR, G.F.: Nasopharyngeal chordoma. Plast.
reconstr. Surg. **16**, 138–144 (1955)

ESSAMMAA, E.: Chordoma of the oropharynx. J. Laryng. **73**, 65–68 (1959)

HANDOUSA-BEY, A.E.: A case of nasopharyngeal chordoma. J. Laryng. **63**, 31–33 (1949)

HARRISON, D.F.N.: A case of primary chordoma of
the sphenoidal sinus. J. Laryng. **75**, 429–432 (1961)

LIVINGSTONE, G.: Chordoma of the base of the skull.
J. Laryng. **50**, 852–855 (1935)

ORTON, H.B.: Chordoma: Final report and re-evalua-
tion of treatment. Ann. Otol. (St. Louis) **62**,
371–391 (1953)

Vertebral

BAKER, H.W., COLEY, B.L.: Chordoma of lumbar vertebra. J. Bone Jt Surg. **35A**, 403 (1953)

CHIARI, H.: Über ein Chordom der Wirbelsäule. Zbl.
allg. Path. path. Anat. **42**, 481 (1928)

DYKE, C.G.: The roentgen-ray diagnosis of spinal cord
tumors in diagnostic roentgenology. GOLDEN, R.
(ed.). New York: Thomas Nelson & Sons, 1941

EPSTEIN, B.: The spine. A radiological text and atlas.
3rd ed. Philadelphia: Lea & Febiger, 1969

HUSAIN, F.: Chordoma of the thoracic spine. J. Bone
Jt Surg. **42-B**, 560 (1960)

IMPERATORI, C.J.: Chordoma of cervical region. Further report of such a condition operated upon two
years previously. Laryngoscope **58**, 1037–1043
(1948)

JONES, R.B.: Chordoma of the third lumbar vertebra
simulating carcinoma of the prostate with vertebral
metastasis. Brit. J. Surg. **208**, 162 (1960)

JOYCE, T.M.: Chordoma of the second and third cervical vertebrae. Surg. Clin. N. Amer. **13**, 85 (1933)

LEMAN, P., COHADEN, F., COHADEN, S.: Les chordomes
vertébraux. J. Chir. **89**, 485 (1965)

MEANEY, T.F., GREENWALD, C.M., PHALEN, G.S.:
Chordoma. Clin. Orthop. **7**, 103 (1956)

OWEN, C.I., HERSHEY, L.N., GURDJIAN, E.S.: Chordoma dorsalis of the cervical spine. Amer. J.
Cancer **16**, 830 (1932)

RAUL, P., DISS, A.: Chordome malin de la colonne
vertébrale lombaire. Bull. Soc. anat. Paris **94**, 935
(1924)

SYME, W.S., CAPPELL, D.F.: A case of chordoma of
the cervical vertebrae with involvement of the pharynx. J. Laryng. (Paris) **41**, 209–222 (1926)

TRELAT, B.: Enchondrome a marche rapide. Gaz. Hôp.
(Paris) **41**, 254 (1868)

Sacrococcygeal

ALEXANDER, W.A., STRUTHERS, J.W.: A sacrococcygeal chordoma. J. Path. Bact. **29**, 61–64 (1922)

LITTMAN, L.: Sacro-coccygeal chordoma – A review and presentation of three additional cases. Ann. Surg. **137**, 80–90 (1953)

Histology

ALEZAIS, M., PEYRON, A.: Sur l'histogenèse et l'origine des chordomes. C.R. Acad. Sci. (Paris) **174**, 419 (1922)

CRAWFORD, T.: The staining reactions of chordoma. J. clin. Path. **11**, 110 (1958)

EVANS, W.R.: Histological appearances of tumors. Chapter VIII, pp. 151–163. Baltimore: Williams & Wilkins Company, 1966

GESCHICKTER, C.F., COPELAND, M.M.: Tumors of bone, 3rd ed. Philadelphia and London: Lippincott, pp. 651, 1949

KNECHTGES, T.C.: Sacrococcygeal chordoma with sarcomatous features (Spindle cell metaplasia). Amer. J. clin. Path. **53**, 612–616 (1970)

RASMUSSEN, T.B., KERNOHAN, J.W., ADSON, A.W.: Pathologic classification with surgical consideration of intraspinal tumors. Ann. Surg. **111**, 513 (1940)

Metastasis

ARGADU, M.R., LESTRADE, A.: II. Sur la precocité de certains chordomes sacro-coccygienne. Bull. Acad. Méd. (Paris) **95**, 375–377 (1926)

CONWAY, C.A.G.: Case of sacro-coccygeal chordoma with extensive metastases. Mag. London (Roy. Free Hosp.). School Med. for Women, **24**, 7–9 (1929)

GRAF, L.: Sacrococcygeal chordoma with metastases. Arch. Path. (Chicago) **37**, 136–139 (1944)

GREENWALD, C.M., MEANEY, T.F., HUGHES, C.R.: Chordoma – Uncommon destructive lesion of cerebrospinal axis. J. Amer. med. Ass. **163**, 1240–1244 (1957)

GUTHERT, H., HENKEL, H.: Ein metastasierendes Chordom der Lendenwirbelsäule. Zbl. allg. Path. **77**, 376–380 (1941)

HIGHINBOTHAM, N.L., PHILLIPS, R.F., FARR, H.W., HUSTU, H.O.: Chordoma. Thirty-five year study at Memorial Hospital. Cancer (Philad.) **20**, 1841–1850 (1967)

McCORMACK, M.P.: Upper lumbar chordoma. J. Bone Jt Surg. **42 B**, 565 (1960)

McSWEENEY, A.J., SHOLL, P.R.: Metastatic chordoma. Use of mechlorenthamine (Nitrogen Mustard) in chordoma therapy. Arch. Surg. (Chicago) **79**, 152–155 (1959)

MAYNARD, R.B.: A case of chordoma with pulmonary metastasis. Aust. N.Z. J. Surg. **22**, 215–219 (1953)

MONTGOMERY, A.H., WOLTMAN, I.J.: Sacrococcygeal chordomas in children. Amer. J. Dis. Child **46**, 1263–1281 (1933)

MORRIS, A.A., RABINOVITCH, R.: Malignant chordoma of the lumbar region. Report of a case with autopsy; comment on usual metastases to the brain, lungs, pancreas, sacrum and axillary and iliac lymph nodes. Arch. Neurol. Psychiat. (Chicago) **57**, 547–564 (1947)

PETERS, W.: Ein rezidivierendes, bösartiges Chordom der sacrococcygealen Gegend mit Metastasen. Dtsch. Z. Chir. **151**, 191–199 (1919)

STOUGH, D.R., HARTZOG, J.T., FISHER, R.G.: Unusual intradural spinal metastasis. J. Neurosurg. **34-4**, 550–562 (1971)

UHR, N., CHURG, J.: Hypertrophic osteoarthropathy; report of a case associated with a chordoma of the base of the skull and lymphangitic pulmonary metastases. Ann. intern. Med. **31**, 681–691 (1949)

Treatment

AUST, J.B., ABSOLON, K.B.: A successful lumbosacral amputation, hemicorporectomy. Surgery **52**, 756 (1962)

CLARKE, T.H., WALSH, W.S.: Treatment of chordoma. In: Treatment of cancer and allied diseases, vol. **8**, 2nd ed., PACK, G.T., ARIEL, I.M. (Ed.). New York: Harper and Row, pp. 490–501, 1964

FRIEDMAN, M.: Technique of treatment of chordoma of a lumbar vertebra with 2 million volt x-rays using the rotation technique. Bull. Hosp. Jt Dis. (N.Y.) **14**, 180–187 (1953)

KENNEDY, C.S., MILLER, E.B., McLEAN, D.C., PERLIS, M.S., DION, R.M., HORVITZ, V.S.: Lumbar amputation or hemicorporectomy for advanced malignancy of the lower half of the body. Surgery **48**, 357 (1960)

MILLER, T.R., MACKENZIE, A.R., RANDALL, H.T., TIGNOR, S.P.: Hemicorporectomy. Surgery **59**, 988–993 (1966)

PATEL, J.C.: Hemicorporectomy. Presse méd. **68**, 2346 (1960)

PEARLMAN, A.W., SINGH, R.K., HOPPENSTEIN, R., WILDER, J.: Chordoma: Combined therapy with radiation and surgery: Case report and new operative approach. Bull. Hosp. Jt Dis. (N.Y.) **33**, 47–57 (1972)

ZOLTAN, L., FENYES, I.: Stereotactic diagnosis and radioactive treatment in case of spheno-occipital chordoma. J. Neurosurg. **17**, 888 (1960)

Adamantinoma (Malignant Angioblastoma) Schwannoma (Neurilemmoma), Neurofibroma

by

Howard F. Faunce

A. Adamantinoma Long Bones and Ameloblastoma—Jaw

I. Nomenclature

Adamantinoma of the appendicular skeleton is a rare but relatively distinctive primary bone neoplasm. This lesion was first described by FISCHER (1913). He was responsible for naming this long bone neoplasm adamantinoma. It was so named because of its close histologic resemblance to the benign, but potentially locally invasive, tumor of the mandible or maxilla, also called adamantinoma. This is a true neoplasm of enamel-type tissue which does not undergo differentiation to the point of enamel formation and is the classical adamantinoma of the jaw. Interestingly enough, aside from a close histologic resemblance, adamantinoma of long bones parallels certain clinical and many roentgenologic characteristics of the classical adamantinoma of the jaw. As it relates to long bones, however, the term ameloblastoma conveys incorrect meaning since it indicates a tumor composed of or originating from, the embryonal enamel forming cells. Enamel has never been found in these tumors. Adamantinoma is even more misleading since it indicates a tumor consisting of enamel.

Because of some significant similarities, it is appropriate to include a brief and basic description of adamantinoma of the mandible and maxilla so that one may be able to draw his own conclusions as to the relationship between this tumor and adamantinoma of long bones. Because this is an odontogenic tumor arising from enamel type epithelium, the preferred and now generally accepted term for this tumor is ameloblastoma. The term adamantinoma should not be used to designate this tumor in the jaw.

Ameloblastoma of the jaw accounts for approximately 1% of all tumors and cysts of the jaws. As is true with most other jaw tumors, these are thought to be more common in Africans than in the white races. In some parts of Africa, ameloblastomas account for 0.3% of all tumors. In general, they are much less common than periodontal cysts, dentigerous cysts, fissural cysts, and odontogenic keratocysts. The average age of onset is approximately 33 years. Half of these tumors occur between the ages of 20 and 30 years. Approximately 80% of ameloblastomas present in the mandible; and 75% of these are in the molar-ramus area. The most frequent clinical presentation is a painless swelling of the jaw. This is the basis for the dictum that all painless swellings of the jaw should be investigated roentgenologically before treatment is instituted. It begins as an asymptomatic central destructive lesion, enlarges slowly and causes progressive expansion of the overlying cortical bone. As the tumor enlarges, however, pain and deformity of the jaw and face occur. Occasionally, the tumor may rupture through the cortical plate and discharge fluid content into the oral cavity. Large tumors may lead to pathologic fracture.

Grossly, the tumor can be a solid or cystic soft tissue mass, depending on its size. The largest tumors tend to undergo degeneration and assume a cystic structure. Histologically it consists of a cellular connective tissue stroma in which there are present islands and strands of epithelial tumor cells. The presence of a connective tissue capsule is variable. The periphery of these structures is formed by cuboidal or columnar cells which resemble ameloblasts. In the central portion, stellate-shaped cells resembling the stellate reticulum of the enamel organ are present. The connective tissue stroma and the epithelial cells may undergo cystic degeneration accounting for occasional microscopic cystlike spaces. The gross cavitation previously mentioned is accounted for by the coalescence of these spaces. Various portions of a singular tumor may have considerable differences in histologic appearance. There are a number of different histologic types of ameloblastomas. These include: follicular, plexiform, acanthomatous, basal cell, and granular cell. The adenoameloblastoma (adenomatoid odontogenic tumor) is a distinct entity and should not be considered a variant of the ordinary ameloblastoma. This tumor contains ductlike structures scattered throughout the tumor mass. These are not true ducts. The lesion is encapsulated. It is seen earlier in life than the ordinary ameloblastoma, nearly always under the age of 30 and often under 20.

The origin of ameloblastoma of the jaw has been attributed to a variety of sources. These include the following: cell rests of the enamel organ (epithelial rests of Malassez), the dental lamina, the outer enamel epithelium, the dental follicle surrounding unerupted teeth, and the oral epithelium. It is important to note that the multi-potential lining epithelium of dentigerous (follicular) cysts has occasionally undergone transformation to an ameloblastoma. Dentigerous cysts are found in association with the crown of an unerupted or impacted tooth, most frequently in the area of the 3rd mandibular molar.

It is generally believed that the ameloblastoma is a benign tumor, although it behaves differently from simple cysts or tumors because it is locally invasive and tends to recur after removal. There have been reports claiming metastasis to the neck, thorax, lymph glands, and lung. In extremely rare instances, ameloblastoma has undergone transformation into a carcinoma. They tend to recur following incomplete surgical removal. The majority of recurrences manifest 10–15 years after surgery. Resection of this tumor, therefore, tends to be a more extensive procedure than the simple enucleation of a benign cyst or tumor. The value of diagnostic radiology, therefore, is to determine which tumors of the jaw are more likely to be an ameloblastoma so that proper preoperative planning of the surgical excision of the tumor can be done. It should be remembered that ameloblastomas account for only 1% of all cysts and tumors of the jaw and, therefore, it should not be considered the most probable diagnosis for all radiolucent jaw lesions.

Certain radiologic features, however, are found rather consistently in ameloblastoma and therefore the radiologic diagnosis can be made with a significant degree of certainty (Fig. 1). These are solitary bone lesions, and as previously stated, are found in the molar-ramus area of the mandible. It is a lytic lesion. The following roentgenographic features which, together, tend to typify this tumor are discussed in order of decreasing frequency as elaborated in a series of cases reported by McIvor (1974). As does any growing tumor or cyst, the ameloblastoma causes eventual expansion of the overlying plate of cortical bone. It appears that this is a more constant finding in ameloblastoma than in other tumors and cysts of the jaw. It was seen in 81% of the cases presented by McIvor (1974). The next most frequently encountered roentgenographic sign is the presence of a scalloped, well-defined cortical margin of the tumor. This is an uncommon feature of simple cysts and tumors of the jaw but was seen in 62% of the cases reviewed by McIvor (1974). In 46% of his cases, the tumor presented a multilocular appearance, again a rare finding in the simple cysts or tumors of the jaw. When the tumor is in association with the root of a tooth, there is frequent resorption of the root of that tooth but there is relatively little displacement of that tooth. Root resorption was seen in 31% of the cases discussed by McIvor (1974). Although it occurs rarely in simple cysts and tumors of the jaws, root resorption, when seen in these entities, is usually accompanied by significant displacement of the affected tooth. The incidence of perforation of the overlying cortical bone plate has probably been underestimated. It is important that this finding be searched for since it is by this means that ameloblastoma becomes locally invasive and spreads into adjacent soft tissues. The recurrent ameloblastomas in the series reported by McIvor (1974) showed perforation of the cortical plate in all instances. In addition, all of these recurrent lesions showed a scalloped cortical margin and a multilocular appearance. Serial roentgenographs are important in these cases for the purpose of demonstrating a progressively enlarging lesion. To summarize, the most important roentgenologic signs in ameloblastoma of the jaw in order of decreasing frequency are as follows: (1) Expansion of the cortical plate. (2) Scalloped cortical margin. (3) Multilocular appearance. (4) Resorption of adjacent tooth roots. When several of these roentgenologic findings are present in a particular tumor, the prebiopsy diagnosis of ameloblastoma can be made with relative certainty. Nevertheless, the roentgenologic differential diagnosis of this lesion would include the following cysts and tumors of the jaw: dentigerous (follicular) cyst, odontogenic keratocyst, fibroma, fibrosarcoma, hemangioma, aneurysmal bone cyst, giant cell tumor, giant cell reparative granuloma, fibrous dysplasia, ameloblastic fibroma, adenoameloblastoma, and ameloblastic sarcoma. The nature of this discussion does warrant a description of how these tumors and cysts differ from one another and more importantly how they can be differentiated from an ameloblastoma. Excellent discussions of this subject can be found in the articles by Robinson et al. (1967) and McIvor (1974).

The treatment of choice for this lesion is wide surgical excision. Ameloblastoma of the jaw is a radioresistant tumor.

In 1913, Fischer first recognized adamantioma of long bone as a separate entity. He described a case involving the tibia. Because of the considerable amount of epithelial

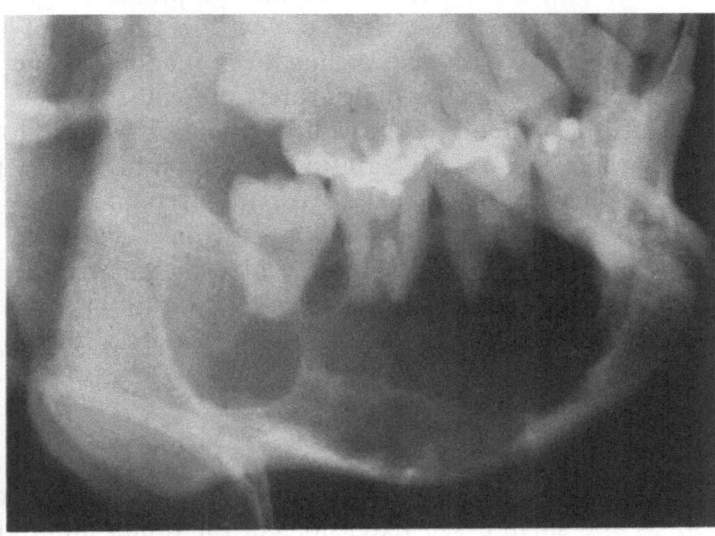

Fig. 1. Typical ameloblastoma of mandible showing expansion of cortical plate, a scalloped cortical margin, a multilocular appearance, and resorption of adjacent tooth roots

components comprising the tumor, he speculated that it arose from abnormal embryonal invagination of fetal epithelium within the bone. Because of the similarities to the adamantinoma (ameloblastoma) of the jaw, FISCHER applied the name adamantinoma of the tibia. Since the first 17 reported cases of this lesion occurred exclusively within the shaft of the tibia, until 1942 it was referred to as adamantinoma of the tibia. Since that time it has become known as adamantinoma of long bones since at least 14 cases have been reported in sites other than the tibia. In 1957, CHANGUS et al. suggested that this tumor was derived from primitive mesenchymal cells, i.e., angioblasts, and that therefore the name be changed to malignant angioblastoma of bone. Recent discussions of this tumor in the literature use both the term adamantinoma of long bones and malignant angioblastoma. There is no apparent consensus of opinion as to the proper nomenclature of this tumor at this time. However, much recent evidence, although subjective, yields fairly convincing evidence that these tumors are in fact of an angioblastic origin and therefore the term malignant angioblastoma would appear more fitting.

II. Clinical

DAHLIN (1957) states that adamantinoma of long bones comprises 0.33% of all primary malignant bone tumors. Approximately 100 cases of this tumor have been reported in the literature.

As reported by MOON (1965), of 91 cases studied, 37 were found in female and 54 in male. The tumor, therefore, tends to have a slight male predominance. The peak age range is between 11 and 50 years. The youngest recorded patient with this tumor was a 10-year-old female. The oldest patient was a 62-year-old female. In females, the peak incidence is between ages 11 and 30. In males, the peak incidence is between ages 31 and 50. By far, the most common site of this tumor is the tibia. It most often is found in the middle or distal one-third of the diaphysis. With the tibia being by far the most common site, the tumor is found in the following long bones in order of decreasing frequency: ulna, fibula, femur, humerus, radius. The short bones in which the tumor has been reported are one case in the carpal capitate and one case in the tarsal 1st cuneiform. The tumor is not found in the vertebral column although a case report by BESEMMAN et al. (1967) suggests the possibility of a metastasis to T12 from a primary adamantinoma in the left humerus.

The outstanding feature of the symptomatology is the extremely long duration of symptoms. This attests to the slow growth rate of these tumors. The most frequent symptom is a painless swelling over the site of the tumor. Less often there will be a painful swelling. The tumor rarely presents with pain alone. The duration of symptoms before the patient seeks medical attention varies from months to years. There is no data which relates the duration of symptoms to the prognosis. Many patients present with a history of trauma to the involved bone but as in many other bone tumors, this appears to be more of an incidental occurrence which merely draws attention to the underlying lesion. On physical examination one usually notes a firm, fixed, and most often, nontender swelling in relation to the bone.

III. Pathology

On gross inspection, adamantinoma of long bones is a pink, fleshy, soft, or firm growth which rarely grows into the soft tissues. There may be an admixture of solid areas and small cysts. Extensions of the tumor along the medullary cavity have a linear configuration. The bone surrounding the tumor has a more dense appearance than normal. In no case has the tumor contained a tooth or enamel. As pointed out by ANDERSON et al. (1942), calcification may be present. BISHOP (1937) described a case where the overlying skin was affected. The external contour of the lesion may be smooth or lobulated. A capsule may or may not be present. In those tumors with cystic cavities, the cavities may be filled with a straw colored fluid or blood.

The typical microscopic appearance is that of small "epithelial" islands contained within a fibrous stroma (Fig. 2). There is considerable variation in the relative amount of these two components in anyone tumor. In addition, the "epithelial" islands vary in structure and shape. They may have a loose central arrangement of cells, forming a microcystic center which is surrounded by peripheral palasading of "basal-appearing" cells. They may also be composed of large masses of small spindle cells which occasionally have a peripheral palisade of cuboidal cells. Other areas may show vascular-appearing channels which are lined with cells similar to those forming the "epithelial" islands. Frequently, one may see a transition between the cellular islands and vascular channels. Two lesions as reported by UNNI et al. (1974) showed mature squamous cells with "keratin pearls." For the most part, the epithelial cells showed rare mitotic figures appearing, therefore, relatively inactive. On rare occasions, the lesions may contain larger cells with frequent mitotic figures. The fibrous areas of the tumor have been described as containing significant numbers of fibroblasts. These tend to arrange themselves in a spiral fashion. In certain areas the tumor may resemble fibrous dysplasia with irregular trabeculae of calcified osteoid contained within the fibrous stroma. In the majority of these cases, however, islands of epithelial cells could be found on careful scrutiny of the histologic sections. The fibrous components of the tumors are not atypical enough to suggest fibrosarcoma. Unusual histologic features have been reported. UNNI

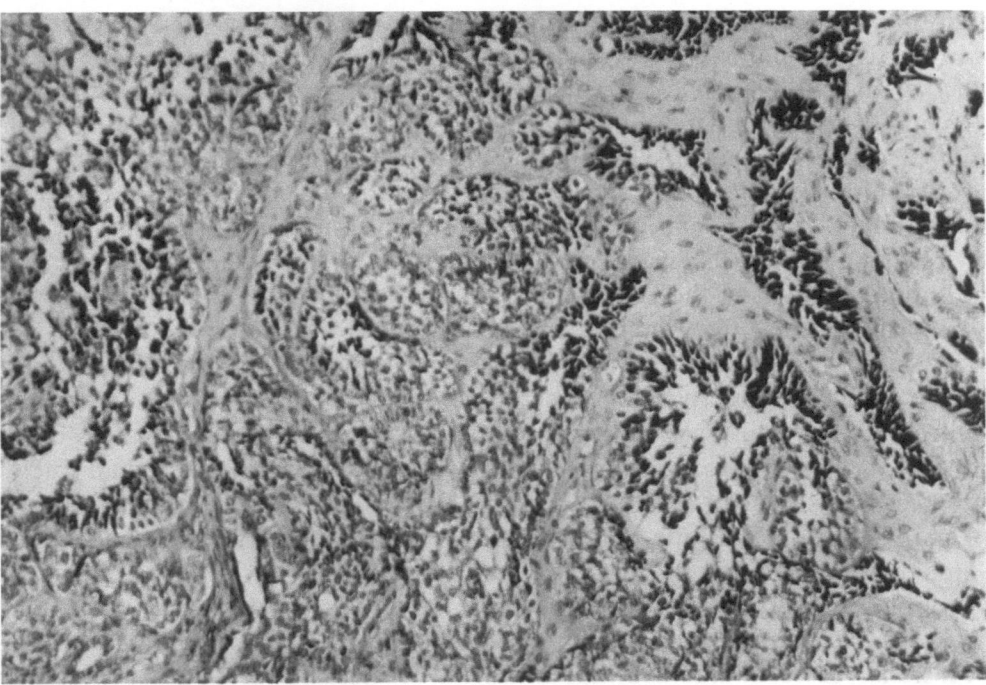

Fig. 2. Photomicrograph of adamantinoma (malignant angioblastoma) of tibia (Figs. 3a, b). Note "epithelial" islands contained in a fibrous stroma; a typical microscopic appearance of this lesion. (Courtesy of Issa Yaghmai, M.D., Medical College of Virginia Hospitals, Richmond, Virginia)

et al. (1974) has described the rare occurrence of benign osteoclastlike giant cells and psammoma bodies in these tumors. BAKER et al. (1954) described a less common pattern characterized by islands of spindle cells which may suggest a diagnosis of spindle cell sarcoma. Variations in the microscopic appearance of this tumor can include the following patterns: basal cell, adenocystic basal cell, squamous cell, ameloblastic, or a sarcomatoid pattern. This pleomorphic picture of the histology is the primary reason that the pathogenesis of this tumor is under considerable controversy. Occasionally, amyloidlike material is seen on light microscopy. Under the electron microscope this has been demonstrated to represent interlacing fibers which form large masses and appear to be tonofibrils. Another important feature of electron microscopy was the presence of tonofilaments and tonofibrils, particularly at the periphery of the cells. Occasionally, the histologic differentiation between adamantinoma and metastatic adenocarcinoma to bone may be quite difficult due to the fact that certain portions of adamantinomas may appear glandular. If sufficient sections are obtained, a thorough search of these will usually reveal more characteristic histologic findings of adamantinoma, making the differentiation possible. To establish a histologic diagnosis of adamantinoma it is necessary to demonstrate "epithelial" islands. It is important to note that these islands may be extremely small in portions of the tumor and therefore an extensive search of the sections may be required to establish the diagnosis. Clinical information is also helpful. Metastatic adenocarcinoma to bone occurs in a generally older age group than adamantinoma. The pleomorphic appearance of adamantinoma may also cause difficulties in differentiating this lesion from synovial sarcoma.

Since FISCHER's (1913) original description of this tumor, multiple theories for the pathogenesis of this tumor have been postulated. As previously noted, FISCHER (1913) originally named this tumor because of noted similarities in the appearance of this an adamantinoma (ameloblastoma) of the jaw. These included the gross appearance, the fibrous connective tissue, and the palisading of the "basal-appearing" cells. He theorized that the tumor represented a primary epithelial tumor which originated from the embryonal epithelium of the enamel germ of the teeth. He stated that the enamel germ in the tibia developed at the time of the formation of the tooth anlage. At this time, the ectodermal elements in the legs of the embryo had the potentiality to develop into enamel epithelial anlage. He felt that this enamel epithelial anlage grew toward and finally sunk into the bone in the tibial location exactly as it does in the jaw. It has been stated that trauma may play a role in stimulating growth of this enamel anlage. RYRIE (1932) felt that basal cells were implanted into bone at the time of injury. Even without a break in the overlying skin, he felt that the trauma caused damage to the deeper structures, resulting in implantation into the underlying bone. Other observers on reviewing (FISCHER's (1913) original material concluded that his case may have, in fact, represented a synovial sarcoma. The theory that the tumor may then represent an intraosseous synovial sarcoma was proposed. It appeared less difficult to explain a tumor derived from mesenchymal tissue arising within bone than one derived from ectodermal tissue. COHEN et al. (1962) pointed out the association of fibrous dysplasia and adamantionoma of long bones. There are similarities in the stroma of adamantinoma and that of fibrous dysplasia. It was then questioned whether the stroma of fibrous dysplasia could be multipotential with the ability to form either adamantinoma or irregular bone trabeculae. If this theory were correct, it is reasonable to assume that occasional cases of adamantinoma would be found in patients with polyostotic fibrous dysplasia. In the many cases of polyostotic fibrous dysplasia reported in the literature, no case of associated adamantinoma has been described. It is therefore felt that the fibrous dysplasia existing in association with adamantinoma is different from that seen in polyostotic fibrous dysplasia. Café au lait spots on the skin, which are seen in polyostotic fibrous dysplasia, have not been present in patients with adamantinoma associated with fibrous dysplasia. Furthermore, studies by UNNI et al. (1974) show that the fibrous areas do not represent classic fibrous dysplasia in that islands of epithelial cells have been demonstrated in these areas reminiscent of fibrous dysplasia. These authors went on to state that the epithelial nature of the cells of the tumor were confirmed on observations from electron microscopy. A more recent theory of the pathogenesis of this tumor has been elaborated by CHANGUS et al. (1957). He showed rather convincing data disploying histochemical and morphologic evidence that the tumor is of angioblastic origin. The term angioblast is used to designate the vascular mesenchyme that is the earliest specialized tissue anlage of the vascular system. On histochemical studies, CHANGUS et al. (1957) showed a similar positive alkaline phosphatase reaction on comparison of unfixed bone-free tissue of these tumors and blood vessel tissue. When the epithelial cells of two proven adamantinomas of the jaw were subjected to this same histochemical test, the alkaline phosphatase reaction was negative. The authors, in this sense, demonstrated a basic difference between the tissue of these tumors and the classical ameloblastoma of the jaw. In addition, by morphologic means CHANGUS et al. (1957) demonstrated that the majority of the normal tissue changes which take place (the process of liquefaction of angioblasts) during the formation of blood vessels are recognizable in adamantinomas of long bones as almost similar changes. The majority of these tumors, which are thoroughly studied, show vascular spaces suggesting angioblastic proliferation. Multiple sections of the tumor, however, must be evaluated to delineate the manifold patterns present within the same tumor. In the histologic diagnosis of this tumor, angiosarcoma should always be ruled out since, in limited fields, this tumor may show histologic patterns resembling rudimentery vessels. It has, therefore, been proposed that this tumor now go under the name of malignant angioblastoma of bone. In the current literature, one still finds the term adamantinoma of long bones and at present there is no clear cut consensus as to which term is more appropriate, although it appears that most authors now agree that the tumor is of a vascular origin. It is important to note that none of the theories on pathogenesis can explain why these tumors tend to occur almost exclusively in the tibia.

Because of the protracted history of adamantinoma of long bones, most early observers considered it benign. This, however, is definitely not the case and the lesion should be considered a formidable one and treated accordingly. As stated by ROSEN and SCHWINN (1966), a long-term follow-up of 27 cases revealed local recurrence in 16 cases and biopsy proven metastasis in 4 cases. Approximately 35% of reported cases show metastasis. Metastasis has been reported to the inguinal lymph nodes by BAKER et al. (1954) and MANGALIK and LAL MEHROTRA (1952), to the lung by NAJI et al. (1964), to the abdominal viscera by BAKER et al. (1954), and to the ribs by MORGAN and MACKENSIE (1956). In one of the cases reported by HUVOS and MARCOVE (1975), a metastasis from the tibia to the humerus was reported. In the case reported by BESEMMAN et al. (1967), a suspected metastatic lesion to the body of the 12th thoracic vertebra from a primary adamantinoma in the left humerus was reported. The recurrence rate of this tumor is nearly 50%.

IV. Roentgenology

The roentgenographic appearance of adamantinoma of long bones is, in general, that of a lesion beginning within bone which is growing at a moderate speed but not showing rapid spread up or down the shaft of the bone (THEROS and ISHAK, 1967).

The roentgenographic appearance, more often than not, is quite suggestive of the diagnosis. Many times, however, identification of the tumor has not been estabilished before surgical intervention. This is probably due to the rarity with which this tumor is encountered. The most frequent site of the tumor is in the distal third of the diaphysis of the tibia. As previously stated, the tumor has been encountered in all of the long bones of the body. The tumor can be multicentric as demonstrated by the simultaneous occurrence in both the tibia and fibula in three cases reported by UNNI et al. (1974). These authors also described one case with a presenting lesion in the humerus. On autopsy, there was also involvement of the ribs, vertebrae, and pubis. These secondary sites may have been metastatic foci. However, in the absence of any evidence of concomitant visceral metastasis, one feels it is more likely that they represented a multifocal origin of the tumor. In most instances, however, the tumor is solitary. Classically the tumor is a sharply defined, eccentric, lobular, lytic lesion. The bone is usually expanded and shows varying amounts of cortical destruction (Fig. 3). Occasionally there is a "sawtoothed" area of cortical bone loss. This finding is quite characteristic of this tumor (Fig. 4). The margin of the tumor is usually quite well-defined and with time becomes rather dense. It is important to note that most times the tumor extends beyond these apparent margins. It can appear as a solitary cystic lesion but more frequently has a multicystic appearance. The intervening bone between the cystic areas is abnormally dense. The tumor may break through the cortex and show various amounts of periosteal reaction and soft tissue mass. As is the case with fibrous dysplasia, periosteal reaction is more common when these undergo pathologic fracture (Fig. 5). Typically, one of

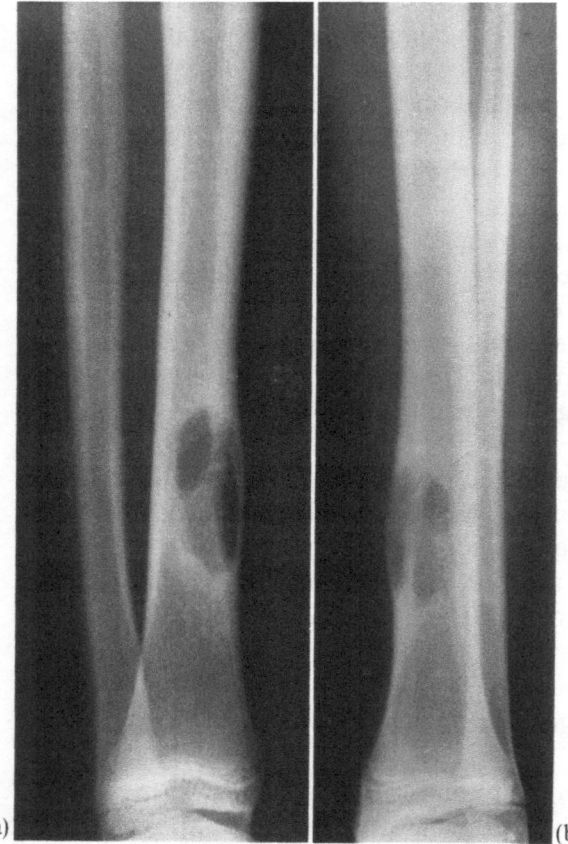

(a)
(b)

Fig. 3. Adamantinoma (malignant angioblastoma) of tibia in 11-year-old female. (a) Anterior view. (b) Lateral view. (Courtesy of Issa Yaghmai, M.D., Medical College of Virginia Hospitals, Richmond, Virginia)

the lytic areas is larger than the rest and the multiplicity of cystic areas occasionally gives these tumors a "soap bubble" appearance. This appearance is said to be more common in long standing lesions. The more malignant the lesion, the less distinctive is this "soap bubble" or "honeycombed" pattern (THEROS and ISHAK, 1967). Occasionally the tumor may involve only the cortical bone, sparing the medullary cavity. More rarely they may arise on the surface of the tibia (THEROS and ISHAK, 1967). The tumor can involve significantly large portions of the shaft of a particular bone. In a case reported by ANDERSON et al. (1942), two-thirds of the shaft of an ulna was involved with the tumor. In such cases, the shaft of the bone may be appreciably widened and deformed. DONNER and DIKLAND (1966) reported a long-standing case with roentgenograms covering a period of 17 years. Initial studies showed a fairly extensive radiopaque lesion. Fibrous dysplasia was originally considered a good possibility. Later roentgenograms revealed a loss of radiopacity with a simultaneous gradual transformation into a multicystic lesion. Metastatic lesions to other bones have similar roentgen features but show a prominent osteoblastic component (EDEIKEN and HODES, 1973). The roentgenologic differential diagnosis includes the following: aneurysmal and other bone cysts, giant cell tumor, nonossifying fibroma, solitary fibrous dysplasia, chondrosarcoma, eosinophilic granuloma, angiosarcoma (hemangioendothelioma), metastatic carcinoma from an unknown primary site, and occasionally reticulum cell sarcoma.

The angiographic findings in a histologically proven case involving the left femoral shaft were reported by ROSEN and SCHWINN (1966). This case showed displacement of the muscular branches of the deep femoral artery about a soft tissue mass in the

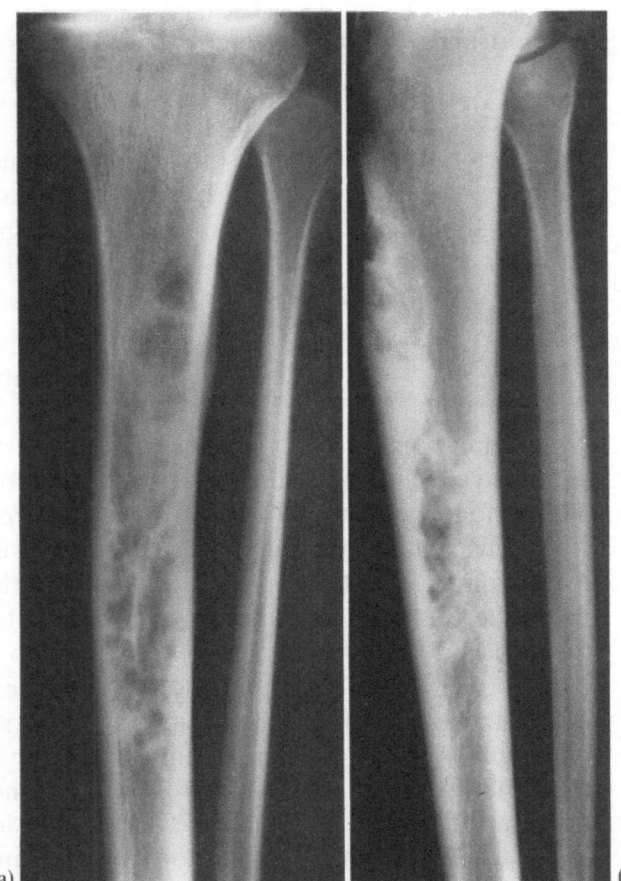

Fig. 4. Adamantinoma (malignant angioblastoma) of tibia. Note "saw tooth" appearance of inner cortical margin, a rather characteristic finding in this lesion. A. Anterior view. B. Lateral view. (Courtesy of Klaus Ranniger, M.D., Medical College of Virginia Hospitals, Richmond, Virginia)

(a)

(b)

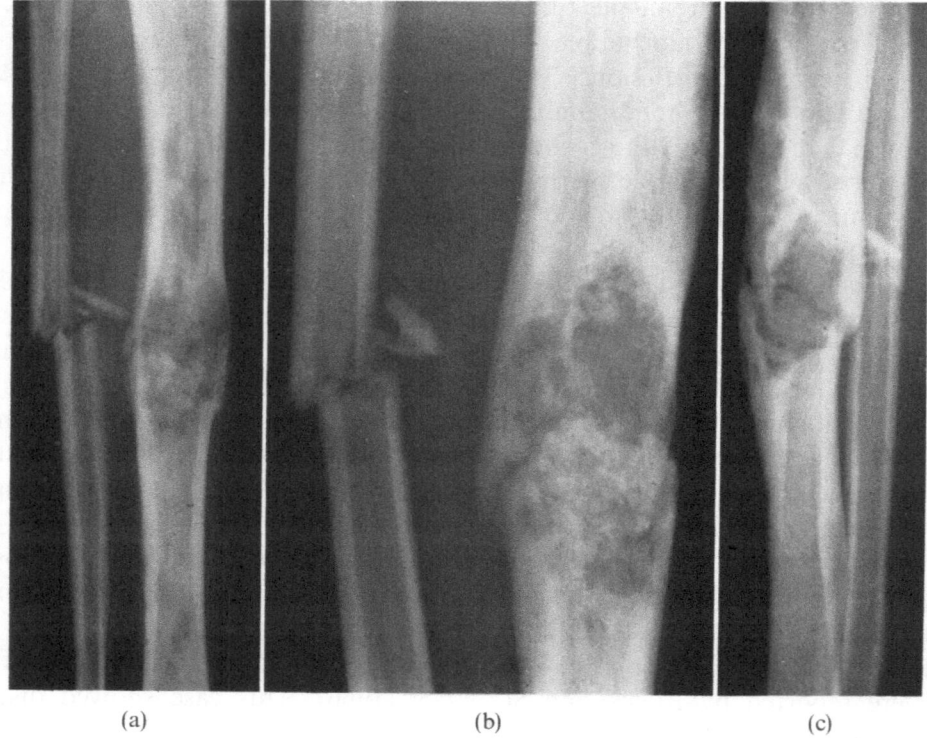

(a)   (b)   (c)

Fig. 5a–c. Adamantinoma (malignant angioblastoma) of tibia with pathologic fracture. Note multicentric involvement of tibia (Figs. a and c). (a) Anterior view. (b) Close-up anterior view. (c) Lateral view. (Courtesy of Department of Pathology and Radiology; W.H. Talbot, M.D., Pathologist, Rockingham Memorial Hospital, Harrisonburg, Virginia)

early arterial phase. Best seen in the parenchymal phase, this soft tissue mass was vascular and contiguous with the periosteum. The vessels supplying this mass were abnormal in extent and number. The areas of greatest bone destruction revealed abnormal vascular channels. The angiography of bone tumors is discussed in greater detail in other sections of this book.

V. Treatment

Adamantinoma of long bones is a low grade malignancy. In the past, this has engendered a feeling of complacency which led to a leisurely approach as regards treatment. This is no longer justified and aggressive treatment should be instituted once the diagnosis is established. Local recurrence and metastasis should be considered almost a certainty if the tumor is not completely removed at the time of initial treatment. It should be remembered that the tumor may be present as long as 17 years without developing metastasis. Although metastasis may develop much later, in 25% of patients it occurs from 1 to 8 years after the onset of symptoms (EDEIKEN and HODES, 1973). Surgery is the treatment of choice. If the lesion is relatively small and localized at the time of diagnosis, bloc excision of the tumor focus is justifiable as an attempt to salvage the limb. In such cases close follow-up is necessary and in the event of recurrence, amputation should be performed. In those lesions which, when found, have invaded too extensively to make resection feasible, amputation proximal to the involved bone is the treatment of choice. These tumors are highly radio-resistant. An isolated case of an apparent cure of the tumor with radiotherapy has been reported by ZAND et al. (1972). MORGAN and MACKENSIE (1956) reported shrinkage of an adamantinoma of the ribs to one-fifth its original size employing a tumor dose of cobalt 60 between 4524 (minimum) and 6032 R (maximum). Other than this, there is little evidence that radiation therapy is of value in treatment of these tumors and it should be stressed that the primary therapeutic modality is aggressive undelayed surgery.

B. Schwannoma (Neurilemmoma)

I. Nomenclature

Schwannoma of bone is one of four tumors of bone which are of nerve origin. The other three include neurofibroma, ganglioneuroma, and malignant schwannoma. The schwannoma (neurilemmoma) is a histologically specific tumor of nerve sheath origin. It is a benign encapsulated tumor arising from the sheath of Schwann, and is found occurring along the course of peripheral, cranial, and sympathetic nerves. As pointed out by FISCHER and VUZEVSKI (1968), the principal cellular elements of this tumor have been proven by tissue culture technique to be of Schwann cell origin. Although it has been popular to also designate this tumor as a neurilemmoma, these authors adhere to the designation of schwannoma since it most aptly describes the true histologic nature of this tumor. The term neurilemmoma actually signifies the sheath of Plenk-Laidlaw or basement membrane of Schwann cells rather than the cells per se. In most of the radiologic literature, the terms schwannoma and neurilemmoma have been used with almost equal frequency. Since the term schwannoma appears more histologically specific, I also prefer the use of this term. Other synonyms for the tumor include: lemmocytoma, neurilemmoblastoma, perineural fibroblastoma, neurinoma, peripheral oligodendrocytoma, and acoustic neuroma. VEROCAY gave the first histologic description of this tumor in 1908, at that time designating it a neurinoma. FAWCETT and DAHLIN (1967) found 31 schwannomas of bone reported in the literature.

II. Clinical

As may be inferred from the preceding paragraph, this tumor is an exceedingly rare primary bone tumor. It comprises a fraction of 1% of neoplasms arising in bone. As reported by FAWCETT and DAHLIN (1967), only 7 schwannomas were identified in a series of 3987 histologically verified primary bone tumors at the Mayo Clinic. All 7 of these were benign. No malignant neurogenic tumors of bone were recognized in this material. These tumors have been found between the age ranges of $2^1/_2$ and 65 years. Most cases fall in the age range between the second and sixth decades of life. By far the most frequent site of involvement is the mandible. This is primarily because of the long segment of the mandibular nerve contained within this bone. For similar reasons, the next most frequent site is the sacrum. Following these two sites, less frequent areas of involvement in order of occurrence include: the humerus, the femur, the ulna, the metacarpals, the phalanges, the fibula, the patella, the ribs, and the scapula. On a percentage basis, the mandible has been involved in approximately 33% of cases, the appendicular skeleton in approximately 33%, the sacrum in approximately 9%, and the ribs in approximately 9.5%. Primary schwannoma in bone has not been reported

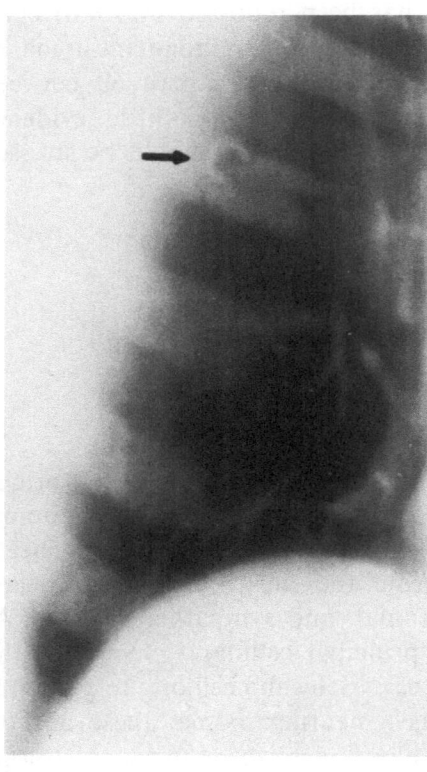

Fig. 6. Intraosseous schwannoma (neurilemmoma) of third anterior rib. (Courtesy of Matthew B. Divertie, M.D., Mayo Clinic,
Rochester, Minnesota; from Divertie, M.B., DAHLIN, D.C.:
Neurilemmoma of rib; Report of a case. Dis. Chest **44**, 635–637
(1963). (With permission of the publisher)

in the calvarium. DICKSON et al. (1971) reported an intraosseous schwannoma of the
third lumbar vertebrae. It has not been reported in the cervical or thoracic spine.

There is no typical clinical symptomatology of patients presenting with this lesion.
For the most part, the tumor is of long duration when first seen. The most common
and often the only symptom is the physical presence of the tumor. Most often this
is manifested only by local pain. Localized swelling and point tenderness may accompany
larger tumors. The patient therefore may have pain alone, swelling, or swelling combined
with pain. Frequently the patient will present with a pathologic fracture through the
lesion. As an example of the long duration of symptoms, AGHA and LILIENFELD (1972)
reported a patient with a 7-year history of a mass on the thenar eminence of the right
hand. The patient only developed pain during the latter 3 months before admission
to the hospital. This lesion proved to be a solitary intraosseous schwannoma of the
distal first metacarpal. Occasionally, the lesion may be found as an incidental finding.
This is especially true in the case of schwannoma involving a rib (Fig. 6). This was
true in cases reported by DIVERTIE and DAHLIN (1963) and FAWCETT and DAHLIN (1967).
Both of these case reports described schwannoma of a rib which was discovered on
chest roentgenography. Neither patient had symptoms referable to the rib lesion, and
in both cases the rib lesion was confused with a pulmonary parenchymal lesion.

III. Pathology

Of the seven cases reported by FAWCETT and DAHLIN (1967), the size of the gross
lesions measured from 6 to 8 cm in diameter. Those lesions which can be removed
in toto are fully encapsulated. They are distinctly separate and well-demarcated from

the adjacent bone. They are basically central tumors although they may perforate through the adjacent cortical bone or more frequently may protrude through a nutrient foramina producing a dumbbell-shaped lesion. Those tumors removed from the mandible show a close association with the mandibular nerve. For the most part, the lesions are solitary. When multiple, they are usually in association with von Recklinghausen's neurofibromatosis. The smaller tumors are usually white and round, oval, or fusiform in shape. They are usually firm in consistency. The larger tumors are irregularly shaped, may appear grayish or yellowish-white on sectioning, and contain occasional cystic areas. Hemorrhagic fluid may occupy these cystic spaces.

On light microscopy, there are two classic histologic patterns that are diagnostic of this lesion. The first of these types is called "Antoni A" tissue. This is characterized by solid appearing nodules of compact bundles and whorls of Schwann cells. The nuclei of these cells are aligned in rows or palisades. Occasionally, these Schwann cells assume an organized arrangement similar to tactile corpuscles. When present, these formations are called Verocay bodies. Between the palisades of Schwann cells, the cell processes are fused into hyaline masses. All of this is set in a matrix of collagen tissue of variable density. The second characteristic histologic pattern is "Antoni B" tissue. This consists of a loose meshwork of edematous myxomatous and microcystic tissue. Dispersed within this are widely separated Schwann cells and lipidic histiocytes. An important component of this pattern is aggregations of dilated blood vessels with thickened hyaline walls, perivascular hyaline deposits and fibrinous mural thrombi. Also seen are areas of old and recent hemorrhage with hemosiderin deposits in macrophages. The entire tumor may consist of either Antoni A or Antoni B tissue. Other tumors show mixed areas of these two histologic tissue types. Nerve fibers may be found in the peripheral portion of the tumor and are often found in the capsule. These, however, are not an integral part of the neoplasm. Histiocytes and lymphocytes may also be found interspersed within the tumor tissue. These are not found in prominent numbers. Some of the cells may show irregular hyperchromatic nuclei. These apparently represent degenerative changes and are present in some areas in the majority of these neoplasms. On cursory examination, these cells may appear malignant. They are not an uncommon finding in extraosseous schwannomas. A helpful feature in the differentiation from a malignancy is the total lack of mitotic activity in the usual schwannoma. The histologic differential diagnosis rests between other benign fibrous lesions of bone. It may mimic fibrous dysplasia but histologically it lacks the metaplastic osteoid tissue found in fibrous dysplasia. It may also mimic fibroma of bone but the histology of the schwannoma lacks the giant cells found in fibroma. Finally, it may mimic desmoplastic fibroma. Schwannoma, however, lacks the whorled dense fibrous tissue found in this lesion.

The principle cellular elements in both Antoni A and B tissue has been established by tissue culture techniques and electron microscopic study as attributed to Schwann cells (FISCHER and VUZEVSKI, 1968). Most observers now believe that these studies provide sufficient evidence to supercede earlier, rather tenuous histologic or embryologic considerations suggesting these tumors have an origin of fibroblastic nature. Most of these tumors arising in the mandible originate from the mandibular nerve. It is not surprising, therefore, that this is the most frequent site of these tumors. For similar reasons, it is also not surprising that the tumor is found quite frequently in the sacrum. It has not been possible to demonstrate direct connection with nerves in tumors in other bones. It is surprising how little attention has been paid in the literature, in both textbooks of anatomy and books devoted solely to bone, to the nerve supply of bone. SCHERMAN (1963) concludes that: (1) Human bones of any age demonstrate a rich nerve supply. (2) The nerves in bone are usually associated with arterial vessels and most of these

nerves are nonmyelinated. (3) The nerves in bone are probably derived from the auto-
nomic nervous system and are concerned with the regulation of blood flow. The sensory
nerves of bone are located in the periosteum. This tends to explain why a small osteoid
osteoma can cause intense throbbing pain, but a sarcoma which arises centrally in
a major bone is often silent until it has grown to a size sufficient to irritate the periosteum.
Considering these facts, therefore, it is not surprising that one of the cases reported
by Samter et al. (1960), which was a rather small schwannoma located subperiosteally
in the humerus presented with pain and tenderness. Although, as stated by Divertie
and Dahlin (1963), no connections between intraosseous nerves and tumors in bone
have been demonstrated, it is logical to postulate that these tumors arise from the
small nerves accompanying nutrient vessels.

Fawcett and Dahlin (1967) stated, that in the seven schwannomas, which were
identified in a series of 3987 histologically verified primary bone tumors, no malignant
neurogenic tumors were recognized. Samter et al. (1960) stated that to their knowledge
no case of malignant change in a schwannoma has been observed. In 1934, a case
of a primary intramedullary neurogenic sarcoma (malignant schwannoma) involving
the ulna was reported by Peers. Roentgenograms of that lesion showed an expanding
fusiform tumor arising within the medullary cavity of the ulna and pushing a fairly
complete thin shell of cortical bone before it. Thin bony septa divided the tissue into
large locules giving it a "soap bubble" appearance. There was no periosteal reaction.
From this description it is evident that the tumor had many features suggesting benignity.
Samter et al. (1960) reviewed the histologic illustrations in this case and felt these were
consistent with a benign schwannoma. Furthermore, metastases were not noted clinically
at the time the case was recorded. Certain reports mention the persistence of the tumor
following surgical removal. For the most part, these have been large tumors and incomplete removal at first operation, not malignant degeneration, has been the cause
of this persistence. Ghosh et al. (1973) reviewed 902 patients with tumors of the peripheral
nervous system which were treated at the Memorial Sloan-Kettering Cancer Center
between 1920 and 1970. Of these cases, 150 fulfilled strict criteria for the clinicopathologic
diagnosis of malignant schwannoma. They described tumors of the peripheral nerves
arising most frequently in the extremities, then trunk, and the head and neck. They
also showed the association of malignant schwannoma with plexiform neuroma or von
Recklinghausen's disease as signifying a more malignant tumor carrying a poorer prognosis. At no point in the article, however, did they describe a malignant schwannoma
of intraosseous origin. Güthert (1952) and Bose et al. (1970) described intraosseous
malignant schwannomas. Other than for these two cases, the paucity in the literature
concerning malignant schwannoma arising in bone is somewhat puzzling. This may,
for the most part, be due to an unfamiliarity with the versatility of Schwann cells.
These, through metaplasia, are said to be capable of producing a wide variety of tissues
(cartilage, bone, fat, striated muscle, etc.), which are not ordinarily thought of as being
derived from them (Stout, 1949). Lichtenstein (1972) stated there has been no comprehensive description of malignant schwannoma in bone. On review of the literature,
it must be concluded that the vast majority of schwannomas arising in bone are benign
tumors.

IV. Roentgenology

Roentgenologically, schwannomas can involve bone in three ways. They may be
central lesions, producing rarefaction of the bone; they may be located in a nutrient
canal producing a dumbbell-shaped lesion; or they may be extraosseous causing erosion

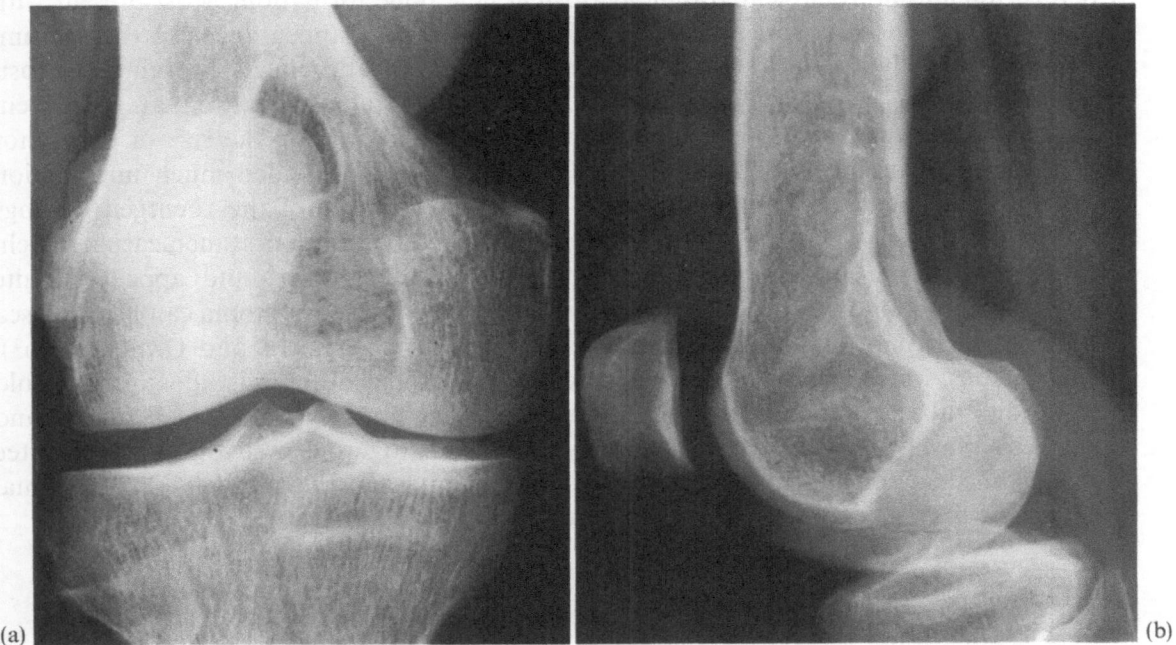

(a)   (b)

Fig. 7a and b. Schwannoma (neurilemmoma) causing a well-demarcated, erosive defect in the distal femur. (a) Anterior view, (b) lateral view. (Courtesy of Klaus Ranniger, M.D., Medical College of Virginia Hospitals, Richmond, Virginia)

of bone (Fig. 7). Central tumors produce roentgenologic findings characteristic of a benign tumor which completely replaces bone and pushes it aside as it grows. It will, therefore, classically produce a discretely demarcated zone of rarefaction sometimes with a thin sclerotic band of immediately adjacent bone (Fig. 6). Basically these are central tumors but occasionally they can be eccentric and proliferate and expand the overlying bone cortex. The tumors can protrude out through a nutrient foramen producing a dumbbell-shaped lesion.

In most cases, the tumor has been less than 6 cm in size at the time of discovery. Lodwick (1965) states that malignant tumors are usually larger than 6 cm when first discovered. He states that although slow growing benign tumors may eventually grow to 6 cm or larger, primary malignant bone tumors are rarely less than 6 cm in size. Occasionally, the lesions have a multilocular appearance. This may be due to reflections or corrugations on the walls of the cavity containing the tumor. When this multilocular appearance is evident in tumors involving the jaw, they may closely simulate ameloblastoma in appearance. In the mandible, the tumor usually presents in or near the angle. It is a nontrabeculated lytic lesion with a well-defined margin at its interface with normal bone. Periosteal reaction is not seen and the tumor lacks any evidence of central calcification. Schwannoma in the appendicular skeleton is a geographic lytic defect within the medullary portion of the shaft. A trabeculated or "soap-bubble" appearance is more frequent than in the mandible. A frequent location in long bones is in the midshaft. These tumors can account for considerable expansion and thinning of the overlying bone. Periosteal reaction is not a finding. Eccentrically located lesions may completely efface the overlying "expanded" cortex. These eccentric lesions are often found at the site of a nutrient foramen. Schwannoma in the metacarpal bones shows almost universal erosion of the cortex and extension into the metaphyses. The lesions show no central calcification and no roentgenographic periosteal new bone formation. Most present with marginal bone sclerosis and a trabeculated "soap-bubble" appearance. In the sacrum, schwannoma is a lytic defect and in most instances is non-trabeculated. Marginal sclerosis may or may not be seen. Periosteal reaction and central calcification are not seen. Erosion of the overlying cortex in this location is dependent upon the size of the tumor and the area of its location. Agha and Lilienfield (1972) provided much information as regards the roentgen features of this tumor in their review of the roentgen findings in 20 reported cases. These authors reported a case involving the first metacarpal which, was geographic in character, had a "soap-bubble" appearance, and appeared quite similar to an enchondroma roentgenographically. In the rib, schwannoma can be confused with a parenchymal lung lesion as in the case reported by Divertie and Dahlin (1963). Other lesions which would enter into a roentgenographic differential diagnosis would be: Brodie's abscess, chondromyxoid fibroma, solitary bone cyst, giant cell tumor, and fibrous dysplasia. In the jaw, the lesion may mimic a dentigerous cyst if non-trabeculated and if trabeculated, an ameloblastoma. If the lesion lacks the more typical marginal sclerosis, it may be confused with a fibrosarcoma.

V. Treatment

The treatment of choice is local surgical excision, owing to the benign nature of this lesion. The majority of these lesions are small enough to be safely and adequately removed. An occasional larger lesion may require sequential excision.

C. Neurofibroma

I. Nomenclature

The terminology of tumors originating in or connected with the perineural fibrous tissue is still in a considerable state of confusion. Terms used synonomously with neurofibroma include: neurinoma, neurogenic fibroma, neurogenic fibroblastoma, and perineural fibroblastoma. Here, the overlap with schwannoma can be appreciated. The solitary neurofibroma is a benign tumor of nerve and connective tissue arising from both peripheral and cranial nerves. It is a slowly growing, relatively circumscribed, but nonencapsulated neoplasm. It is composed principally of Schwann cells. The vast majority of these tumors are found in the soft tissues and they are frequently found in association with the congenital disease of mesodermal and neuroectodermal elements, neurofibromatosis (von Recklinghausen's disease). Solitary intraosseous neurofibromas comparable to those not infrequently observed in soft parts are extremely rare and little information in regards to these is found in the literature. These can develop in bone as a manifestation of neurofibromatosis, although this is by no means as frequent an occurrence as is generally assumed (Lichtenstein, 1972).

Before proceeding with a discussion of solitary intraosseous neurofibroma, it is appropriate that a brief description of the salient clinical and roentgenographic features of neurofibromatosis be presented since some pathologists have argued that solitary intraosseous neurofibroma is a form fruste of neurofibromatosis and that multiple lesions are missed on the first diagnosis or appear later (Prescott and White, 1970).

Neurofibromatosis was first described by Smith. Later in 1882 von Recklinghausen evaluated the histology of the disease and related it to the central nervous system. It is a congenital complex dysplastic condition involving both mesenchymal tissue and neuroectodermal derivatives. Clinically, it is characterized by areas of skin pigmentation (café au lait), cutaneous fibromas (fibroma molluscum) and neurofibromas of peripheral and cranial nerves. LEVIN (1958) has listed the salient skeletal changes as follows: (1) An erosive defect in bone due to the presence of neurofibromas contiguous to bone. (2) Scoliosis. (3) Growth disorders including overgrowth and underdevelopment. (4) Bowing and pseudoarthrosis of the lower leg. (5) Intraosseous cystic lesions. (6) Congenital anomalies. Scoliosis is by far the most common skeletal change, being seen in approximately 50% of patients with the disease (EDEIKEN and HODES, 1973). The scoliosis is usually in the lower dorsal region and is associated with a considerable kyphosis. It may be due to either an adjacent neurofibroma of the dorsal roots eroding the vertebral body or it may be secondary to a discrepancy in leg length due either to underdevelopment or overgrowth of an involved extremity. The posterior portions of the vertebral body may be eroded and the spinal canal may be enlarged. These changes most frequently are due to cysts or dilatation of the spinal canal but can also be the manifestation of bone erosion from a local neurofibroma. Intrathoracic meningoceles are commonly seen in patients with neurofibromatosis. For the most part, these are asymptomatic. They characteristically produce posterior mediastinal masses and have been frequently misinterpreted as neurofibromas. Patients with neurofibromatosis have abnormal periosteum which accounts for several findings. The bones of these patients have been described as "gracile" and the ribs can assume a "twisted ribbon" appearance. These changes are due to abnormal appositional bone growth due to the abnormal periosteum. Due to the abnormal periosteum, there is an abnormal response to trauma which can either manifest as large calcified subperiosteal hemorrhage or pseudoarthrosis. Although pseudoarthrosis occurs as a separate entity, approximately 50% of patients with this entity show the other stigmata of neurofibromatosis. Erosive defects from periosteal or adjacent soft tissue neurofibromas are among the most common bone changes in this entity. These produce a characteristic "pit or concave" defect in long bones which is characteristically long in relation to its depth. It is usually bounded by a sclerotic zone. This area of increased density may extend as much as several centimeters in all directions from the adjacent erosion. The rib notching frequently seen in this disorder is due to erosive changes from neurofibromas in the adjacent intercostal nerves. The bone overgrowth usually involves tubular bones. The bone is usually increased in length and often there is an accompanying increase in width as well. The sites of overgrowth are usually in areas with accompanying soft tissue involvement. The overgrowth is postulated to be due to the increased blood flow in the area with the resultant periosteal hyperemia (LEVIN, 1958). In other instances there may be retardation of the bone growth. These bones show a wavy appearance. They may be abnormally thick or slender. In the skull, orbital defects associated with pulsating exophthalmos may be seen. These may be small or large to the extent that almost an entire sphenoid bone is deficient. The intraosseous cystic lesions are, interestingly enough, for the most part related to osteolytic changes and represent areas of deossification whereas medullary localization of neurofibroma is an unusual cause of these.

It should be remembered that skin manifestations are the most common findings in neurofibromatosis and most of the significant changes occur in the nervous system. Less than 10% of cases show findings in the bones other than in the vertebra. A definite familial incidence has been established. The hereditary factor behaves as a dominant and is transmitted to both sexes (CORNELL and VARGAS, 1955). Males are involved

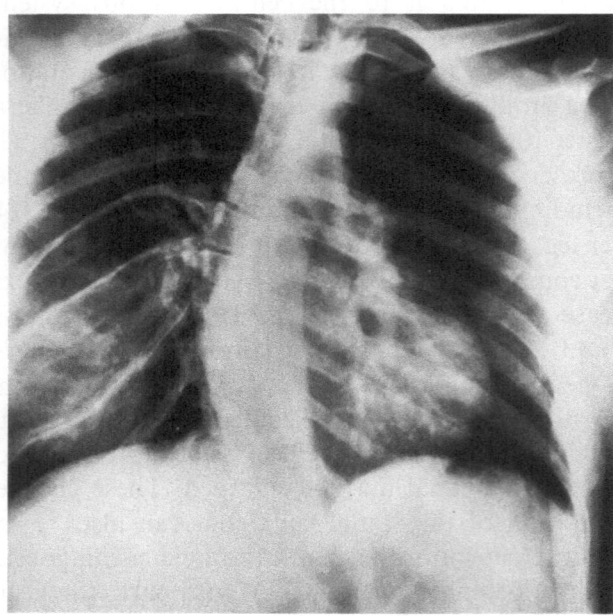

Fig. 8. Chest roentgenogram of a patient with neurofibromatosis (von Recklinghausen's disease). Note thoracic scoliosis, "ribbon" rib deformities, notching of seventh right rib, and nodules in the soft tissues

more often than females. There is no racial predominance. Approximately 10% of neurofibromas may undergo sarcomatous degeneration and this occurs in the joints or soft tissues as neurofibrosarcoma (Edeiken and Hodes, 1973). Mental deficiency is not an infrequent associated clinical finding in these patients. Hyperparathyroidism, acromegaly, and development of pheochromocytoma have been noted in these patients.

II. Clinical

Clinically, the majority of neurofibromas are associated with neurofibromatosis. They can, however, be found as solitary lesions in the skin, the oral cavity, deeper regions of the spine, and in the jaws (Gutman, 1964).

The incidence of solitary intraosseous neurofibroma is extremely low. Very few cases have been reported in the world literature. Of these few reports, the majority of the lesions are in the mandible. In fact, a search of the literature revealed only two reports of primary intraosseous neurofibroma involving bones other than the mandible in patients without the stigmata of von Recklinghausen's disease. The first reported case was seen by Gross et al. (1939). This lesion involved the midshaft of the humerus. The second case was reported by Baldwin and Weiner (1974). This involved the ulna and was associated with congenital bowing of that bone. In these sites there seems to be no age predilection. The tumor involving the humerus was in a 30-year-old woman. The tumor in the ulna was in a 3-year-old girl. At least 17 cases of solitary intraosseous neurofibroma of the mandible have been reported in the oral surgery literature Cundy and Matukas (1972). In a review of the literature by Prescott and White (1970), of the 16 cases reviewed, the age ranged between 4 and 65 years. The average age was 27 years. The sex distribution was exactly equal with 8 lesions occurring in males and 8 in females. There were 11 lesions which occurred in Caucasians, 1 lesion occurred in a Negro, and 4 of the cases had no information as regards to the race. Clinically, the first and most frequent symptoms are a diffuse swelling in the jaw or face. According to CUNDY and MATUKAS (1972), less than 50% of patients with primary intraosseous neurofibroma of the mandible have associated pain. This is a clinical feature which tends to separate these tumors from traumatic neuromas which, for the most part, are associated with pain. When pain is a feature, there may be associated tenderness of the overlying dentition and the pain may be exacerbated on mastication. As the tumor enlarges, a later manifestation is increased intradental spaces and malocclusion. JOHNSON (1959) reported a case involving the inferior alveolar nerve. This case was associated with paresthesia of the lower lip. VILLA et al. (1962) reported a case of a central neurofibroma in the mandible which was associated with occasional spontaneous hemorrhage.

III. Pathology

Grossly, these lesions are of a firm or elastic consistency and are white, grey, or yellow in color. The tumor is not completely encapsulated and the periphery may be irregular and rough. Occasionally on pressure, a yellowish liquid can be expressed from these tumors.

The histologic features of neurofibroma are characterized by the presence of peripheral nerve elements (schwannian cells and neurites) which are arranged in a diffuse, haphazard manner. As previously stated, the majority of these lesions are not encapsulated. There has been considerable confusion as regards the histologic criteria of neurofibroma, neurilemmoma (schwannoma), and traumatic neuroma. WAGGENER (1966) pointed out that neurofibroma and schwannoma have different and distinguishing ultrastructural patterns. The neurofibroma has large extracellular spaces in which there are compact bundles of collagen fibers widely separating the individual tumor cells. The neurofibroma has increased numbers of axon cylinders, histiocytes, fibroblasts, and vascular channels. Traversing the typical neurofibroma are small nerve bundles with axons of normal size and structure originating from these. The principle cells of the tumor show moderate variation in their size and shape. They exhibit a prominent cell body because of the density of the packed microfibrils and organelles. According to WAGGENER (1966), these cells exhibit a limited number of dense cytoplasmic extensions on electron microscopy. The neurofibroma does not form Verocay bodies as does the schwannoma. It, instead, occasionally produces cellular patterns similar to Meissner tactile corpuscles.

Although some pathologists argue that single lesions in the absence of von Recklinghausen's disease are a form fruste of this entity, in light of the significant number of cases involving the mandible and the two cases involving the appendicular skeleton (BALDWIN and WEINER, 1974; GROSS et al., 1934), all of which presented in the absence of any clinical or roentgenographic evidence of von Recklinghausen's disease, it appears that these lesions do in fact exist in a solitary form in rare instances. SCHERMAN (1963) elaborated on the nerves of bone. It is presumed that primary intramedullary neurofibroma of bone originates from the myelinated and nonmyelinated nerve fibers which, in association with blood vessels, enter the bone by various foramina. Neurofibroma can also arise in a subperiosteal or periosteal location from nerves in this region but the tumors in these locations present as subperiosteal cortical cysts and do not extend into the bone. BALDWIN and WEINER (1974) stated that surgical trauma can cause activation of these neoplasms. As to the associated presence of congenital bowing with an intraosseous neurofibroma as reported by BALDWIN and WEINER (1974), it is thought that this asymmetrical bone growth is caused by the presence of the tumor. AEGERTER (1950) postulated that the neurofibroma was not responsible for the bowing but that the bowing and pseudoarthrosis is due to a dysplasia.

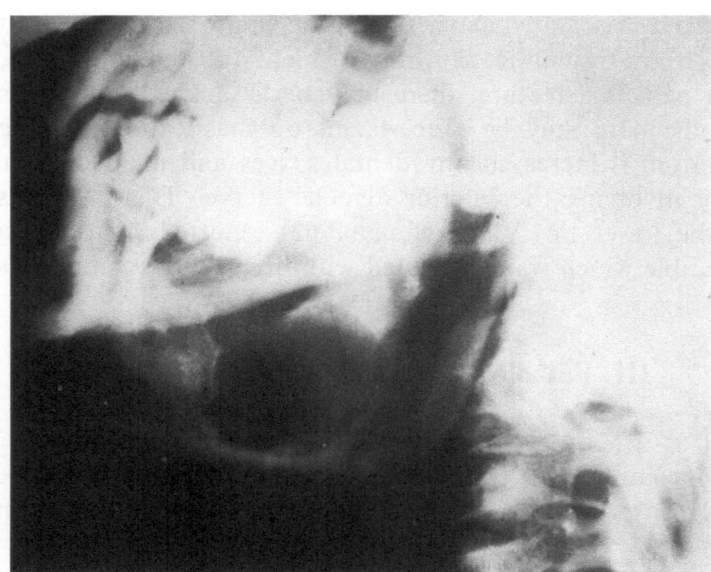

Fig. 9. Intraosseous neurofibroma of mandible. (Courtesy of Richard L. Cundy, M.D., University of Colorado Medical Center, Denver, Colorado; from CUNDY, R.L., MATUKAS, V.J.: Solitary intraosseous neurofibroma of the mandible. Arch. Otolaryngol. **96**, 81–83 (1972) (With permission of publisher)

The solitary intraosseous neurofibroma is considered a benign lesion. Malignant change in this tumor is extremely rare. INGRAM (1962) reported one case of malignant change in a solitary neurofibroma of the mandible. As with other true neoplasms, the tumor has a tendency to recur. It is accepted that intraosseous neurofibroma can and does occur. This, however, is the exception rather than the rule. As stated by CORNELL and VARGAS (1955), occasional neurofibromas in the head and neck can involve nerves diffusely and far beyond the area of growth involvement. Recurrence of these lesions is likely. It may be that the same situation exists in relation to the intraosseous neurofibroma which recurs.

IV. Roentgenology

By far, the most frequent site of this lesion is the mandible with approximately 17 reported cases in this region. Only 2 cases have been found which were apparently unassociated with von Recklinghausen's disease and involved the axial skeleton (BALDWIN and WEINER, 1974; GROSS et al., 1934). Similar to the neurilemmoma of bone, it is felt that the increased incidence of the neurofibroma in the mandible is due to the fact that the mandibular nerve traverses this bone. This assumption is reinforced when one notes that the most frequent location in the mandible is in the premolar region. The typical roentgenographic appearance of a central neurofibroma is that of a benign expanding lesion (Fig. 9). It is a lytic lesion with a geographic appearance denoting benignity. The margins of the lesion, although well-defined, may be sharply irregular and there is usually little to no visible marginal sclerosis. The lesion may appear multiloculated and may contain bony septa and trabeculae. It is not uncommon to see an associated soft tissue mass in proximity to the bony lesion. Expansion of the overlying cortical plate is a frequent finding in the mandible. In PRESCOTT and WHITE'S (1970) review of 16 cases, 14 lesions were found to expand the cortical plate and 8 of the lesions perforated the cortical plate. All of these tumors destroyed bone with varying degrees of severity. In most instances the bone destruction was located distal to the mental foramen and the mandibular canal was usually involved. Occasionally, there may be fluting of the inferior dental canal (CUNDY and MATUKAS, 1972). The radiographic appearance of this lesion in the mandible is suggestive of, but not pathognomonic for, neurofibroma. The radiologic differential diagnosis, according to PRESCOTT and WHITE (1970) consists of primordial cyst, ameloblastoma, dentigerous cyst, and malignant disease. One should also consider the other rare neurogenic bone tumor in this region, the schwannoma.

Periosteal and subperiosteal neurofibromas causing juxtacortical lesions are more common than endosteal lesions. These neurofibromas are also most often associated with von Recklinghausen's disease but several cases have been recorded as arising de novo. It forms a "blisterlike" lesion causing local bone destruction and little reaction. The lesion may be covered with a thin "eggshell" layer of periosteal new bone. The inner surface of the eroded bony cortex may be limited by a thin shell of delicate dense bone. These lesions although more common than the intraosseous neurofibroma are found primarily in relation to the long bones.

V. Treatment

Neurofibroma of bone is considered a benign bone lesion and is treated as such. Primary surgical removal of the lesion is the treatment of choice. Most lesions involving the mandible can be removed intraorally with conservative enucleation. This carries a minimum of morbidity. Those lesions that recur require removal of the parent tissue as well. This is justified to prevent a further recurrence which may manifest malignant changes. When a solitary neurofibroma is found, every effort should be made on the part of the clinician to rule out von Recklinghausen's disease as this entity commonly manifests itself as previously undiagnosed multiple neurofibroma of skin, bone, and viscera with café au lait spots on the skin.

References

Adamantinoma Long Bones and Ameloblastoma — Jaw

ABRAMS, A.M., MELROSE, R.J., HOWELL, F.V.: Adeno-ameloblastoma. a clinical pathologic study of ten new cases. Cancer (Philad.) 22, 176–185 (1968)

ACKERMAN, L.V., DEL REGATO, J.A.: Cancer diagnosis, treatment and prognosis, 4th ed. St. Louis: C.V. Mosby 1970

AGARWAL, S., MANJREKAR, P.S., KOSHAL, K.D., PRASAD, U.S.:Adamantinoma of the tibia. Indian J. Cancer 4, 257–262 (1967)

ANAND, S.V., DAVEY, W.W., COHEN, B.: Tumors of the jaw in West Africa. A review of 256 patients. Brit. J. Surg. 54, 901–917 (1967)

ANDERSON, C.E., SANDERS, J.B., DE, C.N.: Primary adamantinoma of the ulna. Surg. Gynec. Obstet. 75, 351–356 (1942)

BAKER, A.H., HAWKSLEY, L.M.: A case of primary adamantinoma of the tibia. Brit. J. Surg. 18, 415–421 (1931)

BAKER, P.L., DOCKERTY, N.B., COVENTRY, M.B.: Adamantinoma (so-called) of long bones: review of literature and report of 3 new cases. J. Bone Jt Surg. 36-A, 704–720 (1954)

BAUX, S., APOIL, A., ORCEL, L.: Tibial adamantinoma treated with extensive resection followed by a graft. Rev. Chir. orthop. 57, 479–484 (1971)

BECKER, W.: Zum Nomenklaturproblem bei den Knochentumoren. Z. Orthop. 108, 476–490 (1970)

BECKER, R., PERTL, A.: On therapy of ameloblastoma. Dtsch. Zahn-, Mund- u. Kieferheilk. 49, 423–436 (1967)

BELL, A.L.: A case of adamantinoma of the femur. Brit. J. Surg. 30, 81–82 (1942)

BESEMMAN, E.F., PEREZ, M.A.: Malignant angioglastoma, so-called adamantinoma, involving the humerus. Amer. J. Roentgenol. 100, 538–541 (1967)

BISHOP, E.L.: Adamantinoma of the tibia. Sth. med. J. (B'ham, Ala.) 30, 571–573 (1937)

BRAIDWOOD, A.S., McDOUGALL, A.: Adamantinoma of the tibia. Report of two cases. J. Bone Jt Surg. 56B, 735–738 (1974)

BYRNE, M.P., KOSMALA, R.L., CUNNINGHAM, M.P.: Ameloblastoma with regional and distant metastases. Amer. J. Surg. 128, 91–94 (1974)

CHANGUS, G.W., SPEED, J.S., STEWART, F.W.: Malignant angioblastoma of bone: reappraisal of adamantinoma of long bone. Cancer (Philad.) 10, 540–559 (1957)

COHEN, D.M., DAHLIN, D.C., PUGA, D.G.: Fibrous dysplasia associated with adamantioma of long bones. Cancer (Philad.) 15, 515–521 (1962)

COLEY, B.L.: Neoplasms of bone, 2nd ed. New York: Hoeber 1960

CREHALET, Y.L., PUCCENELLI, A.D.: Un adamantinome solitaire du tibia. J. Radiol. Électrol. 50, 517–518 (1969)

CSIBA, A., OKROS, I., DZSINCH, C., SZABO, D.: Virus-like particles in a human ameloblastoma. Arch. oral Biol. 15, 817–826 (1970)

DAHLIN, D.C.: Bone tumors: general aspects and an analysis of 2276 cases. Springfield, Ill.: Charles C Thomas 1957

DAHLIN, D.C.: Bone tumors—general aspects and data on 3987 cases, 2nd ed. Springfield, Ill.: Charles C Thomas 1967

DAHLIN, D.C.: Malignant tumors involving bone of nonosseous origin (myeloma, malignant lymphoma, Ewing's sarcoma, chordoma, adamantinoma, angiosarcoma, liposarcoma). Proc. nat. Cancer Conf. 6, 757–767 (1970)

DAVIDSON, H.B.: Adamantinoma of the tibia. Amer. J. Path. 16, 703 (1940)

DELARUE, J., CHONETTE, G., BROCHERIOU, C.: Adamantinoma du tibia et "dysplasie fibreuse." Ann. Anat. path. 9, 373 (1964)

DIEPEVEEN, W.P., HJORT, G.H., POCKSTEEN, O.C.: Adamantinoma of the capitate bone. Acta radiol. (Stockh.) 53, 377 (1960)

DOCKERTY, M.B., MEYERDING, H.W.: Adamantinoma of tibia: report of 2 new cases. J. Amer. med. Ass. 199, 932–937 (1942)

DONNER, R., DIKLAND, R.: Adamantinoma of the tibia. A long-standing case with unusual histological features. J. Bone Jt Surg. 48B, 138–144 (1966)

DUNNE, R.E.: Primary adamantinoma of the tibia. New Engl. J. Med. 218, 634 (1938)

DUTESCU, N., SAFTA, M., DUTESCU, D.: The potential of malignant degeneration of ameloblastoma. Stomatol. DDR. 24, 448–451 (1974)

EDEIKEN, J., HODES, P.J.: Roentgen diagnosis of diseases of bone, 2nd ed. Baltimore: Williams and Wilkins 1973

ELLIOTT, G.B.: Malignant angioblastoma of long bone—so-called "tibial adamantinoma." J. Bone Jt Surg. 44, 25–33 (1962)

ETCHART, M., VIVIANI, G., BEHN, K.: Adamentinom der Ulna. Fortschr. Roentgenstr. 95, 415–418 (1961)

FISCHER, B.: Über ein primäres Adamantinom der Tibia. Frankf. Z. Path. 12, 422–441 (1913)

GARDNER, A.F.: The pseudoameloblastoma of the long bones of the skeletal system. Oral Surg. 16, 1223 (1963)

GARLAND, S.: Adamantinoma of the tibia. J. Bone Jt Surg. 44B, 961 (1962)

GIKAS, P.W., HEADINGTON, J.T.: Angioblastic tumors of bone and skin. J. Bone Jt Surg. 45A, 554 (1963)

GLAUBER, A., JUHÁSZ, J.: Das Adamantinom der Tibia. Z. Orthop. 96, 523 (1962)

GLOOR, F.: Das sogenannte Adamantinoma der langen Röhrenknochen. Virchows Arch. path. Anat. 336, 489 (1963)

GOLDMAN, H.M.: Odontogenic mixed tumors—observations concerning inductive effects. Surg. Clin. N. Amer. 49, 695–702 (1969)

GOUTALLIER, D., DEBEYRE, J.: Une observation d'adamantinome du Tibia. J. Chir. (Paris) 103, 231–236 (1972)

HALPERT, B., DOHN, H.P.: Adamantinoma in the tibia. Arch. Path. (Chicago) 43, 313 (1947)

HEBBEL, R.: Adamantinoma of the tibia. Surgery 7, 860 (1940)

HERTZ, J.: Adamantinoma. Studies in histopathology and prognosis. Acta med. scand. 142, 529 (1952)

HICKS, J.D.: Synovial sarcoma of tibia. J. Path. Bact. 67, 151 (1954)

HOLDEN, E., JR., GRAY, J.W.: Adamantinoma of the tibia. J. Bone Jt Surg. 16, 401 (1934)

HUVOS, A.G., MARCOVE, R.C.: Adamantinoma of long bones. A clinicopathological study of fourteen cases with vascular origin suggested. J. Bone Jt Surg. 57, 148–154 (1975)

JAFFE, H.L.: Tumors and tumorous conditions of the bones and joints. Philadelphia: Lea and Febiger 1958

JOHNSON, L.C.: Congenital pseudarthrosis, adamantinoma of long bone, and intracortial fibrous dysplasia of the tibia. Lab. Invest. 28, 387 (1973)

JOHNSON, R.H., TOPAZIAN, R.G.: The management of variants of ameloblastoma. Plast. reconstr. Surg. 41, 356–363 (1968)

JURGENS, P.H.: Ameloblastoma of the mandible. J. oral Surg. 24, 325–331 (1966)

KRANZ, D.: On the histology of adamantinomas. Dtsch. Stomat. 19, 17–25 (1969)

KÜHNE, H.H.: Über das sogenannte Adamantinom der langen Röhrenknochen. Singuläre Beobachtung als Beitrag zur Differentialdiagnose. Langenbecks Arch. klin. Chir. 318, 161–177 (1967)

LAW, W.B.: Secondary adamantinoma of the ischium. Aust. N. Z. J. Surg. 38, 265–268 (1969)

LEDERER, H., SINCLAIR, A.J.: Malignant synovioma simulating adamantinoma of the tibia. J. Path. Bact. 67, 163–168 (1954)

LEE, K.W., CHIN, T.C., PAUL, G.: Peripheral ameloblastoma. Brit. J. oral Surg. 8, 150–153 (1970)

LICHTENSTEIN, L.: Bone tumors, 4th ed. St. Louis: C.V. Mosby 1972

MAIER, C.: Ein primäres myelogenes Plattenepithelcarcinom der Ulna. Bruns Beitr. klin. Chir. 26, 552–556 (1900)

MANDARD, J.C., LeGAL, Y., FIEVEZ, M.: L'adamantinome des os longs. Ann. Anat. path. **16**, 483–498
(1971)

MANGALIK, V.S., LAL MEHROTRA, R.N.: Adamantinoma of the tibia. Report of a case. Brit. J. Surg.
39, 429 (1952)

MARCIAL-ROJAS, R.: Adamantinoma of the tibia.
Cancer Semin. **2**, 122 (1958)

McIVOR, J.: The radiological features of ameloblastoma. Clin. Radiol. **25**, 237–242 (1974)

MEFFLEY, W.H., NORTHRUP, S.W.: Adamantinoma of
the tibia. J. int. Coll. Surg. **10**, 291–300 (1947)

MERLE D'AUBIGŃE, R.: Adamantinome du Tibia. Rev.
Chir. orthop. **46**, 92 (1960)

MINCER, H.H., McGINNIS, J.P.: Ultrastructure of
three histologic variants of the ameloblastoma.
Cancer (Philad.) **30**, 1036–1045 (1972)

MOON, N.F.: Adamantinoma of the appendicular skeleton. A statistical review of reported cases and
inclusion of ten new cases. Clin. Orthop. **43**,
189–213 (1965)

MORGAN, A.D., MacKENSIE, D.H.: Metastasing
adamantinoma of tibia. J. Bone Jt Surg. **38B**,
893–898 (1956)

NAJI, A.F., MURPHY, J.A., STASNEY, R.J., NEVILLE,
W.E., CHRENKA, P.: So-called adamantinoma of
long bones. Report of a case with massive pulmonary metastasis. J. Bone Jt Surg. **46A**, 151
(1964)

NELSON, N.A.: So-called adamantinoma of the tibia
(two cases). Proc. roy. Soc. Med. **58**, 171 (1965)

OBERLING, C., VERNES, E., CHEVEREAU, J.: Adamantinome du Tibia. Bull. Ass. franç. Cancer **27**, 373
(1938)

PENNISI, V.R., YOUNG, A., ANLYAN, A.J., GRISEZ,
J.L.: Ameloblastoma with long standing pulmonary metastases. Plast. reconstr. Surg. **38**, 534–540
(1966)

PÉROCHON and VELVET: A propos du diagnostic radiologique d'une tumeur du tibia. J. Radial. Électrol.
12, 178 (1928)

PETROV, N., GLASUNOW, M.: Über die sogenannten
Knochenendotheliome und die primären epithelia-
len Knochengeschwülste. Langenbecks Arch. klin.
Chir. **175**, 589 (1933)

PILZ, G.: The pathogenesis of the adamantoblastoma.
Dtsch. Stomat. **20**, 362–370 (1970)

POLLACK, R.S.: Extraosseous adamantinoma. Arch.
Surg. (Chicago) **70**, 353–358 (1955)

POPOW, K.P.: On the histogenesis of adamantinomas.
Gegenbaurs morph. Jb. **109**, 251–252 (1966)

PUGH, D.G.: Roentgenologic diagnosis of diseases of
bones. New York: Thomas Nelson and Sons 1951

PUGH, D.G.: Unusual form of fibrous dysplasia of
bone: Report of 3 cases. Amer. J. Roentgenol.
71, 632–642 (1954)

RANKIN, J.O.: Adamantinoma of the tibia. J. Bone
Jt Surg. **21**, 425 (1939)

REHBOCK, D.J., BARBER, C.G.: Adamantinoma of tibia. J. Bone Jt Surg. **20**, 187 (1938)

REHRMANN, A.: Pathology and clinical aspects of the
lower jaw tumors. Arch. klin. exp. Ohr-, Nas.- u.
Kehlk.-Heilk. **187**, 302–322 (1966)

RICHTER, C.S.: Ein Fall von adamantinomartiger
Geschwulst des Schienbeins. Z. Krebsforsch. **32**,
272 (1930)

ROBBINS, S.L.: Pathology 3rd ed. Philadelphia-Lon-
don: W.B. Saunders 1967

ROBINSON, H.G.B.: Adamantinoma of the tibia. J.
Amer. med. Ass. **119**, 1524 (1942)

ROBINSON, M., CANTER, S., SHUKEN, R.: Multiple progressive bone cysts of the mandible and maxilla.
Oral Surg. **23**, 483–486 (1967)

ROSAI, J.: Adamantinoma of the tibia: Electron microscopic evidence of its epithelial origin. Amer.
J. clin. Path. **51**, 786–792 (1969)

ROSEN, R.S., SCHWINN, C.P.: Adamantinoma of limb
bone. Malignant angioblastoma. Amer. J. Roentgenol. **97**, 727–732 (1966)

RYRIE, B.J.: Adamantinoma of the tibia: aetiology
and pathogenesis. Brit. med. J. **2**, 1000 (1932)

SALMON, M., PAYAN, H., TRIFAUD, A.: Adamantinome
du tibia, résection large greffe, guérison de six ans.
Rev. Chir. orthop. **46**, 54 (1960)

SCHAFTER, W.G.: Cysts, neoplasms and allied conditions of odontogenic origin. Semin. Roentgenol.
6, No. 4 (1971)

SCHILLING, A.: Das sogenannte Adamantinom des
Schienbeins. Bruns Beitr. klin. Chir. **204**, 265 (1962)

SEWARD, G.R., DUCKWORTH, R.: A review of the pathology of the calcifying odontogenic cysts and tumors. Dent. Practit. (Bristol) **18**, 83–98 (1967)

SHATKIN, S., HOFFMEISTER, F.S.: Ameloblastoma—a
rational approach to therapy. Oral Surg. **20**,
421–435 (1965)

SMITH, J.F.: The controversial ameloblastoma. Oral
Surg. **26**, 45–75 (1968)

SPJUT, H.J., DORFMAN, H.D., FECHNER, R.E., ACKER-
MAN, L.V.: Tumors of bone and cartilage. Atlas
of Tumor Pathology, fasc. 5. Washington, D.C.:
Armed Forces Institute of Pathology 1971

SPOUGE, J.D.: The adenoameloblastoma. Oral Surg.
23, 470–482 (1967)

SPOUGE, J.D., SPRUYT, C.L.: Odontogenic tumors.
Histochemical comparison of the adenoameloblastoma and developing tooth. Oral Surg. **25**, 447–456
(1968)

STOUT, F.W., LUNIN, M.: The ultrastructure of oral
tumors. Oral Surg. **22**, 340–348 (1966)

TAYLOR, B.G.: Ameloblastoma of the mandible. A
clinical study of 25 patients. Amer. Surg. **34**, 57–62
(1968a)

TAYLOR, B.G.: Ameloblastoma. CA **18**, 205–207
(1968b)

The Netherlands Committee on Bone Tumors. Radiological atlas of bone tumors. Baltimore: Williams and Wilkins Company 1973

THEROS, E.G., ISHAK, B.W.: An exercise in radiologic-
pathologic correlation. Radiology **89**, 747–752
(1967)

THOMAS, R.G.: Adamantinoma of the tibia. Brit. J. Surg. **26**, 547 (1939)

TROTT, J.R.: Ameloblastic fibroma – case report. Brit. J. oral Surg. **5**, 11–15 (1967)

UEHLINGER, E.A.: Das Skelettsynoviom (Adamantinom) in Röntgendiagnostik. Ergebnisse 1952–1956, pp. 96–103. Stuttgart: Georg Thieme 1957

UNNI, K.K., DAHLIN, D.C., BEABOUT, J.W., IVINS, J.C.: Adamantinomas of long bones. Cancer (Philad.) **34**, 1796–1805 (1974)

VANDENBUSSCHE, F., DONAZZAN, M., CARLIER, G., BONTE, G.: Ameloblastic tumors of the maxilla. Statistical data. Ann. Radiol. (Paris) **12**, 523–547 (1969)

VICKERS, R.A., GORLIN, R.J.: Ameloblastoma – delineation of early histopathologic features of neoplasia. Cancer (Philad.) **26**, 699–710 (1970)

WILLIAMS, G.: Adamantinoma of the tibia. Radiol. Electrol. Med. Nucl. **52**, 727–728 (1971)

WOLFORT, B., SLOANE, D.: Adamantinoma of the tibia. J. Bone Jt Surg. **20**, 1011 (1938)

ZAND, A., CHAMBERS, G.H., STREET, D.M.: So-called "adamantinoma of long bone." Clin. Orthop. **86**, 178–182 (1972)

Schwannoma (Neurilemmoma)

ACKERMAN, L.V., SPJUT, H.J.: Tumors of bone and cartilage. Atlas of tumor pathology, Section Z, Facile 4. Washington, D.C.: Armed Forces Institute of Pathology 1962

AGHA, F.P., LILIENFELD, R.M.: Roentgen features of osseous neurilemmoma. Radiology **102**, 325–326 (1972)

BAETZ, F.O., SCHACKELFORD, J.: A schwannoma of the inferior alveolar nerve: Report of a case. J. oral Surg. **9**, 331–333 (1951)

BEST, P.V.: Erosion of the petrous temporal bone by neurilemmoma. J. Neurosurg. **28**, 445–451 (1968)

BOSE, K.S., THAKUR, S., CHAKRABARTY, S., BANERJEE, S.: Intra-osseous malignant schwannoma. J. Indian med. Ass. **54**, 328–329 (1970)

BRUCE, K.W.: Solitary neurofibroma (neurilemmoma, schwannoma) of the oral cavity. Oral Surg. **7**, 1150–1159 (1954)

CAHN, L.R.: Traumatic (amputation) neuroma. Amer. J. Orthodont. **25**, 190–193 (1939)

CALDWELL, J.B., HUGHES, K.W., COX, R.S., JR.: Neurofibroma of the mandible: Report of a case. J. oral Surg. **19**, 166–171 (1961)

COWLEY, A.H., MILLER, D.S.: Neurilemmoma of bone: A case report. J. Bone Jt Surg. **24**, 684–689 (1942)

CRACCHIOLOG, A. III, BLAZINE, M.E., MARMOR, L.: Masses at the medial side of the knee joint. Clin. Orthop. **62**, 167–171 (1969)

DAHLIN, D.C.: Bone tumors: General aspects and an analysis of 2276 cases. Springfield, Ill.: Charles C Thomas 1957

DAHLIN, D.C.: Bone tumors: General aspects and data on 3987 cases, 2nd ed. Springfield, Ill.: Charles C Thomas 1967

DEBAIN, J.J., GRIGNON, J.L., CHROME, J.: Two cases of nerve tumors of the jaws. Ann. Oto-laryng. (Paris) **78**, 5 (1961)

DELIGDISH, L., LOWENTHAL, M., FRIEDLANDER, E.: Malignant neurilemmoma (schwannoma) in the lymph nodes. Int. Surg. **49**, 226–230 (1968)

DICKSON, J.H., WALTZ, T.A., FECHNER, R.E.: Intraosseous neurilemmoma of the third lumbar vertebra. J. Bone Jt Surg. **53**, 349–355 (1971)

DIVERTIE, M.B., DAHLIN, D.C.: Neurilemmoma of rib: Report of a case. Dis. Chest **44**, 635–637 (1963)

FAWCETT, K.J., DAHLIN, D.C.: Neurilemmoma of bone. Amer. J. clin. Path. **47**, 759–766 (1967)

FISCHER, E.R., VUZEVSKI, V.D.: Cytogenesis of schwannoma (neurilemmoma), neurofibroma, dermatofibroma, and dermatofibrosarcoma as revealed by electron microscopy. Amer. J. clin. Path. **49**, 141–154 (1968)

GHOSH, B.C., GHOSH, L., HUVOS, A.G., FORTNER, J.G.: Malignant schwannoma. A clinicopathologic study. Cancer (Philad.) **3**, 184–190 (1973)

GRINELS, J.R.: A case report of neurilemmona of the fourth rib anteriorly, resembling a breast tumor. J. Abdom. Surg. **4**, 98–99 (1962)

GÜTHERT, H.: Ein malignes Neurinom des Knochens. Zbl. allg. Path. path. Anat. **88**, 185 (1952)

GUPTRA, T.K. DAS, BRASFIELD, R.O., STRONG, E.W., HAJDU, S.I.: Benign solitary schwannomas (neurilemmomas). Cancer (Philad.) **24**, 355–366 (1969)

GUPTRA, T.K. DAS, BRASFIELD, R.O.: Tumors of peripheral nerve origin – benign and malignant solitary schwannomas. Cancer **20**, 228–233 (1970)

HART, M.S., BASOM, W.C.: Neurilemmoma involving bone. J. Bone Jt Surg. **40A**, 465–468 (1958)

HORI, A.: Intraspinal schwannosis of Lissauer's zone terminalis (formes frustes of Recklinghausen's neurofibromatosis or reactive). Acta Neuropath. (Berl.) **25**, 89–94 (1973)

ILLADES, C.E., GELMA, N.H.: Neurilemmoma of the palate. Eye, Ear, Nose Thr. Monthly **54**, 6, 246–247 (1975)

INGEIS, G.W., CAMPBELL, D.C., JR., GIAMPETRO, A.M., KOZUB, R.E., BENTLAGE, C.H.: Malignant schwannomas of the mediastinum. Report of two cases and a review of the literature. Cancer (Philad.) **27**, 1190–1201 (1971)

JACOBS, R.L., BARMARDA, R.: Neurilemmoma. A review of the literature with six case reports. Arch. Surg. (Chicago) **102**, 181–186 (1969)

JAFFE, H.L.: Tumors and tumorous conditions of the bone and joints. Philadelphia: Lea and Febiger 1958

JONES, H.M.: Neurilemmoma of bone. Brit. J. Surg. **41**, 63–65 (1953)

KAPLAN, M.S., OPITZ, J.M., GOSSET, F.R.: Noonan's syndrome. A case with elevated serum alkaline phosphatase levels and malignant schwannoma of the left forearm. Amer. J. Dis. Child. **116**, 359–366 (1968)

LAPAYOWKER, M.S., CLIFF, M.M.: Bone changes in acoustic neurinomas. Amer. J. Roentgenol. **107**, 652–658 (1969)

LEWIS, H.H., KORBIN, H.I.: Neurilemmoma of the first metacarpal. A case report. Clin. Orthop. **82**, 67–69 (1972)

LICHENSTEIN, L.: Bone tumors, 4th ed. St. Louis: C.V. Mosby 1972

LODWICK, G.S.: A probabilistic approach to the diagnosis of bone tumors. Radiol. Clin. N. Amer. **3**, 487–489 (1965)

LODWICK, G.S.: Tumors of bone and soft tissue. Chicago: Year Book Medical Publishers 1965

MAZINGARBE, A., MAXABRAUD, A.: A case of neurinoma of the tibia. Rev. Chir. orthop. **56**, 83–88 (1970)

MORTADA, A.: Neurilemmoma of the orbital bones causing exophthalmus. Brit. J. Ophthal. **52**, 550–554 (1968)

MORTON, K.S., VASSAR, P.S.: Neurilemmoma in bone. Report of a case. Canad. J. Surg. **7**, 187–189 (1964)

PEERS, J.H.: Primary intramedullary neurogenic sarcoma of ulna. Amer. J. Path. **10**, 811 (1934)

PINEDA, A.: Electron microscopy of the lemmocyte in peripheral nerve tumors (neurolemmomas). J. Neurosurg. **25**, 35–44 (1966)

SAMTER, T.G., VELLIOS, F., SHAFER, W.G.: Neurilemmoma of bone. Report of 3 cases with a review of the literature. Radiology **75**, 215–222 (1960)

SANE, S., YONIS, GREER R.: Subperiosteal or cortical cyst and intramedullary neurofibromatosis—Uncommon manifestations of neurofibromatosis. J. Bone Jt Surg. **53-A**, 1194–1201 (1971)

SANTO, D.A. DE, BURGESS, E.: Primary and secondary neurilemmoma of bone. Surg. Gynec. Obst. **71**, 454–461 (1940)

SETH, H.N., PIAO, B.D.P., KATHPALIA, P.M.L.: Neurilemmoma of bone: Report of a case. J. Bone Jt Surg. **45-B**, 382–383 (1963)

SHERMAN, M.S.: The nerves of bone. J. Bone Jt Surg. **45-A**, 522–528 (1963)

SHIMURA, K., ALLEN, E.C., KINOSHITA, Y., TAKAESU, T.: Central neurilemmoma of the mandible—report of a case and review of the literature. J. oral Surg. **31**, 363–367 (1973)

STOUT, A.P.: Tumors of the peripheral nervous system. J. Mo. med. Ass. (1949)

STURM, K.W., BONIS, G., KOSMAOGLU, V.: On a neurinoma of the cribriform lamina. Zbl. Neurochir. **29**, 217–222 (1968)

SUN, C.N., WHITE, H.J.: An electron-microscopic study of a schwannoma with special reference to banded structures and peculiar membranous multiple-chambered spheroids. J. Path. **114**, 13–16 (1974)

The Netherlands Committee on Bone Tumors: Radiological atlas of bone tumors. Baltimore: The Williams and Wilkins Company 1973

VEROCAY, J.: Festschr. Clinai, 378 (1908)

VITA, U. DE, GUARINO, M.: First findings on the relationship between histologic differentiation and pain in neurinomas. Arch. ital. Chir. **91**, 292–304 (1965)

WAGGENER, J.D.: Ultrastructure of benign peripheral nerve sheath tumors. Cancer (Philad.) **19**, 699–709 (1966)

WALDRUN, C.A.: Nonodontogenic neoplasms, cysts and allied conditions of the jaws. Semin. Roentgenol. **6**, No. 4 (1971)

WHITE, H.R., JR.: Survival in malignant schwannoma. An 18-year study. Cancer (Philad.) **27**, 720–729 (1971)

ZILKENS, K.: Über ein Neurinom am Unterkiefer. Z. Stomat. **35**, 461–467 (1937)

Neurofibroma

ABELL, M.R., HART, W.R., OLSON, J.R.: Tumors of the peripheral nervous system. Hum. Path. **1**, 503–551 (1970)

AEGERTER, E.E.: The possible relationship of neurofibromatosis, congenital pseudarthrosis, and fibrous dysplasia. J. Bone Jt Surg. **32A**, 618–626 (1950)

ANDERL, H.: Malignant degeneration of neurofibromas and neurofibromatosis. Klin. Med. (Wien). **21**, 528–530 (1966)

BALDWIN, D.M., WEINER, D.S.: Congenital bowing and intraosseous neurofibroma of the ulna. A case report. J. Bone Jt Surg. **56**, 803–807 (1974)

BIRD, C.C., WILLIS, R.A.: The histogenesis of pigmented neurofibromas. J. Path. **97**, 631–637 (1969)

BRASFIELD, R.O., DAS GUPTA, T.K.: Von Recklinghausen's disease—a clinicopathological study. Ann. Surg. **175**, 86–104 (1972)

BURTON, D.S., NAGEL, D.A.: Surgical treatment of malignant soft-tissue tumors of the extremities in the adult. Clin. Orthop. **84**, 144–148 (1972)

CALDWELL, J.B., HUGHES, K.W., COX, R.S.: Neurofibroma of the mandible: Report of a case. J. oral Surg. **19**, 166 (1961)

COBB, N.: Neurofibromatosis and pseudarthrosis of the ulna. A case report. J. Bone Jt Surg. **50B**, 146–149 (1968)

CORNELL, C.F., VARGAS, H.A.: Intraosseous neurofibroma of mandible. Oral Surg. **8**, 34 (1955)

CUNDY, R.L., MATUKAS, V.J.: Solitary intraosseous neurofibroma of the mandible. Arch. Otolaryng. (Chicago) **96**, 81–83 (1972)

DE VORE, D.T., WALDRON, C.A.: Malignant peripheral nerve tumors of the oral cavity: Review of the literature and report of a case. Oral Surg. **14**, 56 (1961)

EDEIKEN, J., HODES, P.J.: Roentgen diagnosis of diseases of bone, 2nd ed. Baltimore: Williams and Wilkins 1973

FISCHER, E.R., VUZEVSKI, V.D.: Cytogenesis of schwannoma (neurilemmoma), neurofibroma, dermatofibroma, and dermatofibrosarcoma as revealed by electron microscopy. Amer. J. clin. Path. **49**, 141–154 (1968)

Friedman, M.: Intraosseous neurofibroma of the mandible. Oral Surg. **8**, 34–35 (1955)

Garcia, R.L.: Multiple localized neurofibromas. J. Amer. med. Ass. **215**, 1670 (1971)

Gross, P., Bailey, F.R., Jacox, H.W.: Primary intramedullary neurofibroma of the humerus. Arch. Path. (Chicago) **28**, 716–718 (1939)

Gruszkiewicz, J., Doron, Y., Gelle, I.B.: Plexiform neurofibroma of the lumbar region. Case report. J. Neurosurg. **30**, 69–70 (1969)

Gutman, D.: Solitary neurofibroma of the mandible. Oral Surg. **17**, 1 (1964)

Hardt, N., Hardt, K.U.: Diagnosis and differential diagnosis of neural mandibular neoplasms. ZWR. **80**, 613–616 (1971)

Hosoi, K.: Multiple neurofibromatosis (von Recklinghausen's disease) with special reference to malignant transformation. Arch. Surg. (Chicago) **22**, 258–281 (1931)

Hunt, J.C., Pugh, D.G.: Skeletal lesions in neurofibromatosis. Radiology **76**, 1 (1961)

Ingram, F.L.: Radiology of tumors of the mandible. Clin. Radiol. **13**, 47 (1962)

Johnson, H.S.: Central neurofibroma: Report of a case. Oral Surg. **12**, 379 (1959)

Levin, B.: Neurofibromatosis: Clinical and roentgen manifestations. Radiology **71**, 48–58 (1958)

Lichtenstein, L.: Bone tumors, 4th ed. St. Louis: C.V. Mosby 1972

Mark, H.I.: Central fibroma of the mandible. Oral Surg. **17**, 1 (1964)

Mennel, H.D., Zulch, K.J.: Morphology of malignant tumors of peripheral nerves. Zbl. Neurochir. **32**, 11–24 (1971)

Meszaros, W.T., Guzzo, F., Storsch, H.: Neurofibromatosis. Amer. J. Roentgenol. **98**, 557–569 (1966)

Miller, M.R., Kasahara, M.: Observations on the innervation of human long bones. Anat. Rec. **145**, 13–23 (1963)

Nolan, N.G.: Intense uptake of 99 MTC-diphosphonate by an extraosseous neurofibroma. J. Nucl. Med. **15**, 1207–1208 (1974)

Nürnberger, F., Korting, G.W.: On the occurrence of acid mucopolysaccharides in neurofibromas and neurofibrosarcomas. Arch. klin. exp. Derm. **235**, 97–114 (1969)

Paulsen, H.J.: Neurofibromas and their malignant degeneration. Z. Laryng. Rhinol. **46**, 588–595 (1967)

Prescott, G.H., White, R.E.: Solitary central neurofibroma of the mandible. Report of a case and review of the literature. J. oral Surg. **28**, 305–309 (1970)

Raimondi, A.J., Beckman, F.: Perineural fibroblastomas—their fine structure and biology. Acta Neuropath. (Berl.) **8**, 1–23 (1967)

Reeder, M.M., Gelford, G.J., Robb, P.L.: An exercise in radiologic—pathologic correlation. Radiology **90**, 1023–1029 (1968)

Rio-Hortega, P.D.: Tumors of the peripheral nerves. Springfield, Ill.: Charles C Thomas 1962

Russell, D.S., Rubinstein, L.J.: Tumors of the nerve roots and peripheral nerves. Pathology of tumors of the nervous system, 2nd ed. Baltimore: Williams and Wilkins 1963

Salzer-Kuntschik, M.: Current nomenclature of primary bone neoplasms and tumor-like diseases of the bone (jaw—specific tumors excepted). Wien. klin. Wschr. **83**, 567–572 (1971)

Sands, M.J.: Fatal malignant degeneration in multiple neurofibromatosis. J. Amer. med. Ass. **233**, 1381–1382 (1975)

Schmidt, A.: Tumors in the region of the hand. Zbl. Chir. **96**, 1113–1123 (1971)

Sherman, M.S.: The nerves of bone. J. Bone Jt Surg. **45-A**, 522–528 (1963)

Shklar, G., Meyer, I.: Neurogenic tumors of the mouth and jaws. Oral Surg. **16**, 1076 (1963)

Siegel, M.W.: Intraosseous glomus tumor. A case report. Amer. J. Orthop. **9**, 68–69 (1967)

Stavron, D.: Comparativepathology of nervous system tumors. A morthologic and enzyme—histochemical study on spontaneous, or experimental nervous system tumors of various animal species and comparable tumors in man. Zbl. Vet.-Med. A. **18**, 585–628 (1971)

The Netherlands Committee on Bone Tumors: Radiological atlas of bone tumors. Baltimore: The Williams and Wilkins Company 1973

Villa, V.G., Laico, J.E., Banez, L.O.N.: Central neurofibroma in the mandible associated with occasional spontaneous hemorrhage. Report of a case. Oral Surg. **15**, 836–842 (1962)

Waggener, J.D.: Ultrastructure of benign peripheral nerve sheath tumors. Cancer (Philad.) **19**, 699–709 (1966)

Weber, K., Braun-Falco, O.: Ultrastructure of neurofibromatosis. Hautarzt **23**, 116–122 (1972)

Wilber, M.C., Woodcock, J.A.: Ganglioneuromata in bone. Report of a case. J. Bone Jt Surg. **39A**, 1385 (1957)

Tumor-like Lesions

by

Melvin H. Becker, Nancy Branom Genieser and Amy Goldman

There are a number of lesions which resemble tumors but are not neoplasms. Among these are the solitary bone cyst (simple or unicameral bone cyst), aneurysmal bone cyst, juxta-articular bone cyst (intraosseous ganglion), metaphyseal fibrous defect (nonossifying fibroma), eosinophilic granuloma, fibrous dysplasia, myositis ossificans, and the brown tumor of hyperparathyroidism.

A. The Solitary Bone Cyst

I. Introduction

The solitary bone cyst is usually a single-chambered cystic lesion of bone that is fluid filled. It is a benign lesion of unknown etiology.

Among the various names applied to it are benign bone cyst, juvenile unicameral bone cyst, simple bone cyst, simple unicameral bone cyst, unicameral bone cyst, and localized osteitis fibrosa cystica.

II. History

In the early medical literature, the solitary bone cyst was included with a number of other disorders as localized fibrocystic disease of bone. Probably, the first paper to describe this lesion was by VIRCHOW in 1876. In this article, he described a fluid-filled lesion in the proximal end of the humerus of a 56-year-old woman. The first to describe the roentgenographic appearance was HEINEKE in 1903. Among the other early studies that included discussions as to classification, etiology, and treatment are the reports of VON MIKULICZ (1905), BLOODGOOD (1910), and COLEY and HIGINBOTHAM (1934). In 1942 JAFFE and LICHTENSTEIN firmly established the solitary unicameral bone cyst as an independent and distinctive entity.

III. Clinical

The clinical aspects of the solitary bone cyst can be found described in many textbooks as well as in review articles such as those by JAFFE and LICHTENSTEIN (1942), JAMES et al. (1948), GRAHAM (1952), GARCEAU and GREGORY (1954), LODWICK (1958), NEER et al. (1966 and 1973), SPENCE et al. (1969), and MOURGUES et al. (1974). The solitary bone cyst is a relatively uncommon lesion that is usually found in the long bones of children and adolescents. It is usually asymptomatic until fractured. However, some patients have had mild discomfort in the area at variable times prior to the discovery of the lesion. The lesion may be found either because of a fracture due to insignificant trauma or incidently when the patient was examined roentgenographically for other reasons. Until such time as a fracture occurs, the physical examination is normal.

This lesion is seen predominantly in males, being reported two to three times as frequent as in females. It is seen most often during the first and second decades of life, with the reported cases ranging in age from 2 months to 58 years. Most of the cases are over 7 years of age and under 15 when the cyst is discovered.

The solitary bone cyst is seen mainly in the proximal ends of the long bones near the epiphyseal plate. The most commonly involved bones are the humerus, femur, and tibia. Over 50% of the lesions involve the proximal humerus and about 30% involve the femur. Other areas that have been reported to have this disorder include the distal humerus, the distal femur, the distal tibia, the fibula, the calcaneus, the ulna, the radius, the ilium, the talus, the rib, the metacarpal, and the metatarsal. JAFFE and LICHTENSTEIN (1942) stated in their first paper that the solitary bone cyst is near to the epiphyseal cartilage. It rarely (if ever) transgresses the plate so as to be both in the shaft and in the neighboring epiphysis. HUTTER (1950) has reported a case in which the lesion involved the proximal tibial shaft and its neighboring epiphysis in a $6^1/_2$-year-old girl. BOSEKER et al. (1968) reported another case where a cyst involved the adjacent epiphysis of the neck of the femur in a 22-year-old woman. SADLER and ROSENHAIN (1964) reported the first known instance in which two unicameral bone cysts were found simultaneously; one was in the proximal left humerus and the other was in the lower third of the left tibia of a 10-year-old boy. BOSEKER et al. (1968) reported another patient with two simple cysts; the second appeared in the proximal portion of the humerus after the initial treatment of a cyst in the proximal portion of the femur.

The natural course of the simple bone cyst is one correlated with the growth of the patient. The lesion forms at, or near, the epiphyseal plate in the metaphysis of a long bone. As the patient grows, the lesion tends to move toward the diaphysis. At times the cystic area continues to be near the epiphyseal plate as the cyst enlarges. In other individuals, the cyst seems to move away from the epiphyseal plate and normal bone is seen between the plate and the cyst. JAFFE and LICHTENSTEIN (1942) have divided solitary bone cysts into active and latent stages. When a cyst extends to the immediate vicinity of, or abuts upon, the epiphyseal cartilage plate, it is regarded as having potentiality for growth; this is called the active stage. The latent cyst is one which has moved away from the plate so that there is a reconstructed area of shaft between it and the plate. While ADAMS (1926) has reported a case in which the cyst disappeared completely without surgical intervention, this is not the usual course of events. As a rule, the cyst persists indefinitely unless it has been obliterated by surgery. Pathologic fractures occur frequently and tend to heal with the cyst recurring. Occasionally, after multiple fractures, the cyst may heal. JAFFE (1958) has seen one case in which the cyst was present for 25 years, at which time it was surgically obliterated.

Although these cysts tend to recur after attempts at surgical obliteration, they are considered to be a benign, self-limited disorder. However, GRABIAS and MANKIN (1974) reported a case of a 14-year-old boy who had had a unicameral bone cyst in his humerus. This had been proven by biopsy on two occasions. On the site of the cyst, a chondrosarcoma developed 6 years after the first discovery of the cyst. There may be some doubt as to whether or not the tumor arose from the cyst or was transplanted along with bone chips used in earlier treatment. JOHNSON et al. (1962) reviewed the world literature

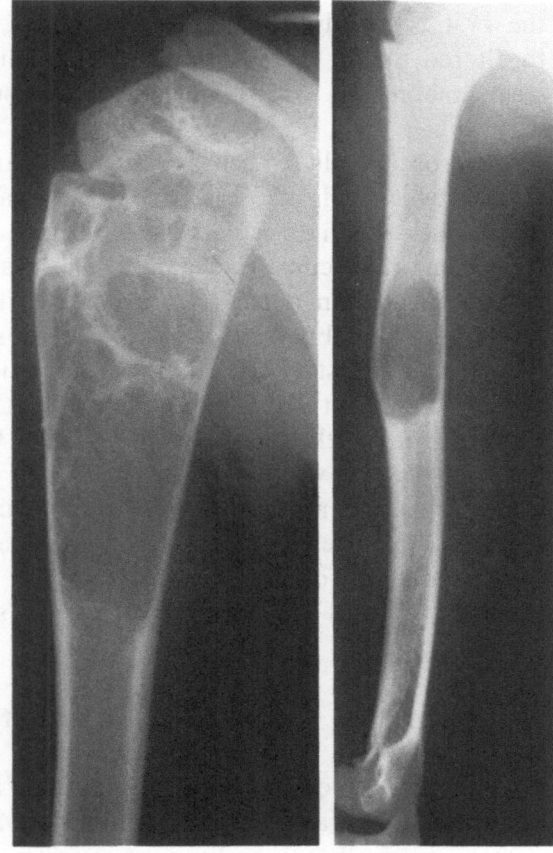

Fig. 1. Simple bone cyst of "active type" in proximal humerus of 6-year-old boy. Ridges in cyst wall give appearance of multiloculations but at time of surgery, unicameral bone cyst was found

Fig. 2. Simple bone cyst, "latent type" of humerus of 7-year-old boy

Fig. 1   Fig. 2

and could find no anatomically or histologically verified case of an unradiated solitary bone cyst in which a sarcoma had developed. In their report, they presented five examples of untreated cystic lesions of bone, roentgenographically resembling simple bone cysts, but histologically unproven, in which sarcomas arose from the walls of the cyst.

IV. Pathology

The description of the pathology of the simple bone cyst or the unicameral bone cyst has been little changed since its classic presentation in 1942 by JAFFE and LICHTENSTEIN. The discussions by AEGERTER and KIRKPATRICK (1968), SPJUT et al. (1971), and others confirm their findings.

The gross pathology of the simple cyst is best described by the surgeon. When exposing the cyst, the muscles surrounding the lesion will be normal unless the cyst has been fractured. If a break in the cyst had been present, the muscle will show changes secondary to the trauma, such as discoloration from hemorrhage. When exposed, the cortical walls of the cyst may present a bluish sheen due to the thinness of the cortex and the translucency of the fluid. The fluid in the cyst may be clear yellow or serosanguinous. If there has been a recent fracture, the fluid may be discolored by the blood and the cyst may contain blood clots. After the fluid is removed, the inside of the cyst will have bony ridges of various sizes and thicknesses, but the ridges will not divide the space into compartments. It is these ridges that may give the roentgenogram a multiloculated appearance to what is a unicameral cyst. The inner surface of the cyst is mostly gray-white, red-brown, or brown. The brown discoloration is due to altered blood. Curettings from the wall of the cyst may be meager. The connective tissue membrane which lines the inner surface of the cortex is usually smooth and very thin.

Microscopically, specific diagnostic features are lacking. The lining membrane varies from a few strands of connective tissue to a rather thick and sometimes vascular connective tissue. At times, isolated osteoid and mature bone may be seen in the membrane. New bone may constitute part of the cyst wall. The bone wall of the cyst is usually less compact than normal cortical bone. The intertrabecular spaces may often contain blood vessels. Subperiosteal bone formation is seen, particularly if the cyst is complicated by a fracture. Osteoblastic and osteoplastic activity may be seen in the areas of injury. Foci of luxuriant repair with many giant cells may be confused with, and diagnosed as cystic giant cell tumor, or aneurysmal bone cyst. The new bone and accompanying fibrosis in a cyst wall have, at times, been mistaken for fibrous dysplasia. Most solitary bone cysts contain foci of granulation tissue, evidence of old hemorrhage, fibrin, calcific deposits, cholesterol slits, macrophages, and a few inflammatory cells. The recurrent cysts frequently contain residuals of the bone chip grafts. The histologic features of the "active" and "latent" bone cysts are similar.

V. Pathogenesis

The etiology of the solitary bone cyst and the mechanism of its formation are not known, but several theories have been advanced. RECKLINGHAUSEN (1891) and SCHMIDT (1901) conceived of the solitary bone cyst as an area of fibrous osteitis that had undergone cystic degeneration. VIRCHOW's (1876) conception was that the solitary bone cyst represents a central bone tumor which has undergone cystic softening. These two theories are not in keeping with the known histology of the lesion.

Another theory, no longer in favor, was that postulated by MONCKEBERG (1904), and supported by KONJETZNY (1922), as well as GESCHICKTER and COPELAND (1949). It suggested that the solitary bone cyst was a healing form of localized osteitis fibrosa.

POMMER (1920) speculated that the solitary bone cyst results from a traumatic hematoma which is not absorbed. This was supported by LANG (1922). However, there is no proof for this either clinically, anatomically, or roentgenographically. PHEMISTER and GORDON's (1926) theory of infection as an etiologic factor also is lacking in verification.

MIKULICZ (1905) felt that the predilection of the solitary bone cyst for the young patient and for regions of active growth of long bones, suggests some local disturbance in bone growth and development as the etiologic factor.

The studies of COHEN (1960 and 1970) on the composition of the fluid contained in the simple cyst have led to the most likely explanation for the cause of the simple cyst. The fluid contained within the cysts was shown to have chemical components similar to that of serum. He has also demonstrated local abnormality in veins adjacent to a bone cyst by injecting aqueous radio-opaque contrast medium into the cyst. BRODER (1968) described two developing femoral cysts; in one patient with a contralateral congenital slipped epiphysis and in another with a contralateral congenital hip dislocation. Both cysts developed in areas with poorly defined lesions (nonossifying fibroma or calcified cartilagenous rests), further suggesting developmental abnormalities, with the cyst representing an expression of vascular abnormality.

VI. Roentgenology

The roentgenographic appearance of the solitary bone cyst has been well described by JAFFE and LICHTENSTEIN (1942), LODWICK (1958) and in various textbooks on roentgenology such as those by AEGERTER and KIRKPATRICK (1968), and EDEIKEN and HODES (1973).

The solitary bone cyst is a sharply demarcated metaphyseal lesion accompanied by expansion and thinning out of the bony cortex. As a rule, it originates adjacent to the epiphyseal plate and does not involve the plate or the epiphysis. The two reported exceptions have been described earlier in this article.

The exact location of cystic lesions of bone is important in the diagnosis and differential diagnosis of these lesions. The solitary bone cyst is centrally, or very rarely, eccentrically situated in the metaphysis. The cyst is elongated in the direction of the shaft, and its transverse diameter at the epiphyseal plate has the same width as the epiphysis. The cyst walls taper from the origin at, or near, the epiphyseal plate to the end of the cyst in the diaphyseal area, thus giving the cystic cavity a shape resembling a truncated cone. The transverse diameter of the cyst almost never exceeds the width of the epiphyseal plate. The gradual increase in the diameter near the plate is probably the result of progressive transverse growth of the plate from which the cyst is believed to have originated. The shape of the cyst is felt to be due to the static retention of the cystic cavity as the bone gets longer. This elongated wedge shape contrasts sharply with the round or oval shape of many central cystic lesions of bone which result from tumor growth (Fig. 3).

As the long bone grows, the relationship between the end of the cyst and the epiphyseal plate ends and normal cancellous bone grows between the epiphyseal plate and the cyst wall. Thus, as the epiphyseal plate grows away from the cyst, the cyst eventually is seen to be in the shaft of the bone. GRAHAM (1952) reported one case in which the cyst seemed to migrate from the proximal epiphyseal plate to the midshaft of the humerus during a period of nine years. JAFFE and LICHTENSTEIN (1942) used this distance between the cystic and the epiphyseal plate to name those at the plate as "active" and those at some distance from the plate as "latent." In general, the "latent" cyst ceases to increase in size and is more amenable to treatment. However, there are a few exceptions to this rule.

The simple bone cyst never extends through the cortex into the soft tissues. This observation will help to differentiate the cyst from most bone tumors.

The roentgenographic pattern of bone destruction seen with the simple bone cyst is of the same unicentric type seen with slowly growing benign cystic tumors. The central spongy bone in the region of the cyst is completely destroyed. In the typical cyst, the regular inner surface of the cortical bone forms a single unilocular cyst with sharply defined edges. Usually the cortex is very thin but never completely destroyed. While the edge of the cyst is quite sharp at the cortex and the epiphyseal plate, the edge near the narrow end may be indistinct. This indistinct area tends to become more sharply delineated as the cyst is separated from the epiphyseal line. The contour of the edge is regular or slightly scalloped where trabeculae traverse the inner wall of the cortex. Sometimes these ridges of bone in the wall of the cyst may be sufficiently prominent to give the roentgenographic appearance of a multilocular cyst, but when opened surgically will still be a single-chambered cyst.

The roentgen patterns of proliferative bone in simple bone cysts are those of a lesion without marginal aggressiveness and of static nature. Where the cyst adjoins cancellous bone, the reactive sclerosis of bone is seen as a sclerotic margin. When

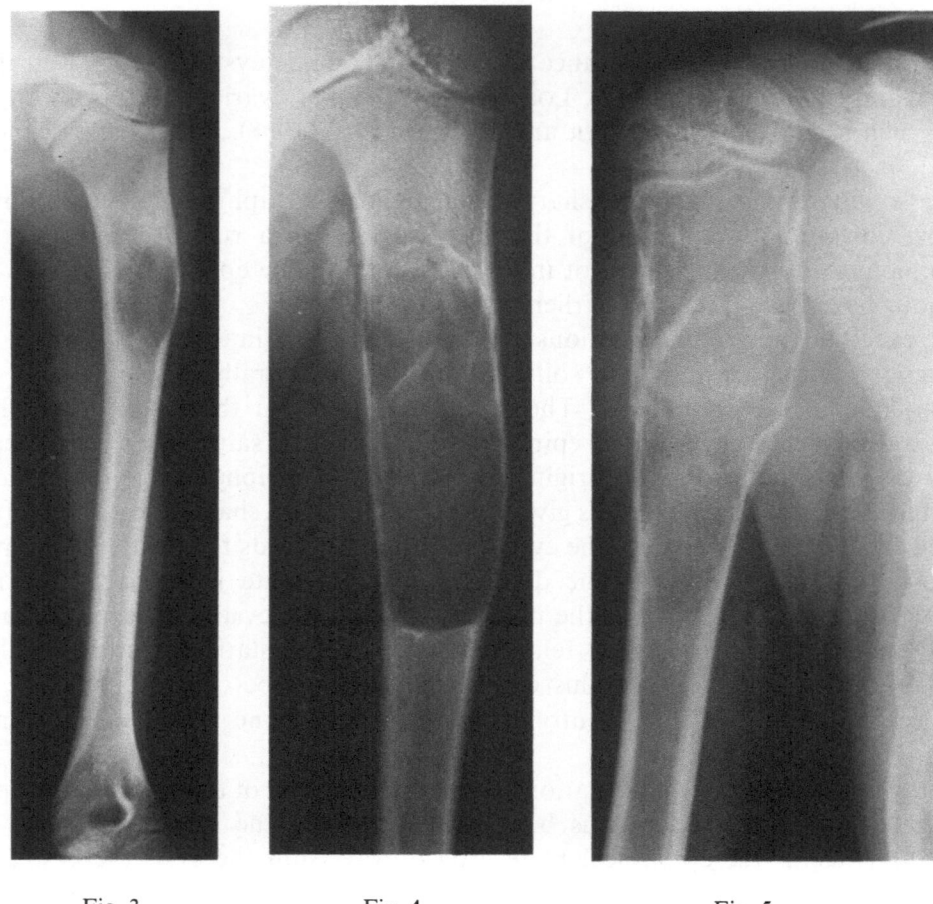

Fig. 3   Fig. 4   Fig. 5

Fig. 3. Simple bone cyst of proximal humerus of 8-year-old girl

Fig. 4. Fracture with "fallen fragment" of simple bone cyst of humerus of 5-year-old boy

Fig. 5. Fracture with "fallen fragment" of simple bone cyst of humerus of 7-year-old boy

fractured, there may be some slight outward pointing or bulging of the thin cortical wall. An excellent roentgenographic sign for this lesion was described by REYNOLDS (1969). This is the "fallen fragment sign" (Figs. 4,5). When a pathologic fracture or infraction of a cyst occurs, one of the fragments of bone can be seen within the cyst. This provides reliable evidence that the lesion is hollow and therefore a true cyst. When the fracture heals there is localized thickening of the cortex, and at times, the end of the cyst adjacent to the epiphyseal plate fills in with new bone. Normally, there is no surface lamina of periosteal new bone, nor laminated periostosis. Codman's triangle and spiculation are absent (Figs. 6–9).

MORCHOISNE and MASSE (1970) reported on the roentgen appearance of the evolution of simple bone cysts. About five years after diagnosis and treatment, there is residual cortical thickening, with or without additional thickened bone toward the medulla. Single or multiple lucent zones surrounded by sclerosis often remain. When the roentgen film is seen at this time, the appearance of the lesion resembles fibrous dysplasia.

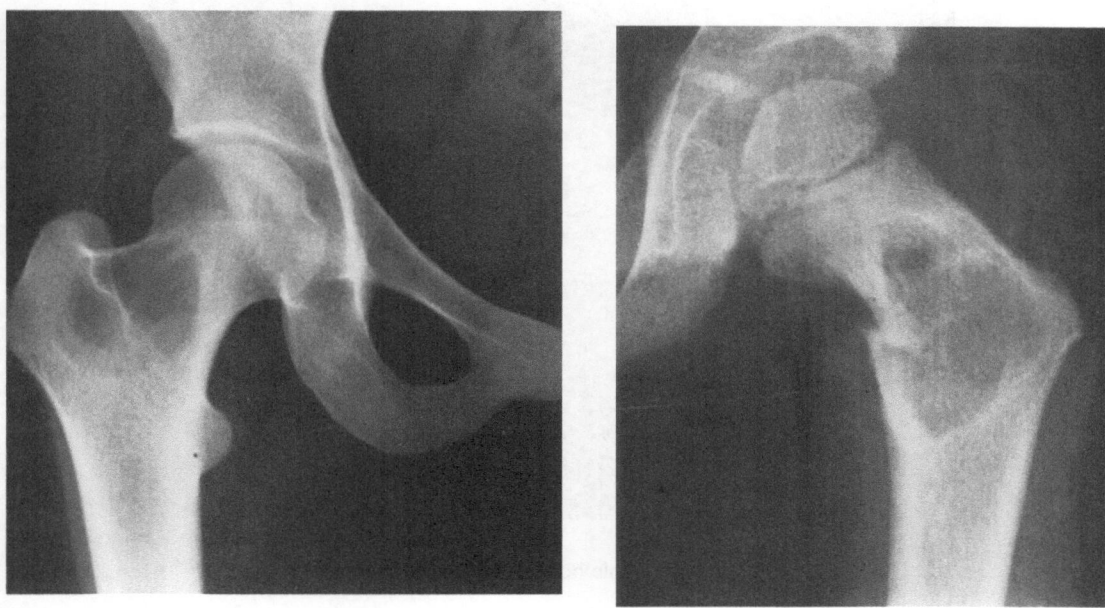

Fig. 6   Fig. 7

Fig. 6. Simple bone cyst in femoral neck of 17-year-old girl

Fig. 7. Fracture through simple cyst of femoral neck of 4-year-old boy

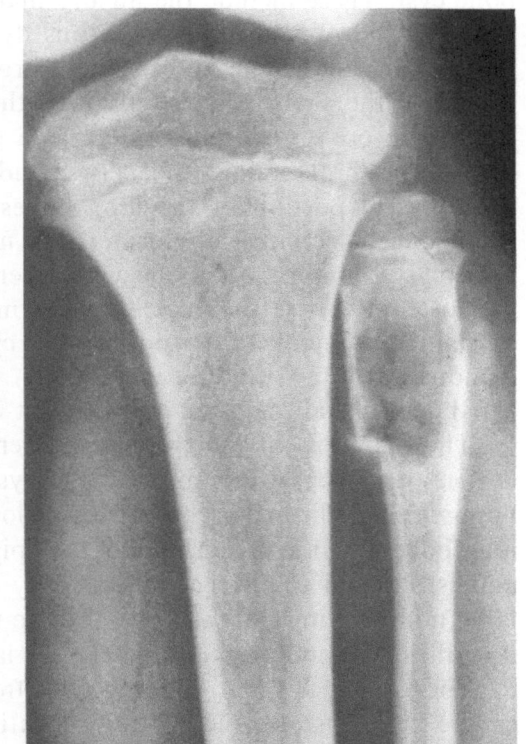

Fig. 8. Fracture of simple bone cyst of proximal fibula

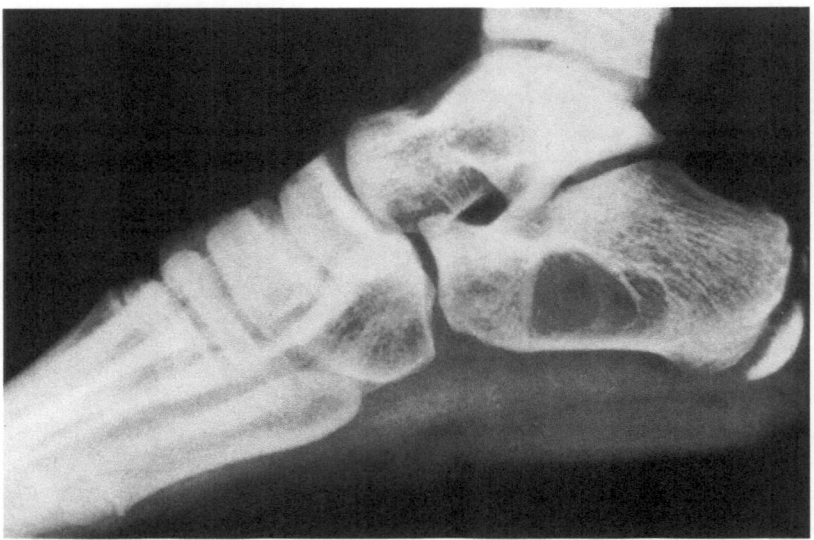

Fig. 9. Simple bone cyst of calcaneus

VII. Differential Diagnosis

There are several lesions to be considered in the differential diagnosis of the simple bone cyst. These include the aneurysmal bone cyst, the benign epiphyseal chondroblastoma, chondromyxofibroma, fibrous dysplasia, enchondroma, eosinophilic granuloma, lipoma, neurofibroma, and osteitis fibrosa cystica resulting from hyperparathyroidism.

While the skeletal distribution of the aneurysmal bone cyst tends to be similar to the simple bone cyst, the former has a greater tendency to develop in flat bones, such as the vertebral bodies, the pelvis, and the scapula. It is also more frequent in the metaphyseal portion of the long bones. It differs from the simple bone cyst in that it tends to be eccentrically located and may penetrate the cortical shell. The aneurysmal bone cyst contains soft tissue with intercellular matrix, especially metaplastic cartilage and osteoid. These may calcify to form flecks and spotty areas of increased density, a finding not seen with the simple bone cyst. There is a moderate marginal aggressiveness demonstrated by smudged or slightly moth eaten margins. The cortex is frequently expanded by trabeculation and the cyst is spherical rather than tapering and elongated.

The major roentgenographic differences between the nonossifying fibroma (benign cortical defect) and the simple bone cyst are the size and location of the lesions. The nonossifying fibroma is eccentrically located in the tapered segment of the end of a long bone at some distance from the epiphyseal plate. Usually, this lesion is quite small and is situated in the cortex but may extend into the medullary spongy bone. The large nonossifying fibroma may involve the entire medullary canal and, in this instance, it is difficult to differentiate from the "latent" simple bone cyst.

The principal roentgenographic differences between the giant cell tumor and the simple bone cyst are the eccentric location, the complete penetration of the cortex and the evidence of active expansion of the cortex in the giant cell tumor. The most common sites for the giant cell tumor are the distal femur and proximal tibia, relatively uncommon locations for the simple cyst. Also, the giant cell tumor will frequently involve the epiphysis.

It is relatively easy to separate the benign epiphyseal chondroblastoma from the simple bone cyst. While both have a cystic appearance, the benign epiphyseal chondroblastoma is primarily an epiphyseal lesion which may at times involve the metaphysis. It is eccentric in location and may break through the cortex to invade soft tissues. Flocculent calcification may be seen within the tumor.

The roentgenographic changes seen in the chondromyxofibroma resemble those of the aneurysmal bone cyst. It is an eccentrically located metaphyseal lesion with a moderate degree of active cortical expansion.

On rare occasions, it may be impossible to separate a localized area of fibrous dysplasia from the simple bone cyst because of the more extensive amount of the bone involved and the "soap bubble" appearance of the lesion on the roentgenogram.

Differentiation of a solitary bone cyst from an enchondroma is usually not difficult because the latter is most commonly seen in the diaphysis of a short tubular bone and punctate radiopacities can be seen within the tumor.

The roentgenographic appearance of the isolated eosinophilic granuloma will rarely suggest a solitary bone cyst. The eosinophilic granuloma starting out as a smaller lesion, may be anywhere in the bone and is frequently painful. The margins tend to be less distinct than those of the solitary bone cyst. Also eosinophilic granuloma frequently elicit a periosteal reaction. A central sequestrum and beveled edges may also be seen with the eosinophilic granuloma.

On rare occasions, the lipoma of bone may simulate the solitary bone cyst. This is especially true when the lesion is in the calcaneus. However, lipomas of bone are seen more often in older age groups than are the simple bone cysts.

While a rare intraosseous neurofibroma may resemble a solitary bone cyst, the usual changes of neurofibromatosis on bone are more like fibrous dysplasia.

The roentgenographic changes seen in osteitis fibrosa cystica resulting from hyperparathyroidism (brown tumor) resemble the giant cell tumor more than they do the solitary bone cyst. The margins of the lesion tend to be indistinct and the bone expanded. The ends of long bones are most frequently involved and the disorder is usually found at an older age than is common for the solitary bone cyst. Also, the serum calcium and the alkaline phosphatase levels are elevated.

VIII. Treatment and Prognosis

In 1942 JAFFE and LICHTENSTEIN recommended that the treatment of choice for the solitary bone cyst (whether active or latent) was to expose the cyst, curette its wall, fill it with autogenous bone chips, collapse the cyst wall, and close the wound. They did not recommend radiation therapy and felt that it would not help to heal the cyst. JAFFE (1958) noted that $6^{1}/_{2}$ years after the irradiation of a solitary bone cyst of the humerus, a fibrosarcoma developed at the site of the lesion.

In general, the technique of curetting the cyst and then packing it with bone chips has become the most common method of treatment. GRAHAM (1952) used autogenous bone chips, bone bank chips, or bone mill. SPENCE et al. (1969) used freeze-dried cancellous bone allografts. However, modifications of this method of treatment have been suggested by various authors. MARCOVE (1975) freezes the cavity with liquid nitrogen prior to packing with bony chips. FAHEY and O'BRIEN (1973) recommend subtotal resection of one-half to two-thirds of the cortex surrounding a cyst, saucerizing the remaining medullary surface and placing a tibial strut in the intramedullary cavity for reinforcement with iliac bone grafts filling the remaining space. AGERHOLM and GOODFELLOW (1965) suggested a treatment of subperiosteal radical excision of the entire cyst bearing part of the diaphysis. BADGLEY (1957) recommended treatment by crushing the cystic walls and filling the space with onlay grafts.

The follow-up of the treatment of solitary bone cysts has been reported by various authors including AGERHOLM and GOODFELLOW (1965), ALLDREDGE (1942), BOSEKER et al. (1968), GARCEAU and GREGORY (1954), GRAHAM (1952), JAMES et al. (1948), MOURGUES et al. (1974), and WILBER and HYATT (1960). NEER et al. (1973) report the largest series and their paper is one of the most recent. A survey of the literature reveals a recurrence rate of solitary bone cyst after treatment ranging 5–50%. The exact figures are difficult to obtain because of the lack of definitive criteria as to what constitutes recurrence. NEER et al. (1973) found that of 47 solitary bone cysts of the proximal humerus watched for 2–15 years, 70% remained adjacent to the epiphyseal plate. In addition, the cure rates for active and latent cysts after surgery was about the same. Their observation that recurrence is more frequent in patients under 10 years of age agrees with the studies of GARCEAU and GREGORY and other authors. Both NEER et al. (1973) and SPENCE et al. (1969) found a higher recurrence rate in males. The graft material used seems to have some influence on the cure rate. NEER et al. (1973) believe that autogenous grafts are superior to the various other types of bone available for grafting.

Several authors have reported on the outcome of pathologic fractures through solitary bone cysts. None of the 31 pathologic fractures reported by GRAHAM (1952) resulted in healing of the bone cyst. However, 15% of the bone cysts healed after a pathologic fracture in GARCEAU and GREGORY's (1954) series. ROBINS and PETERSON (1972), after reviewing the literature and their own experience, recommended that pathologic fractures in solitary bone cysts be managed by immobilization of the fracture until stability in an acceptable alignment is achieved. Then, after the epiphysis has grown a distance away from the cyst, a biopsy be made. After confirmation of the diagnosis, a subperiosteal full cortical thickness excision be done encompassing up to three-fourths of the tubular diameter and the medullary surface of the remaining bone excoriated. Then, the remaining defect is to be packed with autogenous bone. GALASKO's (1974) review of his own experience is in agreement.

Roentgen therapy is not recommended as a treatment for the solitary bone cyst. Not only might it delay healing, but over a period of time, could lead to growth arrest. In addition, JAMES et al. (1948) reported three instances of malignant transformation in areas treated for bone cyst with roentgen therapy 13–15 years earlier. These cases are in addition to others cited earlier in this paper.

B. Aneurysmal Bone Cyst

I. Introduction

The aneurysmal bone cyst is a benign lesion of bone, consisting of a cystic cavity filled with nonendothelial-lined spaces containing blood. It gets its name from its roentgen appearance rather than from its histology, an unusual occurrence among bone lesions.

Prior to 1942, this lesion was called by a variety of names. In 1950 it was definitely established as an entity in separate papers by JAFFE and by LICHTENSTEIN. The names that have been used for this lesion include aneurysmal giant cell tumor, atypical giant cell tumor, benign bone aneurysm, hemorrhagic bone cyst, ossifying hematoma, ossifying subperiosteal hematoma, subperiosteal giant cell tumor, hemangioma of bone, malignant bone aneurysm, and expansile hemangioma.

II. History

Prior to 1942 when JAFFE and LICHTENSTEIN first considered the aneurysmal bone cyst a distinct entity in the description of two cases in their classic paper on solitary bone cysts, this lesion was carried in the literature under various names and often considered a variant of the giant cell tumor. BRAILSFORD (1948), CONE (1928), and VAN ARSDALE (1893) wrote on ossifying hematoma, lesions that at the present time would be considered aneurysmal bone cysts. Also, the lesions called subperiosteal giant-cell tumor by COLEY (1949), GESCHICKTER and COPELAND (1949), HODGEN and FRANTZ (1947), PRESENT (1945), and THOMPSON (1954) by current criteria would be aneurysmal bone cysts. The atypical giant cell tumor of COLEY and MILLER (1942), the aneurysmal giant cell tumor of EWING (1940), the hemorrhagic bone cyst of BLOODGOOD (1923), and the expansile hemangioma of GURI (1948) would all be described as aneurysmal bone cysts by present day standards. Since the articles by JAFFE and LICHTENSTEIN written in 1950, there has been much less confusion in the nomenclature of this lesion.

III. Clinical

The exact incidence of the aneurysmal bone cyst is not known. Since 1950 there have been many isolated case reports of the disorder but few with any significant number of cases. DAHLIN et al. (1955) reviewed the experience of the Mayo Clinic with this lesion and found 26 aneurysmal bone cysts in a series of more than 2000 primary bone tumors. BESSE et al. (1956) reported that the incidence of aneurysmal bone cysts was approximately 1.5% of all primary tumors of bone removed surgically at the Mayo Clinic and that they are one third as common as giant cell tumors of bone.

The relative skeletal distribution of the lesions, the sex and age incidence can be generally summarized from nearly 600 cases reported by BARNES (1956), BEELER et al. (1957), BESSE et al. (1956), BIESECKER et al. (1970), BOOHER (1957), BOSSART and FITZPA-TRICK (1964), CLOUGH and PRICE (1968), CRUZ and COLEY (1956), DABSKA and BURAC-ZEWSKI (1969), DAUGHERTY and EVERSOLE (1971), DAHLIN et al. (1955), DOMINOK et al. (1971), DONALDSON (1962), GODFREY and GRESHAM (1959), KAZAN and KALIMOWA (1965), KOLAR (1958), LICHTENSTEIN (1957), LICHTENSZTAJN and GOLBERT (1960), LINDBOM et al. (1961), LOCHER and KAISER (1975), MC COHEN et al. (1964), PHELAN (1964), SHERMAN and SOONG (1957), SLOWICK et al. (1968), SUBRAMANIAM and MATHIAS (1962), TAYLOR (1956), TILLMAN et al. (1968), VERBIEST (1965), and others. The lesion is slightly more common in females than in males. The youngest patient reported with this disorder was 3-months-old and the oldest was 72-years-old. The vast majority of the lesions was seen in patients under 22 of age and most were 10–20 years-of age. The average age was about 16 years. The aneurysmal bone cyst has been reported to involve practically every bone in the body. It is usually a solitary lesion in any given patient.

The long bones and vertebrae are the most commonly involved sites. The lower extremity is involved 36% of the time, the proximal tibia being the most commonly affected site, then the distal femur. The metaphyseal areas of the bone are the areas of predilection but at times the diaphysis is involved.

The bones of the vertebral column are affected in 19% of the patients. The cervical and lumbar areas are the major sites of the disease. Several cases have been reported in which adjacent vertebrae have been involved by direct extension. The vertebral column is the area where multiple aneurysmal cysts, although an uncommon finding, are most apt to occur.

The upper limb is afflicted with aneurysmal bone cysts 16% of the time. The proximal humerus is the most common site of involvement.

The pelvis and sacrum are the site of disease in about 11% of the patients. The ribs are involved in 4%, the skull in 4%, the maxilla in 2%, the mandible in 3%, the clavicle in 4%, the scapula in 2%, and the sternum in less than 1%.

The presenting complaint of a patient with an aneurysmal bone cyst will vary with the bone involved. When a long bone is involved, the presenting complaint is usually that of local pain of several weeks or months duration. Frequently, a history of local trauma having been sustained shortly prior to the onset of the chronic pain is given. If the lesion is near the end of a long bone, stiffness and pain in the adjacent joint may be present. On physical examination of the area, a tender swelling may be found and a bruit may be heard, especially if the lesion is large. When the vertebral column is involved, pain and stiffness of the affected segment of the spine are the initial complaints. As the lesion increases in size, associated neural complaints are frequent. In the thoracic area, there may be girdle pains or progressive weakness of the lower limbs, possibly with numbness. In the cervical region, there may be neurological changes associated with pressure on the brachial plexus. If the lesion is in the lumbar or sacral area, loss of bladder and bowel control may develop. If the integrity of the affected vertebral body becomes undermined so that it partially collapses, the complaints associated with it will be accentuated and paraplegia may develop. The pain tends to be more severe with rapidly growing tumors.

The natural history of the aneurysmal bone cyst is not known. Some cysts have been observed to grow very slowly and others very rapidly. The finding of aneurysmal bone cysts in adults and the occurrence of cysts which have features of an aneurysmal bone cyst which has regressed into an inactive form, suggests the possibility of a process of natural repair in undetected cysts. SHERMAN (1957) observed 17 cases for periods from 3 months to 3 years prior to the institution of therapy. He found that there were three stages of development. The lytic or early phase was followed by a mature or characteristic appearing cyst, followed finally by a late or calcified stage. The majority of cases that he saw were in the mature stage. The development of the peripheral bone shell and internal septa may take place in a few months. After the appearance of a full blown lesion, several events may take place. First, the cyst may continue to grow at a variable and unpredictable rate. One case was noted to have increased four times in volume in seven months. Yet, another case was noted to increase in volume only 10% in a 3-year period. Second, reactivity may develop following a period of latency. Before the appearance of calcification, there was the possibility of further growth of the lesion although there had been a period of apparent stability of the lesion. Spontaneous regression or transformation from a full blown lesion into a calcified one may occur. There were three regressions in SHERMAN's series. Once the lesion reached the solidified stage (appearance of calcification and ossification) there was no recurrence. GODFREY and GRESHAM (1959) studied six cases at different ages including two in which the lesion was not detected until necropsy. They suggested a natural history of onset in childhood with a period of active growth proceeding in those cysts remaining undetected to an inactive stage with thrombosis and fibrosis.

While in general the aneurysmal bone cyst is a solitary lesion, TILLMAN et al. (1968)

reported multiple involvement of vertebrae in 7 of 15 cases in which the lesion involved the spinal column. They also reported a 10-year-old girl who had an aneurysmal cyst of the talus treated, who developed another lesion in the distal tibia 11 months later. TILLMAN et al., also noted that the aneurysmal bone cyst may involve more than one bone due to expansion. It is the only benign lesion known to extend from one bone to another in the vertebral column.

The aneurysmal bone cyst is a benign lesion. HIRST et al. (1970) reported four cases which they believed to be malignant aneurysmal bone cysts. LICHTENSTEIN (1975) and other authors believe the "malignant aneurysmal bone cyst" to be a telangiectatic osteogenic sarcoma or an angiosarcoma.

BIESECKER et al. (1970) found an intimate relationship between aneurysmal bone cysts and other bone lesions; as evidenced by the presence of both entities in the initial lesion and in the recurrences. Other accompanying primary bone lesions appeared in 21 of 66 aneurysmal bone cysts (32%). The recurrences contained both lesions in seven of eight instances (86%). They believed the relationship of the two lesions to be a cause and effect.

EDEIKEN and HODES (1973) state that aneurysmal bone cysts frequently arise from pre-existing bone lesions, such as chondroblastoma, giant cell tumor, chondromyxoid fibroma, xanthoma, or osteosarcoma. Since the primary lesion may be small and overlooked, aneurysmal bone cysts should be considered with suspicion of an underlying tumor.

IV. Pathology

The pathology of the aneurysmal bone cyst is summarized in many articles with the best descriptions in the papers by LICHTENSTEIN (1950), DAHLIN et al. (1955), and SPJUT et al. (1971).

The gross pathologic findings of the lesion are rarely seen because the treatment is usually by curettage. However, when the lesion is totally resected, the excised part of the bone resembles an inflated balloon with raised periosteum. Underneath the periosteum, a thin osseous shell covers the entire tumor. Under the shell, the bone is completely destroyed and replaced by a labyrinth of rounded cavities of various sizes filled with liquid blood. When sectioned, the aneurysmal bone cyst has the appearance of a cavernous vascular tumor. In the long bones, the tumor is usually eccentrically located. The cavities within it are surrounded by whitish grey or brownish elastic fibrous tissue and vary in size from a few millimeters to a few centimeters. The inner surfaces are smooth and glossy. Some tumors have a strikingly cystic structure with the multiple small cysts divided by a scanty amount of fibrous connective tissue and resemble sponges. Others are more fibrous with few cavities and look more like swiss cheese. Osseous material may be found in the fibrous tissue dividing the cavities.

When seen by the surgeon at the time of the surgical approach, the aneurysmal bone cyst has a very thin outer shell of bone which, when broken through, releases free flow of venous blood. The bleeding may be profuse. When the bleeding is controlled, the gross pathology is as described above. At times, the cysts may contain fluid other than blood. The small aneurysmal bone cysts are usually more solid and less cavernous than are the large ones.

The microscopic anatomy of the aneurysmal bone cyst is variable. Basically, the lesion is formed by large and small blood spaces that may be outlined by trabeculae of fibrous tissue, osteoid, or granulation tissue in which multinucleated giant cells are seen. The trabeculae separating these vascular channels are of different thicknesses and

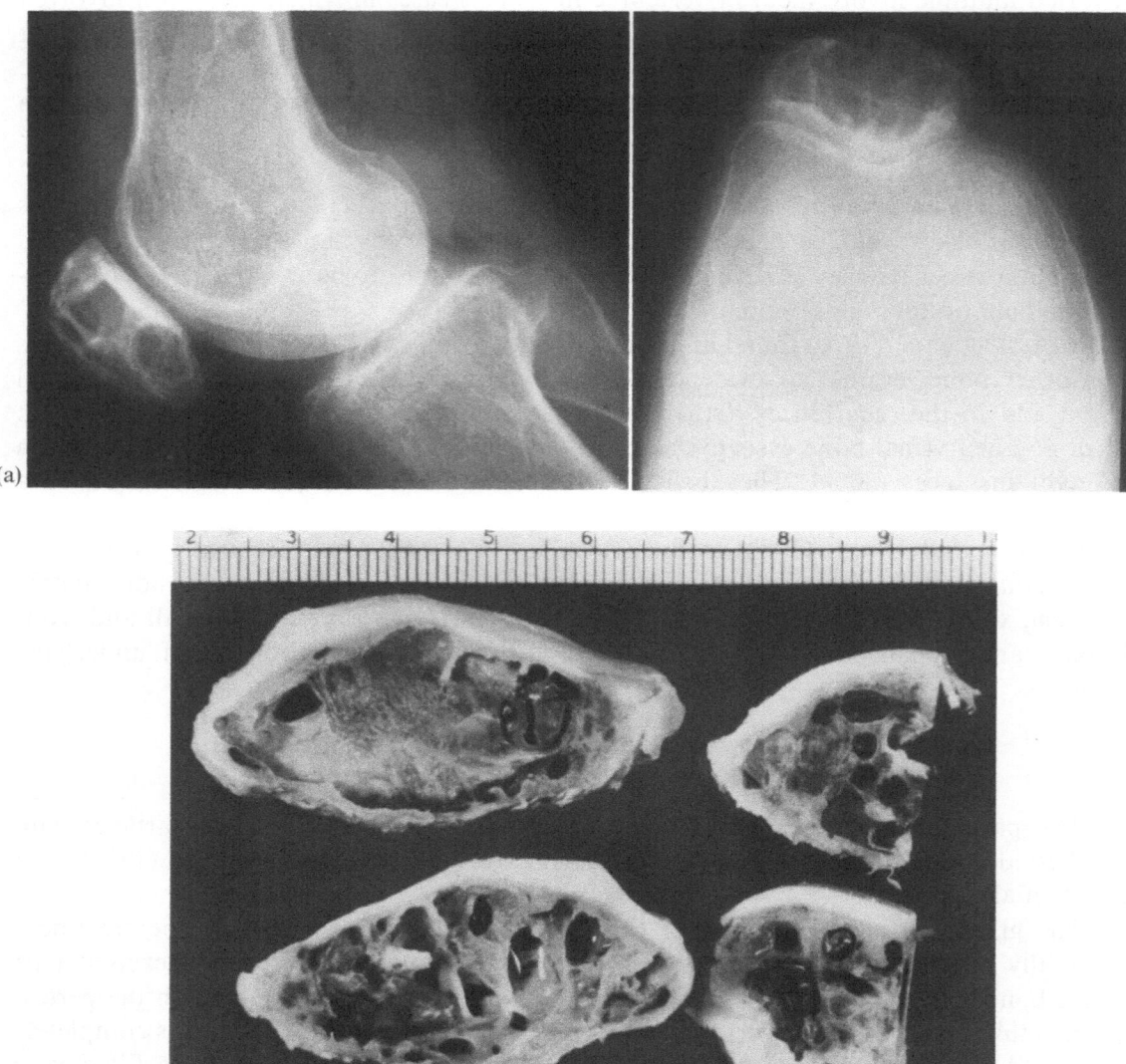

Fig. 10a and b. Aneurysmal bone cyst of patella. (c) Gross pathology of patella lesion. (d) Histopathology of aneurysmal bone cyst. At top of illustration is shown articular cartilage of patella beneath which are trabeculae of subchondral bone. In this section much of cancellus bone of patella has been replaced by stroma resembling poorly organized granulation tissue. Hemorrhagic areas and numerous giant cells are scattered throughout

lengths, but tend to be spindly. Solid areas of fibrous tissue, spindly osteoid, mature bone, and multinucleated giant cells may be seen. In some of the aneurysmal bone cysts, the blood spaces are lined by an indistinct endothelium without a smooth muscle layer. The stroma may contain hemosiderin, extravasated blood, histiocytes, and a variety of inflammatory cells. In the periphery, subperiosteal bone formation may be present while adjacent soft tissues such as skeletal muscle, fat, and connective tissue are compressed (Fig. 10a–d).

When interpreting the histology of a lesion suspected to be an aneurysmal bone cyst, the roentgenographs, and the clinical information should be reviewed. This is necessary because the presence of multinucleated giant cells and blood filled channels

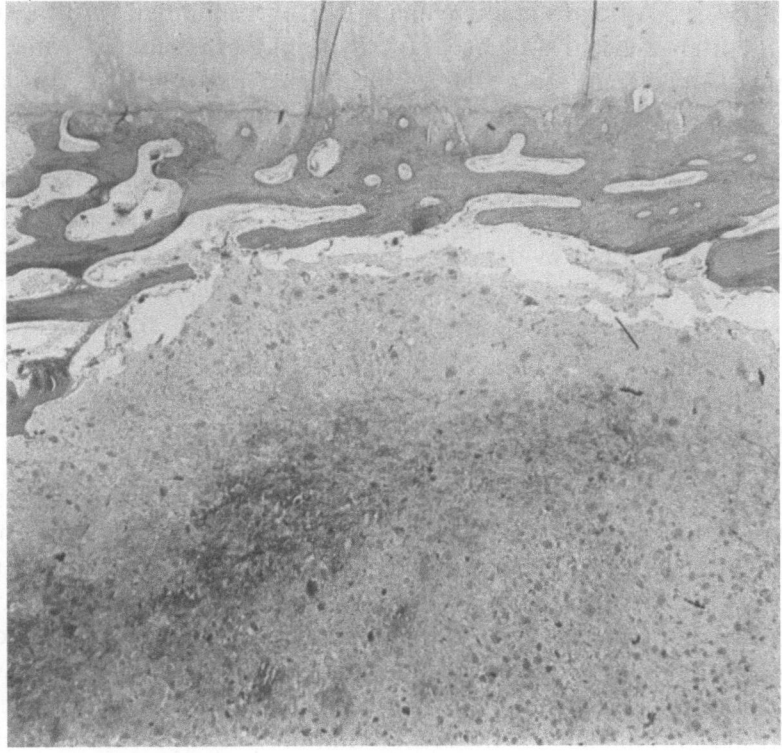

Fig. 10d

may lead to a mistaken diagnosis of giant cell tumor. Also, the reaction of the various tissue components of an aneurysmal bone cyst to fracture may suggest an osteosarcoma.

V. Pathogenesis

The pathogenesis of aneurysmal bone cyst is unknown. Three etiologic concepts have been suggested to explain the development of aneurysmal bone cyst. The first is that the cyst is a secondary manifestation developing in a pre-existing lesion altered by hemorrhage, cystic change, or some other superimposed pathologic process. The second theory, which is the most widely accepted one, is that the lesion is caused by some variation in the vascular supply or hemodynamics of the region. The third is that the disorder is an unusual late result of trauma.

Some authors such as BIESECKER et al. (1970) and BURACZEWSKI and DABSKA (1971) favor the theory that the aneurysmal bone cyst develops in some way from a pre-existing lesion. They base this upon the finding of other lesions in conjunction with the cyst. BIESECKER et al. found aneurysmal bone cysts accompanying primary lesions of bone in 32% (21 of 66) of their cases. BURACZEWSKI and DABSKA suspected that in some of the cases the underlying lesion was fibrous dysplasia and cited two cases in which the two lesions coexisted. Aneurysmal bone cysts have been reported to be found in the same lesion of bone along with chondromyxoid fibroma, benign osteoblastoma, nonossifying fibroma, chondroblastoma, giant cell tumor of bone, giant cell reparative granuloma, fibromyxoma, and unicameral bone cyst. However, most of the reported cases do not have histologic evidence of any lesion other than aneurysmal bone cyst.

The concept of a local vascular change was proposed by LICHTENSTEIN (1950) as the underlying cause leading to reactive changes in the bone that result in the aneurysmal bone cyst. The often marked and occasionally rapid extension of some of these cysts, and the common operative finding of a blood filled cyst with the blood often welling up to the extent as to give rise to some concern, are bits of evidence which tend to support this theory. The arteriographic studies of DOS SANTOS (1950), LINDBOM et al. (1961) RING et al. (1972) and SCHOBINGER and STOLL (1957) which show changes suggesting a vascular lesion and the possibility of an arteriovenous shunt add further support for this concept. Additional evidence is the manometric studies showing elevation of cyst pressure to arteriolar levels in some cysts (BIESECKER et al., 1970). Thus, it appears reasonable that the aneurysmal bone cyst originates as the result of a local change in hemodynamics, usually in the more vascular active tissues of the immature skeleton, i.e., the metaphyses, and that some arise secondarily in a pre-existing bone lesion. The cause of this vascular change is subject to debate and some believe that trauma may play a role.

Some support is given to trauma as an etiologic factor in the case reported by GINSBURG (1974). This was a newborn boy who was found to have a healing fracture of the radial diaphysis and a destructive lesion in the distal radial metaphysis, 6 hours following birth. The fracture healed normally, but, although the child was, 3 months old, the progressive increase in size of the metaphyseal lesion led to a surgical exploration. An aneurysmal bone cyst was found and curetted. Six months later there was no evidence of the cyst remaining. However, most authors discount trauma as the sole etiologic factor and feel that trauma may be the reason that the patient seeks medical care, resulting in the discovery of the aneurysmal bone cyst.

VI. Roentgenology

The roentgenographic features of the aneurysmal bone cyst are described in many papers and textbooks. Probably the best descriptions are those by DAHLIN et al. (1955), LICHTENSTEIN (1953), and SHERMAN and SOONG (1957).

The roentgenographic appearance of the aneurysmal bone cysts varies to some degree depending upon the bone in which it resides. It has its "classic" picture when seen in the long bones. In the flat bones and small tubular bones its appearance is much less unique. The aneurysmal bone cyst when seen in the long bones may be eccentric, central, or parosteal types (SHERMAN and SOONG). The eccentric and central types may be seen in either the metaphysis or diaphysis of the bone.

The "classic" aneurysmal bone cyst (as seen in long bones) is eccentric in position and diaphyseal in location (Figs. 11, 12a, b, 13a, b, 14, 15). It has an ovoid configuration with an expanding, ballooned-out, rarefied area containing fine and incomplete ridges or septa, producing a honeycomb appearance. The borders are well-demarcated, with a thin layer of new bone in continuation with the thinned out and expanded cortex. While the location is most often metaphyseal, it frequently extends into the diaphysis and at times is purely diaphyseal. As a rule, the epiphysis is never affected when the epiphyseal plate is still visible. Following the cessation of endochondral bone growth, the epiphyseal part of the bone may be invaded by direct extension. The long axis of this ovoid lesion coincides with the long axis of the bone. The inner or intraosseous margin of the aneurysmal bone cyst is smooth and distinct with occasional sclerotic areas. The outer or extraosseous border is a thin layer of new bone resembling an "eggshell" which becomes thicker and denser with growth of the cyst. In spite of bulky extension of the lesion beyond the bone, there is usually no local soft tissue reaction. At times, a minimal, smooth, laminated periosteal elevation with triangular or cufflike appearance at both ends of the cyst is present. The internal picture of the lesion is relatively characteristic. The ballooned-out lytic area contains fine and incomplete lines forming many small loculations, which are more numerous at the periphery of the

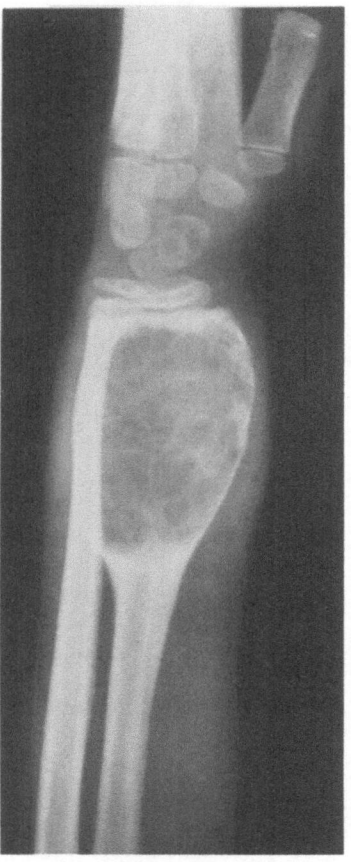

Fig. 11. Aneurysmal bone cyst of distal radius with marked "ballooning" of cortex

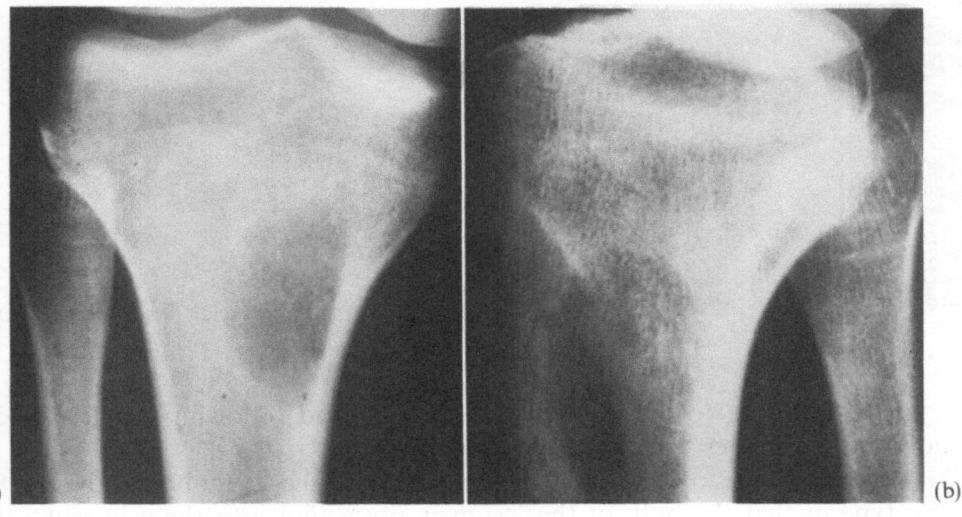

(a)   (b)

Fig. 12a and b. Early changes in proximal tibia of aneurysmal bone cyst in frontal and lateral views

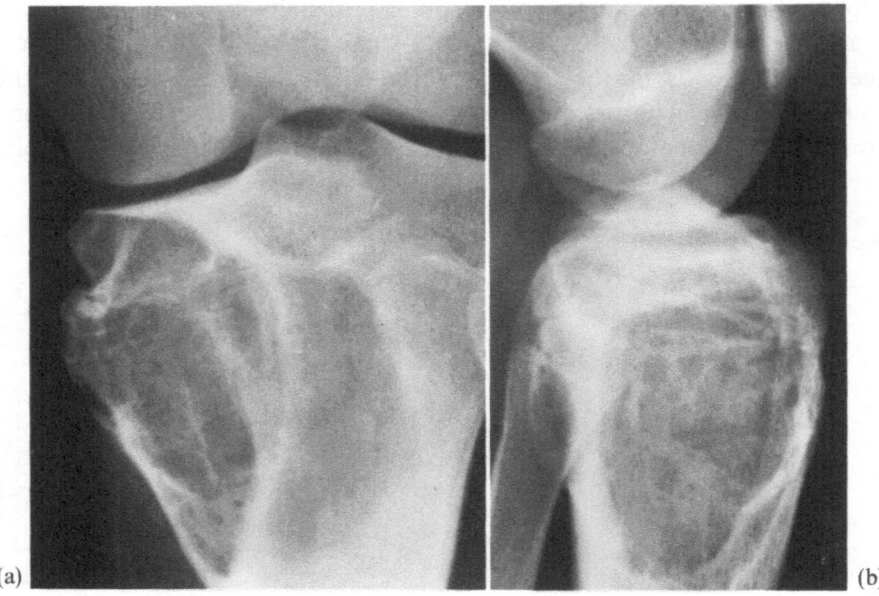

(a)   (b)

Fig. 13a and b. Frontal and lateral views of aneurysmal bone cyst of proximal tibia. Note eccentric location

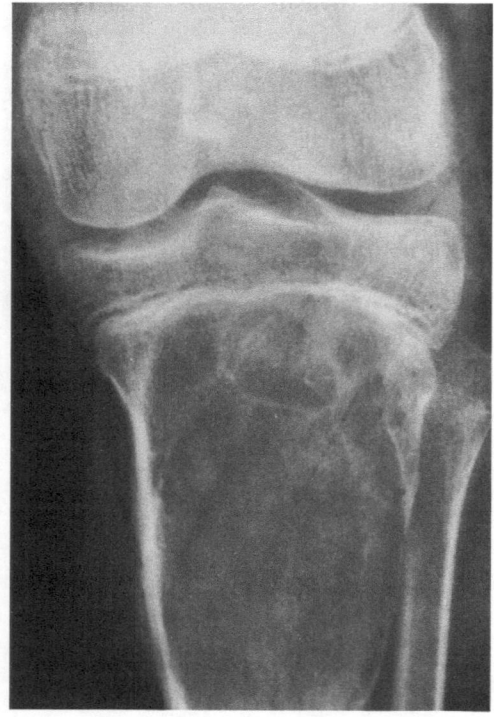

Fig. 14. Large aneurysmal bone cyst of proximal tibia

lesion. In the late stage of development of the cyst and following surgical intervention or irradiation, the ridges become denser and coarser.

The parosteal type of aneurysmal bone cyst of the long bones differs from the eccentric type in that the bulk of the lesion is projecting into the adjacent soft tissues with only minimal erosion of the outer cortex.

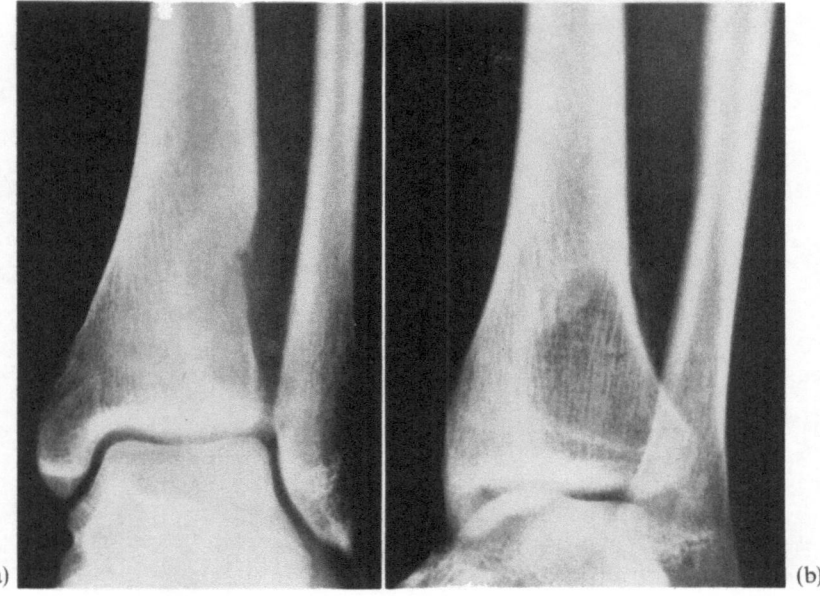

(a)   (b)

Fig. 15a and b. Aneurysmal bone cyst of distal tibia

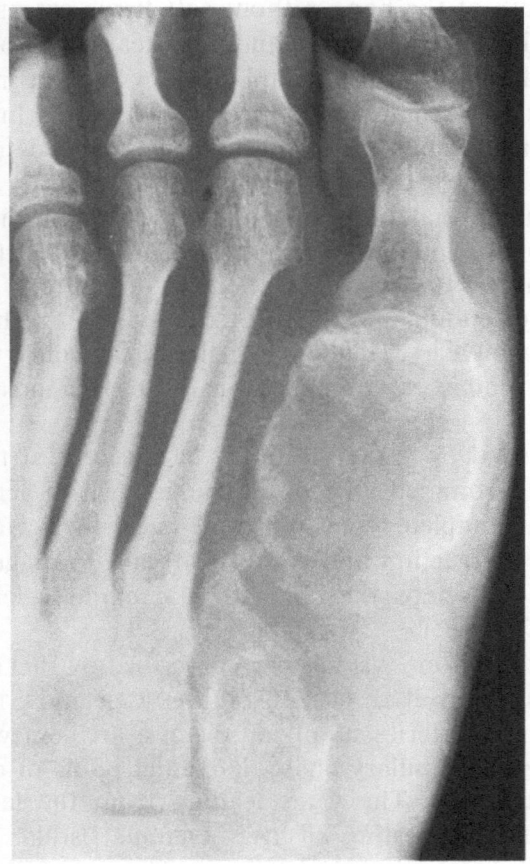

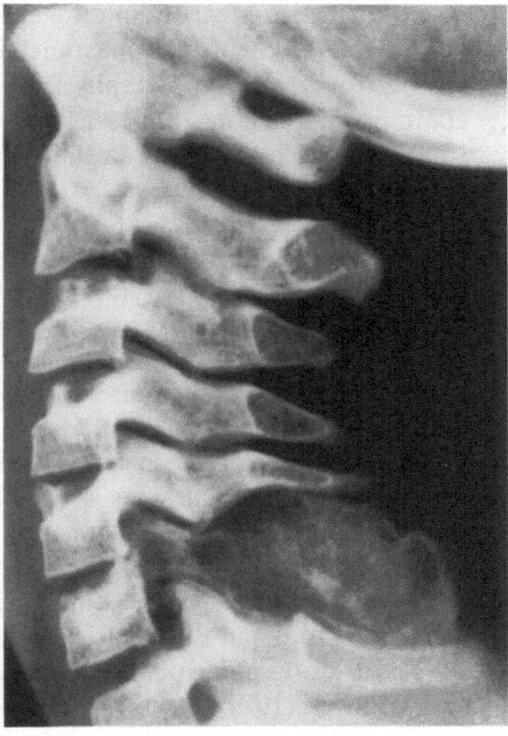

Fig. 17. Classical appearance of aneurysmal bone cyst involving posterior elements of sixth cervical vertebra. Note expansion and thinning of spinous process. (Figures 17 and 18 are from the Department of Radiology, Hospital for Special Surgery, New York, N.Y.)

Fig. 16. Aneurysmal bone cyst of first metatarsal

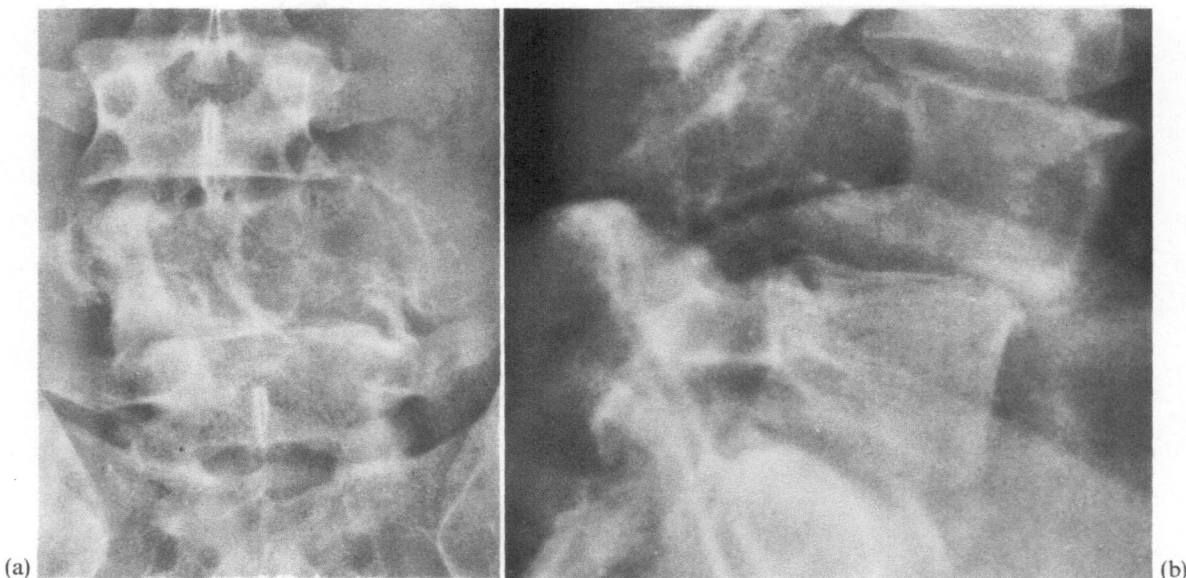

Fig. 18a and b. Frontal and lateral views of aneurysmal bone cyst involving posterolateral aspects of fourth lumbar vertebra. Note predominant involvement of posterior elements and mild spondylolisthesis

In the central type, the aneurysmal bone cyst is a symmetrically located, pear-shaped or fusiform lesion expanding the entire width of the bone without soft tissue extension. Otherwise, the roentgen appearance is similar to the eccentric and parosteal. The central type is found in the metaphysis or the diaphysis. The metaphyseal cysts were most common in the long bones such as the tibia, femur, and humerus. The cysts in the small tubular bones such as the metacarpals, metatarsals, and phalanges tended to be diaphyseal in location (Fig. 16).

When the vertebra is involved, the aneurysmal bone cyst almost always is in the lamina and extends to other parts of the bone. The lesion is usually eccentric in location, beginning as an area of rarefaction with barely discernable borders. Eventually, an expanding multiloculated process is noted, extending into the soft tissues with "eggshell" borders. If the vertebral body becomes involved, it tended to collapse at some time in the course of the disease. If the body collapses completely, roentgen diagnosis is almost impossible (Figs. 17, 18a, b).

In the bones of the pelvis, the aneurysmal bone cyst tends to be the central type. When seen in the iliac wing it presents as a rounded area of rarefaction with sclerotic borders, containing faint calcifications and incomplete septa. When seen near the acetabulum, it starts as an area of irregular bone destruction and is most difficult to diagnose accurately. As the cyst becomes bigger, it develops the characteristic ovoid calcified structure and diagnosis is easier (Figs. 19, 20a, b).

The arteriographic picture of the aneurysmal bone cyst has been described by BILLINGS and WERNER (1972), LINDBOM et al. (1961), RING et al. (1972), SCHOBINGER and STOLL (1957), and ZUCCHI and ALLEGRINI (1962). The arteries supplying the cyst are somewhat dilated and peripherally distributed. During the capillary phase, indistinct pools of contrast medium are seen within the cyst structure. The veins leading from the lesion are filled slightly earlier than the other veins suggesting an arteriovenous fistula. The degree of the shunt is less than that seen in most malignant tumors. The angiographic findings in the patient described by RING et al. had features usually associated with

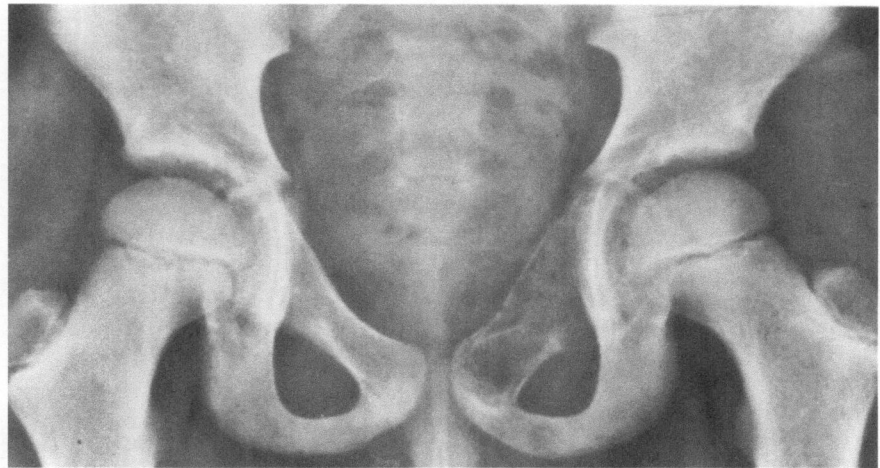

Fig. 19. Aneurysmal bone cyst of pubic bone

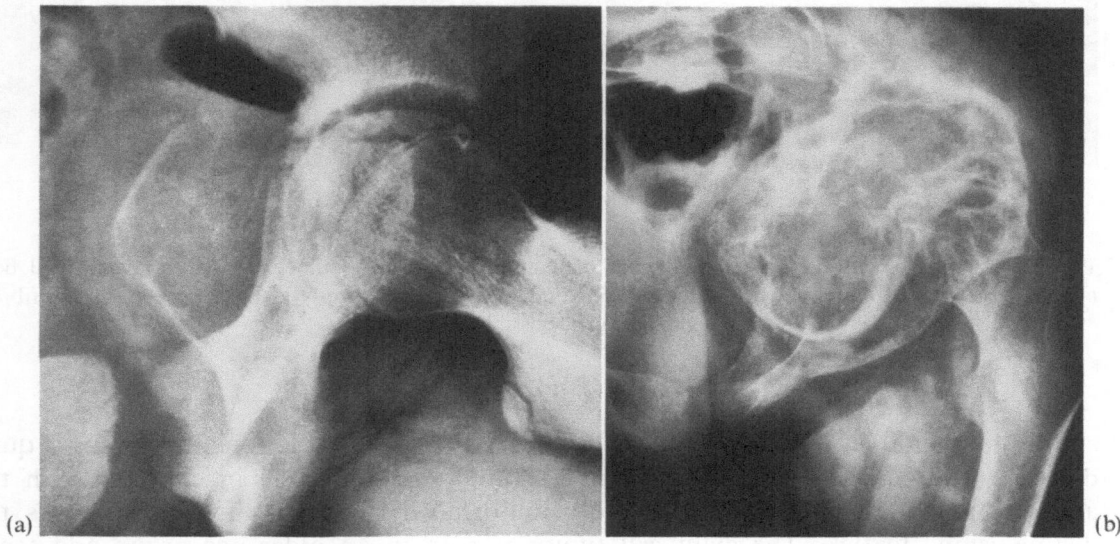

Fig. 20. (a) Aneurysmal bone cyst of pubic bone of 12-year-old girl. (b) Four months later. Note increase in size and extent of lesion

sarcomas of bone, i.e., an intense vascularity, early and rapid venous shunting, and soft tissue extension of the tumor. Angiographic studies do not seem to be helpful in the diagnosis of aneurysmal bone cysts.

VII. Differential Diagnosis

The differential diagnostic possibilities of the aneurysmal bone cyst include the giant cell tumor, fibrous dysplasia of bone, simple bone cyst, ossifying hematoma, some forms of myositis ossificans, cavernous hemangioma of bone, chondroma, chondromyxoid fibroma, malignant highly vascularized tumors metastatic to bone (renal carcinoma or thyroid carcinoma), and primary bone tumors including angiosarcoma, hemangioendothelioma, and teleangiectatic osteogenic sarcoma (Fig. 21 a–d).

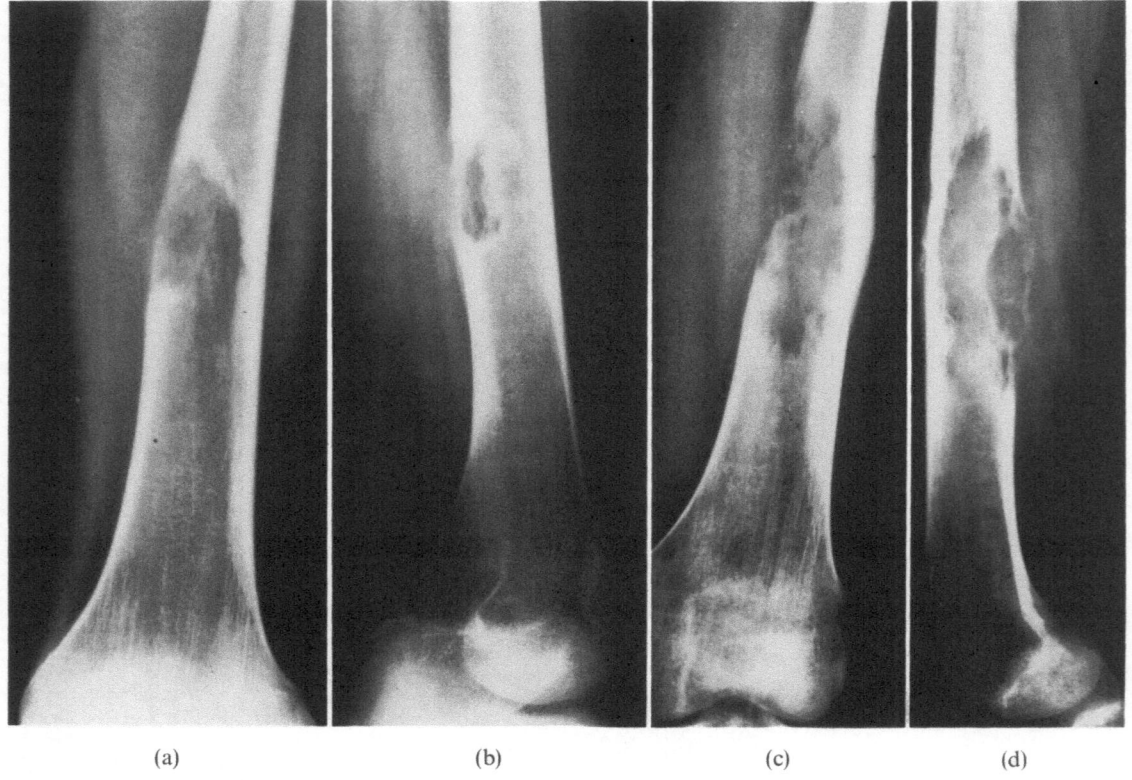

(a)　　　　　　　　(b)　　　　　　　　(c)　　　　　　　　(d)

Fig. 21a–d. Note eccentric lytic lesion of shaft of femur. Biopsy at this time reported as aneurysmal bone cyst. Recurrence 3 months later following curetting and bone grafting. Biopsy as this time reported as fibrous histiocytoma, possibly malignant

In the mandible, roentgenographic differentiation of cystic lesions that occur is quite difficult. The central giant cell reparative granuloma has much in common with the aneurysmal bone cyst but may be more uniformly radiolucent. The histology is the distinguishing feature. The giant cell tumor is seen in an older age group and tends to be more aggressive. The "brown" tumor of hyperparathyroidism is diagnosed from the appearance of other bones in the skeleton and by the alterations of the serum calcium, serum phosphorus, and alkaline phosphatase levels.

The giant cell tumor may at times be very difficult to distinguish from the aneurysmal bone cyst roentgenographically. However, the separation can frequently be done. The giant cell tumors usually occur in the long bones, where they almost invariably arise in the epiphysis. They are rare in persons under 20 years of age. They recur more often than the aneurysmal bone cyst and metastasize 10% of the time. The histologic features are decidedly different. Giant cell tumors have a homogenous cellular stroma with numerous multinuclear cells and lack the cavernous blood spaces of the aneurysmal bone cast.

Fibrous dysplasia is usually easy to separate from the aneurysmal bone cyst roentgeno-graphically by the absence of the cystic spaces. However, on rare occasions, the roentgen picture may defy differentiation. The microscopic features are entirely diagnostic.

Differentiation of the simple bone cyst is usually not difficult and is discussed earlier in this chapter.

The chondromyxoid fibroma may resemble an aneurysmal bone cyst in its expansion, eccentric location, and reticulated internal pattern. However, the chondromyxoid fibroma has more scalloped margins and denser, thicker, and more complete septation.

The roentgen characteristics of the aneurysmal bone cyst (i.e. eccentricity, characteristic expansion, and internal pattern) are such that nonossifying fibroma, chondroma, chondroblastoma and enchondroma are easily ruled out.

At times the malignant lesions may be difficult to distinguish from the aneurysmal bone cyst; but the fuzzy indistinct margins of the malignant lesions, and the pattern of periosteal reaction adjacent to them will make the differential diagnosis easier.

Ossifying hematomas and myositis ossificans sometimes have a roentgenographic image that suggests the aneurysmal bone cyst. Shell-like ossification may be present. The ossification is more intense in the final phase and is always spontaneous, thus compact bone is formed outside the bone. A tangential roentgenogram can help by showing the separation between the ossification and the bone.

The roentgenographic picture of the cavernous hemangioma of bone is quite different than that of the aneurysmal bone cyst. The former has dense, regular septae, sometimes in a parallel arrangement. There is no expansile effect on bone and the lesion is rare in long bones; being seen most often in vertebral bodies.

VIII. Treatment and Prognosis

Treatment is generally advised for the aneurysmal bone cyst soon after the diagnosis is established. This is because of the rapid potential for growth of the lesion and especially in the lesion of the spine where occasionally paraplegia has resulted from pressure of the cyst.

The treatment is usually surgical but may be roentgen therapy (NOBLER et al., 1968) or cryotherapy (BIESECKER et al., 1970; MARCOVE and MILLER, 1969), or any combination of these techniques. The surgery may be resection of the involved section of the bone, the whole bone, or excision of the lesion from the involved bone. Another surgical approach is that of curettage, either partial or complete.

Cryotherapy (BIESECKER et al., MARCOVE and MILLER) is a treatment technique which involves the introduction of liquid nitrogen into the cyst after curettage, to freeze the tissues 1–2 cm deep to the periphery of the cyst. This is done because of the feeling that curettage alone fails since it often does not deal with the underlying vascular abnormality in the bone outside the cyst wall.

Roentgen therapy has been used successfully in the management of the aneurysmal bone cyst. NOBLER et al. recommend a tumor dose of 2000–3000 rads, given in 2–3 weeks. This was the most successful dose in their experience. They feel that roentgen therapy is the treatment of choice.

Determination of the effectiveness of the different forms of treatment is difficult because of the relative rarity of the aneurysmal bone cyst, the many methods of treatment used and the dilemma in knowing how thorough the curettage or excision has been.

Treatment may fail to stop the growth and expansion of the aneurysmal bone cyst; or after a period of quiescence further growth or recurrence may occur. CLOUGH and PRICE (1973) found that recurrences are unusual after 2 years, and quite rare after 4 years. TILLMAN et al. (1968) reported a recurrence 13 years following treatment.

The anatomical site, the size of the cyst, its speed of growth, and the presence or the imminent threat of pathologic fracture or spinal cord involvement are factors which determine the method of therapy. Additional points to be considered are whether the lesion is a primary or recurrent one. Complete resection of the involved area of bone (such as a cyst of the proximal fibula) is a dependable method of achieving a cure. However, since the aneurysmal bone cyst is a benign lesion, more conservative methods are recommended if resection could interfere with function. It is in this instance where the decision to use curettage or roentgen therapy must be made. The recurrence rate (CLOUGH and PRICE, 1973) after resection is zero, after curettage 28.7%, and after roentgen therapy 16.6%. Although, roentgen therapy seems to have a better cure rate, curettage is often the treatment used. This is done because an open biopsy to establish the diagnosis is necessary prior to therapy and no further risk is incured by extending this to a full curettage if the macroscopic diagnosis is certain. In addition, roentgen therapy introduces the additional potential risk of interference with the growth plate and more remotely of post-irradiation sarcoma (DABSKA and BURACZEWSKI, 1969; LICHTENSTEIN, 1953, and TILLMAN et al., 1968). Roentgen therapy, probably, should be used in those cysts which are surgically inaccessible and where the operative risk is judged greater than the risk of post-irradiation sarcoma. It should also be considered to treat those cysts which are so big or so situated as to be difficult to curette completely; which continue to grow after curettage; or which recur repeatedly. Roentgen therapy is often used to treat lesions of the pelvis, sacrum, and spine. In the spine, surgical decompression and/or fusion may be necessary.

Recurrences are more likely in patients under 15 years than in those over 15 years of age (TILLMAN et al., BIESECKER et al.). If a lesion recurs, it should be rebiopsied to check for the possibility of another coexisting lesion. Failure to control growth of the original cyst or definite recurrence is an indication for further treatment. Recurettage and/or roentgen therapy will often control the lesion.

Despite their high recurrence rate, aneurysmal bone cysts have, with treatment, an excellent prognosis.

C. Juxta-Articular Bone Cyst (Intraosseous Ganglia)

I. Introduction

1. Other terms that have been used in the literature for this entity are: synovial cyst, bursal cyst, and degenerative cyst.

2. The juxta-articular bone cyst is currently defined as a primary bone lesion of unknown etiology, which is identical on pathologic specimens to the far commoner soft tissue ganglion (JOHNSON et al., 1965). A rare lesion, the largest reported series of biopsy proven intraosseous ganglia, included 38 cases (FELDMAN and JOHNSTON, 1973), and a review of the literature by the latter authors revealed only 40 other documented cases. However, the incidence of this lesion in the population may be falsely low due to the confusing nomenclature.

Although most juxta-articular bone cysts are present in young adults, the age range varies considerably, with cases reported from 14 years of age to 73 years of age (FELDMAN and JOHNSTON, 1973). There is a slight male predominence and the lesions occur predominently in the lower extremities.

II. Etiology

Juxta-articular bone cysts or intraosseous ganglia have been referred to in the literature variously as synovial cysts, bursal cysts, or degenerative cysts. The variation in the nomenclature reflects the numerous theories concerning the origin of these lesions. The basic question which remains unanswered is whether these benign cysts arise as primary bone lesions, or whether they are a secondary manifestation of pathology in the neighboring joint space. Their predilection for occurring in the subchondral areas of a bone has led to the investigation of the joint as the site of the inital abnormality.

Current investigators (KING, 1932; MORRIS and GOLDMAN, 1960) support the hypothesis that the juxta-articular bone cyst is a primary bone lesion, and that it is the result of metaplasia of nonspecific mesenchymal cells into fibroblasts. These fibroblasts become capable of mucin production and their proliferation is postulated to produce pressure atrophy resulting in cyst formation (GOLDMAN and FRIEDMAN, 1969; JOHNSON et al., 1965). The latter theory of intramedullary metaplasia is supported by histochemical studies indicating that: (1) the proliferating cell type is fibroblastic (KING, 1932; MORRIS and GOLDMAN, 1960), and (2) that the fibroblasts are the source of the high concentration of hyaluronic acid which is found in the myxoid cysts (MORRIS and GOLDMAN, 1960). Pathologic evidence of hypervascularity around the periphery of juxta-articular bone cyst, active secretion of mucin, and recurrences after surgical excision, all suggest that the intraosseous ganglion is an active lesion, as opposed to a secondary degenerative process (FELDMAN and JOHNSTON, 1973).

Other theories attribute these lesions to synovial abnormalities. The proximity of these lesions to a joint space, the identification of synovial-like cells in the cyst lining, and the fact that pain tends to increase with exercise suggest a relationship to an intra-articular abnormality. Herniation of synovium through a traumatic defect in the joint capsule, or an increase in joint pressures forcing fluid into the bone through a cartilage disruption have been suggested as mechanisms for the formation of intraosseous ganglia (CRANE and SCARANO, 1967). Ectopic synovial tissue has also been postulated as the etiology (FELDMAN and JOHNSTON, 1973). The evidence against the primary abnormality originating in the adjacent joint space includes (1) the incompleteness of the cyst lining, (2) the fact that no particular cell type predominates, (3) only rarely can communications with a joint be demonstrated on arthrography or pathologic specimens (BYERS and WADSWORTH, 1970; CARP and STOUT, 1928), and even if joint communications are present, they may represent physiologic defects which are present normally and do not lead to cyst formation (ONDROUCH, 1963), and (4) in a series of 38 cases (FELDMAN and JOHNSTON, 1973), only 8 patients had either degenerative or productive changes in the neighboring joint.

The extension of a parosteal ganglion into the adjacent bone has also been considered. Three such cases were reported by FELDMAN and JOHNSTON (1973) but this cannot be invoked to explain all of the lesions. A purely traumatic origin is unlikely due to the absence of blood or respiratory pigments within the cysts. An inflammatory process is difficult to support in the absence of granulation tissue or giant cells.

III. Clinical

The chief complaint is usually of dull aching joint pain, which is exacerbated by motion. The patient's history frequently extends over a period of months to years. Physical examination may be completely negative or there may be an area of localized swelling, associated with tenderness on palpation. The treatment of these lesions is curettage and packing with bone chips. Recurrences, although not a common problem, have been reported (FELDMAN and JOHNSTON, 1973).

IV. Pathology

Juxta-articular bone cysts or intraosseous ganglia are identical, histologically, to cutaneous myxoid cysts. The gross specimens are smooth, bluish in color, and round or oval in shape. They may be either unilocular or multilocular. The cysts contain a viscous gelatinous material which has a high content of hyaluronic acid and other mucopolysaccarides. This mucin-like material was analyzed by Soren (1966) and contains 96–245 mg/100 ml glucosamine, 2850–3240 mg/100 ml of albumen, and 1200–1900 mg/100 ml of globulin.

Microscopic sections show that the lining consists predominantly of fibroblasts, with an occasional "synovial type" of cell and interstitial mucopolysaccharide secretion. High concentrations of hyaluronic acid are found within the cytoplasm of the cells, in the cellular membranes, and within the extracellular spaces. This substance is probably responsible for the enlargement of the osseous cysts (Feldman and Johnston, 1973).

The major clinical and roentgenographic differential diagnosis is that of subchondral cysts, which are secondary to degenerative joint disease. Grossly, the latter lesions are usually multiple and smaller in size than intraosseous ganglia. In addition, cysts secondary to "osteoarthritic" changes are associated with disruption of the adjacent articular cartilage, whereas intraosseous ganglia are usually near a normal joint. Communications with the joint space are commonly identified in the presence of cysts related to degenerative changes in the articular cartilage. However, such communications are rarely demonstrable between an intraosseous ganglion and the synovial space. The microscopic findings are also a differential point. Degenerative cysts characteristically contain a combination of cartilage, fibrous tissue, giant cells, and debris.

V. Roentgen Appearance

Juxta-articular bone cysts or intraosseous ganglia occur most frequently in the bones of the lower extremities. In Feldman and Johnston's (1973) series of 38 cases, the commonest location was the femoral head and neck (37%), while the lower tibia was second in frequency, and the proximal tibia third. Of the lesions in this study, 23% occurred in the upper extremity (usually in the ulna and carpal bones). Other clinical studies (Crabbe, 1966; Sim and Dahlin, 1971) reported the distal tibia as the most frequent site, with a predilection for the medial malleolus (Fig. 22).

On roentgenograms, intraosseous ganglia are usually epiphyseal in location, although they can occur in the metaphyses. In the tubular bones they are usually eccentric in position. The size can vary from 2 mm–7 cm, with the larger lesions usually located in the hip. The intraosseous ganglion appears on x-ray as a totally lytic, nonaggressive lesion. The zone of transition is short and frequently there is a sclerotic margin (Figs. 22, 23). The adjacent joint is usually normal and arthrography only rarely demonstrates a communication with the joint space (Fig. 24).

The most difficult roentgen differential diagnosis is the subchondral cyst of degenerative joint disease. "Osteoarthritic cysts" are almost invariably associated with a roentgenographically abnormal joint space (Fig. 25), while intraosseous ganglia are usually adjacent to normal joints, however, ganglia can produce secondary hypertrophic changes. This problem occurs most frequently when myxoid cysts are located in the femoral head. In Feldman and Johnston's (1973) series, all eight cases of intraosseous ganglia associated with abnormal joints occured in the hip. In these latter cases, identification of the primary abnormality may be difficult. Clinically, ganglia can occur at any age but if the

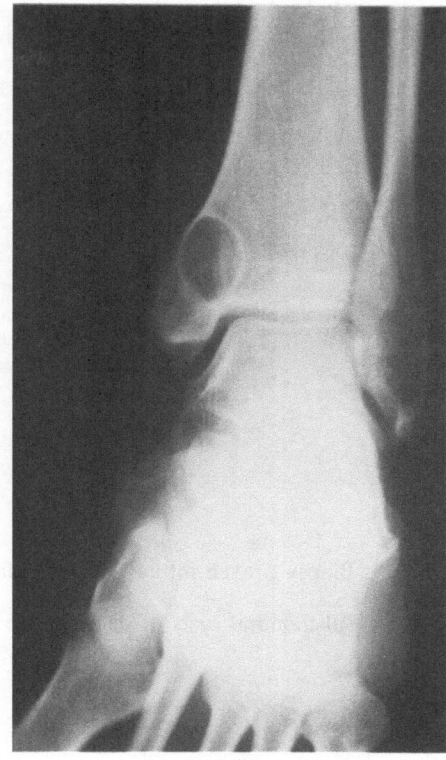

Fig. 22. Intraosseous ganglion, located in medial malleolus, demonstrating short zone of transition and sclerotic margin

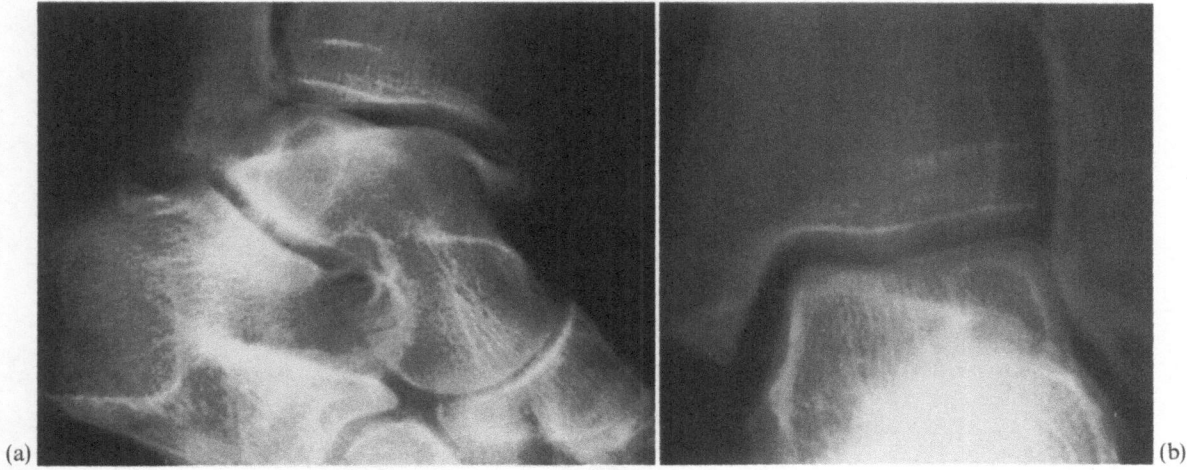

(a)   (b)

Fig. 23. Lytic lesion of talus, which proved to be intraosseous ganglion

patient is young, it favors a diagnosis of myxoid cyst, as opposed to primary degenerative joint disease. Roentgenographic criteria include (1) the size of the lesion, since the intraosseous ganglion tends to be larger than osteoarthritic cysts, (2) the location of the lesions, because in general the subchondral cysts of degenerative joint disease occur in the area of greatest weight bearing, e.g., under the anterior inferior iliac spine of the hip, where as a ganglion is more frequently located medially (EGGERS et al., 1963), (3) the number of multiple cysts degenerative joint disease produces, usually on both sides of the joint, ganglia may occur either within the acetabulum or femoral head but are usually single, and

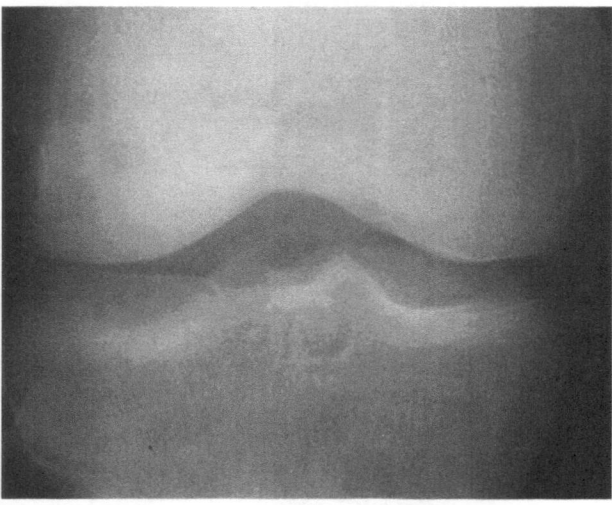 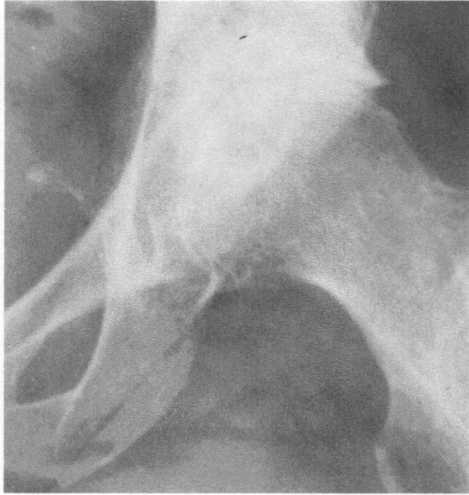

Fig. 24   Fig. 25

Fig. 24. Biopsy proven intraosseous ganglion in subarticular region of tibia. Adjacent joint space is intact

Fig. 25. Subchondral cysts of degenerative joint disease. Cysts are small, multiple, occur in area of greatest weight bearing, and are associated with abnormal joint

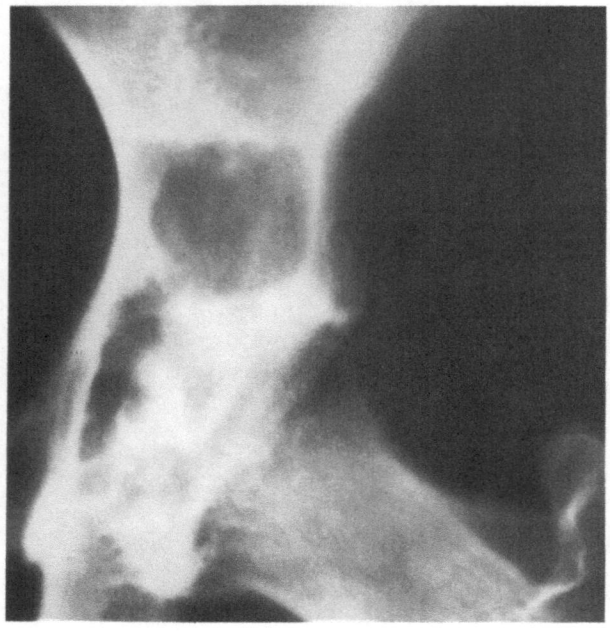

Fig. 26. Pigmented villonodular synovitis producing multiple erosions on both sides of joint space

(4) the presence of associated roentgen findings related to the adjacent joint space. Cystic lesions occur relatively late in the course of the joint disease and are preceded by loss of joint space, osteophyte formation, and flattening of the femoral head. If available, serial films can help to distinguish the initial event which produced the hip abnormalities.

Other arthritides can produce bone destruction. Pigmented villonodular synovitis (Fig. 26), like degenerative joint disease, can produce multiple erosions on both sides of the joint. However, the latter process is also characterized by large intra-articular

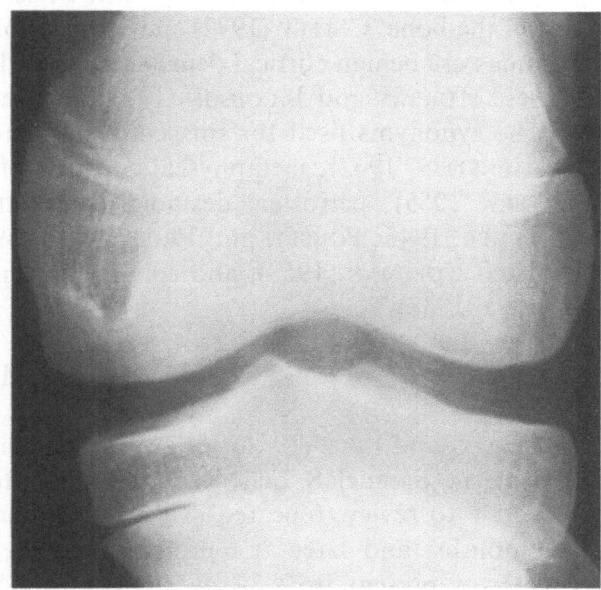

Fig. 27. Uncalcified chondroblastoma

soft tissue masses, which have an increased roentgen density due to hemosiderin deposits. The latter soft tissue findings are not present in association with intraosseous ganglia. The synovial cysts of rheumatoid arthritis are also multiple, tend to have irregular margins, and are associated with fusiform soft tissue swelling. In addition, the monoarticular form of rheumatoid arthritis is rare.

Primary lesions of bone may also be in the differential diagnosis of the juxta-articular bone cyst or intraosseous ganglion. Prior to the fusion of the growth plate, a chondroblastoma may produce a similar roentgen appearance (Fig. 27), but 50% of the latter lesions are calcified (EDEIKEN and HODES, 1973). In older individuals, in the third and fourth decades, giant cell tumors may produce eccentric epiphyseal lesions, although they tend to be more expansile and rarely have a sclerotic margin. A recurrent intraosseous ganglion would be more difficult to distinguish on x-ray appearance, since they may appear more aggressive. A Brodie abscess is also in the roentgen differential diagnosis. In the small bones of the wrist and hand, enchondromas may mimic intraosseous ganglia, although the former are frequently calcified.

D. The Fibrous Cortical Defect or Nonosteogenic Fibroma

I. Introduction

The fibrous cortical defect is a superficial, well-demarcated, cortical based, nonneoplastic, fibrotic lesion in the metaphyseal ends of long bones. When this process enlarges and extends into the marrow cavity, causing destruction of the spongiosa, it is referred to as a nonosteogenic or nonossifying fibroma of bone. Both lesions are identical histologically. The confusion arises in that only rarely has anyone observed a fibrous cortical defect mature (JAFFE, 1958) and develop into a nonossifying fibroma. Hence, some people separate the lesions purely on the basis of size and involvement of the medullary part of the bone. CAFFEY (1972) states that probably in their earlier stage, all nonossifying fibromas are benign cortical defects and that these lesions are the same entity in different phases. MURRAY and JACOBSON (1971) believe them to be the same entity.

The synonyms used for this entity are: nonosteogenic fibroma of bone (JAFFE and LICHTENSTEIN, 1942); metaphyseal cortical defects (SELBY, 1961); fibrous cortical defects (CAFFEY, 1955); periosteal desmoids (KIMMELSTIEL, 1951); metaphyseal fibrous defect (HATCHER, 1945; PONSETI and FRIEDMAN, 1949; MAUDSLEY and STANSFELD, 1956; COMPERE and COLEMAN, 1957), and solitary xanthoma of bone (PHELIP, 1935; BURMAN and SINBERG, 1938).

II. Incidence

SONTAG and PYLE (1941) reviewed roentgenograms of the femora taken on 101 children at the Samuel S. Fels Research Institute in Yellow Springs, Ohio, U.S.A. They were able to review repeated skeletal examinations on children from the day of birth, at 3 months, and later at 6 month intervals until the age of 8. The fibrous cortical defect was present in 22% of girls, with 54 being studied, and 53% of boys, with 47 being studied. The area of skeletal roentgenographic review was confined to the femur.

CAFFEY (1955) studied 154 children who were part of an annual clinical and roentgenographic study by the New York State Board of Health and its Committee on Fluoridation of Water Supply. The children were examined over a period of 6–8 years. He found that 33 boys, or 42% showed defects and 23 girls, or 31% showed defects. CAFFEY'S roentgenologic examinations were limited to frontal projections of both knees and a single hand and forearm frontal projection. He states that it is possible to have missed short-lived defects because of the 12 months interval between examinations. He feels that the incidence would have increased if all tubular bones had been included.

SELBY (1961), again working at the Fels Research Institute, studied 151 children, with 88 boys and 63 girls; and found that 24 boys and 18 girls had defects, making an incidence of 27% in boys and 29% in girls. He concluded that the overall total population incidence would be 27%.

PONSETI and FRIEDMAN (1949) report having observed three fibrous defects arising at various time intervals from the same area of the epiphyseal plate. We have observed similar findings.

SELBY (1961) states that there is a definite familial incidence. In his series if one child had a defect, there was a 50% chance that a sibling would also have a defect. No genetic or hereditary pattern has been established.

SONTAG and PYLE (1941) felt that sex and age influenced the defects. Their youngest child was 22 months. They felt that the defects did not occur after 10 years of age; however, CAFFEY (1955) and HATCHER (1945) have observed defects after 10 years. Defects, however, have never been shown for the first time during adult life. SONTAG and PYLE found an overall percentage of 22% in girls and 53% in boys.

CAFFEY (1955) found no fibrous cortical defects in the 0–21 month age group. In examining 90 children in their third year, he found an overall incidence of 7.7% with 12% being boys and 4% being girls. The overall incidence in children then was between 15 and 17% from age 4–12. There was then a decline from years 13 and 14 respectively. The highest years for boys were 7, 8 and 10, with approximately 23% of the boys examined being affected. For girls 6, 8 and 11 years of age had a 15% maximum. The defects appeared earlier and lasted longer in boys. In 12 boys and 2 girls the defects lasted 5–8 years. The average duration of a defect in girls was 2.1 years and in boys 4.4 years.

SELBY (1961) records an incidence of 27% in boys and 29% in girls. His figures have not been observed by others.

LICHTENSTEIN (1972) states that there is no predilection for either sex. However, DAHLIN (1970) in his series of 50 metaphyseal fibrous defects, found 30 males and 20 females, with the oldest being 25 years of age.

KITAGAWA et al. (1964) reported a 20% incidence in boys and an 8% incidence in girls.

III. Clinical Manifestations

The small fibrous cortical defects are totally asymptomatic and are diagnosed during roentgenographic examination for some other abnormality. CAFFEY (1955), in looking at data on 1000 healthy children, found no evidence of any abnormal local or general reaction in a child from this defect. The larger nonosteogenic fibroma may present pain when it becomes large enough to weaken the integrity of the underlying bone. There is nothing characteristic about the clinical history (LICHTENSTEIN, 1972). In most cases the history of discomfort and swelling is brief, and trauma is usually attributed to the difficulty. There may be a fracture through the attenuated cortex. Often, however, this lesion, like the smaller fibrous cortical defect, is a coincidental finding.

1. Laboratory Findings

In the cases of fibrous cortical defect the serum phosphorus, calcium, and phosphatase were normal (SONTAG and PYLE, 1941). In nonosteogenic fibromas all lab values are normal except in the case of pathological fracture, in which the alkaline phosphatase would be elevated.

2. Other Clinical Findings

HATCHER (1945) found epiphyseal disorders in 14 of his 45 patients. He also mentioned the presence of osteochondritits of the tibial epiphysis, patella and femoral epiphysis. It was because of these findings that he postulated a vascular defect in the region of the epiphyseal plate.

IV. Location and Bilaterality

The fibrous cortical defect statistical work has been confined to the knees. In CAFFEY's series (1955) of 154 children, the distal femora were affected 254 times, the proximal tibia 25 times, and the proximal fibulae 4 times. Bilateral defects were almost as common as unilateral defects. When femoral defects were unilateral, they were more common on the right than the left. Most of the femoral defects were on the medial side of the midsagittal plane of the distal femoral shaft. Lateral femoral defects were not seen before the seventh year. Multiple defects in a single bone were observed.

Defects in the upper extremities are rare; however, they have been identified in the humerus, radius, and ulna. LICHTENSTEIN (1972) reported a nonosteogenic fibroma in the iliac bone.

Fibrous cortical defects have never been observed in the epiphysis. MAUDSLEY and STANSFIELD (1956) reported 10 cases, all with lesions in the lower limbs.

V. Pathogenesis

It is believed by some (Spjut, 1971; Hatcher, 1945) that the lesion is a result of a developmental disturbance in the epiphyseal plate. They cite the following observations to support this theory. The lesion is found only in the metaphyseal region of the bone. The lesion moves away from the epiphyseal area as the bone grows in length. The defect tends to be elliptical in the long axis of the bone, indicating that the change is occurring over a period of time. Murray and Jacobson (1971) believe that nonossifying fibromas are capable of arising de novo, which precludes solely the possibility of a metaphyseal origin. Some authors have considered the nonosteogenic fibroma to be the outcome of a circulation disturbance (Hatcher, 1945; Aegerter and Kirkpatrick, 1958), others a dysplasia of bone (Ponseti and Friedman, 1949) and an abnormal response to injury (Schlumberger, 1946). Delvin et al. (1955), in reporting six cases of nonossifying fibroma, believed the defect to have arisen from the bone marrow connective tissue. Cunningham and Ackerman (1956) feel that there is no evidence of malignant transformation or unusual mitotic activity. Note should be made of a report by Bhagwandeen (1966) of a nonossifying fibroma which was curetted in a 21-year-old male. An aggressive fibrosarcoma appeared at the curetted site 18 months after curettage. Jaffe (1958) has observed a patient who presented a cortical defect in the femur at the age of $9^1/_2$ years which converted to a nonosteogenic fibroma $3^1/_2$ years later radiographically. Katz and Marek (1950) and Lichtenstein (1972) have reported instances of osteogenic sarcoma and coexistent but unrelated nonosteogenic fibroma in the same patient. We have observed similar cases (Fig. 28).

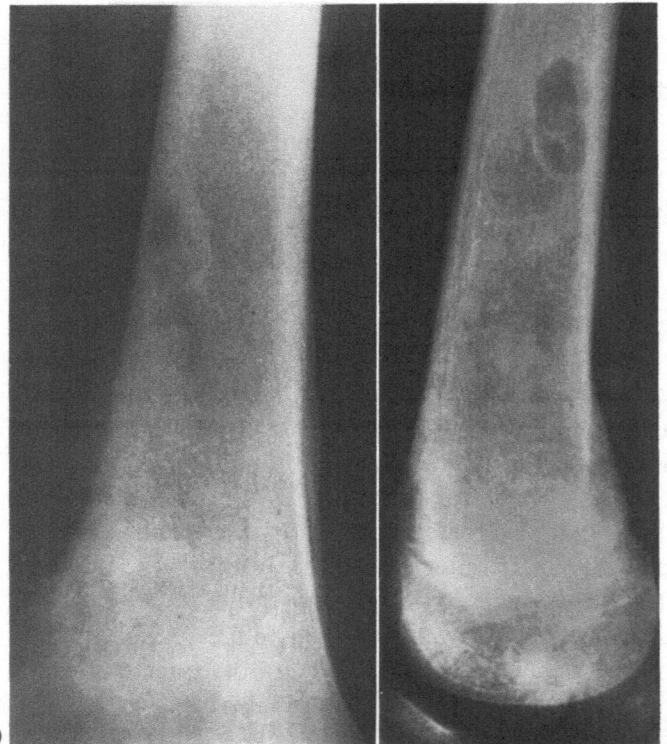

Fig. 28. (a) AP roentgenogram of distal femur with osteogenic sarcoma in proximal portion and fibrous cortical defect above. (b) AP roentgenogram of femur with osteogenic sarcoma in proximal metaphysis and fibrous cortical defect above

VI. Pathology

JAFFE and LICHTENSTEIN in 1942 were the first to separate this lesion from the giant cell tumor variants. HATCHER (1945) presented microscopic findings in 17 cases and proposed the designation of metaphyseal fibrous defect. The cases of PHELIP (1935) and of BURMAN and SINBERG (1938) reported as solitary xanthoma of bone were felt to be similar to those of HATCHER (1945) and probably represent cases of fibrous cortical defects in a stage of partial lipidization.

Grossly the cortex is felt to be intact without any periosteal reaction unless a fracture has occurred (SPJUT et al., 1971; LICHTENSTEIN, 1972). MAREK (1955), however, describes grayish-white thickening of the periosteum over the site of the cortical defect. The lesion may be eccentric in position, abutting the cortex or extending across the entire shaft. It is yellowish-gray-brown, depending on the amount of lipid, and varies from soft to firm. The areas can be separated by areas of sclerotic spongiosa. The overlying cortex may be thick or thin.

Microscopic. The lesion consists of whorled bundles of connective tissue with a variation of the cellular stroma. There is a variation of the vascularity, and the giant cells are scattered or form a nest (SPJUT et al., 1971). If the lesion is brown, the connective tissue cells are spindle-shaped and compacted with scant intercellular material (LICHTENSTEIN, 1972). Hemosiderosis is present in the cytoplasm of stromal cells; hence the brown color (Figs. 29, 30).

If the lesion is yellow, nests of lipid-containing foam cells are seen encircled by stromal tissue. Connective tissue cells are present in strands or whorled bundles. It

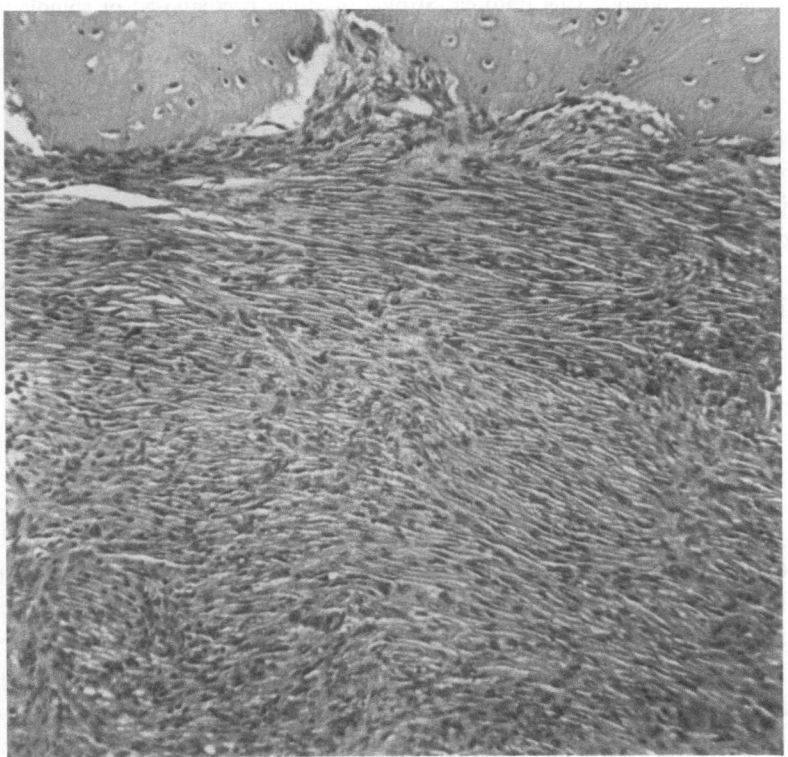

Fig. 29. Histopathology of nonossifying fibroma. At top of illustration is shown dense compact bone corresponding to sclerotic border or rim of lesion. Tissue consists of irregularly disposed fibroblasts interspersed with collagen fibers

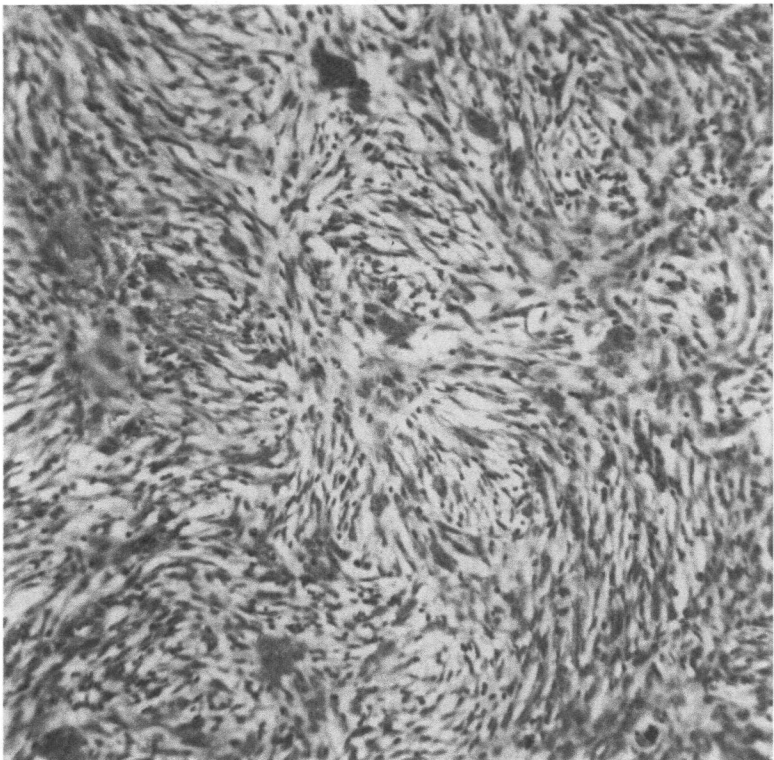

Fig. 30. Histopathology of nonossifying fibroma. Stroma of lesion is composed of spindle-shaped fibroblasts disposed in whorled pattern. Numerous giant cells are present

is because of this lipid that the lesion was originally called a xanthoma or xanthofibroma (PHELIP, 1935; BURMAN and SINBERG, 1938). Osteogenesis is not a feature of this lesion. Bone formation represents a response of neighboring tissue and not the lesion itself. However, MORTON (1964) believes that there is bone production in nonosteogenic fibromas. Bone is present as the lesion heals. AEGERTER and KIRKPATRICK (1958) say that in its fully developed state, the metaphyseal cortical defect appears to be composed of several confluent areas of compact and deossification cancellous bone.

VII. Roentgenology

The roentgenographic changes are distinctive. The fibrous cortical defect shows an area of increased radiolucency in the metaphyseal area of long bones, especially the femur and tibia (Figs. 31 and 32). When the bone shaft is seen in two projections, the lesion is superficial, being located in the cortical wall. The lucent area is sharply defined, has an elliptical shape in the longitudinal bone axis, and measures approximately 1–3 cm. The area of bone in continuity with the defect may be sclerotic or of normal density. There may be a bulging of the thin shell of bone just under the periosteum and next to the spongiosa, but cortical destruction is the sign of fibrous cortical defect. When the defect is larger and the spongiosa destroyed, the medullary cavity dilated and the cortex thinned, this is referred to as a nonosteogenic fibroma. Trabeculation in the mass may cast a reticulated multilocular shadow. The terminal third of the shaft

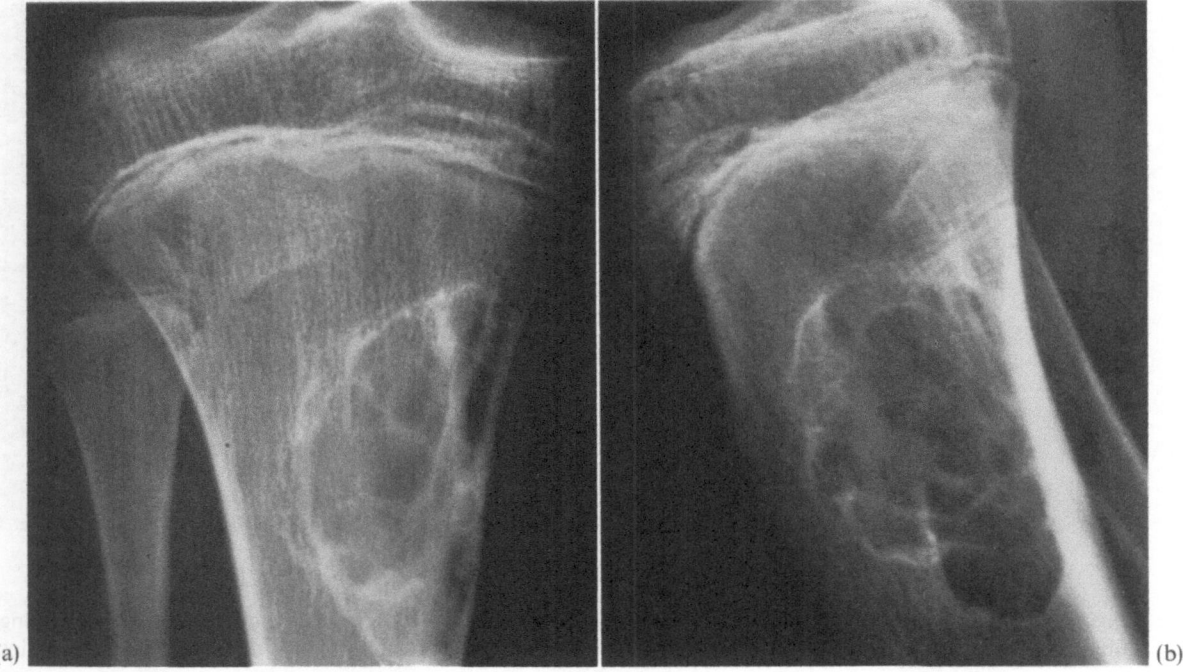

Fig. 31. (a) AP roentgenogram, Nonossifying fibroma of the tibia. (b) Lateral roentgenogram, Nonossifying fibroma of proximal tibia

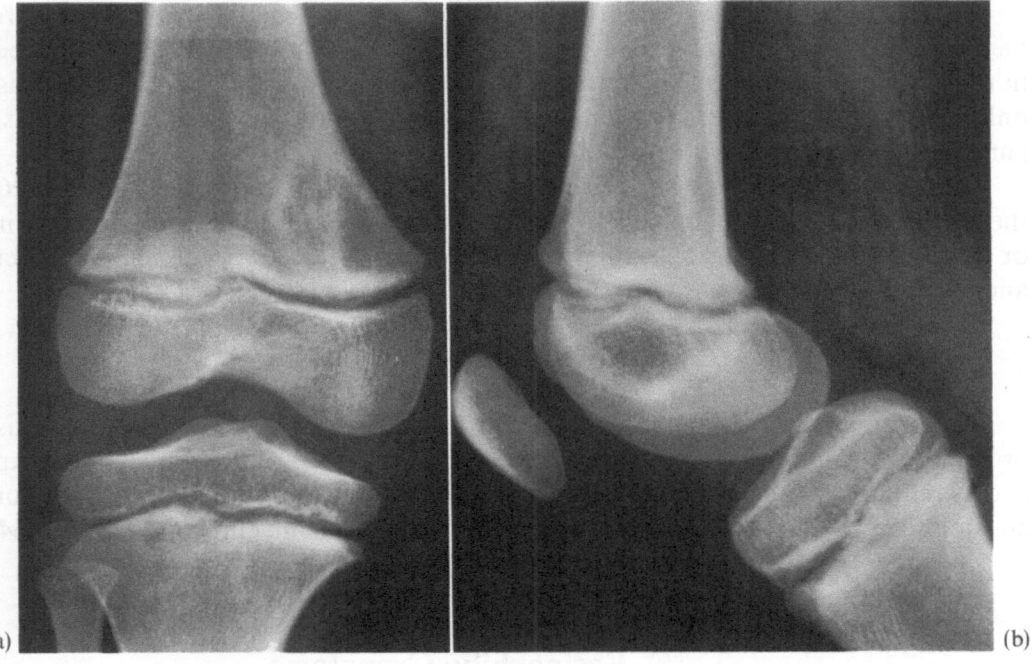

Fig. 32. (a) AP roentgenogram, fibrous cortical defect proximal tibia. (b) Lateral roentgenogram of fibrous cortical defect distal femur

is the predilected site, with 1–2 in. of normal bone interspersed between the epiphyseal plate and the edge of the fibroma. When the lesion develops in the fibula or ulna, it tends to occupy the entire width of the bone.

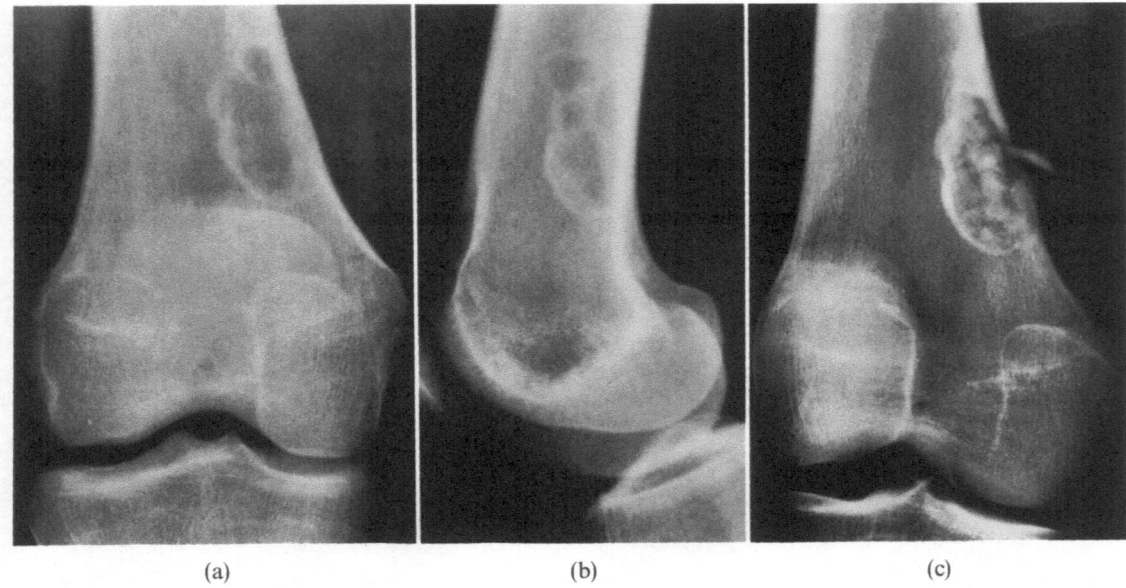

(a)   (b)   (c)

Fig. 33. (a) AP roentgenogram prior to biopsy. Nonossifying fibroma. (b) Lateral roentgenogram of nonossifying fibroma prior to biopsy. (c) AP roentgenogram of nonossifying fibroma after biopsy and packing with bone chips

VIII. Roentgenologic Course and Prognosis

The course is highly variable for fibrous cortical defect. Most shift away from the metaphysis, shrink in size and disappear. Others become sclerotic, sclerosis beginning in the more cephalad part. Some fragment, becoming multiple lesions. Others disappear, only to recur in the exact site. For the larger nonossifying fibromas, curettage is usually curative (Fig. 33).

DEVLIN (1955) reports six cases which he cured by surgery. BERKIN (1966) feels the condition to be benign and to require treatment only if the diagnosis is in doubt or if the defect is so large as to weaken the bone. He feels treatment to be curettage and bone chips.

IX. Differential Diagnosis

The roentgen appearance is so typical that differential diagnosis is not usually a problem. If the lesion is in a slender bone in which there is marked medullary expansion, a differential diagnosis is in order. This would include fibrous dysplasia, bone cyst, eosinophilic granuloma, aneurysmal bone cyst, and osteomyelitis (GORDON, 1964).

E. Eosinophilic Granuloma

I. Introduction

Eosinophilic granuloma is a nonneoplastic, benign, solitary lytic lesion of bone which is believed to arise from the reticuloendothelial system. This lesion is grouped with the reticuloendothelial proliferative disorders, which include Letterer-Siwe disease and

Hand-Schüller-Christian disease, on the basis of histologic similarity. From a clinical standpoint the lesions behave differently.

The names used for this disorder are: eosinophilic granuloma (LICHTENSTEIN and JAFFE, 1940); histiocytosis X, which includes eosinophilic granuloma, Letterer-Siwe disease and Hand-Schüller-Christian disease, all single-entity phases (LICHTENSTEIN, 1953; FARBER, 1941); solitary granuloma (OTANI and EHRLICH, 1940); eosinophilic myeloma (FINZI, 1929) and destructive granuloma of bone (GREEN and FARBER, 1942).

II. History

Eosinophilic granuloma was described as a specific entity in 1940 by LICHTENSTEIN and JAFFE and by OTANI and EHRLICH. This lesion was believed to represent a myeloma or an osteomyelitis (FITZPATRICK, 1967). FARBER (1941) described the nature of "solitary or eosinophilic granuloma" of bone and suggested the relationship of Hand-Schüller-Christian disease and Letterer-Siwe disease. LICHTENSTEIN (1953) suggested the name histiocytosis X to include all three entities in different phases. OTANI (1957) believes eosinophilic granuloma is a separate entity, and this concept is supported by SPJUT et al. (1971).

FARBER'S idea of interrelation between Hand-Schüller-Christian and Letterer-Siwe was not new, this having been suggested by FLORI and PARENTI (1937), GLANZMANN (1940), and WALLGREN (1940).

III. Clinical Manifestations

FOWLES and BOBECHKO (1970) report an equal frequency of eosinophilic granuloma in both sexes. SPJUT et al. (1971), WHITEHEAD (1972), and SCHAJOWICZ and SLULLITEL (1973) reported a male predominance.

SPJUT et al. (1971) reported cases from infants to the sixth decade, with a peak incidence of 5–10 years. In GREEN and FARBER'S group (1942) the average age was 5 years 1 month. SCHAJOWICZ and SLULLITEL (1973) reported 76 cases of eosinophilic granuloma, with 62% being 1–15 years of age. They noticed a peak between years 5–10. Their oldest patient was 53 years old, and their youngest was 1. FOWLES and BOBECHKO (1970) believed most people to be under 20, with age being evenly distributed between 7 months and 14 years.

Complaints vary from a few days to several months of localized bone pain. Usually the pain is solitary, but at times it may be disseminated and polyostotic. In cases with multiple bone involvement, only one lesion may be symptomatic, with the others being silent (JAFFE and LICHTENSTEIN, 1944). This mandates that all bones should be examined radiographically for signs of disease. The lesion, however, may be totally asymptomatic and only recognized when a pathologic fracture occurs. A lowgrade fever may be present for several days. If the temporal bone is involved, otitis media may be the main clinical complaint. A nodule in the scalp may reflect skull involvement.

Leukocytosis of moderate severity with no differential shift may be present (JAFFE and LICHTENSTEIN, 1944). There may be an increase in the eosinophil count. SCHAJOWICZ and SLULLITEL (1973) reported an elevated sedimentation rate with a Katz index of 25. In one case, in which a sternal marrow was performed, there was a 15% eosinophilic count. WELLS (1956) cites two cases in which there was a peripheral eosinophilia of 9 and 8%. FOWLES and BOBECHKO (1970) had 4 children out of 26 studied with a 6–8% eosinophilia. The 24 children who had sedimentation rates ranged from 16–59 mm in the first hour. Blood cholesterol, cholesterol esters, and total lipids were normal. Viral and bacterial cultures were normal (Jaffe and Lichtenstein, 1944).

Leiken et al. (1973) studied the immunologic parameters in patients with histiocytosis X. His group found no evidence that would support a combined immunodeficiency disorder in patients with clinical Letterer-Siwe disease or in seven older children with various phases of histiocytosis.

Eosinophilic granuloma has been found in all the bones of the body (Jaffe and Lichtenstein, 1944). The most frequent bones affected by eosinophilic granuloma are the frontal and parietal bones, mandible, humerus, rib, and femur. If a long bone is involved, the lesion may be in either the metaphysis or diaphysis, with no predilection for either (Spjut et al., 1971). Rarely, eosinophilic granuloma may involve the epiphysis (Ochsner, 1966). Fowles and Bobechko (1970) state that in the older patient the lesions are most common in the ribs, mandible, clavicle, scapula, and skull. In the younger patient it is the skull.

Dundon et al. (1946) state the most common area of involvement to be the ribs, vertebrae, humerus, skull, femur, and mandible. In our experience, the most common areas have been the skull and femur.

When treatment for a solitary lesion is being given, other bones may become involved (Fitzpatrick, 1967).

IV. Pathogenesis

The pathogenesis is unknown (Spjut et al., 1971). A study by McGavran and Spady (1960) of 28 cases with eosinophilic granuloma showed no transition of this entity to either Letterer-Siwe disease or Hand-Schüller-Christian disease. Lieberman et al. (1969) reviewed 82 cases of eosinophilic granuloma and found no reason for classifying the three entities together. Spjut et al. (1971) support the concept that eosinophilic granuloma, Hand-Schüller-Christian disease and Letterer-Siwe disease are separate entities, at least clinically. Otani (1957) supports this view along with Fowles and Bobechko (1970) and McGavran and Spady (1960).

However, others believe these entities to be different stages of the same disease process (Gross and Jacox, 1942; Jaffe and Lichtenstein, 1944; Schajowicz and Polak, 1947; Ponsetti, 1948; Nezelof and Guibert, 1963; Enriquez et al., 1967; Cheyne, 1971; Schajowicz and Slullitel, 1973). They classify Letterer-Siwe as acute or disseminated histiocytosis X and Hand-Schüller-Christian disease as a chronic disseminated histiocytosis X (Lichtenstein, 1964). Both these diseases can have visceral and soft tissue involvement.

This difference of opinion rests on the fact that the etiology is unknown. There are some who believe that this represents a type of immunoallergic process (Schajowicz and Polak, 1947; Avioli et al., 1963). Lichtenstein felt that this might be infectious, possibly viral.

V. Radiographic Findings

In general, the radiographic findings of eosinophilic granuloma consist of destructive, punched-out lesions which vary in size from a few millimeters in diameter to several centimeters in diameter. Eosinophilic granuloma occurs in both membranous and long bones. The borders of the lesion are well-defined, and less than half reveal marginal reactive sclerosis (Takahashi et al., 1966; Avery et al., 1957; Hodgson et al., 1951; Dundon et al., 1946; Hamilton et al., 1946).

1. Skull

The lesions consist of sharply defined, punched-out areas of bone with no margin of reactive bone (Figs. 34, 35). An irregular margin may be seen if the lesion is early (ENNIS et al., 1973) or if the patient has Letterer-Siwe (TAKAHASHI et al., 1966). On rare occasions there may be small peripheral lesions. The lesions develop in the diploë

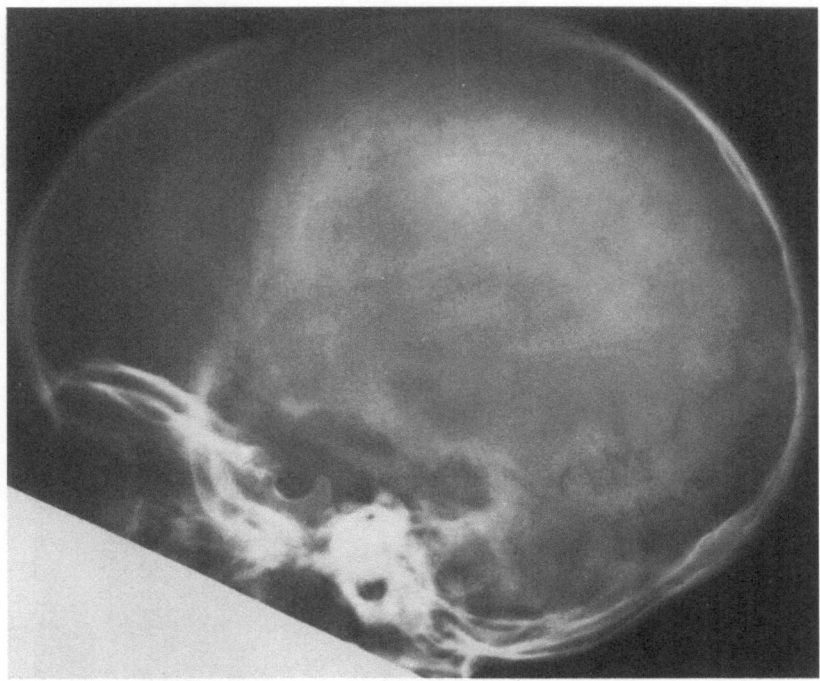

Fig. 34. Lateral roentgenogram of 8-year-old girl revealing osteolytic punched out area at base of skull involving temporal bone due to eosinophilic granuloma. Patient did not have diabetes insipidus but did have draining ear on affected side

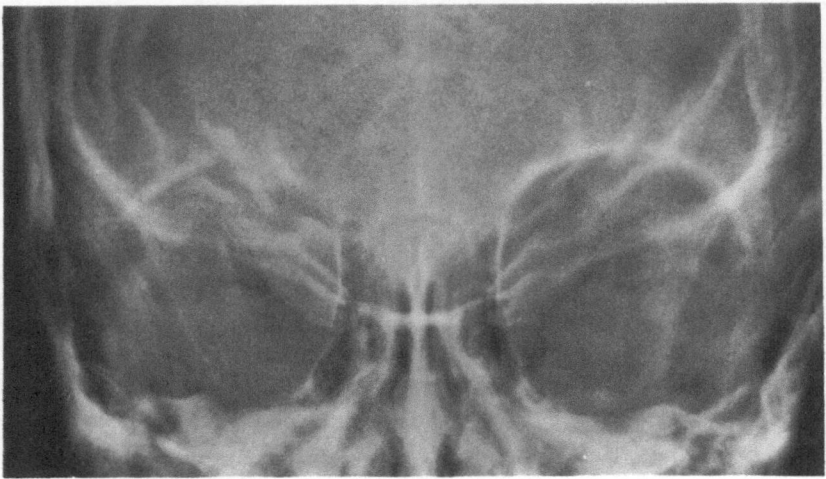

Fig. 35. Frontal view of skull showing destructive lesion of eosinophilic granuloma of right superior orbit and its roof

and usually destroy both the inner and outer tables. There is no periosteal reaction (Wells, 1956). The outer table is usually more extensively involved, producing a characteristic double contour with beveling of the margin. If several areas coalesce, a geographic skull develops. Syphilis and tuberculosis must be considered (Tirona, 1954). Wells (1956) described a characteristic sequestrum which appears as a "button of intact bone in the center of the bony osteolytic skull lesions" (Fig. 36a–c). He cites four cases. Soft tissue masses are frequently palpable overlying the lytic process. The lesions can occur in a 6-week period (Avery et al., 1957). Platybasia can result if the lesion at

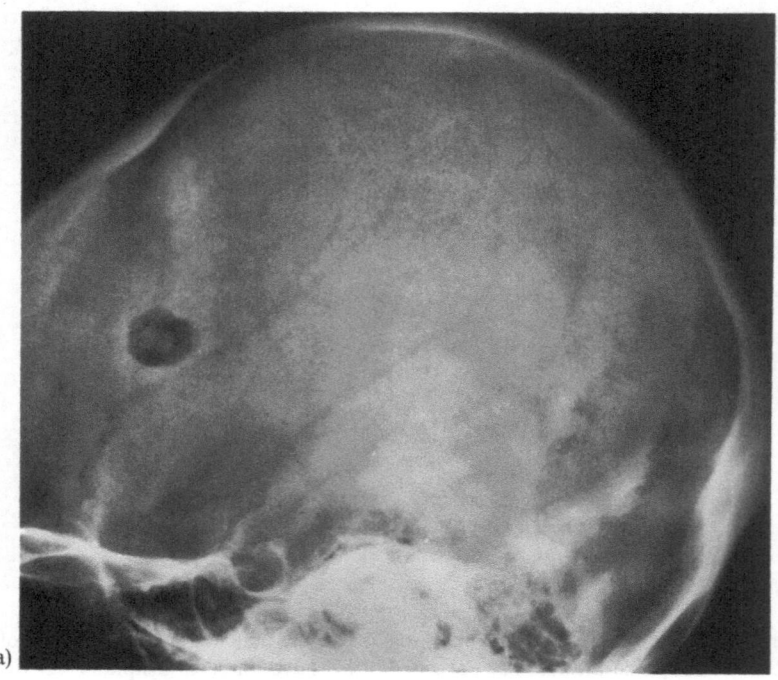

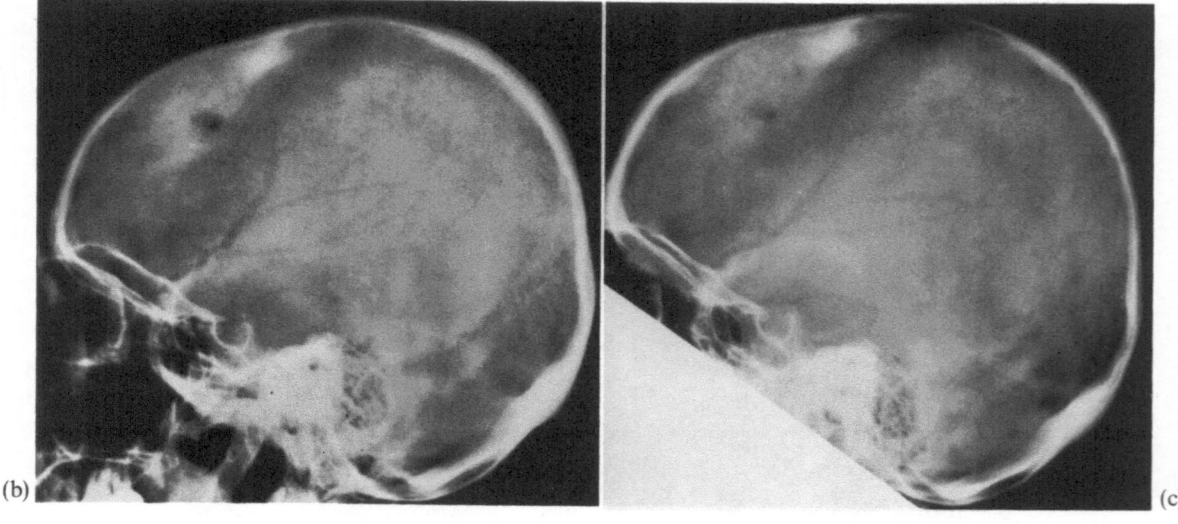

Fig. 36. (a) Eosinophilic granuloma seen on lateral roentgenogram. Note punched out lucent lesion in frontal area with sequestrum in middle. (b) One year later, note that lesion is no longer as sharply defined and that "button sequestrum" is not visible. (c) Two years later, lesion is much smaller and less distinct

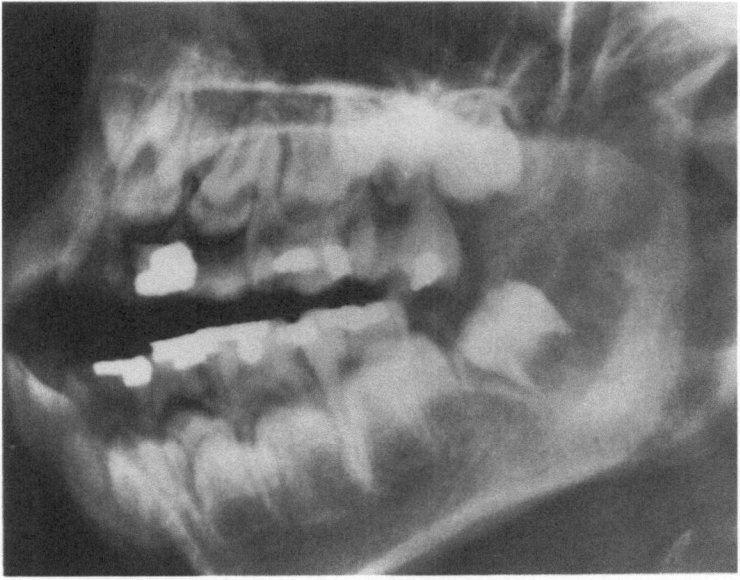

Fig. 37. Lateral roentgenogram of mandible of ten-year-old boy with expanding lucent area in posterior angle giving posterior molar tooth appearance of floating. Pathologic study of biopsy of this area revealed eosinophilic granuloma

the base is large enough (CHRISTIAN, 1919). The sella turcica may be destroyed. Diabetes insipidus associated with Hand-Schüller-Christian disease can occur with or without sellar destruction. The orbit may be destroyed. When it heals, it frequently resembles fibrous dysplasia as a thickened, dense bone, causing asymmetry.

2. Mandible

There is destruction of the lamina dura and supporting alveolar bone, which gives the teeth a floating appearance (Fig. 37). If the teeth are not erupted, there is erosion of the dense margin surrounding the tooth follicle (ENNIS et al., 1973). ALBERS et al. (1973) describe a case of the mandible in which following curetting and removal of the first molar tooth bud and lower left deciduous second molar, the patient was free of disease $2^1/_2$ years later. The presence of floating teeth is not pathognomonic and is seen in reticulum cell sarcoma, Ewing sarcoma, and familial dysproteinemia (ALBERS et al., 1973).

3. Spine

A single vertebra may collapse, causing a vertebra plana (Fig. 38 a, b). On rare occasions a vertebra may become lytic and expansible, involving the body and arch (KAYE and FREIBERGER, 1969). BUCHMAN (1927) coined the expression vertebra plana. CALVE (1925) had felt that this was caused by aseptic necrosis or osteochondritis. COMPERE et al. (1954) presented four cases of vertebra plana caused by eosinophilic granuloma. It is now generally accepted that any patient under 15 years of age with vertebra plana has eosinophilic granuloma until proven otherwise (ENNIS et al., 1973). As the patient improves, the vertebral body regains its height, but this is rarely complete. TAKAHASHI et al. (1966) and KEIFFER et al. (1969) noted that the growth spurt in repair is faster

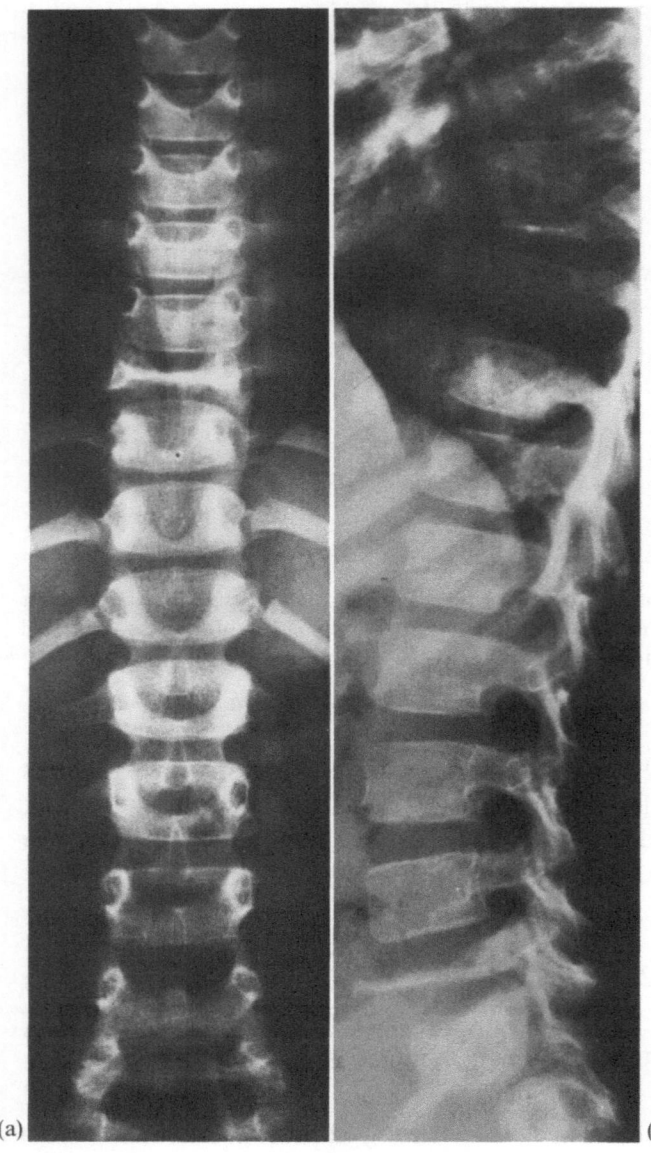

(a)

(b)

Fig. 38a and b. Antero-posterior and lateral roentgenograms of thoracolumbar spine showing vertebra plana of T9 and L5 secondary to eosinophilic granuloma

than the normal adjacent vertebral bodies, but it never regains full height. A bone-in-bone appearance may sometimes be seen if new bone is laid down around the vertebral body (ENNIS et al., 1973). Scoliosis can occur at the deformity. Patients with vertebral involvement, even those with total collapse, rarely exhibit neurologic involvement. GREEN and FARBER (1942) reported six patients with a total of eight vertebral lesions who had local pain and tenderness and no neurologic signs. KEIFFER et al. (1969) reported 35 involved vertebral bodies in 10 patients, none of whom had neurologic involvement. There are other cases of similar nature reported (COMPERE et al., 1954; DAVIES, 1949; EPSTEIN, 1969; SBARARO and FRANCIS, 1961; FRIPP, 1958; LINDENBAUM and GOTTES, 1970; MATSON, 1969; NELSON, 1969). OBERMAN (1961) had a patient with vertebral collapse and cauda equina signs. DAVIDSON and SHILLITO (1970) reported six cases of eosinophilic granuloma of the cervical spine; two had neurologic manifestations. GIBSON and EISEN (1963) reported adjacent thoracic vertebrae with eosinophilic granuloma.

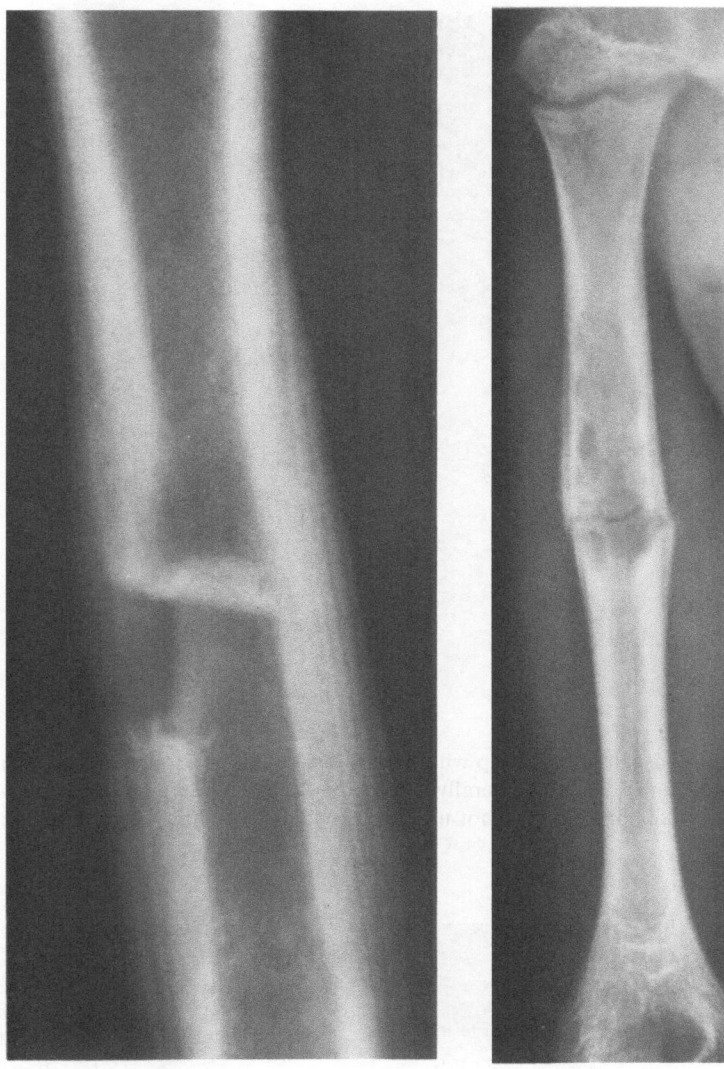

Fig. 39   Fig. 40

Fig. 39. Frontal roentgenogram of femur demonstrating lamillated or "onion skin" periosteal reaction of eosinophilic granuloma. Note presence of defect due to biopsy that was taken

Fig. 40. Frontal roentgenogram of right humerus with eosinophilic granuloma in 8-year-old girl. There is osteolytic process with pathological fracture in upper $^1/_3$ of diaphysis with endosteal scalloping and periosteal reaction. Margins are discrete and beveled edge is present in distal portion of lesion

4. Long and Flat Bones

In the long bones there are mottled lytic areas of destruction in the medullary cavity. If large enough, the lesion erodes the cortex from the endosteal side and may progress to destroy it locally and induce periosteal new bone formation (Figs. 39–42). The periosteal reaction is linear, usually layered, with an "onion skin" appearance. ENNIS et al. (1973) state that in all cases in which periosteal reaction was noted, there eventually was destruction of the medulla and in some cases of the cortex. Osteoporosis may be present. The long bone lesions do not affect the joint but may involve the bones on either side. Pathologic fracture is uncommon (HODGSON et al., 1951).

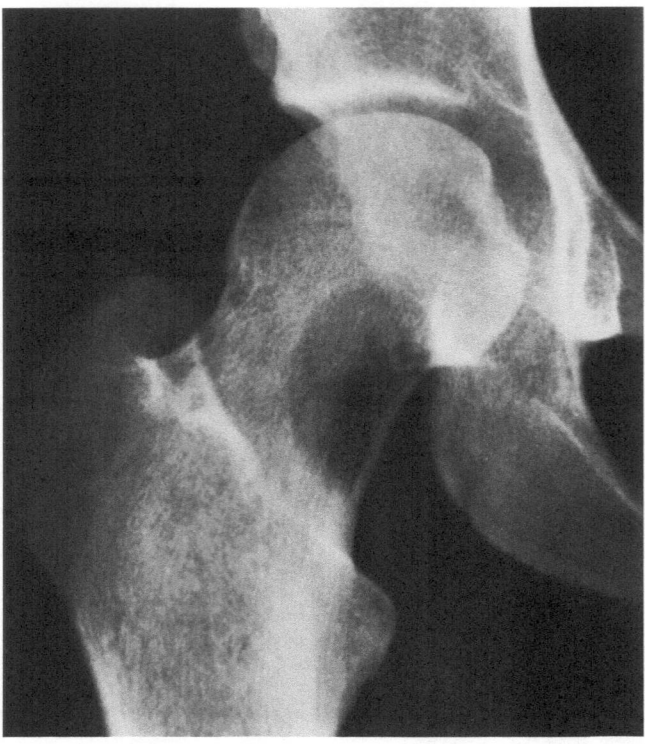

Fig. 41. Frontal roentgenogram of right hip with lucent area due to eosinophilic granuloma in medial femoral neck. Margin is sharp superiorly and laterally but border is not clear inferiorly. No periosteal reaction is seen. Lesions in femoral neck do not usually show typical findings of eosinophilic granuloma

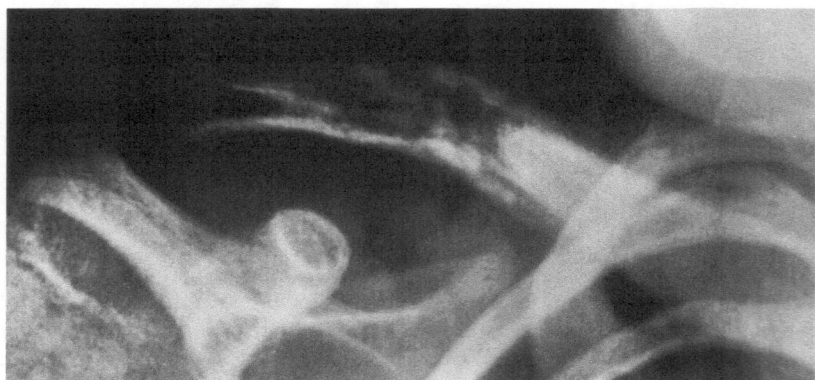

Fig. 42. Frontal roentgenogram of right clavicle with eosinophilic granuloma demonstrating expansile osteolytic lesion with periosteal reaction

It is rare to see periosteal reaction in the ribs. In the flat bones there may be expansion. This indicates a long-standing process in the long bones. In the flat bones there may be a multilocular lytic pattern caused by the process's advancing unevenly. The ilium is involved just above the acetabulum margin or adjacent to the sacroiliac joint (Moseley, 1963). A soft tissue mass is usually present.

VI. Pathology

1. Gross

The tissue is soft light yellow and has some areas of focal hemorrhage (SPJUT et al., 1971).

2. Microscopic

Microscopically there are moderately large reticulum cells which have an indented nucleus that is vesicular. The cell has an amphophilic centrally placed nucleolus. The cytoplasm is mildly granular and eosinophilic. The cell background is what has caused the lesion to be mistaken for a reticulum cell sarcoma. OTANI (1957) believes that he can differentiate Hand-Schüller-Christian disease and Letterer-Siwe disease on the basis of the foam cells in the former (SPJUT et al., 1971) (Fig. 43).

JAFFE and LICHTENSTEIN (1944) believe that the histiocytes constitute the basic component of the lesion. The histiocyte is derived from the adventitia of the blood vessels situated in the marrow.

SMITH (1969) classifies the lesion as early or late, based on the amount of lipid seen. Many eosinophils are seen in early lesions, and more mature lesions show large amounts of lipoid in the histiocytes. Late lesions are fibrous, and there are few eosinophils. The electron microscope has been of little value in studying histiocytosis (RITTER, 1966).

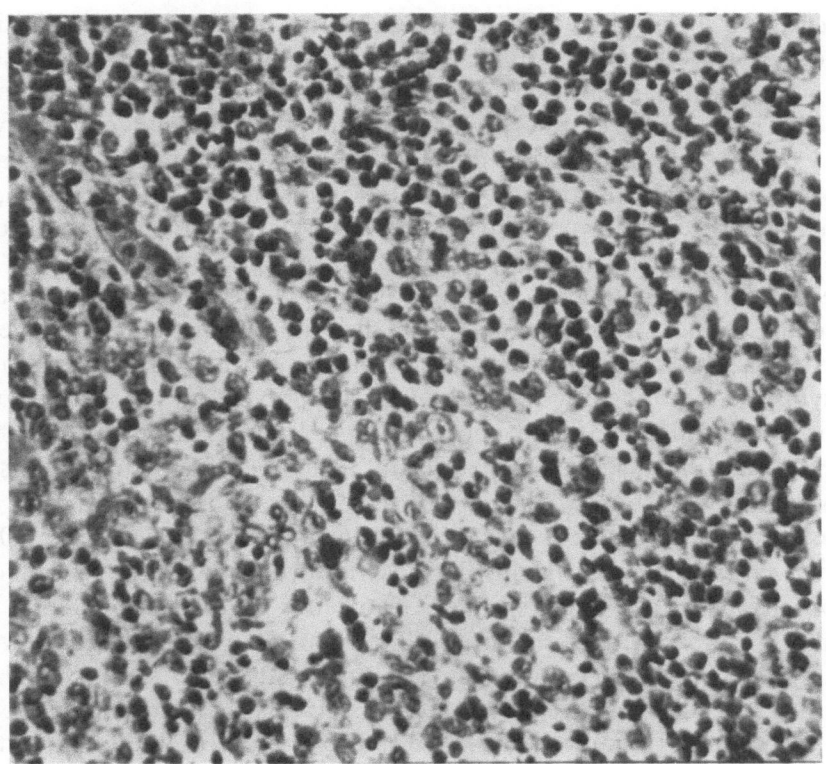

Fig. 43. Histopathology of eosinophilic granuloma. Numerous eosinophils are scattered throughout lesion mainly composed of histocytes

VII. Differential Diagnosis

The bony lesion of Letterer-Siwe and Hand-Schüller-Christian disease are radiologically similar to solitary eosinophilic granuloma, although bony lesions in Letterer-Siwe are uncommon. Ewing tumor, osteomyelitis, osteogenic sarcoma, fibrous dysplasia, epidermoid, reticulum cell, or metastatic carcinoma must also be considered in the differential.

VIII. Treatment and Course

Eosinophilic granuloma can be cured. It responds to radiation or curettage. AVERY et al. (1957) reviewed 40 cases of eosinophilic granuloma presenting as a solitary lesion. They found a recurrence rate of 20%. FOWLES and BOBECHKO (1970), in reporting 40 cases of eosinophilic granuloma, reported additional bony lesions in 10% of cases. Expansion of a lesion following biopsy may be indicative of widespread involvement (ALBERS et al., 1973).

F. Fibrous Dysplasia

I. Introduction

Fibrous dysplasia of bone is a pathologic entity of bone characterized by extensive proliferation of fibrous tissue replacing normal bone elements. Prior to 1930 much confusion was present as to nomenclature and many disorders were clumped together under the category of fibrocystic disease of bone. During that era many names were applied to what is now called fibrous dysplasia of bone. Among these titles are cystofibromatose, osteodystrophia fibrosa, juvenile Paget disease, leontiasis ossea, osteogenesis imperfecta tarda, osteitis fibrosa, von Recklinghausen disease of bone, fibrocystic disease of bone, osteitis deformans juvenilis, osteitis fibrosa cystica, and morbo di Jaffe-Lichtenstein. These terms may have been modified with the adjectives as localizata, monostotic, polyostotic, disseminata, multiple foci, or by the addition of the extra skeletal manifestations. Currently, the most commonly used synonyms are Albright syndrome, McCune-Albright syndrome, monostotic fibrous dysplasia, polyostotic fibrous dysplasia, and osteitis fibrosa disseminata. Other terms that have been used but are not recommended as synonyms are fibroma ossificans, fibrous osteoma, focal area of osteodystrophia fibrosa, focal fibrosis of bone, focal osteitis fibrosa, ossifying fibroma, and osteofibroma.

Fibrous dysplasia of bone has a varied spectrum of manifestations. Only one bone may be involved (monostotic fibrous dysplasia). Several bones may be involved (polyostotic fibrous dysplasia). There may be extraosseous manifestations such as pigmented skin lesions or endocrine dysfunction. When there is osseous disease, with cutaneous pigmentation and precocious puberty, the disorder is called Albright syndrome.

According to LICHTENSTEIN (1975), fibrous dysplasia is probably the second most frequently encountered anomaly of skeletal development (hereditary multiple exostosis being first). JACOBSON (1971), reported that the Netherlands Committee on bone tumors found 78 cases of fibrous dysplasia among its 1569 tumors and tumor-like diseases of bone.

II. History

In 1891 von RECKLINGHAUSEN wrote on three groups of bone disorders, all of which had a common denominator, the production of fibrocystic changes in bone. Among the disorders are fibrous dysplasia of bone, neurofibromatosis, and hyperparathyroidism. Thereafter many articles were written on fibrocystic bone disease. After the discovery of parathormone, about 1925, the literature became more specific about the types of fibrocystic disease of bone, and fibrous dysplasia was established as an entity apart from hyperparathyroidism. Among these articles are those by WIELAND (1922), on osteitis fibrosa cystica, by WEISS (1924), by WINTER (1929), on a case of generalized osteitis fibrosa cystica in the absence of a parathyroid tumor, and IVIMEY (1929) on bone dystrophy with characteristics of leontiasis ossium, osteitis deformans, and osteitis fibrosa cystica in a child. In 1931 TELFORD published the gross and microscopic pathology of osteitis fibrosa. In the same year, HUNTER and TURNBULL included a probable case of fibrous dysplasia in their report on hyperparathyroidism. BRAID (1932, 1939), ELMSLIE (1914, 1934, 1935), FAIRBANK (1934), FREEDMAN (1933), FREUND (1934), FREUND and MEFFERT (1936), GARLOCK (1938), HIRSCH (1929), HUMMEL (1934), HUNTER and TURNBULL (1931), HORWITZ and CANTAROW (1939), KNAGGS (1926), LEADER and GRAND (1932), MANDL (1926), MORTON (1922), PRIESEL and WAGNER (1932), RYPINS (1933), SALZER (1933), SNAPPER and PARISEL (1933), TOBLER (1926), VON BEUST (1920), WINTER (1929) and others wrote papers contributing to the early knowledge of fibrous dysplasia. Then in 1942, LICHTENSTEIN and JAFFE reported on 90 cases that they were able to collect from their own experience and the literature. In this paper they titled the disorder fibrous dysplasia of bone, inferring that the skeletal lesions were not necessarily polyostotic. Since then fibrous dysplasia of bone has been the preferred name for the disorder.

In 1914, ELMSLIE published a case of fibrous dysplasia with a nevus on the nape of the neck of the patient. This was probably the first report of the disorder with extraskeletal manifestations. The first known description of the syndrome of precocious puberty, skin pigmentation, and spontaneous fractures of bone in a 9-year-old girl was written by WEIL in 1922. Similar cases were published in the next several years by GAUPP (1932), FREEDMAN (1932), STALMANN (1933), GOLDHAMER (1934), BORAK and DOLL (1934), and FREUND (1934). The syndrome has become known as the Albright syndrome or the McCune-Albright syndrome since the publication of the now classic articles by ALBRIGHT et al. (1937, 1938) and MCCUNE (1936, 1937). The autopsy findings on the patient first reported by MCCUNE were published in 1942 by STERNBERG and JOSEPH.

III. Clinical

The manifestations of fibrous dysplasia of bone are variable. Patients with this disorder may be divided into three groups. In the first group are the patients with only one bone involved (monostotic fibrous dysplasia); in the second group more than one bone is involved (polyostotic fibrous dysplasia); and in the third group there are skeletal and extraskeletal changes, as well as precocious puberty (Albright syndrome or McCune-Albright syndrome).

Fibrous dysplasia has been estimated to comprise 2.5% of the tumefactions and similar anomalies of the skeleton by COLEY (1960). While many cases have been reported, many others have not been and the literature tends to report the more spectacular forms. However, most authors believe that the incidence of the monostotic group exceeds that of the polyostotic group by several times and that of Albright syndrome by tenfold or more. JAFFE (1958) estimated that the ratio of the incidence of Albright syndrome to monostotic fibrous dysplasia is as 1:30–40.

The description of the clinical manifestations of this disorder can be drawn from the excellent review articles by ALBRIGHT and REIFENSTEIN (1948), BELAVAL and SCHNEIDER (1953), DAVES and YARDLEY (1957), EVERSOLE et al. (1972), FALCONER et al. (1942), FIRAT and STUTZMAN (1968), GIBSON and MIDDLEMISS (1971), HARRIS et al. (1962), HENRY (1969), LICHTENSTEIN and JAFFE (1942), MCCART (1952), MOORE (1969), PRIT-CHARD (1951), REED (1963), SANTE et al. (1948), SCHLUMBERGER (1946), SHERMAN and STERNBERGH (1948), STEWART et al. (1962), VALLS et al. (1950), VAN HORN et al. (1963), VINES (1957), WARRICK (1973), WELLS (1949), ZIMMER et al. (1956) and selected case reports.

1. Monostotic Fibrous Dysplasia

The clinical complaints of patients with monostotic fibrous dysplasia are either absent or rather mild. Frequently, the lesion is discovered when the bone is examined roentgenographically because of trauma or other reasons. In other cases, a local swelling, a pathologic fracture, pain, or functional disturbance may lead to the detection of the lesion. Skin lesions are rarely seen with the monostotic form of fibrous dysplasia. Laboratory studies are normal. However, when a fracture has been sustained, the serum alkaline phosphatase may be elevated.

Practically all bones have been described to have been involved with monostotic fibrous dysplasia. In a group of 259 cases collected from the literature (SCHLUMBERGER, 1946; HADDERS, 1957; HARRIS et al., 1962; STEWART et al., 1962; REED, 1963; FIRAT and STUTZMAN, 1968; HENRY, 1969; TALBOT et al., 1974), the ribs were involved in 65, the femur in 45, the tibia in 36, the maxilla in 33, the mandible in 32, the calvarium in 16, the humerus in 11, the radius and ulna in 7, the fibula in 7, the base of the skull in 3, the pelvis in 3, the clavicle in 3, the tarsi in 3, the zygoma in 2, the vertebrae in 2, and the metatarsals in 1. However, if isolated case reports and the dental literature is reviewed, the craniofacial area would seem to be the most common site of involvement. EVERSOLE et al. (1972) reviewed the literature on fibro-osseous lesions of the jaws and found 841 cases and reported 75 additional cases. Of these cases 228 were listed as monostotic fibrous dysplasia, 40 as craniofacial fibrous dysplasia, 41 as occurring with polyostotic fibrous dysplasia, and 225 as ossifying fibroma. In the remaining 307 cases, data was insufficient to distinguish between ossifying fibroma and fibrous dysplasia. In those cases classified as monostotic fibrous dysplasis 64% were in the maxilla and 36% were in the mandible.

The sex incidence of monostotic fibrous dysplasia seems to be equal in most series, but in a survey of the literature males tend to predominate because the cases were reported from army studies. In EVERSOLE's (1972) collection of monostotic fibrous dysplasia of the jaws 38% were in males and 62% in females.

Fibrous dysplasia seems to be primarily a disease of growing bone. Most of the cases are discovered between the ages of 10 and 20 years with the range extending from under 1 year of age to 70 years of age. The lesions of fibrous dysplasia tend to progress slowly and usually stop growing when the period of adolescence is over. There have been reported cases in which growth of the lesion was resumed or accelerated by pregnancy (HENRY, 1969; HUNTER and TURNBULL, 1931; DOCKERTY et al., 1945; BONDUELLE and CLAISSE, 1948).

In searching the literature, no cases have been found where the monostotic form of fibrous dysplasia developed into the polyostotic form.

When the craniofacial area is involved with fibrous dysplasia, it is frequently limited to that area with one or more bones being involved. However, in the polyostotic form the craniofacial area is frequently involved. There are other differences to be considered when the jaws are involved. Several authors have considered the expansile delineated lesions called ossifying or cementifying fibroma to be variants of monostotic fibrous dysplasia (GEORGIADE et al., 1955; HADDERS, 1957, 1967; MAMMEL, 1948; PANDERS, 1967; SCHLUMBERGER, 1946; ZEGARELLI et al., 1963; ZIMMERMAN et al., 1958). Others feel that only those lesions comprised of woven bone should be considered fibrous dysplasia (FRIES, 1957; LICHTENSTEIN, 1938; REED, 1963; SCHMAMAN et al., 1971; SMITH and SCHMAMAN, 1970). Nonossifying fibroma of bone is considered by some to be a variant of monostotic fibrous dysplasia (BINGOLD, 1956; MORTON, 1954). A distinction is made by some authors between fibrous dysplasia and ossifying fibroma on the basis of radiographic appearance, contending that the lesions with defined boundaries are ossifying fibromas, whereas the lesion with diffuse blending boundaries are monostotic fibrous dysplasia (COOKE et al., 1949; SHERMAN et al., 1948; SMITH and ZAVALETA, 1952; WALDRON, 1970, 1973). EVERSOLE et al. (1972) contend that monostotic fibrous dysplasia and ossifying fibroma are distinct entities and should be distinguished primarily on a clinical and roentgenographic basis, if the histology is fibro-osseous in nature.

Diffuse involvement of the face and possibly the skull may give the patient the appearance of leontiasis ossea. This term was used by VIRCHOW to describe leontine facies associated with facial hyperostotic bone disease. While fibrous dysplasia is one of the disorders associated with this appearance, a variety of other disorders such as Paget disease, osteomyelitis, craniometaphyseal dysplasia, and others may also have a similar appearance (CAHN, 1953; EVANS, 1953; FAIRBANK, 1950; PUGH, 1945; REISZ, 1936; TENNENT, 1946; LEEDS and SEAMAN, 1962).

Cherubism, or familial fibrous swelling of the jaws, may resemble fibrous dysplasia roentgenographically and to some pathologically. It will not be considered in this discussion of fibrous dysplasia. It is a separate disease and is characterized by its hereditary nature, being autosomal dominant (ANDERSON and McCLENDON, 1962; CORNELIUS and McCLENDON, 1969; CAFFEY and WILLIAMS, 1951; JONES, 1933; THOMA, 1956; LAWRENCE et al., 1970; Mc DONALD and SHAFER, 1955).

The clinical aspects will vary with the bone involved. In the long bones there may be deformities, especially if the femur is involved. Pathologic fracture may be the presenting complaint. When the skull is involved cranial nerves may be affected, especially the optic nerve. Seizures may also be found in these patients (SASSIN and ROSENBERG, 1968; MOORE, 1969).

Congenital pseudo-arthrosis is sometimes due to fibrous dysplasia (AEGERTER, 1950; JOHNSON, 1972).

2. Polyostotic Fibrous Dysplasia and Albright Syndrome

There is some debate as to whether monostotic fibrous dysplasia and polyostotic fibrous dysplasia should be considered as the same disorder. While both have similar pathologic changes in the bone, the extraskeletal changes, such as skin lesions and endocrine changes, are much more common in the polyostotic form. The Albright syndrome tends to have extensive bone involvement and is separated from the other forms of fibrous dysplasia by the presence of precocious puberty. It is our feeling that the three forms represent different degrees of severity of the disease.

In the polyostotic form of fibrous dysplasia, the multiple bones involved may be limited to one limb (monomelic) or to one side of the body, but often the bones involved are scattered throughout the body and practically all bones have been described to have been involved. In 66 cases collected from the articles by FURST and SHAPIRO (1943); HOBOEK (1951); STEWART et al. (1962); REED (1963); VAN HORN et al. (1963); FIRAT and STUTZMAN (1968); GIBSON and MIDDLEMISS (1971), the femur was involved 45 times, the skull 45, the tibia 35, the humerus 22, the ribs 17, the fibula 16, the radius and ulna 15, the mandible 13, the vertebrae 11, the calvarium 8, the scapula 6, the sacrum 5, the maxilla 4, the metacarpals 4, the carpals 3, the clavicle 3, the zygoma 2, phalanges 2, metacarpals 2, and the tarsal bone 1. In HARRIS's et al (1962) review of 37 patients (some of which had Albright syndrome) the femur was involved in 92%, the tibia in 81%, the pelvis 78%, the metatarsals 73%, the fibula 62%, the toes 61%, the metacarpals 56%, the ribs 55%, the occiput 53%, the base of the skull 50%, the humerus 50%, the radius 43%, the frontal bone 43%, the facial bones 40%, the fingers 39%, the ulna 33%, the scapula 33%, the tarsal bones 30%, the lumbar spine 14%, the clavicle 10%, the carpal bones 10%, and the cervical spine 7%.

In FALCONER's et al. (1942) review of 15 cases of Albright syndrome, the femur was involved in 15, the tibia and fibula in 14, the pelvis in 13, the humerus in 12, the radius and ulna in 12, the foot in 12, the calvarium in 11, the base of the skull and the face in 10, the hand in 10, the thorax in 10, the vertebral column in 9, and the shoulder girdle in 7.

Polyostotic fibrous dysplasia and Albright syndrome are usually diagnosed in childhood (PRITCHARD, 1951; STEWART et al., 1962; HARRIS et al., 1962; VAN HORN et al., 1963). Polyostotic fibrous dysplasia is seen almost as often in males as in females. In Albright syndrome, the females are affected much more often than the males. The presenting symptom of these patients is usually related to the skeletal lesions. Common among these complaints are pain, repeated fractures, deformities especially of the face and/or skull, and unequal length of the limbs (most often the legs). Often a limp or a waddling gait may be the first sign (HARRIS et al., 1962; VAN HORN et al., 1963). Skin pigmentation may be present in infancy, but vaginal bleeding of sexual precocity of the Albright syndrome is its most common presenting complaint. Later in life, other endocrine disturbances may be the presenting complaint. When the skull is involved, dizziness, visual abnormalities, or cranial nerve palsies may be the cause of the visit to the physician. The deformities may cripple a patient if severe polyostotic fibrous dysplasia started early in life (HARRIS et al., 1962). During life new lesions tend to form and existing ones spread. In general, the progress of the disease stabilizes at puberty but exceptions have been reported (DAHLMANN, 1955; HARRIS et al., 1962; RAMSEY et al., 1970). Reactivation may occur during pregnancy (HUNTER and TURNBULL, 1931; DOCKERTY et al., 1945; BONDUELLE and CLAISSE, 1948).

The most common extraskeletal lesion is cutaneous pigmentation. It is rarely seen with monostotic fibrous dysplasia but is present in over 50% of the patients with polyostotic fibrous dysplasia. It is seen in most of the patients with Albright syndrome (JAFFE, 1946; PROFFIT et al., 1949; RUSSEL and CHANDLER, 1950; FAIRBANK, 1951; HARRIS et al., 1962; LICHTENSTEIN and JAFFE, 1942; ALBRIGHT and REIFENSTEIN, 1948). These lesions are patches of brown, café-au-lait, or yellow color. They are flat and frequently unilaterally situated. The margins of the lesions tend to be more irregular than those seen in VON RECKLINGHAUSEN neurofibromatosis. ALBRIGHT et al. (1937) referred to them as "coast of Maine" in fibrous dysplasia and "coast of California" in neurofibromatosis. However, we have seen both types of lesions in both disorders. The skin pigmentations of fibrous dysplasia tend to be few in number and tend to be smaller than those of neurofibromatosis. These lesions are mainly scattered about the trunk, buttocks, and legs. While at times the skin lesions tend to coincide with the areas of bone involvement, this is not always the case (BENEDICT et al., 1968). Usually pigmentation is stated to have been present from the time of birth, but the patches have been observed to develop as the child gets older and new ones may appear (PRITCHARD, 1951). The skin lesions sometimes precede both the onset of the bone lesions and the development of sexual precocity. The pigmented skin areas do not differ histologically from the unaffected adjacent skin areas (JAFFE, 1958). The discoloration is thought by many authors to be caused by the presence of an abnormal amount of melanin pigment in the basal cells of the epidermis, some cells of the granulosa layer and pigment bearing cells in the corium. In 1968 BENEDICT et al. introduced a new diagnostic criterion. They stated that the most salient cytological feature of the pigmentary disturbance in neurofibromatosis was the presence of giant pigment granules in either malpighian cells or melanocytes, and that such granules were demonstrated in both café-au-lait spots and in normal skin. Of the patients with neurofibromatosis, there was only one in whom giant granules were not found, and these granules were identified in only one of the patients with Albright's syndrome. Thus the presence of these giant granules seemed to be a criterion for differential diagnosis. However, SILVERS et al. (1974) found that these giant granules may not be found in all cases of neurofibromatosis and that they may be less common in children.

The laboratory findings in the polyostotic form of fibrous dysplasia are usually normal. But, at times, the serum alkaline phosphatase has been elevated (PRITCHARD, 1951; HARRIS et al., 1962). CHANGUS (1957) found elevated levels of alkaline phosphatase in the bone lesions of fibrous dysplasia. This may be due to osteoclastic resorptive processes. In a few patients the calcium content of the blood was found to be increased (PRITCHARD, 1951).

The neurologic symptoms seen in patients with fibrous dysplasia usually are secondary to the bone lesion of the skull or spinal column. Deformities of the skull and face should lead one to suspect that the patient may have neurologic complications of fibrous dysplasia. This was found in 52 of 85 cases reported by FRIES (1957) and LEEDS and SEAMAN (1962). In 20 cases abnormalities of the orbit occurred, where the frontal, sphenoid, or ethmoid bones were involved. The eyeball may be abnormally situated. Exophthalmus, displacement of the orbit and/or globe, and orbital hypertelorism may develop. Exophthalmus was also noted to be associated with fibrous dysplasia by ALBRIGHT et al. (1938), STAUFFER et al. (1941), FALCONER et al. (1942), PUGH (1945), FEIRING et al. (1951), PRITCHARD (1951), and MOORE (1969). The fundus of the eye may show varying anomalies including congested veins, papilledema, and optic atrophy (FEIRING et al., 1951). FALCONER et al. (1942) described one patient in whom optic atrophy was combined with heterolateral papilledema and a central scotoma. They also, described a patient with bilateral optic atrophy and a bitemporal hemianopsia. SASSIN and ROSENBERG (1968) reported 50 patients with cranial fibrous dysplasia, 10 with optic canal involvement and of these 3 were bilaterally affected. In these patients, visual symptoms included failing eyesight, scintillating scotoma, diplopia, and optic atrophy.

Fibrous dysplasia can cause problems in the ears and nose. The temporal bone has been involved (COHEN and ROSSENWASSER, 1969; KINNMANN et al., 1969; VENKER, 1971). The bone lesion may take the form of an exostosis obstructing the external auditory meatus. The eighth cranial nerve may be affected by the narrowed internal canal (KANAVEL, 1907; FAIRBANK, 1951; EVANS, 1953; LEEDS and SEAMAN, 1962; SASSIN and ROSENBERG, 1968). The patients may have tinnitus, hearing loss (often conductive), vertigo, postauricular swelling, otitis media, and cholesteatoma (KINNMANN et al., 1969). Other symptoms such as visual disorders, and signs of a pyramidal lesion may be the result of the fibrous dysplasia causing thickening of the base of the skull. When the nasal bones are involved, the patient may have nasal obstruction and/or a nasal discharge which is sometimes bloody. The tear duct may be obstructed and lead to epiphora. Obliteration of the openings of the paranasal sinus, tear ducts, and nose may result in inflammatory disorders.

Neurologic problems can arise when the spinal column (especially the cervical and dorsal areas) is involved. In 8 of 29 cases reviewed by ROSENCRANTZ (1965), there was a variable degree of paraplegia from involvement of the spinal cord or nerve roots. In three of these cases, the symptoms were due to compression fractures (TENG et al., 1951; SKANSE et al., 1956; JIROUT and LEWITT, 1957). In the remaining five, expansion either of a vertebral body or of arches and articular processes were the cause of the symptoms (JAFFE, 1946; LEDOUX-LEBARD, 1953; LECOCO, 1956; ROSENDAHL-JESSEN, 1956). MONTOYA et al. (1968) reported a case of polyostotic fibrous dysplasia of the thoracic spine with spinal cord compression which responded favorably to a decompression laminectomy.

MCINTOSH et al. (1962) studied the circulatory dynamics of six patients with polyostotic fibrous dysplasia. Cardiac enlargement was present in half of the cases. The resting cardiac index exceeded normal values in five of six patients. Small arteriovenous oxygen level differences were noted across areas of extensive skeletal involvement when measured by selective venous sampling. They concluded that the osseous lesions of fibrous dysplasia contain functioning arteriovenous fistulae and that polyostotic fibrous dysplasia may be accompanied by high output cardiac failure.

3. Associated Disorders

In many patients, polyostotic fibrous dysplasia has been found associated with cutaneous pigmentation and manifestations of endocrine disturbance. In the descriptions of ALBRIGHT et al. (1937) and of MCCUNE (1936), the association was also in conjunction with precocious puberty. Thus, to the purist the terms Albright's syndrome or McCune-Albright's syndrome should be limited to those patients who exhibit the premature development of secondary sex characteristics and the others as polyostotic fibrous dysplasia with whatever endocrine dysfunction coexists with it (Fig. 44a–f). While sexual precocity occurs in about one-third of the female patients with polyostotic fibrous dysplasia, it is rare in males (WARRICK, 1949, 1973; BENEDICT, 1966; FALCONER et al., 1942; and HACKETT and CHRISTOPHERSON, 1949). They have advanced skeletal age and the epiphyses close early with a resultant short stature. Sometimes menstruation begins in the first year of life and often before the 10th year. It is frequently preceeded by the development of secondary sex characteristics. The ovaries and adrenals are usually normal, but ovarian cysts have been seen (BOENHEIM and MCGAVACK, 1952; PETERMAN, 1956; DOCKERTY et al., 1944). MCCUNE and BRUCH (1937) reported increased estrogen excretion in the urine of their patient. In the few women with Albright's syndrome who have become pregnant, the gestation and children have been normal (PRITCHARD, 1951). Menopause comes at the normal age. In the affected males, sexual precocity may occur but osseous precocity is frequent (FALCONER et al., 1942; ALBRIGHT et al., 1938; WARRICK, 1949). Gynecomastia, adiposogenital dystrophy, or acromegalic features may be seen (PRITCHARD, 1951; FALCONER et al., 1942). In BENEDICT's (1966) patient, a testicular biopsy taken at the age of 6 years, revealed active spermatogenesis and mature Leydig cells.

There have been many other disorders reported to be associated with polyostotic fibrous dysplasia. There have been several reports of coexistent hyperthyroidism (ALBRIGHT et al., 1937; MCCUNE and BRUCH, 1937; MOLDAWER and RABIN, 1966; KIM and KBERA, 1961; BENEDICT, 1962; SAMUEL et al., 1972). It may develop in either sex

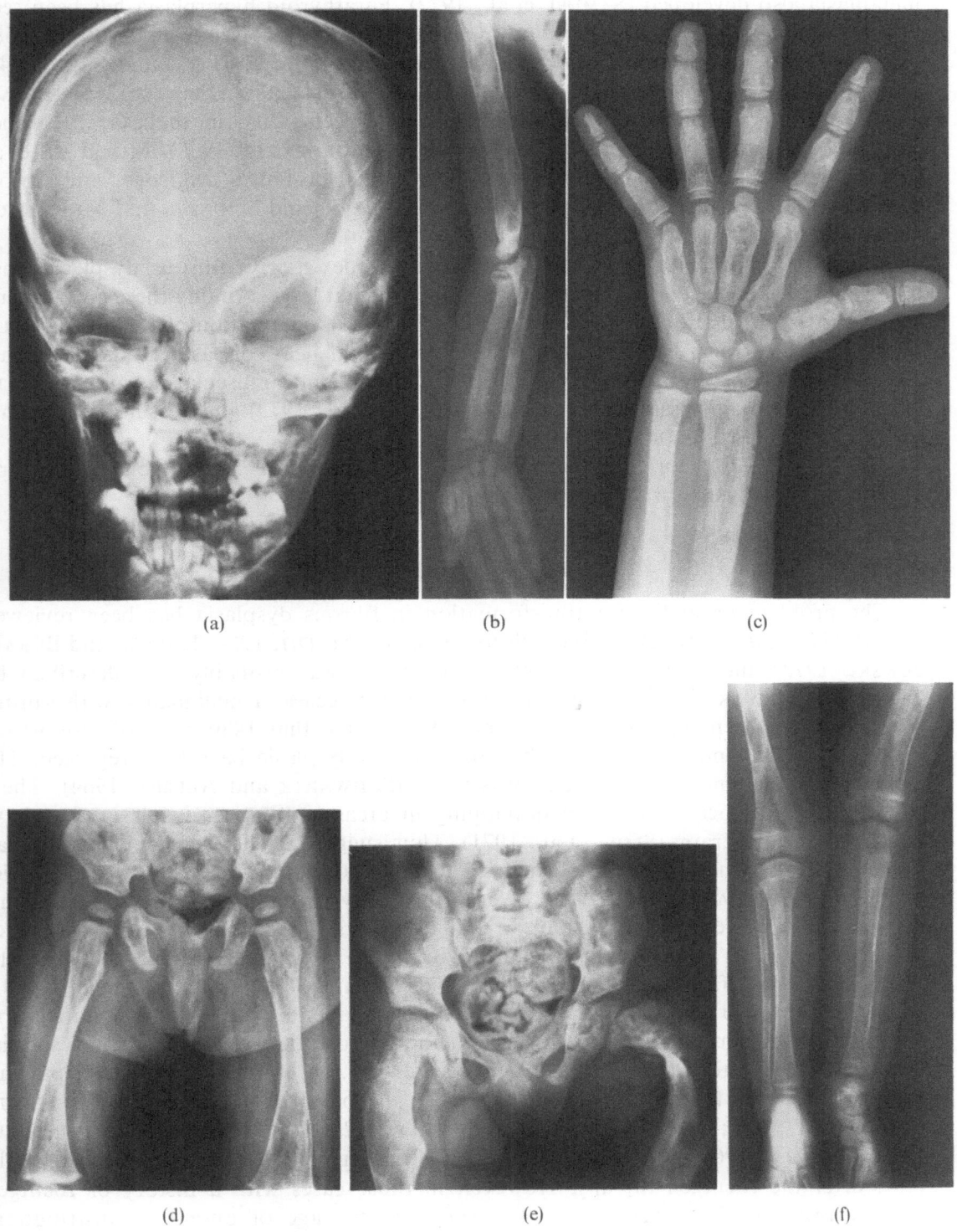

Fig. 44a–f. McCune-Albright's syndrome in girl. (a) Sclerotic area of skull involving supraorbital areas, left ethmoid and sphenoid bone due to fibrous dysplasia. (b) Diffuse involvement of humerus, radius, ulna, and hand with fibrous dysplasia. (c) Close-up view of hand and wrist to show areas involved with fibrous dysplasia. (d) Frontal view of pelvis and femora showing diffuse areas of fibrous dysplasia. (e) Frontal view of pelvis and femora 4 years later, after weighting bearing. Note deformities of femora. (f) Femora, tibiae, fibulae, left foot, and ankle are also involved

before or after the appearance of the bone lesions. In one of these patients, myeloid metaplasia also developed (SAMUEL et al., 1972). Parathyroid hyperplasia has been seen in a few patients with fibrous dysplasia (BENEDICT, 1962; FIRAT and STUTZMAN, 1968). The combination with diabetes mellitus has also been reported (PECK and SAGE, 1944; FEIRING et al., 1951; FRIES, 1957; MOLDAWER and RABIN, 1966; FIRAT and STUTZMAN, 1968). Acromegaly or acromegaloid features have been noted in the cases described by FALCONER et al. (1942), PECK and SAGE (1944), MORGENSON (1958), MCINTOSH et al. (1962), and SCURRY et al. (1964). The association of Cushing's syndrome and fibrous dysplasia was reported by AARSKOG and TVETERAAS (1968) and BENJAMIN and MCROBERTS (1973).

While many other extraskeletal manifestations coexist with fibrous dysplasia, they are probably no more common than in the population at large. Among these are congenital arteriovenous malformations (STAUFFER et al., 1941), coarctation of the aorta (COLEMAN, 1939), dextrocardia (VERGHESE, 1962), congenital heart disease (DOCKERTY et al., 1945), angio-osteohypertrophy (DANTAS, 1973), multiple intramuscular myxomas (WIRTH et al., 1971), myositis ossificans progressiva (FRAME et al., 1972) and esosinophilic granuloma of bone (GATEWOOD and ESTERLY, 1956).

JOHNSON (1972) reported the coexistence of adamantinoma of long bones with intracortical fibrous dysplasia and pseudarthrosis of the tibia.

4. Malignant Transformation

The problem of malignant transformation in fibrous dysplasia has been reviewed by several authors (SETHI et al., 1962; SCHWARTZ and ALPERT, 1964; DABSKA and BURACZEWSKI, 1972; and HUVOS et al., 1972) (Fig. 45). It was probably first described by COLEY and STEWART in 1945. Since that time, over 48 cases of malignancy with fibrous dysplasia have been reported. SLOW et al. (1971) noted that 1480 cases of monostotic fibrous dysplasia and 37 cases of polyostotic fibrous dysplasia have been reported. The incidence of malignant degeneration was 0.5% (SCHWARTZ and ALPERT, 1964). There is a higher incidence of sarcoma developing in areas of fibrous dysplasia that have had irradiation therapy (SLOW et al., 1971). Thus suggesting that roentgen therapy can potentiate a tendency for fibrous dysplasia to undergo malignant change. In the series reviewed by SCHWARTZ and ALPERT (1964), fibrous dysplasia was diagnosed in patients between 4 and 39 years of age, the mean being 16 years. The age of onset of malignancy ranged from 8–61 years of age, the mean being 32 years. The interval between the diagnosis and the finding of the sarcoma varied from 2–30 years with a mean of 13.5 years. The sex distribution was equal. A few less patients with the monostotic form developed a sarcoma than did patients with the polyostotic from of fibrous dysplasia. Four of the polyostotic cases had Albright's syndrome. Of 48 cases reported, 19 patients had had roentgen therapy to the area prior to the onset of the sarcoma (SCHWARTZ and ALPERT, 1964; DABSKA and BURACZEWSKI, 1972; HUVOS et al., 1972; FEINTUCH, 1973; RIDDELL, 1964; SLOW et al., 1971). The malignancy was noted to appear 6–18 years after the roentgen therapy. However, in those cases with a history of roentgen therapy prior to the development of a sarcoma, the age of onset, sex distribution, lag period, and prognosis were not significantly different than those cases in which therapy had not been given (SCHWARTZ and ALPERT, 1964). The distribution of the sarcomas in the skeleton paralleled the distribution of the fibrous dysplasia. The bones of the craniofacial area were involved 15 times, the femur 15, the tibia 6, the humerus 4, the scapula 3, the pelvis 2, and the fibula, rib, metatarsal one each. The histology of the sarcoma was osteogenic in 27, fibrosarcoma in 12, chondrosarcoma in 5, and giant

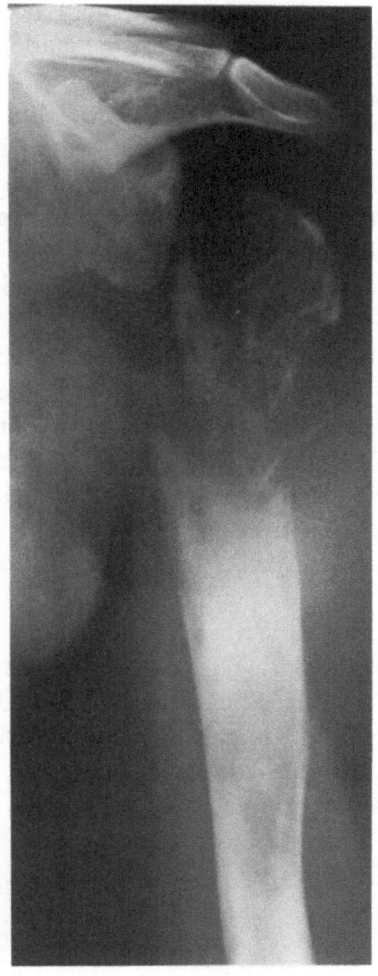

Fig. 45. Fibrosarcoma arising from site of fibrous dysplasia in humerus

cell or mixed sarcoma in 4. The most significant findings indicating the malignant transformation were pain, swelling, and a definite change in the roentgenogram image. In some patients, the initial diagnosis of fibrous dysplasia was made at the same time as the diagnosis of the sarcoma (HUVOS et al., 1972).

IV. Pathology

The pathology of fibrous dysplasia has been studied by many investigators (LICHTENSTEIN and JAFFE, 1942; SCHLUMBERGER, 1946; VALLS et al., 1950; STRASSBURGER et al., 1951; PRITCHARD, 1951; CHANGUS, 1975; JAFFE, 1958; HARRIS et al., 1962; STEWART et al., 1962; REED, 1963; KWEE, 1964; PANDERS, 1970; EVERSOLE et al., 1972). Autopsy findings were reported by COLEMAN (1939), STERNBERG and JOSEPH (1942), JERVIS and SCHEIN (1951), WIGGINS (1955), MOLDAWER and RABIN (1966), and BENJAMIN and McROBERTS (1973).

The gross pathologic examination of this disorder will show a solid mass of fibrous-like tissue replacing the bone marrow. This tissue usually leaves the bone intact, but in advanced cases, it will be found to thin the cortex of a long bone, frequently causing the contours of the bone to bulge. The cortex may not be seen, but the periosteum remains intact and may be thickened (Harris et al., 1962). In these cases the whole width of the bone is made up of a tough, soft, or firm, white to brownish fibrous tissue which is vascular. It is usually gritty due to the new bone formation within it. While the texture of this fibrous-like tissue varies in different areas, it usually cuts easily with a scalpel. Small hemorrhages, islands of cartilage, and cysts may be found. When cut, the surface is flat and incompressible. If rubbed with a finger, it may feel as if one is rubbing a fine grade of sand paper. The lesions are usually found in the diaphysis or the metaphysis. Rarely the epiphysis may be involved.

Microscopically, the basic components of fibrous dysplasia are fibrous tissue and associated bony trabeculae (Fig. 46). The fibrous tissue is usually composed of spindle cells formed into strands and whorls. At times, the fibrous constituent is made up of more loosely arranged cells, similar to those seen in embryonic fibrous tissue. In other areas or lesions, a paucity of cells, and large amounts of collagen will be seen. As a rule, the osteoid is scattered through the fibrous tissue as isolated deposits that are irregular in shape, variable in size, and show no specific pattern of arrangement. Large areas may contain no osseous component. However, in the radio-opaque lesions that involve the skull and face, large interconnecting trabeculae can be the main feature. Poorly oriented trabeculae of bone may be semicalcified and separated by cellular fibrous tissue. With reticulum stains under polarized light, the bone appears woven rather than lamellar. This finding aids in distinguishing fibrous dysplasia from other fibro-osseous lesions (Spjut et al., 1971). On rare occasions, cartilage may be found. Van Horn et al. (1963) described finding cartilage in the microscopic sections studied in 10% of their patients who were less than 11-years-old. Bone formation, one of the components of

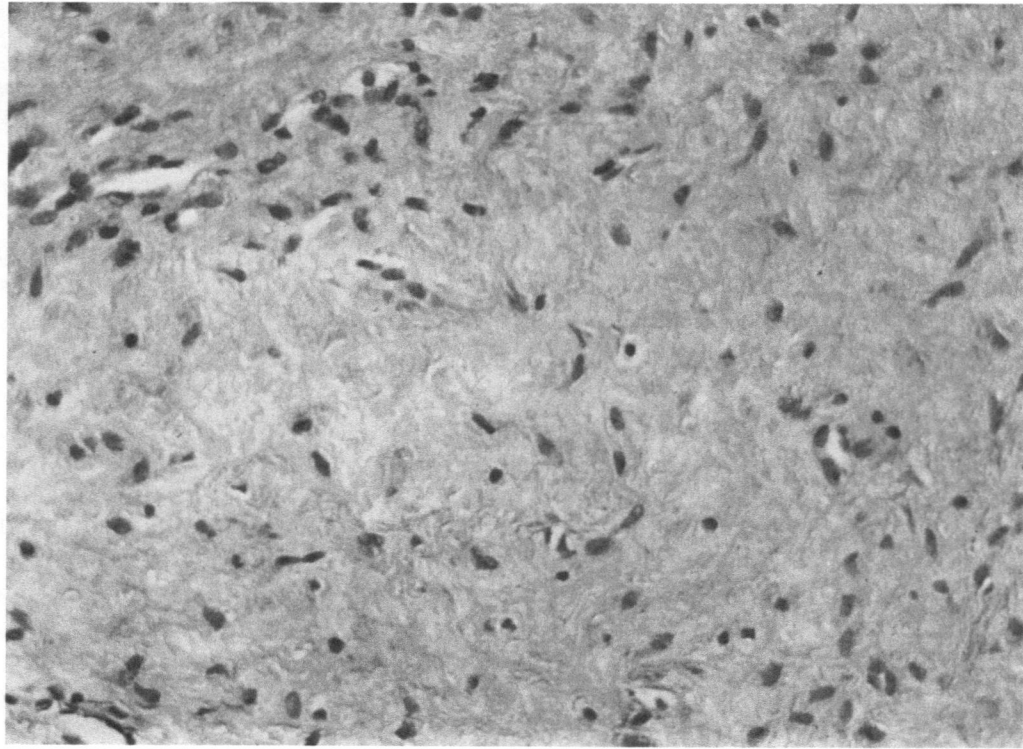

Fig. 46. Histopathology of fibrous dysplasia. Nuclei of fibrocysts distributed throughout densely collagenous extracellular substance

fibrous dysplasia, is believed by many to be metaplasia of connective tissue. Using the Hortega technique, VALLS et al. (1950) demonstrated formation of trabeculae from reticulo-histiocytic elements of the lesion. The new bony trabeculae are seen in many forms such as circles and C-shapes. They are irregular in size, shape, and distribution. The lack of osteoblastic rimming of the bone trabeculae is an important feature in the diagnosis of fibrous dysplasia. Near areas of degeneration, foci of macrophages and multinucleated giant cells may be found. Fibrous dysplasia is generally believed to be a defect in the conversion of woven bone to lamellar bone.

V. Etiology

The cause of fibrous dysplasia is unknown. LICHTENSTEIN and JAFFE (1942) believe it to be a developmental abnormality of the bone forming mesenchyme. ALBRIGHT and REIFENSTEIN (1948) felt that the disorder may be an expression of an embryologic defect or of a disseminated neurologic disturbance, the gonadal anomaly resulting from afferent nerve impulses from the hypothalamus to the anterior pituitary. SCHLUMBERGER (1946) felt that fibrous dysplasia was a disturbance of the normal reparative process following bone injury. AEGERTER et al. (1963) suggested that in fibrous dysplasia the physiologic metabolism of the bone is deranged, in that catabolism takes place, but not anabolism, due to an unknown disturbance, probably of a local nature. HALL and WARRICK (1972) and WARRICK (1973) postulated that a congenital abnormality of the hypothalamus causes overproduction of one or more releasing hormones, thus simulating the anterior pituitary to produce the hormones which cause the endocrine disturbances seen in some patients with polyostotic fibrous dysplasia.

VI. Roentgenology

The roentgenographic manifestations of fibrous dysplasia have been described by many authors (ALBRIGHT et al., 1937; LICHTENSTEIN and JAFFE, 1942; FURST and SHAPIRO, 1943; SCHLUMBERGER, 1946; SANTE et al., 1948; WELLS, 1949; FAIRBANK, 1950; PRITCHARD, 1951; DAVES and YARDLEY, 1957; HARRIS et al., 1962; GIBSON and MIDDLEMISS, 1971; WARRICK, 1973; and in the various textbooks on roentgenology). According to WARRICK (1973), the skeletal changes of fibrous dysplasia vary to some degree with age. In infancy, the earliest changes are small foci of either cyst-like lesions in the cortex of the bone or of a ground-glass change in an expanded cortex. Coarsening of trabeculae or ground-glass areas in the medulla may also be seen. Hyperostosis of the base of the skull may be present. Prior to weight bearing, deformities of the lower limbs usually do not develop. Most of the skeletal lesions seem to appear during childhood, and rapid extension into normal bone may be noted during the first decade of life. Epiphyseal involvement with lesions of fibrous dysplasia is rare prior to fusion, but may occur (NIXON and CONDON, 1973). Early fusion of epiphyses is common in the involved bones. Occasionally, an individual lesion may increase in size during adult life. This is more apt to be seen with monostotic lesions. When the focal area of fibrous dysplasia expands, there is absorption of the cortex and the differentiation between cortex and medulla is lost. The normal bony structure is replaced by a more or less uniform appearance often likened to ground glass. In the older patient, lesions which have been present for many years acquire a dense spotty or linear calcification, a picture that resembles that seen with bone infarcts.

The roentgen appearance of fibrous dysplasia has often been referred to as cystic, due to a focal thinning of the cortex with a smooth bordered radiolucent area. This is not a fluid-filled cavity as the term cyst would infer. The basic change due to fibrous dysplasia is a solid fibro-osseous mass, which occasionally contains degenerated zones with fluid-filled cavities. Change in the cortical thickness is a result of slow resorption of the endosteal surface or endosteal erosion. The periosteum is smooth. Periosteal reaction is seen only after fracture.

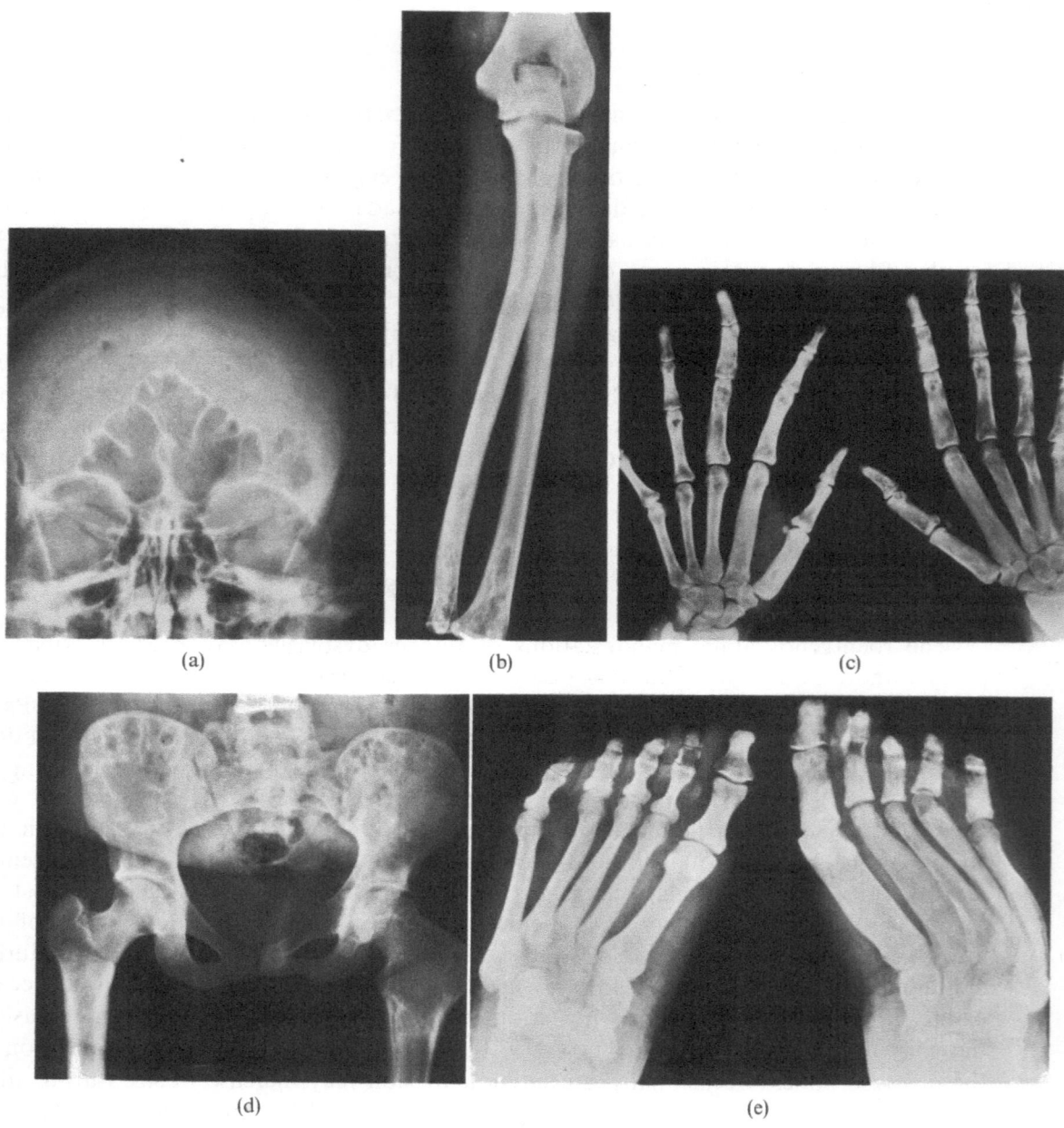

(a)   (b)   (c)

(d)   (e)

Fig. 47a–e. Polyostotic fibrous dysplasia in 19-year-old girl. (a) There is mixed cystic and blastic lesion of fibrous dysplasia involving left supraorbital area. (b) Sequestrum like areas of fibrous dysplasia in distal radius and ulna. These lesions resemble bone infarcts. (c) Diffuse involvment of hands with fibrous dysplasia. (d) Pelvis and femora are also involved with lesions of fibrous dysplasia. (e) Diffuse involvement of feet with fibrous dysplasia. Note that one side of body is more severely affected

The multilocular picture seen with some lesions of fibrous dysplasia is an illusion brought about by the scalloped endosteal erosions, and the transverse lines of preserved normal cortex between areas of cortical erosion. Sometimes blunt septa project from the endosteum and do not cross the medullary canal. Usually, however, individual lesions tend to be unicameral and medullary.

When the ground-glass appearance is seen in bones afflicted with fibrous dysplasia, it is a manifestation of an intrinsic property of the disease tissue. It is the result of superimposition of myriad, thin calcified trabeculae.

Deformities in bones with fibrous dysplasia, such as extreme degrees of expansion, bowing, increase in length, distortion of shape, cystic formation, and hyperostosis are usually associated with repeated fractures or infractions.

PRATT et al. (1969) described two patients in whom a sequestrum was seen in the medullary cavity of a long bone within a sclerotic zone of fibrous dysplasia. In both patients, the diagnosis was confirmed histologically and neither patient had any evidence of osteomyelitis.

GIBSON and MIDDLEMISS (1971) in their review of 55 cases of fibrous dysplasia, point out that while monostotic and polyostotic forms have almost identical roentgen manifestation in the involved bones, there are some differences. A fusiform expansion of bone, gradually merging with normal bone, is a feature of the polyostotic form. The monostotic form usually has a well-defined, often sclerotic, border. The monostotic lesion is usually medullary with the cortex involved as a result of growth of the lesion. The polyostotic lesion more frequently involves the entire bone and gross bending of long bones is much more common than in the monostotic lesions (Fig. 47a–e). A ground-

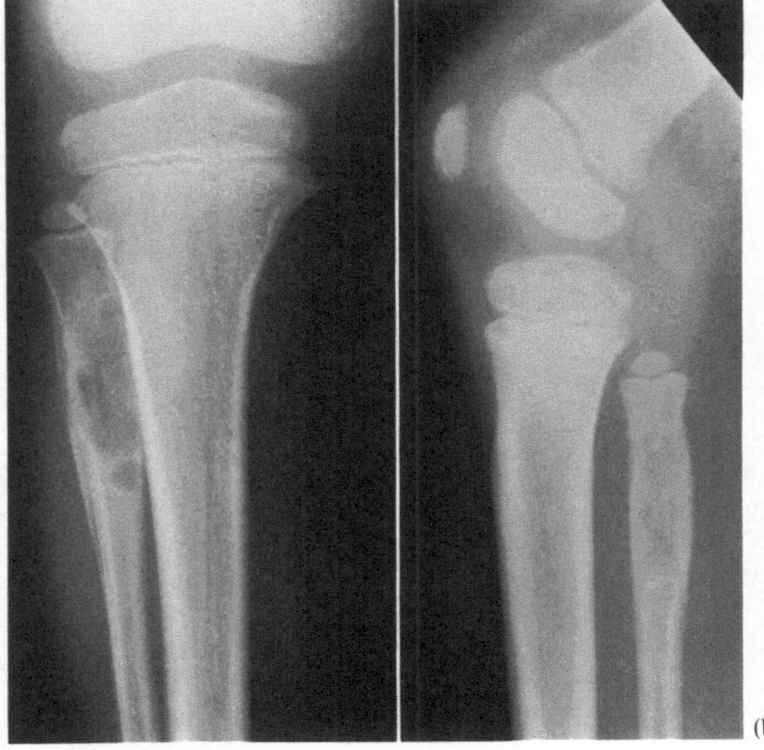

(a)   (b)

Fig. 48a and b. Frontal and lateral views of area of fibrous dysplasia of proximal fibula. Periosteal new bone is result of healing of minor pathologic fracture which had been present in this monostotic lesion two months earlier

glass appearance is more apt to be found in the polyostotic form, whereas trabeculation is a more common feature in the monostotic. Also, fractures are more common in the polyostotic lesion.

When the long bones are involved with fibrous dysplasia, the major change is replacement of the medullary cavity with lesions varying in appearance from completely radiolucent to homogeneous ground-glass (Figs. 48a, b, 49–52). The density of the lesion depends upon the amount of fibrous or osseous tissue deposited in the medulla and upon its calcium content. In the radiolucent lesion, the cortex is thinned from the medullary side and shows well-defined sclerotic margins. However, following fractures the cortex may be thickened. When the lesion of fibrous dysplasia is a dense one, normal cortical definition is lost and the entire area of the bone appears to be of one texture. When the bones of the lower half of the body are involved, the femur is almost always diseased. Bowing deformities are usually the result of healed fractures. Coxa vara is prominent and the "shepherd's crook" deformity may be present. Bowing of the tibia and of the humerus may be present.

When the small bones such as the carpi or tarsi are involved, the lesion of fibrous dysplasia is either homogeneous ground-glass or pseudo-cystic in appearance.

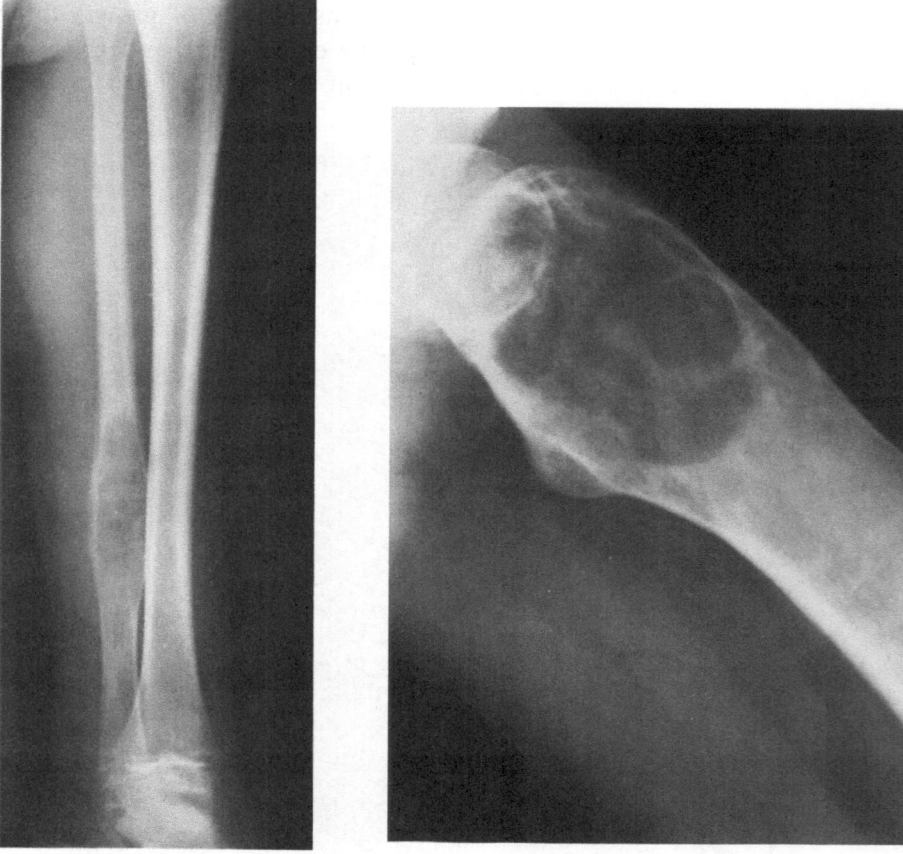

Fig. 49   Fig. 50

Fig. 49. Monostotic fibrous dysplasia in middle of fibula having appearance suggestive of sequestrum formation

Fig. 50. Monostotic involvement of femur with fibrous dysplasia. There is cystic appearing area in intertrochanteric area. Upper shaft of femur is widened and there is "ground glass" appearance to medulla

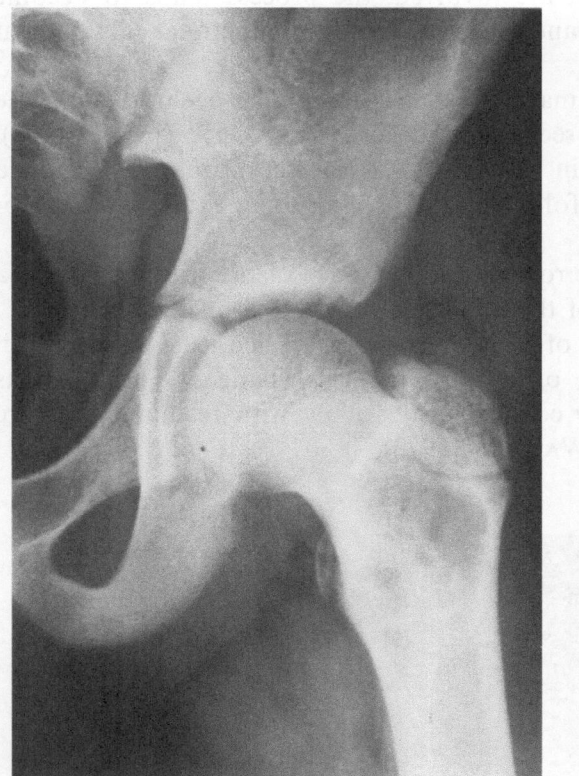 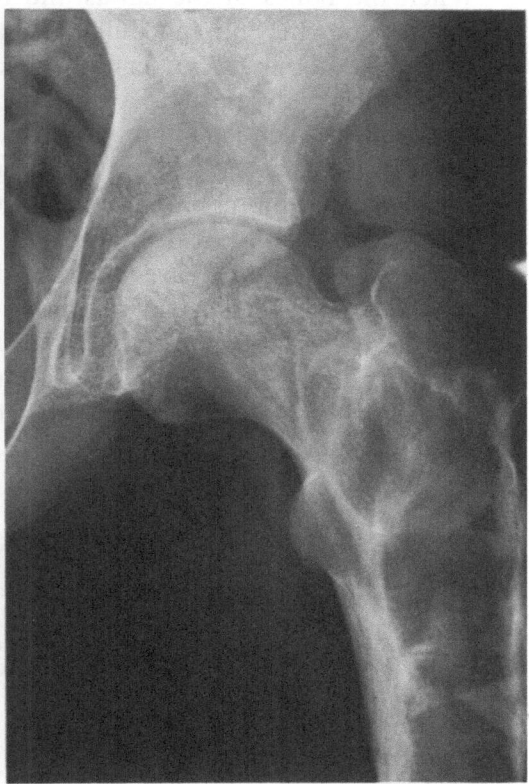

Fig. 51   Fig. 52

Fig. 51. Isolated area of fibrous dysplasia in proximal portion of femur

Fig. 52. Fibrous dysplasia in medullary area of upper femoral shaft. Note pseudo-cystic appearance

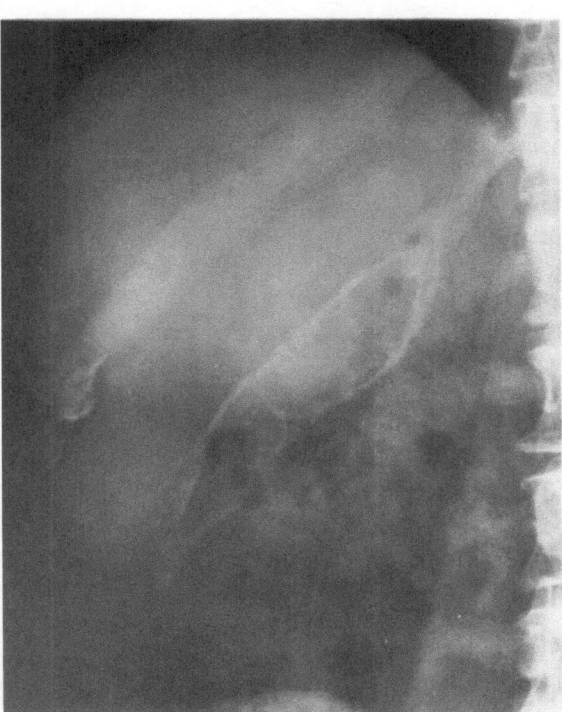

Fig. 53. Twelfth rib is expanded and has "ground glass" appearance to its medullary area. Pathologic examination revealed this to be fibrous dysplasia. This was isolated lesion

When the bones of the hands and feet are involved, the process tends to become confluent, filling the entire medullary canal and causing uniform symmetrical enlargement of the involved bone (Sante et al., 1948).

When fibrous dysplasia involves a rib, marked expansion tends to occur. The degree of enlargement is much more than that seen in other involved bones (Figs. 53, 54). The involvement of the ribs may result in a collapse of the chest wall producing a chest roentgenogram resembling that seen following the healing of an extensive thoracoplasty (Daves and Yardley, 1957).

When the pelvic bones are involved, the roentgen appearance of the fibrous dysplasia tends to be cystic. Intrapelvic protrusion of the acetabula may develop (Fig. 55).

The vertebral body is not often the site of fibrous dysplasia. When it is, the roentgen image takes the form of cyst-like lesions or of ground glass changes. These lesions may degenerate into cysts. Vertebral body collapse may follow with resultant pressure on the spinal cord producing paraplegia (Warrick, 1973).

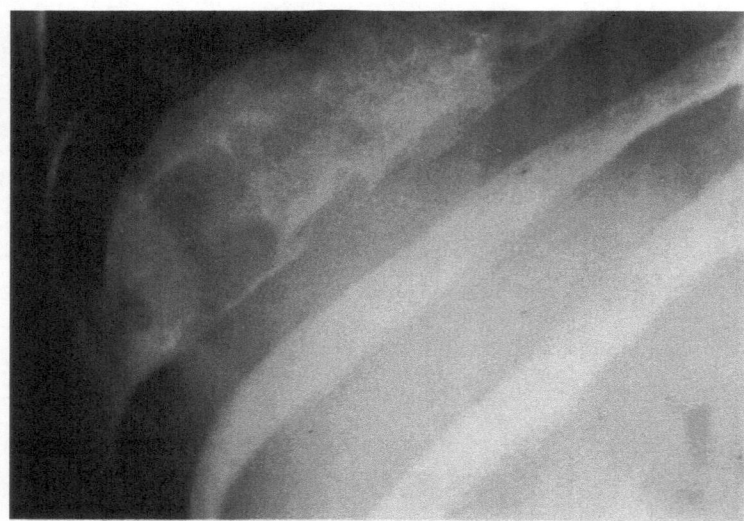

Fig. 54. Extensive involvement of tenth rib in case of monostotic fibrous dysplasia

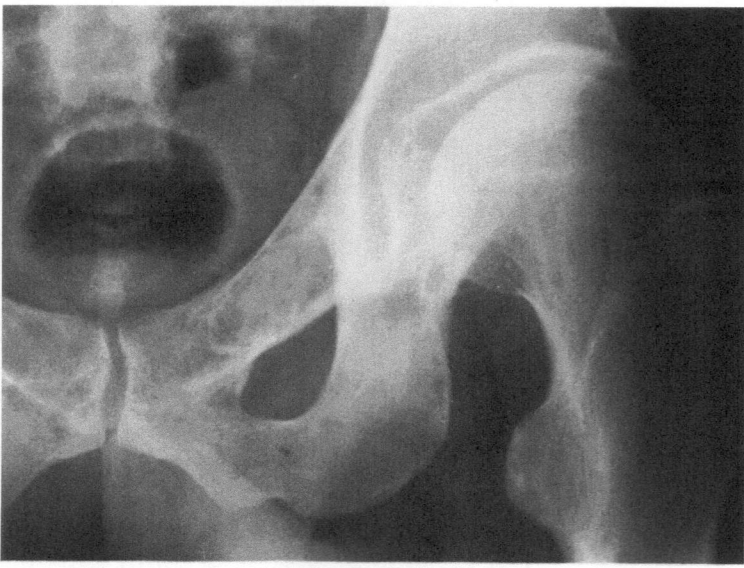

Fig. 55. Pubic bone contains isolated area of fibrous dysplasia

The roentgenographic changes of fibrous dysplasia in the craniofacial area present three major forms, the pagetoid type, the sclerotic type, and the cyst-like type (FRIES, 1957). In the pagetoid type, the involved area is expanded and has alternate areas of density and radiolucency. The calvarium may be quite thick and has been noted to be up to 7 cm thick. The expansion is outward, with thinning erosion and disappearance of the outer table. In FRIES' (1957) patients, 56% had the pagetoid type of involvement, 23% the sclerotic, and 21% the cystic type. The experience of LEEDS and SEAMAN (1962) is similar. The sclerotic type tends to involve the face and the base of the skull while the cystic type tends to be found in the calvarium. The pagetoid type is found in the older patients and possibly is the end result of the cystic and sclerotic types. Patchy areas of sclerosis may occur in the calvarium (LEEDS and SEAMAN, 1962; KWEE, 1964). The sclerotic form usually exhibits a diffuse homogenous enlargement of the base of the skull mostly involving the frontal, sphenoid, maxillary, and zygomatic bones. Sometimes a broad zone of basal extension, from the supraorbital to the suboccipital region, may be seen, several centimeters in width and being very dense. Often the process is unilateral. When the supraorbital region is involved the frontal sinus does not develop and the orbit on the involved side is small (TCHANG, 1973). The cystic type occurs mostly in the bones of the calvarium; FRIES (1957) found it once in the facial bones. The lesion is often solitary, with a dense, thin, and distinct border. The whole skull may be involved and the calvarium thickened (WINDHOLZ, 1947; FRIES, 1957). The extension of the lesion is not limited by the suture lines and both outer and inner tables may be involved.

The facial lesions of fibrous dysplasia are of the sclerotic type with homogenous structure and rather blurred outlines. The lesion is usually unilateral, involves several bones, and often is associated with involvement of the base of the skull. The mandible, however, is more apt to have a cystic appearance (Figs. 56, 57a, b, 58). The bones of the face and the orbits may be involved in a dense fibrotic process and resemble leontiasis ossea (Fig. 59). The expansion of the disease process often leads to facial asymmetry and ocular proptosis.

LIN et al. (1969) described the angiographic features of fibrous dysplasia of the skull. When the bony changes involved the outer table of the skull, no evidence of intracranial space-occupying lesion nor abnormal vasculature was found (Fig. 60). In a patient with thickening of the floor of the anterior fossa due to fibrous dysplasia, there was a slight

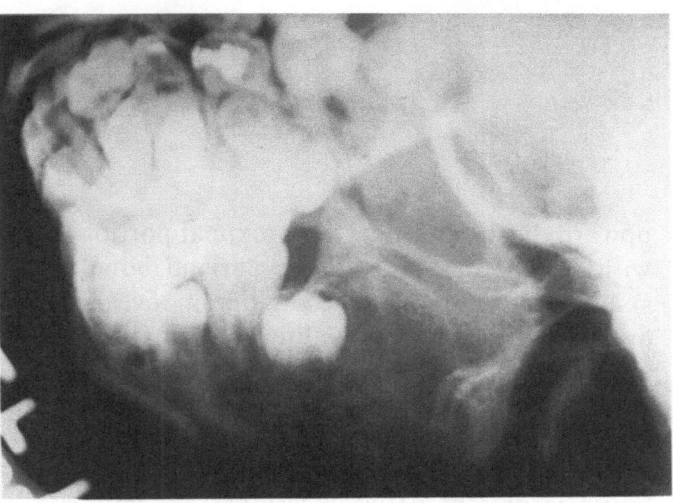

Fig. 56. Fibrous dysplasia in angle of mandible

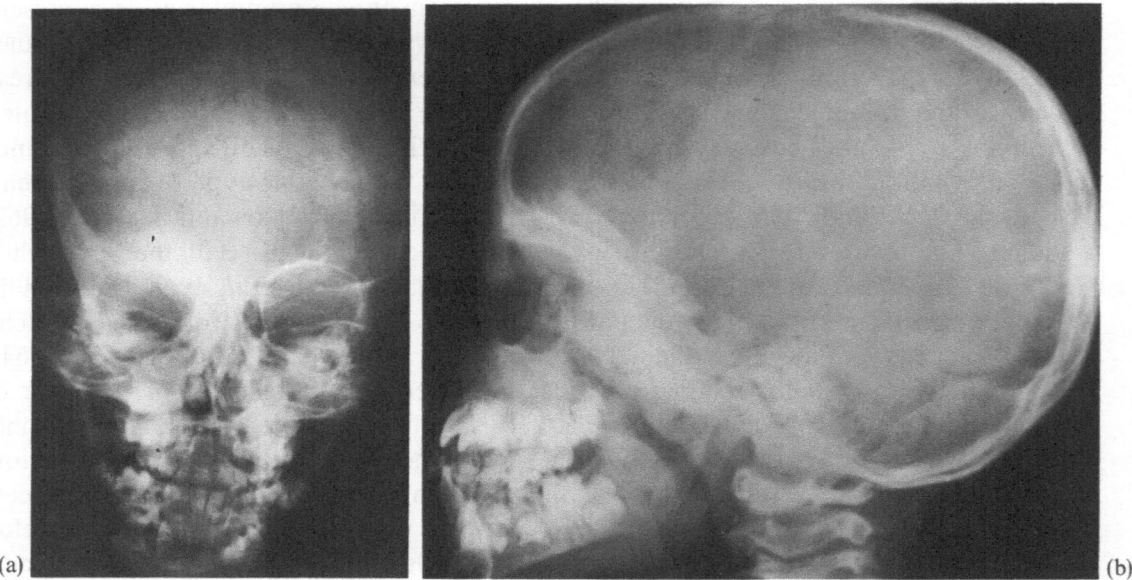

Fig. 57a and b. Fibrous dysplasia involving orbit and base of skull. Note displaced orbit and its decreased size

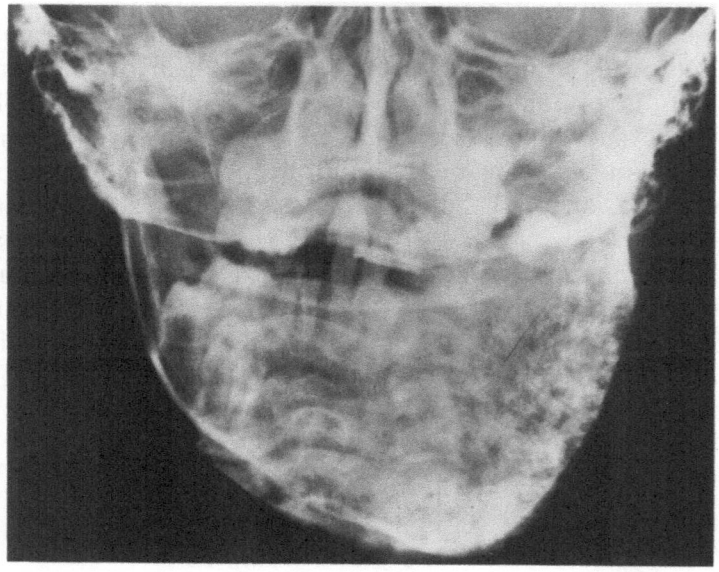

Fig. 58. Extensive asymmetrical involvement of mandible with fibrous dysplasia

upward displacement of the proximal portion of the anterior cerebral artery. In a patient with fibrous dysplasia of the parietal bone, large vascular channels were seen on the skull roentgenograms. The angiogram revealed an abnormally dilated superficial temporal artery and its branches, abnormal small beaded vessels, large early filling veins, and arterial and venous aneurysms.

BELEVAL and SCHNEIDER (1953) summarized the diagnostic roentgenographic features of fibrous dysplasia. These included: a well-demarcated radiolucent area within a bone; the lesion usually being in the diaphysis when a long bone is affected; normal osseous fabric is present between lesions; a "smudged" or "ground glass" appearance seen

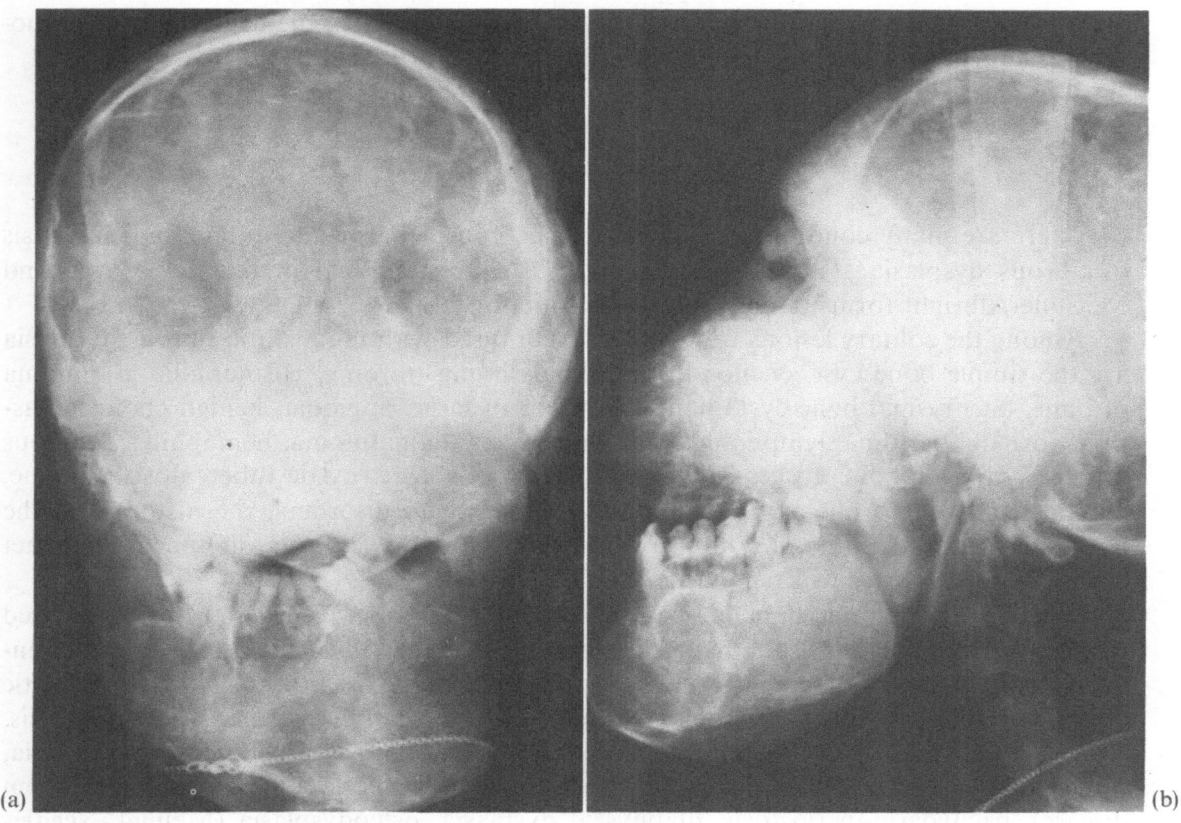

Fig. 59a and b. Diffuse involvement of face, mandible, and skull with fibrous dysplasia. This type is referred to as leontiasis ossea

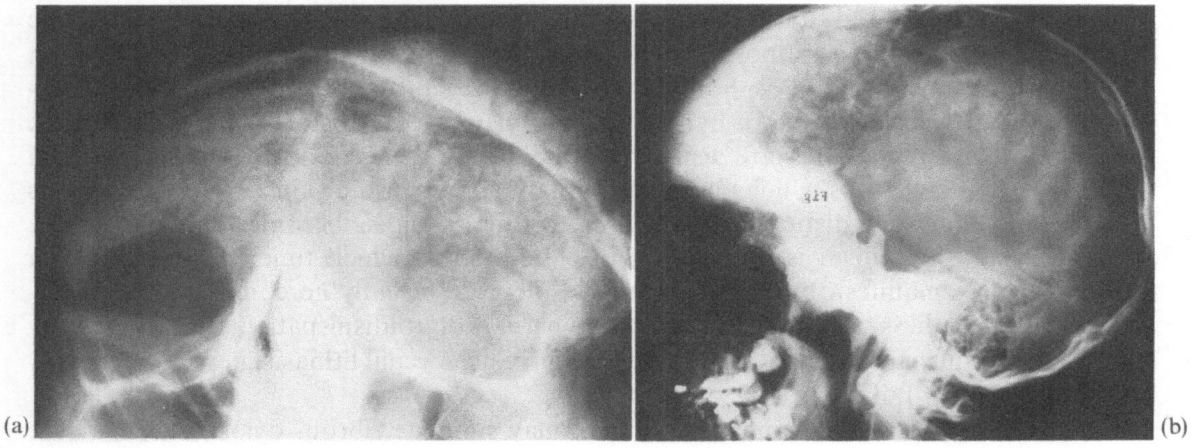

Fig. 60a and b. Extensive fibrous dysplasia of base of skull and frontal bone. If frontal bone were sole site of disease, meningioma would also have to be considered

in the medullary portion of the affected long bones due to intrinsic calcification; the presence of ridge formation and trabeculation suggesting cystic changes and often producing a multilocular appearance; the cortex of the bone is broadened or expanded with frequent marked deformities; periosteal reaction is absent except in the presence of a healing fracture; the presence of osteosclerotic skull lesions (besides rarefaction) with consequent disfigurement; early epiphyseal closure and frequently accelerated osseous growth in childhood resulting in dwarfism or deficient stature; the occurrence of pathologic fractures with frequent shortening and gross distortion of bone.

VII. Differential Diagnosis

There are many conditions which should be considered in the differential diagnosis of fibrous dysplasia. The diagnosis is more easily established in the polyostotic and McCune-Albright forms than in the monostotic form.

Among the solitary lesions which may be confused with monostotic fibrous dysplasia are the simple bone cyst, enchondroma, nonossifying fibroma, eosinophilic granuloma of bone, aneurysmal bone cyst, giant cell tumor of bone, angioma, benign chondroblastoma, osteoid osteoma, lymphoblastoma, myeloma, adamatinoma, hemophilia, tuberous sclerosis, chronic bone abscess, sclerosis, osteitis of Garre, cystic tuberculosis of bone, gumma, and fungus infection of bone. Usually, in these disorders, the history and the pathologic examination will establish the diagnosis; and even then, at times, the exact nature of the disorder will remain in doubt.

When more than one bone is involved, the most common disorders to be considered in the differential diagnosis are hyperparathyroidism, neurofibromatosis, skeletal enchondromatosis, osteogenesis imperfecta, Paget disease of bone, histiocytosis, and metastatic disease. Among the rare conditions are dysosteosclerosis, sclerosteosis, melorheostosis, craniometaphyseal dysplasia, craniodiaphyseal dysplasia, frontometaphyseal dysplasia, osteoectasia with hyperphosphatasia, endosteal hyperostosis recessive type (van Buchem disease), pachydermoperiostosis, diaphyseal dysplasia, osteodysplasia (Melnick-Needles syndrome), idiopathic hypercalcemia, and metaphyseal chondrodysplasia (Jansen type) (Spranger et al., 1974).

Prior to the establishment of fibrous dysplasia as a definite entity, many cases of hyperparathyroidism and fibrous dysplasia were grouped into the disorders of fibrocystic disease of bone. Now it is possible to separate these two disorders. A high serum calcium level, a low serum phosphorus level, generalized osteoporosis, and demineralization of bone are characteristic of hyperparathyroidism. In polyostotic fibrous dysplasia, the blood chemistry studies are usually normal; and there is normal bone between the fibrocystic-like lesions which tend to be unilateral. When the skin lesions, precocious puberty, and endocrine disturbances are present, the diagnosis becomes easier to make. Also hyperparathyroidism is uncommon in childhood at which time fibrous dysplasia usually becomes manifest. In fibrous dysplasia, there are usually no constitutional symptoms except for the skeletal disabilities. In hyperparathyroidism patients are frequently distressed with muscular weakness, digestive disturbances, renal lithiasis, nephrocalcinosis, and possibly renal failure.

Neurofibromatosis with bone involvement may simulate fibrous dysplasia. However, it is usually relatively easy to separate the two. In neurofibromatosis the bone lesion is secondary to erosion of the fibrous nodule from the periosteal surface into or through the cortex. There are soft-tissue tumors in the skin or subcutaneous tissues. The pigmented area of the skin tends to have smooth edges as compared to the irregular margins of somewhat similar lesions in fibrous dysplasia. Neurofibromatosis tends to be a hereditary diesease while fibrous dysplasia is not.

Skeletal enchondromatosis (dyschondroplasia or Ollier's disease) begins early in life and is associated with dwarfism and may be unilateral thus resembling fibrous dysplasia. However, the bone lesions tend to be very different roentgenographically. There is a characteristic involvement of the bones of the hands and feet by cartilagenous lesions giving rise to a typical punched-out appearance with bulging of the bone contours. The bones involved are those that start from cartilage, and skull changes are almost unknown. Sexual precocity and skin pigmentation are not identified with Ollier's disease. In the skeletal enchondromatosis, the pathology of the bone lesion is distinctive, with hyaline cartilage bascially being involved.

The roentgenographic changes seen with Paget's disease of bone resemble those of fibrous dysplasia, especially in the skull. In the calvarium, both conditions may show dense, fibrous, circumscribed areas, along with regions of rarefaction and a spongy, blotchy appearance, with blurring of the outline of the inner and outer tables. The long bone changes are not nearly as identical. In Paget's disease, there is thickening of the shaft, increase in the size of the bone, and involvement of both the cortex and medullary canal. The histologic appearance of bone is distinctive. Also there is a marked age difference in the patients with Paget's disease of bone usually occurring in elderly people.

Histiocytosis X (eosinophilic granuloma of bone, Hand-Schüller-Christian Disease, etc.), has an occasional resemblance to fibrous dysplasia roentgenographically. There may be large, circumscribed radiolucent areas in the calvarium in both disorders. The other osseous lesions, however, as a rule are quite different. Also, the clinical manifestations are dissimilar and pathology will readily separate the diseases.

The type of osteogenesis imperfecta found in infants with multiple fractures, blue sclerae, and deafness does not usually present a problem in differential diagnosis. However, the type, which is not noted until childhood, adolescence, or adult life, with the occurrence of pain or pathologic fracture, may resemble fibrous dysplasia to some degree. The roentgenologic study of these patients will help to separate the conditions; with osteogenesis imperfecta showing generalized osteoporosis, usually with some bowing of the long bones; as contrasted to the spotty distribution of either cystic appearing lesions or the ground-glass appearance of fibrous dysplasia.

When the craniofacial area is involved, the differential diagnosis includes those conditions which cause cranial hyperostosis such as the disorders mentioned above, in addition to meningioma. Usually fibrous dysplasia in the craniofacial area is easily identified on the roentgenogram. However, the wide range of roentgenographic changes of fibrous dysplasia may simulate many disorders (LEEDS and SEAMAN, 1962). Among the conditions to be considered are craniometaphyseal dysplasia, craniodiaphyseal dysplasia, frontometaphyseal dysplasia, metaphyseal chondrodysplasia Jansen type, dysosteosclerosis, sclerosteosis, osteopetrosis, metaphyseal dysplasia of Pyle, osteoectasia with hyperphosphatasia, endosteal hyperostosis, neurofibromatosis, pachydermoperiostosis, diaphyseal dysplasia of Camurati-Englemann, osteodysplasia of Melnick-Needles, idiopathic hypercalcemia, cherubism, tuberous sclerosis, rickets, syphilis, tuberculosis, chronic osteomyelitis, sinusitis, hemolytic anemias such as thalassemia and sickle cell anemia, iron deficiency anemia, cyanotic congenital heart disease, healed cephalhematomas, postirradiation necrosis, ossified subdural hematomas, acromegaly, hyperparathyroidism, pseudohypoparathyroidism, Paget's bone disease, hyperostosis of the skull, meningioma, osteoma, osteogenic sarcoma, hemangioma, metastatic carcinoma, metastatic neuroblastoma, and ossifying fibroma.

The ossifying fibroma, or fibro-osteoma is a sharply outlined monostotic lesion. It may be radiolucent or somewhat sclerotic. It is found in the maxilla, maxillary antrum, and the mandible. The sharp outline tends to separate this from fibrous dysplasia, but there are times when the distinction between the two is in doubt.

The osteoma is a sharply outlined tumor with homogenous dense sclerosis and a lobulated shape. It is a benign, slowly growing tumor of the membranous bones of the face and skull. It is eburnated and may project into the paranasal sinuses or it may arise from the outer table of the calvarium (KWEE, 1964). When it is associated with colonic polyps, it is a part of the Gardner's syndrome.

Chronic sinusitis may result in increased bone density and thickening along the floor of the anterior fossa and into the cranial vault. When this happens the differentiation between it and fibrous dysplasia is difficult.

The differential diagnosis between fibrous dysplasia and meningioma is often difficult to make. This is especially true when the sphenoid bone is involved; even pneumoencephalography and angiography may be negative (WAGMAN et al., 1960). According to LEHRER (1969), intraosseous meningiomas of the "en plaque" type have to be differentiated from the "blistering" meningioma which resembles the ossifying fibroma of the orbital roof or sphenoid bone. When the roentgenograph shows a ballooning of the orbital root, surrounded by slight to moderate reactive bone sclerosis, the appearance may resemble that of a dermoid or mucocele of the frontal sinus. The changes also should be separated from those of fibrous dysplasia in the same area. The age of the patient may help, since fibrous dysplasia usually starts in early youth and meningiomas in adult life. The bony reactions of meningioma are circumscribed; first involving the inner table and later the diploë and outer table. Enostosis may develop. In fibrous dysplasia, the diploë is the primary localization of the disease which is usually cystic and expands outward. However, when the lesions of the calvarium are sclerotic, it is very difficult to discriminate between meningioma, fibrous dysplasia, and osteoma (LEEDS and SEAMAN, 1962; KWEE, 1964). ROSENCRANTZ (1969) described widened vascular grooves in fibrous dysplasia of the skull which are similar to those seen, at times, with meningioma.

Another lesion which at times resembles fibrous dysplasia of the skull is the hemangioma. It may appear as a diffuse lesion with enlarged vascular channels, or as a honeycomb appearance to the calvarium.

When osteosarcoma arises from the jaws, the walls of the paranasal sinuses, or the temporal bones, it may cause erosions in the cranial bones, or it may produce a bone network with nodular areas, spicules, and shell-like areas. This, occasionally, results in a roentgenogram that suggests fibrous dysplasia. Also metastatic growths involving the calvium with destructive and, at times productive, bone lesions can simulate fibrous dysplasia.

The skull lesions of histiocytosis X are lytic at their onset, but when they are healing, hyperostosis and sclerosis may develop and thus resemble the lesions of fibrous dysplasia.

When there is a sclerotic lesion of the skull, in addition to fibrous dysplasia, one must consider the congenital types of hyperostosis such as osteopetrosis, progressive diaphyseal dysplasia, craniometaphyseal dysplasia, craniodiaphyseal dysplasia, frontometaphyseal dysplasia, other congenital dysplasia as listed above, infections, tuberous sclerosis, melorheostosis, and other rare conditions.

Roentgenographically, Paget's disease of bone involving the skull is one of the most difficult lesions to separate from fibrous dysplasia. Some of the differences that may be helpful in the differentiation are that Paget's disease tends to develop at a later age; it usually results in a comparatively uniform thickening and enlargement of the skull; circumscript bulges do not occur; absence of large, ground glass-like translucencies; and the cottonwool appearance, with gradual change from pathologic to normal bone. Other conditions to be considered in the differential diagnosis of Paget's disease and fibrous dysplasia are osteoectasia with hyperphosphatasia and endosteal hyperostosis of von Buchem.

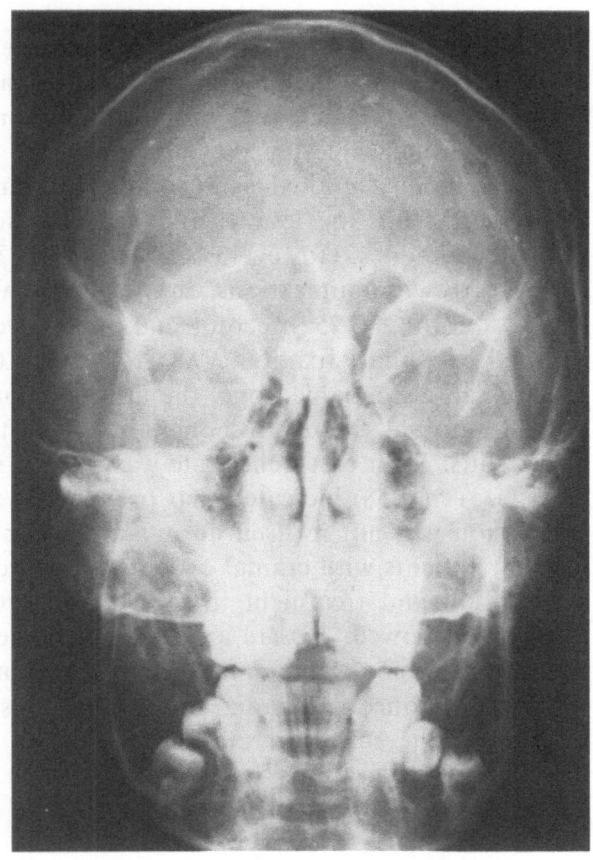

Fig. 61. Cherubism. Note symmetrical involvement of mandible

When the face is involved with cystic type lesions, one of the conditions to be considered is cherubism (Fig. 61). This was described as "familial fibrous dysplasia" of the jaws (JONES, 1933). It is a hereditary disease involving the mandible and frequently the maxilla. The children with this disorder are described as having a chubby face with a "heavenward gaze." It is a nonosteogenic fibrous lesion which sometimes contains many giant cells and tends to regress spontaneously. These features are sufficient to separate it from fibrous dysplasia.

When there is diffuse symmetrical involvement of the face and at times the skull, a gross deformity of the face develops and the appearance is that of leontiasis ossea. While this may be due to fibrous dysplasia, other disorders such as craniodiaphyseal dysplasia, craniometaphyseal dysplasia, dysosteosclerosis, frontometaphyseal dysplasia, endosteal hyperostosis of von Buchem, metaphyseal chondrodysplasia of Jansen, and sclerosteosis may have a similar facial involvement (SPRANGER et al., 1974). Paget's disease of bone, congenital gigantism, pituitary gigantism, cranioostosis, syphilitic osteoperiostitis, and tumors of the nose and paranasal sinuses have been referred to as false or symptomatic leontiasis ossea (EVANS, 1953).

To establish the diagnosis of fibrous dysplasia when one area is identified, the whole skeleton should be examined roentgenographically. If the lesion is solitary and a doubt exists, a biopsy may establish the diagnosis. When the lesions are multiple, the typical distribution of the lesions and the triad of the McCune-Albright's syndrome will facilitate the diagnosis. In addition, the fact that the disease is rarely, if ever, familial or hereditary is helpful.

VIII. Treatment

The major considerations in the management of patients with fibrous dysplasia, are those concerned with the skeletal manifestations of the disease. In general, indications for surgical treatment are continued pain in the region of a localized bone lesion; fracture through a lesion; severe bowing of a long bone; impending narrowing of a foramen about a cranial nerve or of the spinal canal or neurologically, deficient due to pressure from the lesion; and cosmetic surgery for disfiguring swellings especially of the facial bones. However, various authors have different approaches to management. In the early communications, the tendency was to treat only when necessary. ROBERT and DUCROGUET (1952) recommend preventive surgery for femoral lesions causing pain, with intramedullary fixation. VAN HORN et al. (1963) believed that if the fibrous dysplasia involves an expendable bone, the affected portion of the bone should be resected and possibly grafted. In major bones, bone grafting after a thorough curettage, gave the best results. Their recurrence rate was 21% in monostotic lesions and 36% in polyostotic cases. JAFFE (1958) indicated that prognosis was usually good and felt that the presence of a lesion was not in itself an indication for treatment. SASSIN and ROSENBERG (1968) felt that patients with cranial or vertebral fibrous dysplasia should be kept under careful observation and treatment instituted if neurologic changes developed or if the optic foramen narrowed. ROSENCRANTZ (1965) recommended early diagnosis and treatment of vertebral lesions which may give rise to complications.

While at one time radiation therapy was suggested, the current feeling is that it is of no value in the treatment of fibrous dysplasia and may be a potentiator for malignant degeneration (SCHWARTZ and ALPERT, 1964).

G. Myositis Ossificans

I. Introduction

Myositis ossificans progressiva and myositis ossificans circumscripta are two different clinical entities in which there is nonneoplastic heterotopic bone formation in the collagenous supporting tissues. The classification which is based on these two clinical syndromes is illustrated in Table 1. The circumscripta form was further subdivided by NOBLE in 1924 according to the presence or absence of a history of preceding trauma. 60% of the cases reviewed by NORMAN and DORFMAN (1970) and 75% of the cases reported by PATERSON (1970) have a clearly traumatic origin. The remaining patients either have one of the systemic diseases associated with myositis ossificans circumscripta (Table 1),

Table 1. Classification of myositis ossificans

A. Myositis ossificans progressiva: hereditary, fatal
B. Myositis ossificans circumscripta: acquired, self-limited
   1. Myositis ossificans traumatica (60%)
   2. Myositis ossificans circumscripta without a history of trauma (40%)
     a. associated with systemic diseases, e.g., paraplegia, burns, tetanus
     b. idiopathic—the "pseudomalignant" osseous tumor oft soft tissue

or develop the heterotopic ossification independently. The localized lesions without any known etiology have been referred to as the "pseudomalignant" osseous tumor of soft tissue (JEFFREYS and STILES, 1966), because without history this lesion may be mistaken both roentgenographically and pathologically for a malignancy.

1. Other Terms

Other terms that have been used in the literature for myositis ossificans circumscripta are myo-osteosis; extra osseous localized nonneoplastic bone; fibrositis ossificans.

2. Etiology

The association of myositis ossificans circumscripta with trauma was not clearly established until 1832. At that time a doctor in the Prussian infantry noted ossification of the deltoid and pectoralis muscles in recruits who were drilling with bayonets. While the infantry may have brought this entity to the attention of the medical community, it was the cavalry who popularized it. The term "charley-horse" originated from the gymnastic exercise of jumping onto the back of a padded wooden horse: an exercise which in novices frequently resulted in the formation of a firm painful mass in the adductor muscles of the thigh.

After the establishment of the relationship between trauma and the subsequent ossification of the injured striated muscles, tendons, and/or fascae, little definitive information as to the etiology has been added. Most investigators agree that soft tissue disruption and hemorrhage are of primary importance. This observation was confirmed by a clinical study of 548 cases of elbow injuries. In this group, the incidence of myositis ossificans was five times greater in those cases which sustained a combination of fracture and dislocation, as opposed to those with uncomplicated fractures (THOMPSON and GARCIA, 1967).

Several unanswered questions remain as to the pathophysiology of post-traumatic myositis ossificans. First, the mechanism by which soft tissue trauma stimulates localized bone or cartilage formation is a matter of conjecture. Following trauma, both interstitial hemorrhage and muscle necrosis release respiratory pigments: hemoglobin and myoglobin. It has been postulated that the protein moieties in these substances act as activators to stimulate heterotopic bone formation (PATERSON, 1970). A change in the pH of the interstitium, toward alkalinity, has also been invoked as the stimulant for heterotopic bone formation (FLYNN and GRAHAM, 1964).

A second unanswered question is the source of the osteoblastic cells. It is not known whether they originate in the damaged periosteum or whether pleuripotent cells are already present in the damaged connective tissues. The latter theory of fibro-osseous metaplasia is currently favored since myositis ossificans circumscripta had been produced experimentally by isolated damage to skeletal muscle (CLASSEN et al., 1960). Another area of dispute is the site of injury. ADAMS et al. (1962) believe that the name "myositis" is incorrect and that it is the damage to the interstitium which produces the heterotopic ossification. These authors postulate that the muscle fibers are merely compressed secondary to the proliferation of connective tissue, and that the fibrosing and calcifying interstitium is the primary abnormality. Indeed, undamaged muscle fibers can be identified even in well-advanced ossified lesions. Metabolic studies have yielded no consistent abnormality in patients with post-traumatic heterotopic bone formation (LIBERMAN et al., 1967; KALES and PHANG, 1970) (Table 2).

Table 2. Locations of myositis ossificans circumscripta

LIBERMAN et al. (1967) — 124 cases	
Flexors of the arm	64
Quadriceps femoris	43
Adductors of the thigh	13
Other	23

The etiology of the cases of myositis ossificans circumscripta without a pre-existing history of trauma is even more obscure. There are certain common features in all the systemic diseases associated with myositis ossificans (Table 1). First, the patients are immobilized. Second, pain, proprioception, and motion are impaired and third, lesions occur in the most easily traumatized areas, the elbows, hips, and shoulders. Thus, soft tissue trauma may be the common denominator in this group as well, the trauma being produced by the disease itself, e.g., as in tetanic spasms or it can be produced by the inadvertent injury done to those who cannot help themselves.

The last category of subjects with myositis ossificans circumscripta are those patients who have no history of trauma and no evidence of a systemic disease. The latter cases may be secondary to minor trauma which went unnoticed by the patient and indeed the common locations of these so-called pseudo-tumors correspond to the locations of the clearly traumatic lesions.

3. Clinical

Myositis ossificans circumscripta occurs most frequently in young men, with 80% of the cases occuring in the large muscle groups of the thighs and upper arms (SPJUT et al., 1970). Statistically, the brachialis muscles, the quadriceps femoris, and the adductor of the thigh account for the majority of cases.

Clinically, the initial insult may be of any type; a single episode of major trauma, recurrent episodes of minor trauma, or sustained irritation. Careful questioning may be needed to elicit the history, as in one reported case in which the damage was produced by the impact of loose coins in a pocket (FLYNN and GRAHAM, 1964). Another patient developed myositis ossificans circumscripta adjacent to his elbow after the strain of a long cross country drive with his forearm resting on the open window (FREEMAN, 1966). However, history alone cannot be relied on to establish the benignity of a lesion, since in a series of 16 cases of parosteal osteogenic sarcomas, 6 cases recalled trauma to the area in question (VAN DER HEUL and VON RONNEN, 1967).

The classical complaint is of a localized, painful swelling which becomes more severe 24 hours after the initial trauma. The pain is frequently associated with limitation of motion of the adjacent joint. Physical examination reveals a firm tender mass in the soft tissues, but at this time the x-ray examination will be negative. Over a 4-week period the palpable mass becomes firmer and more discrete, and the roentgenograms will begin to show calcific densities in the soft tissues. The area of myositis ossificans undergoes a period of active growth lasting about 10 weeks. The mass then becomes stagnant or regresses spontaneously. The younger the patient, the more likely regression is to take place.

Fig. 62a–d. Gross and histological sections of patient with myositis ossificans circumscripta, (a) surgical specimen demonstrating well-encapsulated area of myositis ossificans, (b) microscopic section of central portion of lesion with rapidly proliferating fibroblasts, (c) middle zone of area of myositis ossificans with osteoblasts and islands of osteoid, (d) periphery of lesion containing mature trabeculae which are clearly separated from surrounding tissues

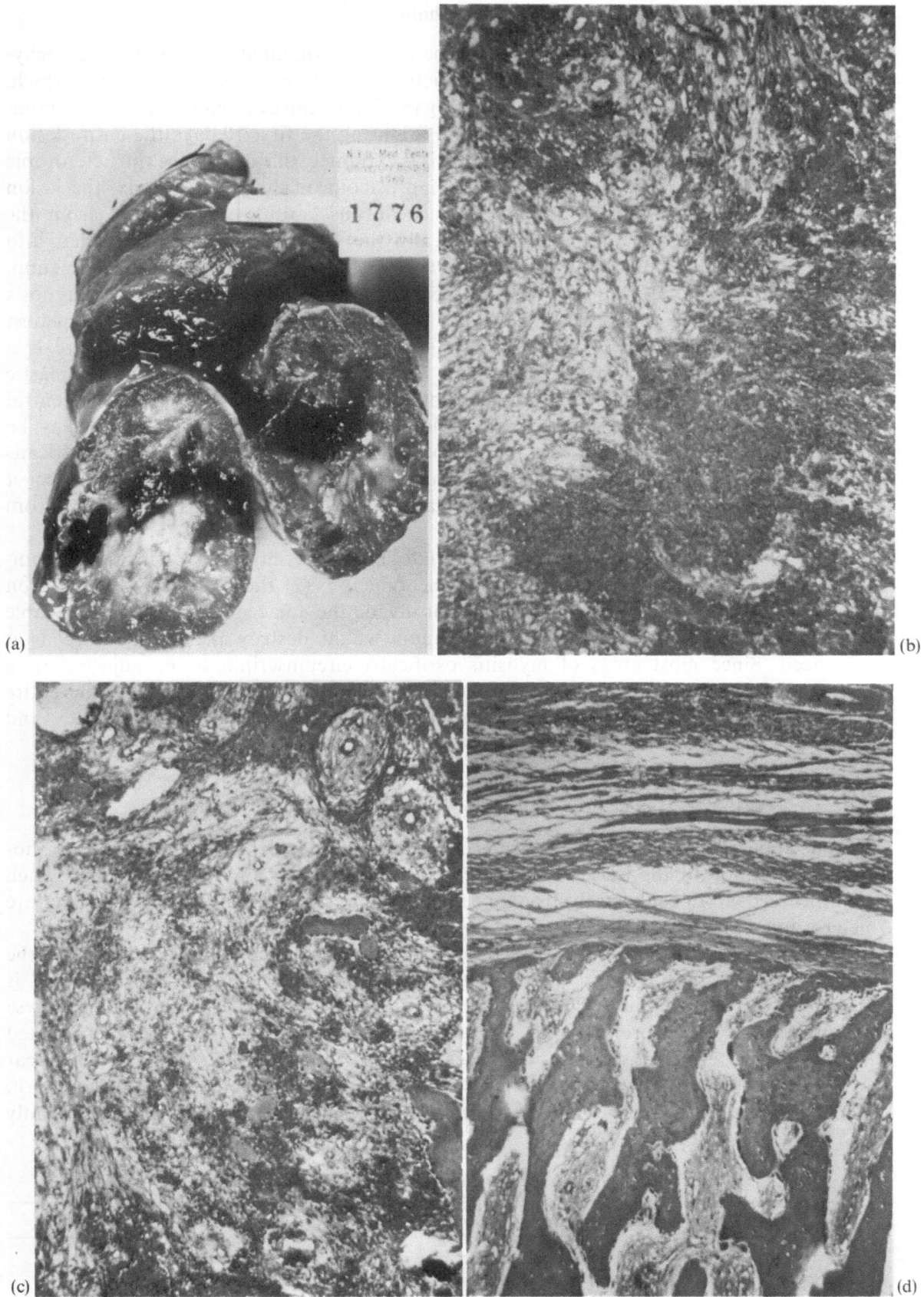

Fig. 62a–d

4. Pathology

The earliest pathologic findings are edema and an inflammatory exudate. Mesenchymal proliferation then results in the production of a large mass of collagen, which, unlike normal collagen, is capable of accepting the deposition of calcium salts — a phenomenon referred to as "dystrophic calcification." During the first 10 days the entire lesion is poorly differentiated and definitive diagnosis is extremely difficult. Once the heterotopic osteoblasts and chondroblasts begin producing osteoid or chondroid matrix, the lesion becomes grossly well-defined and develops a fibrous capsule separating it from the surrounding tissues (Fig. 62a). Microscopically the developing lesion is divided into three zones, which gradually blend into one another (Fig. 62b). This zonal phenomenon, which was first described by ACKERMAN (1958) is an important criteria for the diagnosis of immature myositis ossificans. The center of the lesion, which is the area of greatest damage, is occupied by rapidly proliferating fibroblasts. More peripherally there is a zone of osteoblasts with islands of osteoid. In the presence of the florid osteoblastic activity, the functioning cells may appear young and hyperchromatic and if the central zones are the ones to be biopsied a pathologic differentiation from sarcoma may be difficult. It is for this reason FINE and STOUT (1956) have labeled myositis ossificans circumscripta in its formative stages a pseudo-tumor (Fig. 62c). The third and most peripheral zone contains mature, normal trabeculae which are clearly separated from the surrounding connective tissue (Fig. 62d).

The pathologic criteria which differentiate immature myositis ossificans circumscripta from a sarcoma are (1) the zonal phenomenon, (2) the periphery of the lesion composed of mature trabeculae which do not invade the adjacent tissues, and (3) viable muscle fibers within the lesion itself — a tumor would destroy the musculature as it advanced. Since most areas of myositis ossificans circumscripta occur adjacent to a long bone, the major differential is parosteal osteogenic sarcoma. Eventually, the entire area of myositis ossificans is transformed into mature bone with a clear cortex and medullary space and trabeculae oriented to lines of stress.

5. Roentgen Appearance

The appearance of myositis ossificans circumscripta on serial x-rays reflects the pathologic maturation of the lesion. The three general steps are: soft tissue swelling, which then proceeds to flocculated dystrophic calcification, which is finally replaced by mature heterotopic bone (Fig. 63).

The roentgenographic findings in the first 4 weeks depend on the location of the initial trauma. One of the roentgen classifications (GILMER and ANDERSON, 1959) is based on the site of injury. The first group (Table 3) are the parosteal lesions. These lesions arise in close proximity to the shaft of a bone and are frequently associated with an early periosteal reaction. The second type (Table 3) results from a direct tear of the periosteum and within the first 2 weeks produces a layered periosteal pattern. The third category (Table 3) are the extraosseous lesions. These cases will show only

Table 3. Roentgenographic classification of myositis ossificans

GILMER and ANDERSON (1959)

A. Parosteal —	adjacent to the shaft of a bone: may produce a periosteal reaction	
B. Periosteal —	produced by a direct tear of the periosteum: layered periosteal reaction	
C. Extraosseous —	early roentgen findings consist only of soft tissue swelling	

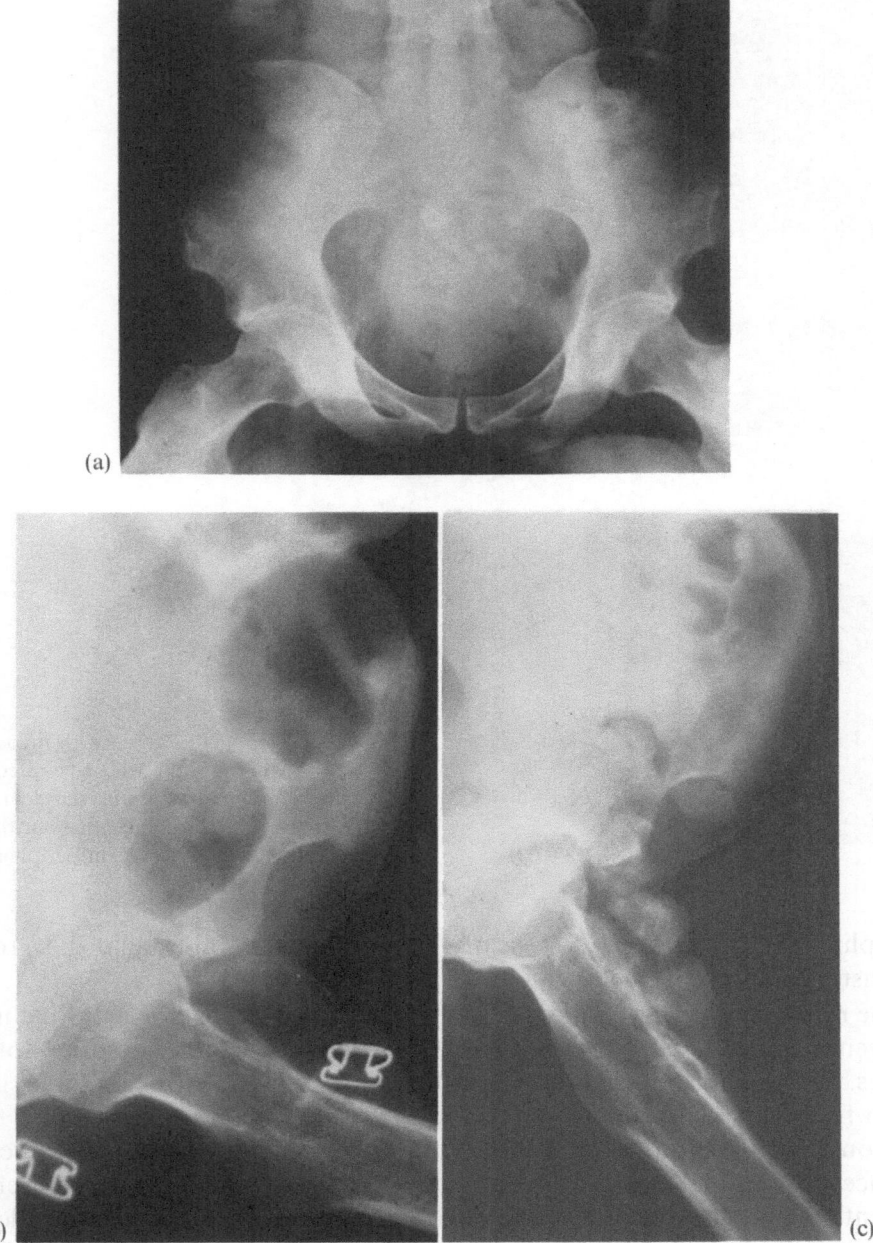

Fig. 63a–c. Roentgenographic progression of myositis ossificans, (a) roentgenogram of patient's pelvis at time he became paraplegic, (b) six months after initial roentgenogram calcific densities are seen adjacent to left hip, (c) 12 months following onset of paraplegia, well-defined osseous lesions are present

soft tissue swelling on early x-ray examinations. The early x-ray findings, like the early pathologic findings, are nonspecific and diagnosis is extremely difficult.

Approximately 1 month after the initial trauma, flocculated calcific densities can be recognized on x-rays, but their appearance can vary from 11 days to 6 weeks. Osteoid can usually be recognized pathologically at 2 weeks (HOUGHSTON et al., 1962). Immobilization apparently delays the deposition of mineral salts. The calcific densities gradually enlarge and coalesce and the centrifugal maturation of the lesion proceeds roentge-

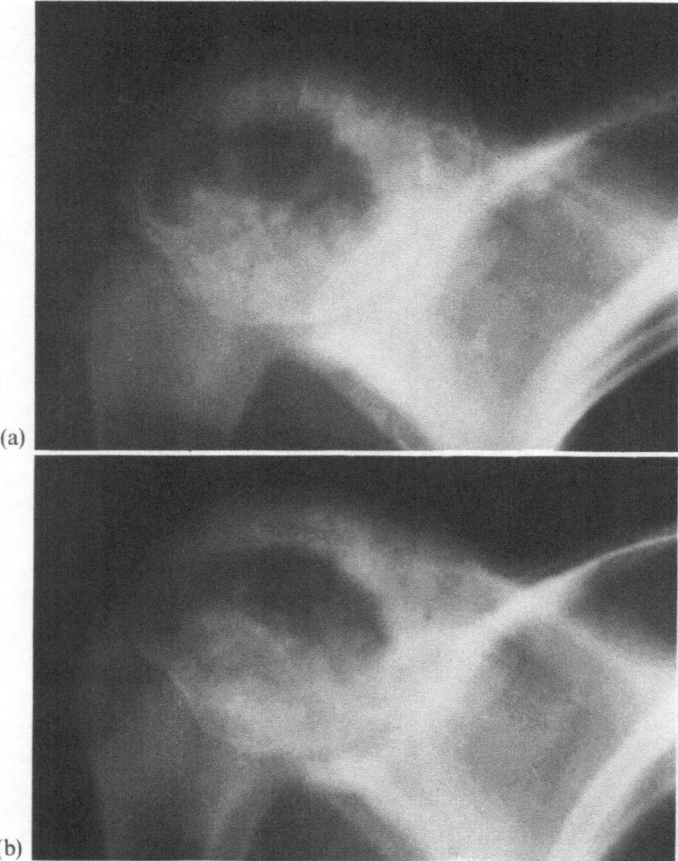

(a)

(b)

Fig. 64. Patient with myositis ossificans circumscripta who presented chief complaint
of hard mass in shoulder. Tomograms revealed calcified mass with greatest density
in periphery

nographically as it does pathologically. The roentgenograms, like the gross specimens,
demonstrate the zonal phenomenon (Fig. 64).

The roentgen differential diagnosis of immature myositis ossificans includes: parosteal
osteogenic sarcoma, extraosseous osteogenic sarcoma, or other calcified soft tissue malignancies. The roentgenographic criteria for differentiation of myositis ossificans circumscripta from sarcomas include: (1) a lucent zone between the lesion and the underlying
bone on multiple projection, (2) the underlying cortex should be intact even in the
presence of periosteal new bone formation, (3) myositis ossificans circumscripta is usually
adjacent to the shaft of the long bone as opposed to a sarcomatous lesion which is
more likely to be metaphyseal in location, (4) in contrast to malignancies the densest
calcification is peripheral and not at the base of the lesion, and (5) after maturation
bone trabeculae can be differentiated from calcification (Figs. 65, 66). Serial x-rays are
also helpful since myositis ossificans will shrink as it matures. Synovial tumors present
a difficult differential problem since one-third of these lesions calcify and they may
arise in the intramuscular spaces at some distance from a joint. The use of angiography
in differentiating immature myositis ossificans circumscripta from malignant lesions has
not been widely investigated. A single study reported in the roentgenologic literature
(HUTCHESON et al., 1972) revealed hypervascularity without A–V shunting, venous lakes,
or amputated vessels. The areas of greatest stain corresponded to the areas of calcification.

When the lesion has matured into trabecular bone, the differential diagnosis becomes
simplified. Mature heterotopic bone has two x-ray appearances. The "dotted veil" or
"feathery" pattern (Fig. 67a), which results from the dissection of a hematoma along

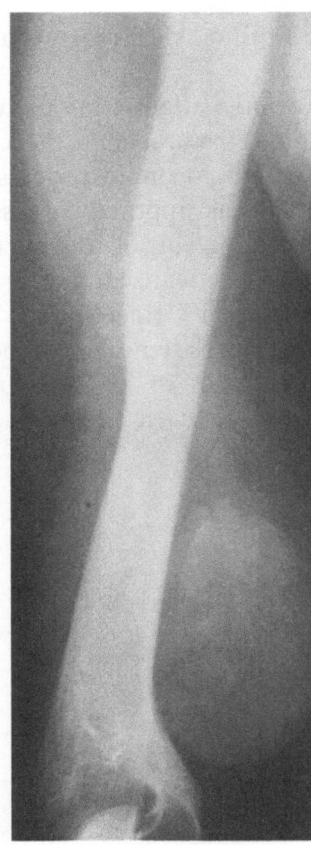

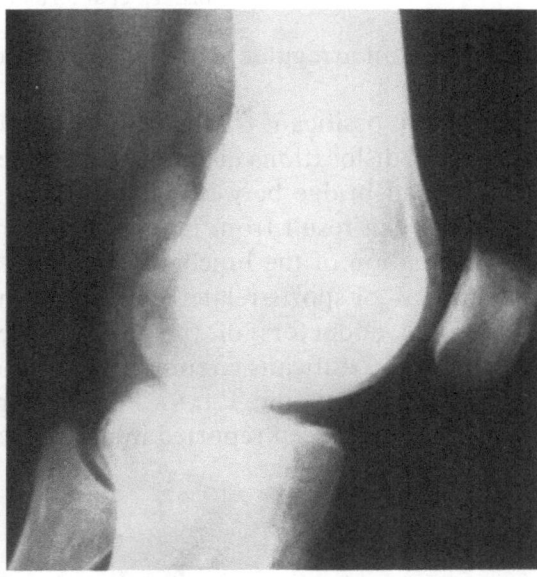

Fig. 66. Parosteal osteogenic sarcoma. There is no lucent zone between lesion and underlying bone in this projection. Greatest density of calcifications is at base of lesion

Fig. 65. This patient's roentgenograms demonstrate several criteria for diagnosis of myositis ossificans: lucent zone between lesion and adjacent bone; normal underlying bone; dense peripheral calcification

Fig. 65

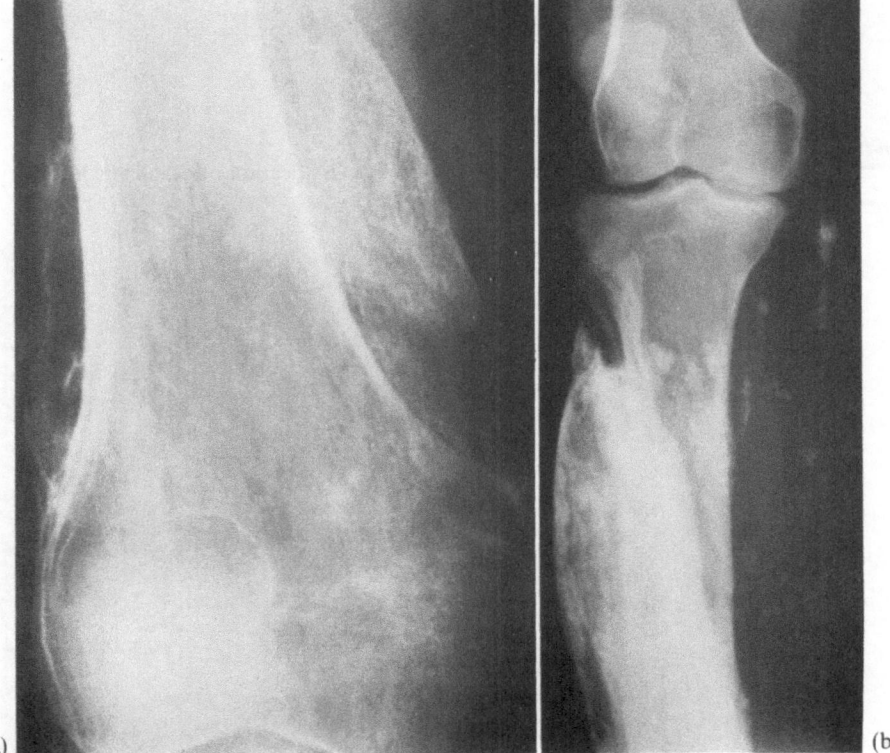

(a)

(b)

Fig. 67a and b. Roentgen appearances of mature myositis ossificans; (a) "dotted veil" pattern, (b) dense mass of bone with its own cortex and medullary space

fascial planes, or an irregular dense mass of bone with a clear cortex and marrow space (Fig. 67 b).

Mature myositis ossificans traumatica does have several distinct x-ray pictures. Radial head fractures and dislocations may result in ossification of the brachialis muscle (Fig. 68), which forms a solid bridge between the humeral shaft and coronoid process. The same roentgen findings can result from repetitive minor trauma as opposed to a single severe insult, e.g., ossification of the brachialis muscle may be the result of fencing or baseball. Other occupational- or sports-related patterns of myositis ossificans circumscripta include ossification of the adductors of the thigh, which is called "rider's bone" (Fig. 69), and isolated myositis ossificans circumscripta of the quadriceps femoris — an occupational hazard in football (Ellis and Frank, 1966) (Fig. 70). Cases of myositis ossificans in the gluteal muscles have been reported in motorcycle riders. Muscle necrosis secondary to

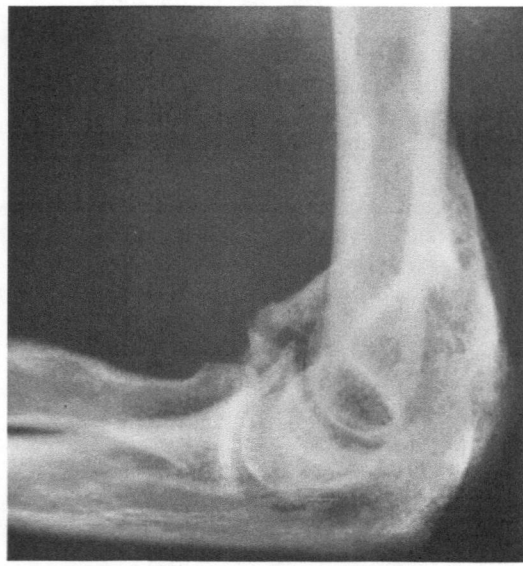

Fig. 68. Ossification of brachialis muscle

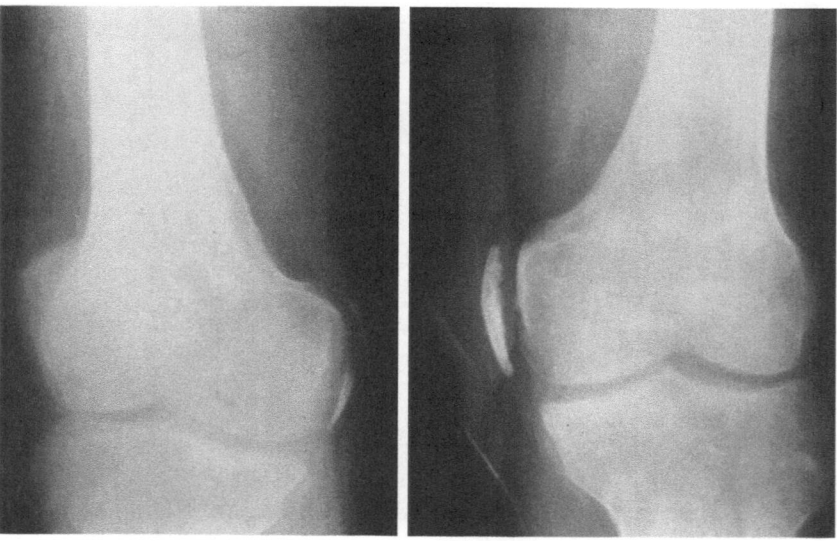

Fig. 69. Ossification of adductor muscles of thigh

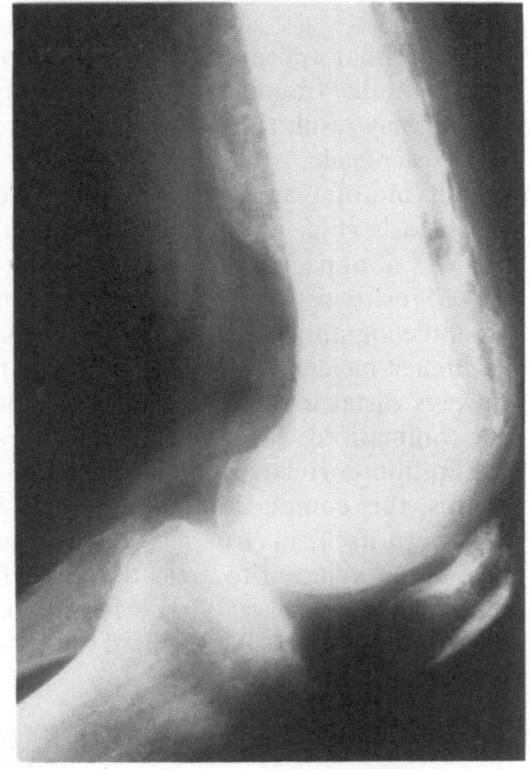

Fig. 70. Ossification of quadriceps femoris

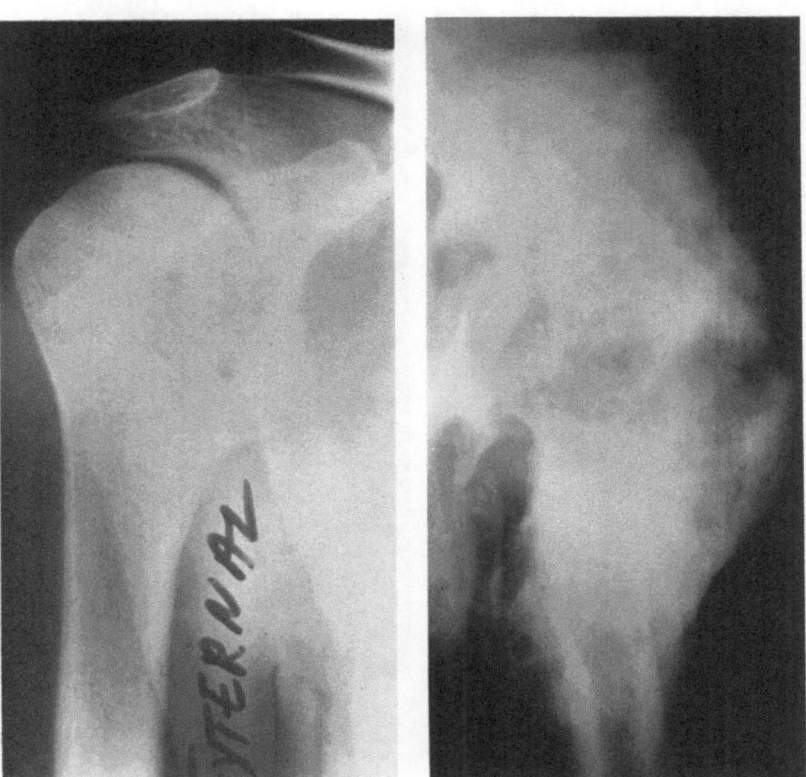

Fig. 71   Fig. 72

Fig. 71. Exostotic lesion resulting from isolated injury to tendon

Fig. 72. Ankylosis of joint produced by ossification of surrounding ligaments

narcotic abuse has also been implicated in the formation of heterotopic bone (DEUTSCH, 1971).

The final appearance of myositis ossificans traumatica is related to the area which was initially traumatized. If the injury was isolated to a single tendon, an exostotic lesion may result (Fig. 71), which must be differentiated from osteochondromas or parosteal osteogenic sarcomas. Ossification of the ligaments surrounding a joint space may result in total ankylosis (Fig. 72). Longstanding myositis ossificans may produce a synostosis (Fig. 73). If the periosteum was originally involved, the late result may be a mass of appositional bone distorting the cortex (Fig. 74).

Myositis ossificans circumscripta associated with systemic diseases also has certain roentgenographic characteristics. Of paraplegics 40–50% have myositis ossificans, with a higher incidence in those whose paralysis resulted from trauma. The ossification is always distal to the cord lesion (CODDINGTON, 1961) and in the areas most likely to be traumatized: the elbows, hips, and shoulders (Figs. 75, 76). Spasticity and soft tissue ulceration correlate with the location of the heterotopic bone. In patients with severe burns, this complication occurs in 2–3% of cases, usually involving the elbows, while the burn itself, may or may not involve the elbows. Hemosiderin deposits and fibrosis are found adjacent to areas of ossification. Therefore, it is felt that trauma is the likely etiology (GRISWOLD, 1963). Myositis ossificans circumscripta is also a rare complication of tetanus (FENNI-PEARSE and OLOWU, 1971; PITTS, 1964). In a series of 160 cases

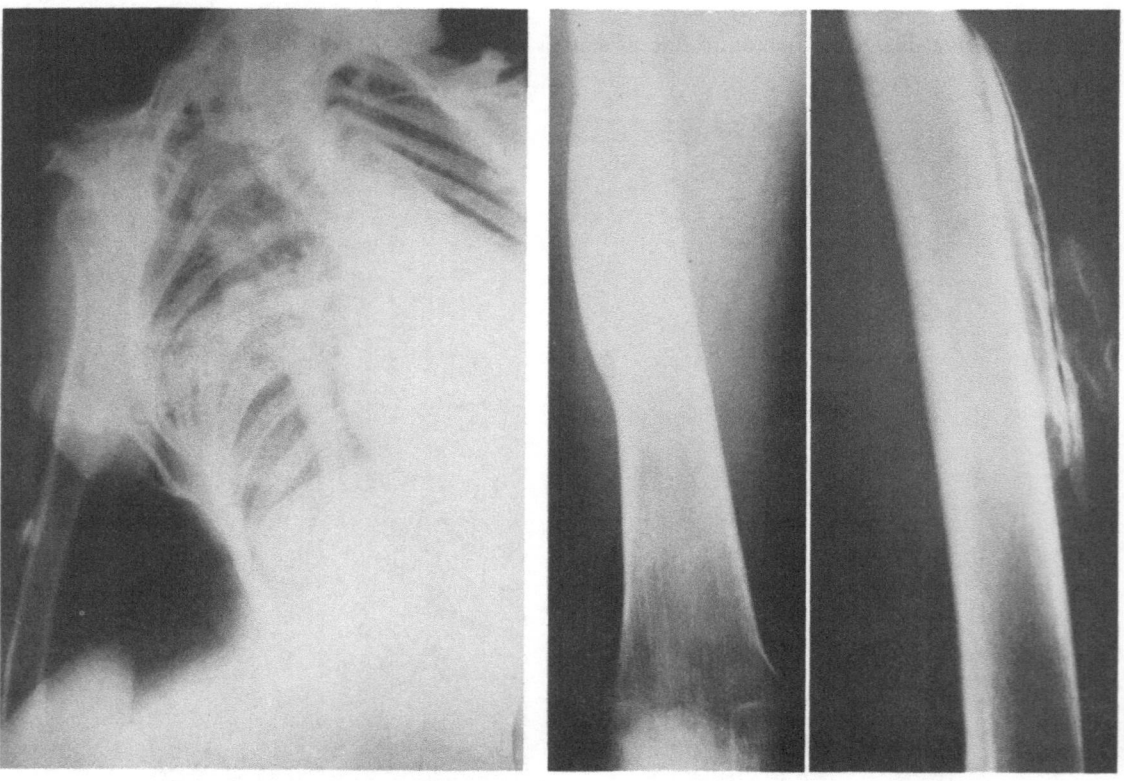

Fig. 73   Fig. 74a   Fig. 74b

Fig. 73. Synostosis of adjacent ribs secondary to myositis ossificans

Fig. 74a and b. Mature myositis ossificans producing appositional mass of bone with resultant distortion of cortex

of tetanus from Africa, two patients developed myositis ossificans circumscripta (FENNI-PEARSE and OLOWU, 1971). Ossification occurs in the extensor muscles secondary to extensor spasm, which dominates the clinical picture. The lesions again correlate with areas of muscle trauma and necrosis.

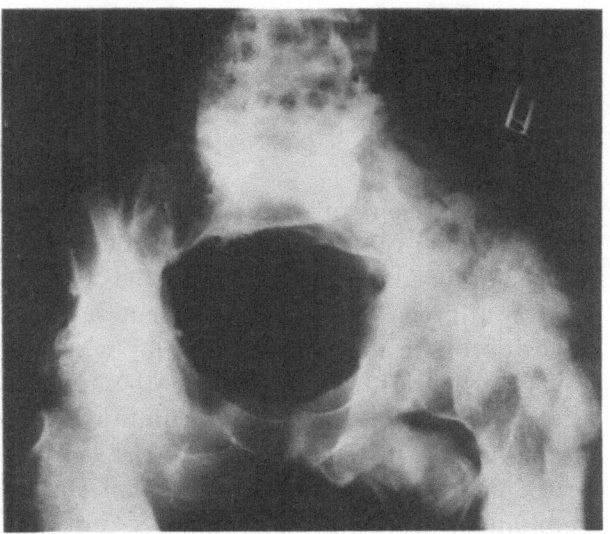

Fig. 75. Pelvis and lumbar spine of paraplegic patient. All areas of myositis ossificans circumscripta are distal to cord lesion

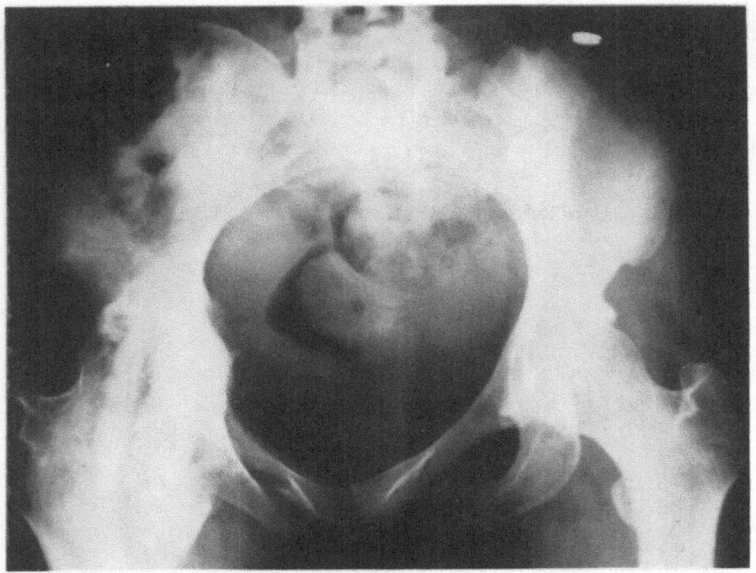

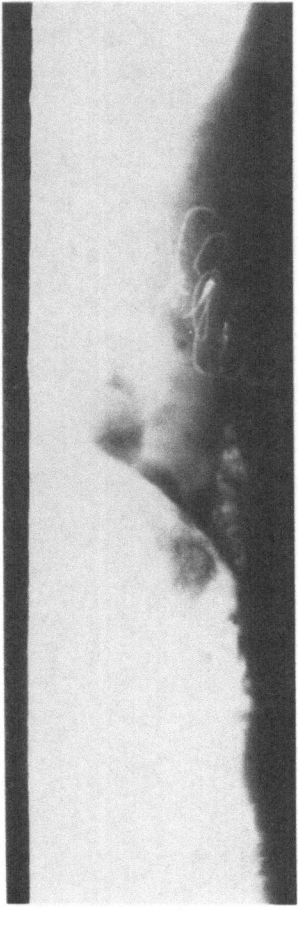

Fig. 76. Patient with multiple sclerosis demonstrating myositis ossificans circumscripta in only one hip—corresponding to paralyzed limb

Fig. 77. Ossification of longitudinal surgical incision of abdomen following bowel surgery. Patient had no history of wound infection

Another form of myositis ossificans circumscripta is the ossification of surgical scars. It usually occurs in adult males with longitudinal incisions that terminate on bony or cartilagenous surfaces (CLASSEN et al., 1960). CLASSEN et al. postulated that longitudinal incisions produce greater disruptive forces. There is no statistical correlation with any primary disease and in recent studies there is apparently no correlation with postoperative infections. The recognition of this entity is important in that it must be differentiated from recurrence of malignant disease at the surgical site (Fig. 77).

6. Treatment

The treatment of myositis ossificans circumscripta is in two stages, depending on the acuteness of the process. Following recognition of the entity, the acute therapy consists of bedrest until the pain has resolved. Massage and/or physiotherapy should not be utilized. The latter treatments actually increase the incidence of post-traumatic myositis ossificans (THOMPSON and GARCIA, 1967; MOHAN, 1972). ELLIS and FRANK (1966) reviewed the value of radiotherapy in reducing the initial inflammatory response. These authors felt that while resolution was more rapid, the results were not sufficiently dramatic to justify the dangers of the radiation exposure.

Of patients with myositis ossificans circumscripta, 12% will have lesions that regress spontaneously. Of the remaining group some will require surgical intervention. The

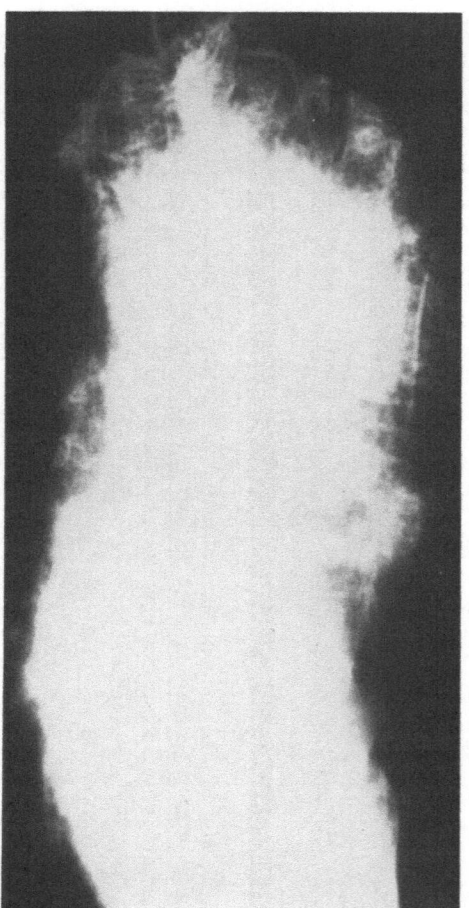

Fig. 78. This patient sustained occupational injury to his foot 20 years prior to admission. Multiple surgical procedures were performed in order to remove osseous tissue which had ankylosed foot. Pathologic specimens were interpreted as myositis ossificans circumscripta. Due to repeated recurrences, final procedure was performed and diagnosis of parosteal osteogenic sarcoma was based on amputation specimen. It would be difficult to determine if this case represents malignant degeneration of benign lesion or extremely well-differentiated low-grade malignancy

criteria for surgery include: restriction of joint motion, a pointed end producing pain, or a large mass of heterotopic bone which may predispose to further injury. Definitive therapy should be postponed for 6–12 months because surgery performed prior to complete maturation of the lesion will frequently result in recurrence. There is a possibility of recurrence even after an adequate interval has elapsed prior to excision. Bone scanning has been attempted as a means of evaluating the activity of the lesion prior to surgery (GOLDMAN and BRAUNSTEIN, 1975). However, the results obtained at our institution have not been consistent. Radionuclide uptake studies, such as those which have been used in the evaluation of the activity of pagetic lesions of bone, may provide a more sensitive indication of the decreasing osteoblastic activity (GOLDMAN and BRAUNSTEIN, 1975). Pharmaceutical agents such as Na EDPA have been used in conjunction with surgery to prevent recurrences (LIBERMAN et al., 1967).

The potential danger of malignant degeneration of myositis ossificans circumscripta had led some authors to advocate the surgical removal of all areas of heterotopic bone. This opinion is based on series of 12 cases reported by FINE and STOUT (1956), and one case published by SHANOFF et al. (1967). However, the true incidence of malignant degeneration is extremely difficult to evaluate since myositis ossificans circumscripta can mimic a sarcoma clinically, radiologically, and pathologically (SPJUT et al., 1970). Figure 78 demonstrates a case, where even in retrospect, the differentiation between a slow growing malignancy and the transformation of a benign lesion into a malignant one cannot be determined.

II. Myositis Ossificans Progressiva

1. Other Terms

Other terms used in the literature for this entity are: Munchmeyer disease, fibrositis ossificans progressiva.

2. Etiology

Myositis ossificans progressiva is a mesodermal disorder which is characterized by progressive ossification of striated muscle, tendons, ligaments, and fasciae. It is a rare disease, with only 280 documented cases in the literature (LUDWAK, 1964). The diagnosis can be made by roentgenographic studies.

Historically, this syndrome was first described in 1692 by PATIN who reported a case of a young woman, who in his words "turned to wood." However, it was MUNCH-MEYER (1971) who published the first series of 12 cases of this disease.

Myositis ossificans progressiva is classified as a hereditary disorder on the basis of two pieces of evidence. First, there have been two sets of homozygous twins with the disorder (LETTS, 1969). Second, there is a high association of congenital digital abnormalities. Of the cases, 75% have bilateral microdactyly of the first toe with absence of the distal phalanx and synostosis of the remaining phalanges, as well as 5% of their families (Fig. 79). Other associated congenital abnormalities include: microdactyly of the thumbs, hallux valgus, broad femoral necks, abnormal teeth, hypogonadism, and absence of the ear lobes. The etiology of myositis ossificans progressiva is unknown. Blood chemistries, serum alkaline phosphatase, renal function, and parathormone levels are all within normal limits (LUDWAK, 1964). Calcium kinetic studies, using radioactive

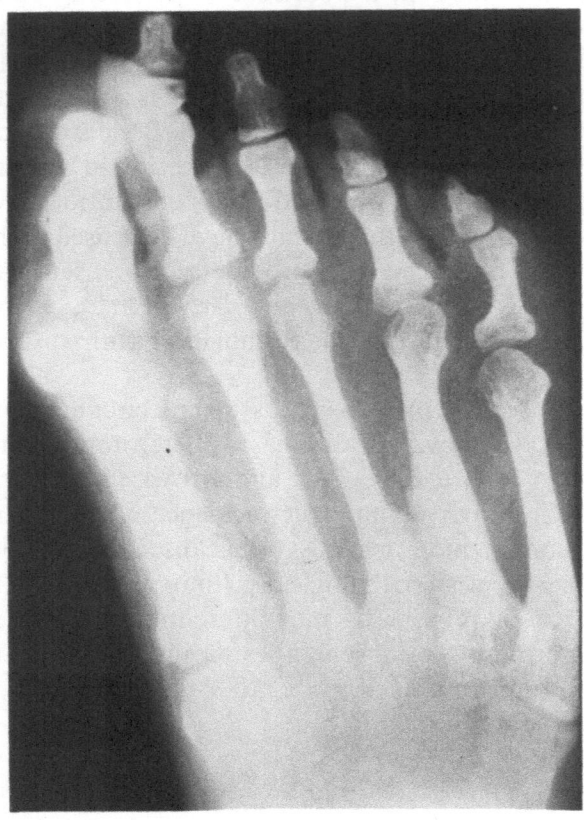

Fig. 79. Roentgenogram of patient with myositis ossificans progressiva demonstrating microdactyly of first digit of foot with synostosis of phalanges and hallux valgus deformity

calcium, indicate only an expected increase in the rates of bone deposition and reabsorption, with a disproportionate increase in deposition (LUDWAK, 1964). The prevailing theory supported by McKUSICK (1960) is that the disease primarily affects the interstitial tissues and that muscle damage is secondary to pressure atrophy. The abnormal deposition of calcium salts has been attributed to either the absence of a circulating inhibitor, or a primary defect in the collagen fiber itself. The localized increase in the alkaline phosphatase supports this concept. However, more recently, electromyelogram studies on the unossified muscles of these patients revealed abnormalities consistent with a myopathy, and histochemical examination shows variability in muscle fiber size and a decreased ATPase activity predating ossification (SMITH et al., 1966; FLETCHER and Moss, 1965). Thus, the location of the metabolic error is still unknown.

3. Clinical

Clinically there is no sex prevalence. In 98% of the cases, the onset of symptoms is in the first two decades of life. The presenting symptom is usually torticollis and or a painful mass within the sternocleidomastoid muscle. The disease usually progresses from the shoulder girdle, to the upper arms, spine, and then the pelvis (Fig. 80). The heart, diaphragm, larynx, tongue, and sphincters are spared as are all smooth muscle structures. The course of the disease is one of remissions and exacerbations. An exacerbation may be precipitated by trauma. As an area becomes involved, the first symptoms are of heat, edema, and a painful mass. The pain gradually decreases and the mass

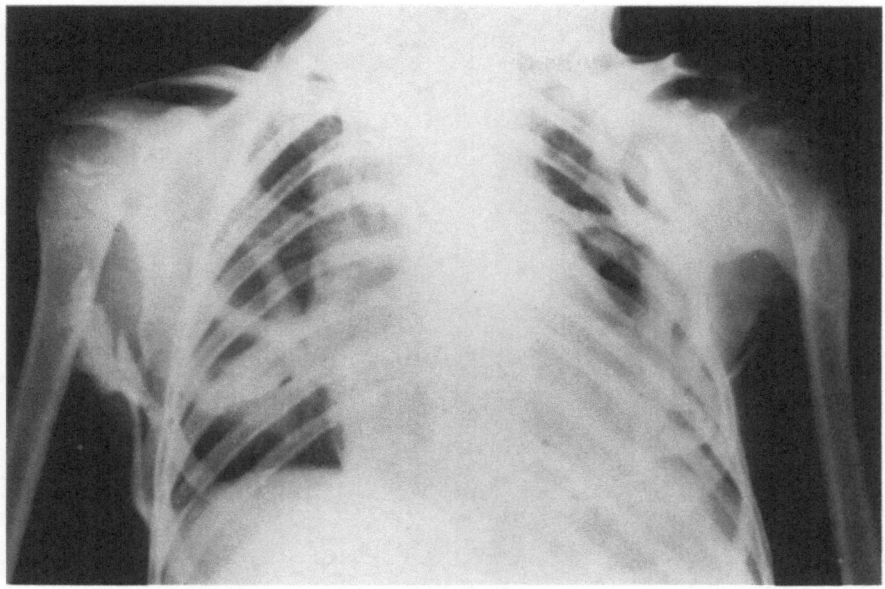

Fig. 80. Myositis ossificans progressiva involving central skeleton

gradually hardens as bone formation takes place. Joint ankylosis and conductive hearing loss are complications. Death is inevitable and may be secondary to respiratory disease due to constriction of the chest wall or it may result from starvation after ossification of the masseter muscles.

4. Pathology

Pathologically, the individual lesions are identical to myositis ossificans circumscripta, with the same progression from inflammatory exudate, to dystrophic calcification, and finally to heterotopic bone formation.

5. Roentgen Appearance

Digital abnormalities are present at birth. The commonest anomaly (75%) is bilateral microdactyly of the first toes with synostosis of the remaining phalanges. There is a high association of hallux valgus deformities. On occasion, the entire first digit is absent, and 30–50% of subjects have similar findings in the thumbs.

After the onset of symptoms, the roentgen findings in the individual locations are identical to those of the circumscripta form of myositis ossificans, with progression from soft tissue swelling to dystrophic calcification which extends centrifugally, and finally to ossification. The neck and shoulders are usually the first areas to ossify and the disease then progresses to the remainder of the spine, pelvis, and limbs.

The neural arches of the spine are usually the first to fuse (Fig. 81). The sesamoid bones of the hands and feet frequently become fused and resemble small exostoses.

The roentgen differential diagnosis includes the gamut of metastatic calcifications, e.g., calcinosis universalis, dermatomyositis, calcium metabolic disorders. However, in all these conditions the densities remain calcific and do not proceed to the roentgenographic appearance of mature bone.

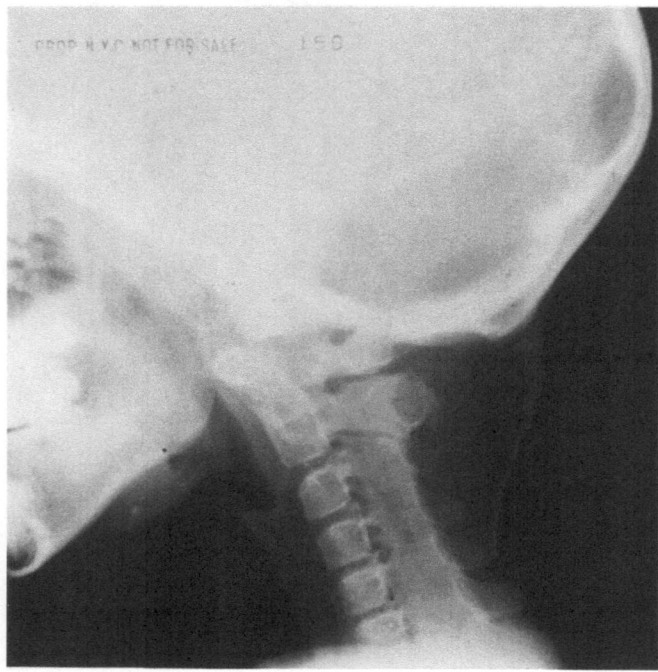

Fig. 81. Spinal fusion in myositis ossificans progressiva with fusion of neural arches

6. Treatment

The success of therapeutic agents has been difficult to evaluate since the disease frequently has temporary spontaneous remissions. Steroids have been used in an attempt to reduce the inflammatory response. The current treatment of choice is disodium etidronate, which inhibits the rate of turnover of hydroxyapatite crystals both by decreasing the rate of production and retardation of the absorption of pre-existing crystals. This agent is used most effectively in conjunction with surgery to prevent recurrences (RUSSELL et al., 1972; KAMMERMAN, 1975).

H. Brown Tumors of Hyperparathyroidism

I. Introduction

Other terms that have been used in the literature for this entity are: osteoclastoma and osteitis fibrosa cystica generalisata of von Recklinghausen. "Osteitis fibrosa cystica generalisata of von Recklinghausen," is applied to the bone changes which result from hypersecretion of parathormone. The word "osteitis" is actually misleading since this disorder is not the end result of an inflammatory process. The term "fibrosa" refers to the marked increase of the supporting cells within the bone marrow which characterizes this disease, and "generalisata" indicates that the process is a metabolic one (ALBRIGHT and REIFENSTEIN, 1948). The bone changes of hyperparathyroidism are characterized by a generalized decalcification of the osseous structures with superimposed cysts and tumors (ALBRIGHT and REIFENSTEIN, 1948).

II. History

The history of hyperparathyroidism has been reviewed in several publications (COPE, 1966; ROWLANDS, 1972). The relationship between the parathyroid glands and bone physiology was identified in 1880 by SANDSTROM. In 1891, VON RECKLINGHAUSEN, a pathologist at Strasbourg, described a bone disease which now bears his name. He postulated that this demineralizing disease, which he called osteitis fibrosa cystica, was the result of a primary bone abnormality, possibly related to osteomalacia. The publication in which his description appeared was dedicated to the 71st birthday of Rudolf Virchow.

In 1903, ASKANAZY, a pathologist at Tübingen, described a patient with both a parathyroid tumor and von Recklinghausen demineralizing bone disease. However, when ERDHEIM (1907), a leading pathologist in Vienna, became aware of the coexistence of these two entities, he incorrectly postulated that the changes in the endocrine system were a secondary result of the disordered bone metabolism. The theory that osteitis fibrosa cystica was a primary bone disease persisted until 1926. At that time, another Viennese pathologist, MANDL (1926), devised an experiment to substantiate ERDHEIM's (1907) premise that the changes in the parathyroid glands were a secondary phenomenon in von Recklinghausen disease. He transplanted parathyroid glands into a patient with demineralizing bone disease, expecting to see no change in the patient's status but hyperplasia of the glandular tissue. Instead, the patient's condition was severely exacerbated. During the process of removing the transplanted glands he, serendipitously, found a parathyroid tumor. Once the tumor was removed the patient's bone disease remitted. The same year COLLIP (1925) in Alberta and AUB et al. (1925) in Massachusetts successfully isolated parathormone. Early animal experiments performed with this hormone indicated that it produced an elevation in the serum calcium, a reduction in the serum phosphorus level, and an increase in the urinary calcium excretion. The first clinical application of parathormone was in the treatment of lead poisoning. This group of patients demonstrated identical changes in the serum and urinary electrolytes to those described in experimental animals.

The evidence which confirmed that parathyroid disease was the etiology of osteitis fibrosa cystica can be attributed to the perseverance of a sea captain named Charles Martell. In 1928, he presented to Dr. Du Bois of Bellevue hospital, with a chief complaint of loss of stature. His height had decreased from 6 feet to 5 feet 6 inches, and he had noted limb deformities, protrusion of the jaw, as well as multiple fractures resulting from trivial injuries. Further examination revealed that he had a diffuse bone disease accompanied by abnormal serum electrolytes which resembled those of AUB et al.'s (1925) patients who were being treated with parathormone. With a presumptive diagnosis of abnormally increased parathyroid function, he was transferred to the Massachusetts General Hospital. After seven exploratory procedures, the parathyroid adenoma was found in his anterior mediastinum. Unfortunately, Capt. Martell died 6 weeks after the surgery as a result of tetany.

The combined experience of AUB et al. (1925) in America and MANDL (1926) in Europe led to the identification of an increasing number of patients with hyperparathyroidism. COPE (1966) and CASTLEMAN and MALLORY (1935) at Harvard, performed 30 postmortem dissections to determine the normal anatomy of the parathyroid glands. These authors found that the parathyroids could be located in the entire area where these glands can be found in embryonic development, extending from the upper neck to the mediastinum.

ALBRIGHT and REIFENSTEIN (1948) were responsible for the recognition of the importance of renal disease in patients with hyperparathyroidism. Of their cases, 80% with osseous disease had coexisting renal calculi. Later, they reviewed the records of patients with renal calculi at the Massachusetts General Hospital and found several undiagnosed cases of parathyroid pathology. They concluded that osseous changes were not invariably present in this disorder.

Incidence. Primary hyperparathyroidism is twice as common in females (Aegeter and Kirkpatrick, 1968), and is most frequently the result of a solitary adenoma (Aegeter and Kirkpatrick, 1968). In recent clinical studies of primary hyperparathyroidism, approximately 30% of cases presented with osseous disease (Steinbach et al., 1961, Edeiken and Hodes, 1973). Earlier studies reported the incidence of bone disease to be higher, with figures of 70% to 90% (Pugh, 1958; Albright and Reifenstein, 1948). This change in the incidence of osseous findings may be the result of earlier diagnosis.

III. Etiology

The location of the four parathyroid glands is extremely variable due to their embryonic origin. The upper pair of glands arise in relation to the thyroid gland. If one of this set becomes abnormally heavy it may be pushed down by swallowing or pulled down by the negative pressure of the chest, into the posterior mediastinum, close to the esophagus (Cope, 1966). The lower two glands arise within the thymus and migrate downward. They descend so far that they may rest in the anterior mediastinum instead of the neck. This variability in location frequently creates a problem in the surgical therapy of hyperparathyroidism.

Parathormone is secreted by the chief cells of the parathyroid glands. The hormone has two separate and independent effects, (1) the regulation of phosphate homeostasis by increasing the inhibition of phosphorus reabsorption in the distal convoluted tubules of the kidneys, and (2) regulation of the serum calcium level by mobilization of mineral from bone by directly stimulating osteoclasts (McLean and Urist, 1955; Steinbach et al., 1961). In hyperparathyroidism these two normal effects are intensified.

Hyperparathyroidism affects the entire skeleton. The earliest and severest lesions appear at sites of bone production and remodeling, e.g., in children the metaphysis is the area which is affected first. In both adults and children early lesions appear along the periosteal surfaces of the cortex, especially at tendon and ligament attachments. The latter areas are again sites of high bone turnover. Sites of injury and mechanical pressure also have high osteoclastic activity with coexisting osteoblastic repair. Thus, traumatized bone is more sensitive to the parathormone effect (Steinbach et al., 1961). This phenomenon may be responsible for patients with hyperparathyroidism who present with brown tumors before the onset of roentgenographically detectable subperiosteal reabsorption. Dent (1975) has seen two patients in whom brown tumors of hyperparathyroidism appeared at sites of previously documented trauma.

1. Primary Hyperparathyroidism

Overproduction of parathormone is most frequently due to a solitary adenoma (Table 4). In 1935 Castleman and Mallory indentified multiple adenomas in 2 of 19 patients with primary hyperparathyroidism. The phenomenon of multiple adenomas has also been noted in subsequent large clinical studies (Black, 1953; Cope, 1966; and Wolner et al., 1952). Aegerter and Kirkpatrick (1968) theorize that the parathyroid adenoma consists of increased number of functioning cells, which mature and

Table 4. Causes of primary hyperparathyroidism

	BLACK (1953) (112 cases)	COPE (1966) (343 cases)	WOOLNER[a] et al. (1952) (140 cases)
Single adenoma	92	263	115
Multiple adenomas	10	13	6
Hyperplasia	9	53	12
Carcinoma	1	15	2

[a] Five cases had multiple endocrine abnormalities

secrete like normal cells but fail to respond to either stimulation or depression. The reason for the loss of control is not known. The parathyroid glands are independent of other ductless glands and normally respond to a low serum calcium (MCLEAN, 1958; AEGERTER and KIRKPATRICK, 1968).

A less frequent cause of primary hyperparathyroidism is diffuse hyperplasia of all of the parathyroid glands (Table 4). There are two cellular types of hyperplasia. The commoner entity is clear cell hyperplasia (COPE, 1966). The appearance of each gland is identical to a solitary adenoma. Recognition of the diffuse nature of the hyperplasia depends on careful surgical exploration with identification of all four glands (COPE, 1966). Chief cell hyperplasia is a rarer form but easier to identify surgically since the glands appear dark brown with pseudopod extensions (COPE, 1966).

True tumors of the parathyroid glands are rare and usually don't function. On occasion, a carcinoma may produce primary hyperparathyroidism (Table 4).

2. Secondary Hyperparathyroidism

The excessive secretory activity which characterizes this syndrome, is the result of prolonged stimulation of the parathyroid glands by continuously low serum calcium. The skeletal changes occur only in long standing disease and are identical to those described in primary hyperparathyroidism.

IV. Clinical

Primary hyperparathyroidism occurs most frequently in the third, fourth, and fifth decades of life. The ratio of females to males has been reported as 2:2 (AEGERTER and KIRKPATRICK, 1968) or 3:1 (TSENG and NATHAN, 1960).

Serum electrolyte abnormalities consist of a calcium exceeding 12 mg/100 ml. Hypoproteinemia may produce a falsely low serum calcium due to a decrease in the protein bound fraction. Cases of normocalcemic hyperparathyroidism have been reported but usually present with renal disease. Rare cases of osteitis fibrosa cystica generalisata, in the presence of a normal serum calcium, have appeared in the literature (HEATH and WILLS, 1971; WATSON, 1973; FRAME et al., 1970). Localized lytic lesions, especially when they are isolated to the jaw, may present in the absence of abnormal chemistries (WATSON, 1973). The increase in serum alkaline phosphatase in patients with hyperparathyroidism is due to reparative attempts by the osteoblasts.

Hyperparathyroidism is characterized by three sets of symptoms. The calcium ion normally acts as an insulator to nerve impulses and symptoms referable to the motor system may result from a high serum calcium. This group of symptoms includes lethargy, loss of muscle tone, anorexia, and constipation. Psychic disturbances may also be due to the action of the calcium ion. The second group of clinical problems results from the ectopic deposition of calcium salts, in the soft tissues, cartilage, and within the urinary system. Third, the decrease in bone mineralization leads to symptoms referable to the osseous system. Approximately 50% of patients with hyperparathyroidism complain of bone pain (Edeiken and Hodes, 1973) with 30% of cases having roentgenographically detectable lesions (Edeiken and Hodes, 1973; Steinbach et al., 1961). Albright and Reifenstein (1948) characterized the early complaints as "bone tenderness" which was frequently mistaken for an arthritic process. The decreased mineralization of the skeleton produces abnormal stress and is responsible for the pain (Aegerter and Kirkpatrick, 1968). Steinbach et al. (1961) stress that fractures which result from minor injuries may be the earliest manifestation of osteitis fibrosa cystica generalisata, as opposed to pain or tenderness. Limb deformities occur with more advanced disease and result from both fractures and local areas of expansion (Steinbach et al., 1961). Rarely a patient may present with only an expansile lesion which had deformed the jaw or other bone (Watson, 1973).

Urinary tract disease is statistically the commonest presentation of primary hyperparathyroidism (Cope, 1966; Hellstrom, 1957). Dietary variation may explain why some patients fail to exhibit roentgen changes referable to the osseous system. A high calcium diet may prevent the progression of bone lesions.

V. Pathology

The name osteitis fibrosa cystica generalisata is applied to the severe osseous changes of hyperparathyroidism. There is a generalized replacement of normal bone by proliferating fibroblasts. The high osteoclastic activity which characterizes hyperparathyroidism produces reparative fibrosis accompanied by poorly calcified new bone (Steinbach et al., 1961) (Fig. 82). In addition, the extravasation of blood which results from multiple infractions also leads to a fibrotic response within the marrow (Aegerter and Kirkpatrick, 1968). Other histologic findings are: increased lacunar absorption of bone (Anderson, 1966), bone reabsorption along the surfaces of finer structures (Steinbach et al., 1961), aggregates of giant cells in the areas of hemorrhage, lamellation of new bone over old which produces a mosaic pattern resembling Paget's disease, wide seams of recently formed osteoid (Aegerter and Kirkpatrick, 1968), and fluid collections in the marrow spaces which may be generalized or well-defined cysts (Edeiken and Hodes, 1973).

Brown tumors are localized collections of fibrous tissue and cells which occur secondary to necrosis and liquifaction. Hunter and Turnbull, in 1931, designated them as "osteoclastomata" but the increase in the number of osteoblasts is equally dramatic (Camp, 1932; Albright and Reifenstein, 1948). Sections through brown tumors reveal a matrix of proliferation fibroblasts along with a large number of giant cells (Aegerter and Kirkpatrick, 1968). Large areas of hemorrhage and hemosiderin deposits are also found within these lesions. The differentiation of giant cell tumors from the brown tumor of hyperparathyroidism may be extremely difficult on the basis of the pathologic specimens. Theoretically, the stromal nuclei of giant cell tumors are younger and less uniform than those of the brown tumor. In addition, the nuclei in the giant cells of the primary giant cell tumor are less likely to be arranged peripherally and are fewer in number.

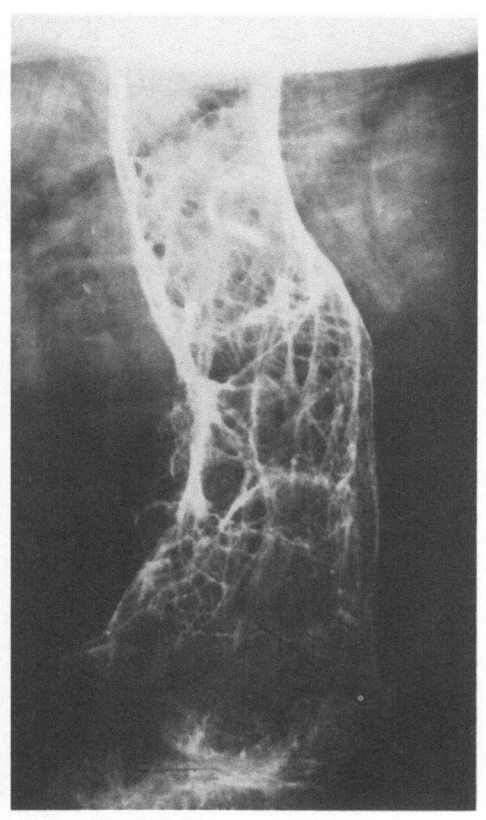

Fig. 82. Advance changes of osteitis fibrosa cystica genera-lisata. Roentgen changes of decreased density, coarsened trabeculae, and softening due to replacement of bone by fibrous tissue, reflect the pathologic changes of hyperparathyroidism

VI. Roentgen Findings

The serum calcium and phosphorus levels of patients with hyperparathyroidism do not correlate with the severity of bone reabsorption. However, the elevation of the serum alkaline phosphatase does indicate an increase in osteoblastic activity and does correlate with the presence of osseous findings and with their severity (STEINBACH et al., 1961; EDEIKEN and HODES, 1973). Alkaline phosphatase levels averaged about 5.4 Bo-dansky units in patients without bone changes on roentgenograms, while this value rose to an average level of 23.1 Bodansky units in patients with positive bone x-rays (EDEIKEN and HODES, 1973; STEINBACH et al., 1961). The weight of the parathyroid adenoma is also proportional to the osseous roentgen changes. Patients with roentgen evidence of osteitis fibrosa cystica generalisata had tumors that were five times heavier than those with normal studies (STEINBACH et al., 1961; HELLSTROM, 1957).

In most patients with brown tumors, subperiosteal reabsorption is present at the time the lytic lesion is diagnosed (CAMP, 1932; PUGH, 1958). In STEINBACH et al's (1961) series, the 11 subjects with brown tumors all had subperiosteal reabsorption, although diffuse demineralization was not invariably present. However, there are documented cases in which the single lytic lesion was the first and only roentgen finding of hyperpara-thyroidism (EDEIKEN and HODES, 1973). The variability of roentgen findings at the time of diagnosis may be due to diet, and/or the temporal progression of the disease process (DENT, 1975). Those patients with an acute onset are diagnosed quickly and the bone changes reflect the rapid mobilization of bone. However, longstanding mild disease predisposes to the formation of localized lytic lesions at the sites of high osteoblastic activity (DENT, 1975).

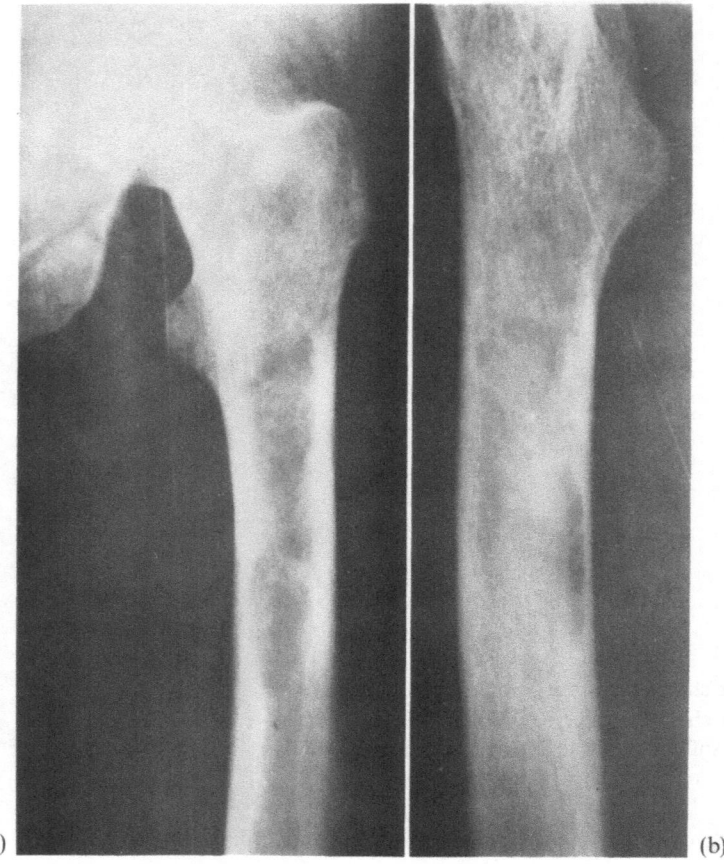

Fig. 83. (a) Multiple lytic lesions in medullary portion of femur of middle-aged female proved to be brown tumors, (b) after therapy, brown tumors of hyperparathyroidism are replaced by areas of sclerotic bone

Brown tumors appear roentgenographically as localized areas of destruction (Fig. 83a, b). They have the density of soft tissue and frequently have indistinct margins (AEGERTER and KIRKPATRICK, 1968). The lesions may be multilocular or small and cystic. Larger lesions are usually expansile (STEINBACH et al., 1961) (Fig. 84), and may produce periosteal new bone formation (AEGERTER and KIRKPATRICK, 1968).

The commonest location of brown tumors is in the metaphysis of long bones (AEGERTER and KIRKPATRICK, 1968; TSENG and NATHAN, 1960; CAMP, 1932), especially at sites of rapid bone turnover: the medullary portion (Fig. 83) or below the periosteum (Fig. 85) (CAMP, 1932). The roentgen appearance, like the pathologic findings, closely resembles a primary giant cell tumor (Fig. 86). However, a subperiosteal or eccentric location may suggest the correct diagnosis (ALBRIGHT and REIFENSTEIN, 1948; EDEIKEN and HODES, 1973; STEINBACH et al., 1961). Another differential point may be the presence of other changes of hyperparathyroidism: granular osteoporosis (ELLIS and HOCHSTIM, 1960), subperiosteal reabsorption (CAMP, 1932; PUGH, 1958), ectopic calcium deposition in soft tissues or cartilage (LLOYD, 1971; WANG et al., 1969), and periosteal new bone formation (MEEMA et al., 1974).

The roentgen differential diagnosis between giant cell tumors and the brown tumor is simplified if the lesion occurs in the mandible (STEINBACH et al., 1961; HELLSTROM, 1957), facial bones (STEINBACH et al., 1961; CAMP, 1932), or within the small bones of the hands and feet (SPJUT et al., 1971). In these locations the presence of a lytic

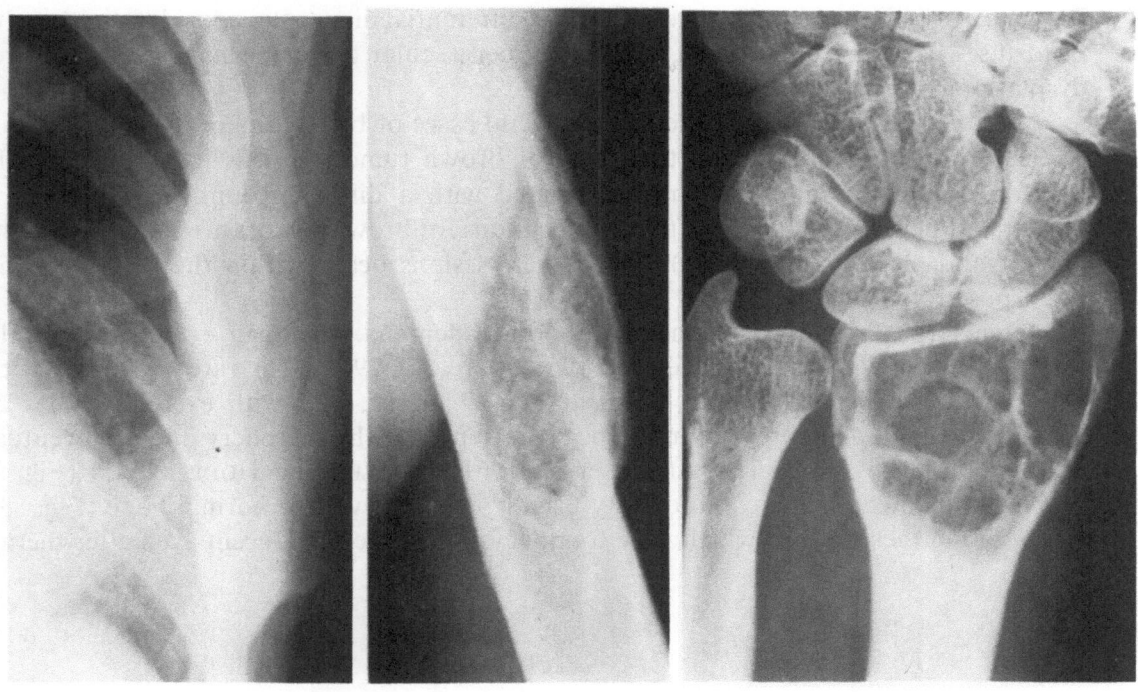

Fig. 84   Fig. 85   Fig. 86

Fig. 84. Expansile lytic lesion in rib which was proven by biopsy to be brown tumor

Fig. 85. Eccentric expansile lytic lesion in humerus of patient with advanced hyperparathyroidism

Fig. 86. Classic roentgen appearance of giant cell tumor, located in distal epiphysis of radius

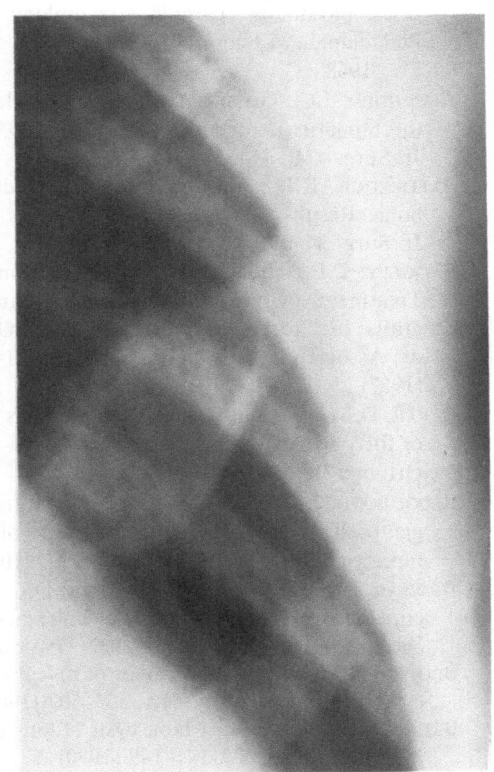

Fig. 87. Healing brown tumor of rib with sclerosis beginning in periphery of lesion

(Films courtesy of Dr. J. Zausner)

lesion resembling a giant cell tumor should suggest the possibility of a diagnosis of brown tumor of hyperparathyroidism. Other differential diagnostic considerations include metastases from thyroid, kidney, or other hypervascular tumors, plasmacytoma, fibrous dysplasia, and aneurysmal bone cyst.

Ellis and Hochstim (1960) reviewed several cases of brown tumors in the calvarium. The latter authors emphasized the rarity of brown tumors in this location, and when they do occur, they are frequently associated with a diffuse ground glass appearance or granular densities. Other less frequent locations for brown tumors are the ribs, vertebral bodies, and pelvis (Camp, 1932). When these lesions occur within the spine they may predispose to vertebral collapse.

After surgical removal of the parathyroid adenoma, roentgen evidence of healing can be appreciated within 4–6 weeks (Steinbach et al., 1961). The rate of reconstruction varies with the dietary calcium, with vitamin D intake, and with exercise (Ellis and Hochstim, 1960). The brown tumors begin to repair at the periphery and are eventually filled in with dense bone (Steinbach et al., 1961; Edeiken and Hodes, 1973) (Fig. 87). The resulting areas of increased density usually do not revert to normal bone (Fig. 83 b). Areas within these lesions which were totally cystic may remain lucent even after therapy.

References

The Solitary Bone Cyst

Adams, A.W.: Report of a case of solitary fibrocystic disease of the humerus exhibiting spontaneous resolution. Brit. J. Surg. 13, 734–741 (1926)

Aegerter, E., Kirkpatrick, J.A.: Orthopedic diseases, physiology, pathology, radiology, 3rd. ed. Philadelphia, London, Toronto: W.B. Saunders Co., 1968

Agerholm, J.C., Goodfellow, J.W.: Simple cysts of the humerus treated by radical excision. J. Bone Jt. Surg. 47 B, 714–717 (1965)

Alldredge, R.H.: Localized fibrocystic disease of bone. Results of treatment in 152 cases. J. Bone Jt. Surg. 24, 795–804 (1942)

Badgley, C.E.: Unicameral cysts of the long bones. Treatment by crushing cystic walls and onlay grafts. In: Proceedings of the American Orthopaedic Association. J. Bone Jt. Surg. 39 A, 1429–1430 (1957)

Baker, D.M.: Benign unicameral bone cysts. A study of forty-five cases with long term follow-up. Clin. Orthop. 71, 140–151 (1970)

Bloodgood, J.C.: Benign bone cysts, osteitis fibrosa, giant cell sarcoma, and bone aneurysms of the long pipe bones. Ann. Surg. 52, 145–185 (1910)

Boseker, E.H., Bickel, W.H., Dahlin, D.C.: A clinicopathologic study of simple unicameral bone cysts. Surg. Gynec. Obstet. 127, 550–560 (1968)

Broder, H.M.: Possible precursor of unicameral bone cysts. J. Bone Jt. Surg. 50 A, 503–507 (1968)

Brunschwig, A.: Solitary bone cysts of long duration. J. Bone Jt. Surg. 12, 141–149 (1930)

Cohen, J.: Simple bone cysts, studies of cyst fluid in 6 cases with a theory of pathogenesis. J. Bone Jt. Surg. 42 A, 609–616 (1960)

Cohen, J.: Etiology of simple bone cysts. J. Bone Jt. Surg. 52 A, 1493–1497 (1970)

Coley, B.L., Higinbotham, N.L.: Solitary bone cysts. Ann. Surg. 99, 432–448 (1934)

Copleman, B., Vidoli, M.F., Crimmings, F.J.: Solitary bone cyst of the calcaneus. Radiology 47, 142–148 (1946)

Dahlin, D.C.: Bone tumors, 2nd ed. Springfield, Ill., Charles C. Thomas, 1967

Edeiken, J., Hodes, P.J.: Roentgen diagnosis of diseases of bone, 2nd ed. Baltimore: Williams and Wilkins, 1973

Ehrlich, M.G., Chaglassian, J.H.: Unicameral bone cyst in the scapula. Clin. Orthop. 103, 80–81 (1974)

Elmslie, R.C.: Fibrocystic disease of the bones, benign cysts, osteitis fibrosa, osteitis fibrosa with formation of tumors and giant cell sarcomata (von Recklinghausen) and mollities ossium with giant cell sarcomata. Brit. J. Surg. 2, 17–67 (1914)

Fahey, F.F., O'Brien, E.T.: Subtotal resection and grafting in selected cases of solitary unicameral bone cyst. J. Bone Jt. Surg. 56 A, 59–68 (1973)

Francisco, C.B., Pubitz, M.E., Gerundo, M.: Malignant degeneration in benign bone cyst? Arch. Surg. (Chicago) 32, 669–678 (1936)

Freund, E., Meffert, C.B.: On the different forms of non-generalized fibrous osteodystrophy. Surg. Gynec. Obstet. 62, 541–563 (1936)

Galasko, C.S.B.: The fate of simple bone cysts which fracture. Clin. Orthop. 101, 302–304 (1974)

Garceau, G.J., Gregory, C.F.: Solitary unicameral bone cysts. J. Bone Jt. Surg. 36 A, 267–280 (1954)

GESCHICKTER, C.F., COPELAND, M.M.: Tumors of bone, 3rd ed. Philadelphia: J.B. Lippincott, 1949

GIESEKING, H.: Das familiäre Auftreten von jugendlichen Knochencysten. Chirurg 21, 670–672 (1950)

GRABIAS, S., MANKIN, H.J.: Chondrosarcoma arising in histologically proved unicameral bone cyst. A case report. J. Bone Jt. Surg. 56A, 1501–1509 (1974)

GRAHAM, J.J.: Solitary unicameral bone cyst. A follow-up study of 31 cases with proven pathological diagnosis. Bull. Hosp. Jt. Dis. (N.Y.) 13, 106–130 (1952)

HAGBERG, S., MANSFELD, L.: The solitary bone cyst. A follow-up of 24 cases. Acta. chir. scand. 133, 25–29 (1967)

HEINEKE, H.: Ein Fall von multiplen Knochencysten. Bruns' Beitr. klin. Chir. 40, 481–498 (1903)

HEUBLEIN, G.W., BAIRD, C.L.: Solitary unicameral bone cyst of right ilium. Amer. J. Roentgenol. 59, 699–704 (1948)

HUNDLEY, J.M.: Solitary bone cyst of the os calcis (a form of osteitis fibrosa). J. Ark. med. Soc. 45, 7–8 (1948)

HUTTER, C.G.: Unicameral bone cyst. Report of unusual case. J. Bone Jt. Surg. 32A, 430–432 (1950)

JAFFE, H.L., LICHTENSTEIN, L.: Solitary unicameral bone cyst with emphasis on the roentgen picture, the pathologic appearance and the pathogenesis. Arch. Surg. (Chicago) 44, 1004–1025 (1942)

JAFFE, J.L.: Tumors and tumerous conditions of the bones and joints. Philadelphia: Lea and Febiger, 1958

JAMES, A.G., COLEY, B.L., HIGINBOTHAM, N.L.: Solitary (unicameral) bone cyst. Arch. Surg. (Chicago) 57, 137–147 (1948)

JANES, J.M.: Localized bone cyst of the os calcis. J. Bone Jt. Surg. 28, 182 (1946)

JOHNSON, L.C., VETTER, J., PUTSCHAR, W.G.J.: Sarcomas arising in bone cysts. Virchows Arch. path. Anat. 335, 428–451 (1962)

KINGSBERRY, L.B.: Solitary cyst of the os calcis in adults or children. Report of eight cases. J. int. Coll. Surg. 27, 83–91 (1957)

KLEINBERG, S.: The solitary bone cyst report of a case of twenty-five years duration. J. Bone Jt. Surg. 26, 337–343 (1944)

KONJETZNY, G.E.: Die sogenannte lokalisierte Ostitis fibrosa. Arch. klin. Chir. 121, 567–634 (1922)

LANG, F.J.: Beiträge zu den mikroskopischen Befunden bei Knochenzysten. Dtsch. Z. Chir. 172, 193–210 (1922)

LANG, F.J.: Über Knochencysten. Zbl. Chir. 58, 1618–1621 (1931)

LASTHAUS, M.: Jugendliche Knochencyste und Unfall. Chirurg 21, 672–679 (1950)

LICHTENSTEIN, L.: Bone tumors, 3rd ed. St. Louis: C.V. Mosby, 1965

LODWICK, G.S.: Juvenile unicameral bone cyst. A roentgen reappraisal. Amer. J. Roentgenol. 80, 495–504 (1958)

MARCOVE, R.C.: Unpublished report at New York State Medical Society Meeting (1975)

MC LACHLIN, A.D.: Treatment and results in localized osteitis fibrosa cystica (The solitary bone cyst). J. Bone Jt. Surg. 25, 777–790 (1943)

MIKULICZ, J. VON: Über cystische Degeneration der Knochen. Verh. Ges. Dtsch. Naturforsch. u. Ärzte. 76th meeting 2nd half — part II 107 (1905)

MONCKEBERG: Über Cystenbildung bei Ostitis fibrosa. Verh. dtsch. path. Ges. 7, 232–234 (1904)

MORCHOISNE, P., MASSE, P.: Radiological evolution of simple bone cysts. Ann. Radiol. 13, 811–826 (1970)

MOURGUES, G., DE FISCHER, I., CARRET, J.P., MOYEN, B.: Le kyste essentiel le l'os. A propos de huit observations revues après long recul et d'une revue de 310 cas de la littérature. Acta orthop. belg. 40, 45–70 (1974)

NEER, C.S., FRANCIS, K.C., MARCOVE, R.C., TERZ, J., CARBONARA, P.N.: Treatment of unicameral bone cyst. J. Bone Jt. Surg. 48A, 731–745 (1966)

NEER, C.S., FRANCIS, K.C., JOHNSTON, A.D., KIERNAN, H.A.: Current concepts on the treatment of solitary unicameral bone cyst. Clin. Orthop. 97, 40–51 (1973)

OGDEN, J.A., GRISWOLD, D.M.: Solitary cyst of the talus. J. Bone Jt. Surg. 55A, 1309–1310 (1974)

PFEIFFER, C.: Über cystische Degeneration der Knochen. Beitr. klin. Chir. 53, 473–495 (1907)

PHEMISTER, D.B., GORDON, J.F.: Etiology of solitary bone cyst. J. amer. med. Ass. 87, 1429–1433 (1926)

PLATT, H.: Cysts of the long bones of the hand and foot. Brit. J. Surg. 18, 20–37 (1930)

POMMER, G.: Zur Kenntnis der progressiven Hematom- und Phlegmasieveränderungen der Röhrenknochen. Arch. orthop. Unfall-Chir. 17, 17–69 (1920)

RECKLINGHAUSEN, F. VON: Die Fibrose oder deformierende Ostitis, die Osteomalacie, und die osteoplastische Carzinose in ihren gegenseitigen Beziehungen. Festschrift Rudolf Virchow zu seinem 71. Geburtstag gewidmet. Berlin G. Reimer (1891)

REYNOLDS, J.: The fallen fragment sign in the diagnosis of unicameral bone cysts. Radiology 92, 949–953 (1969)

ROBINS, P.R., PETERSON, H.A.: Management of pathologic fractures through unicameral bone cysts. J. amer. med. Ass. 222, 80–81 (1972)

SADLER, A.H., ROSENHAIN, F.: Occurrence of two unicameral bone cysts in the same patient. J. Bone Jt. Surg. 46-A, 1557–1560 (1964)

SCHMIDT, M.B.: Allgemeine Pathologie und pathologische Anatomie der Knochen. Ergebn. allg. Path. path. Anat. 7, 221 (1901)

SMITH, N.R.: Cyst of the os calus. J. Bone Jt. Surg. 12, 416 (1930)

SMITH, R.W., SMITH, C.F.: Solitary unicameral bone cyst of the calcaneus. A review of twenty cases. J. Bone Jt. Surg. 56A, 49–56 (1974)

SPENCE, K.F., SELL, K.W., BROWN, R.H.: Solitary bone cyst. Treatment with freeze-dried cancellous bone allograft. J. Bone Jt. Surg. **51A**, 87–96 (1969)

SPJUT, H.J., DORFMAN, H.D., FECHNER, R.E., ACKERMAN, L.V.: Atlas of tumor pathology, second series, fascicle 5, Tumors of bone and cartilage. Washington, D.C., Armed Forces Institute of Pathology (1971)

STEWART, M.J., HAMEL, H.A.: Solitary bone cyst. Sth. med. J. **43**, 927–934 (1950)

SWIFT, W.E., HALLOCK, H.: Treatment of localized fibrocystic cavities in bone by curettage and packing with bone chips. J. Bone Jt. Surg. **20**, 411–418 (1938)

TACHDJIAN, M.O.: Pediatric orthopedics. Philadelphia, London, Toronto: W.B. Saunders, 1972

VERSTANDIG, C.C.: Clinical Note. Solitary unicameral cyst of the os calcis. New Engl. J. Med. **237**, 21–22 (1947)

VIRCHOW, R.L.L.: Über die Bildung von Knochencysten. Akad. Mber. 369–381 (1876)

WILBER, M.C., HYATT, G.W.: Bone cysts. Results of surgical treatment in 200 cases. In Proceedings of the American Academy of Orthopaedic Surgeons. J. Bone Jt. Surg. **42A**, 879 (1960)

Aneurysmal Bone Cyst

ANDREJEW, J.: Angiographie bei Knochentumoren. Z. Orthop. **16**, 35 (1969)

ANJARIA, P.D.: Paraplegia due to aneurysmal bone cyst of rib. A case report. J. postgrad. Med. **19**, 102–109 (1973)

ARSDALE, W.W. VAN: Ossifying haematoma. Ann. Surg. **18**, 8–17 (1893)

BARNES, R.: Aneurysmal bone cyst. J. Bone Jt. Surg. **38-B**, 301–311 (1956)

BECKMANN, Z.M.: Beitrag für röntgenologische Differentialdiagnostik zystischer und pseudozystischer Aufhellungen im Knochen. Z. Orthop. **91**, 26 (1959)

BEELER, J.W., HELMAN, C.H., CAMPBELL, J.A.: Aneurysmal bone cyst of spine. J. amer. med. Ass. **163**, 914–918 (1957)

BERNIER, J.L., BHASKAR, S.N.: Aneurysmal bone cysts of the mandible. Oral Surg. **11**, 1018–1028 (1958)

BERRY, M.: An aneurysmal bone cyst of the mandible. A case report. Aust. Radiol. **17**, 196–198 (1973)

BESSE, B.E., JR., DAHLIN, D.C., PUGH, D.G., GHORMLEY, R.K.: Aneurysmal bone cysts: Additional considerations. Clin. Orthop. **7**, 93–102 (1956)

BHASKAR, S.N., BERNIER, J.L., GODBY, F.: Aneurysmal bone cyst and other giant cell lesions of the jaws: Report of 104 cases. J. oral Surg. **17**, 30–41 (1959)

BHENDE, G.M., KOTHARE, S.N.: Aneurysmal bone cyst. Indian med. Gaz. **85**, 544–546 (1950)

BIESECKER, J.L., MARCOVE, R.C., HUVOS, A.G., MIKE, V.: Aneurysmal bone cysts. A clinicopathologic study of 66 cases. Cancer (Philad.) **26**, 615–625 (1970)

BILLINGS, K.J., WERNER, L.G.: Aneurysmal bone cyst of the first lumbar vertebra. Radiology **104**, 19–20 (1972)

BINSWANGER, U.: Zur Klinik der aneurysmatischen Knochencyste der Wirbelsäule. Schweiz. Arch. Neurol. Psychiat. **92**, 44–63 (1963)

BLOCK, C., PECK, H.M.: Radiological notes. Aneurysmal bone cyst with documented subperiosteal origin. J. Mt. Sinai Hosp. **35**, 192–195 (1968)

BLOODGOOD, J.C.: Bone tumors, benign bone cysts due to central osteitis fibrosa of the unhealed latent type. J. Radiol. **4**, 345–351 (1923)

BOLLMANN, L., MOBIUS, G., HENNEBERG, H.: Zur Klinik und Pathologie der aneurysmatischen Knochenzyste. Chirurg **38**, 171–176 (1967)

BOOHER, R.J.: Aneurysmal bone cyst of a metatarsal. J. Bone Jt. Surg. **39A**, 435–440 (1957)

BOSSART, R.A., FITZPATRICK, H.F.: Aneurysmal bone cyst of rib. Arch. Surg. (Chicago) **88**, 229–232 (1964)

BRAILSFORD, J.F.: Ossifying haematomata and other simple lesions mistaken for sarcomata; the responsibility of biopsy. Brit. J. Radiol. **21**, 157–170 (1948)

BUCK, R.E., BAILEY, R.W.: Replacement of a cervical vertebral body for aneurysmal cyst. J. Bone Jt. Surg. **51A**, 1656–1658 (1969)

BURACZEWSKI, J., DABSKA, M.: Pathogenesis of aneurysmal bone cyst. Relationship between the aneurysmal bone cyst and fibrous dysplasia of bone. Cancer (Philad.) **28**, 597–604 (1971)

BURMEISTER, H.: Zur Kenntnis aneurysmatischer Knochenzysten der Wirbelsäule. Chirurg **35**, 420–424 (1964)

BURNS-COX, C.J., HIGGINS, A.T.: Aneurysmal bone cyst of the frontal bone. J. Bone Jt. Surg. **51B**, 344–345 (1969)

BYRD, D.L., ALLEN, J.W., KINDRICK, R.D., DEWITT, J.D.: Aneurysmal bone cyst of the maxilla. J. oral Surg. **27**, 296–300 (1969)

CADAC, M.A., MALIS, L.I., ANDERSON, P.J.: Aneurysmal parietal bone cyst. Case report. J. Neurosurg. **37**, 237–240 (1972)

CAMPANACCI, M., ZANOLI, S.: Osservagioni morfologiche ed istomeccaniche sulla cisti aneurysmatica dello scheletro. Arch. ital. Anat. Istol. pat. **36**, 251–273 (1962)

Case Reports of the Massachusetts General Hospital. New Engl. J. Med. **254**, 430–433 (1956)

CHITKARA, N.L., GREWAL, K.S., SING, H.: Aneurysmal bone cyst. Indian J. Surg. **22**, 98 (1960)

CLOUGH, J.R., PRICE, C.H.G.: Aneurysmal bone cyst. Review of twelve cases. J. Bone Jt. Surg. **50B**, 116–127 (1968)

CLOUGH, J.R., PRICE, C.H.G.: Aneurysmal bone cyst: Pathogenesis and long term results of treatment. Clin. Orthop. **97**, 52–63 (1973)

COLEY, B.L.: Neoplasms of bone and related conditions: Their etiology, pathogenesis, diagnosis and treatment. New York: Paul B. Hoeber, Inc., 1949

COLEY, B.L., MILLER, L.E.: Atypical giant cell tumor. Amer. J. Roentgenol. **47**, 541–548 (1942)

CONE, S.M.: Ossifying hematoma. J. Bone Jt. Surg. **10**, 474–482 (1928)

CRUZ, M., COLEY, B.L.: Aneurysmal bone cyst. Surg. Gynec. Obstet. **103**, 67–77 (1956)

DABSKA, M., BURACZEWSKI, J.: Aneurysmal bone cyst. Pathology, clinical course and radiologic appearances. Cancer (Philad.) **23**, 371–389 (1969)

DAHLIN, D.C., BESSE, B.E., PUGH, D.G., GHORMLEY, R.K.: Aneurysmal bone cysts. Radiology **64**, 56–65 (1955)

DAS, A.K., BASN MALLICK, K.C.: Aneurysmal bone cyst. Indian J. Surg. **22**, 325 (1960)

DAUGHERTY, J.W., EVERSOLE, L.R.: Aneurysmal bone cyst of the mandible. Report of case. Oral Surg. **29**, 737–741 (1971)

DAWSON, G.R., JR.: Giant cell tumor of the pelvis at the acetabulum, ilium, ischium, and pubis. J. Bone Jt. Surg. **45A**, 1537–1538 (1963)

DOMINOK, G.W., KNOCH, H.G., MANJA, B., SCHULZE, K.J.: Die aneurysmatische Knochencyste. Bericht über 7 eigene und 344 Fälle der Literatur. Langenbecks Arch. klin. Chir. **328**, 153–168 (1971)

DONALDSON, W.F., JR.: Aneurysmal bone cyst. J. Bone Jt. Surg. **44-A**, 25–39 (1962)

DOS SANTOS, R.: Arteriography in bone tumors. J. Bone Jt. Surg. **32B**, 17–29 (1950)

EBLING, H., WAGNER, J.E.: Aneurysmal bone cysts of the mandible: Report of a case. Oral Surg. **18**, 646–652 (1964)

EDEIKEN, J., HODES, P.J.: Roentgen diagnosis of disease of bone. 2nd ed. Baltimore: Williams and Wilkins, 1973

EDLING, N.P.G.: Is the aneurysmal bone cyst a true pathologic entity? Cancer (Philad.) **18**, 1127–1130 (1965)

ELLIS, D.J., WALTERS, P.J.: Aneurysmal bone cyst of the maxilla. Oral Surg. **34**, 26–32 (1972)

EWING, J.: Neoplastic diseases: A treatise on tumors. 4th ed. Philadelphia and London: W.B. Saunders, 1940

FUCHS, G., HOFBAUER, J.: Zur Röntgentherapie des Osteoklastoma. Krebsarzt **18**, 313–323 (1963)

GARNJOBST, W., HOPKINS, R.: Aneurysmal bone cyst of pubis. Report of a case presenting as an abdominal mass. J. Bone Jt. Surg. **49A**, 971–975 (1967)

GESCHICKTER, C.F., COPELAND, M.M.: Tumors of bone, 3rd ed. Philadelphia: J.B. Lippincott, 1949

GINSBURG, L.D.: Congenital aneurysmal bone cyst. Report with comments of the role of trauma in the pathogenesis. Radiology **110**, 175–176 (1974)

GODFREY, L.W., GRESHAM, G.A.: The natural history of aneurysmal bone cyst. Proc. roy. Soc. Med. **52**, 900–905 (1959)

GRUSKIN, S.E., DAHLIN, D.C.: Aneurysmal bone cysts of the jaws. J. oral Surg. **26**, 523–528 (1968)

GURI, J.P.: Tumors of the vertebral column. Surg. Gynec. Obstet. **87**, 583–598 (1948)

HADDERS, H.N., OTERDOOM, H.J.: The identification of aneurysmal bone cyst with hemangioma of the skeleton. J. Path. Bact. **71**, 193–200 (1956)

HIRST, E., McKELLAR, C.C., ELLIS, J.M., VINER SMITH, K.: Malignant aneurysmal bone cyst. J. Bone Jt. Surg. **53B**, 791 (1970)

HODGEN, J.T., FRANTZ, C.H.: Subperiosteal giant-cell tumor. J. Bone Jt. Surg. **29**, 781–784 (1947)

HOPPE, W.: An aneurysmal bone cyst of the mandible: Report of a case. Oral Surg. **25**, 1–5 (1968)

JAFFE, H.L.: Aneurysmal bone cyst. Bull. Hosp. Jt. Dis. (N.Y.) **11**, 3–13 (1950)

JAFFE, H.L.: Discussion following a paper by DONALDSON, W.F. JR. Aneurysmal bone cyst. J. Bone Jt. Surg. **44-A**, 40 (1962)

JAFFE, H.L., LICHTENSTEIN, L.: Solitary bone cyst with emphasis on the roentgen picture, the pathologic appearance and the pathogenesis. Arch. Surg. (Chicago) **44**, 1004–1025 (1942)

JAMES, E.S.: Subtotal removal of the scapula for aneurysmal bone cyst. J. Bone Jt. Surg. **39B**, 128–130 (1957)

KAZAN, J.M., KALIMOWA, M.K.: Anewrizmaticzeskije cysty kostej. Wiestnik Rentgenologii i Radiologii **2**, 3–9 (1965)

KOLAR, J.: Aneurysmaticky kostni cysta Čsl. Roentgenol. **11**, 40–42 (1958)

KOTICHA, H.K.: Aneurysmal bone cyst. Indian J. med. Sci. **19**, 315–319 (1965)

LICHTENSTEIN, L.: Aneurysmal bone cyst. A pathological entitiy commonly mistaken for giant-cell tumor and occasionally for hemangioma and osteogenic sarcoma. Cancer (Philad.) **3**, 279–289 (1950)

LICHTENSTEIN, L.: Aneurysmal bone cysts, further observations. Cancer (Philad.) **6**, 1228–1237 (1953)

LICHTENSTEIN, L.: Aneurysmal bone cyst. Observations on fifty cases. J. Bone Jt. Surg. **39A**, 873–882 (1957)

LICHTENSTEIN, L.: Diseases of bone and joint. St. Louis: C.V. Mosley, 1975

LICHTENSZTAJN, J.A., GOLBERT, Z.W.: Aneurizmatoczeskaja kista kosti. Wiestnik Radiologii **2**, 74–77 (1960)

LIEBEGOTT, G.: Die Morphologie der primären Knochengeschwülste. Verh. dtsch. orthop. Ges. **47**, 101 (1959/60)

LINDBOM, A., SODERBERG, O., SPJUT, H.J., SUNNQUIST, O.: Angiography of aneurysmal bone cyst. Acta radiol. (Stockh.) **55**, 12–16 (1961)

LINSCHEID, R.L., DAHLIN, D.C.: Unusual lesions of the patella. J. Bone Jt. Surg. **48A**, 1359–1366 (1966)

LIVOTI, P.: Contributo allo studio delle neoplasie primitive delle vertebra. Oncologia **2**, 161–176 (1949)

LOCHER, G.W., KAISER, G.: Giant cell tumors and aneurysmal bone cysts of ribs in childhood. J. pediat. Surg. **10**, 103–108 (1975)

Mach, J.: Bemerkungen zur Differentialdiagnose von Beckentumoren 18. Tag. Ges. Ostop., Erfurt 7, 10, 5 (1969)

Mayer, L., Kestler, O.C.: Aneurysmal bone cyst of spine. Bull. Hosp. Jt. Dis. (N.Y.) 5, 16–22 (1944)

Marcove, R.C., Miller, T.R.: Treatment of primary and metastatic bone tumors by cryosurgery. J. amer. med. Ass. 207, 1890–1894 (1969)

Mc Cohen, D.M., Dahlin, D.C., Mac Carty, C.S.: Vertebral giant cell tumor and varients. Cancer (Philad.) 17, 461–473 (1964)

Mittelmeier, H.: Prognose und Therapie der gutartigen Knochengeschwülste. Verh. Dtsch. orthop. Ges. 7, 229 (1959/1960)

Nobler, M.P., Higinbotham, N.L., Phillips, R.F.: The cure of aneurysmal bone cyst. Radiology 90, 1185–1192 (1968)

Ochsner, S.F.: Aneurysmal bone cyst in the humerus. J. Louisiana med. Soc. 126, 369–371 (1974)

Oliver, L.P.: Aneurysmal bone cyst: Report of a case. Oral Surg. 35, 67–76 (1973)

Parrish, F.F., Pavey, J.K.: Surgical management of aneurysmal bone cyst of the vertebral column. A report of three cases. J. Bone Jt. Surg. 49-A, 1597–1604 (1967)

Phelan, J.T.: Aneurysmal bone cyst. Surg. Gynec. Obstet. 119, 979–983 (1964)

Potts, W.J.: Subperiosteal giant cell tumor. J. Bone Jt. Surg. 22, 417–420 (1940)

Prakash, B., Banerji, A.K., Tandor, P.N.: Aneurysmal bone cyst of spine. J. Neurol. Neurosurg. Psychiat. 36, 112–117 (1973)

Present, A.J.: So-called subperiosteal giant cell tumor. Radiology 44, 77–79 (1945)

Reed, R.J., Rothenberg, M.: Lesions of bone that may be confused with aneurysmal bone cyst. Clin. Orthop. 35, 150–162 (1964)

Ring, S.M., Beranbaum, E.R., Madayag, M.A.: Angiography of aneurysmal bone cyst. Bull. Hosp. Jt. Dis. (N.Y.) 33, 1–7 (1972)

Roukkula, M., Salovaara, E.: Aneurysmal bone cyst of the fourth thoracic vertebra with compression of the spinal cord. Acta radiol. (Stockh.) 57, 373 (1962)

Sabanas, A.O., Dahlin, D.C., Childs, D.S., Jr., Ivris, J.C.: Postradiation sarcoma of bone. Cancer (Philad.) 9, 528–542 (1956)

Schobinger, R., Stoll, H.C.: The arteriographic picture of benign bone lesions containing giant cells. J. Bone Jt. Surg. 39A, 953–960 (1957)

Sherman, R.S., Soong, K.Y.: Aneurysmal bone cyst: Its roentgen diagnosis. Radiology 68, 54–64 (1957)

Shoji, H., Koshino, T., Marcove, R.C., Thompson, T.C.: Subperiosteal resection of the distal portion of the fibula for aneurysmal bone cyst. J. Bone Jt. Surg. 52A, 1472–1476 (1970)

Sirsat, M.V.: Aneurysmal bone cyst. Indian J. Path. Bact. 1, 90 (1958)

Slowick, F.A., Campbell, C.J., Kettelkamp, D.B.: Aneurysmal bone cyst. An analysis of thirteen cases. J. Bone Jt. Surg. 50A, 1142–1151 (1968)

Sowinski, J.: Tetniakowa torbiel kostna (cystis aneurismatica ossis). Chir. Narząd Ruchu 30, 329–332 (1965)

Spjut, H.J., Dorfman, H.D., Fechner, R.E., Ackerman, L.V.: Atlas of tumor pathology, second series, Fascicle 5, Tumors of bone and cartilage. Washington, D.C., Armed Forces Institute of Pathology (1971)

Srivastava, K.K.: Aneurysmal bone cyst of the patella. Aust. N.Z. J. Surg. 43, 54–64 (1973)

Steimlé, R., Pageaut, G., Gehin, Ph., Tropet, Y.: Kyste anévrismal de l'occipital. Acta neurochir. 30, 139–148 (1974)

Subramaniam, C.S.V., Mathias, P.F.: Aneurysmal Bone Cyst. J. Bone Jt. Surg. 44B, 93–101 (1962)

Taylor, F.W.: Aneurysmal bone cyst: Report of three cases. J. Bone Jt. Surg. 38-B, 293–300 (1956)

Thompson, P.C.: Subperiosteal giant-cell tumor. Ossifying subperiosteal hematoma-aneurysmal bone cyst. J. Bone Jt. Surg. 26-A, 281–306 (1954)

Tillman, B.P., Dahlin, D.C., Lipscomb, P.R., Steward, J.R.: Aneurysmal bone cyst: An analysis of ninety-five cases. Mayo Clin. Proc. 43, 478–495 (1968)

Tillmann, K., Torklus, D.: Die aneurysmatische Knochenzyste. Z. Orthop. 101, 73 (1966)

Verbiest, H.: Giant-cell tumors and aneurysmal bone cysts of the spine with special reference to the problems related to removal of a vertebral body. J. Bone Jt. Surg. 47B, 699–713 (1965)

Vianna, M.R., Horizonte, B.: Aneurysmal bone cysts in maxilla: Report of case. J. oral Surg. 20, 432–434 (1962)

Waldron, C.A.: Nonodontogenic neoplasm cysts and allied conditions of the jaws. Semin. Roentgenol. 6, 414–425 (1971)

Waldron, C.A., Shafer, W.G.: The central giant cell reparative granuloma of the jaws. An analysis of 38 cases. Amer. J. clin. Path. 45, 437–447 (1966)

Wang, S.Y.: An aneurysmal bone cyst in the maxilla. Plast. reconstr. Surg. 25, 62–72 (1960)

Winter, A., Firtel, S.: Aneurysmal bone cyst of vertebra with compression. J. amer. med. Ass. 177, 870–871 (1961)

Witwicki, T., Beskid, M.: Aneurysmatische Knochenzyste. Chir. Narzad. Ruchu. 28, 529–531 (1963)

Yarington, C.T., Abbott, J., Raines, D.: Aneurysmal bone cyst. Arch. Otolaryng. (Chicago) 80, 313–317 (1964)

Zucchi, V.: Aneurysmal osseous cysts. Angiographic study. Arch. Orthop. 76, 27–42 (1963)

Zucchi, V., Allegrini, R.: Angiographic diagnosis in the eccentric subperiosteal variety of aneurysmal bone cyst. Atti. Acad. Med. Lombard. 22, 197–207 (1962)

Juxta-Articular Bone Cyst

BYERS, P.D., WADSWORTH, T.: Parosteal ganglion. J. Bone Jt. Surg. (Br.) **52**, 290–295 (1970)

CARP, L., STOUT, A.P.: Study of ganglion with special reference to treatment. Surg. Gynec. Obstet. **47**, 56–78 (1928)

CARTER, T.E., DETENBECK, L.C.: Intraosseous ganglion cyst of the patella: report of a case. Texas Med. **70**, 95–96 (1974)

CRABBE, W.A.: Intra-osseous ganglia of bone. Brit. J. Surg. **53**, 15–17 (1966)

CRANE, A.R., SCARANO, J.J.: Synovial cysts, ganglia of bone. J. Bone Jt. Surg. (Am.) **49**, 355–361 (1967)

EDEIKEN, J., HODES, P.J.: Roentgen Diagnosis of Disease of Bone, 2nd ed. Baltimore: Williams and Wilkens, 1973

EGGERS, G.W., EFANS, E., BLUMEL, J., BUTLER, J.: Cystic change in iliac acetabulum. J. Bone Jt. Surg. (Am.) **45**, 669–686 (1963)

FELDMAN, F., JOHNSTON, A.: Intraosseous ganglion. (Amer. J. Roentgenol. Med. **118**, 328–343 (1973)

GOLDMAN, R.L., FRIEDMAN, N.B.: Ganglia and synovial cysts arising in unusual locations. Clin. Orthop. **63**, 184–189 (1969)

JOHNSON, W.C., GRAHAM, J.H., HELWIG, E.B.: Cutaneous myxoid cyst. J. amer. med. Ass. **191**, 109–114 (1965)

KING, E.S.: Pathology of ganglia. Australian and New Zealand. J. Surg. **1**, 367–381 (1932)

MORRIS, C.C., GOLDMAN, G.C.: Production of acid mucopolysaccharides by fibroblasts in cell cultures. Nature **188**, 407–409 (1960)

ONDROUCH, A.S.: Cyst formation in osteoarthritis. J. Bone Jt. Surg. (Br.) **45**, 755–760 (1963)

PAABY, H.: Solitary cysts of the talus. Report of two operated cases. Acta orthop. scand. **44**, 560–563 (1973)

SEYMOUR, N.: Intraosseous ganglia. J. Bone Jt. Surg. **50**, 134–137 (1968)

SIM, F.H., DAHLIN, D.C.: Ganglion cysts of bone. Mayo Clin. Proc. **46**, 484–488 (1971)

SOREN, A.: Pathogenesis and treatment of ganglion. Clin. Orthop. **48**, 173–179 (1966)

SPJUT, H.J., DORFMAN, H.D., FECHNER, R.E., ACKERMAN, L.V.: Tumors of Bone and Cartilage. Armed Forces Institute of Pathology, Washington, D.C., second series (1971)

The Fibrous Cortical Defect or Nonostogenic Fibroma

AEGERTER, E., KIRKPATRICK, J.A., JR.: Orthopedic Diseases. Philadelphia: W.B. Saunders Co. 1958, pp. 563–566

BERKIN, C.R.: Nonossifying fibroma of bone. Brit. J. Radiol. **39**, 469–471 (1966)

BHAGWANDEEN, S.B.: Malignant transformation of a nonosteogenic fibroma of bone. J. Path. Bact. **92**, 562–564 (1966)

BURMAN, M.S., SINBERG, S.F.: Solitary xanthoma lipoid granulomatosis of bone. Arch. Surg. (Chicago) **37**, 1017–1032 (1938)

CAFFEY, J.: On fibrous defects in cortical walls of growing tubular bones. In: Advances in Pediatrics. Chicago: Year Book 1955, Vol 7, pp. 13–51

CAFFEY, J.: Pediatric X-Ray Diagnosis, 6th ed. Chicago: Year Book 1972

COMPERE, C.L., COLEMAN, S.S.: Nonosteogenic fibroma of bone. Surg. Gynec. Obstet. **105**, 588–598 (1957)

CUNNINGHAM, J.B., ACKERMAN, L.V.: Metaphyseal fibrous defects. J. Bone Jt. Surg. **38A**, 797–808 (1956)

DAHLIN, D.C.: Bone Tumors, Springfield, Ill.: Charles C. Thomas. 1970, pp. 90–99

DEVLIN, J.A., BOWMAN, H.E., MITCHELL, C.L.: Nonosteogenic fibroma of bone: A review of the literature with the addition of six cases. J. Bone Jt. Surg. **37A**, 472–486 (1955)

GORDON, I.R.S.: Fibrous lesions of bone in childhood. Brit. J. Radiol. **37**, 253–259 (1964)

HATCHER, C.H.: The pathogenesis of localized fibrous lesions in the metaphyses of long bones. Ann. Surg. **121**, 1016–1030 (1945)

JAFFE, H.L.: Fibrous cortical defect and nonossifying fibroma, Tumors and Tumorous Conditions of the Bones and Joints, Philadelphia: Lea & Febiger, 1958, pp. 76–91

JAFFE, H.L., LICHTENSTEIN, L.: Nonosteogenic fibroma of bone. Amer. J. Path. **18**, 205–221 (1942)

KATZ, J.F., MAREK, F.M.: Case of coexistent benign and malignant bone tumors. J. Mt. Sinai Hosp. **17**, 187–191 (1950)

KIMMELSTIEL, P., RAPP, I.: Cortical defect due to periosteal desmoids. Bull. Hosp. Jt. Dis. (N.Y.) **12**, 286–297 (1951)

KITAGAWA, T., YAMASHITA, S., KONDO, M.: Metaphyseal cortical defects in the lower femur metaphysis of Japanese children. Kumamoto med. J. **17**, 1–431 (1964)

LICHTENSTEIN, L.: Nonosteogenic fibroma of bone, Bone Tumors, St. Louis: C.V. Mosby, 1972, pp. 121–134

MAREK, F.M.: Fibrous cortical defect (periosteal desmoid). Bull. Hosp. Jt. Dis. (N.Y.), **16**, 77–87 (1955)

MAUDSLEY, R.H., STANSFELD, A.G.: Nonosteogenic fibroma of bone (fibrous metaphyseal defect). J. Bone Jt. Surg. **38B**, 714–733 (1956)

MORTON, K.S.: Bone production in nonosteogenic fibroma: An attempt to clarify nomenclature in fibrous lesions of bone. J. Bone Jt. Surg. **46B**, 233–243 (1964)

MURRAY, R.O., JACOBSON, H.G.: The Radiology of Skeletal Disorders: Exercises in Diagnosis, Baltimore: Williams & Wilkins, 1971, pp. 356–360

PHELIP, J.A.: Ostéite kystique vacuolaire juvenile xanthomateuse de l'extrémité du fémur. Bull. Soc. nat. Chir. **61**, 443–446 (1935)

PONSETTI, I.V., FRIEDMAN, B.: Evolution of metaphyseal fibrous defects. J. Bone Jt. Surg. **31A**, 582–585 (1949)

SCHLUMBERGER, H.G.: Fibrous dysplasia of single bones (monostotic fibrous dysplasia). Milit. Surg. **99**, 504–527 (1946)

SELBY, S.: Metaphyseal cortical defects in the tubular bones of growing children. J. Bone Jt. Surg. **43A**, 395–400 (1961)

SONTAG, L.W., PYLE, S.I.: The appearance and nature of cystlike areas in the distal femoral metaphyses of children. Amer. J. Roentgenol. **46**, 185–188 (1941)

SPJUT, H., DORFMAN, H., FECHNER, R., ACKERMAN, L.: Atlas of Tumor Pathology. Fascile 5, Tumors of Bone and Cartilage. Armed Forces Institute of Pathology, Washington, D.C., 1971

Eosinophilic Granuloma

ALBERS, S., FRANCIS, D., ALBERT, B., LASKIN, D.: Eosinophilic granuloma of the mandible. J. oral Surg. **31**, 841–843 (1973)

AVERY, M.E., McAFEE, J.G., GUILD, H.G.: The course and prognosis of reticuloendotheliosis (eosinophilic granuloma), Schüller-Christian disease and Letterer-Siwe disease: A study of 40 cases. Amer. J. Med. **22**, 636–652 (1957)

AVIOLI, L.V., LASERSOHN, J.T., LOPRESTI, J.M.: Histiocytosis X (Schüller-Christian disease) Medicine **42**, 119–147 (1963)

BUCHMAN, J.: Osteochondritis of vertebral body. J. Bone Jt. Surg. **9**, 55–56 (1927)

CALVE, J.: Localized affection of spine suggesting osteochondritis of vertebral body with clinical aspect of Pott's disease. J. Bone Jt. Surg. **7**, 41–46 (1925)

CHEYNE, C.: Histiocytosis X. J. Bone Jt. Surg. **53B**, 366–382 (1971)

CHRISTIAN, H.A.: Defect in membranous bones exophthalmos and diabetes insipidus: Unusual syndrome of dyspituitarism. Med. Contrib. Biol. Res. **1**, 391–401 (1919)

COMPERE, E., JOHNSON, W., CONVENTRY, M.: Vertebra plana (Calve's disease) due to eosinophilic granuloma. J. Bone Jt. Surg. **36**, 969–980 (1954)

DAVIDSON, R.I., SHILLITO, J.: Eosinophilic granuloma of the cervical spine in children. Pediatrics **45**, 746–752 (1970)

DAVIES, P.M.: Xanthomatosis associated with vertebra plana. Brit. J. Radiol. **22**, 725–728 (1949)

DUNDON, C.C., WILLIAMS, H.A., LAIPPLY, T.C.: Eosinophilic granuloma of bone. Radiology **47**, 433–444 (1946)

ENNIS, J.T., WHITEHOUSE, G., ROSS, M.G.F., MIDDLEMISS, J.H.: The radiology of bone changes in histiocytosis X. Clin. Radiol. **24**, 212–220 (1973)

ENRIQUEZ, P., DAHLIN, D.C., HAYLES, A.B., HENDERSON, E.D.: Histiocytosis X: a clinical study. Mayo Clin. Proc. **42**, 88–99 (1967)

EPSTEIN, B.: The Spine. 3rd ed. Philadelphia: Lea & Febiger 1969, p. 698

FARBER, S.: The nature of solitary or eosinophilic granuloma of bone. Amer. J. Path. **17**, 625–629 (1941)

FINZI, O.: Mieloma con orevalenza delle cellude eosinofile circoscritto all'osso frontale in un giovane di 15 anni. Minerva med. (Torino) **9**, 239–241 (1929)

FITZPATRICK, B.: Eosinophilic granuloma in an infant mandible. Brit. J. oral Surg. **4**, 243–246 (1967)

FLORI, A.G., PARENTI, G.C.: Reticuloendoteliosi iperplasia infettiva ad evoluzione, granulo-xantomatosa (tipo Hand-Schüller-Christian). Riv. Clin. pediat. **35**, 193 (1937)

FOWLES, J.V., BOBECHKO, W.P.: Solitary eosinophilic granuloma in bone. J. Bone Jt. Surg. **52**, 238–251 (1970)

FRIPP, A.T.: Vertebra plana. J. Bone Jt. Surg. **40**, 378–384 (1958)

GIBSON, R.M., EISEN, A.A.: Eosinophilic granuloma of bone in two adjacent thoracic vertebrae: report of a case. J. Bone Jt. Surg. **45**, 566–569 (1963)

GLANZMANN, E.: Infektiöse Retikuloendotheliose (Abt-Letterer-Siwe'sche Krankheit) und ihre Beziehungen zum Morbus Schüller-Christian. Ann. Paediat. **155**, 1–8 (1940)

GREEN, W.T., FARBER, S.: Eosinophilic or solitary granuloma of bone. J. Bone Jt. Surg. **24**, 499–526 (1942)

GROSS, P., JACOX, H.W.: Eosinophilic granuloma and certain other reticuloendothelial hyperplasias of bone. Amer. J. med. Sci. **203**, 673–687 (1942)

HAMILTON, J.B., BARTHER, J.L., KENNEDY, P.C., McCORT, J.J.: The osseous manifestations of eosinophilic granuloma: report of nine cases. Radiology **47**, 445–456 (1946)

HODGSON, J.R., KENNEDY, R.L., CAMP, J.D.: Reticuloendotheliosis. Radiology **57**, 642–652 (1951)

JAFFE, H., LICHTENSTEIN, L.: Eosinophilic granuloma of bone. Arch. Path. (Chicago) **37**, 99–118 (1944)

KAYE, J.J., FREIBERGER, R.H.: Eosinophilic granuloma of the spine without vertebra plana: a report of two unusual cases. Radiology **92**, 1188–1191 (1969)

KEIFFER, S.A., NESBIT, M.E., D'ANGIO, G.J.: Vertebral plana due to histiocytosis X: serial studies. Acta radiol (Stockh.) **8**, 241–250 (1969)

LEIKEN, S., PUROGANAN, G., FRANKEL, A., STEERMAN, R., CHANDRA, R.: Immunologic parameters in histiocytosis X. Cancer (Philad.) **32**, 796–802 (1973)

LICHTENSTEIN, L.: Histiocytosis X: Integration of eosinophilic granuloma of bone, Letterer-Siwe disease and Schüller-Christian disease as related manifestations of a single nosologic entity. Arch. Path. (Chicago) **56**, 84–102 (1953)

LICHTENSTEIN, L.: Histiocytosis X (eosinophilic granuloma of bone, Letterer-Siwe disease, and Schüller-Christian disease): Further observations of pathology and clinical importance. J. Bone Jt. Surg. **46**, 76–90 (1964)

LICHTENSTEIN, L., JAFFE, H.L.: Eosinophilic granuloma of bone, with report of a case. Amer. J. Path. **16**, 595–604 (1940)

LIEBERMAN, P.H., JONES, C.R., DARGEON, H.W., BEGG, C.F.: A reappraisal of eosinophilic granuloma of bone, Hand-Schuller-Christian syndrome and Letterer-Siwe syndrome. Medicine **48**, 375–400 (1969)

LINDENBAUM, B., GOTTES, N.I.: Solitary eosinophilic granuloma of the cervical region. Clin. Orthop. **68**, 112–114 (1970)

MATSON, D.D.: Neurosurgery of Injury in Childhood. 2nd ed. Springfield, Ill.: Charles C. Thomas, 1969, p. 612

McGAVRAN, M.H., SPADY, H.A.: Eosinophilic granuloma of bone: a study of twenty-eight cases. J. Bone Jt. Surg. **42A**, 979–992 (1960)

MOSELEY, J.E.: The reticuloendothelioses-eosinophilic granuloma, Letterer-Siwe disease and Schüller-Christian disease. In: Bone Changes in Hematologic Disorders: Roentgen Aspects. New York: Grune & Stratton 1963

NELSON, W.E., VAUGHAN, V.C. III, McKAY, R.J. (eds.): Textbook of Pediatrics, 9th ed. Philadelphia: W.B. Saunders Co., 1969, pp. 1479–1482

NEZELOF, C., GUIBERT, C.: L'Histiocytose X: Nosologie et prognostic. Arch. franl. Pédiat. **20**, 1063–1103 (1963)

OBERMAN, H.: Idiopathic histiocytosis X: a clinicopathologic study of 40 cases. Pediatrics **28**, 307–327 (1961)

OCHSNER, S.F.: Eosinophilic granuloma of bone: experience with 20 cases. Amer. J. Roentgenol. **97**, 719–726 (1966)

OTANI, S.: A discussion on eosinophilic granuloma of bone, Letterer-Siwe disease and Schuller-Christian disease. J. Mt. Sinai Hosp. **24**, 1079–1092 (1957)

OTANI, S., EHRLICH, J.C.: Solitary granuloma of bone simulating primary neoplasm. Amer. J. Path. **16**, 479–490 (1940)

PONSETTI, I.V.: Bone lesions in eosinophilic granuloma Hand-Schüller-Christian disease, and Letterer-Siwe disease. J. Bone Jt. Surg. **30A**, 811–833 (1948)

RITTER, R.A., JR.: Histiocytosis X: A case report with electron microscopic observations. Cancer **19**, 1155–1164 (1966)

SBARARO, J.L., FRANCIS, K.C.: Eosinophilic granuloma of bone. JAMA **178**, 706–710 (1961)

SCHAJOWICZ, F., POLAK, M.: Contribucion al estudio del denominado granuloma eosinofilico y sus relaciones con la xantomosis osea. Rev. Asoc. méd. argent. **61**, 218–226 (1947)

SCHAJOWICZ, F., SLULLITEL, J.: Eosinophilic granuloma of bone and its relationship to Hand-Schüller-Christian and Letterer-Siwe Syndromes. J. Bone Jt. Surg. **55**, 545–565 (1973)

SMITH, I.: A report of three cases of solitary eosinophilic granuloma of the mandible. J. dent. Ass. S. Afr. **24**, 321–323 (1969)

SPJUT, H., DORFMAN, H., FECHNER, R., ACKERMAN, L.: Atlas of Tumor Pathology. Fascile 5, Tumors of Bone and Cartilage. Armed Forces Institute of Pathology, Bethesda, Md. 1971

TAKAHASHI, M., MARTE, W., OBERMAN, H.A.: The variable roentgenographic appearance of idiopathic histiocytosis. Clin. Radiol. **17**, 48–53 (1966)

TIRONA, J.: The roentgenological and pathological aspects of tuberculosis of the skull. Amer. J. Roentgenol. **72**, 762–768 (1954)

WALLGREN, A.: Systemic reticuloendothelial granuloma. Amer. J. Dis. Child. **60**, 471–500 (1940)

WELLS, P.: The button sequestrum of eosinophilic granuloma of the skull. Radiology **67**, 746–747 (1956)

WHITEHEAD, F.I.H.: Histiocytosis X. Brit. J. oral Surg. **10**, 199–204 (1972)

F. Fibrous Dysplasia

AARSKOG, D., TVETERAAS, E.: McCune-Albright's syndrome following adrenalectomy for Cushing's syndrome in infancy. J. Pediat. **73**, 89–96 (1968)

AEGERTER, E.E.: The possible relationship of neurofibromatosis, congenital pseudoarthrosis and fibrous dysplasia. J. Bone Jt. Surg. **32A**, 618–626 (1950)

AEGERTER, E.E., KIRKPATRICK, J.A., JR.: Orthopedic Diseases, 2nd ed. Philadelphia: W.B. Saunders Co., 1963

ALBRIGHT, F., BUTLER, A.M., HAMPTON, A.O., SMITH, P.H.: Syndrome characterized by osteitis fibrosa disseminata, areas of pigmentation and endocrine dysfunction, with precocious puberty in females. Report of five cases. New Engl. J. Med. **216**, 727–746 (1937)

ALBRIGHT, F., REIFENSTEIN, F.C.: The parathyroid glands and metabolic bone disease. Selected studies. Baltimore: Williams and Wilkins, 1948

ALBRIGHT, F., SCOVILLE, W.B., SULKOWITCH, H.W.: Syndrome characterized by osteitis fibrosa disseminata, areas of pigmentation and gonadal dysfunction: further observations including report of two more cases. Endocrinology **22**, 411–421 (1938)

ANDERSON, D.E., MC CLENDON, J.L.: Cherubism-hereditary fibrous dysplasia of the jaws. 1. Genetic considerations. Oral Surg. **15**. Suppl. 2, 5–16 (1962)

BASEK, M.M.: Fibrous dysplasia of the middle ear. Arch. Otolaryng. (Chicago) **85**, 4–7 (1967)

BELEVAL, G.S., SCHNEIDER, R.W.: Fibrous dysplasia of bone. Cleveland Clinic Quart. **21**, 158–168 (1953)

BENEDICT, P.H.: Endocrine features in Albright's syndrome (fibrous dysplasia of bone). Metabolism **11**, 30–45 (1962)

BENEDICT, P.H.: Sexual precocity and polyostotic fibrous dysplasia. Amer. J. Dis. Child. **111**, 426–431 (1966)

BENEDICT, P.H., SZABO, G., FITZPATRICK, TH.B., SINEST, S.J.: Melanotic macules in Albright's syndrome and in neurofibromatosis. J. Amer. med. Ass. **205**, 618–627 (1968)

BENJAMIN, D.R., MC ROBERTS, J.W.: Polyostotic fibrous dysplasia associated with Cushing syndrome. Arch. Path. (Chicago) **96**, 175–178 (1973)

BEUST, A.T. VON: Osteitis fibrosa and bone cysts in congenital fracture of lower leg. Dtsch. Z. Chir. **152**, 60–89 (1920)

BINGOLD, A.C.: Benign fibrous tumors of single bones. Ann. roy. Coll. Surg. Engl. **18**, 28–45 (1956)

BOENHEIM, F., McGAVACK, T.H.: Polyostotische fibröse Dysplasie: Ergebn. inn. Med. Kinderheilk. **3**, 157–184 (1952)

BONDUELLE, M., CLAISSE, R.: Dysplasie fibreuse des os et syndrome d'Albright. Leur place nosologique. Sem. Hôp. Paris **24**, 514–521 (1948)

BORAK, J., DOLL, B.: Unilateral von Recklinghausen's disease of bone with precocious puberty. Wien. klin. Wschr. **47**, 540 (1934)

BRAID, F.: Osseous dystrophy following icterus gravis neonatorum. **7**, 313–320 (1932)

BRAID, F.: Osseous dystrophy following icterus gravis neonatorum. Generalized osteitis fibrosa with areas of pigmentation of skin and precocious puberty in female. Arch. Dis. Child. **14**, 181–202 (1939)

BUCHEM, F.S.P. VAN, HADDERS, H.N., HANSEN, J.F., WOLDRING, M.G.: Hyperostotis corticalis generlisata. Ned. T. Geneesk. **107**, 64–74 (1963)

CAFFEY, J., WILLIAMS, J.L.: Familial fibrous swelling of the jaws. Radiology **56**, 1–14 (1951)

CAHN, L.R.: Leontiasis ossea. Oral Surg. **6**, 201–212 (1953)

CHANGUS, G.W.: Osteoblastic hyperplasia of bone: histochemical appraisal of fibrous dysplasia of bone. Cancer. (Philad.) **10**, 1157–1165 (1975)

COHEN, A., ROSENWASSER, H.: Fibrous dysplasia of the temporal bone. Arch. Otolaryng. (Chicago) **89**, 447–459 (1969)

COLEMAN, M.: Osteitis fibrosa disseminata. Report of a case. Brit. J. Surg. **26**, 705–713 (1939)

COLEY, B.L.: Neoplasms of bone and related conditions, 2nd ed. New York: P.B. Hoeber, 1960

COLEY, B.L., STEWART, F.W.: Bone sarcoma in polyostotic fibrous dysplasia. Ann. Surg. **121**, 872–881 (1945)

COOKE, S.L., POWERS, W.H.: Monostotic fibrous dysplasia: report of two cases. Arch. Otolaryng. (Chicago) **50**, 319–329 (1949)

CORNELIUS, E.A., MC CLENDON, J.L.: Cherubism-hereditary fibrous dysplasia of the jaws. Amer. J. Roentgenol. **106**, 136–143 (1969)

DABSKA, M., BURACZEWSKI, J.: On malignant transformation in fibrous dysplasia of bone. Oncology **26**, 369–383 (1972)

DAHLMANN, J.: Zur Kenntnis der Albright's disease. Fortschr. Röntgenstr. **82**, 723–740 (1955)

DANTAS, C.: Angio-osteohypertrophy syndrome with fibrous dysplasia. J. Laryng. **87**, 77–83 (1973)

DAVES, M.L., YARDLEY, J.H.: Fibrous dysplasia of bone. Amer. J. med. Sci. **234**, 590–606 (1957)

DIECKMANN, H., TANZER, A.: Zur Klinik der Fibrosen Dysplasie und des Albright-Syndromas. Dtsch. Z. Nervenheilk. **176**, 617–636 (1957)

DOCKERTY, M.B., MEYERDING, H.W., WALLACE, G.T.: Albright's syndrome. Proc. Mayo Clin. **19**, 81–88 (1944)

DOCKERTY, M.B., GHORMLEY, R.K., KENNEDY, R.L.J., PUCH, D.G.: Albright's syndrome. Arch. intern. Med. **75**, 357–375 (1945)

ECHLIN, F.: Cranial osteomas and hyperostoses produced by meningeal fibroblastomas. A clinical pathological study. Arch. Surg. (Chicago) **28**, 357–405 (1934)

EDEIKEN, J., HODES, P.J.: Roentgen diagnosis of diseases of bone. Baltimore: Williams and Wilkins 1967

ELMSLIE, R.C.: Fibrocystic disease of bone. Brit. J. Surg. **2**, 17–67 (1914)

ELMSLIE, R.C.: Fibrocystic disease of bone. Brit. J. Surg. **2**, 17–67 (1967)

ELMSLIE, R.C.: Discussion of fibrocystic disease of bone. Proc. roy. Soc. Med. **27**, 973–975 (1934)

ELMSLIE, R.C.: Fibrosis of bone: generalized osteitis fibrosa cystica not due to hyperparathyroidism. St. Bart.'s Hosp. Rep. **68**, 147–158 (1935)

ETTER, L.E., HURST, J.W.: Polyostotic fibrous dysplasia. Radiology **41**, 70–74 (1943)

EVANS, J.: Leontiasis ossea. Critical review with reports of 4 original cases. J. Bone Jt. Surg. **35 B**, 229–234 (1953)

EVERSOLE, L.R., SABES, W.R., ROVIN, S.: Fibrous dysplasia: A nosologic problem in the diagnosis of fibro-osseous lesions of the jaws. J. oral Path. **1**, 189–220 (1972)

FAIRBANK, H.A.T.: Discussion on fibrocystic disease of bone. Proc. roy. Coll. Med. **27**, 977–978 (1934)

FAIRBANK, H.A.T.: Fibrocystic disease of bone. J. Bone Jt. Surg. **32 B**, 403–423 (1950)

FAIRBANK, H.A.T.: An atlas of general affections of the skeleton. Edinburgh: E. and S. Livingstone, 1951

FALCONER, M.A., COPE, C.L., ROBB-SMITH, A.H.T.: Fibrous dysplasia of bone with endocrine disorders and cutaneous pigmentation (Albright's disease). Quart. J. Med. **11**, 121–154 (1942)

FEINTUCH, T.A.: Chondrosarcoma arising in a cartilaginous area of previously irradiated fibrous dysplasia. Cancer (Philad.) **31**, 877–881 (1973)

FEIRING, W., FEIRING, E.H., DAVIDOFF, L.M.: Fibrous dysplasia of the skull. J. Neurosurg. **8**, 377–397 (1951)

FIRAT, D., STUTZMAN, L.: Fibrous dysplasia of the bone. Amer. J. Med. **44**, 421–429 (1968)

FONTAINE, R., WARTER, P., MÜLLER, J.N., STOLL, G., GANDAR, P.: Syndrome d'Albright. Ostéite fibro-géodique disséminée à prédominance unilatérale avec pigmentations cutanées et puberté précoce. J. Radiol. Électrol. **35**, 893–987 (1954)

FRAME, B., AZAD, N., REYNOLDS, W.A., SAEED, S.M.: Polyostotic fibrous dysplasia and myositis ossificans progressiva. A report of coexistence. Amer. J. Dis. Child. **124**, 120–122 (1972)

FREEDMAN, E.: Leontiasis ossea. Radiology **20**, 8–13 (1933)

FREEDMAN, H.J.: Disturbances of function of the suprarenal glands in children. Amer. J. Dis. Child. **44**, 1285–1294 (1932)

FREUND, E.: Osteodystrophia fibrosa unilateralis. Report of a case. Arch. Surg. (Chicago) **28**, 849–866 (1934)

FREUND, E., MEFFERT, C.B.: On the different forms of non-generalized fibrous osteodystrophy. Surg. Gynec. Obstet. **62**, 541–561 (1936)

FRIES, J.W.: The roentgen features of fibrous dysplasia of the skull and facial bones. A critical analysis of thirty-nine pathologically proved cases. Amer. J. Roentgenol. **77**, 71–88 (1957)

FURST, N.J., SHAPIRO, R.: Polyostotic fibrous dysplasia: review of literature with two additional cases. Radiology **40**, 501–515 (1943)

GARLOCK, J.H.: Differential diagnosis of hyperparathyroidism with special reference to polyostotic fibrous dysplasia. Ann. Surg. **108**, 347–361 (1938)

GATEWOOD, O.M.B., ESTERLY, J.R.: Coexistent polyostotic fibrous dysplasia and eosinophilic granuloma of bone. An unique association. Amer. J. Roentgenol. **97**, 110–117 (1966)

GAUPP, V.: Pubertas praecox bei Osteodystrophia fibrosa. Mschr. Kinderheilk. **53**, 312–322 (1932)

GEORGIADE, N., MASTERS, F., HORTON, C., PICKRELL, K.: Ossifying fibromas (fibrous dysplasia) of the facial bones in children and adolescents. J. Pediat. **46**, 36–43 (1955)

GIBSON, M.J., MIDDLEMISS, J.H.: Fibrous dysplasia of bone. Brit. J. Radiol. **44**, 1–13 (1971)

GOLDHAMER, K.: Osteodystrophia fibrosa unilateralis. Fortschr. Röntgenstr. **49**, 456–481 (1934)

HACKETT, J.J., JR., CHRISTOPHERSON, W.M.: Polyostotic fibrous dysplasia. J. Pediat. **35**, 767–780 (1949)

HADDERS, H.N.: Dysplasia fibrosa monostotica. Ned. T. Geneesk. **101**, 378–380 (1957)

HADDERS, H.N.: Fibreuze dysplasie, cementofibroom en cementoom. Ned. T. Tandheelk. **74**, 721–742 (1967)

HALL, R., WARRICK, C.K.: Hypersecretion of hypothalamic releasing hormones. A possible explanation of the endocrine manifestations of polyostotic fibrous dysplasia (Albright's syndrome). Lancet **1**, 1313–1316 (1972)

HARRIS, W.J., DUDLEY, H.R., BARRY, R.J.: The natural history of fibrous dysplasia. J. Bone Jt. Surg. **44A**, 207–233 (1962)

HENRY, A.: Monostotic fibrous dysplasia. J. Bone Jt. Surg. **51B**, 300–306 (1969)

HIBBS, R.E., RUSH, H.P.: Albright's syndrome. Ann. intern. Med. **37**, 587–597 (1952)

HIRSCH, I.S.: Generalized osteitis fibrosa. Radiology **13**, 44–84 (1929)

HOBOEK, A.: Polyostotic fibrous dysplasia of bone. Acta radiol. (Stockh.) **36**, 145–153 (1951)

HOBOEK, A.: Polyostotische fibröse Dysplasie des Knochens. Fortschr. Röntgenstr. **76**, 132 (1959)

HORN, P.E. VAN, JR., DAHLIN, D.C., BICKEL, W.H.: Fibrous dysplasia: a clinical pathologic study of orthopedic surgical cases. Proc. Mayo Clin. **38**, 175–189 (1963)

HORWITZ, T., CANTAROW, A.: Polyostotic fibrous dysplasia. Arch. intern. Med. **64**, 280–285 (1939)

HOUSTIN, W.O.J., JR.: Fibrous dysplasia of maxilla and mandibula: Clinicopathologic study and comparison of facial bone lesions with lesions affecting general skeleton. J. oral Surg. **23**, 17–29 (1965)

HUMMEL, R.: Zwei Fälle von Ostitis deformans Paget juvenilis. Röntgenpraxis **6**, 513–519 (1934)

HUNTER, D., TURNBULL, H.M.: Hyperparathyroidism: generalized osteitis fibrosa. Brit. J. Surg. **31**, 203–284 (1931)

HUSBAND, P., SNODGRASS, G.J.A.: McCune-Albright syndrome with endocrinological investigations. Amer. J. Dis. Child. **119**, 164–167 (1970)

HUVOS, A.G., HIGINBOTHAM, N.L., MILLER, T.R.: Bone sarcomas arising in fibrous dysplasia. J. Bone Jt. Surg. **54A**, 1047–1066 (1972)

IVIMEY, M.: Bone dystrophy with characteristics of leontiasis ossea, osteitis deformans and osteitis fibrosa cystica. Amer. J. Dis. Child. **38**, 348–369 (1929)

JACOBSON, S.A.: The comparative pathology of the tumors of bone. Springfield, Ill.: Charles C. Thomas, 1971

JAFFE, H.L.: Fibrous dysplasia of bone. A disease entity and specifically not an expression of neurofibromatosis. J. Mt. Sinai Hosp. **12**, 364–381 (1945)

JAFFE, H.L.: Fibrous dysplasia of bone. Bull. N.Y. Acad. Med. **22**, 588–604 (1946)

JAFFE, H.L.: Fibrous dysplasia. Tumors and tumorous conditions of the bones and joints. Philadelphia: Lea and Febiger, 1958

JERVIS, G.A., SCHEIN, H.: Polyostotic fibrous dysplasia (Albright's syndrome); case showing central nervous system changes. Arch. Path. (Chicago) **51**, 640–650 (1951)

JIROUT, J., LEWITT, K.: Cases of fibrous dysplasia with disturbances of the nervous system. Csl. Roentgenol. **10**, 163; Zbl. ges. Radiol. **54**, 161 (1957)

JOHNSON, L.C.: Congenital pseudarthrosis, adamantinoma of long bones and intracortical fibrous dysplasia of the tibia. J. Bone Jt. Surg. **54A**, 1355 (1972)

JOHNSON, R.P., MOHNAC, A.M.: Polyostotic fibrous dysplasia. J. oral Surg. **25**, 521–533 (1967)

JONES, W.A.: Familial multilocular cystic disease of the jaws. Amer. J. Cancer **17**, 946–950 (1933)

KANAVEL, A.B.: Surgical intervention in leontiasis ossea. Surg. Gynec. Obstet. **4**, 719–734 (1907)

KANTHAK, F.F., HAMM, W.G., YARU, C.P.: Fibrous dysplasia of facial bones. Plast. reconstr. Surg. **15**, 41–55 (1955)

KIM, J.P., KBERA, S.A.K.: Polyostotic fibrous dysplasia associated with hyperthyroidism. J. Bone Jt. Surg. **43A**, 897–904 (1961)

KINNMANN, J.E.G., HONG, C.E., LEE, E.B., SHIN, H.S.: Fibrous dysplasia of the face and skull. Pract. oto-rhino-laryng. (Basel) **31**, 11–21 (1969)

KNAGGS, R.H.: The inflammatory and toxic diseases of bone. Bristol: John Wright and sons, 1926

KWEE, T.H.: Fibreuze osteodysplasie. Academisch proefschrift. Amsterdam: Jacob van Campen, 1964

LAWRENCE, D., NOGRADY, M.B., CLOUTIER, A.M.: Cherubism. A case report. Amer. J. Roentgenol. **108**, 468–472 (1970)

LEADER, S.D., GRAND, M.J.H.: Von Recklinghausen's disease in children: Report of a case presenting cutaneous pigmentation and bone changes. J. Pediat. **1**, 754–763 (1932)

LECOCO, M.: Un cas de localisation vertébrale de la dysplasie fibreuse des os ou maladie de Jaffé-Lichtenstein. J. belge Méd. phys. Rhum. **11**, 17 (1956)

LEDOUX-LEBARD, G.: Les localisations vertébrales de la dysplasie fibreuse des os ou maladie de Jaffé-Lichtenstein (à propos de deux observations). Presse méd. **61**, 272 (1953)

LEEDS, N., SEAMAN, W.B.: Fibrous dysplasia of the skull and its differential diagnosis. Radiology **78**, 570–583 (1962)

LEHRER, H.Z.: Ossifying fibroma of the orbital roof. Its distinction from "blistering" or "intraosseous" meningeoma. Arch. Neurol. (Paris) **20**, 536–541 (1969)

LICHTENSTEIN, L.: Polyostotic fibrous dysplasia. Arch. Surg. (Chicago) **36**, 874–898 (1938)

LICHTENSTEIN, L.: Bone tumours. 3rd ed. St. Louis: C.V. Mosby Co., 1965

LICHTENSTEIN, L.: Diseases of bone and joints. St. Louis: C.V. Mosby Co., 1975

LICHTENSTEIN, L., JAFFE, H.L.: Fibrous dysplasia of bone: a condition affecting one, several or many bones, the gravest cases of which may present abnormal pigmentation of skin, premature sexual development, hyperthyroidism, or still other extraskeletal abnormalities. Arch. Path. (Chicago) **33**, 777–816 (1942)

LIN, J.P., GOODKIN, R., CHASE, N.E., KRICHEFF, I.I.: The angiographic features of fibrous dysplasia of the skull. Radiology **92**, 1275–1280 (1969)

MACMAHON, H.E.: The pathology of the endocrine system in Albright's syndrome. Amer. J. Path. **26**, 747–758 (1950)

MAMMEL, C.K.: Histologic comparisons of localized fibrous dysplasia of bone and ossifying fibroma. J. oral Surg. **6**, 27–37 (1948)

MANDL, F.: Klinisches und experimentelles zur Frage der lokalisierten und generalisierten Ostitis fibrosa. Arch. klin. Chir. **143**, 1–46 (1926)

McCART, H.: Fibrous dysplasia. Laryngoscope **62**, 496–513 (1952)

McCUNE, D.J.: Osteitis fibrosa cystica: the case of a nine year old girl who also exhibits precocious puberty, multiple pigmentation of the skin and hyperthyroidism. Amer. J. Dis. Child. **52**, 745 (1936)

McCUNE, D.J., BRUCH, H.: Osteodystrophia fibrosa: report of a case in which the condition was combined with precocious puberty, pathological pigmentation of the skin and hyperthyroidism, with review of the literature. Amer. J. Dis. Child. **54**, 806–848 (1937)

McDONALD, R.E., SHAFER, W.G.: Disseminated juvenile dysplasia of the jaws. Amer. J. Dis. Child. **89**, 354–358 (1955)

McINTOSH, H.D., MILLER, D.E., GLEASON, W.L., GOLDNER, J.L.: The circulatory dynamics of polyostotic fibrous dysplasia. Amer. J. Med. **32**, 393–403 (1962)

MEYERSOHN, S., GREK, I.J.: Polyostotic fibrous dysplasia. Brit. J. Radiol. **24**, 629–632 (1951)

MOEHLIG, R.C., SCHREIBER, F.: Polyostotic fibrous dysplasia. Amer. J. Roentgenol. **44**, 181–202 (1939)

MOEHLIG, R.C., SCHREIBER, F.: Polyostotic fibrous dysplasia. Report of a case with unilateral involvement. Amer. J. Roentgenol. **44**, 17–23 (1940)

MOLDAWER, M., RABIN, E.R.: Polyostotic fibrous dysplasia with thyrotoxicosis. Report of a complete autopsy and skeletal reconstruction. Arch. Intern. Med. **118**, 379–385 (1966)

MONTOYA, G., EVARTS, C.M., KOHN, D.F.: Polyostotic fibrous dysplasia and spinal cord compression. Care report. J. Neurosurg. **29**, 102–106 (1968)

MOORE, R.T.: Fibrous dysplasia of the orbit. Surv. Ophthal. **13**, 321–334 (1969)

MORGENSON, E.G.: Fibrous dysplasia of bone. Report of an unusual case with endocrine disorders. Acta Med. Scand. **161**, 453–458 (1958)

MORTON, J.J.: Generalized type of osteitis fibrosa cystica. Arch. Surg. (Chicago) **4**, 534–566 (1922)

MORTON, K.S.: Bone production in non-osteogenic fibroma. J. Bone Jt Surg. **46B**, 233–243 (1954)

MURRAY, R.C., KIRKPATRICK, H.J.R., PORRAT, E.: Albright's syndrome (osteitis fibrosa disseminata). Brit. J. Surg. **34**, 48–56 (1946)

NIXON, G.W., CONDON, V.R.: Epiphyseal involvement in polyostotic fibrous dysplasia. Radiology **106**, 167–170 (1973)

PANDERS, A.K.: Fibreuze dysplasie cementofibroom en cementom. II. Klinick en differentiele diagnose. Ned. T. Tandheelk. **74**, 794–800 (1967)

PANDERS, A.K.: Fibro-osseuze en fibro-osseuzecementeuze dysplasie van de kaken. Groningen: Thesis 1970

PECK, F.B., SAGE, C.V.: Diabetes mellitus associated with Albright's syndrome. Amer. J. Med. Sci. **208**, 35–46 (1944)

PERKINSON, N.G., HIGHINBOTHAM, N.L.: Osteogenic sarcoma arising in polyostotic fibrous dysplasia. Cancer (Philad.) **8**, 396–402 (1955)

PETERMAN, M.G.: Polyostotic fibrous dysplasia (with precocious puberty and pigmentation). J. Pediat. **49**, 719–727 (1956)

PRATT, A.D., FELSON, B., WIOT, J.F., PAIGE, M.: Sequestrum formation in fibrous dysplasia. Amer. J. Roentgenol. **106**, 162–165 (1969)

PRIESEL, R., WAGNER, R.: Osteitis fibrosa cystica generalisata (osteodystrophia fibrosa). Z. Kinderheilk. **53**, 146–161 (1932)

PRITCHARD, J.E.: Fibrous dysplasia of the bones. Amer. J. med. Sci. **222**, 313–332 (1951)

PROFFIT, J.N., McSWAIN, B., KALMON, F.H.: Fibrous dysplasia of bone. Ann. Surg. **130**, 881–895 (1949)

PSENNER, L., HECKERMANN, F.: Beitrag zur röntgenologischen Diagnose und Differentialdiagnose der fibrösen Dysplasie des Skelettsystems. Fortschr. Röntgenstr. **74**, 265–288 (1951)

PUGH, D.G.: Fibrous dysplasia of the skull: a probable explanation for leontiasis ossea. Radiology **44**, 548–555 (1945)

RAMSEY, H.E., STRONG, E.W., FRAZELL, E.L.: Progressive fibrous dysplasia of the maxilla. J. Amer. dent. Ass. **81**, 1388–1391 (1970)

RECKLINGHAUSEN, F.D. VON: Die Fibrose oder deformierende Ostitis. Die Osteomalacie und die osteoplastische Carcinose in ihren gegenseitigen Beziehungen. Berlin: Festschr. Rudolf Virchow (1891)

REED, R.J.: Fibrous dysplasia of bone. Arch. Path. (Chicago) **75**, 480–495 (1963)

REISZ, M.: Über die bisher in der Literatur beschriebenen Fälle von Leontiasis ossea. Langenbecks Arch. klin. Chir. **184**, 320–348 (1936)

RIDDELL, D.M.: Malignant change in fibrous dysplasia. J. Bone Jt. Surg. **46B**, 251–255 (1964)

ROBERT, J., DUCROGUET, P.: Traitement chirurgical des localisations fémorales de 6 cas de syndrome d'Albright a Presse méd. **23**, 602–603 (1952)

ROSENCRANTZ, M.: A case of fibrous dysplasia (Jaffe-Lichtenstein) with vertebral fracture and compression of the spinal cord. Acta orthop. scand. **36**, 435–440 (1965)

ROSENCRANTZ, M.: Widened vascular grooves in fibrous dysplasia of the skull. Acta radiol. (Stockh.) **9**, 95–100 (1969)

ROSENDAHL-JESSEN, S.V.: Fibrous dysplasia of the vertebral column. Acta chir. scand. **6**, 490 (1956)

RUSSELL, L.W., CHANDLER, F.A.: Fibrous dysplasia of bone. J. Bone Jt. Surg. **32A**, 323–337 (1950)

RYAN, W.G.: Fibrous dysplasia of bone with vitamin D resistant rickets: a case study. Metabolism **17**, 988–998 (1968)

RYPINS, E.L.: Osteitis fibrosa cystica at unusual age. J. Bone Jt. Surg. **15**, 509–512 (1933)

SALZER, H.: Case of unilateral osteitis fibrosa cystica generalisata. Wien. klin. Wschr. **27**, 862 (1933)

SAMUEL, S., GILMAN, S., MAURER, H.S., ROSENTHAL, I.M.: Hyperthyroidism in an infant with McCune-Albright Syndrome: Report of a case with myeloid metaplasia. J. Pediat. **80**, 275–278 (1972)

SANTE, R.L., BAUER, W.M., O'BRIEN, R.M.O.: Polyostotic fibrous dysplasia (Albright's syndrome) and its comparison with dyschondroplasia (Ollier's disease). Radiology **51**, 676–690 (1948)

SASSIN, J.F., ROSENBERG, R.N.: Neurological compli-

cations of fibrous dysplasia of the skull. Arch. Neurol. (Paris) **18**, 363–369 (1968)

SCHLUMBERGER, H.G.: Fibrous dysplasia of single bones (monostotic fibrous dysplasia). Milit. Surg. **99**, 504–527 (1946)

SCHMAMAN, A., SMITH, I., ACKERMAN, L.V.: Benign fibro-osseous lesions of the mandible and maxilla: A review of 35 cases. Cancer (Philad.) **26**, 303–312 (1971)

SCHWARTZ, D.T., ALPERT, M.: The malignant transformation of fibrous dysplasia. Amer. J. med. Sci. **247**, 1–20 (1964)

SCURRY, M.T., BICHNELL, J.M., FAJANS, S.S.: Polyostotic fibrous dysplasia and acromegaly. Arch. intern. Med. **114**, 40–45 (1964)

SETHI, R.S., CLIMIE, A.R.W., TUTTLE, W.M.: Fibrous dysplasia of the rib with sarcomatous change. J. Bone Jt. Surg. **44A**, 193–198 (1962)

SHERMAN, R.S., STERNBERGH, W.C.A.: The roentgen appearance of ossifying fibroma of bone. Radiology **50**, 595–609 (1948)

SILVERS, D.N., GREENWOOD, R.S., HELWIG, E.B.: Cafe au lait spots without giant pigment granules. Occurrence in suspected neurofibromatosis. Arch. Derm. (Chicago) **110**, 87–88 (1974)

SINHA, A.: Monostotic fibrous dysplasia affecting the skull and facial bones. J. Laryng. **79**, 526–533 (1965)

SKANSE, B., LANGELAND, P., VON ROSEN, S.: Polyostotisk fibros dysplasi—Albrights syndrom. Nord. Med. **55**, 833–836 (1956)

SLOW, I.N., STERN, D., FRIEDMAN, E.W.: Osteogenic sarcoma arising in pre-existing fibrous dysplasia: Report of a case. J. oral Surg. **29**, 126–129 (1971)

SMITH, A.G., ZAVALETA, A.: Osteoma, ossifying fibroma and fibrous dysplasia of facial and cranial bones. Arch. Path. (Chicago) **54**, 507–527 (1952)

SMITH, I., SCHMAMAN, A.: Benign fibro-osseous lesions of the mandible and maxilla. Clinical features. S. Afr. med. J. **44**, 1423–128 (1970)

SNAPPER, I., PARISEL, C.: Xanthomatosis generalisata ossium. Quart. J. Med. **2**, 407–417 (1933)

SPJUT, H.J., DORFMAN, H.D., FECHNER, R.E., ACKERMAN, L.V.: Atlas of tumor pathology, second series, fascicle 5, Tumors of bone and cartilage. Washington, D.C. Armed Forces Institute of Pathology (1971)

SPRANGER, J.W., LANGER, L.O., WIEDEMANN, H.R.: Bone dysplasias, an atlas of constitutional disorders of skeletal development. Philadelphia, Toronto: W.B. Saunders Co., 1974

STALMANN, A.: Nerven-, Haut-, und Knochenveränderungen bei der Neurofibromatosis Recklinghausen und ihre entstehungsgeschichtlichen Zusammenhänge. Virchows Arch. path. Anat. **289**, 96–126 (1933)

STAUFFER, H.M., ARBUCKLE, R.K., AEGERTER, E.: Polyostotic fibrous dysplasia with cutaneous pigmentation and congenital arteriovenous aneurysms. J. Bone Jt. Surg. **23**, 323–334 (1941)

STERNBERG, W.H., JOSEPH, V.: Osteodystrophia fibrosa combined with precocious puberty and exophthalmic goiter. Pathologic report of a case. Amer. J. Dis. Child. **63**, 748–783 (1942)

STEWART, M.J., GILMER, W.S., EDMONTON, A.S.: Fibrous dysplasia of bone. J. Bone Jt. Surg. **44A**, 302–318 (1962)

STRASSBURGER, P., GARBER, C.Z., HALLOCK, H.: Fibrous dysplasia of bone. J. Bone Jt. Surg. **33A**, 407 (1951)

TALBOT, I.C., KEITH, D.A., LORD, I.J.: Fibrous dysplasia of the craniofacial bones. A clinico-pathological survey of seven cases. J. Laryng. **88**: 429–443 (1974)

TAVERAS, J.M., WOOD, E.H.: Diagnostic neuroradiology. Baltimore: Williams and Wilkins, 1964

TCHANG, S.P.K.: The small orbit sign in supraorbital fibrous dysplasia. J. Canad. Ass. Radiol. **24**, 65–69 (1973)

TELFORD, E.D.: Case of osteitis fibrosa, with formation of hyaline cartilage. Brit. J. Surg. **18**, 409–414 (1931)

TENG, P., GROSS, S.W., NEWMAN, C.M.: Compression of spinal cord by osteitis deformans (Paget's disease), giant-cell tumor and polyostotic fibrous dysplasia (Albright's syndrome) of vertebrae: a report of four cases. J. Neurosurg. **8**, 482–493 (1951)

TENNENT, W.: Leontiasis ossea. Brit. J. Radiol. **19**, 388–391 (1946)

THANNHAUSER, S.J.: Neurofibromatosis (VON RECKLINGHAUSEN) and osteitis fibrosa cystica localisata et disseminata (VON RECKLINGHAUSEN); a study of a common pathogenesis of both diseases. Differentiation between hyperparathyroidism with generalized decalcification and fibrocystic changes of the skeleton and osteitis fibrosa cystica disseminata. Medicine **23**, 105–149 (1944)

THOMA, K.H.: Differential diagnosis of fibrous dysplasia and fibro-osseous neoplastic lesions of the jaws and their treatment. J. oral Surg. **14**, 185–194 (1956)

TOBLER, W.: Ostitis fibrosa cystica generalisata im Kindesalter. Z. Kinderheilk. **41**, 334–335 (1926)

VALLS, J., POLAK, M., SCHAJOWICZ, F.: Fibrous dysplasia of bone. J. Bone Jt. Surg. **32A**, 311–322 (1950)

VENKER, H.: Monostotische fibreuze dysplasie uitgaande van het mastoid. Ned. T. Geneesk. **115**, 327–329 (1971)

VERGHESE, A.: Albright's syndome in the male with situs inversus. Proc. roy. Soc. Med. **55**, 357–358 (1962)

VINES, R.H.: Polyostotic fibrous dysplasia. Arch. Dis. Child. **27**, 351–355 (1957)

VIRCHOW, R.: Die krankhaften Geschwülste. **2**, 21 Berlin: A. Hirschwald, 1864

WAGMAN, A.D., WEISS, E.K., RIGGS, H.E.: Hyperplasia of the skull associated with intraosseous meningioma in the absence of gross tumor: report of three cases. J. Neuropath. exp. Neurol. **19**, 111–115 (1960)

WALDRON, C.A.: Fibroosseous lesions of the jaws. J. oral Surg. **28**, 58–64 (1970)

WALDRON, C.A., GIANSANTI, J.S.: Benign fibro-osseous lesions of the jaws: A clinical-radiologic-histologic review of sixty-five cases. Part I. Fibrous dysplasia of the jaws. Part II. Benign fibro-osseous lesions of periodontal ligament origin. Oral Surg. **35**, 190–201, 340–350 (1973)

WARRICK, C.K.: Polyostotic fibrous dysplasia — Albright's syndrome; a review of the literature and report of four male cases, two of which were associated with precocious puberty. J. Bone Jt. Surg. **31B**, 175–183 (1949)

WARRICK, C.K.: Some aspects of polyostotic fibrous dysplasia. Possible hypothesis to account for the associated endocrinological changes. Clin. Radiol. **24**, 125–138 (1973)

WEIL, A.: Pubertas praecox und Knochenbrüchigkeit. Klin. Wschr. **1**, 2114–2115 (1922)

WEISS, K.: Über den Halbseitentypus des multiplen Chondromes. Fortschr. Roentgenstr. **31**, 615 (1924)

WELLS, P.O.: Fibrous dysplasia of bone (monostotic). Radiology **52**, 642–654 (1949)

WIELAND, E.: Über Osteodysplasia cystica congenita. Monatsschr. f. Kinderh. **22**, 356–363 (1922)

WIGGINS, J.C.: Polyostotic fibrous dysplasia with extraskeletal features. New med. J. **16**, 520–527 (1955)

WINDHOLZ, F.: Cranial manifestations of fibrous dysplasia of bone. Amer. J. Roentgenol. **58**, 51–63 (1947)

WINDHOLZ, F., CUTTING, W.C.: Leontiasis ossea. Stanf. med. Bull. **3**, 69–81 (1945)

WINTER, H.: Über einen Fall von Ostitis fibrosa generalisata ohne Epithelkörperihentumor. Zbl. Chir. **56**, 2647–2649 (1929)

WIRTH, W.A., LEAVITT, D., ENZINGER, F.M.: Multiple intramuscular myxomas. Cancer (Philad.) **27**, 1167–1173 (1971)

WYATT, G.M., RANDALL, W.S.: Monostotic fibrous dysplasia. Amer. J. Roentgenol. **61**, 354–364 (1949)

YETTRA, C.M., STARR, P.: Polyostotic fibrous dysplasia associated with hyperthyroidism. J. clin. Endocr. **2**, 312–321 (1951)

ZANGENEH, F., LULEJIAN, G.A., STEINER, M.M.: McCune-Albright syndrome with hyperthyroidism. Amer. J. Dis. Child. **111**, 644–648 (1966)

ZEGARELLI, E.V., KUTSCHER, A.H.: Fibrous dysplasia of the jaws. Dent. Radiog. Photog. **36**, 27–32 (1963)

ZIMMER, J.F., DAHLIN, D.C., PUGH, D.G., CLAGETT, O.T.: Fibrous dysplasia of bone: analysis of 15 cases of surgically verified costal fibrous dysplasia. J. thorac. Surg. **31**, 488–496 (1956)

ZIMMERMAN, D.C., DAHLIN, D.C., STAFNE, E.C.: Fibrous dysplasia of the maxilla and mandible. J. oral. Surg. **11**, 55–86 (1958)

Myositis Ossificans

ACKERMAN, L.V.: Extraosseous localized non-neoplastic bone and cartilage formation (so-called myositis ossificans). Clinical and pathological confusion with malignant neoplasms. J. Bone Jt. Surg. **40**, 279–298 (1958)

ADAMS, R.C., DENNY-BROWN, D., PEARSON, C.M.: Diseases of Muscle: a Study of Pathology, 2nd ed. New York: Harper 1962

ANGERVALL, L., STENER, B., STENER, I., AHREN, C.: Pseudomalignant osseous tumor of soft tissue. J. Bone Jt. Surg. **51**, 654–663 (1969)

CLASSEN, K.L., WIEDERANDERS, R.E., HERRINGTON, J.L.: Heterotopic bone formation developing in abdominal scars. Surgery **47**, 918–923 (1960)

CODDINGTON, R.C.: Neurogenic ossifying fibromyositis in paraplegia. J. Indiana med. Ass. **54**, 484–487 (1961)

DEUTSCH, I.: Myositis ossificans: a complication of tetanus. Clin. Radiol. **22**, 1035 (1971)

DICKERSON, R.C.: Myositis ossificans in early childhood. Report of an unusual case. Clin. Orthop. **79**, 42–43 (1972)

ELLIS, M., FRANK, H.G.: Myositis ossificans traumatica: with special reference to the quadriceps femoris muscle. J. Trauma **6**, 724–738 (1966)

FENNI-PEARSE, D., OLOWU, A.O.: Myositis ossificans—a complication of tetanus. Clin. Radiol. **22**, 89–92 (1971)

FINE, G., STOUT, A.P.: Osteogenic sarcoma of extraskeletal soft tissues. Cancer (Philad.) **9**, 1027 (1956)

FLETCHER, E., MOSS, M.S.: Myositis ossificans progressiva. Ann. rheum. Dis. **24**, 267–272 (1965)

FLYNN, J.E., GRAHAM, J.H.: Myositis ossificans. Surg. Gynec. Obstet. **118**, 1001–1005 (1964)

FREEMAN, R.H.: Myositis ossificans. Proc. roy. Soc. Med. **59**, 710–711 (1966)

GILMER, W.S., ANDERSON, L.D.: Reactions of soft somatic tissue which may progress to bone formation: circumscribed (traumatic) myositis ossificans. Sth. med. J. **52**, 1432–1438 (1959)

GOLDMAN, A.B., BRAUNSTEIN, P.: Personal experience (1975)

GRISWOLD, M.L., JR.: Extra articular bone formation as a burn complication. Plast. reconstr. Surg. **32**, 544–548 (1963)

GWINN, J.L.: Radiological case of the month. Progressive myositis ossificans. Amer. J. Dis. Child. **116**, 655–656 (1968)

HAIT, G., BOSWICK, J.A., STONE, N.H.: Heterotopic bone formation secondary to trauma. J. Trauma **10**, 405–411 (1970)

HEUL, R.O. VAN DER, RONNEN, J.R. VON: Juxtacortical osteosarcoma, diagnosis, differential diagnosis: an analysis of 80 cases. J. Bone Jt. Surg. **49**, 415–439 (1967)

HOUGHSTON, J.C., WHATLEY, G.S., STONE, M.M.: Myositis ossificans traumatica (myo-osteosis). Sth. med. J. **55**, 1167–1170 (1962)

HUTCHESON, J., KLATTE, E.C., KREMP, R.: The angiographic appearance of myositis ossificans circumscripta. A case report. Radiology **102**, 57–58 (1972)

ILLINGWORTH, R.S.: Myositis ossificans progressiva (Munchmeyer's disease). Brief review with report of 2 cases treated with corticosteroids and observed for 16 years. Arch. Dis. Child. **46**, 264–268 (1971)

JEFFREYS, T.E., STILES, P.J.: Pseudomalignant osseous tumor of soft tissue. J. Bone Jt. Surg. **48**, 488 (1966)

KALES, A.N., PHANG, J.M.: Dietary calcium perturbances in patients with abnormal calcium deposition. J. clin. Endocr. **31**, 204–212 (1970)

KAMMERMAN, S.: Personal communication (1975)

KATZ, S.: Bone formation in abdominal scars. G.P. **35**, 119 (1967)

KNAPP, M.E.: Late treatment of fractures and complications. Postgrad. Med. **40**, 113–118 (1966)

LETTS, R.M.: Myositis ossificans progressiva: a report of two cases with chromosome studies. Canad. med. Ass. J. **99**, 856–862 (1968)

LETTS, R.M.: Myositis ossificans progressiva. Canad. med. Ass. J. **100**, 133 (1969)

LIBERMAN, U.A., BARZEL, U., DEVRIES, A., ELLIS, H.: Myositis ossificans traumatica Ca^{++} PO_4 = manganese excretion. Amer. J. med. Sci. **254**, 35–47 (1967)

LUDMAN, H., HAMILTON, E.B.D., EADE, A.W.T.: Deafness in myositis ossificans progressive. J. Laryng. **82**, 57–63 (1968)

LUDWAK, L.: Myositis ossificans progressiva. Mineral, metabolic and radioactive calcium studies of the effects of hormones. Amer. J. Med. **37**, 269–293 (1964)

MCKUSICK, V.A.: Fibrodysplasia ossificans progressiva. In: Hereditable Disorders of Connective Tissue. St. Louis: C.V. Mosby Co., 1960

MOHAN, K.: Myositis ossificans traumatica of the elbow. Int. Surg. **57**, 475–478 (1972)

MUNCHMEYER: As sited by ILLINGWORTH, R.S.: Myositis ossificans progressiva (Munchmeyer's disease). Brief review with report of 2 cases treated with corticosteroids and observed for 16 years. Arch. Dis. Child. **46**, 264–268 (1971)

NOBLE, T.P.: Myositis ossificans. A clinical and radiological study. Surg. Gynec. Obstet. **39**, 795–802 (1924)

NORMAN, A., DORFMAN, H.D.: Juxtacortical circumscribed myositis ossificans: evolution and radiographic features. Radiology **96**, 301–306 (1970)

PATERSON, D.C.: Myositis ossificans circumscripta. Report of four cases without a history of injury. J. Bone Jt. Surg. **52**, 296–301 (1970)

PATIN, G.: as sited by ILLINGWORTH, R.S.: Myositis ossificans progressiva (Munchmeyer's disease). Brief review with report of 2 cases treated with corticosteroids and observed for 16 years. Arch. Dis. Child. **46**, 264–268 (1971)

PITTS, N.C.: Myositis ossificans as a complication of tetanus. JAMA **189**, 237–239 (1964)

RUSSELL, R.G., SMITH, R., BISHOP, M.C., PRICE, D.A.: Treatment of myositis ossificans progressiva with a diphosphonate. Lancet **1**, 10–11 (1972)

Shanoff, L.B., Spira, M., Hardy, S.B.: Myositis ossificans: evolution to osteogenic sarcoma. Report of a histologically verified case. Amer. J. Surg. **113**, 537–541 (1967)

Shea, T.E.: Calcified soft tissue mass in the medical aspect of the thigh. JAMA **200**, 1050–1052 (1967)

Simpson, A.J., Friedman, S.: Myositis ossificans progressiva. Mt. Sinai J. Med. **38**, 416–422 (1971)

Skajaa, T.: Myositis ossificans. Acta chir. scand. **116**, 68–72 (1958)

Smith, D.M., Zeman, W., Johnston, C.C., Deiss, W.P.: Myositis ossificans progressiva. Case report with metabolic and histochemical studies. Metabolism **15**, 521–528 (1966)

Spjut, H.J., Dorfman, H.D., Fechner, R.E., Ackerman, L.V.: Tumors of Bone and Cartilege, second series. Washington D.C.: Armed Forces Institute of Pathology (1970)

Thompson, N.C. III, Garcia, A.: Myositis ossificans: aftermath of elbow injuries. Clin. Orthop. **50**, 129–134 (1967)

Venerables, C.: An unusual case of myositis ossificans. Proc. roy. Soc. Med. **60**, 5 (1967)

Yoslow, W., Becker, M.H.: Osseous bridges between the transverse processes of the lumbar spine. J. Bone Jt. Surg. **50**, 513–520 (1968)

Zaccaline, P.S., Urist, M.R.: Traumatic periosteal proliferation in rabbits. The enigma of experimental myositis ossificans traumatica. J. Trauma **4**, 344–357 (1964)

Brown Tumors

Aegerter, E.E., Kirkpatrick, J.A.: Orthopedic Diseases: Physiology, Pathology, Radiology. 3rd ed. Philadelphia: W.B. Saunders, 1968

Albright, F.C., Reifenstein, E.C.: The Parathyroid Glands and Metabolic Bone Disease. Baltimore: Williams and Wilkins, 1948

Anderson, W.A.D.: Pathology. 5th ed. St. Louis: C.V. Mosby Co. 1966

Askanazy, M.: Über Ostitis deformans ohne osteides Gewebe. Arch. path. Anat. Inst. Tübingen **4**, 398–422 (1904)

Aub, J.C., Fairhall, L.T., Minot, A.S., Reznikoff, P.: Lead poisoning. Medicine **4**, 1–250 (1925)

Black, B.M.: Hyperparathyroidism. Springfield, Ill.: Charles C. Thomas, 1953

Camp, J.D.: Osseous changes in hyperparathyroidism. A roentgenographic study. J. Amer. med. Ass. **99**, 1913–1917 (1932)

Camp, J.D., Ochsner, H.C.: The osseous changes in hyperparathyroidism associated with parathyroid tumor: a roentgenologic study. Radiology **17**, 63–69 (1931)

Castleman, B., Mallory, T.B.: Pathology of parathyroid gland in hyperparathyroidism; study of 25 cases. Amer. J. Path. **11**, 1–72 (1935)

Collip, J.B.: The extraction of a parathyroid hormone which will prevent or control parathyroid tetany and which regulates the level of blood calcium. J. biol. Chem. **63**, 395–438 (1925)

Collip, J.B.: The parathyroid glands. Medicine **5**, 1–57 (1926)

Cope, O.: The story of hyperparathyroidism at the Massachusetts General Hospital. New Engl. J. Med. **274**, 1174–1182 (1966)

Dent, C.E.: Metabolic bone disease, radiology of hyperparathyroidism, osteomalacia, and osteoporosis. Presented at the second refresher course on skeletal disorders, London (1975)

Edeiken, J., Hodes, P.J.: Roentgen Diagnosis of Diseases of Bone, 2nd ed. Baltimore: Williams and Wilkens 1973

Ellis, K., Hochstim, R.J.: The skull in hyperparathyroidism bone disease. Amer. J. Roentgenol. **83**, 732–743 (1960)

Erdheim, J.: Über Epithelkörperbefunde bei Osteomalacie. S.-B. Akad. Wiss. Wien, math.-nat. Kl. **116**, 311–370 (1907)

Frame, B., Foroozanfar, F., Patton, R.B.: Normocalcemic primary hyperparathyroidism with osteitis fibrosa. Ann. intern. Med. **73**, 253–257 (1970)

Friedenberg, R.M., Sayegh, V.: Advanced skeletal changes in hyperparathyroidism. Amer. J. Roentgenol. **83**, 743–747 (1960)

Heath, D.A., Wills, M.R.: Normocalcemic primary hyperparathyroidism with osteitis fibrosa. Postgrad. med. J. **47**, 815–817 (1971)

Hellstrom, J.: Experience from 105 cases of hyperparathyroidism. Acta chir. scand. **113**, 501–505 (1957)

Hunter, D., Turnbull, H.M.: Hyperparathyroidism: generalized osteitis fibrosa. Brit. J. Surg. **31**, 213–284 (1931)

Lloyd, H.M.: Calcification of primary hyperparathyroidism. Ann. intern. Med. **74**, 798–799 (1971)

Luck, V.J.: Bone and Joint Diseases. Springfield, Ill.: Charles C. Thomas 1950

Mandl, F.: Klinisches und Experimentelles zur Frage der lokalisierten und generalisierten Ostitis fibrosa. Arch. klin. Chir. **143**, 1–46 (1926)

Mandl, F.: Zur Technik der Parathyreoidektomie bei Ostitis fibrosa aufgrund neuer Beobachtungen. Dtsch Z. Chir. **240**, 362–375 (1933)

McLean, F.C.: Ultrastructure and function of bone. Science **127**, 451–456 (1958)

McLean, F.C., Urist, M.R.: Bone: An Introduction to the Physiology of Skeletal Tissue. Chicago: University of Chicago, Press 1955

Meema, H.E., Oreopoulos, D.G., Rabinovich, H.H., Rapoport, A.: Periosteal new bone formation in renal osteodystrophy. Relationship to osteosclerosis, osteitis fibrosa, and osteoid excess. Radiology **110**, 513–522 (1974)

Melvin, K.E.W.: Clinicopathological excercises. Case 50. New Engl. J. Med. **285**, 1422–1429 (1971)

Pugh, D.G.: Roentgenographic Diagnosis of Diseases of Bone. In: R. Golden Diagnostic Roentgenology. Baltimore: Williams and Wilkens, Vol. II, 1952

PUGH, D.G.: The roentgenographic diagnosis of hyperparathyroidism. Surg. Clin. N. Amer. **32**, 1017–1030 (1958)

RECKLINGHAUSEN, F.D. VON: Die Fibrose oder deformierende Ostitis, die Osteomalacie und die osteoplastische Carcinose in ihren gegenseitigen Beziehungen. Festschr. Rudolf Virchow 1–89 (1891)

ROWLANDS, B.C.: Hyperparathyroidism: an early historical survey. Ann. roy. Coll. Surg. Engl. **51**, 81–90 (1972)

SANDSTROM, I.: Om en ny kortel hos menniskan och atskilliga daggdjur. Upsla Ladaref. Forh. **15**, 441–471 (1880)

SPJUT, H.J., DORFMAN, H.D., FECHNER, R.E., ACKERMAN, L.V.: Tumors of Bone and Cartilege. Armed Forces Institute of Pathology, Washington, D.C., second series (1971)

STEINBACH, H.L., GORDON, G.S., EISENBERG, E.,

CRANE, J.T., SILBERMAN, S., GOLDMAN, L.: Primary hyperparathyroidism: a correlation of roentgen, clinical and pathologic features. Amer. J. Roentgenol. **86**, 329–343 (1961)

STRAUSS, M.B.: Clinicopathological exercises. Case 15. New Engl. J. Med. **282**, 799–806 (1970)

TSENG, T.C., NATHAN, M.H.: Primary hyperparathyroidism: Amer. J. Roentgenol. **83**, 716–731 (1960)

WANG, C.A., MILLER, L.M., WEBER, A.L., KRANE, S.M.: Pseudogout. A diagnostic clue to hyperparathyroidism. Amer. J. Surg. **117**, 558–565 (1969)

WATSON, L.: Endocrine bone disease. Practitioner **210**, 376–383 (1973)

WOOLNER, L.B., KEATING, F.R., BLACK, B.M.: Tumors and hyperplasia of the parathyroid glands; review of pathological findings in 140 cases of primary hyperparathyroidism. Cancer (Philad.) **5**, 1069–1088 (1952)

Metastatic Bone Disease

by

Jerry P. Petasnick

A. Incidence

Metastatic cancer is the most common malignant tumor of bone and the skeleton is one of the most common sites of metastatic disease. The incidence of skeletal metastases is greatly underestimated as most lesions are clinically silent and escape detection until pain, pathologic fracture, soft tissue mass or neurologic symptoms occur. Roentgenologic surveys may reveal a number of unsuspected lesions, however, there are inherent limitations in the roentgenographic examination and the full extent of skeletal involvement may not be appreciated. The reported frequency of skeletal metastases varies widely depending on the duration and stage of disease in the population sampled as well as on the manner and extent of sampling (ABRAMS et al., 1950; JOHNSTON, 1970; WARREN and MEISSNER, 1966). The actual incidence and distribution of skeletal metastases can be made only after careful study of many bones in cases which have run their full course. The more thoroughly one investigates the bones at autopsy the greater the probability that skeletal metastases will be found. JAFFE (1958) has stated that the overall chance of finding skeletal metastases in patients dying of a malignant neoplasm is 70% if the bones are adequately sampled. In those patients with carcinomas that commonly metastasize to bone such as breast, lung, or prostate, the chance of finding skeletal metastases will approximate 85%.

Any malignant tumor is potentially liable to metastasize to the skeleton, however, the great majority of skeletal metastases are from carcinomas of the breast, lung, prostate, kidney, and gastrointestinal tract (DELCLOS, 1965; JOHNSTON, 1970; LODWICK, 1965; WARREN and MEISSNER, 1966). LODWICK (1965) estimated that these sources account for 80% of all metastatic disease. Although metastases from soft tissue sarcomas are unusual, primary bone sarcomas metastasize to the skeletal system at a surprisingly high rate (MCNEIL et al., 1973). In children, neuroblastoma is the most frequent source of bone metastases, however, osteosarcoma, Ewing's sarcoma, retinoblastoma, and embryonal rhabdomyosarcoma may also give rise to skeletal lesions (CAFFEY, 1973).

Certain tumors have a definite predilection to involve bone. The incidence of skeletal metastases from carcinoma of the breast has been variously reported as 49% (WARREN and MEISSNER, 1966), 57% (JOHNSTON, 1970) and 74% (ABRAMS et al., 1950). Similar figures for carcinoma of the lung are 23% (WARREN and MEISSNER, 1966), 44% (JOHNSTON, 1970) and 32% (ABRAMS et al., 1950). At autopsy, skeletal metastases have been found in 55% of patients with carcinoma of the prostate (JOHNSTON, 1970) and 32% of patients with carcinoma of the kidney (WARREN and MEISSNER, 1966). Cancers least likely to metastasize to bone originate in the rectosigmoid colon, pancreas, cervix, stomach, or head and neck region (Johnston, 1970; Warren and Meissner, 1966). Although carcinoma of the thyroid is frequently included with those tumors having a high incidence of bone metastases, Warren and Meissner (1966) found skeletal metastases in only 14% of patients with carcinoma of the thyroid coming to autopsy.

B. Localization

The most common sites of involvement in metastatic disease are those parts of the skeleton which are important in hematopoietic function. In order of frequency, skeletal metastases localize in the vertebral column, particularly the lumbosacral region, pelvis, proximal femur, skull, ribs, and proximal humerus (Copeland, 1970). Metastases distal to the knee or elbow are rare, however, half of those encountered in the hands or feet are from carcinoma of the lung (Kerin, 1958; Trachtenberg and Roswit, 1961). When vertebral metastases from all primary sites are considered together, the thoracic region is most often affected followed by the lumbar region. However, for carcinoma of the prostate, the sites of predilection are the lumbar and sacral regions (Jaffe, 1958).

Metastatic disease generally affects multiple sites. Lodwick (1965) found this to be true in 75% of patients evaluated roentgenographically while Johnston (1970) found that only 9% of autopsied patients with skeletal metastases had solitary lesions.

C. Method of Diagnosis

I. Clinical Evaluation

Pain and pathologic fracture are the most common presenting complaints in metastatic disease. The development of "bone pain" is significant in patients with cancer and usually indicates the presence of skeletal metastases. Ariel and Lehman (1965) noted that roentgenographic evidence of metastases was present within 1 month in 49% of patients with carcinoma of the breast and within 6 months in 90%. Pathologic fractures occur most often with metastases from carcinoma of the breast, lung, or prostate (Parrish, 1965). Clinical evidence of suspected bone involvement often precedes the roentgenographic appearance of metastases by several months, however, bone lesions may be present without giving rise to clinical complaints and in some instances may be the first sign of neoplastic disease (Chute et al., 1958; Jaffe, 1958; Legier and Tauber, 1968; Sherman and Ivker, 1950; Sherman and Pearson, 1948). Solitary metastases frequently mimic primary bone tumors and differentiation from nonneoplastic diseases such as Paget's disease, fibrous dysplasia, and hyperparathyroidism may be difficult. Examination of a biopsy specimen from the presenting lesion usually resolves the problem and in many cases provides a diagnosis as to the primary lesion. Occasionally the primary tumor is clinically obscure at the time of death and in rare occasions may not be found at autopsy. Secondary deposits may lie quiescent within bone for years and it is not unusual to find metastases manifesting themselves many years after a radical mastectomy for breast cancer (AEGERTER and KIRKPATRICK, 1968), or nephrectomy for carcinoma of the kidney (AGGARWAL et al., 1972).

Alterations in the serum levels of acid and alkaline phosphatase, although unreliable, have been used as indices of metastatic bone disease. Elevation of alkaline phosphatase occurs as a result of osteoblastic activity regardless of the etiology. Metastatic bone disease would be expected to produce an increase in alkaline phosphatase levels, however, similar increases are seen in Paget's disease and metabolic bone diseases characterized by increased osteoblastic activity. Alkaline phosphatase levels are also increased as a result of liver disease or biliary obstruction.

Elevation in the serum acid phosphatase level was initially thought to indicate the presence of metastatic carcinoma of the prostate (GUTMAN et al., 1936). Acid phosphatases have been described in highest concentration in the cells and secretions of the prostate, however, they are also found in erythrocytes, liver, kidney, spleen, pancreas, bile, bone, and urine (DOE and SEAL, 1965; LEPOW et al., 1962). Methods are available to separate the prostatic and erythrocytic fractions, however, the serum level of acid phosphatase is unreliable as an index of skeletal metastasis in carcinoma of the prostate. It is claimed that an elevation in serum acid phosphatase is indicative of extension beyond the prostatic capsule, however, the correlation is far from perfect. Undifferentiated cell types may be incapable of acid phosphatase production and chance extension into a venous channel may give a false elevation in serum levels. DOE and SEAL (1965), in a review of the literature, noted that approximately 20% of patients with roentgenographically demonstrable metastases had normal serum acid phosphatase levels whereas approximately 30% of patients with normal roentgenographic surveys had elevated serum acid phosphatase levels. LONDON et al. (1954) similarly noted the high incidence of normal values in patients with skeletal metastases and postulated that substances normally present in the serum inhibit the prostatic acid phosphatase with resultant false negative normal values. Serum levels may be elevated in many other diseases as a result of destruction or impairment of tissues rich in acid phosphatase or as a result of impaired secretion of the enzyme because of intrahepatic or extrahepatic biliary obstruction (DOE and SEAL, 1965; LEPOW et al., 1962).

II. Roentgenographic Examination

Roentgenologic evaluation of the skeleton has been widely used as a means of detecting skeletal metastases, however, this does not provide an accurate index of the incidence or extent of metastatic disease. Roentgenographic examinations may be normal in spite of extensive osseous involvement and widespread metastases, particularly in the spine, may not be detected even on roentgenograms obtained shortly before death (BACHMAN and SPROUL, 1955; BORAK, 1942; YOUNG and FUNK, 1953). Where roentgenographic findings are present, the extent of skeletal involvement may not be appreciated. Roentgenographic surveys are a relatively insensitive technique for detecting early bone metastases as numerous reports have indicated that marrow aspiration may demonstrate tumor cells prior to the roentgenographic appearance of skeletal metastases (FINKELSTEIN et al., 1970; FLOCKS, 1963; HANSEN et al., 1971; MENDOZA et al., 1969; NELSON et al., 1973). SLAGER and REILLY (1967) found marrow involvement in 41 of 410 patients with histologically proven cancer subjected to routine marrow aspiration in the course of their workup. Of these patients, 16 (39%) had normal roentgenographic examinations at the time of marrow aspiration. Although a large number of patients with carcinoma of the breast eventually develop metastatic disease, GIBBONS et al. (1961) found that fewer than 2%

of patients with operable tumors had roentgenographic evidence of bone involvement on skeletal surveys taken within 6 weeks of a radical mastectomy in spite of the fact that 35% of these patients had positive axillary nodes. The overall incidence of marrow involvement in reported series ranges from 7 to 14%, however, in carcinoma of the breast the reported incidence has been as high as 29% (MENDOZA et al., 1969). This latter series includes all stages of disease, however, the majority of patients had advanced disease with metastases. HANSEN et al. (1971) found marrow involvement in 14% of patients with unresectable carcinoma of the lung. Roentgenographic evidence was present in only 1 of 14 patients with positive marrow findings. Although the overall incidence of marrow involvement was 14%, the incidence in oat cell carcinoma was 45%. In children, FINKELSTEIN et al. (1970) found malignant cells in the marrow in 49 of 90 patients with neuroblastoma, 5 of 25 with embryonal rhabdomyosarcoma and 3 of 13 with retinoblastoma. MENDOZA et al. (1969) have demonstrated a pronounced shortening of the survival time in patients with carcinoma of the breast or lung who had tumor cells in the bone marrow at the time the primary tumor was diagnosed. These findings emphasize the difficulty in staging patients by roentgenographic examination alone.

III. Bone Scanning

Bone scanning as currently employed has resulted in earlier detection of skeletal metastases and has proven to be the best method of determining the extent and distribution of bone involvement at varying stages of disease. Bone scans have demonstrated that a significant number of patients with early carcinoma of the breast may have metastases at the time of surgery. GALASKO (1971) found that 24% of patients with early carcinoma of the breast had positive Fluorine-18 scans but negative roentgenographic surveys. In patients with advanced carcinoma of the breast, 84% of patients had positive scans while only 68% had roentgenographic evidence of skeletal disease. In 28% of the patients additional lesions not seen on roentgenographic examination were detected on Fluorine-18 scans.

The bone scan is capable of detecting reactive osteoid before roentgenographic changes occur since the scan reflects the rate of new bone formation whereas the roentgenogram depicts cumulative concentration (CHARKES, 1972). In most large series of patients with metastatic bone disease studied by both techniques the frequency of bone lesions visualized by scanning but not by roentgenography ranges between 14 and 34% (CHARKES, 1972). The initial clinical studies with ^{85}Sr indicated a high percentage of positive scans in histologically or roentgenologically proven metastases (CHARKES and SKLAROFF, 1964; CHARKES et al., 1966). Fluorine-18 and ^{99m}Tc-polyphosphonate have increased the accuracy of bone scanning and have provided the major impetus for its routine use in the evaluation of patients with suspected or proven malignant neoplasms (HARMER et al., 1969; HOPKINS et al., 1972; PENDERGRASS et al., 1973; SILBERSTEIN et al., 1973).

The detection of metastases by bone scan depends upon the preferential incorporation of the scanning agent into the crystalline matrix. Increased activity is a reflection of increased metabolic activity. Consequently, bone production is detected before it is evident roentgenographically. Although the distribution of bone involvement is best evaluated by bone scan, this must be supplemented by roentgenographic examinations since any process in which there is bone production such as Paget's disease, osteomyelitis or healing fracture will produce a positive scan. In some cases rapidly growing metastases may not be detected on scans since the lesions are growing too rapidly to produce new bone (BECKER and SCHWARTZ, 1973; HARMER et al., 1969; HOPKINS et al., 1972).

Retrospective evaluation of the roentgen examination and use of pleurodirectional tomography may result in identification of metastases at sites initially interpreted as normal.

CHARKES et al. (1966) have compared the histologic changes with the findings on ^{85}Sr scans. They found a high degree of correlation between ^{85}Sr deposition and the presence of immature reactive bone. Initially the scan would be expected to be positive while the roentgenographic findings are minimal. As the bone matures and osteoid seams become mineralized the osteoblastic changes appear roentgenographically. The fully mineralized bone takes up little additional ^{85}Sr despite its great density on roentgenograms and the scan at this time could be negative in spite of the presence of extensive osteoblastic metastases. The ^{85}Sr scan correlates well with the histologic activity of the bone lesion. Areas of tumor growth may give rise to pain and hot scans despite normal roentgenograms, whereas, older, quiescent lesions may appear normal on scan but radiodense. As has been pointed out, false-positives may occur with any process in which there is increased bone metabolic activity or increase in reactive new bone formation. Similarly, false-negative examinations may also occur when there is no reactive bone formation.

D. Mechanisms of Metastasis

The location of skeletal metastases is influenced by the manner of extension, filtering barriers encountered by the tumor cells, the status of the capillary bed receiving the tumor cells, and the variations in the growth potentials of primary tumors (COPELAND, 1970). Cancer cells metastasize to bone almost exclusively by the hematogenous route. The lymphatic system is of little importance in transporting tumor cells to bone since the marrow is relatively devoid of lymphatic channels, however, tumor cells may spread to the periosteum by lymphatic extension and then into the adjacent bone by direct extension. Where such extension occurs, bones near the primary site have a higher incidence of involvement.

Extension of tumor via the hematogenous route is usually the result of invasion of draining venous channels with resultant spread to the first capillary bed. Tumor cells are usually arrested in the vascular network of the first organ encountered, however, experiments with transplanted tumors indicate that some tumor cells may pass through the liver, lungs, kidney, or spleen without being arrested (ZEIDMAN, 1957). The mechanisms involved in the passage of tumor cells through the vascular beds or organs is not known, however, the demonstration that tumor emboli may pass through organs is of clinical interest in explaining unusual distribution of metastases. It may also explain the observation that patients with bony metastases are often free of visceral metastases and vice versa.

Sites of metastatic involvement are not determined solely by blood flow. If this were true, the kidney, which is more richly perfused than other organs, would be expected to have the highest incidence of metastases, whereas, the frequency of renal metastases is disproportionately low (ABRAMS et al., 1950; WARREN and MEISSNER, 1966). Similarly, one would expect areas in the bone with increased vascularity such as Paget's disease to have a higher incidence of metastases. Although Paget's disease occurs in the same age distribution as metastatic disease, there does not appear to be an increased incidence of metastatic disease in areas of Paget's disease.

Tumor emboli may be deposited anywhere within bone, but the hematopoietic marrow appears to be the most fertile for survival and growth. The morphologic pattern of the skeletal vasculature partially explains the high incidence of bone metastasis relative to the low percentage distribution of cardiac output and provides an understanding of the preferential localization of metastasis to the red or hematopoietic marrow (Turner and Jaffe, 1940). The peripherally directed branches of the nutrient artery subdivide into capillaries as they near the endosteal margin of bone. The capillaries, in turn, are continuous with a rich sinusoidal system that communicates with the central veins. The capacity of these venous and sinusoidal channels is 6–8 times that of the osseous arterial system making them more vulnerable to metastases (Johnston, 1970). This vulnerability is further reinforced by the pattern of venous return which is subjected to reflux with muscle contraction thereby providing a system in long bones very much like Batson's vertebral plexus (Batson, 1940).

Hematogenous skeletal metastases may occur as the result of tumor embolization via the vertebral venous plexus which consists of a network of valveless veins surrounding the lumbar vertebrae with connections to the brain, abdominal wall, and extremities (Batson, 1940, 1942). There are also connections with the inferior and superior vena cava allowing tumor emboli to seed directly into the skeleton bypassing the liver and lungs. The prostatic venous plexus drains into the vertebral plexus explaining the frequency with which prostatic cancer involves the spine when it metastasizes. Skeletal metastases probably occur most often as a result of spread via the vertebral venous system, however, tumors may also spread via the arterial system. This may result from passage of tumor cells through the lung capillary bed or invasion of a lung tumor into the pulmonary veins. Such tumor cell emboli may lodge in bones of the axial skeleton or extremities.

E. Roentgenographic Diagnosis

Metastatic lesions can be subdivided into osteolytic, osteoblastic or mixed types depending on whether the dominant roentgenographic appearance is the result of bone destruction, bone production, or a combination of the two. When the dominant process is bone destruction, metastases present roentgenographically as osteolytic lesions when there has been sufficient destruction of the trabeculae and/or cortex to allow detection of the lesion. Osteoblastic metastases are indicative of repair irrespective of the site of origin of the primary tumor and appear roentgenographically as areas of increased density as a result of trabecular and subperiosteal new bone formation. The designation of metastatic disease as predominantly osteolytic or osteoblastic may help in predicting the possible site of the primary tumor, however, any malignant tumor is potentially liable to metastasize to the skeleton and produce lesions that are purely lytic, blastic or mixed.

The roentgenographic appearance of skeletal metastases is too varied to permit the formulation of any comprehensive description. The diagnosis of metastatic disease is usually simple when multiple lesions are present, however, since the roentgenographic patterns produced by metastatic and primary tumors are similar it may be difficult to clearly distinguish a solitary metastasis from a primary malignant bone tumor. Furthermore, since the manner in which bone can react is limited, similar roentgenographic patterns may be found with metastases from any primary tumor.

I. Patterns of Destruction

The majority of skeletal metastases are predominantly destructive (JAFFE, 1958; MILCH and CHANGUS, 1956). Osteolytic metastases present roentgenographically as solitary or multiple areas of destruction which generally reflect the aggressiveness of the primary tumor. The rate of growth is best characterized by three patterns of bone destruction; geographic, moth-eaten, and permeative (LODWICK, 1964, 1965). Each may occur alone in pure form or two or all three may be found together.

Geographic bone destruction is characterized by a relatively large, well-defined lucent defect with clearly delineated edges (LODWICK, 1964). The destructive process begins in the spongiosa, however, no lesion is identified until there is destruction of sufficient trabeculae or until the cortex is involved. The rate of growth of these lesions is slow enough to allow time for complete destruction of bone to occur in the involved areas (Figs. 1–8). The sharpness of the edges is related to the rate of growth. Lesions with wide zones of transition between normal and abnormal bone (Figs. 4–6) have a more rapid rate of growth than lesions with sharply demarcated margins (Figs. 1–3).

Moth-eaten bone destruction indicates a moderately aggressive lesion and is characterized by multiple lucent areas of moderate size which tend to coalesce (LODWICK, 1964). The edges of the individual lesions are rarely punched out and are usually irregular and ill-defined (Figs. 9–13). This pattern reflects cortical involvement and is best appreciated in the diaphysis of long bones. The involved cortex may be totally destroyed or may appear scalloped (Fig. 10).

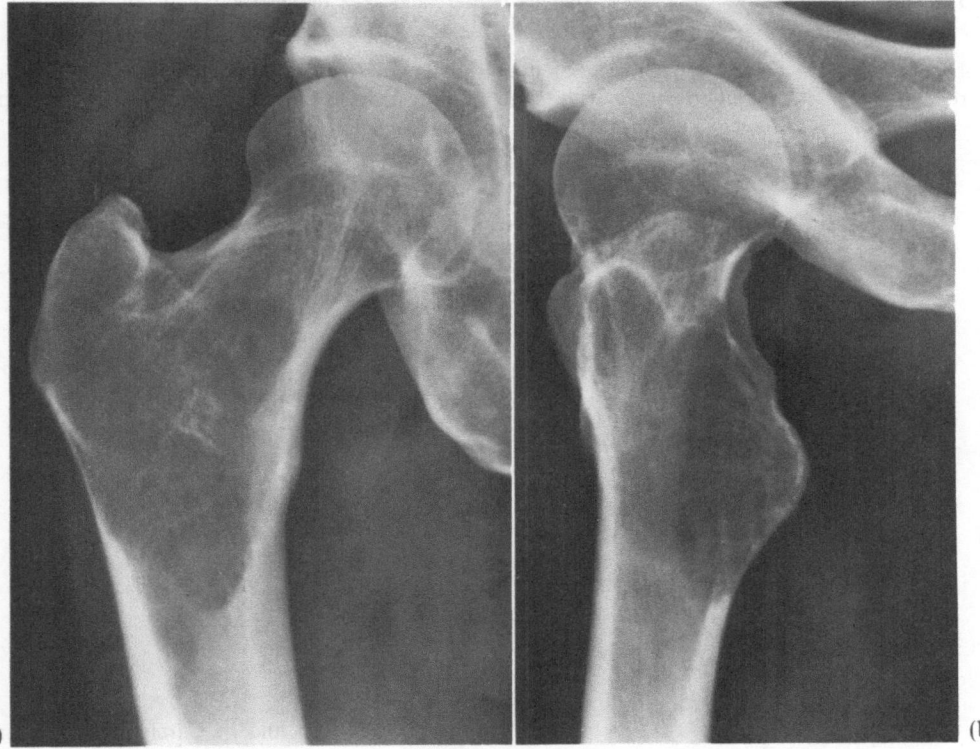

(a)   (b)

Fig. 1a and b. Carcinoma of lung. (a) and (b) demonstrate large, sharply demarcated area of destruction involving intertrochanteric region of femur. There is destruction of cortex, however, no periosteal reaction is identified. Coarse trabecular pattern identified on lateral projection (b) is produced by en face viewing of irregular cortical destruction

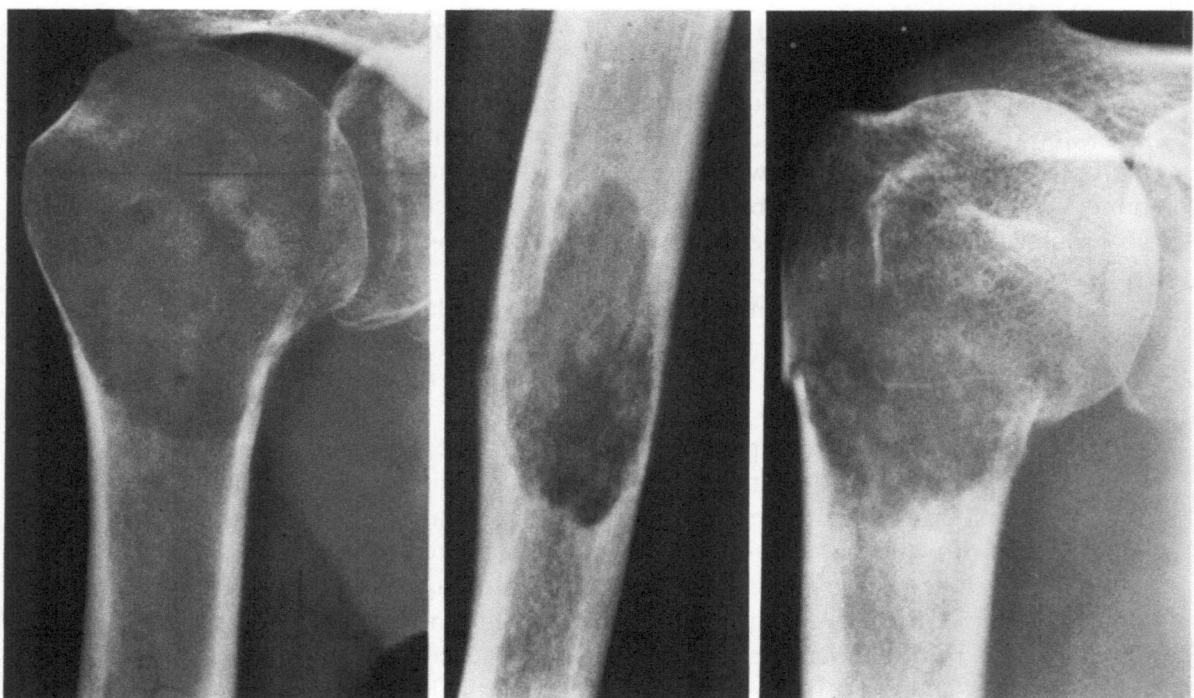

Fig. 2   Fig. 3   Fig. 4

Fig. 2. Ameloblastoma. Large, clearly demarcated area of destruction involving proximal humerus with cortical destruction identified superiorly in region of greater tuberosity

Fig. 3. Carcinoma of kidney. Elongated, sharply demarcated area of destruction in midshaft of left humerus with erosion of endosteal surface of cortex

Fig. 4. Carcinoma of kidney. Destructive lesion in proximal humerus with ill-defined margins. This is particularly apparent in distal end of lesion where wide zone of transition is identified between normal and abnormal bone. There is cortical destruction as well as pathologic fracture

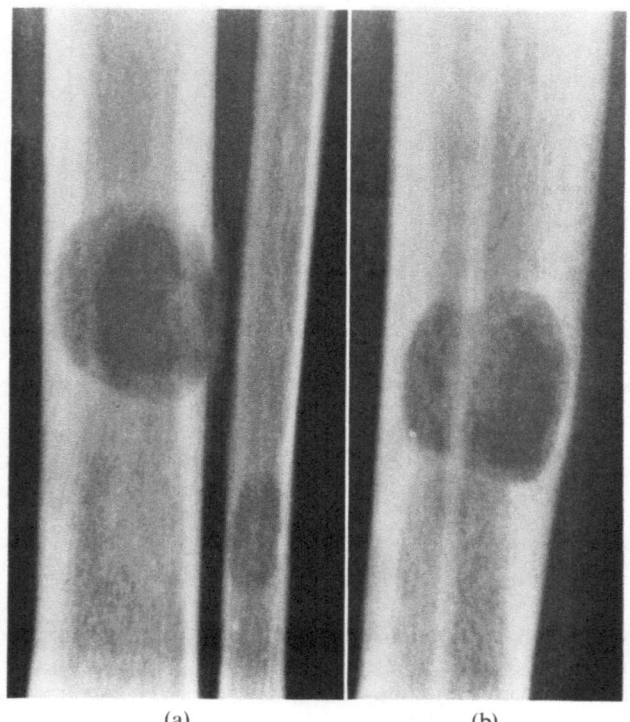

(a)   (b)

Fig. 5a and b. Carcinoma of breast. (a) and (b) demonstrate destructive lesions in diaphysis of tibia and fibula. Note wide zone of transition in tibial lesion. Laterally cortex is destroyed and there is minimal periosteal new bone formation. (Courtesy of Dr. JEROME BROSNAN, University of Chicago, Chicago Illinois)

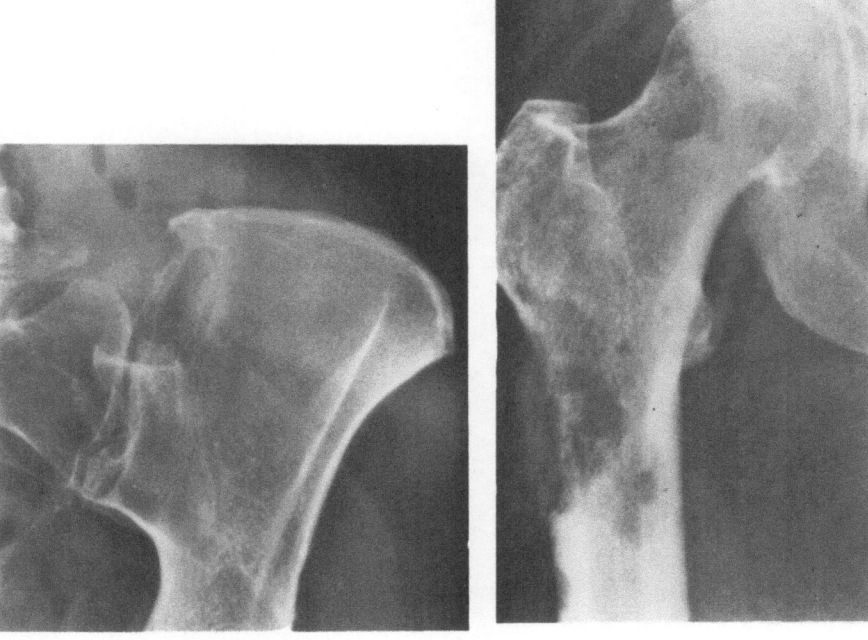

Fig. 6   Fig. 7

Fig. 6. Carcinoma of breast. Well-defined area of destruction with irregular margins in medial aspect of left ilium. There is destruction of cortex superiorly and wide zone of transition between lesion and normal bone

Fig. 7. Carcinoma of breast. Large destructive lesion in subtrochanteric region of femur with ill-defined margins and extensive cortical destruction. There is wide zone of transition between lesion and normal bone. Several smaller satellite lesions are present distally

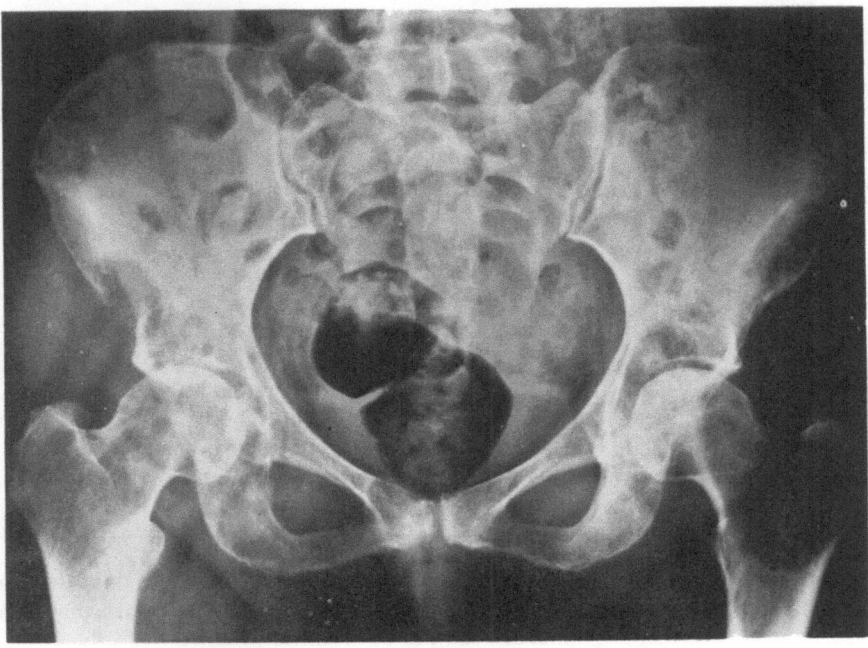

Fig. 8. Carcinoma of breast. Multiple large destructive lesions are present in pelvis and proximal femurs. Lesions have wide zones of transition and there is destruction of cortex. This is particularly apparent in lesion just above right acetabulum

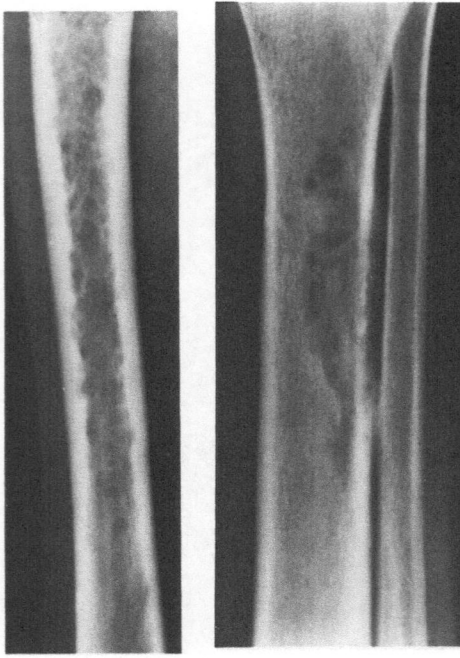

Fig. 9   Fig. 10

Fig. 9. Carcinoma of breast. Moth-eaten pattern of destruction characterized by multiple small radiolucent lesions in
femoral shaft. There is cortical involvement as reflected by
scalloped endosteal margins

Fig. 10. Carcinoma of breast. Multiple small confluent areas
of destruction are noted in distal tibia with involvement of
lateral cortex

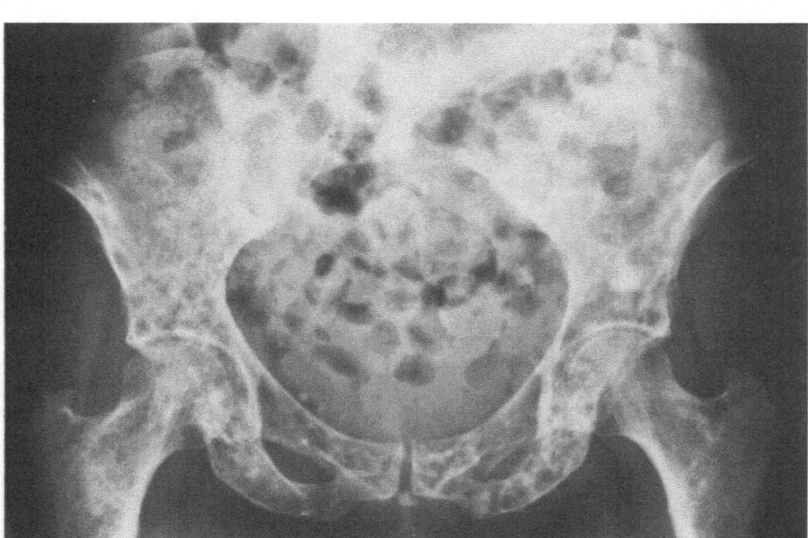

Fig. 11. Carcinoma of breast. There are multiple osteolytic lesions scattered throughout pelvis and proximal
femurs. Lesions are best indentified in superior and inferior pubic rami and proximal femoral shafts. Radio-dense
areas separate osteolytic lesions indicating presence of bony repair

Fig. 14a and b. Carcinoma of kidney. AP and lateral views of femoral shaft demonstrate permeative lesion
involving midshaft with extensive involvement of cortex. In spite of extensive destruction of cortex, cortical
margins can still be identified

Fig. 15a and b. Carcinoma of breast. AP and lateral views of left proximal femur demonstrate an extensive
permeative area of destruction in subtrochanteric region of left femur. Medially, on AP projection, there
is evidence of periosteal new bone formation at site of maximum cortical destruction

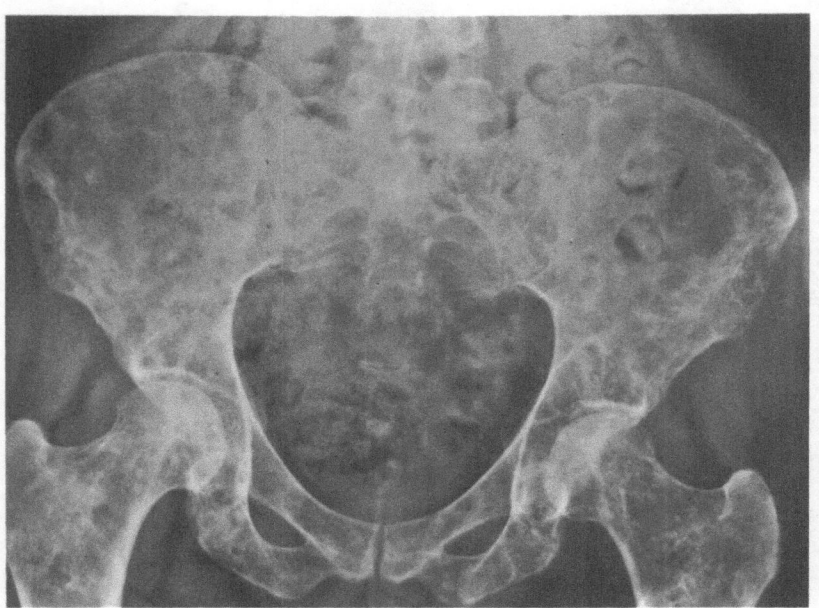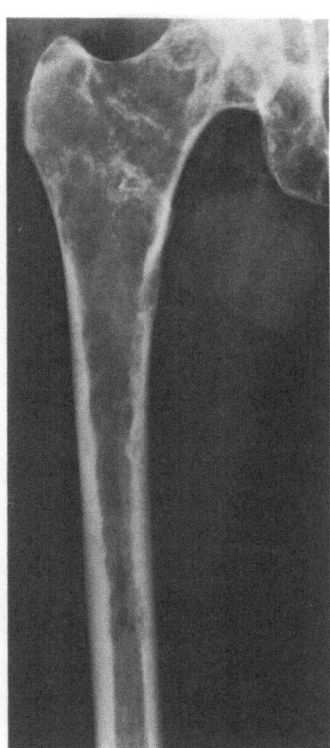

Fig. 12   Fig. 13

Fig. 12. Carcinoma of breast. There are multiple destructive lesions present in pelvis and proximal femurs. Margins are indistinct, making it difficult to clearly delineate lesions. Linear radio-dense areas lying between lesions probably represent areas of remaining normal bone although differentiation from osteoblastic metastases may be difficult

Fig. 13. Carcinoma of breast. Extensive destruction of femoral shaft with coalescence of lesions. There is complete loss of trabecular pattern in proximal femoral shaft and femoral neck, and endosteal surface of cortex is scalloped indicating cortical destruction

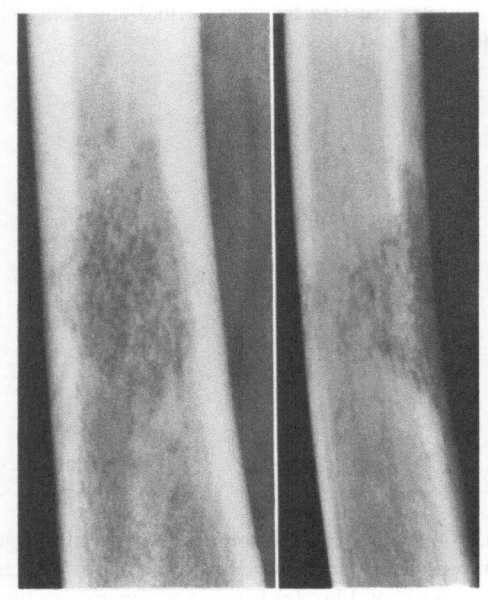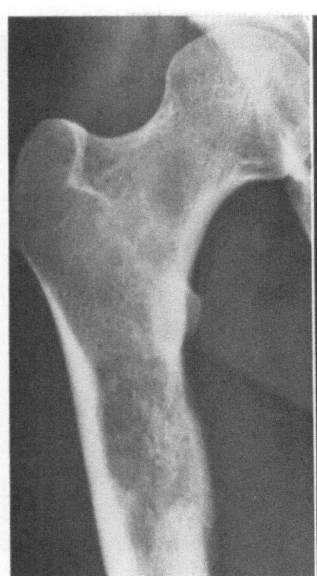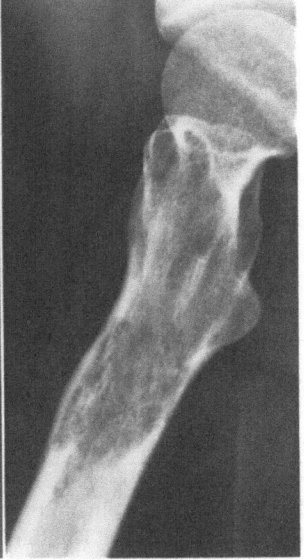

Fig. 14a   Fig. 14b   Fig. 15a   Fig. 15b

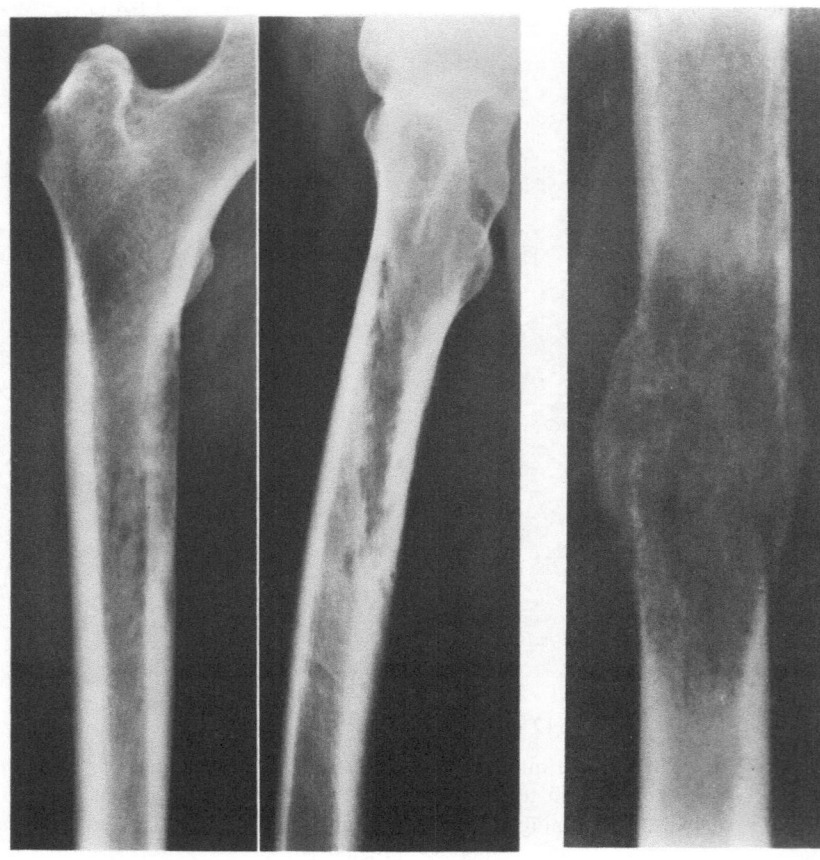

Fig. 16a   Fig. 16b   Fig. 17

Fig. 16a and b. Carcinoma of lung. AP and lateral projections demonstrate extensive destruction of proximal third of femoral shaft. Cortex is irregularly destroyed, however, endosteal margins are smooth, and cortex can still be delineated

Fig. 17. Malignant melanoma. Ill-defined destructive lesion with pathologic fracture in midshaft of humerus. There is extensive cortical destruction at midportion of lesion and demarcation between normal and abnormal bone is ill-defined

Fig. 20a–c. Carcinoma of breast. (a) Extensive permeative destruction of proximal femoral shaft with pathologic fracture. (b) and (c) Tomograms of proximal femoral shaft, more clearly delineate destruction of trabeculae and cortex. Extent of trabecular involvement was not appreciated on plain film, (a) because of superimposition of remaining normal trabeculae

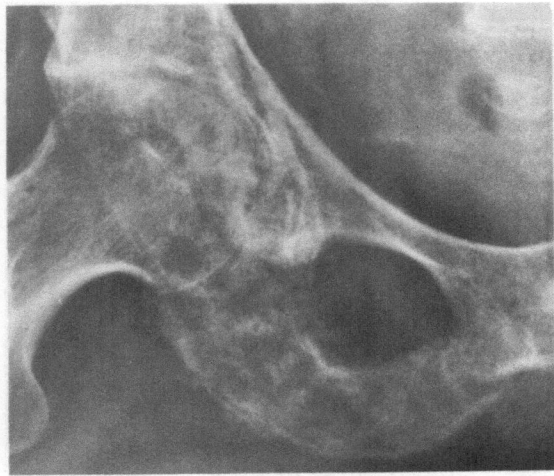

Fig. 18

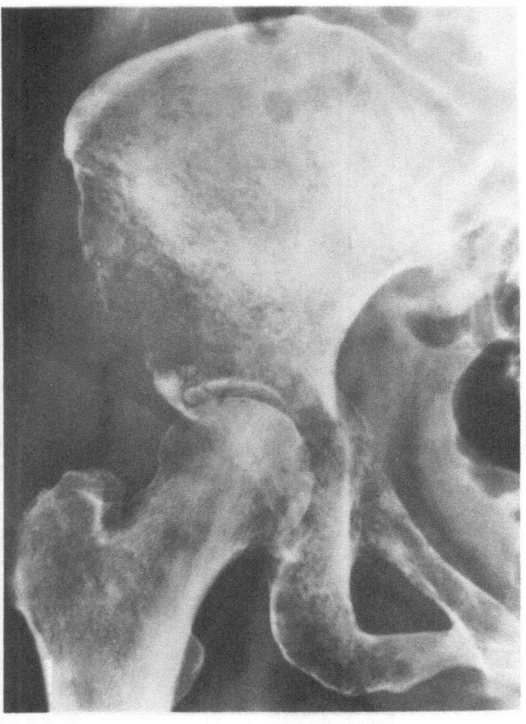

Fig. 18. Rhabdomyosarcoma. There is extensive destruction of permeative type involving inferior ramus of pubis and ischium. Cortex is destroyed and periosteal new bone formation is present. There is disuse osteoporosis of right femur

Fig. 19. Carcinoma of breast. There is extensive destruction of right side of pelvis. A soft tissue mass extends into pelvis displacing bladder medially

Fig. 19

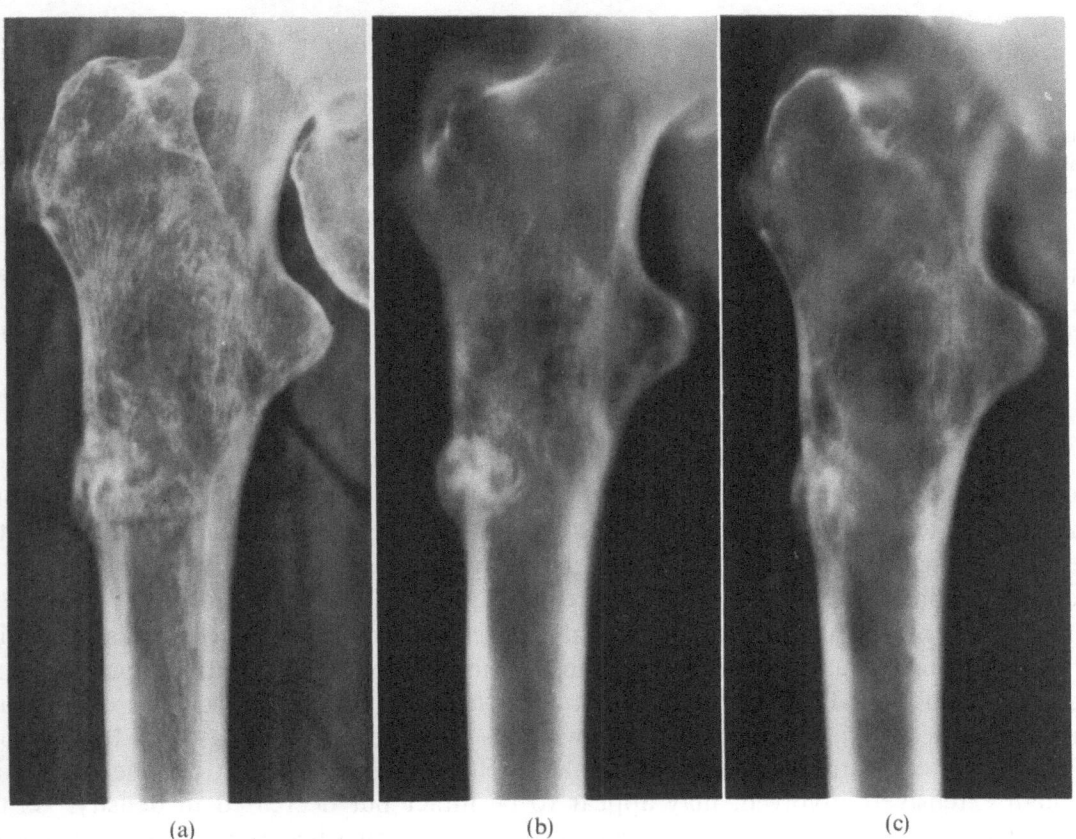

(a)   (b)   (c)

Fig. 20

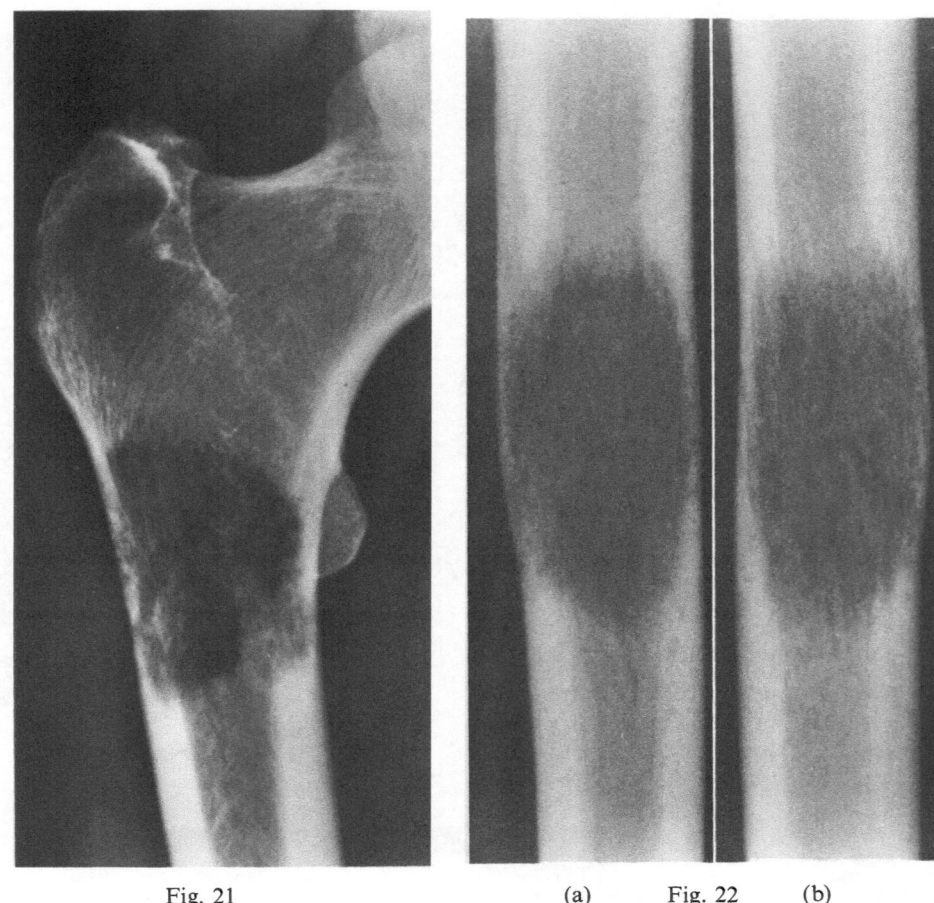

Fig. 21   (a)   Fig. 22   (b)

Fig. 21. Carcinoma of lung. Large destructive lesion involving subtrochanteric region of femur. There is extensive cortical destruction. Margins are ill-defined and numerous small areas of destruction superimposed on lesion indicate presence of cortical involvement. This pattern indicates that growth at margins is occurring at a fairly rapid rate

Fig. 22a and b. Carcinoma of thyroid. AP and lateral views of humerus demonstrate a localized area of destruction in midshaft. There are numerous small areas of destruction superimposed on larger lesions. These areas represent extensive cortical destruction which can be identified on both frontal and lateral projections

Permeative bone destruction is characterized by numerous, tiny, poorly defined lucent defects which run parallel to the long axis of the bone. The defects are usually uniform in size but tend to become smaller and more scattered toward the periphery of the lesion (Lodwick, 1965). There is no sharp line of demarcation between intact and destroyed bone and there is usually extensive involvement of the cortex (Figs. 14–20). This pattern of destruction reflects a highly aggressive growth rate and tumors presenting with this pattern usually show extensive infiltration of tumor beyond the apparent roentgenographic lesion. The rapid spread of tumor through the intertrabecular spaces results in irregular destruction of the trabeculae which is often best demonstrated by tomography (Fig. 20). In contradistinction to the moth-eaten pattern of destruction, the cortex, although extensively involved, may appear to be intact but decreased in density. As the lesion becomes more extensive, however, cortical definition is lost and soft tissue extension becomes apparent.

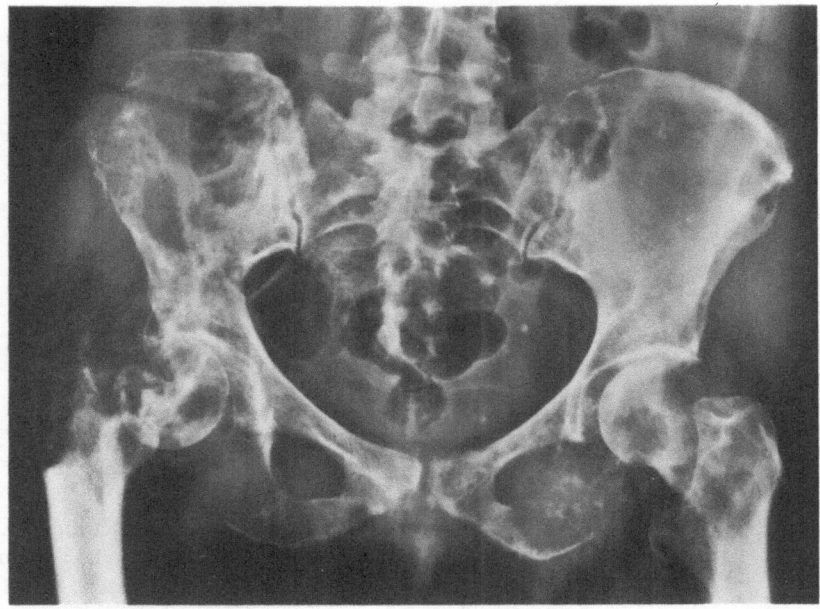

Fig. 23. Carcinoma of breast. Multiple large areas of destruction are present in pelvis and proximal femurs. There is extensive destruction of cortex and lesions, particularly in right and left ischia are ill-defined. There is a pathologic fracture through right femoral neck

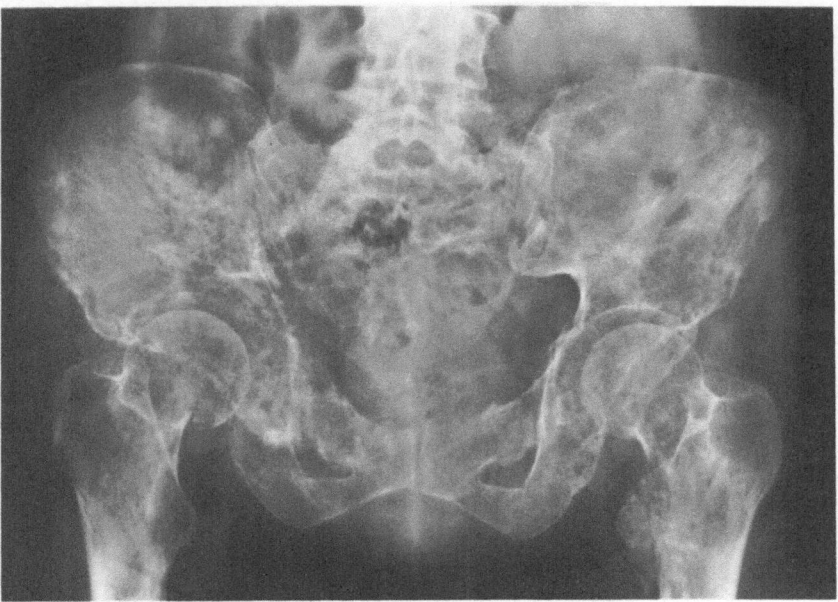

Fig. 24. Carcinoma of breast. Extensive osteolytic involvement of pelvis and proximal femurs with almost complete loss of normal trabecular pattern. There is complete loss of cortex along inferior and right side of pelvic brim and pathologic fractures are present through superior rami of right and left pubis, as well as in intertrochanteric region of left femur

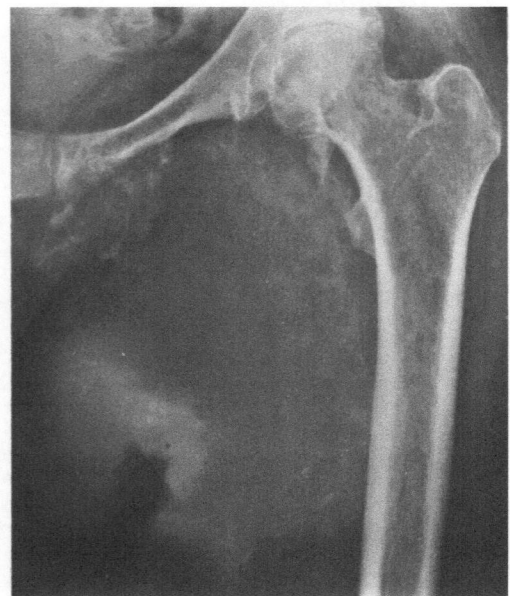

Fig. 25. Carcinoma of endometrium. Extensive destruction of inferior ramus of pubis and ischium with extension
into soft tissues. Note extensive, ill-defined soft tissue
calcification

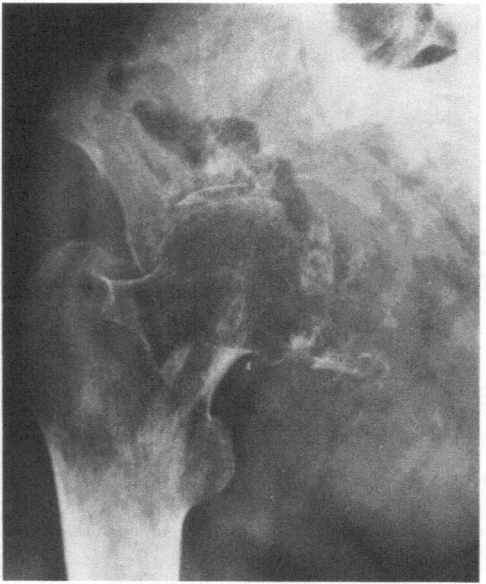 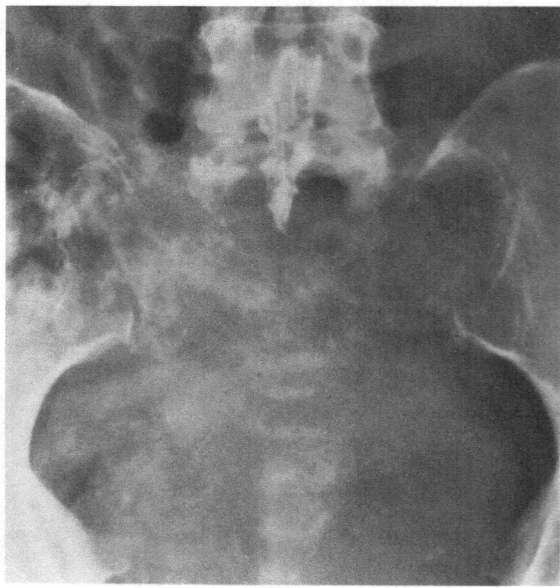

Fig. 26   Fig. 27

Fig. 26. Carcinoma of kidney. Extensive destruction of right side of pelvis with complete loss of margins
of ischium, pubis, and acetabulum. There is large soft tissue mass extending into pelvis and femoral head
is displaced medially

Fig. 27. Carcinoma of breast. Extensive destruction of sacrum with almost complete loss of bony margins

Fig. 29. Myeloma. Irregular expanded lesion involving tip of scapula. Roentgenographic appearance is characteristic of slow growing tumors

Fig. 30. Carcinoma of lung. A large expanding lesion involves iliac crest. Curvilinear calcifications in soft
tissue represent margins of tumor

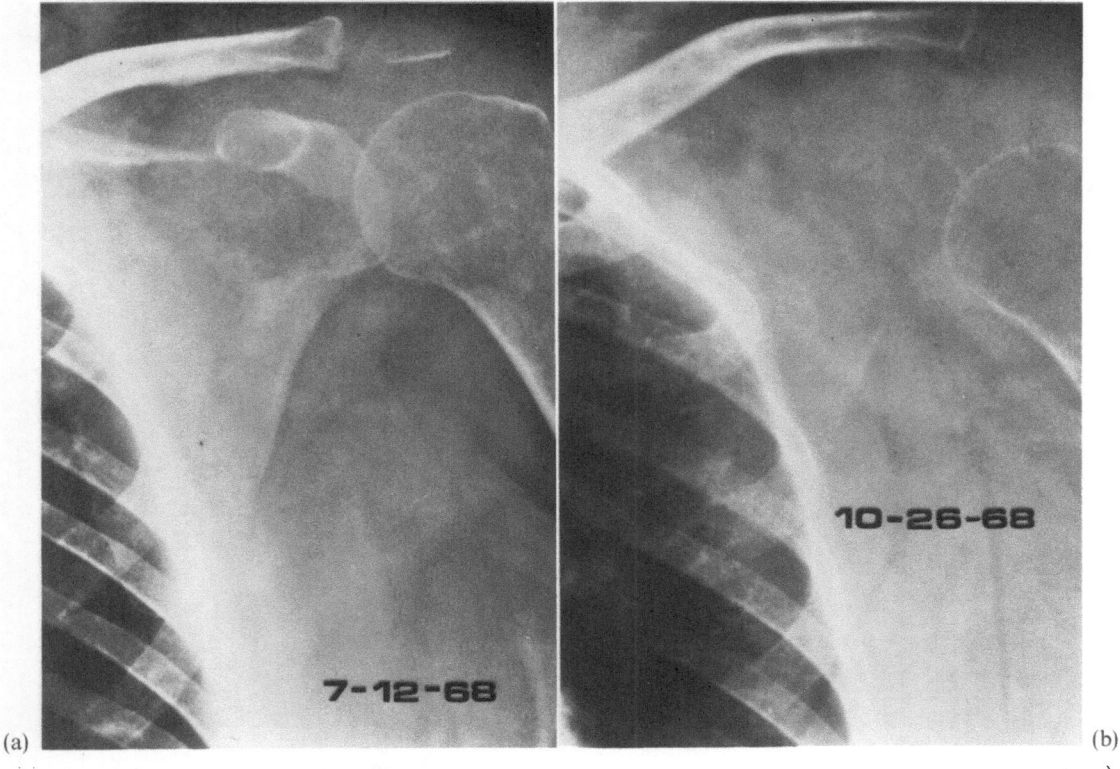

(a)   (b)

Fig. 28a and b. Carcinoma of kidney. AP views of shoulder demonstrate extensive and progressive destruction of scapula with eventual loss of bony margins

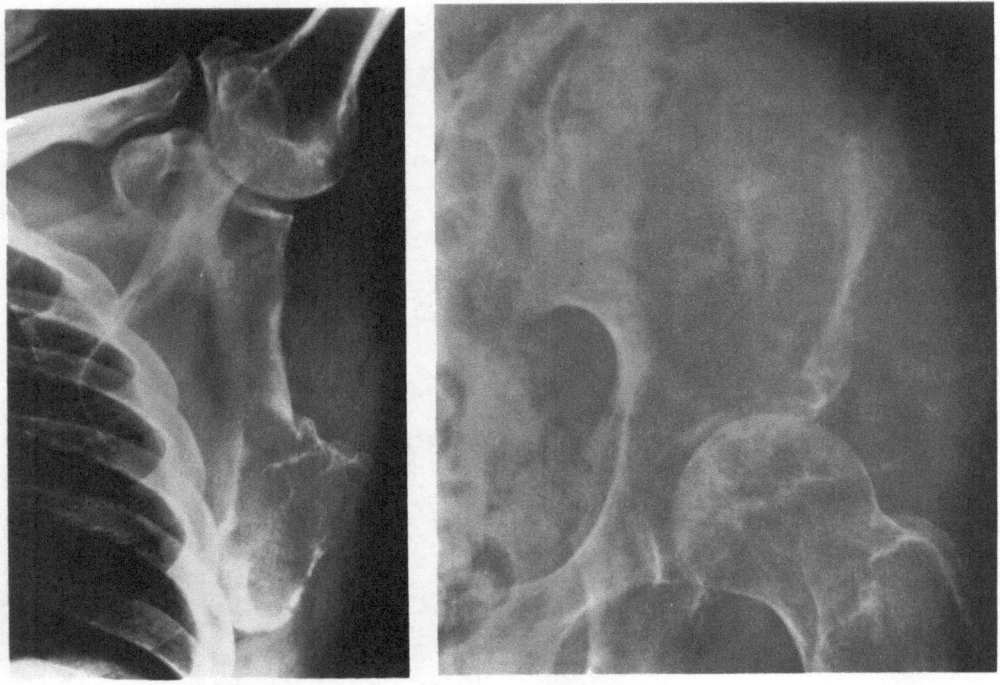

Fig. 29   Fig. 30

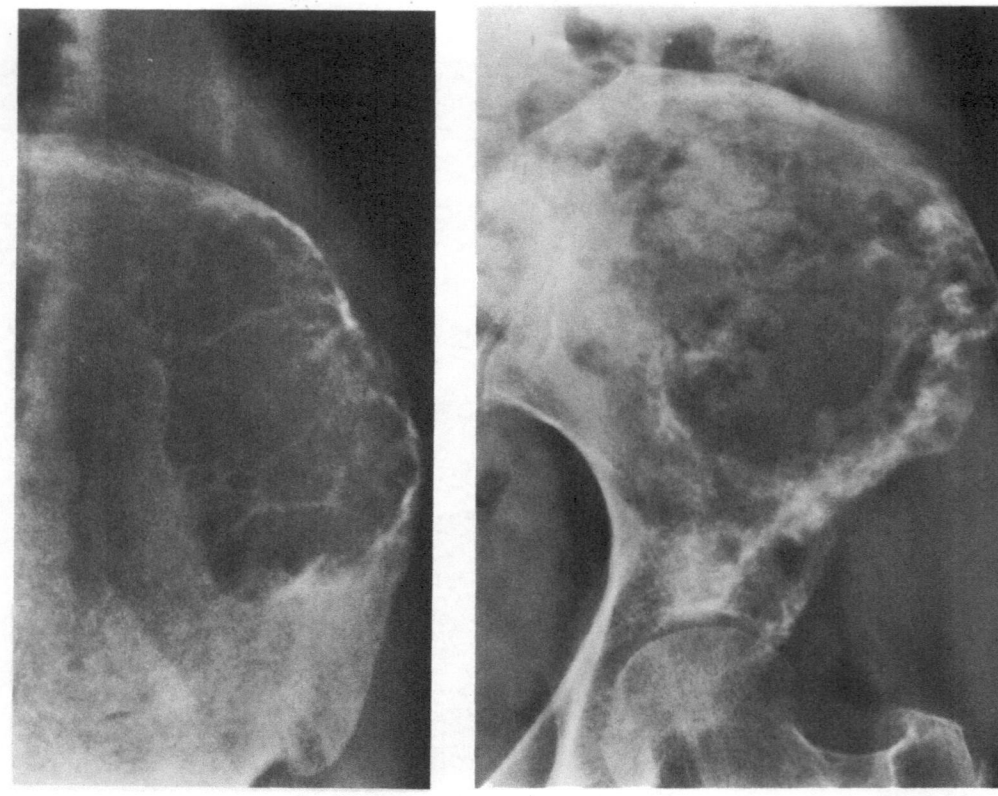

Fig. 31

Fig. 32

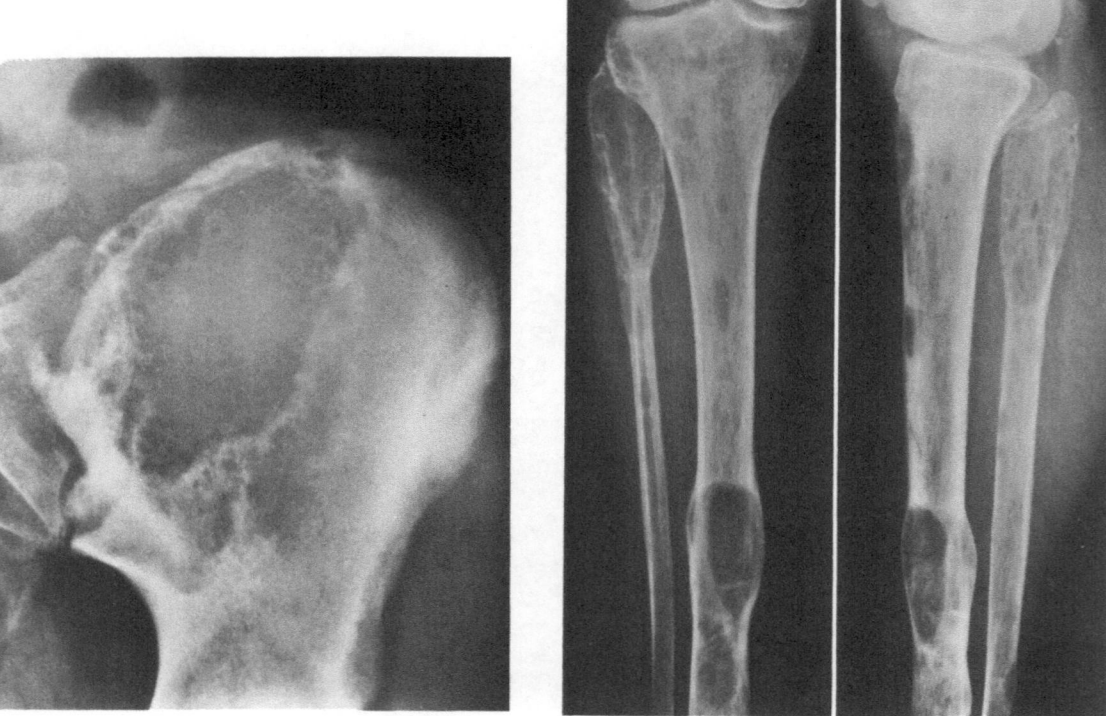

Fig. 33

Fig. 34a

Fig. 34b

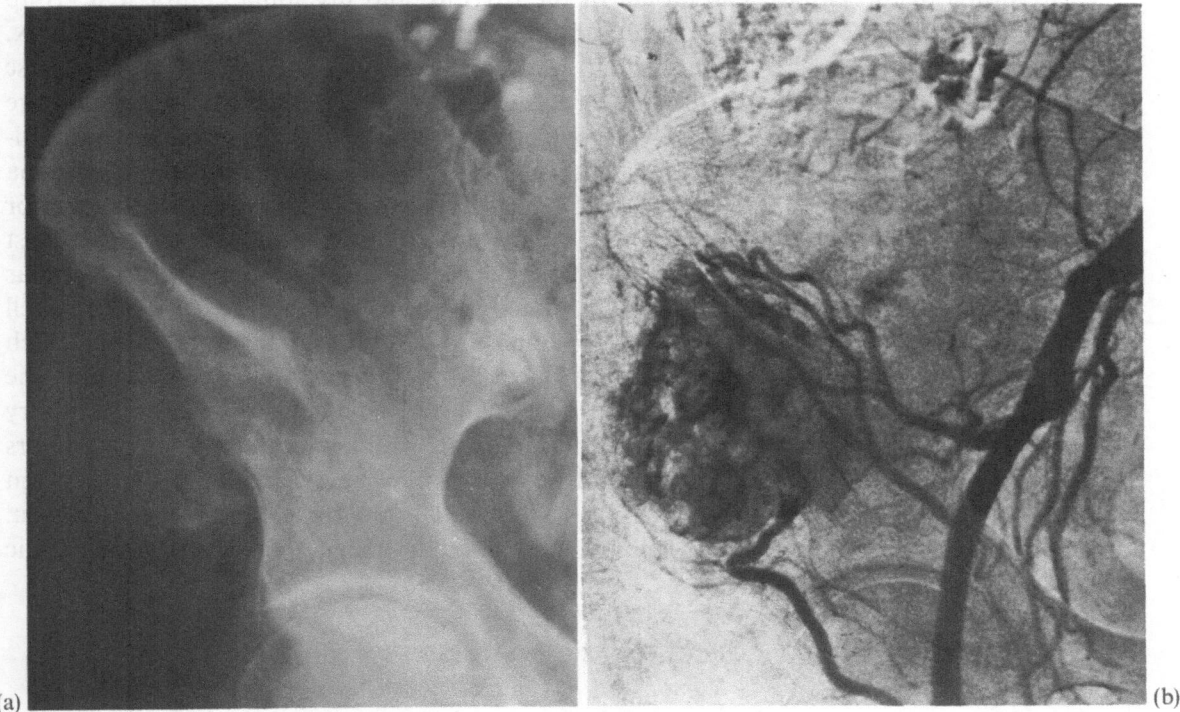

(a)   (b)

Fig. 35a and b. Carcinoma of kidney. (a) There is destruction of lateral margin of right ilium. There is periosteal new bone formation and large soft tissues mass is present. (b) Femoral arteriogram demonstrates marked vascularity of metastatic lesion. Tumor stain is identical to that observed in primary renal tumor. (Courtesy of Dr. WILLIAM WAYNE, Hinsdale, Illinois)

Combinations of these patterns of destruction may occur. Large osteolytic lesions are frequently noted to have poorly defined margins in which there are multiple small osteolytic defects (Figs. 21–22). These changes usually imply that destruction is occurring at a more rapid rate. In some cases destruction may be occurring so rapidly at the margins of large osteolytic lesions that the cortex is completely destroyed and there are no definable borders (Figs. 23–35). In these lesions there is complete penetration of the cortex with extension of the tumor into the soft tissues beyond the projected surface of the cortex. In some cases the destruction may be so extensive that there is complete loss of bony detail (Figs. 26–28).

Fig. 31. Myeloma. Large destructive lesion with lobulated margins involving iliac crest

Fig. 32. Carcinoma of breast. Large destructive lesion involving entire right ilium with evidence of bony repair laterally and superior to acetabulum

Fig. 33. Ewing's sarcoma. Large destructive lesion in left ilium with ill-defined margins. Lesions of this type produce problems in differential diagnosis between metastases and primary bone tumors

Fig. 34a and b. Carcinoma of breast. AP and lateral views of tibia and fibula demonstrate expanded lesions involving distal tibia and proximal fibula. Proximal fibular lesions has expanded trabecular shell characteristic of slow-growing tumors. (Courtesy of Dr. JEROME BROSNAN, University of Chicago, Chicago, Illinois)

Carcinoma of the kidney, carcinoma of the thyroid, and myeloma comprise a group of tumors which may grow very slowly at the primary and secondary sites (Jackson, 1968; Lodwick, 1965; Sherman and Ivker, 1950; Sherman and Pearson, 1948). Because such slow and insidious growth usually causes very few symptoms, the metastases are characteristically large when initially discovered and mimic primary bone tumors. Although large expanded lesions are most frequently seen with myeloma and carcinoma of the kidney or thyroid, this type of lesion may occur with any slow growing tumor and has been observed with carcinoma of the lung and carcinoma of the breast (Figs. 29–35). When located in the long bones or pelvis these lesions may present as large spherical or ovoid lesions encapsulated by an expanded trabecular shell (Figs. 29–30). These metastases may be vascular to the point of being pulsatile which may explain their roentgenographic appearance. Angiography may be helpful in the diagnosis of these unusual lesions (Gooding et al., 1966) particularly when the primary tumor is in the kidney (Fig. 35). Differentiation from primary malignant bone tumors such as Ewing's sarcoma (Fig. 33) or chondrosarcoma may be difficult. At times, benign bone tumors such as aneurysmal bone cyst, giant cell tumor, chondromyxoid fibroma, and brown tumor of hyperparathyroidism may present with similar roentgenographic findings.

II. Osteolytic Metastases

Primary tumors commonly responsible for osteolytic metastases include carcinomas of the (1) lung (Meyer, 1957; Turner and Jaffe, 1940; Watson, 1968); (2) breast (Deemarsky and Chernomordikova, 1971; Meyer, 1957); (3) kidney (Sherman and Pearson, 1948); (4) thyroid (McCormack, 1966; Sherman and Ivker, 1950), and (5) gastrointestinal tract (Turner and Jaffe, 1940). Metastases from primary squamous cell carcinoma of the cervix, oral cavity, or larynx are usually osteolytic as are metastases from the uterus and bladder. Although carcinoma of the breast most frequently produces osteolytic metastases (Deemarsky and Chernomordikova, 1971), osteoblastic or mixed lesions may be seen particularly following hormonal or radiation therapy (Cole, 1965; Copeland, 1970; Deemarsky and Chernomordikova, 1971; Johnston et al., 1970; Prohaska et al., 1966).

Histologically, osteolytic lesions are characterized by a decrease in the number and thickness of bone trabeculae. A number of hypotheses have been offered to account for bone destruction after invasion by tumor cells (Milch and Changus, 1956). These include destruction as a result of (1) the action of cells derived from the tumor stroma; (2) the action of specific bone-destroying cells, so-called osteoclasts, (3) the elaboration by the cancer cell of bone-resorptive substances; or (4) the mechanical effect of compression of bone by tumor.

The major anatomical reason for the appearance of osteolytic metastases is felt to be the result of direct mechanical pressure exerted by the tumor as it fills the intertrabecular spaces (Jaffe, 1958; Johnston, 1970; Milch and Changus, 1956; Murray and Jacobson, 1971). The role of the osteoclast in the resorption of osseous structures is unknown. Lodwick (1964) has demonstrated the presence of osteoclasts along the margin of resorption and feels that destruction occurs as the result of stimulation of the osteoclasts to remove bone. Jaffe (1958), on the other hand, has stated that if osteoclasts have a role in the resorption of bone they are sparse in the areas of metastases. Multinucleated cells are present in the areas of bone resorption (Milch and Changus, 1956), however, it is not known whether these cells are responsible for bone destruction or appear as a response to bone destruction. No direct evidence has been presented to support the hypothesis that specific resorptive substances are elaborated by cancer cells, however, GOLDHABER (1962) has suggested that the osteoclasts secrete a chelating agent which dissolves the mineral salts of the bony matrix and that this is followed closely by enzymatic reduction of the remaining osteoid.

III. Osteoblastic Metastases

Osteoblastic metastases are indicative of bone repair. The concept that new bone formation may develop in a metastasis of any origin has not been generally appreciated, however, osteoblastic lesions appear when new bone production predominates over any bone destruction that is or has been occurring. The extent of osteoblastic activity observed in a given metastatic lesion may vary considerably. So much new bone may have formed that the area appears densely sclerotic. By and large, osteoblastic metastases are much more likely to appear roentgenographically at an earlier stage of their development than osteolytic metastases. In some cases, extensive osteoblastic metastases are demonstrable prior to the development of clinical complaints (JAFFE, 1958).

The roentgenographic demonstration of osteoblastic activity is related to the deposition of new bone along pre-existing trabeculae and/or the presence of periosteal new bone formation. Osteoblasts deposit new bone on the surface of bone trabeculae or in the intertrabecular spaces with resultant increase in the density or thickness of the trabeculae. Ultimately, the intertrabecular spaces may become filled with new bone producing a dense, solid lesion. Progressive roentgenographic opacity of a skeletal metastasis is indicative of repair, irrespective of the site of origin of the primary neoplasm (MILCH and CHANGUS, 1956).

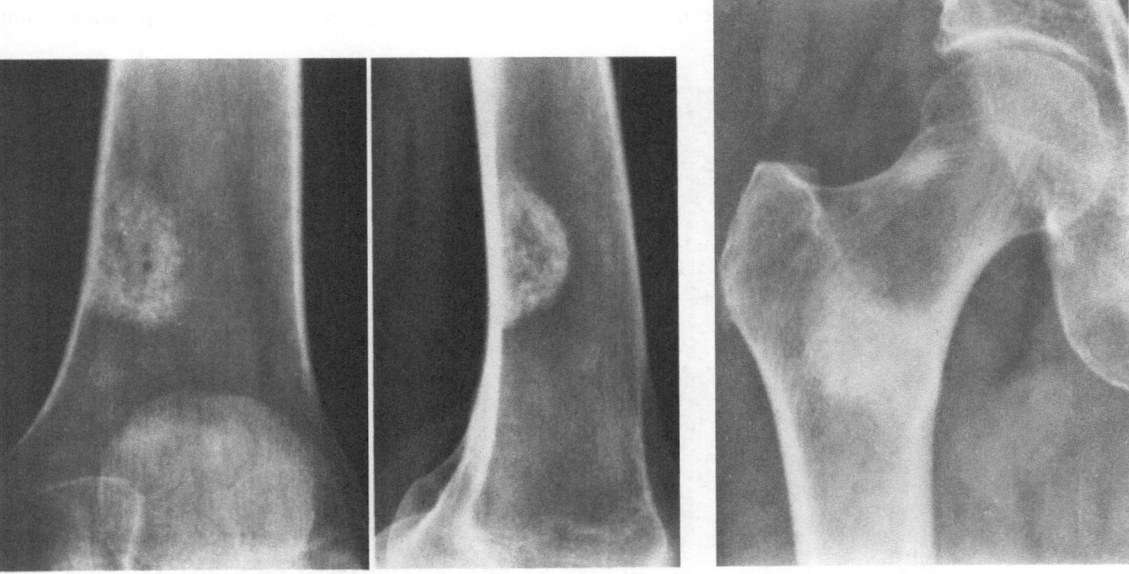

Fig. 36a   Fig. 36b   Fig. 37

Fig. 36a and b. Carcinoma of breast. AP and lateral views of femur demonstrate solitary osteoblastic lesion in distal femoral shaft with accentuation of coarse trabeculae. This type of lesion is frequently seen following hormonal or radiation therapy

Fig. 37. Carcinoma of breast. Osteoblastic lesions are present in proximal femur. Lesions are uniformly dense and trabeculae are no longer identified

Osteoblastic metastases may present initially as poorly defined areas of increased density (Figs. 36 and 37). The trabeculae within the lesions initially appear thickened, however, as the osteoblastic activity progresses the individual trabeculae are no longer identified and the lesions assume an uniformly dense appearance. As the metastatic disease becomes more extensive the lesions tend to coalesce and the bone becomes increasingly dense (Figs. 38–41). In some cases the osteoblastic activity is so extensive that the entire

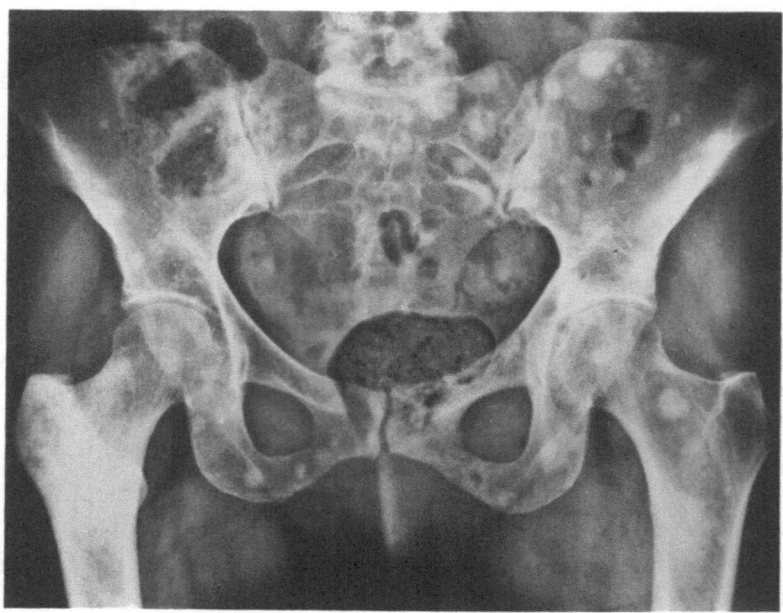

Fig. 38. Carcinoma of breast. Multiple osteoblastic lesions of varying size in pelvis and proximal femurs

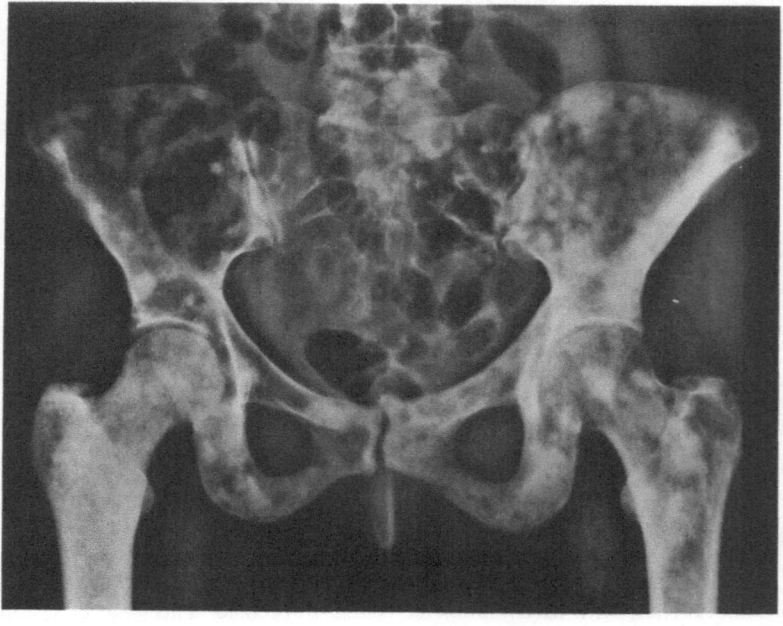

Fig. 39. Carcinoma of breast. (Same case as Figs. 37 and 38). Extensive osteoblastic metastases are present in pelvis and proximal femurs. Lesions clearly delineated on earlier examinations (Figs. 37 and 38) have now become confluent

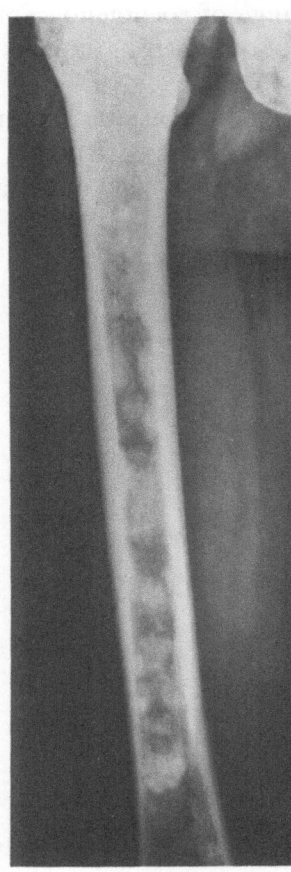

Fig. 40

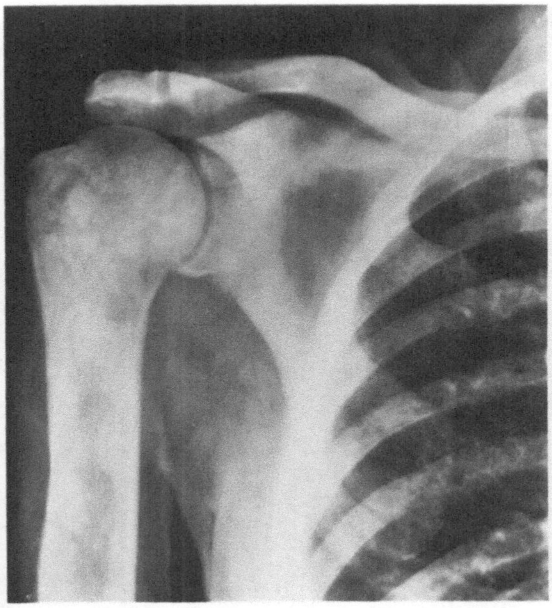

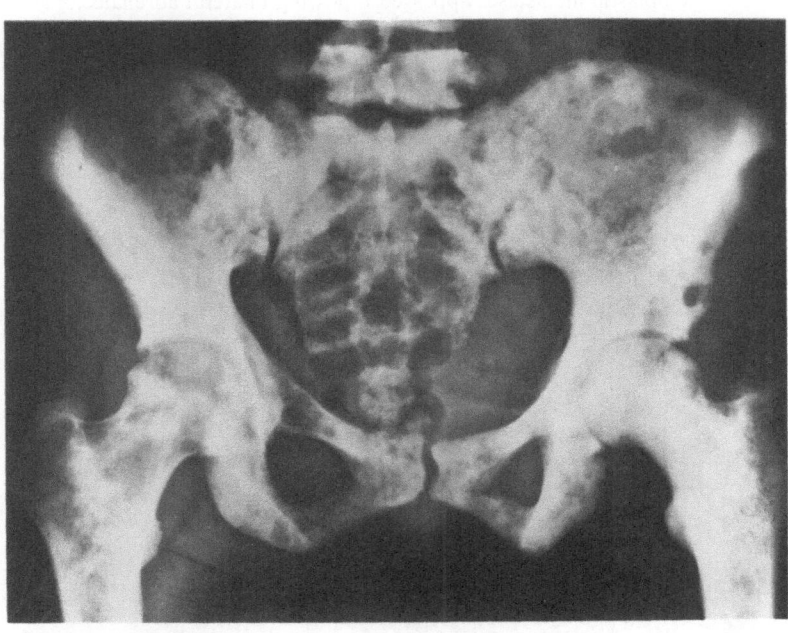

Fig. 41

Fig. 40. Carcinoma of breast. Extensive osteoblastic metastases are present in femoral shaft. Proximally bone appears uniformly dense, and cortical margins are obliterated

Fig. 41. Carcinoma of prostate. Extensive osteoblastic metastases are present. Ribs, scapula, clavicle, and proximal humerus appear uniformly dense

Fig. 42. Carcinoma of breast. Extensive osteoblastic involvement of lumbar spine, pelvis, and proximal femurs with expansion of left ilium. These changes developed after bilateral adrenalectomy. Roentgenographic appearance is identical to that observed with extensive metastases from carcinoma of prostate

skeleton may appear uniformly dense (Fig. 42). The range of roentgenographic changes occurring with osteoblastic metastases is most frequently observed in patients with carcinoma of the breast or prostate.

The extent of osteoblastic activity observed in a given metastatic lesion may vary considerably depending on whether the dominant feature is bone destruction or production. When there is roentgenographic evidence of destruction, the metastatic disease

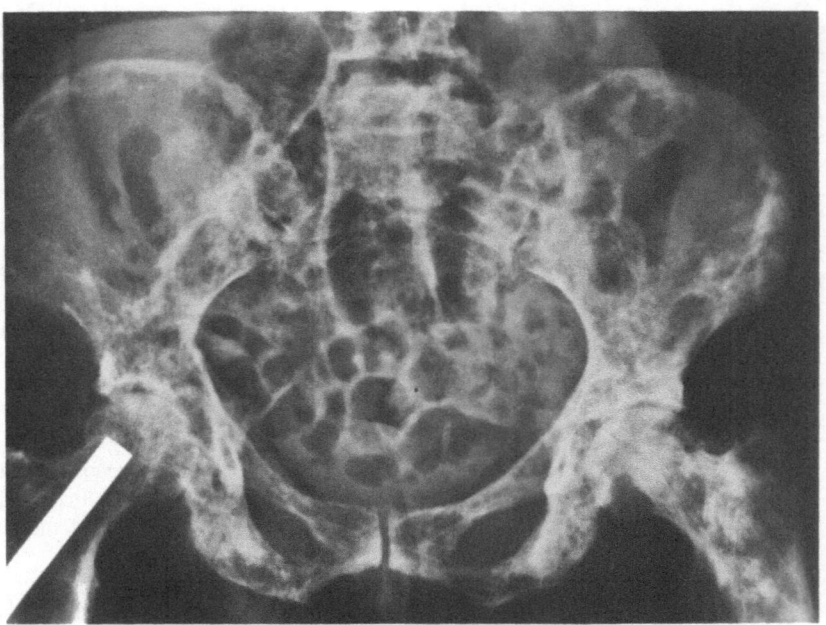

Fig. 43. Carcinoma of breast. Mixed type of metastatic disease characterized by coarsening of bony trabeculae in pelvis. In addition, larger areas of osteoblastic activity are identified in left ilium and proximal femurs. Osteoblastic metastases appeared following bilateral adrenalectomy

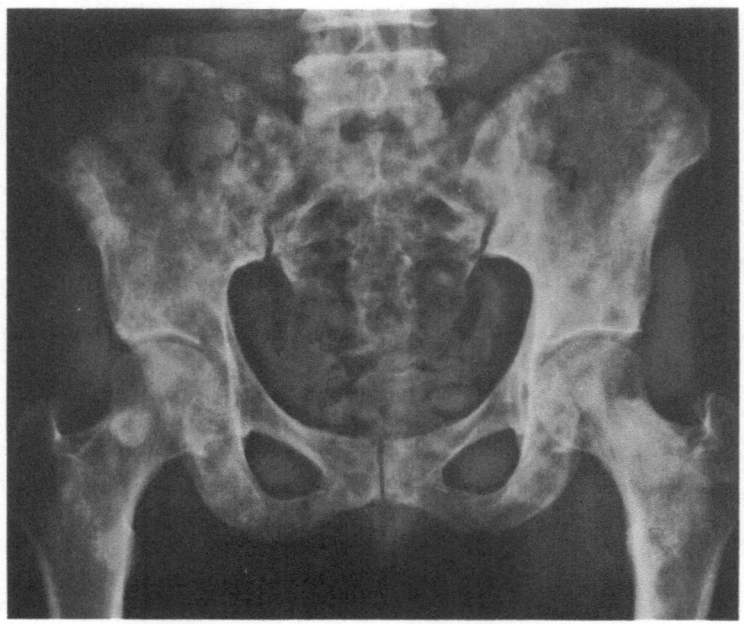

Fig. 44. Carcinoma of breast. Mixed type of metastases

is described as mixed. There may be marginal sclerosis (Fig. 31), or an ill-defined pattern of sclerosis throughout the areas of involvement (Figs. 32, 43, 44). At times it may be difficult to identify specific lesions and the appearance may be confused with extensive ill-defined osteolytic metastases separated by normal bone.

Diffuse metastatic disease may present as sclerosis of remaining trabeculae (Fig. 45). This usually occurs when there is extensive involvement of the intertrabecular spaces, particularly in the ribs, pelvis, and long bones. In some patients, the extent of destruction may not be sufficient to be recognized roentgenographically, however, treatment, particularly when the primary tumor is carcinoma of the breast, may stimulate sufficient new bone formation along the trabeculae to enhance the roentgenographic appearance of the metastatic lesions.

Carcinoma of the prostate is the most common cause of osteoblastic metastases in males while carcinoma of the breast is most frequently responsible in females (COPELAND, 1931; ELKIN and MUELLER, 1954; FRIED, 1946; TURNER and JAFFE, 1940). Any malignant neoplasm can stimulate bone production, however, the neoplasms other than carcinoma of the prostate or breast most frequently responsible for osteoblastic metastases are: (1) gastrointestinal and bronchial carcinoids (HYMAN and WELLS, 1964; PEAVY et al., 1973; TOOMEY and FELSON, 1960); (2) small cell or oat cell carcinomas of the lung (MUGGIA and HANSEN, 1972; NAPOLI et al., 1973); (3) adenocarcinoma of the lung (BEER et al., 1964); (4) mucin-secreting adenocarcinoma of the stomach (MEYER, 1957; TURNER and JAFFE, 1940); and (5) carcinoma of the colon (SEIFE, 1973). Osteoblastic metastases have also been reported with medulloblastoma (DEBNAM and STAPLE, 1973), seminoma (SUM et al., 1960), and pancreas (GILLISON et al., 1970). Lymphomas, particularly Hodgkin's disease (DRESSER and SPENCER, 1936; VIETA et al., 1942), may produce osteoblastic lesions and several non-neoplastic diseases may present problems in differential diagnosis. These include Paget's disease (Fig. 46), tuberous sclerosis, mastocytosis (urticaria pigmentosa) (Fig. 47), and the osteosclerotic form of multiple myeloma (LOWBEER, 1969).

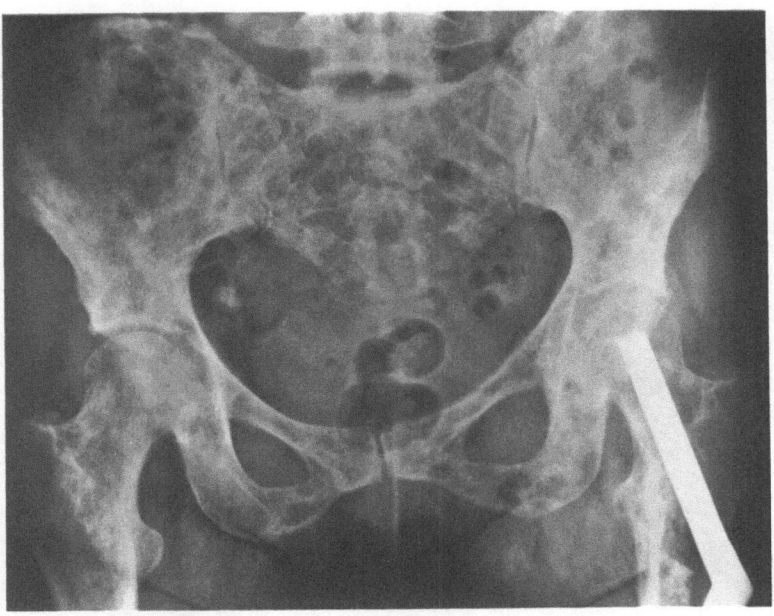

Fig. 45. Carcinoma of breast. Prominent trabeculae are present throughout pelvis. Osteolytic lesions, although poorly defined, are present throughout pelvis and proximal femurs

Osteoblastic lesions are characterized histologically by an irregular interlacing network of moderately to markedly thickened trabeculae, subperiosteal new bone formation, increased numbers of osteoblasts and clumps or isolated islands of tumor cells (MILCH and CHANGUS, 1956). The actual mechanism of osteoblastic activity is unknown. New bone formation occurs as a nonspecific reactive process of the local osteogenic tissue (LODWICK, 1964). If the process of destruction is not too rapid or if there is some stimulus to decrease the rate of destruction, osteoblasts will respond by repairing the

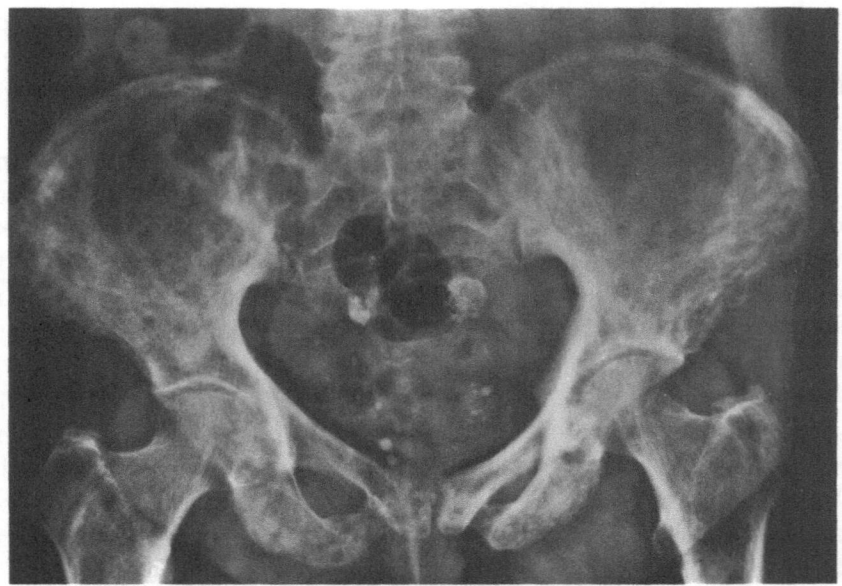

Fig. 46. Paget's disease. Trabecular pattern is accentuated and irregular. As result, left ilium appears to contain large osteolytic lesion. Cortex is thickened and width of left ilium is increased

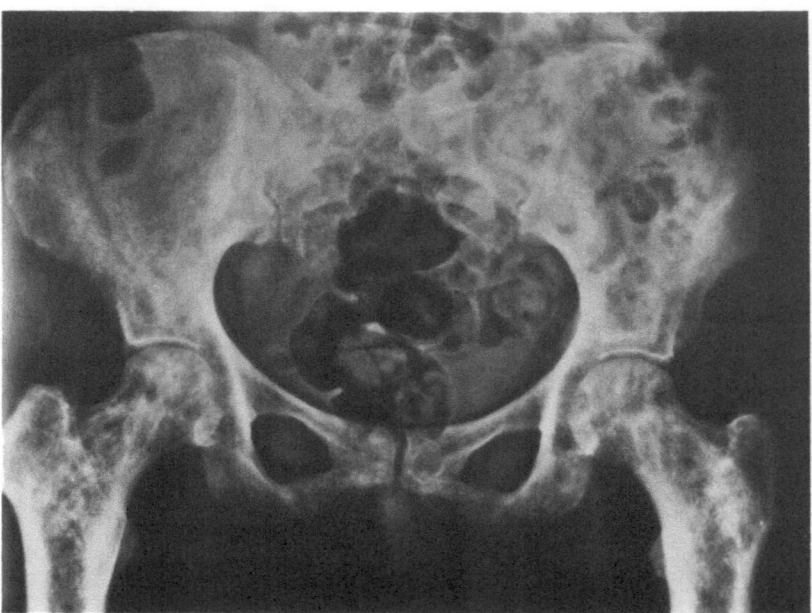

Fig. 47. Mastocytosis. There is diffuse thickening of trabeculae, however, trabecular pattern is otherwise normal. These changes could easily be mistaken for diffuse metastatic disease

destroyed bone (JAFFE, 1958). This may explain the appearance of osteoblastic lesions in prostatic metastases as well as following hormonal or radiation therapy of breast metastases (COLE, 1965; DEEMARSKY and CHERNOMORDIKOVA, 1971; JOHNSTON et al., 1970; MILCH and CHANGUS, 1956). The initiating and modifying stimuli responsible for new bone production is unclear, however, the tumor cells play no direct role in osteogenesis (JAFFE, 1958; LODWICK, 1964; MILCH and CHANGUS, 1956).

IV. Periosteal New Bone Formation

Periosteal reaction occurs much more frequently with metastatic disease than one would gather from the literature and its presence may lead to a mistaken diagnosis of a primary malignant bone tumor. EDEIKEN and HODES (1967) make little mention of metastatic disease in the differential diagnosis of periosteal new bone formation whereas NORMAN and ULIN (1969) found periosteal reaction in 37% of solitary metastasis. The type of periosteal response is non-specific and of no help in differentiating a metastatic neoplasm from a primary malignant bone tumor. The changes observed with osteolytic lesions are often scanty (Fig. 48), however, extensive periosteal reaction identical to

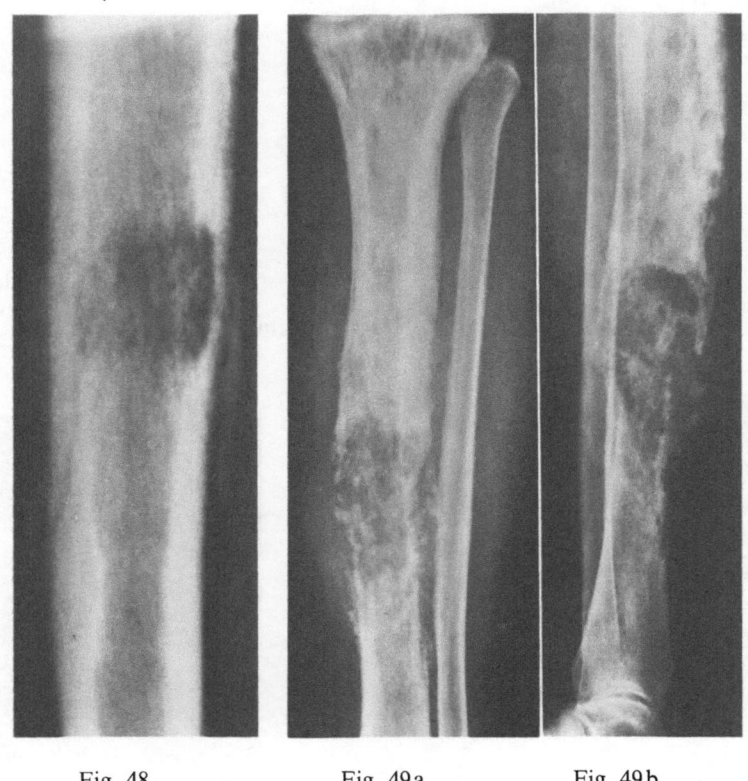

Fig. 48   Fig. 49a   Fig. 49b

Fig. 48. Carcinoma of lung. Ill-defined permeative metastatic lesion in proximal femur. Irregular periosteal new bone formation is present

Fig. 49a and b. Squamous cell carcinoma of lung. AP and lateral views of tibia and fibula demonstrate large, irregular destructive lesion in midshaft of tibia, with extensive periosteal reaction. This lesion was initially diagnosed as primary bone sarcoma because of presence of Paget's disease in tibial shaft. (Courtesy of Dr. THOMAS SONDAG, Oak Park, Illinois)

that seen with primary malignant bone tumors may be present (Figs. 49–54). This is particularly true when osteoblastic metastases are present (JAFFE, 1958; LEGIER and TAUBER, 1968; LEHRER et al., 1970; NORMAN and ULIN, 1969; PEAVY et al., 1973). At times the extensive periosteal reaction seen with hypertrophic pulmonary osteoarthropathy (Fig. 55) may be mistaken for metastatic disease.

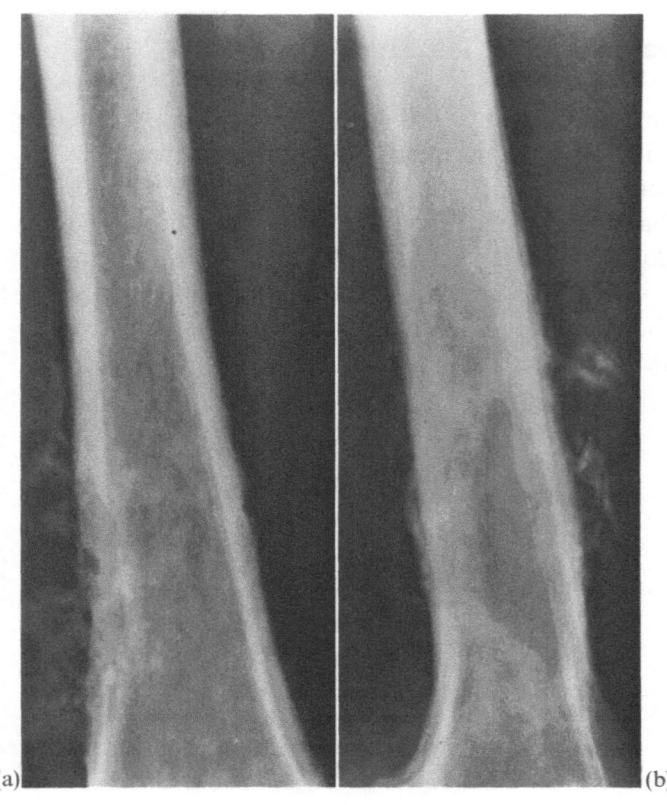

(a)   (b)

Fig. 50a and b. Carcinoma of lung. AP and lateral views demonstrate ill-defined destructive lesion in distal third of femur with exuberant periosteal new bone formation

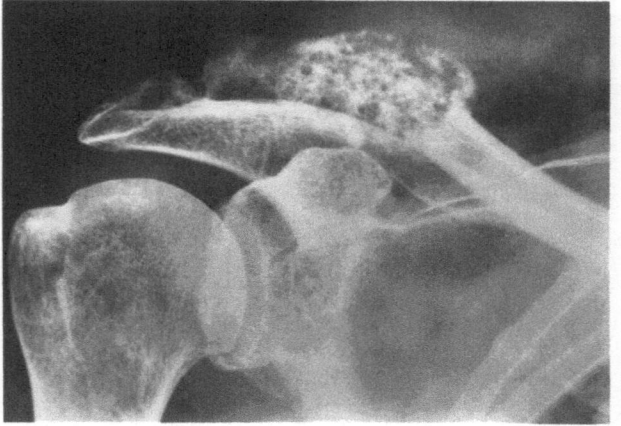

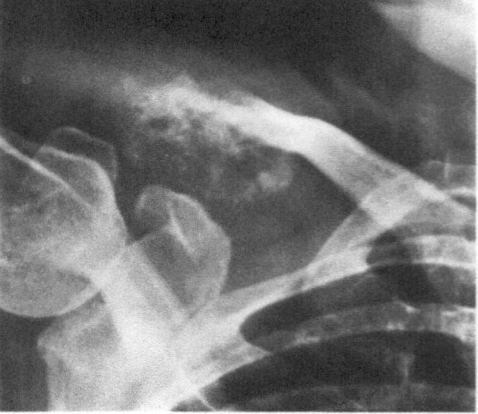

Fig. 51   Fig. 52

Fig. 51. Carcinoma of prostate. Destructive lesion in distal clavicle with extensive periosteal new bone formation

Fig. 52. Angiosarcoma. Destructive lesion with extensive periosteal new bone formation involving distal right clavicle

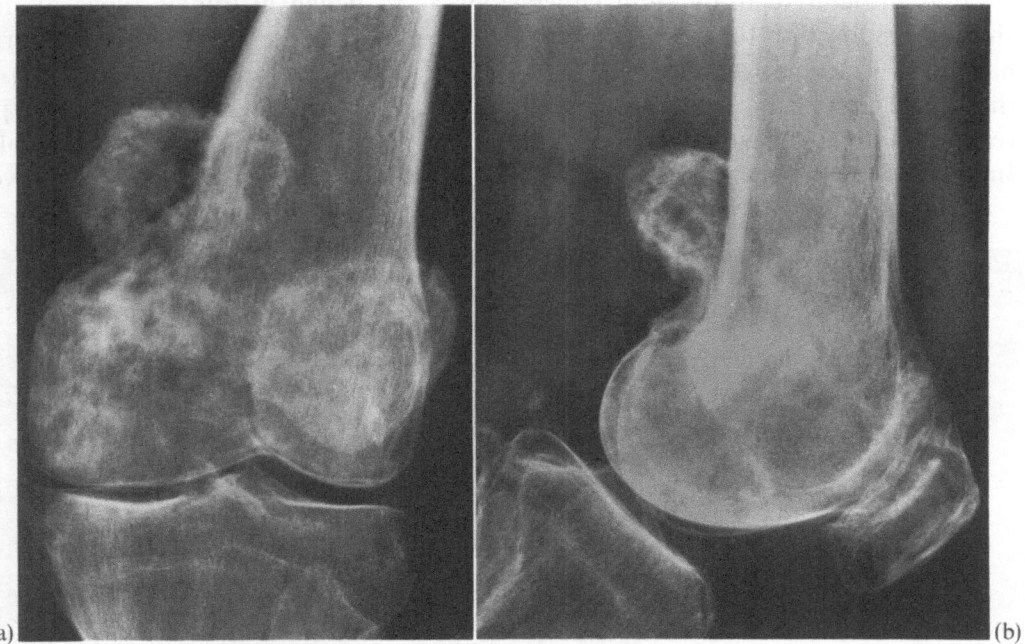

Fig. 53a and b. Metastatic papillary adenocarcinoma, primary site unknown. AP and lateral views of femur demonstrate an ill-defined destructive lesion in distal femur with extensive periosteal new bone formation

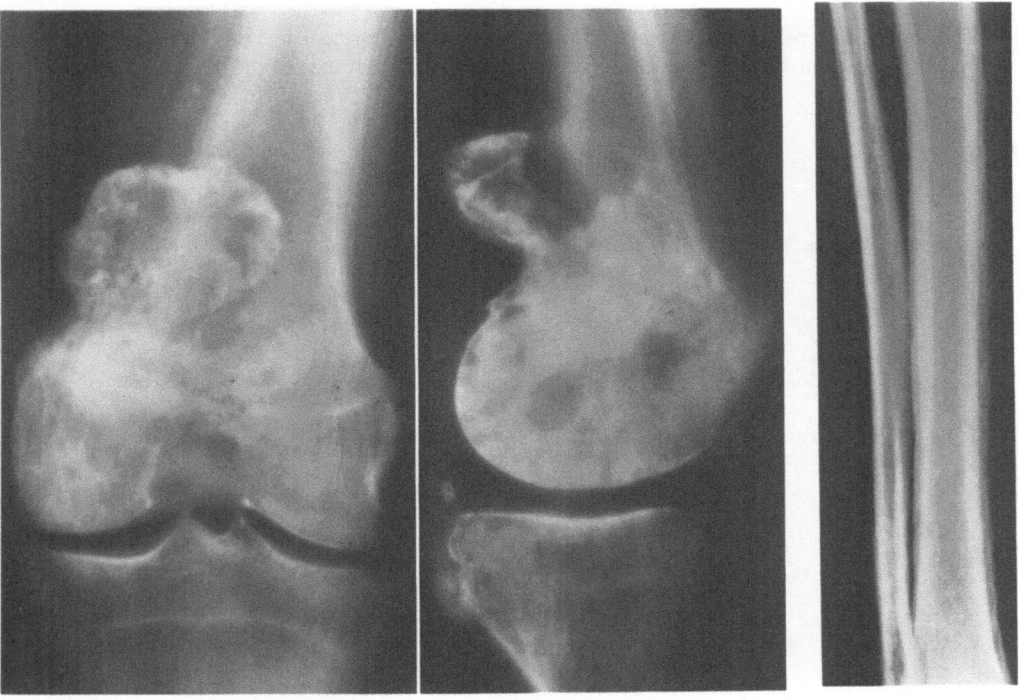

Fig. 54a   Fig. 54b   Fig. 55

Fig. 54a and b. Tomograms of lesion in Fig. 53 more clearly delineate the destructive changes in distal femur, as well as irregular periosteal reaction

Fig. 55. Hypertrophic pulmonary osteoarthropathy in patient with alveolar cell carcinoma of lung

It is difficult to draw valid conclusions as to which histologic types of metastases show a predilection for exuberant periosteal reaction since a variety of primary tumors have been reported to have metastases of this type. NORMAN and ULIN (1969) observed that the primary tumors most frequently responsible for metastatic lesions with periosteal reaction were in metastasis from carcinomas in the colon and prostate or neuroblastomas. In our series, the metastases responsible for exuberant periosteal response were from

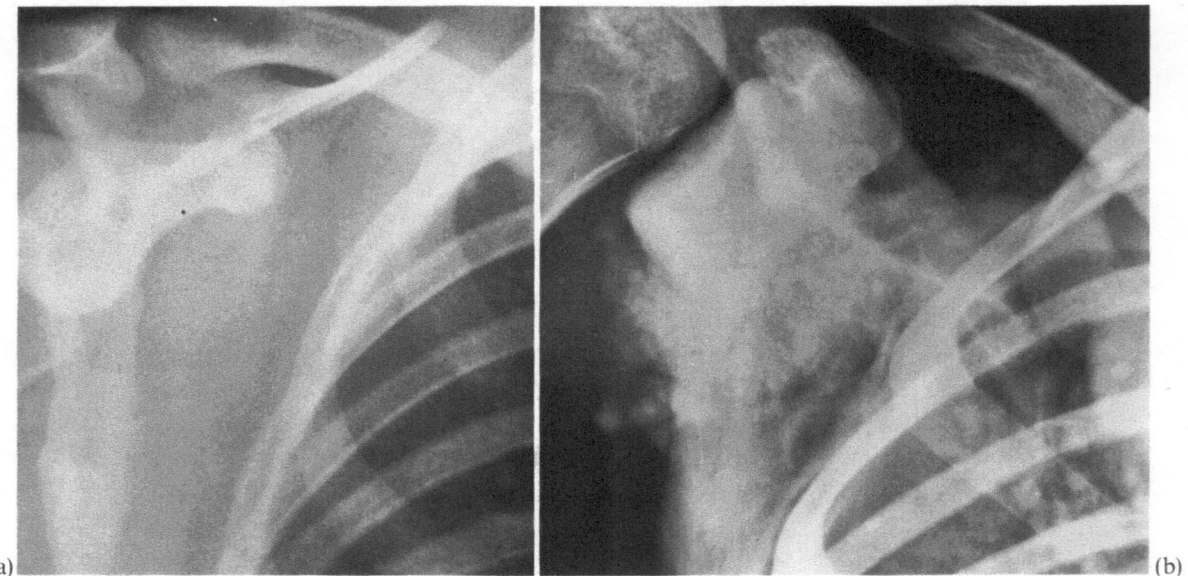

(a)   (b)

Fig. 56a and b. Osteosarcoma. Extensive metastatic disease is present in lung. In (b) metastasis has appeared in right scapula which has roentgenographic appearance of primary osteosarcoma

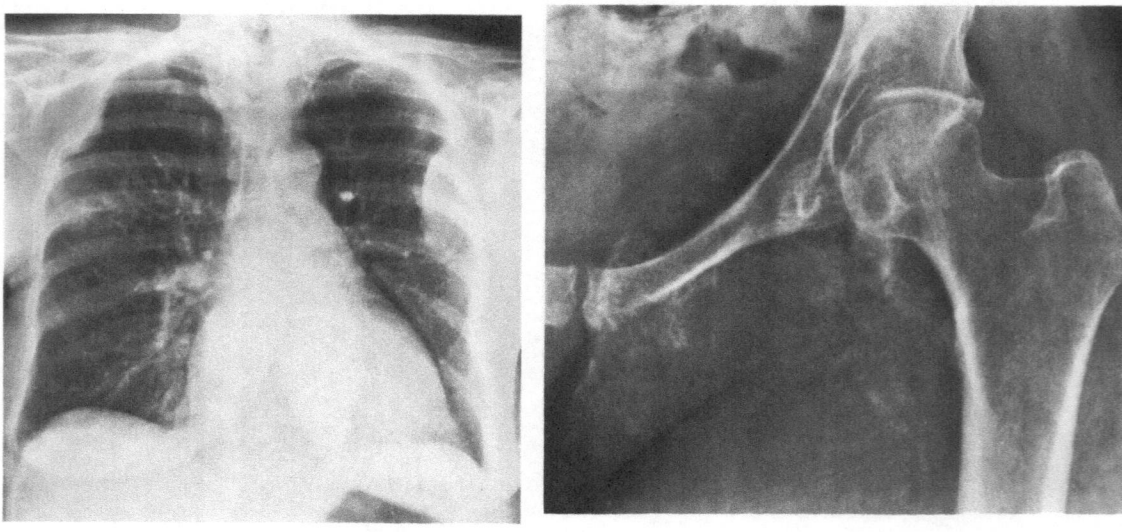

Fig. 57   Fig. 58

Fig. 57. Metastatic adenocarcinoma, primary site unknown. There are extensive destructive changes in ribs with associated subpleural soft tissue masses

Fig. 58. Endometrial carcinoma. Destruction of inferior ramus of pubis and ischium. There is large soft tissue mass containing irregular calcifications. (Same case as Fig. 25)

carcinomas of the lung or prostate with the exception of one patient with metastatic papillary adenocarcinoma (Fig. 54), and one patient with metastatic angiosarcoma (Fig. 52).

Carcinoma of the prostate may produce metastases with a sunburst periosteal pattern similar to that occurring with primary bone sarcomas (JAFFE, 1958; LEGIER and TAUBER, 1968; LEHRER et al., 1970). Extensive periosteal reaction has also been reported with carcinoid tumors in the lung or gastrointestinal tract (PEAVY et al., 1973), carcinoma of the colon (SEIFE, 1973) and retinoblastoma (LEHRER et al., 1970). Osteosarcomas may metastasize to bone producing lesions identical to the primary tumor (Fig. 56). In the skull, periosteal spiculation can occur with invasive meningiomas (JACOBSON et al., 1959; TAVERAS and WOOD, 1964) or neuroblastomas (CAFFEY, 1973).

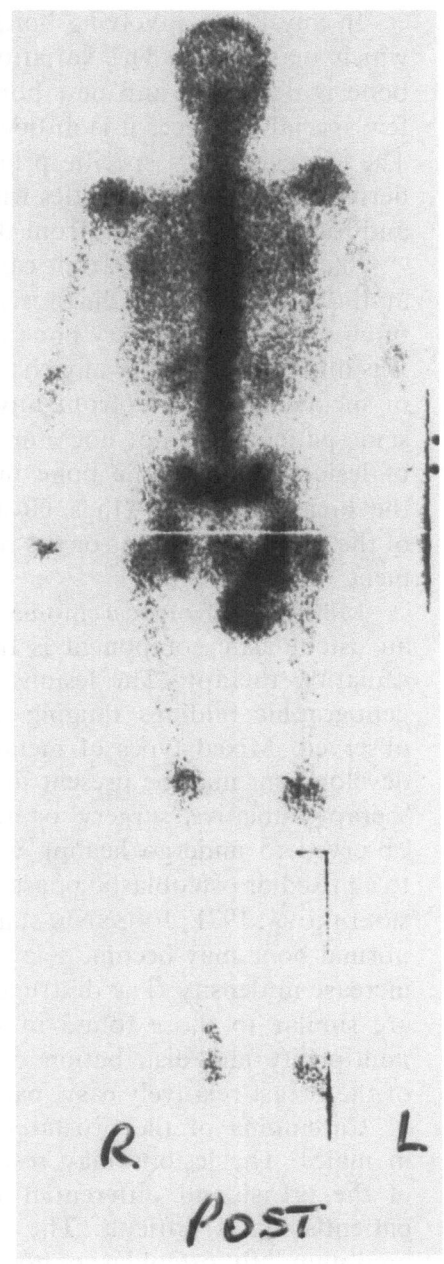

Fig. 59. Endometrial carcinoma. (Same case as Fig. 58). Flourine-18 bone scan demonstrates extensive uptake in soft tissue mass noted in previous figure

Metastatic bone tumors are much less likely to extend into the surrounding soft tissue, however, in some areas such as the ribs, pelvis, or distal portions of the extremities there may be a considerable soft tissue component (Fig. 57). Tumor matrix ossification or calcification is usually observed only in primary bone tumors or their metastases (Lodwick, 1965), however, Figure 58 demonstrates a metastatic lesion from an endometrial carcinoma in which there is extensive destruction of the pubis and ischium as well as a large soft tissue mass containing irregular calcification. Interestingly, the lesion demonstrated increased Flourine-18 uptake in the soft tissues at the time of its initial detection and several months prior to the appearance of soft tissue calcification (Fig. 59).

V. Roentgenographic Characteristics

In any lesion involving bone there are inherent limitations in the kind of response which may occur. The variations are in the combinations or the patterns in which bone is destroyed and new bone deposited (Lodwick, 1965). Therefore, except for a few special instances it is difficult to determine the primary site of any given metastasis. The evidence for a specific primary tumor as a source of metastatic disease is usually derived from the peculiarities within the patterns of lesions as well as from their number and location rather than from the appearance of any given lesion.

Skeletal metastases from carcinoma of the breast or prostate are usually multifocal at the time of initial diagnosis whereas it is not unusual to find solitary metastasis, often mimicking primary bone tumors, from carcinomas of the thyroid, kidney or lung. It is difficult to identify any characteristic pattern since the roentgenographic appearance of metastatic disease from any given neoplasm may vary considerably, even in the same patient. It is not uncommon to observe destructive, osteoblastic, and mixed types of lesions in the same bone in several types of metastatic cancer, particularly from the breast and lung (Figs. 60 and 61). This may be related to the relative maturity of the individual lesions or the result of treatment of lesions at varying stages of development.

Metastases from carcinoma of the breast are predominantly destructive, however, an osteoblastic component is frequently observed, particularly following hormonal or radiation therapy. The lesions are usually multifocal and a wide spectrum of roentgenographic findings ranging from extensive destruction to diffuse sclerosis may be observed. Mixed types of metastases are common and metastases at varying stage of development may be present in the same bone (Figs. 60 and 61). Following hormonal therapy, ablative surgery or radiation therapy, osteolytic metastases are frequently observed to undergo healing with resultant change in the character of the metastases to a mixed or osteoblastic phase (Cole, 1965; Copeland, 1970; Deemarsky and Chernomordikova, 1971; Johnston et al., 1970; Prohaska et al., 1966). In some cases apparently normal bone may become sclerotic as undetected lesions undergo healing with resultant increase in density. The destructive or reparative processes observed in any given lesion are similar to those found in metastases from any primary neoplasm, however, the multiplicity and distribution of lesions makes the diagnosis of metastatic carcinoma of the breast relatively easy, particularly in a female.

Carcinoma of the prostate is the most common cause of osteoblastic metastases in males. The lesions may resemble the osteoblastic metastases seen with carcinoma of the breast and differentiation of these two neoplasms without knowledge of the patient's sex is difficult. The metastatic lesions from carcinoma of the prostate are predominantly osteoblastic, however, the metastases may be mixed or purely lytic (Jor-

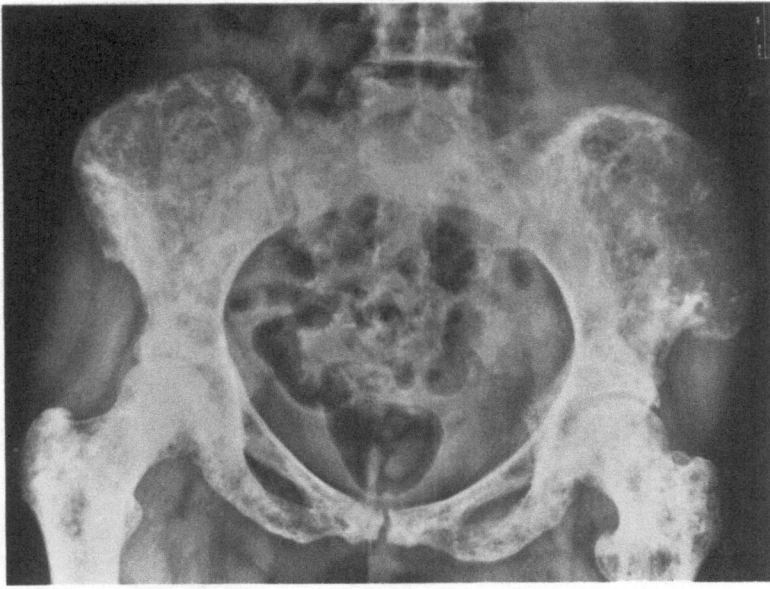

Fig. 60. Carcinoma of breast. Extensive metastatic disease involving spine, pelvis, femurs. Lesions at varying stages of development are present. There is large, irregular area of destruction in left ilium. Destructive lesions are also present in right ilium and left femur. Diffuse osteoblastic lesions at varying stages of development are present in remainder of the pelvis

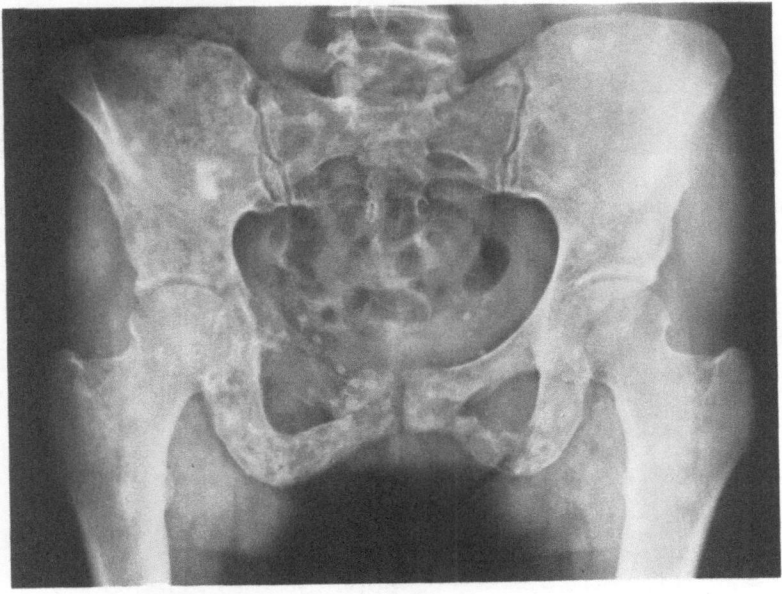

Fig. 61. Carcinoma of breast. Scattered osteoblastic lesions are present in pelvis. Extensive destruction is noted in superior ramus of right pubis, and there are smaller areas of destruction in inferior ramus of left pubis. There is mixed-type of metastatic pattern present in inferior ramus of right pubis and ischium

GENS, 1965). The osteoblastic lesions initially are either sharply delineated areas of increased density or poorly demarcated. As the metastatic disease progresses there may be diffuse sclerosis of the entire skeleton. The bones are rarely increased in size since the new bone formation is primarily endosteal, however, if the periosteum has been stimulated to produce new bone the width of the bone may be increased simulating the changes seen with Paget's disease. Differentiation is usually easy since the trabecular pattern in Paget's disease is distorted and the cortex is thickened. In some cases, the periosteal response may mimic that seen with primary bone tumors (LEHRER et al., 1970; LEGIER and TAUBER, 1968; NORMAN and ULIN, 1969) and localized expansion of bone may occur as a result of this exuberant periosteal response (Figs. 62 and 63).

Metastatic lesions from bronchogenic carcinomas are predominantly osteolytic (WATSON, 1968), however, osteoblastic lesions are frequently found in patients with small cell carcinomas (oat cell) or adenocarcinomas of the lung (BEER et al., 1964; NAPOLI et al., 1973). Osteoblastic lesions have also been observed with bronchial carcinoids (HYMAN and WELLS, 1964; PEAVY et al., 1973; THOMAS, 1968; TOOMEY and FELSON, 1960). The metastatic lesions themselves have no distinguishing characteristics and resem-

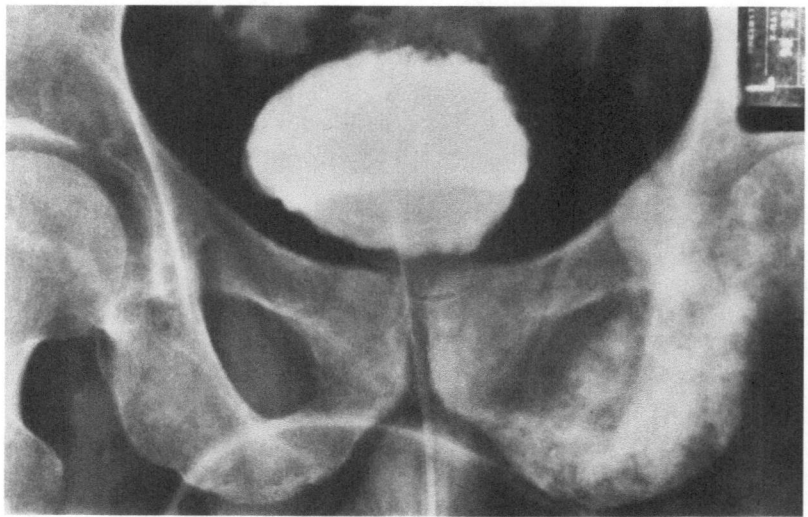

Fig. 62. Carcinoma of prostate. Osteoblastic metastases are present in inferior ramus of pubis and ischium with expansion of bone

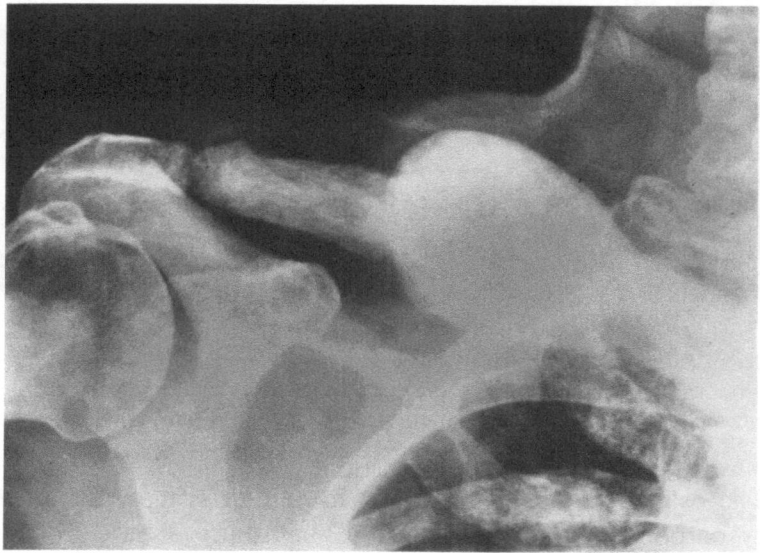

Fig. 63. Carcinoma of prostate. Extensive osteoblastic involvement of clavicle with marked expansion of middle third

ble the metastases from other neoplasms. The lesions are usually multiple, however, the extensive involvement observed with carcinoma of the breast or prostate is seldom found with metastases from lung tumors. On occasion, the metastatic lesion may grow slow enough to produce a large expanded lesion (Fig. 30) or the metastasis may mimic a primary bone tumor (Figs. 48–50).

Metastases from renal cell carcinoma are almost always osteolytic and frequently present as solitary lesions (ARKLESS, 1965; FREID, 1946; SHERMAN and PEARSON, 1948; WEIGENSBERG, 1971). Bone metastases are frequently found in the absence of lung metastases since the tumors usually metastasize via the paravertebral plexus. As a result, the greatest incidence of metastases is in the axial skeleton (ARKLESS, 1965) and those areas connected to the paravertebral plexus (BATSON, 1940, 1942). Renal cell carcinomas may grow slowly at the primary site giving rise to large expanded metastatic lesions, however, most frequently there are no distinguishing features.

VI. Spinal Metastases

Metastatic involvement of the spine is frequent, however, correlative studies comparing the anatomic and roentgenographic appearance of metastases indicate that the roentgen examination may be normal in spite of extensive osseous involvement (BACHMAN and SPROUL, 1955; BORAK, 1942; JAFFE, 1958; YOUNG and FUNK, 1953). The extent of metastatic involvement is variable and no characteristic pattern can be described

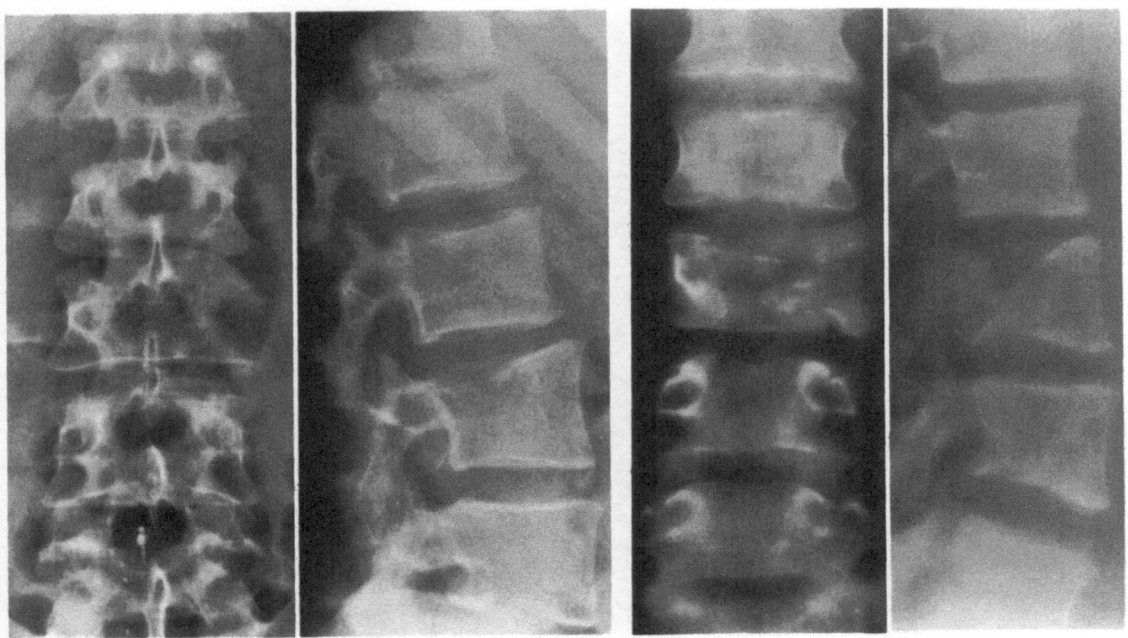

Fig. 64a   Fig. 64b   Fig. 65a   Fig. 65b

Fig. 64a and b. Carcinoma of lung. AP and lateral views of spine demonstrate destruction of left side of centrum of L3 with loss of normal contour. This is best appreciated on AP view. On lateral view only appreciable change is loss in definition of posterior aspect of superior end-plate of body of L3

Fig. 65a and b. Carcinoma of lung. (Same case as Fig. 64). Frontal and lateral tomograms of spine clearly delineate extent of destructive process involving centrum of L3

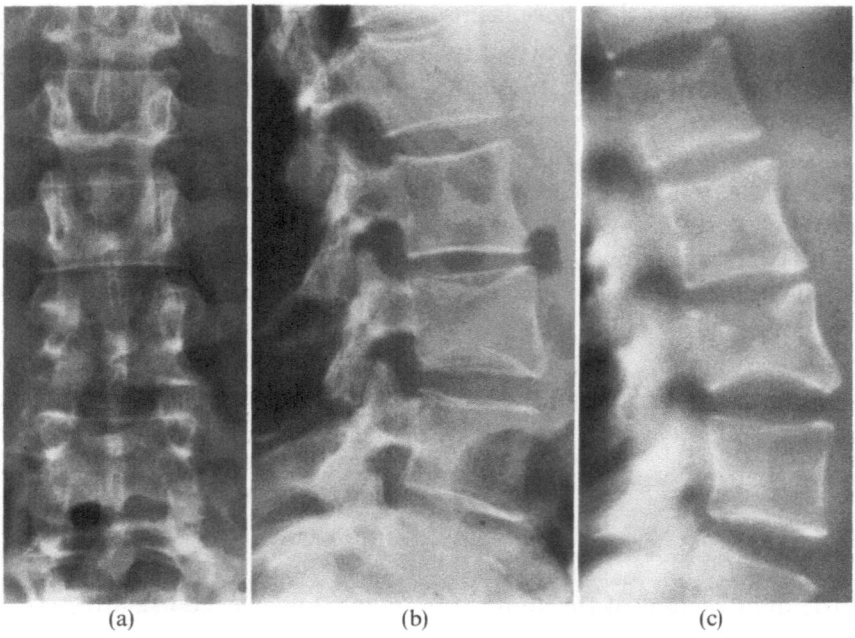

(a)   (b)   (c)

Fig. 66a and b. Carcinoma of breast. Frontal and lateral views of spine demonstrate change in contour of centrum of L3. There is partial compression of right side of vertebral centrum. On lateral view this has resulted in separation of two sides of superior and inferior end-plates. (c) Lateral tomogram of spine clearly delineates change in contour of centrum of L3

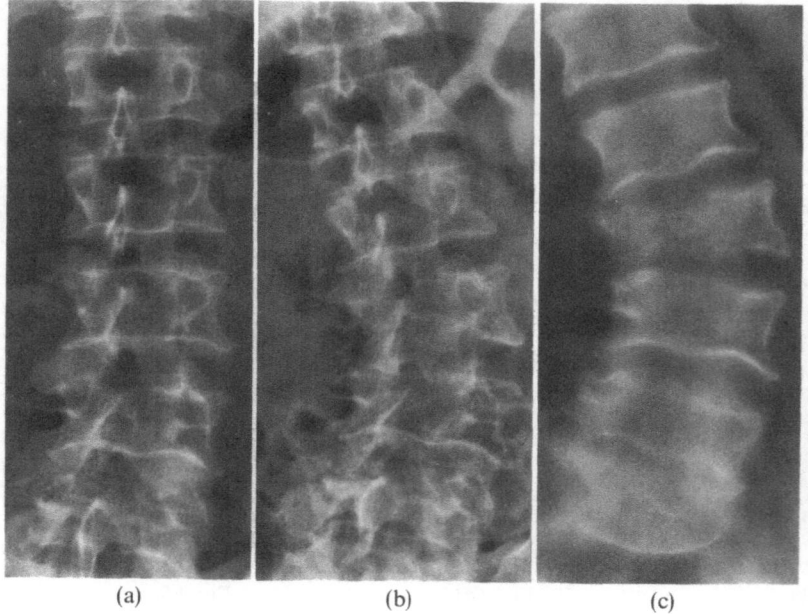

(a)   (b)   (c)

Fig. 67a–c. Carcinoma of prostate. (a) and (b) AP views of spine obtained 4 months apart, demonstrate change in contour of spine as result of compression of centrum of L3. (c) Tomogram of spine demonstrates extensive destruction of centrum of L3. Adjacent intervertebral disc spaces are normal although there is extensive destruction of superior and inferior end-plates

for any specific tumor. Carcinomas of the breast, prostate, kidney, thyroid, and lung commonly metastasize to the spine, however, spinal metastases may occur with any tumor (EPSTEIN, 1969).

The roentgenographic detection of metastases depends upon the identification of bone destruction or production. The earliest sign of metastatic involvement is spotty decalcification of trabeculae or cortex, however, a metastatic lesion in the spine is not likely to become evident until there is considerable osteolytic or osteoblastic activity in the affected area or the contour of the involved bone has been changed (Figs. 64–68). Metastases may develop in any portion of the vertebra and involvement of a pedicle, transverse process or a portion of the neural arch is common (Figs. 69–73). Tomography is often helpful in detecting the lesions at this stage and determining the extent of involvement (Figs. 64, 65, 66, 71, and 72). In some cases there may be extensive destruction

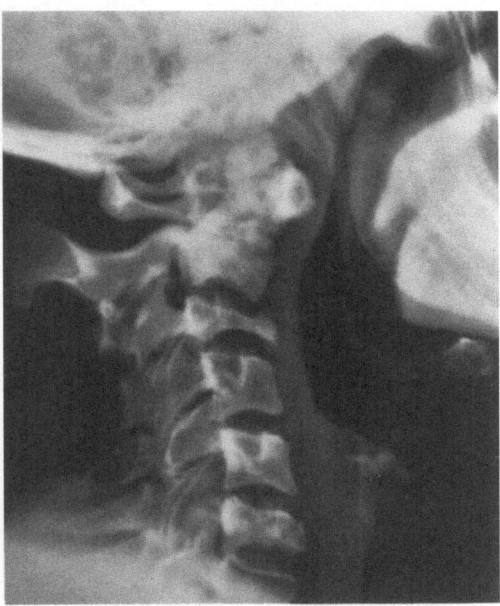

Fig. 68. Carcinoma of breast. There is compression of centra of C3 and C6. Metastatic involvement of base of odontoid process has resulted in subluxation of C1 on C2

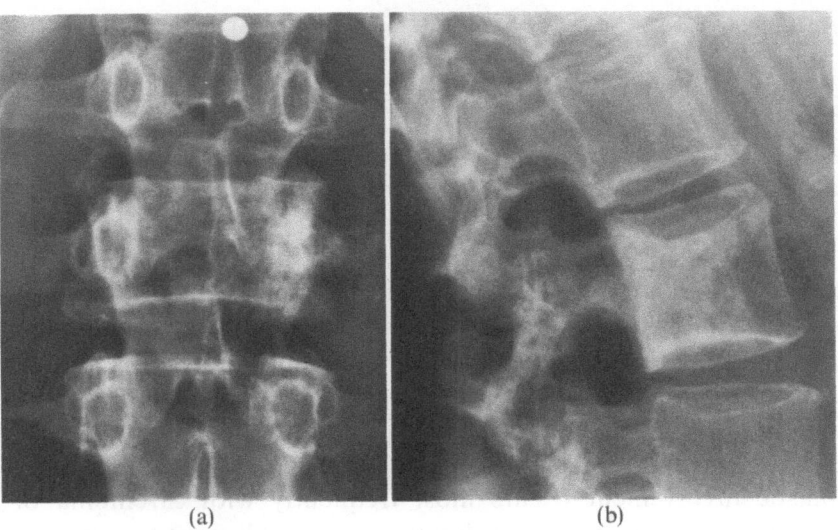

(a)   (b)

Fig. 69. Carcinoma of prostate. Osteoblastic metastases involving pedicle and left side of centrum of L2. There is also involvement of left transverse process. Cortex of pedicle has been completely destroyed

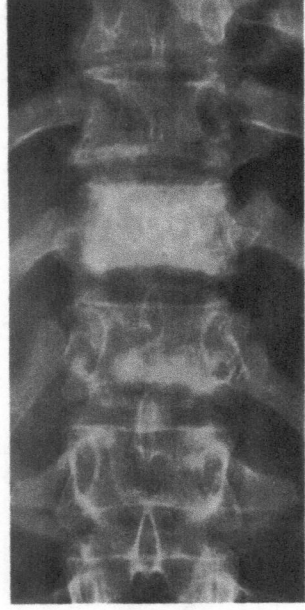

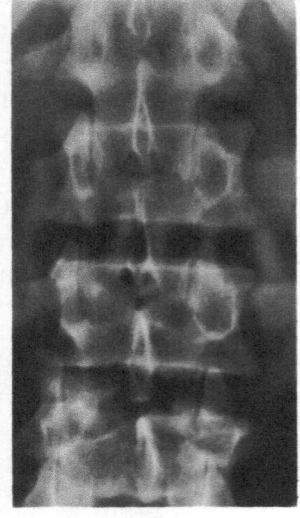

Fig. 70.   Fig. 71.

Fig. 70. Carcinoma of breast. Osteoblastic metastases are present in centra of T11 and T12. In spite of extensive involvement of T11, there is no apparent change in contour

Fig. 71. Carcinoma of lung. There are four non-rib-bearing vertebrae. Right pedicle of the 3rd lumbar vertebra is absent

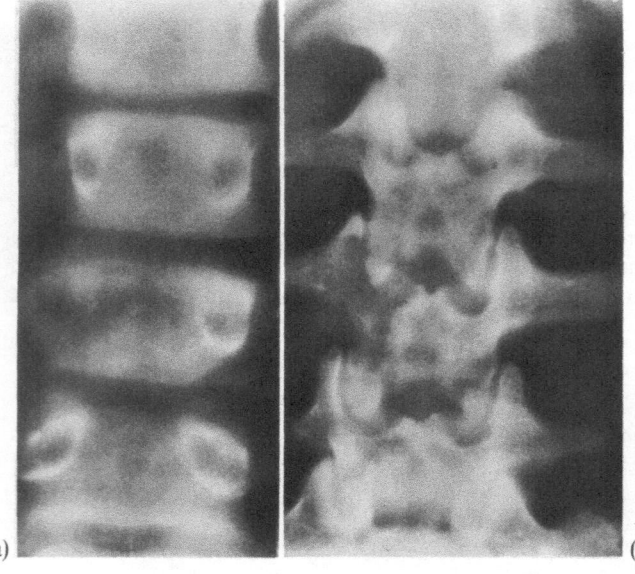

(a)   (b)

Fig. 72a and b. Carcinoma of lung. (Same case as Fig. 71). AP tomograms of spine clearly delineate destruction of pedicle of 3rd lumbar vertebra. In addition there is destruction of transverse process and superior articular facet. These changes are not clearly identified on regular views of spine

of trabeculae without appreciable change in the roentgenographic appearance of the spine, however, compression of the vertebral body eventually occurs. Multiple vertebrae may be involved with resultant kyphosis as the result of multiple pathologic fractures. Metastases to the odontoid process may result in pathologic fracture and atlantoaxial subluxation (Figs. 68 and 74). Tomograms are often necessary to evaluate the extent of metastatic disease in this region (Figs. 75–76).

Osteoblastic involvement occurs most frequently with carcinoma of the breast or prostate, particularly after treatment, however, any malignant tumor can produce osteoblastic metastases. The lesions initially present as localized areas of increased density similar to that seen elsewhere in the skeleton. Osteolytic lesions may undergo evidence

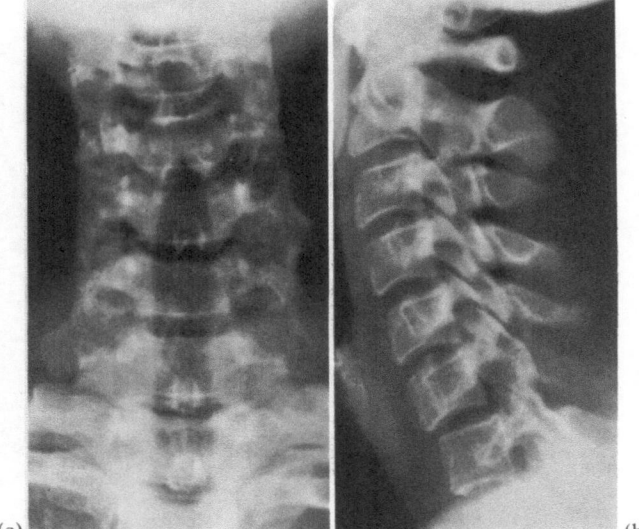

Fig. 73a and b. Carcinoma of breast. There is destruction of spinous process of C6. This is clearly seen on lateral view. On AP view contour of spinous process is completely absent when compared with spinous processes of C5 and C7. Spinous processes should be carefully examined, particularly in lower cervical and thoracic regions as metastases to spinous processes are frequently overlooked

(a)   (b)

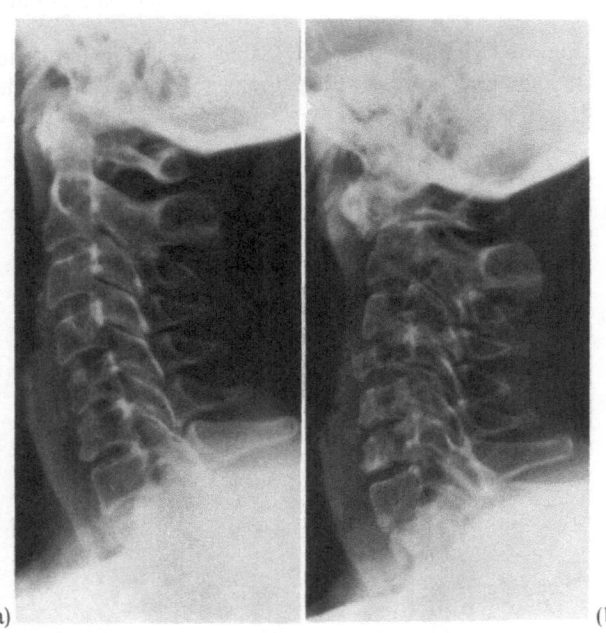

Fig. 74a and b. Carcinoma of breast. Lateral views of spine obtained 6 months apart demonstrate presence of extensive metastatic disease in cervical spine with pathologic fracture of odontoid, subluxation of C1 on C2, and compression of vertebral centra

(a)   (b)

of healing and collapsed vertebra may become sclerotic (Figs. 77 and 78). In some cases, the entire vertebra may become densely sclerotic (Figs. 79 and 80).

Although metastases may develop in any portion of the vertebra, JACOBSON et al. (1958) have pointed out that the pedicles are less frequently involved in myeloma (20%) than in metastatic disease (80%). Preservation of the pedicles in the face of extensive destruction elsewhere in the spine is strongly suggestive of myeloma although the pedicles may be destroyed in myeloma or intact in metastatic carcinoma. The difference in the incidence of pedicle involvement is felt to be related to the lack of red marrow in the pedicles. Multiple myeloma is a disease of marrow and destruction occurs at the site of involvement. Thus, the pedicles are initially spared, whereas metastatic disease

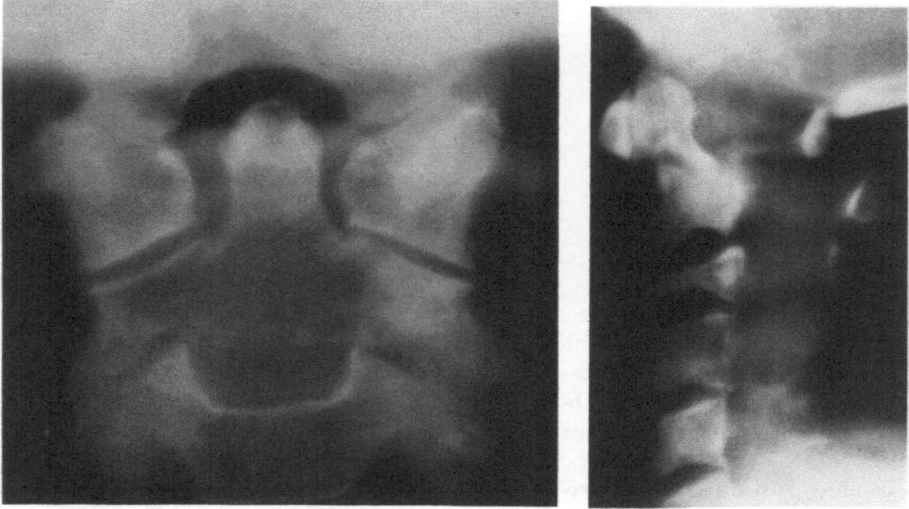

Fig. 75   Fig. 76

Fig. 75. Carcinoma of breast. Tomogram of upper cervical spine demonstrating destruction of body of C2 and base of odontoid process

Fig. 76. Carcinoma of breast. (Same case as Fig. 68). Lateral tomograms demonstrating metastatic involvement of odontoid process with pathologic fracture and subluxation of C1 on C2. There is also compression of centrum of C3

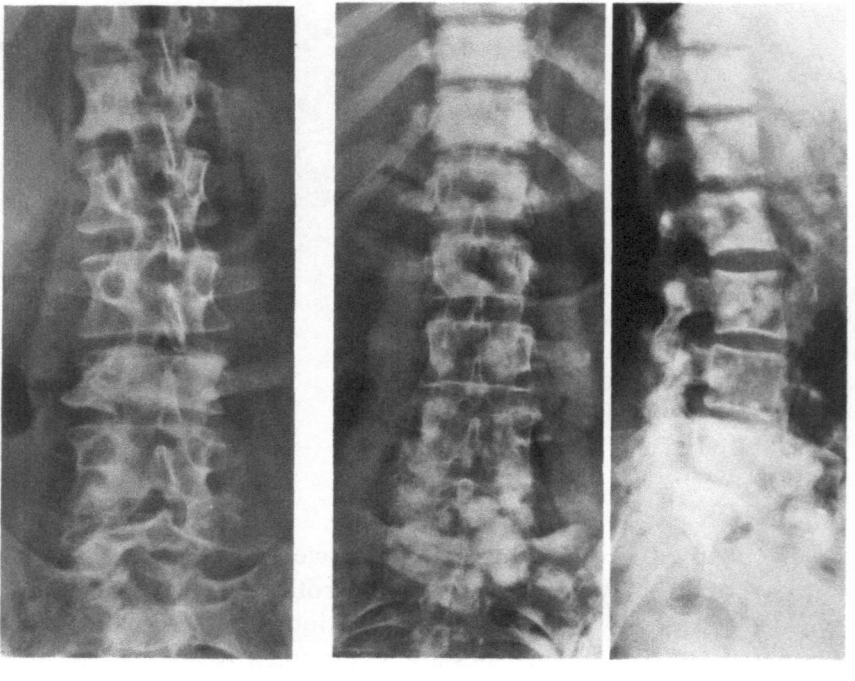

Fig. 77   Fig. 78a   Fig. 78b

Fig. 77. Carcinoma of prostate. Osteoblastic metastases are present in centrum of L1 and L4, with partial collapse of centrum of L4

Fig. 78a and b. Carcinoma of breast. AP and lateral views of spine demonstrate extensive osteoblastic metastases throughout the spine. In spite of extensive involvement there is no change in contour of involved vertebrae

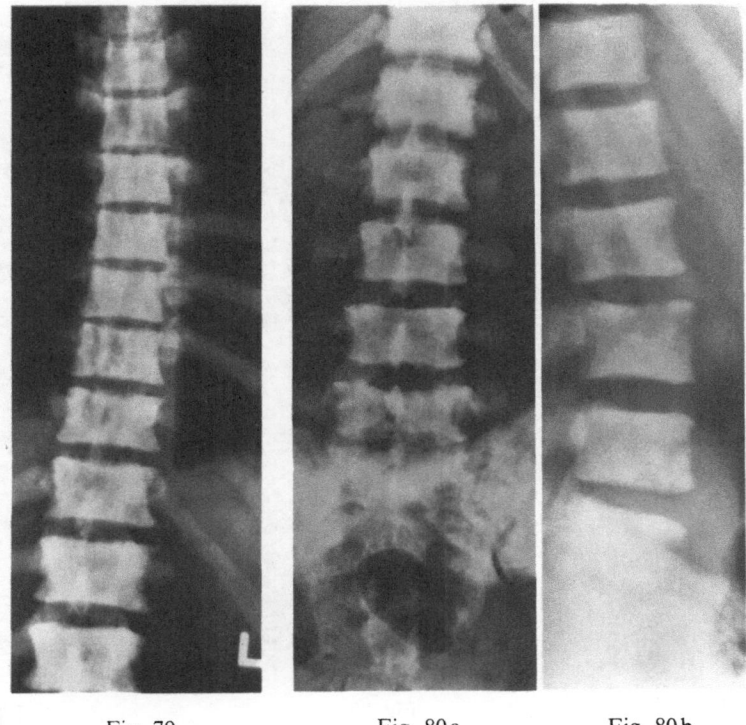

Fig. 79   Fig. 80a   Fig. 80b

Fig. 79. Carcinoma of breast. There is extensive osteoblastic involvement of spine resulting in uniformly dense vertebral centra

Fig. 80a and b. Carcinoma of breast. AP and lateral views of lumbosacral spine demonstrating extensive osteoblastic metastases

may easily spread to the pedicles. Since the pedicles are small and destruction of the cortex easily appreciated, metastases are frequently detected there at an early stage. In spite of extensive destruction of the vertebral bodies, the intervertebral disc spaces are characteristically spared (EPSTEIN, 1969; NORMAN and KAMBOLIS, 1964).

VII. Rib Metastases

Metastatic involvement of the ribs is common, however, the spectrum of roentgenographic changes observed wih rib metastases is less extensive than that observed in other areas. Tumor infiltrates the intertrabecular spaces, however, by the time sufficient destruction has occurred to allow roentgenographic demonstration the involved area of the rib has been destroyed. The spongiosa is thin and it is difficult to detect cortical involvement in most portions of the rib. Metastases to the ribs usually present roentgenographically as multiple areas of destruction (Fig. 81), however, at times the involved area may undergo expansion (Fig. 82), and soft tissue masses may be present (Fig. 83). Osteoblastic involvement usually is manifest as dense sclerosis with loss of trabeculae (Fig. 84), however, osteoblastic metastases, particularly from carcinomas of the prostate and colon or carcinoids, may produce expansion of the rib (Fig. 85).

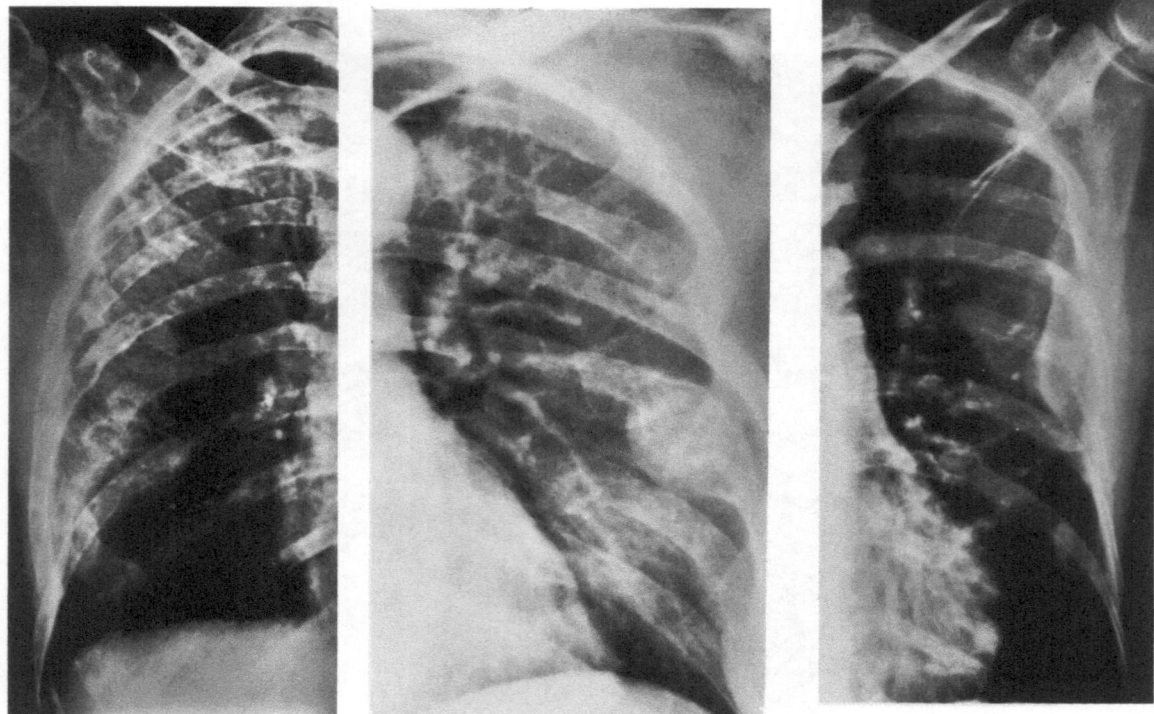

Fig. 81   Fig. 82   Fig. 83

Fig. 81. Carcinoma of breast. Multiple areas of destruction are noted in ribs, right scapula, and clavicle. There is almost complete loss of bony margins at site of maximum destruction

Fig. 82. Carcinoma of breast. Destructive lesions are noted in ribs with associated areas of expansion. This is particularly apparent in left 6th and 7th ribs

Fig. 83. Carcinoma of breast. Destructive lesions are present in left ribs with associated subpleural soft tissue masses

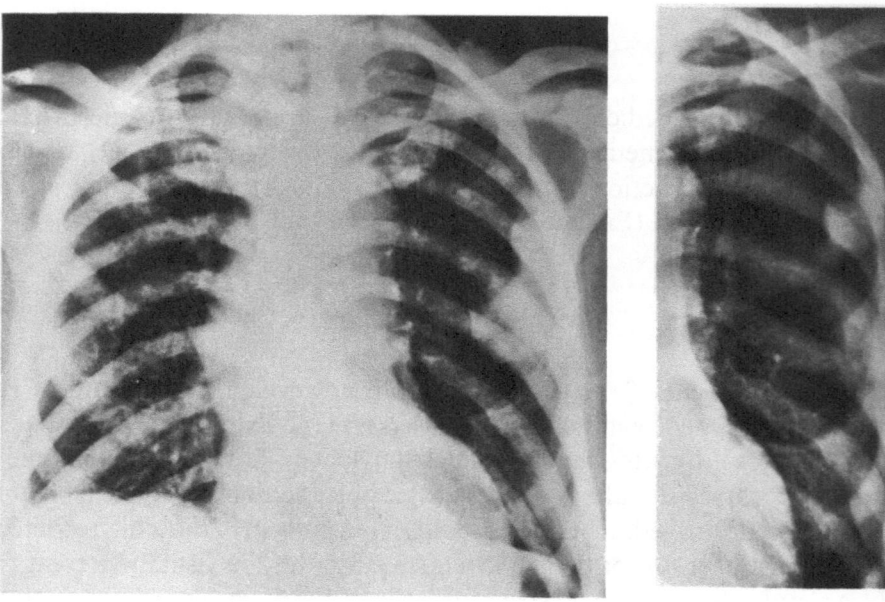

Fig. 84   Fig. 85

Fig. 84. Carcinoma of prostate. Ribs, clavicles, and scapulae are uniformly dense indicating presence of extensive osteoblastic metastases

Fig. 85. Carcinoma of prostate. Extensive osteoblastic involvement of ribs with expansion of anterior ends of ribs

VIII. Skull Metastases

Metastases to the skull are predominantly osteolytic. The roentgenographic findings range from small, sharply demarcated lesions, to large, confluent, ill-defined areas of destruction (Figs. 86–90). At times target lesions may be observed in which the center consists of bone of normal or increased density (Fig. 86). Similar lesions have been found with lymphomas, tuberculosis, or other chronic infections and eosinophilic granuloma. Extensive metastatic involvement may result in almost complete destruction of the inner and outer tables with extension into the adjacent soft tissues (Fig. 90).

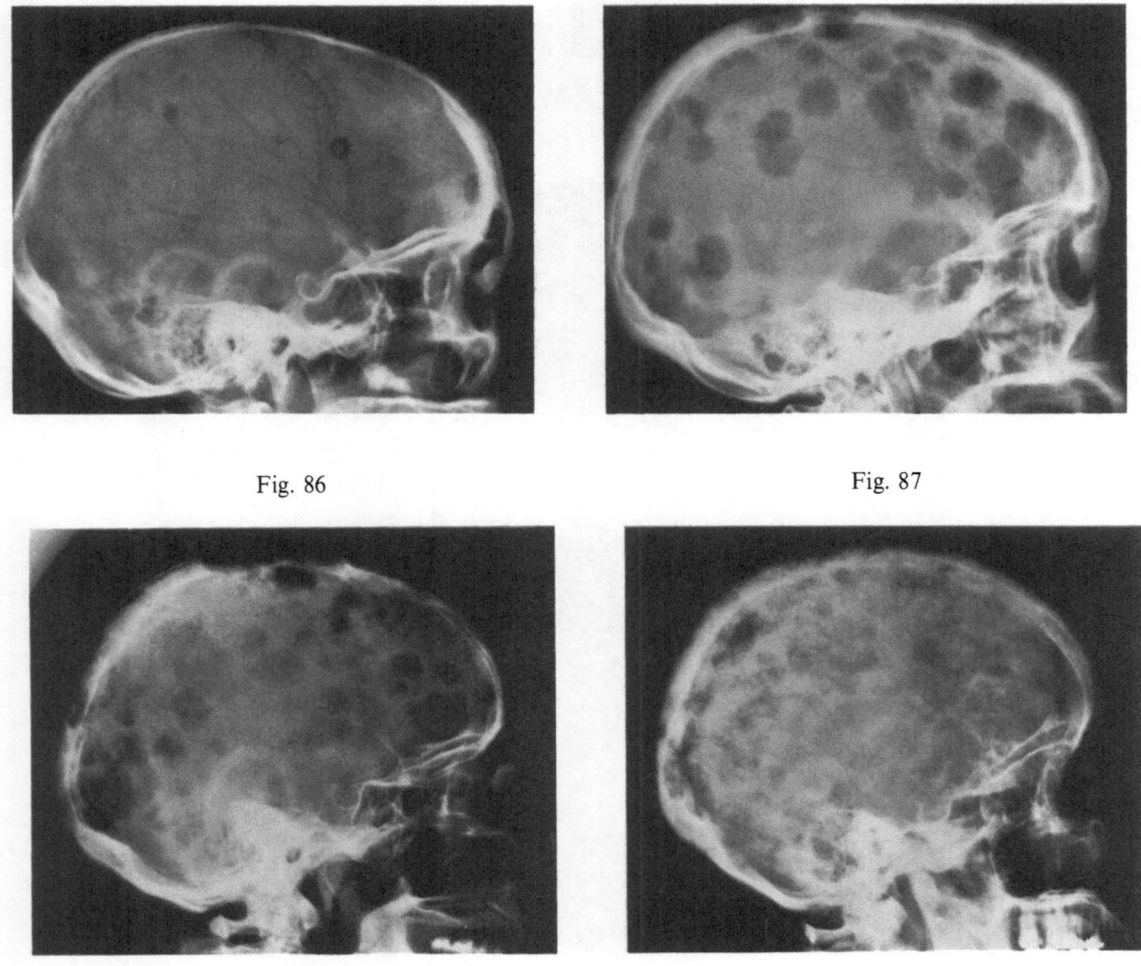

Fig. 86   Fig. 87

Fig. 88   Fig. 89

Fig. 86. Metastatic adenocarcinoma, primary unknown. Multiple small osteolytic lesions are present in calvarium. In posterior frontal region there is small target lesion in which center of normal bone is identified within osteolytic lesion

Fig. 87. Carcinoma of breast. Multiple large osteolytic lesions are present throughout calvarium. Margins are irregular and there is involvement of both inner and outer tables

Fig. 88. Carcinoma of breast. There are extensive confluent osteolytic lesions noted throughout calvarium with involvement of inner and outer tables. Individual lesions are less distinctly identified than those in Fig. 87

Fig. 89. Carcinoma of breast. There is diffuse involvement of entire calvarium. Individual lesions are difficult to identify, and only small portions of normal bone remain

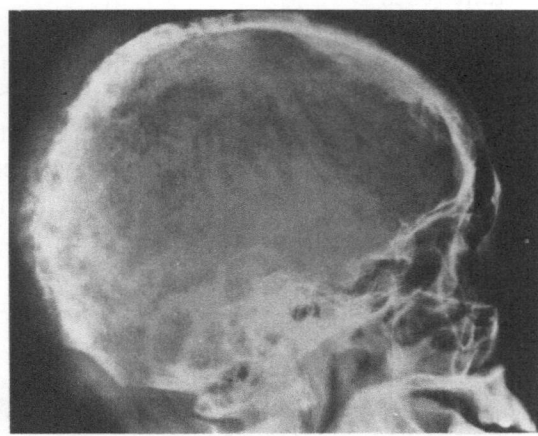

Fig. 90. Lymphoepithelioma. There is extensive destruction of inner and outer tables of parietal and occipital regions with involvement of overlying soft tissues

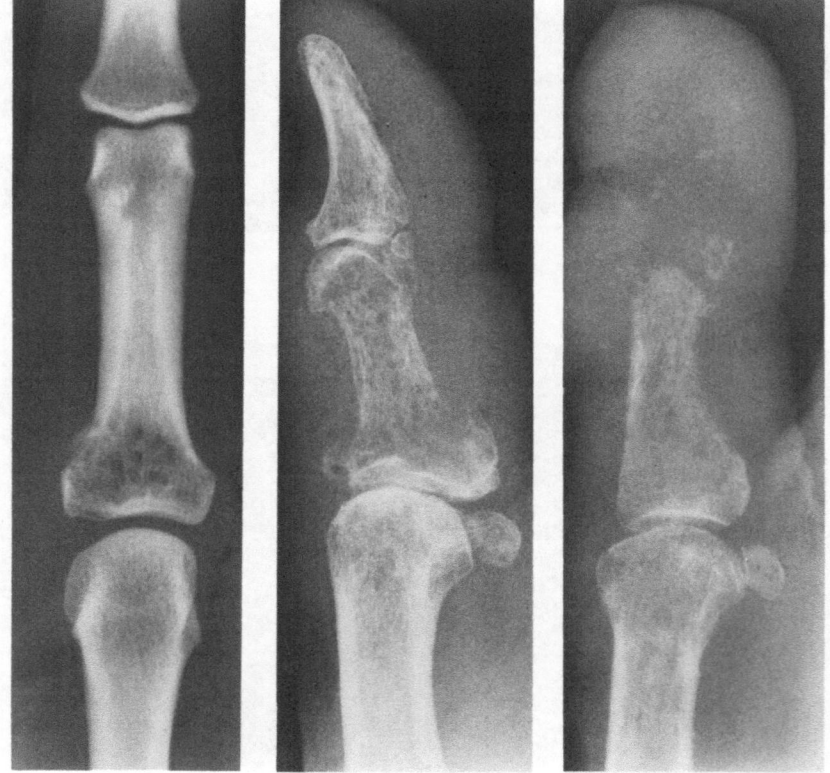

Fig. 91   Fig. 92   Fig. 93

Fig. 91. Carcinoma of breast. There is destructive lesion involving proximal end of proximal phalanx of second digit. Metacarpophalangeal joint is spared

Fig. 92. Carcinoma of lung. Extensive permeative destruction of proximal phalanx of first digit with cortical destruction and soft tissue swelling. In spite of fact that articular cortex is destroyed proximally, metacarpophalangeal joint appears normal

Fig. 93. Metastatic hepatoma. Destruction of distal phalanx of first digit with extensive soft tissue swelling. Tumor in this instance has crossed proximal interphalangeal joint and involves distal end of proximal phalanx. (Courtesy of Dr. JEROME BROSNAN, University of Chicago, Chicago, Illinois)

IX. Peripheral Metastases

Peripheral bone metastases are rare, however, their incidence has increased as a result of earlier detection of metastatic lesions by bone scanning. Peripheral metastases are thought to occur as a late manifestation of widespread skeletal involvement, however, they may occur as isolated lesions and, at times, may be the presenting complaint. The bones of the feet are involved more often than those of the hand and multiple lesions may be present (MULVEY, 1964). The lesions usually occur in the distal phalanges, however, involvement of the proximal phalanges as well as the carpal and tarsal bones may occur (GOLD and REEFE, 1963; KERIN, 1958; LEVINE and SHEINKOP, 1973; SMITH, 1963).

The roentgenographic appearance is usually that of a predominantly destructive lesion with little bone reaction (Figs. 91–93), however, we have seen a case of prostatic metastasis involving the talus with typical osteoblastic lesions (Fig. 94). The metastatic site characteristically appears inflamed and may be painful, swollen, and discolored. The major problem is differentiation from osteomyelitis. Reactive bone is rarely seen with metastatic disease, and the soft tissue involvement is localized, homogeneous, and well-defined. Joint involvement rarely occurs. Osteomyelitis, on the other hand, results in new bone formation and the soft tissue changes are characterized by diffuse swelling, reticulation, and loss of soft tissue planes. The ballooned-out effect on the remaining cortical shell produced by the expanding neoplastic mass is not seen with osteomyelitis.

Bronchogenic carcinoma accounts for approximately 50% of all peripheral metastases (TRACHTENBERG and ROSWIT, 1961; KERIN, 1958). This is probably related to the increased

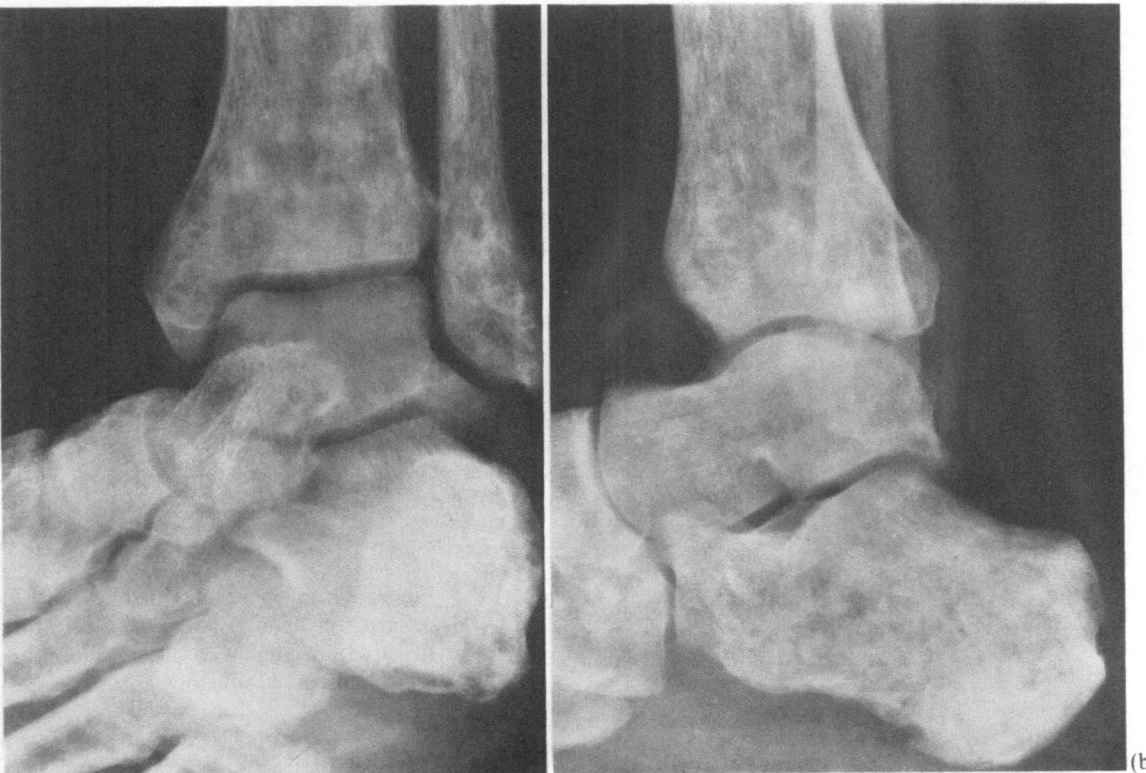

(a)   (b)

Fig. 94a and b. Carcinoma of prostate. AP and lateral views of ankle demonstrating osteoblastic metastases in distal tibia, fibula, and calcaneus

likelihood of a lung tumor invading the pulmonary veins and thus entering the systemic circulation. The arterial dissemination of tumor cells in this manner may account for the rapid appearance of bone metastases in the usual areas as well as in the peripheral bones. The remaining primary sites reported in the literature include the kidney, breast, prostate, uterus, bladder, nasopharynx, and parotid, although theoretically any tumor that reaches the arterial circulation could spread to the hands or feet (Gold and Reefe, 1963; Kerin, 1958; Levine and Sheinkop, 1973). Murray and Jacobson (1970) state that peripheral lesions in the hand or foot usually have their origins in the lung, kidney, breast, uterus, esophagus, or melanoma of the skin. We have observed metastatic lesions with carcinomas in the lung, thyroid, breast, prostate, and liver.

X. Metastatic Disease in Children

The vast majority of skeletal metastases occur in adults over 40, however, it is not unusual to find disseminated metastases from carcinoma of the breast and lung in patients under 30. In children, metastatic lesions most commonly come from neuroblastomas, retinoblastomas, embryonal rhabdomyosarcomas, and primary bone tumors such as Ewing's sarcoma or osteosarcoma (Caffey, 1973). These tumors tend to involve areas of active hematopoiesis and usually produce extensive destruction. In the long bones, ill-defined areas of destruction, often associated with periosteal new bone formation, are found in the metaphysis (Figs. 95–99). At times it may be difficult to differentiate these lesions from the bone changes of acute leukemia. Involvement of the spine likewise results in extensive destruction with vertebral collapse.

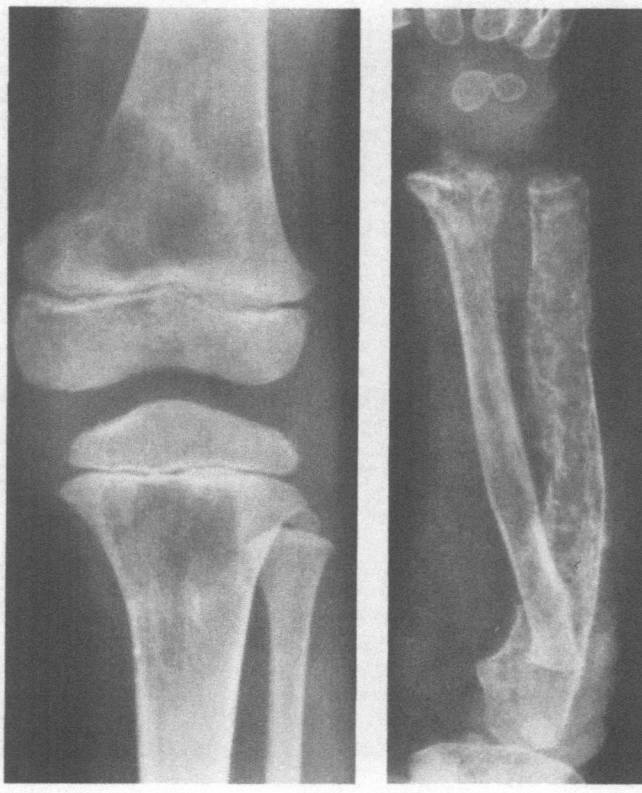

Fig. 95. Embryonal rhabdomyosarcoma. Ill-defined osteolytic lesions with cortical destruction are present in distal femoral and proximal tibial metaphysis

Fig. 96. Metastatic neuroblastoma. There is extensive destruction in radius and ulna. Shaft of ulna is expanded and there is cortical destruction in midshaft of ulna and distal radius

Fig. 95   Fig. 96

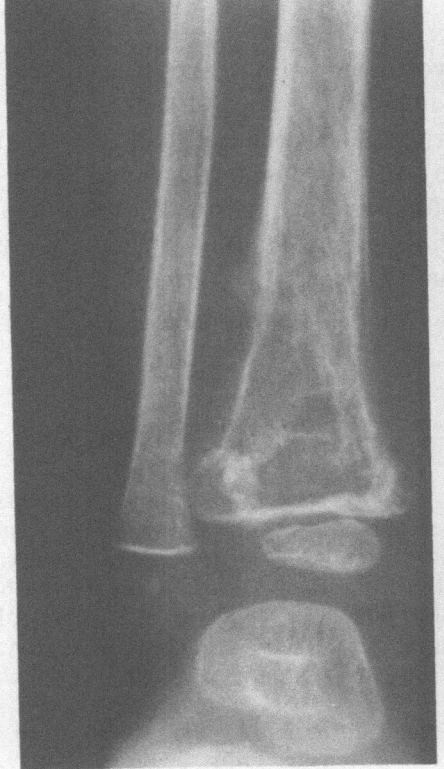
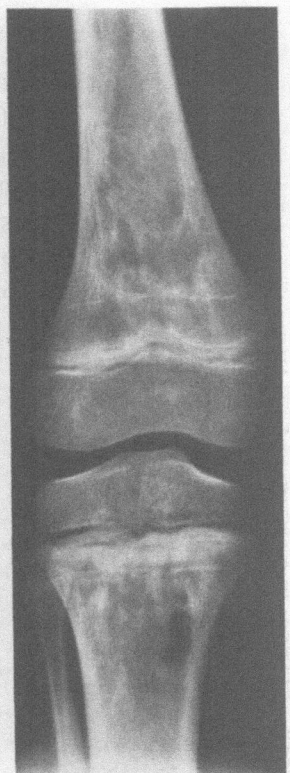

Fig. 97. Metastatic neuroblastoma. There is irregular destruction of distal tibia with associated periosteal reaction

Fig. 98. Metastatic neuroblastoma. There are ill-defined areas of destruction with intervening sclerotic trabeculae present in distal femur and proximal tibia. Radiolucent growth-arrest lines are present in distal femoral and proximal tibial metaphyses. Similar lesions may be seen in acute leukemia

Fig. 97   Fig. 98

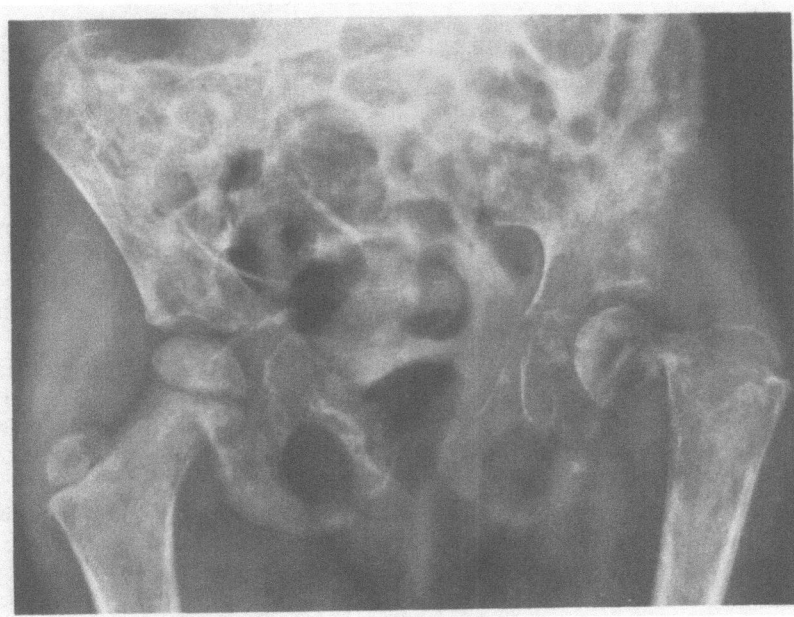

Fig. 99. Embryonal rhabdomyosarcoma. Extensive destruction is present in pelvis and proximal right femur. There is pathologic fracture of right femoral neck with displacement of distal fragment. Sclerotic trabeculae are identified in pelvis indicating that there is some evidence of osteoblastic activity

Conclusion

Metastatic involvement of the skeleton is common with many types of neoplasms, however, except in a few special instances, there are no specific criteria to indicate the responsible primary neoplasm. Bone can react in only a few ways to any malignant neoplasm and any tumor can produce metastatic lesions of similar appearance. The preceding discussion has been an attempt to understand the characteristics of metastatic disease and provide an insight into the clinical problems surrounding the evaluation of metastatic bone lesions.

References

ABRAMS, H.L., SPIRO, R., GOLDSTEIN, N.: Metastases in carcinoma. Cancer (Philad.) **3**, 74–85 (1950)

AEGERTER, E., KIRKPATRICK, J.A.: Orthopedic diseases, 3rd ed. Philadelphia: W.B. Saunders 1968

AGGARWAL, N.O., MITTAL, R.L., BHALLA, R.: Delayed solitary metastasis to the radius of renal cell carcinoma. J. Bone Jt Surg. **54A**, 1314–1316 (1972)

ARIEL, I.M., LEHMAN, W.B.: Prognosis in patients with metastases to bone from primary breast cancer. Bull. Hosp. Jt Dis. (N.Y.) **26**, 40–46 (1965)

ARKLESS, R.: Renal carcinoma: How it metastasizes. Radiology **84**, 496–501 (1965)

BACHMAN, A.L., SPROUL, E.E.: Correlation of radiographic and autopsy findings in suspected metastases in the spine. Bull. N.Y. Acad. Med. **31**, 146–148 (1955)

BATSON, O.V.: The function of the vertebral veins and their role in the spread of metastases. Ann. Surg. **112**, 138–149 (1940)

BATSON, O.V.: The vertebral vein system as a mechanism for the spread of metastases. Amer. J. Roentgenol. **48**, 715–718 (1942)

BECKER, F.O., SCHWARTZ, T.B.: Normal Fluorine-18 bone scans in metastatic bone disease. J. Amer. Med. Ass. **225**, 628–629 (1973)

BEER, D.T., DUBOWY, J., JIMENEZ, F.A.: Osteoblastic metastases from bronchogenic carcinoma. Amer. J. Roentgenol. **91**, 161–166 (1964)

BORAK, J.: Relationship between the clinical and roentgenological findings in bone metastases. Surg. Gynec. Obstet. **75**, 599–604 (1942)

CAFFEY, J.: Pediatric x-ray diagnosis, 6th ed. Chicago: Year Book 1973

CHARKES, N.D.: Radioisotope scanning of roentgenologically occult disorders of bone. In: Clinical uses of radionuclides. GOSWITZ, F.A., ANDREWS, G.A., VIAMONTE, M.KR. (eds.). Washington, U.S. Atomic Energy Commission, 1972

CHARKES, N.D., SKLAROFF, D.M.: Early diagnosis of metastatic bone cancer by photoscanning with strontium-85. J. Nuclear Med. **5**, 168–179 (1964)

CHARKES, N.D., SKLAROFF, D.M., YOUNG, I.: A critical analysis of strontium bone scanning for detection of metastatic cancer. Amer. J. Roentgenol. **96**, 647–656 (1966)

CHUTE, R., IRELAND, E.F., JR., HOUGHTON, J.D.: Solitary distant metastases from unsuspected renal carcinomas. J. Urol. (Baltimore) **80**, 420–424 (1958)

CLAIN, A.: Secondary Malignant Disease of Bone. Brit. J. Cancer **19**, 15–29 (1965)

COLE, J.O.Y.: Bone metastases in advanced breast cancer: Radiological appearances following hypophysectomy. Clin. Radiol. **16**, 295–301 (1965)

COPELAND, M.M.: Bone metastases. Radiology **16**, 198–210 (1931)

COPELAND, M.M.: Metastases to bone from primary tumors in other sites. Proc. nat. Cancer Conf. **6**, 743–756 (1970)

DEBNAM, J.W., STAPLE, T.W.: Osseous metastases from cerebellar medulloblastoma. Radiology **107**, 363–365 (1973)

DEEMARSKY, L.Y., CHERNOMORDIKOVA, M.F.: Clinical and roentgenologic picture of the alterations obtained in the treatment of breast cancer osseous metastases. Cancer (Philad.) **28**, 282–288 (1971)

DELCLOS, L.: The place of radiotherapy in the palliative treatment for bone metastases. In: Tumors of bone and soft tissue. University of Texas M.D. Anderson Hospital and Tumor Institute, Chicago, Year Book. 1965, 243–249

DOE, R.P., SEAL, U.S.: Acid phosphatase in urology. Surg. Clin. N. Amer. **45**, 1455–1466 (1965)

DRESSER, R., SPENCER, J.: Hodgkin's disease and allied conditions of bone. Amer. J. Roentgenol. **36**, 809–815 (1936)

EDEIKEN, J., HODES, P.J.: Roentgen diagnosis of diseases of bone. Baltimore: Williams and Wilkins, 1967

ELKIN, M., MUELLER, H.P.: Metastases from cancer of the prostate. Cancer (Philad.) **7**, 1246–1248 (1954)

EPSTEIN, B.S.: The spine. Philadelphia: Lea and Febiger 1969

FABER, D.D., WAHMAN, G.E., BAILEY, T.A., FLOCKS, R.H., CULP, D.A., MORRISON, R.T.: An evaluation of the strontium[85] scan for the detection and localization of bone metastases from prostate carcinoma. J. Urol. (Baltimore) 97, 526–532 (1967)

FINKELSTEIN, J.Z., EKERT, H., ISAACS, H., JR., HOGGINS, G.: Bone marrow metastases in children with solid tumors. Amer. J. Dis. Child. 119, 49–52 (1970)

FLOCKS, R.H.: Combination therapy for localized prostatic cancer. J. Urol. (Baltimore) 89, 889–894 (1963)

FORT, W.A.: Cancer metastatic to bone. Radiology 24, 96–98 (1935)

FRIED, J.R.: Skeletal and pulmonary metastasis from cancer of kidney, prostate and bladder. Amer. J. Roentgenol. 55, 153–164 (1946)

GALASKO, C.S.B.: The detection of skeletal metastases from carcinoma of the breast. Surg. Gynec. Obstet. 132, 1019–1024 (1971)

GIBBONS, J., HOLLEB, A.I., FARROW, J.H.: An evaluation of routine preoperative skeletal survey for the patients with operable breast cancer. N.Y. J. Med. 61, 4219–4220 (1961)

GILLISON, E.W., GRAINGER, R.G., FERNANDEZ, M.B.: Osteoblastic metastases in carcinoma of pancreas. Brit. J. Radiol. 43, 818–820 (1970)

GOLD, G.L., REEFE, W.E.: Carcinoma and metastases of the bones of the hand. J. Amer. med. Ass. 184, 171–173 (1963)

GOLDHABER, P.: Some current concepts of bone physiology. New Engl. J. Med. 266, 870–877 (1962)

GOODING, C.A., O'CONNOR, J.F., DEALY, J.B., JR.: Angiographic manifestations of osseous metastases from renal cell carcinoma. Vasc. Dis. 3, 208–220 (1966)

GUTMAN, E.B., SPROUL, E.E., GUTMAN, A.B.: Significance of increased phosphates activity of bone at site of osteoblastic metastases secondary to carcinoma of the prostate gland. Amer. J. Cancer 28, 485–495 (1936)

HANSEN, H.H., MUGGIA, F.M., SELAWRY, O.S.: Bone marrow examination in 100 consecutive patients with bronchogenic carcinoma. Lancet 443–445 (28 Aug. 1971)

HARMER, C.L., BURNS, J.E., SAMS, A., SPITTLE, M.: The value of Fluorine-18 for scanning bone tumors. Clin. Radiol. 20, 204–212 (1969)

HOPKINS, G.B., KIRSTENSEN, K.A.B., BLICKENSTAFF, D.E.: Flourine-18 bone scans in the detection of early metastatic bone tumors. J. Amer. med. Ass. 222, 813–814 (1972)

HYMAN, G.A., WELLS, J.: Bronchial carcinoid with osteoblastic metastases. Arch. intern. Med. 114, 541–546 (1964)

JACKSON, D.M.: Myeloma and carcinoma metastatic to bone. Clin. Radiol. 19, 318–322 (1968)

JACOBSON, H.G., LUBETSKY, H.W., SHAPIRO, J.G., CARTON, C.A.: Intracranial meningiomas: roentgen study of 126 cases. Radiology 72, 356–367 (1959)

JACOBSON, H.G., POPPEL, M.H., SHAPIRO, J.G., GROSSBERGER, S.: The vertebral pedicle sign. Amer. J. Roentgenol. 80, 817–821 (1958)

JAFFE, H.L.: Tumors and tumorous conditions of bones and joints. Philadelphia: Lea and Febiger 1958

JOHNSTON, A.D.: Pathology of metastatic tumors in bone. Clin. Orthop. 73, 8–32 (1970)

JOHNSTON, M.J., LIPSETT, J.A., DONOVAN, A.J.: Osseous metastases in mammary cancer: Response to therapy. Arch. Surg. (Chicago) 101, 578–581 (1970)

JORGENS, J.: The radiographic characteristics of carcinoma of the prostate. Surg. Clin. N. Amer. 45, 1427–1440 (1965)

KERIN, R.: Metastatic tumors of the hand. J. Bone Jt Surg. 40A, 263–278 (1958)

LEGIER, J.F., TAUBER, L.N.: Solitary metastasis of occult prostatic carcinoma simulating osteogenic sarcoma. Cancer (Philad.) 22, 168–172 (1968)

LEHRER, H.Z., MAXFIELD, W.S., NICE, C.M.: The periosteal "sunburst" pattern in metastatic bone tumors. Amer. J. Roentgenol. 108, 154–161 (1970)

LEPOW, H., SCHOENFELD, M.R., MESSELOFF, C.R., CHU, F.: Non-prostatic causes of acid hyperphosphatasia: Report of a case due to multiple myeloma. J. Urol. (Baltimore) 87, 991–993 (1962)

LEVINE, A.N., SHEINKOP, M.S.: Metastatic carcinoma from the cervix to the calcaneus. Rush Presbyterian-St. Luke's med. Bull. 12, 234–237 (1973)

LODWICK, G.S.: Reactive response to local injury in bone. Radiol. Clin. N. Amer. 2, 209–219 (1964)

LODWICK, G.S.: The radiologic diagnosis of metastatic cancer in bone. In: Tumors of bone and soft tissue. University of Texas M.D. Anderson Hospital and Tumor Institute. Chicago: Year Book 1965, 253–268

LODWICK, G.S.: The bones and joints. Chicago: Year Book 1971

LONDON, M., MCHUGH, R., HUDSON, P.B.: On low acid phosphatase values of patients with known metastatic cancer of the prostate. Cancer Res. 14, 718–724 (1954)

LOWBEER, L.: Multiple myeloma with osteosclerosis. Amer. J. clin. Path. 52, 757 (1969)

MCCORMACK, K.R.: Bone metastases from thyroid carcinoma. Cancer (Philad.) 19, 181–184 (1966)

MCNEIL, B.J., CASSADY, J.R., GEISER, C.F., JAFFE, N., TRAGGIS, D., TREVES, S.: Flourine-18 bone scintigraphy in children with osteosarcoma or Ewing's sarcoma. Radiology 109, 627–631 (1973)

MENDOZA, C.B., JR., MOORE, G.E., CROSSWHITE, L.H., SANDBERG, A.A., WATNE, A.L.: Prognostic significance of tumor cells in the bone marrow. Surg. Gynec. Obstet. 129, 483–488 (1969)

MEYER, P.C.: A statistical and histological survey of metastatic carcinoma in the skeleton. Brit. J. Cancer 11, 511–518 (1957)

Milch, R.A., Changus, G.W.: Response of bone to tumor invasion. Cancer (Philad.) **9**, 340–351 (1956)

Muggia, F.M., Hansen, H.H.: Osteoblastic Metastasis in small cell (oat cell) carcinoma of the lung. Cancer (Philad.) **30**, 801–805 (1972)

Mulvey, R.B.: Peripheral bone metastases. Amer. J. Roentgenol. **91**, 155–160 (1964)

Murray, R.O., Jacobson, H.G.: The radiology of skeletal disorders. Baltimore: Williams & Wilkins 1971

Napoli, L.D., Hansen, H.H., Muggia, F.M., Twigg, H.L.: The incidence of osseous involvement in lung cancer with special reference to the development of osteoblastic changes. Radiology **108**, 17–21 (1973)

Nelson, C.M.K., Boatman, D.L., Flocks, R.H.: Bone marrow examination in carcinoma of the prostate. J. Urol. (Baltimore) **109**, 667–670 (1973)

Norman, A., Kambolis, C.P.: Tumors of the spine and their relationship to the intervertebral disc. Amer. J. Roentgenol. **92**, 1270–1274 (1964)

Norman, A., Ulin, R.: A comparative study of periosteal new-bone response in metastatic bone tumors (solitary) and primary bone sarcomas. Radiology **92**, 705–708 (1969)

Parrish, F.F.: The management of pathologic fractures. In: Tumors of bone and soft tissue. University of Texas M.D. Anderson Hospital and Tumor Institute. Chicago: Year Book 1965, 250–253

Peavy, P.W., Rogers, J.V., Jr., Clements, J.L., Burns, J.B.: Unusual osteoblastic metastases from carcinoid tumors. Radiology **107**, 327–330 (1973)

Pendergrass, H.P., Potsaid, M.S., Castronovo, F.P., Jr.: The clinical use of ^{99m}Tc-Diphosphonate (HEDSPA). Radiology **107**, 557–562 (1973)

Prohaska, J.V., Houttuin, E., Kocandrle, V.: Mammary carcinoma metastases: Response to bilateral adrenalectomy and oophorectomy. Arch. Surg. (Chicago) **92**, 530–536 (1966)

Seife, B.: Osseous metastases from carcinoma of the large bowel. Amer. J. Roentgenol. **119**, 414–418 (1973)

Sherman, R.S., Ivker, M.: The roentgen appearance of thyroid metastases in bone. Amer. J. Roentgenol. **63**, 196–203 (1950)

Sherman, R.S., Pearson, T.A.: The roentgenographic appearance of renal cancer metastasis in bone. Cancer **I**, 276–285 (1948)

Silberstein, E.B., Saenger, E.L., Tofe, A.J., Alexander, G.W., Jr., Park, H.: Imaging of bone metastases with ^{99m}Tc-Sn-EHDP (Diphosphonate), ^{18}F, and skeletal radiography: A comparison of sensitivity. Radiology **107**, 551–555 (1973)

Slager, U.T., Reilly, E.B.: Value of examining bone marrow in diagnosing malignancy. Cancer (Philad.) **20**, 1215–1220 (1967)

Smith, R.J.: Involvement of the carpal bones with metastatic tumor. Amer. J. Roentgenol. **89**, 1253–1255 (1963)

Sum, P.W., Roswit, B., Unger, S.M.: Skeletal metastases from malignant testicular tumors. Amer. J. Roentgenol. **83**, 704–708 (1960)

Taveras, J.M., Wood, E.H.: Diagnostic neuroradiology. Baltimore: Williams and Wilkins Co. 1964

Thomas, B.M.: Three unusual carcinoid tumors with particular reference to osteoblastic bone metastases. Clin. Radiol. **19**, 221–225 (1968)

Toomey, F.B., Felson, B.: Osteoblastic bone metastasis in gastrointestinal and bronchial carcinoids. Amer. J. Roentgenol. **83**, 709–715 (1960)

Trachtenberg, A.S., Roswit, B.: Bronchogenic carcinoma metastatic to the hand. Amer. J. Roentgenol. **85**, 886–890 (1961)

Turner, J.W., Jaffe, H.L.: Metastatic neoplasms: A clinical and roentgenological study of involvement of skeleton and lungs. Amer. J. Roentgenol. **43**, 479–492 (1940)

Vieta, J.O., Friedell, H.L., Craver, L.F.: A survey of Hodgkin's disease and lymphosarcoma in bone. Radiology **39**, 1–14 (1942)

Warren, S., Meissner, W.A.: Neoplasms. In: Textbook of pathology. Anderson, W.A., D. (ed.). St. Louis: C.V. Mosby Co. 1966, 400–429

Watson, W.L.: Lung cancer. St. Louis: C.V. Mosby 1968

Weigensberg, I.J.: The many faces of metastatic renal carcinoma. Radiology **98**, 353–358 (1971)

Young, J.M., Funk, F.J.: Incidence of tumor metastases to the lumbar spine. J. Bone Jt Surg. **35A**, 55–64 (1953)

Zeidman, I.: Metastasis: A review of recent advances. Cancer Res. **17**, 157–162 (1957)

Study of Bone Tumors with Radionuclides

by

Ernest W. Fordham and Panolil C. Ramachandran

Evaluation of the patient with osseous neoplasm has depended on the analysis and correlation of data gained from the patient's history, physical examination, biochemical determinations, roentgenography, and microscopic examination of biopsy material, occasionally with less than conclusive results. With the recent development of appropriate instrumentation and radiopharmaceuticals, radionuclide imaging has emerged as an additional powerful tool in the study and evaluation of most pathologic processes involving the skeleton.

A. Radionuclides

The first published observation that some radioactive elements could accumulate in human tissues (particularly bone) causing pathologic change was made by BLUM in 1923 in describing a case of radiation osteitis of the mandible. In 1925 several authors (HOFFMAN, 1925; MARTLAND et al., 1925) described radium-mesothorium poisoning, elaborating on the etiology, clinical symptomatology, pathologic changes, and prognosis of this condition, pointing out particular affinity for jaw bones. In 1929 MARTLAND and HUMPHRIES described a case of osteogenic sarcoma of the mandible secondary to radium-mesothorium poisoning, correctly concluding that alpha radiation from radium-mesothorium deposition in bones caused radiation osteitis and osteogenic sarcoma.

Artificially induced radioactivity was discovered by CURIE and JOLIOT (1934) and JOLIOT and CURIE (1934). CHIEWITZ and HEVESY (1935) first used an artificially produced nuclide in the study of animal metabolism, demonstrating deposition of ^{32}P in bones of rats. JONES et al. (1940) showed increased uptake of ^{32}P in soft tissue tumor cells. BOHR and SORENSEN (1950) found increased accumulation of ^{32}P at fracture sites in animals. WILKINSON and LEBLOND (1953) demonstrated increased deposition of ^{32}P in rat fractures employing autoradiography and external Geiger-Mueller counting. TUBIANA et al. (1958) documented increased ^{32}P levels in fractures and in Paget's disease in humans by external Bremsstrahlung counting.

I. Isotopes of Calcium

CAMPBELL and GREENBERG (1940) reported the first biologic application of ^{45}Ca; while measuring absorption and excretion of ^{45}Ca in rats they found the highest concentration in bones and teeth. GREENBERG (1945) reported on the use of radioactive calcium (and strontium) for studies on the mechanism of vitamin D action in rachitic rats. CARLSSON (1951, 1952) reported extensive studies of the metabolism of radiocalcium. KARSHER (1953) demonstrated increased calcium uptake in rat fractures. BAUER (1954) utilized radiocalcium to study rates of bone salt formation in healing fractures. BELLIN and LASZLO (1953) were the first to use ^{45}Ca in human cancer subjects, measuring clearance under normal conditions and after infusion with Na-EDTA. BAUER et al. (1957a) reported their extensive studies of human bone salt metabolism utilizing radiocalcium.

While isotopes of calcium utilized as tracers yielded much of the information available on the physiology and pathophysiology of bone, no isotope of calcium has physical characteristics suitable for skeletal imaging.

II. Isotopes of Strontium

STEWART et al. (1937) and DUBRIDGE and MARSHALL (1940) described the various isotopes of strontium. ERF and PECHER (1940) measured the secretion in milk of ^{89}Sr administered intravenously to lactating cows. While measuring skeletal uptake of ^{45}Ca and ^{89}Sr, PECHER (1941) and PECHER and PECHER (1941) demonstrated transfer of these nuclides to fetuses during the last days of pregnancy and to offsprings through lactation. TREADWELL et al. (1942) demonstrated increased accumulation of ^{89}Sr in metabolically active normal bone and to a greater extent in a variety of primary bone tumors. BAUER and WENDEBERG (1959) and BAUER and SCOCCIANTI (1961), by external counting of ^{47}Ca and ^{85}Sr, demonstrated elevated uptakes of several magnitudes in fractures of long bones and vertebrae. GYNNING et al. (1961) demonstrated increased uptake of ^{85}Sr in spinal metastases from breast cancer. In a series of reports published in the mid-1960's, CHARKES and SKLAROFF (1964, 1965), CHARKES et al. (1966), and SKLAROFF and CHARKES (1964) effectively established ^{85}Sr imaging in a primary role for the detection of skeletal abnormalities related to metastatic disease, confirmed by the experience described in another series of reports by DE NARDO (1966, 1968) and DE NARDO and VOLPE (1966). The cumulative experience with ^{85}Sr scanning clearly showed that radionuclide imaging consistently detected osseous lesions months before roentgenography became abnormal.

Although sensitive and reliable, ^{85}Sr bone imaging was a long and cumbersome procedure with poor resolution and low information density (Fig. 1) at rather high absorbed radiation doses.

MEYERS (1960) investigated ^{87m}Sr obtained from the ^{87}Y generator. MARTY and HOFFMAN (1972) and STAHELI et al. (1972) demonstrated the efficacy of ^{87m}Sr scanning in detecting metastatic and infectious disorders of bone and joint. With a short half-life and low absorbed radiation dose, ^{87m}Sr was appropriate for use in benign disease and in the pediatric population; poor target background ratios obtained with this nuclide prevented its widespread use.

Fig. 1a–f. Comparison of bone seeking radiopharmaceuticals. (a) Anterior and (b) posterior ^{85}Sr scans of 14-year-old female 1 year post radiation for Ewing's sarcoma in right tibia. Anterior (c) and posterior (d) ^{18}F scans 20 months later and anterior (e) and posterior (f) ^{99m}Tc-EHDP scans 44 months later show diminished activity in proximal right tibia secondary to radiation. Note increasing stature and diminishing degree of uptake in epiphysis with advancing age. ^{85}Sr scan required $3^1/_2$ h, while high cost ^{18}F and low cost ^{99m}Tc-EHDP scans required 1 h scanning time. Note improving resolution of bony detail with later radiopharmaceuticals

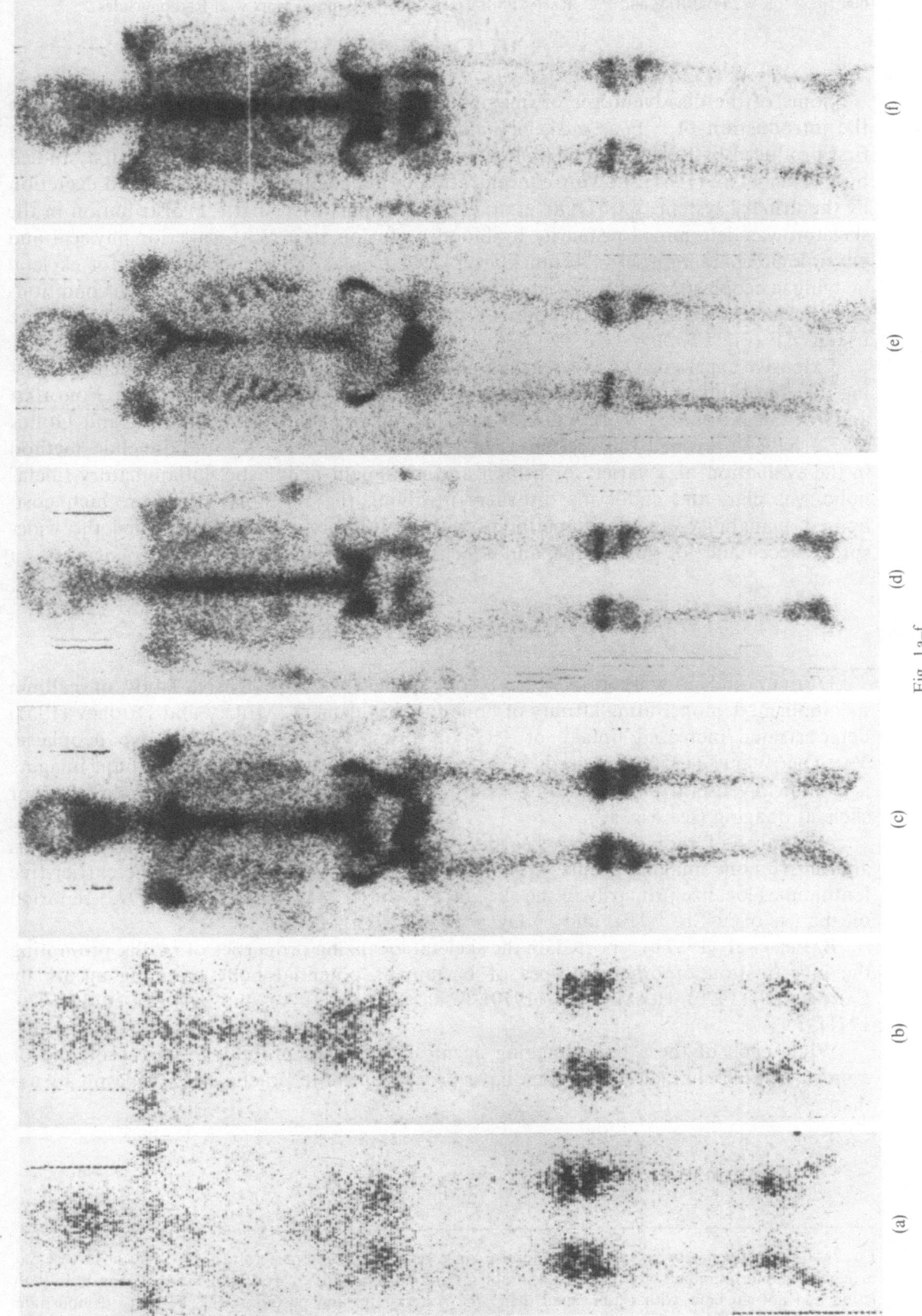

Fig. 1a–f

III. Fluorine-18

Some of the disadvantages of imaging with strontium isotopes were overcome with the introduction of ^{18}F as a skeletal imaging agent by Blau et al. (1962). ^{18}F was first produced by Snell (1937); biologic distribution of ^{18}F in animals was first studied by Volker et al. (1941) showing concentration of nuclide in skeletal tissues and excretion by the urinary system. Van Dyke et al. (1965) demonstrated that ^{18}F distribution in the skeleton was determined primarily by blood perfusion rate. With superior physical and physiologic characteristics, ^{18}F quickly replaced ^{85}Sr as the agent of choice for skeletal imaging in neoplastic conditions and rapidly gained acceptance for use in benign conditions and pediatric patients. Visualization of the entire skeleton became practical with the use of ^{18}F (Figs. 1, 2).

Extensive experience has been accumulated in the study of skeletal abnormality utilizing ^{18}F. In a number of large series Blau et al. (1968), Shirazi et al. (1974a, b), Fordham and Ramachandran (1974), French and McCready (1967) and Sharma and Quinn (1972) have confirmed the usefulness of osseous imaging by the radionuclide method in the evaluation of a variety of benign and malignant neoplastic, inflammatory, metabolic, vascular, and endocrine disorders involving the skeleton. However, high cost, limited availability, and incompatibility with scintillation cameras precluded the widespread acceptance of this reliable and effective radionuclide.

IV. Miscellaneous Radionuclides

Dudley and co-workers (1949a, b, c) reported on an extensive study of gallium metabolism, demonstrating affinity of bone for this element. Mulry and Dudley (1951) demonstrated increased uptake of ^{72}Ga in primary and metastatic bone neoplasia. Van Der Werff (1954) first used ^{66}Ga and ^{67}Ga in the same manner. Gallium imaging is a clinically useful procedure but is not specific for either malignant disease or for skeletal imaging (see Fig. 12).

A number of radioactive rare earths and alkaline earths have been investigated as alternative bone imaging agents. Durbin et al. (1956) demonstrated that the carrier-free lanthanines localize primarily in the skeletal system. O'Mara et al. (1969, 1972) reported on the use of ^{153}Sn, ^{171}Er, and ^{157}Dy.

Bauer et al. (1957b) reported on the skeletal localizing properties of ^{140}Ba, prompting the investigation of other isotopes of barium as potential bone scanning agents by Lange et al. (1970), Hosain et al. (1970), Subramanian (1970), and Spencer et al. (1970, 1971).

While each of these bone imaging agents has offered promise by virtue of one or more favorable characteristics, they have proved no more practical for widespread use than ^{18}F.

Fig. 2a–f. Bone and marrow imaging of chondrosarcoma. Anterior (a) and posterior (b) ^{18}F scans of 11-year-old male with chondrosarcoma of left ileum. Anterior (c) and posterior (d) ^{99m}Tc-EHDP scans demonstrate both lesion and normal bone with better detail than ^{18}F. Anterior (e) and posterior (f) ^{52}Fe scans demonstrate distribution of hematopoietic marrow; note diminished hematopoietic activity in marrow at site of chondrosarcoma

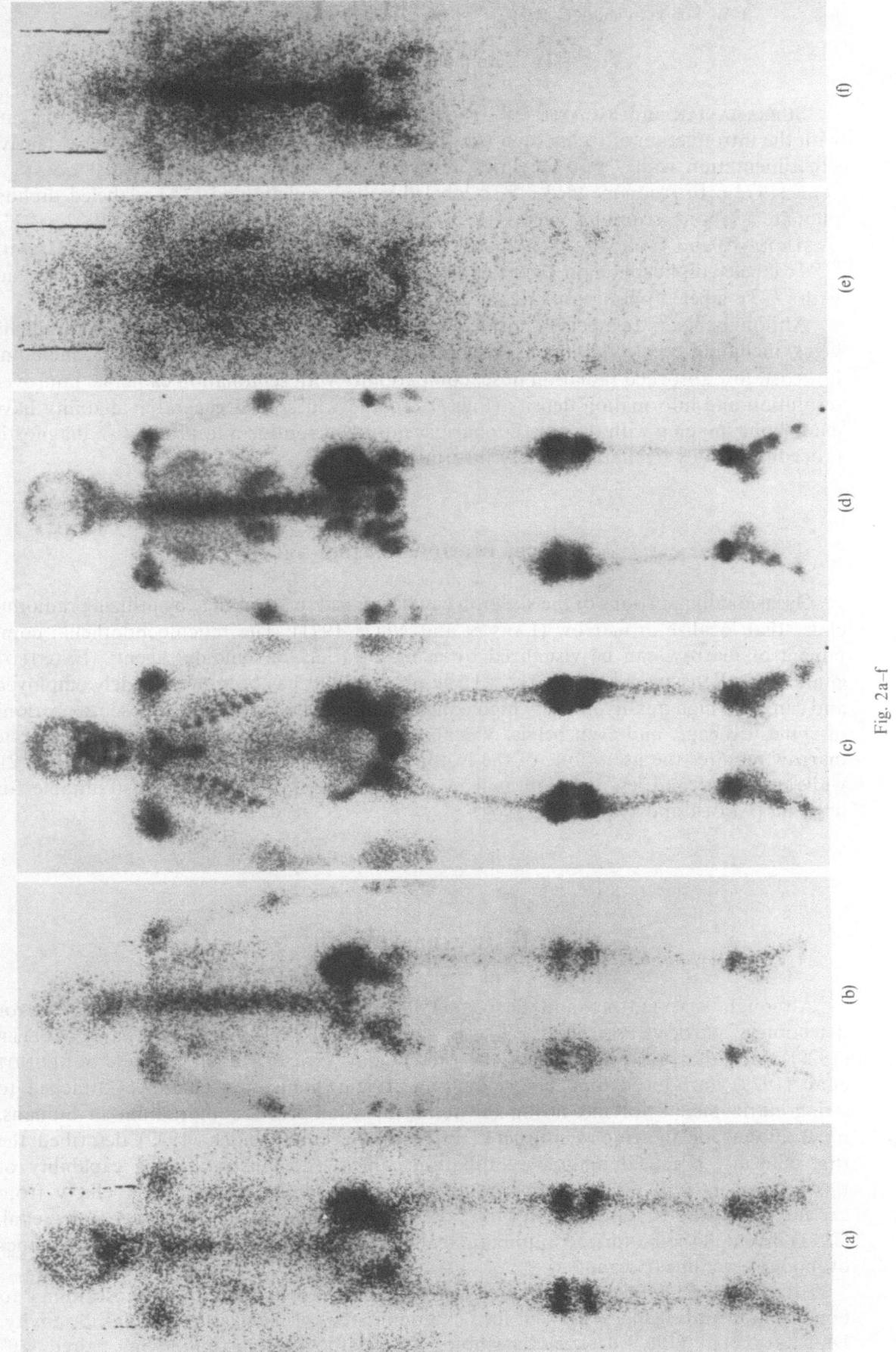

Fig. 2a–f

V. ^{99m}Tc Labeled Phosphate Compounds

SUBRAMANIAN and MCAFEE (1971) achieved a major breakthrough in bone imaging with the introduction of technetium (stannous) sodium tripolyphosphate. After extensive experimentation with ^{99m}Tc labeling of various phosphate compounds. SUBRAMANIAN et al. (1972a, b) recommended ^{99m}Tc labeled polyphosphate and ^{99m}Tc labeled diphosphonate as bone scanning agents. Working independently YANO et al. (1972, 1973), CASTRONOVO and CALLAHAN (1972) and PENDERGRASS et al. (1973) reported success with ^{99m}Tc labeled diphosphonate. PEREZ et al. (1972) conducted initial studies of bone imaging with ^{99m}Tc labeled pyrophosphate.

Although the ^{99m}Tc labeled phosphate compounds suffer from certain minor disadvantages, including occasional inconsistent reproducibility, the major advantages, including low cost, low absorbed radiation dose, compatibility with scintillation cameras, improved resolution and information density (Figs. 1, 2), and widespread general availability have made bone imaging with these radiopharmaceuticals a routine and productive diagnostic procedure readily available in every institution.

VI. Bone Marrow Imaging Agents

Occasionally, portions of the skeleton can be imaged to advantage by utilizing radionuclides that localize in marrow (LARSON and NELP, 1971). The reticuloendothelial component of marrow can be visualized by using a variety of colloidal agents (ENGSTEDT et al., 1958; KNISELY et al., 1966). ^{99m}Tc sulphur colloid has been most widely employed and can yield high quality images; high concentration in liver and spleen obscure portions of spine, rib cage, and even pelvis. Visualization of hematopoietic component of bone marrow requires the use of one of the isotopes of iron (NELP et al., 1966); ^{52}Fe (Fig. 2), while expensive and less than optimal in many respects, is probably most suitable for imaging (ANGER and VAN DYKE, 1964).

B. Instrumentation

Although RUTHERFORD and GEIGER (1908) had constructed the first counters for detection of particles as early as 1906, it was not until 1928 that GEIGER and MÜLLER (1929) made the first prototype of the present day Geiger-Müller counter. SCHLUNDT et al. (1929) introduced total body counting utilizing ionization chambers attached to string electrometers for measuring the retained radon fraction of radium in humans.

Radionuclide imaging was ushered in by two events. ANGER (1949) described the first clinically practical pinhole scintillation camera, demonstrating the capability of this instrument with an in vivo scintigraph of an osseous metastasis in elbow from carcinoma of the thyroid detected by ^{131}I accumulation in the tumor. CASSEN et al. (1951) invented the motorized automatic scanner with recorder which was the forerunner of modern rectilinear scanners.

FLEMING et al. (1961) are credited with the first application of photoscanning to bone, demonstrating increased ^{85}Sr localization in areas of increased osteoblastic activity. DE NARDO et al. (1967) described a whole body profile scanning employing paired 180°

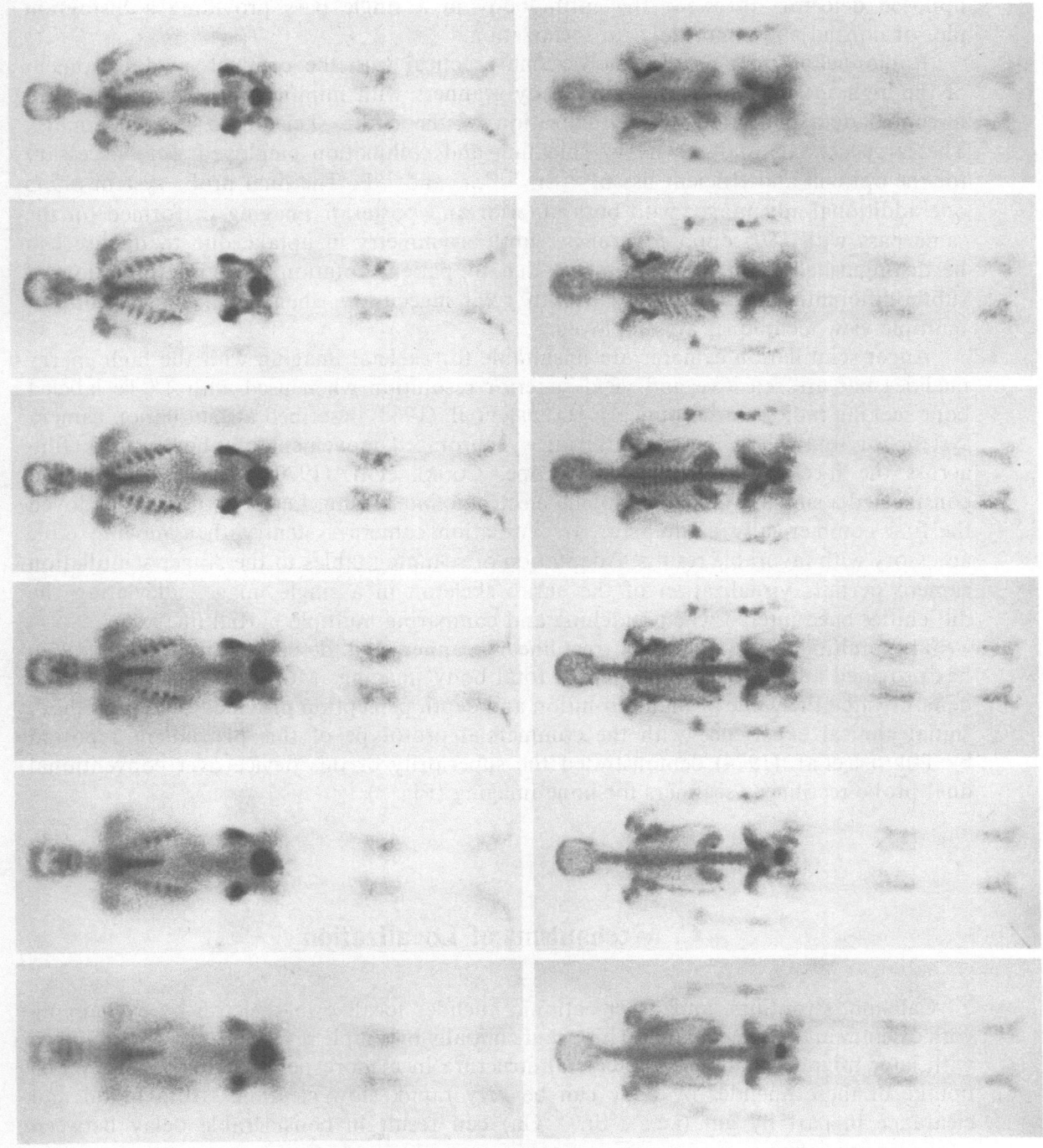

Fig. 3. Tomographic imaging of hereditary chondromatosis. Multiple cartilaginous exostoses in 17-year-old male are well demonstrated on multiple planes obtained during a single pass with Anger tomographic rectilinear scanner utilizing ^{99m}Tc-EHDP. Planes are arranged from superficial anterior (top left) serially through to superficial posterior (lower right). Multiple lesions are present at ankles, knees, iliac crests, scapulae, proximal humeri, and wrists

opposed detectors to sweep the entire body in a single pass providing a histogram plot of normal and abnormal ^{85}Sr localization.

Radionuclide imaging of bone became practical with the commercial development of the high speed, dual probe, total body scanners with minification, permitting uninterrupted data collection and visualization of the entire skeleton in a single image. The large crystals and the heavy shielding and collimation employed were necessary for the optimal and efficient use of ^{85}Sr, ^{87m}Sr, and ^{18}F. The dual probe system offers one additional advantage; with both anterior and posterior imaging performed on the same pass with 180° opposed probes, subtle asymmetry in uptake due to disease can be distinguished from the asymmetry due to patient rotation. The interpretation of subtle differential uptake is fraught with great inaccuracy when either single probe or multiple view techniques are employed.

Anger scintillation cameras are unsuitable for skeletal imaging with the high energy nuclides but are sensitive and yield superior resolution when used with ^{99m}Tc labeled bone seeking radiopharmaceuticals. HARPER et al. (1968) described a scintillation camera system for total body imaging utilizing synchronized movement of photographic film across the face of a display oscilloscope. COOKE et al. (1970, 1972) proposed and constructed a similar system employing electronic interfacing. LEE et al. (1973) employed the first commercially manufactured scintillation camera system with a moving table accessory with favorable results. Adaptation of scanning tables to the Anger scintillation camera permits visualization of the entire skeleton in a single image, alleviating the difficulties encountered when matching and comparing multiple partial images.

The multiplane, tomographic rectilinear scanner first described by ANGER (1968) has provided an alternate approach to total body imaging. McRAE and ANGER (1974) demonstrated the value of high resolution and depth perception provided by this method. Initial clinical experience with the commercial prototype of this instrument reported by TURNER et al. (1974) demonstrated the superiority of this device over conventional dual probe rectilinear scanners for bone imaging (Fig. 3).

C. Mechanisms of Localization

Calcium, strontium, and other cationic nuclides localize in skeleton by exchanging with calcium in the bone matrix. This occurs initially by simple reversible surface exchange with later migration into deeper crystal structure in a more permanent fashion. While uptake of these nuclides by bone can be very rapid, slow clearance from blood and clearance in part by gut (i.e., ^{85}Sr, ^{67}Ga) can result in considerable delay between nuclide administration and scanning, requiring cumbersome patient preparation.

^{18}F localizes in bone rapidly and rather permanently, replacing hydroxyl groups in hydroxyapatite to form fluorapatite crystal. Blood clearance of ^{18}F via the urinary system is extremely rapid. ^{18}F localization in nonosseous tissue is seldom encountered but

Fig. 4a–d. Radionuclide uptake in metastatic osteosarcoma. Soft tissue uptake of ^{18}F (a) is rather specific for metastatic osteosarcoma in lungs (b) of 11-year-old male with amputation for osteosarcoma. ^{99m}Tc-EHDP (c) demonstrates lesions to· better advantage but is not as specific as shown by uptake in lungs of patient (d) in renal failure with diffuse microscopic calcification in lungs

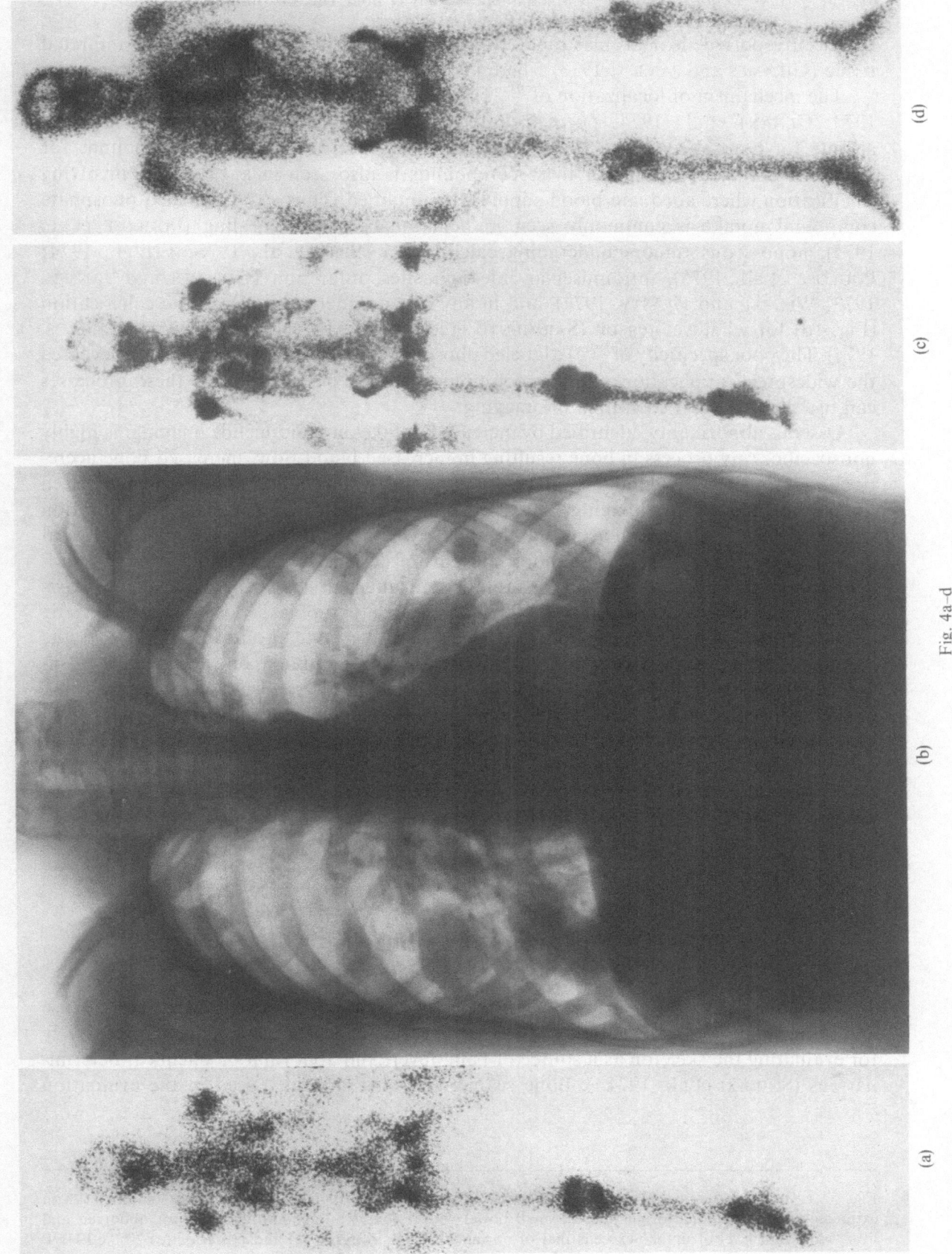

Fig. 4a–d

has been reported in neuroblastoma (ROSENFIELD and TREVES, 1974) and in infarcted tissue (GIRAMES and JANSEN, 1973) where hydroxyapatite is formed.

The mechanism of localization of ^{99m}Tc labeled phosphate compounds (TILDEN et al., 1973; GENANT et al., 1974, ZIMMER et al., 1974) is not entirely clear despite obvious affinity for bone. KAYE et al. (1975) demonstrated the affinity of these compounds for immature collagen. Uptake of these compounds is also seen in any process involving calcification where adequate blood supply is maintained. Thus, ^{99m}Tc labeled phosphate compound uptake is commonly seen in hematomas, wound healing (POULOSE et al., 1975), nonosseous tumors undergoing calcification (BERG et al., 1973; FITZER, 1974; POULOSE et al., 1975), intramuscular injection sites, infarction (GIRAMES and JANSEN, 1973; WENZEL and HEASTY, 1974), and in any organ undergoing metastatic calcification (Fig. 4d) for whatever reason (SARMIENTO et al., 1974; MCLAUGHLIN, 1975; RICHARDS, 1974). The poor specificity of ^{99m}Tc labeled phosphate compound uptake has not prevented the widespread application of these compounds to osseous imaging as these processes can usually be clearly identified on imaging.

Osseous abnormality, identified by increased uptake on radionuclide imaging, is highly nonspecific. Any process in bone resulting in increased blood flow, increased bone accretion, or arousing any kind of a reactive response will produce abnormally increased uptake on radionuclide imaging. Increased bone production and nuclide incorporation will be apparent on the scan as increased uptake whether it be due to growth (epiphyseal plates), repair (healing fractures, and at margins of destructive metastatic lesions), remodeling (seen in Paget's disease and adaptation to unusual stress), or on a diffuse basis to metabolic causes. Thus, the net effect of roentgenographically osteolytic metastatic disease is one of bone destruction, but the reparative bone producing activity at the margins of these lesions yields striking lesions of increased uptake on radionuclide imaging. Similarly, overall mineral content of bone in hyperthyroidism is close to normal, or slightly decreased, but radionuclide imaging will often demonstrate strikingly increased generalized uptake which reflects the increased perfusion and bone turnover rates. Poor specificity of the individual lesion can be overcome in great part by careful attention to the general pattern of involvement which often permits differentiation of the disease process involved.

D. Indicates for Radionuclide Imaging of the Skeleton

The bone scan has been used extensively for staging nonosseous malignant disease and for evaluation of metastatic disease under treatment. It has also been used extensively for evaluating the skeleton as a source of pain, fever, and abnormal biochemical determinations (SHIRAZI et al., 1974a). Bone scanning is also currently used in the evaluation

Fig. 5a–e. Extraosseous bone producing tumors. (a) Anterior and (b) posterior ^{18}F scans of patient with extraosseous osteosarcoma originating in small bowel with lesions scattered through anterior abdomen and liver. Note that level of uptake exceeds that of normal skeleton. Anterior (c) and posterior (d) ^{99m}Tc-EHDP scans show striking uptake in abdominal malignant fibrohistiocytoma with osseous metaplasia. (Courtesy of Nuclear Medicine Department, Lutheran General Hospital, Chicago, Illinois, U.S.A.) (e) Bone producing component of metastatic adenocarcinoma destroying ischial ramus is well demonstrated on ^{18}F scan

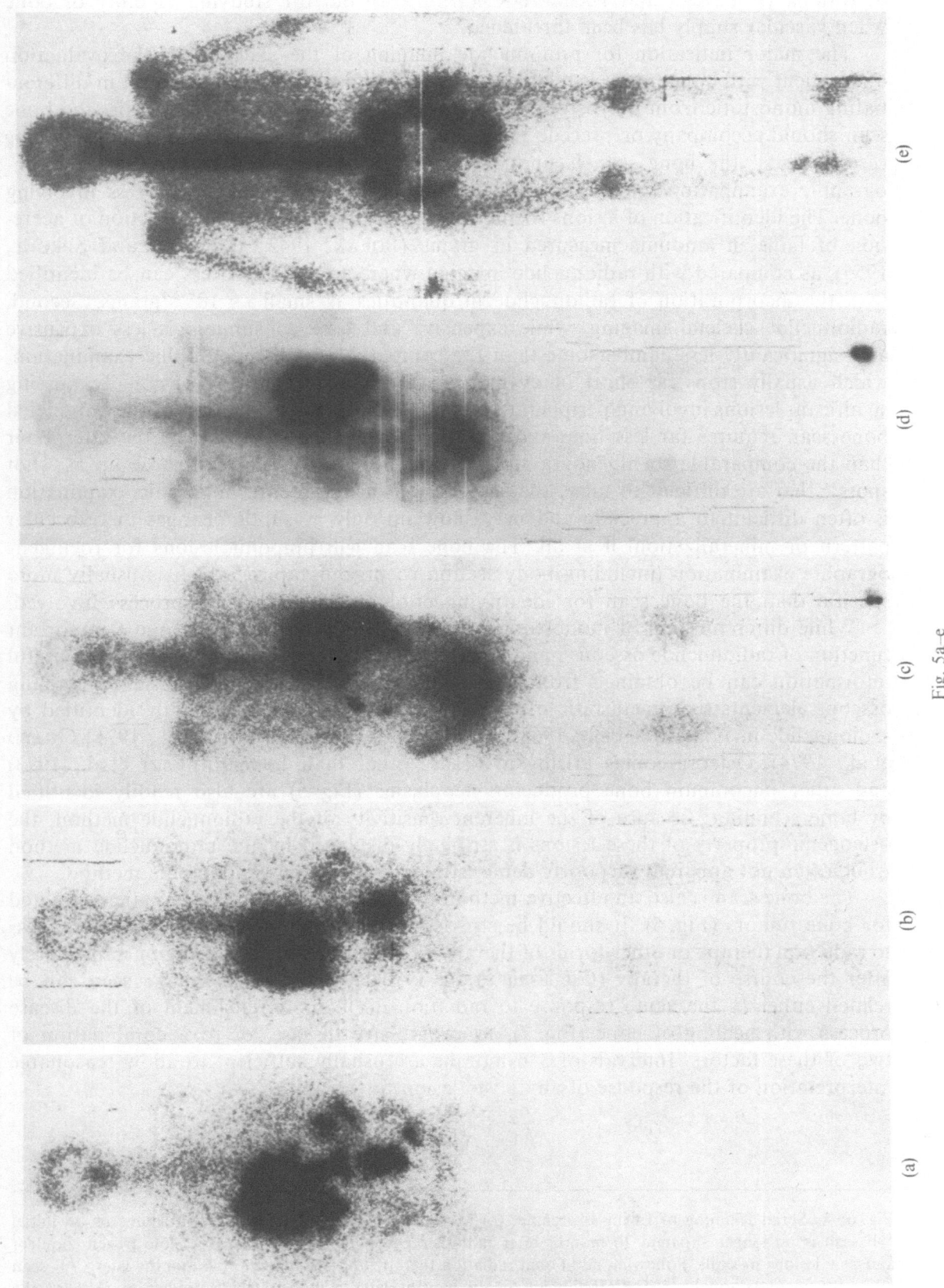

Fig. 5a–e

of trauma (FORDHAM and RAMACHANDRAN, 1974) and for studying viability of bone when vascular supply has been threatened.

The major indication for radionuclide imaging of the skeleton in the evaluation of a patient with bone tumor is related to the exquisite sensitivity of this tool in differentiating monostotic from polyostotic disease. Where the above indications exist the bone scan should accompany or precede the roentgenographic examination for the following resons: First, the bone scan is unquestionably far more sensitive than the roentgenographic examination for the identification of an active pathologic process involving bone. The identification of lesions roentgenographically requires the destruction or accretion of bone in amounts measured in grams (BORAK, 1942; BACHMAN and SPRONL, 1955), as compared with radionuclide imaging where an active process can be identified with the incorporation of radionuclide in quantities as small as 10^{-14}grams. Second, radionuclide skeletal imaging, while expensive and time consuming, is less expensive and significantly less cumbersome than the comparable roentgenographic examination, which usually stops far short of evaluating the entire skeleton, occasionally missing significant lesions involving peripheral skeleton. Finally, the evaluation of the completed bone scan requires far less time and attention to detail on the part of the interpreter than the comparable roentgenographic survey; lesions on bone scan show up as "hot spots" that are difficult to miss; the same lesion on the roentgenographic examination is often difficult to appreciate and may show up only as subtle changes in trabecular pattern or mineralization, if at all. The bone scan will pinpoint lesions for roentgenographic examination (including body section roentgenography) which is usually more specific than the bone scan for identifying etiology of the disease process involved.

While differentiation of monostotic from polyostotic disease is the most important function of radionuclide osseous imaging of patients with bone tumors, additional useful information can be obtained from the bone scan. Soft tissue metastases containing osseous elements (i.e., metastatic osteogenic sarcoma—Fig. 4) are readily identified by radionuclide imaging (SAMUELS, 1968; SCHALL et al., 1971; O'MARA et al., 1971; GHAED et al., 1974). Osteosarcomas arising in tissues other than bone (SHIRAZI et al., 1973) and other uncommon bone producing neoplasms (Fig. 5) are also readily identified by bone scanning. Because of the inherent sensitivity of the radionuclide method, the osteogenic property of these lesions is strikingly displayed by the radionuclide method while often not apparent or poorly demonstrated by the roentgenographic method.

The bone scan is also an effective method for long term follow up of patients treated for bone tumors (Fig. 6). It should be stressed that the response of the disease process to radiation therapy or other forms of therapy cannot be evaluated during or immediately after the course of therapy (GILLESPIE et al., 1975); the increased uptake seen can be related either to the acute response to radiation itself, to retrenchment of the disease process with healing of bone (Fig. 7), to progressive disease, or to a combination of two of these factors. Intervals of 3–6 months are usually sufficient to allow reasonable interpretation of the response of any given lesion to therapy.

Fig. 6a–e. Serial scanning of Ewing's sarcoma. (a) Monostotic Ewing's sarcoma of right humerus on initial ^{18}F scan is no longer apparent 10 months after radiotherapy on repeat ^{18}F scan (b). Note frozen shoulder and new lesions in skull. Following additional radiation therapy and chemotherapy 6 months later, ^{18}F scan (c) is considered normal. ^{99m}Tc-EHDP scan (d) 10 months later demonstrates recurrence at primary site and in skull with questionable abnormality in pelvis and proximal right femur. At 5 months later, ^{99m}Tc-EHDP scan (e) demonstrates additional disease in spine, pelvis, proximal right femur, and distal left femur

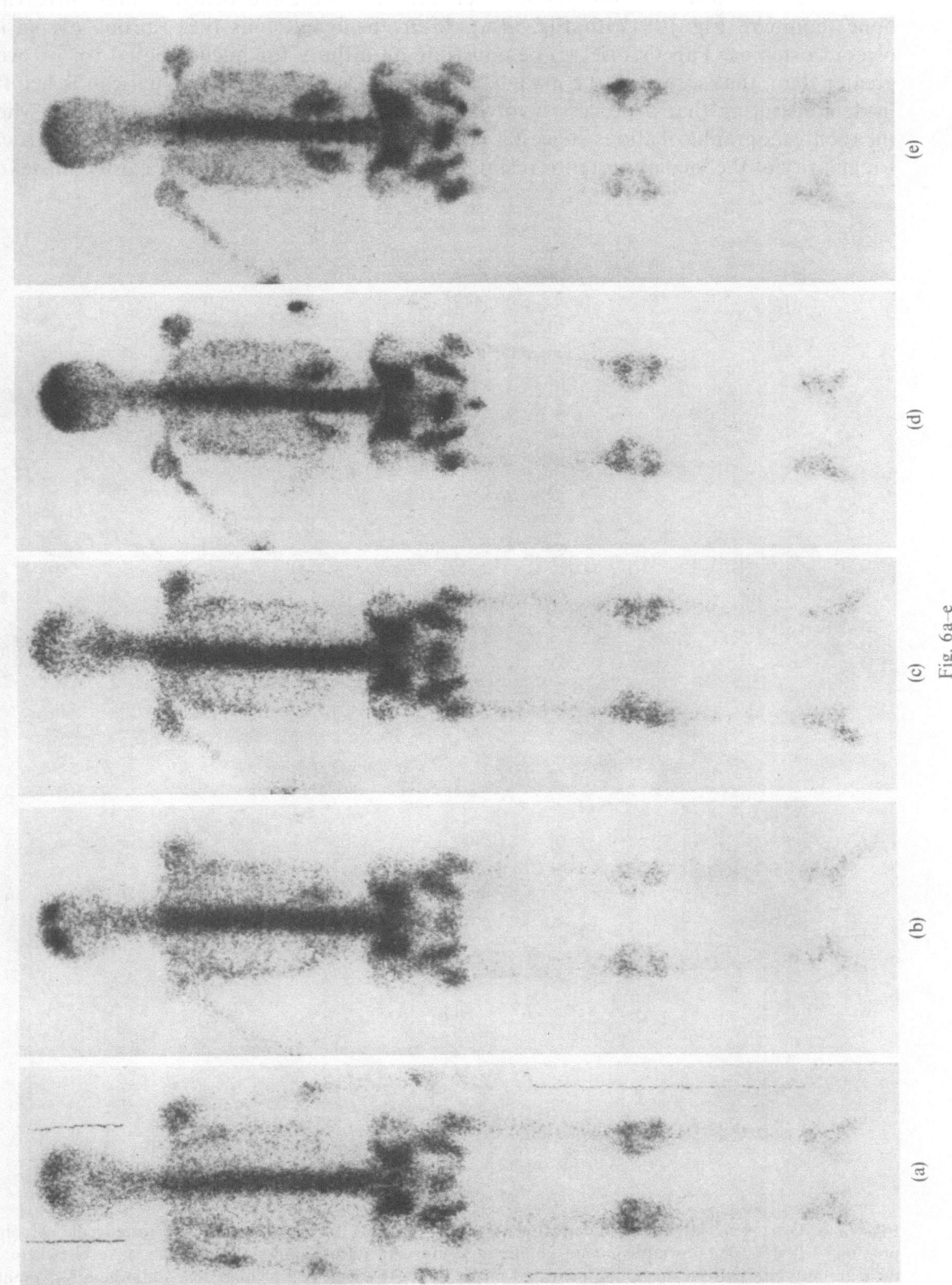

Fig. 6a–e

Contrary to published reports (SAMUELS, 1971; WANKEN et al., 1973) the bone scan cannot be used to reliably differentiate between malignant and benign tumors involving bone (compare Fig. 10a with Fig. 14a.). Many benign lesions (i.e. fibrous dysplasia, osteoid osteoma, Paget's disease) demonstrate an affinity for nuclide equal to, or even greater than, that seen with the malignant tumors. Occasionally the bone scan is helpful in demonstrating that a process involving bone is inactive and therefore benign when the roentgenographic features suggest a possibly malignant process. For example, cortical irregularity of the medial posterior distal femoral metaphysis in children can be mistaken

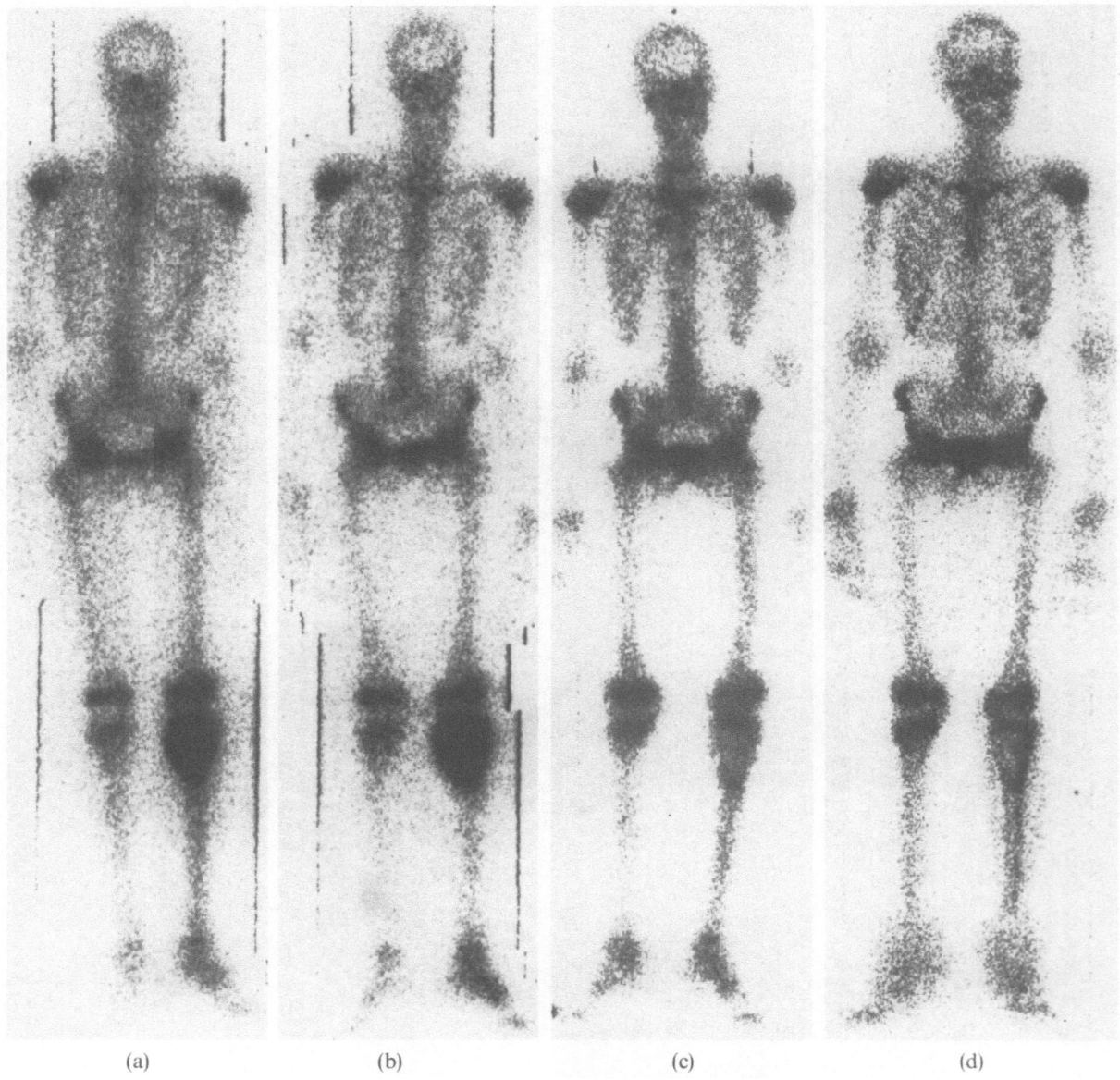

(a)   (b)   (c)   (d)

Fig. 7a–d. Osteogenic sarcoma under treatment. (a) ^{18}F scan of 14-year-old male with osteogenic sarcoma proximal left tibia demonstrates intense uptake in lesion with diffuse, mildly increased uptake elsewhere in the extremity in a pattern suggesting increased blood flow. At conclusion of high dose radiotherapy 1 month later, ^{18}F scan (b) shows no interval change. Repeat ^{18}F scan (c) 3 months later shows marked decrease in activity of tibial lesion with minimal residual abnormality at inferior aspect of original lesion which is better demonstrated on ^{99m}Tc-EHDP scan (d) immediately prior to amputation

roentgenographically for malignant neoplasm, particularly osteosarcoma (SIMON, 1968; BROWER et al., 1971); lack of radionuclide uptake effectively distinguishes this common benign lesion from the malignant process with which it can be confused (CONWAY, 1975).

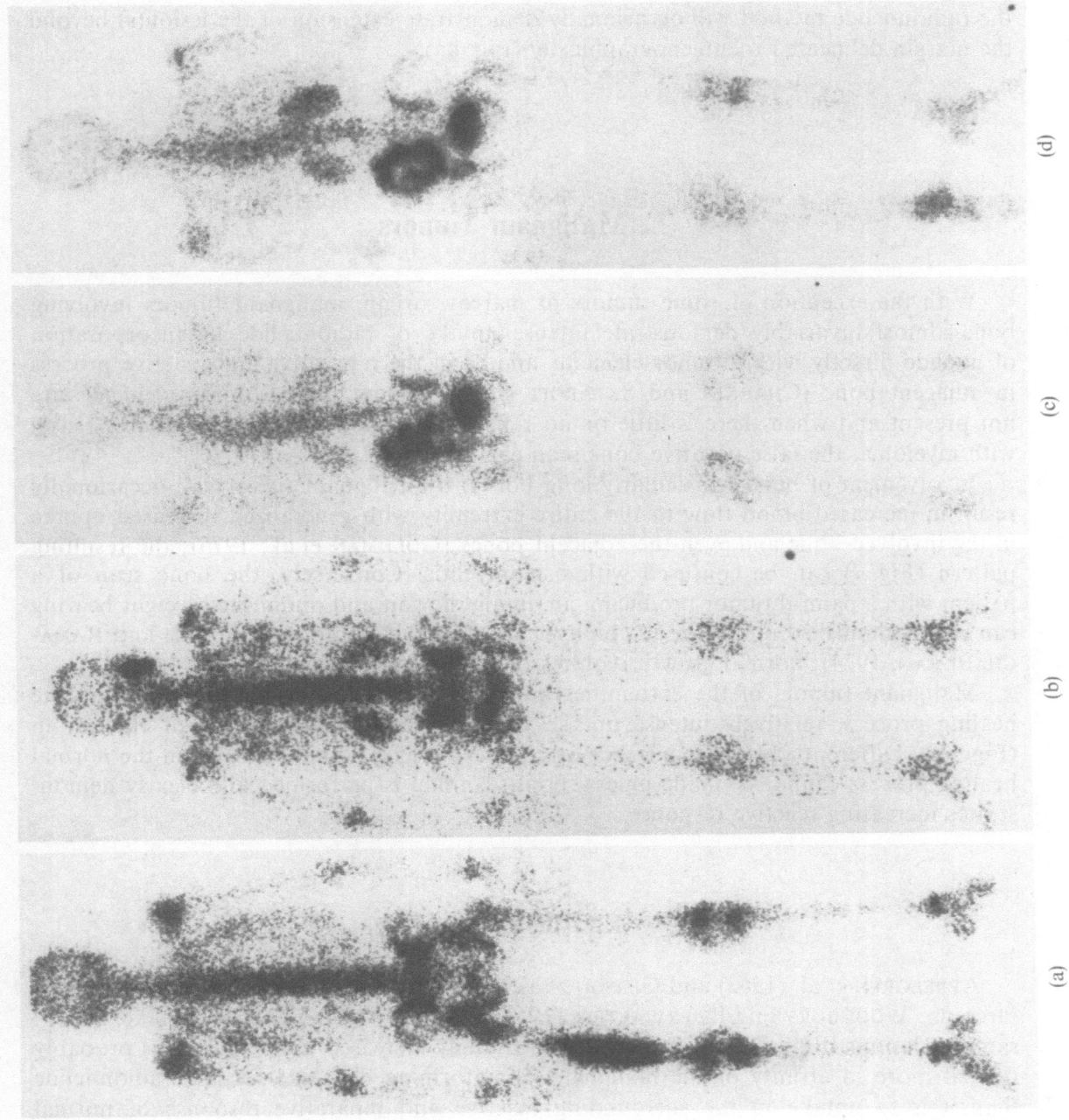

Fig. 8a–d. Unusual cases of osteosarcoma. (a) Lesion of femoral diaphysis mimicking Ewing's sarcoma proved to be osteosarcoma on biopsy. Second lesion in proximal femur demonstrated by scan but not identified roentgenographically was confirmed at amputation. (b) Osteosarcoma of left mandible in 40-year-old female; apparent lesion in right hemipelvis is urinary ^{99m}Tc-EHDP in bladder diverticulum. (c) Irregular exophytic monostotic osteosarcoma right ileum demonstrates peculiar change 10 months post radiation (d) with extension into acetabulum and polyostotic or metastatic disease appearing in distal right tibia, proximal left tibia, and left shoulder

Moreover, the radionuclide method will not differentiate with any reliability the histologic types of malignant or benign tumors. Except for a few tumors or tumorlike conditions which demonstrate characteristic patterns of involvement, the differentiation of any given lesion by the radionuclide method is frequently fraught with error.

Although there is usually excellent correlation (GOLDMAN et al., 1975) between the roentgenographic study and the bone scan in defining the extent of a local tumor, the radionuclide method will occasionally demonstrate extension of the lesion(s) beyond the margin delineated roentgenographically (Fig. 8a).

E. Malignant Tumors

With the exception of some tumors of marrow origin, malignant tumors involving bone almost invariably demonstrate intense uptake of radionuclide by incorporation of nuclide directly within tumor elements and/or in the reparative and reactive process in adjacent bone (CHARKES and SKLAROFF, 1965). Where bone-forming elements are not present and when there is little or no reparative response to tumors, such as seen with myeloma, the false negative bone scan can result.

Involvement of bone (particularly long bones) by malignant tumor will occasionally result in increased blood flow to the entire extremity with generalized increased uptake in the involved bone and even the adjacent bones (GOLDMAN et al., 1975); the resulting pattern (Fig. 7) can be confused with osteomyelitis. Conversely, the bone scan of a patient with a painful tumor producing an antalgesic gait and diminished weight bearing can show diminished uptake in all epiphysis of the afflicted limbs (FORDHAM and RAMACHANDRAN, 1974); normal growth requires the appropriate normal stress.

Malignant tumors of the extremities are often treated by amputation. During the healing process, relatively intense uptake is seen in and near the end of the stump (Fig. 9d). Differentiation of recurrence or complications (i.e., infection) from the normal healing process cannot be made unless serial scanning is performed and clearly demonstrates increasing reactive response.

I. Osteosarcoma

APPELGREN et al. (1963) and GERSON et al. (1972) demonstrated ^{85}Sr uptake in osteosarcoma; WOODBURY and BEIERWALTERS (1967) demonstrated similar ^{18}F uptake. Osteosarcoma lesions (Figs. 7, 8, 9) demonstrate strikingly increased uptake which is probably related more to affinity of the malignant bone-forming elements for the radionuclide than it is to uptake in the surrounding reactive and reparative response of normal bone. This phenomenon is responsible for demonstration of metastatic osteosarcoma lesions in soft tissues (see Figs. 4, 16d).

In a study of 14 patients with osteosarcoma, MC NEIL et al. (1973) suggested that radionuclide imaging was of limited value in following patients with osteosarcoma; with the known predilection of osteosarcoma for pulmonary metastases, these investigators suggested chest roentgenography as the more appropriate follow-up modality. Our own experience suggests that polyostotic lesions without pulmonary metastases occur frequently enough to warrant routine radionuclide imaging (Fig. 8d). Only too often polyostotic disease has been demonstrated shortly after treatment of the primary or most obvious lesion in patients treated without benefit of preoperative radionuclide imaging.

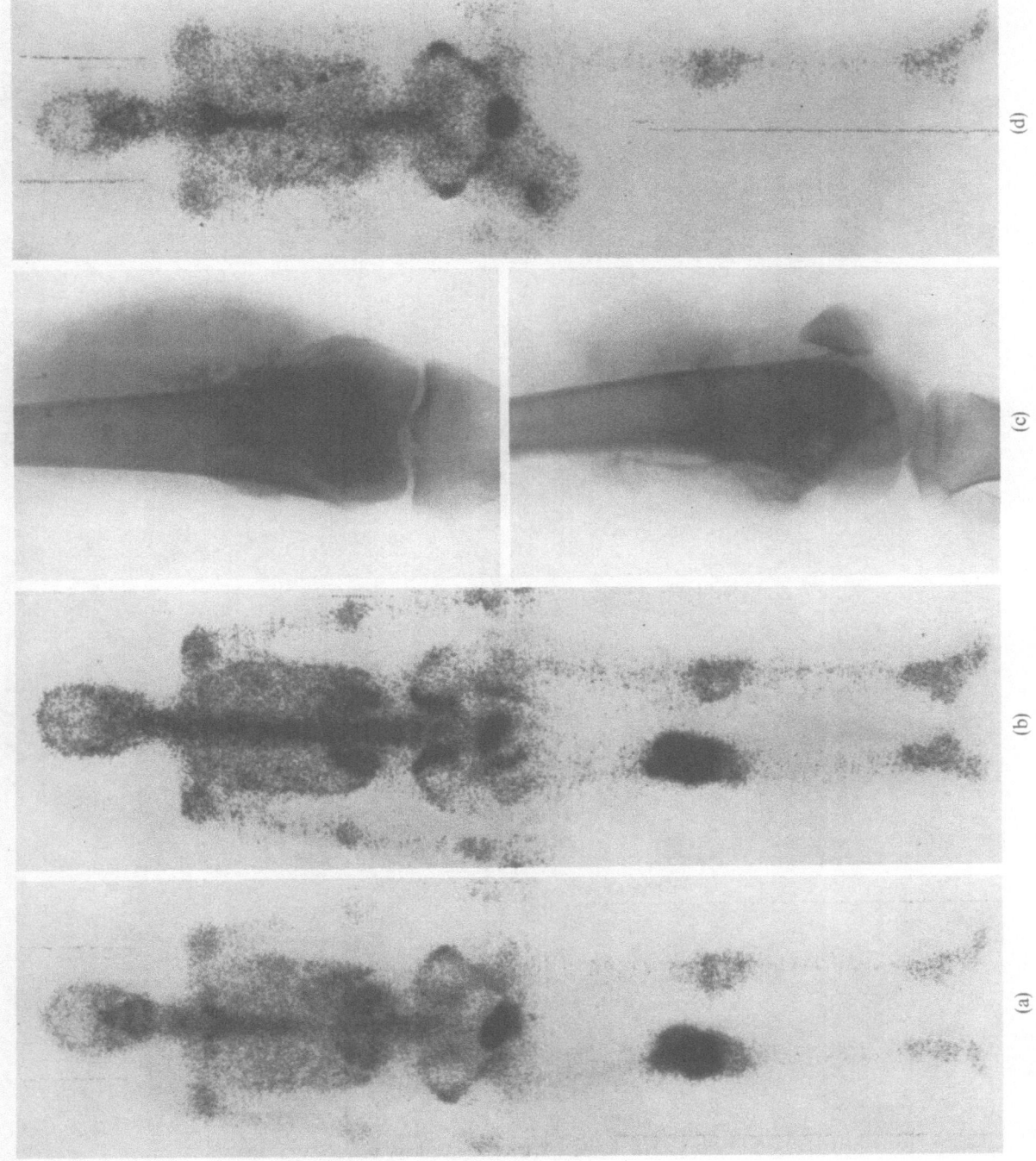

Fig. 9a–d. Osteosarcoma, pre- and postoperative. Anterior (a) and posterior (b) ^{99m}Tc-EHDP scans of 17-year-old female with osteosarcoma of distal right femur clearly demonstrate exophytic nature of lesion shown roentgenographically (c). Postoperative anterior ^{99m}Tc-EHDP scan (d) demonstrates generalized soft tissue increased uptake and greater increased uptake at distal end of stump in a normal healing pattern 1 month post amputation

II. Malignant Tumors of Cartilaginous Origin

SINGHER and MARINELLI (1945) first demonstrated increased uptake of ^{35}S in normal cartilage; LAYTON (1949) showed increased incorporation of ^{35}S in neoplastic disease of cartilaginous origin when grown in tissue culture. Uptake of radionuclide sulphur

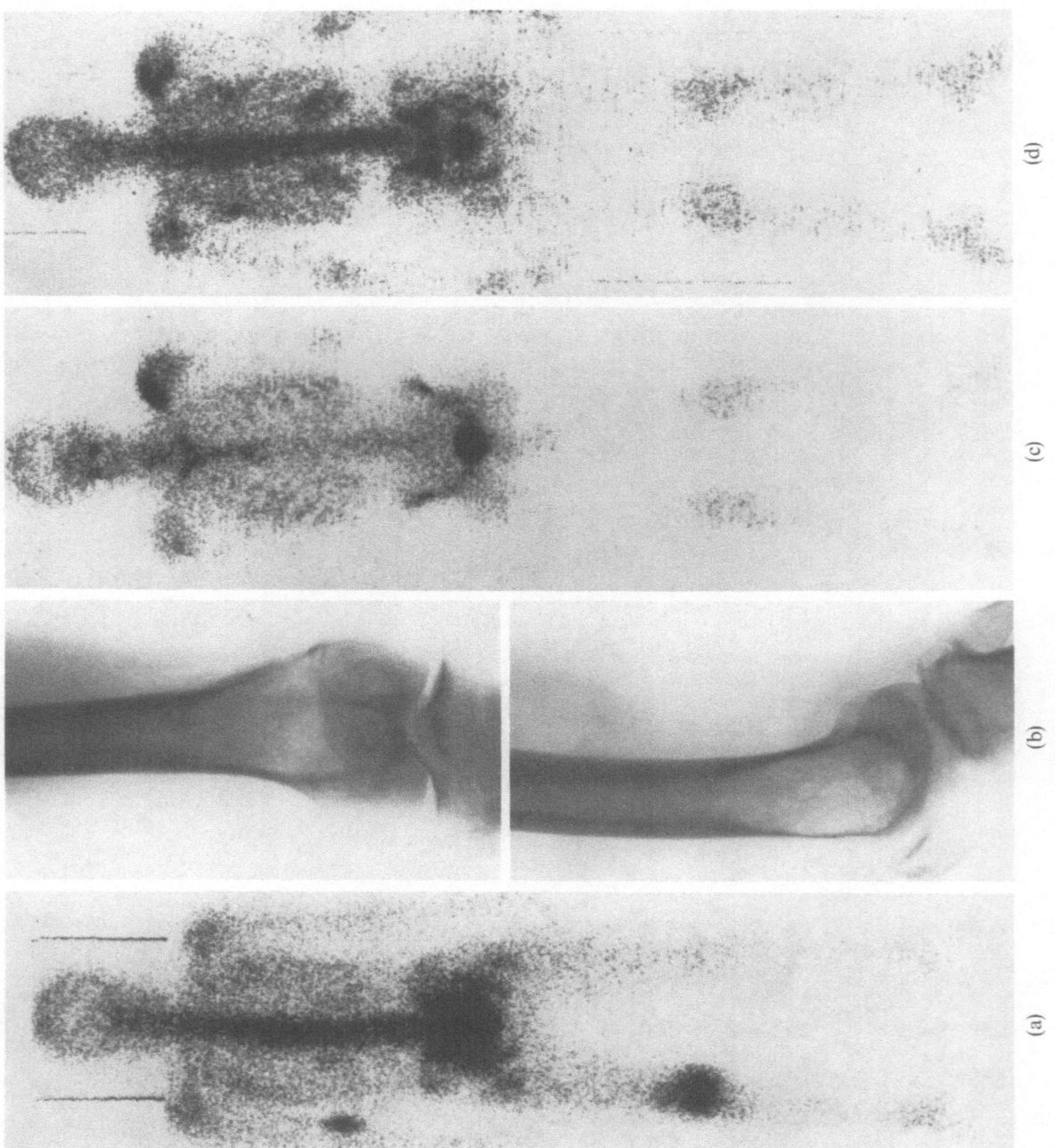

Fig. 10a–d. Malignant tumors of connective tissue origin. (a) Posterior ^{18}F scan of 17-year-old male with fibrosarcoma distal right femur demonstrates nonspecific increased uptake in lesion corresponding well with roentgenography (b). Anterior (c) and posterior (d) ^{99m}Tc-EHDP scans show malignant mixed mesenchymal lesion of left shoulder invading scapula and distal clavicle

by chondrosarcomas in man was demonstrated by GOTTSCHALK and ALLEN (1952). RUBIN et al. (1957) suggested the possible use of ^{35}S labeled sodium sulfate for the treatment of chondrosarcoma. While this beta-emitting nuclide is appropriate for tracer studies and can be rationally considered for therapeutic purposes, it is not appropriate for imaging due to the lack of appropriate photon emission. However, LASA and PEREZ-MO-DREGO (1965) successfully used ^{75}Se (a sulphur analogue) in the imaging of cartilaginous tumors. Imaging of the chondrosarcomas, however, can be appropriately performed with the standard bone-seeking radiopharmaceuticals (Fig. 2). The mechanism of uptake is similar to that seen with the osteosarcomas; these lesions are locally destructive, arousing the usual reactive response, and also undergo ossification resulting in direct radionuclide uptake by the tumor.

III. Malignant Tumors of Vascular and Connective Tissue Origin

There have been no reports of significant levels of experience with radionuclide imaging of malignant tumors arising from vascular and connective tissue components of bone. The few fibrosarcomas, angiosarcomas, and malignant mesenchymal tumors originating in bone that we have seen are easily demonstrable on radionuclide imaging (Fig. 10) with rather intense uptake at the site of the tumor. This affinity for nuclide is probably related to the reactive reparative response of bone to the invasive, destructive process much as is seen with destructive metastatic disease. Apart from possible uptake of the ^{99m}Tc labeled phosphate compounds in areas of calcification, one would not expect significant uptake of the other radiopharmaceuticals directly within tumor elements.

IV. Malignant Tumors of Marrow Origin

1. Ewing's Sarcoma

This disease typically produces strikingly abnormal scans with intense uptake corresponding with the tumor involvement of flat bones and diaphyseal portions of the afflicted long bones. Reactive bone proliferation, as shown roentgenographically by a classic "onion skin" appearance, is undoubtedly responsible for the intense level of activity commonly seen by radionuclide imaging. Because of frequent polyostotic involvement at the time of initial diagnosis (SHIRAZI et al., 1974a), radionuclide skeletal imaging is mandatory in the initial evaluation of the patient. Long-term evaluation of therapy by this method (Fig. 11) is appropriate because of the predilection for metastases to other bones. FRANKEL et al. (1974) demonstrated the superiority of standard radionuclide bone imaging and ^{67}Ga imaging over the roentgenographic method for follow-up evaluation of skeletal metastases.

2. Myeloma

High false negative rates are supposedly seen with radionuclide imaging of osseous myeloma. In our experience only a small fraction of the total number of patients with myeloma demonstrate totally normal bone scans. However, in roughly 50% of the patients with myeloma, the bone scan will demonstrate less striking or fewer abnormalities than can be demonstrated by roentgenographic imaging. The lack of uptake at the margins of this destructive lesion can be explained by the frequent absence of reactive reparative response by bone. Unlike roentgenographically similar lytic lesions from metastatic disease, the myeloma lesion on pathologic examination will frequently show lack of osteoblast activity at the interface between myeloma and normal bone.

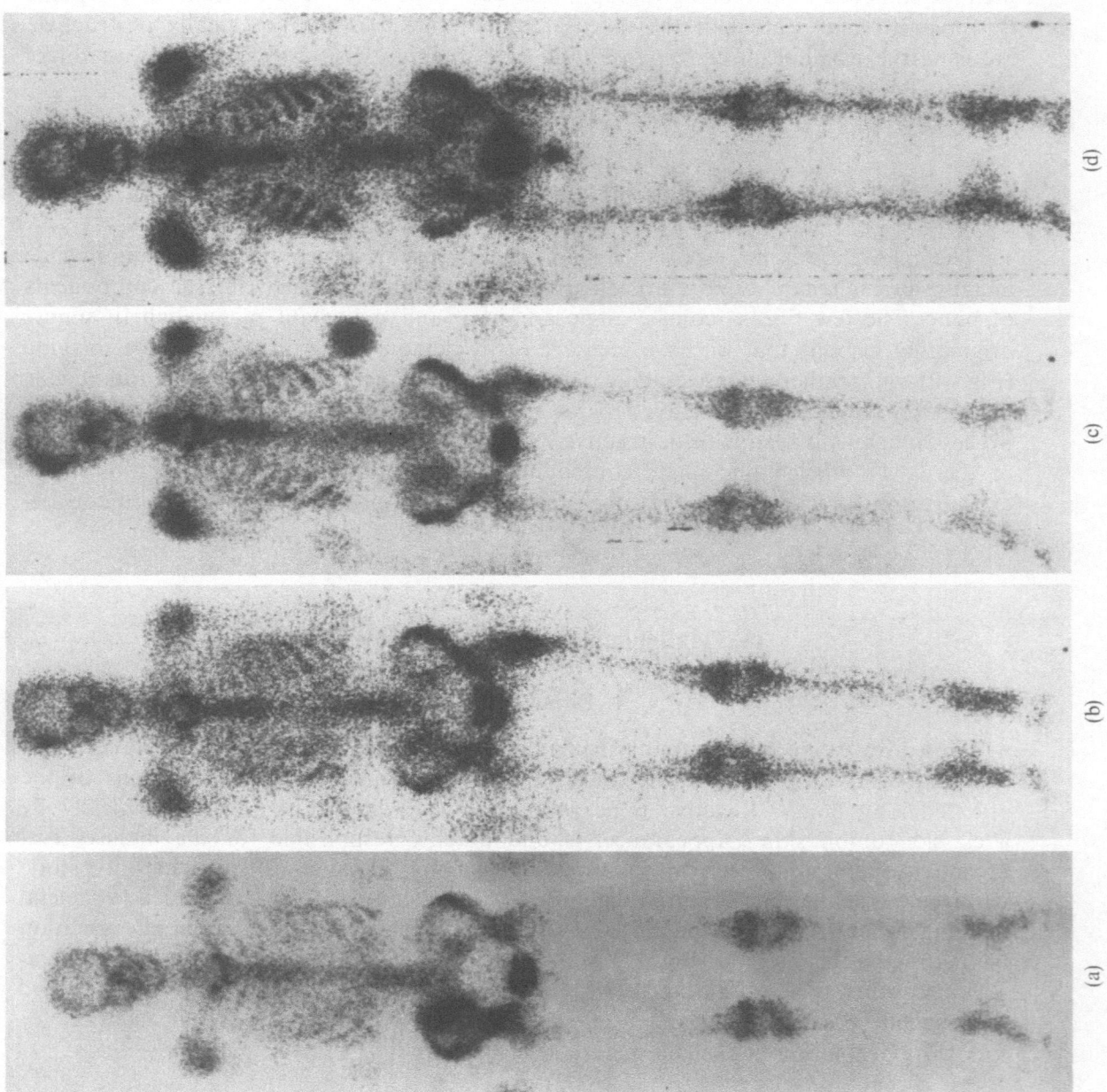

Fig. 11a–d. Ewing's sarcoma under treatment. (a) Monostotic Ewing's disease involving right ileum is no longer apparent (b) 5 months after radiation therapy; note, however, new lesions in skull and proximal left femur. Note progression of untreated skull lesion (c) 3 months later, improvement of treated femoral lesion and appearance of striking disease in both shoulders and subtle disease in rib cage. Despite chemotherapy, 3 months later more generalized disease is apparent (d). Asymmetry of uptake in pelvis on later scans is related to right hemipelvis radiation

3. Leukemia

Discrete or diffuse abnormality can frequently be identified by skeletal radionuclide imaging (Fig. 12); while this procedure is occasionally helpful in the evaluation of the patient with leukemia, it is rarely instrumental in making the initial diagnosis.

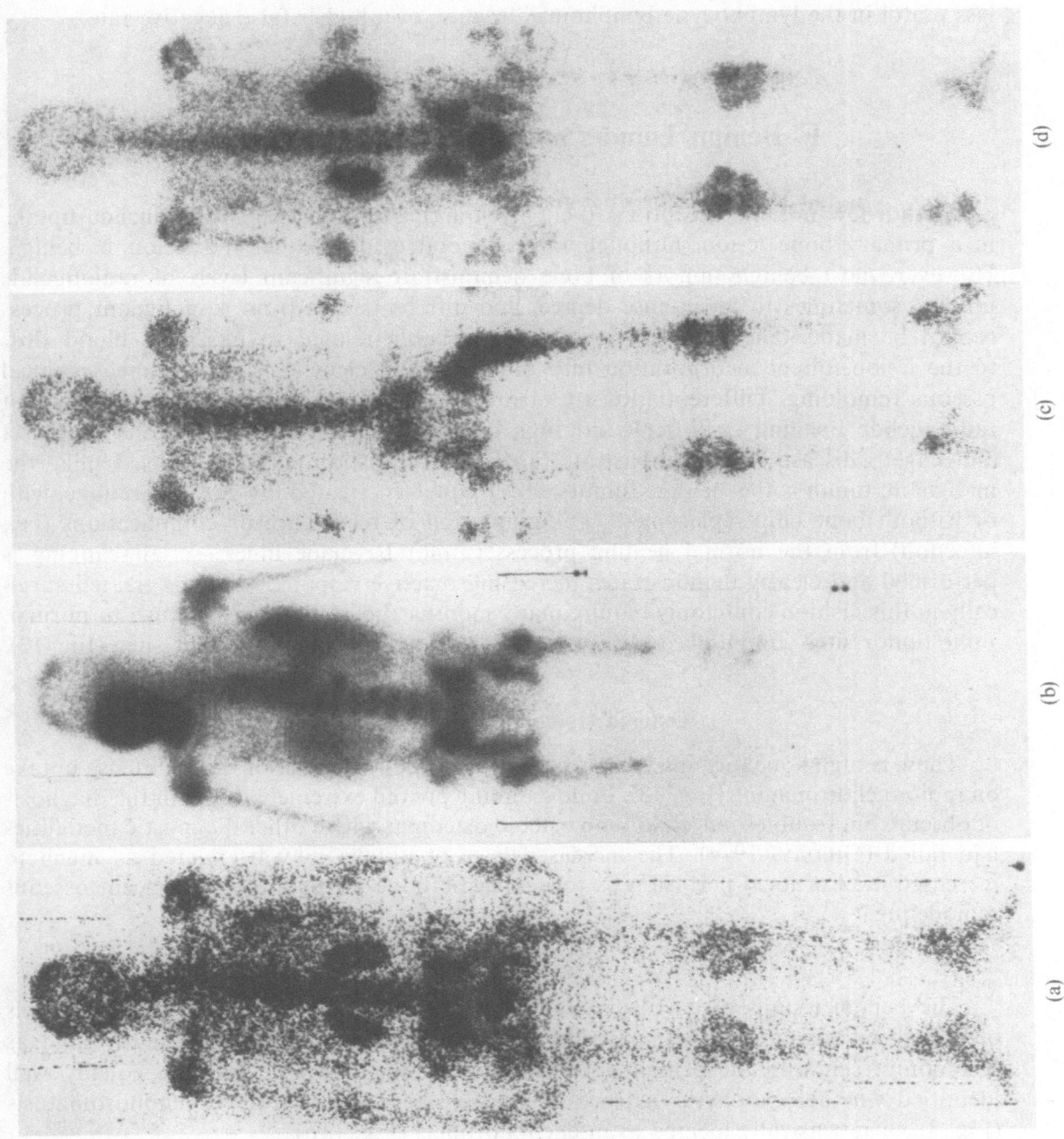

(d)

(c)

(b)

(a)

Fig. 12a–d. Malignant tumor of marrow origin. (a) ^{99m}Tc-EHDP scan, while abnormal, shows less osseous abnormality than is apparent on ^{67}Ga scanning (b) in a patient with chronic granulocytic leukemia with "chloroma" formation. Primary reticulum cell sarcoma of proximal left femur (c) is indistinguishable on ^{99m}Tc-EHDP scan from other neoplasms. ^{99m}Tc-EHDP scan (d) of patient with Hodgkin's disease demonstrates osseous involvement in shaft of right humerus with additional nonosseous disease obstructing and enlarging kidneys

4. Lymphoma

Despite a significant false negative rate, radionuclide imaging of bone is useful in the evaluation of lymphoma patients (particularly in Hodgkin's disease and the histiocytic lymphomas—Fig. 12) since this modality is far more accurate than skeletal roentgenography, serum alkaline phosphatase determination, or even marrow biopsy (Weber et al., 1968; Harbert and Ashburn, 1968; Ferrant et al., 1975). The bone scan is somewhat less useful in the lymphocytic lymphomas because of a higher false negative rate.

F. Benign Tumors and Tumorlike Abnormalities

With a few notable exceptions (i.e., myeloma), the absence of radionuclide uptake in a primary bone lesion, although rare, is good evidence that the lesion is benign. However, most benign tumors of bone demonstrate significant levels of radionuclide uptake, sometimes to an intense degree, and differentiation from a malignant process cannot be made. The increased uptake is probably related to increased blood flow to the lesion, direct incorporation into bone forming elements and/or increased local osseous remolding. Differentiation of various types of benign tumors on the basis of radionuclide imaging is difficult although certain disorders such as fibrous dysplasia and Paget's disease often demonstrate fairly characteristic uptake patterns. Unlike the malignant tumors, the benign tumors are frequently treated by local curettage with or without bone chip replacement. Differentiation of recurrence or complications (i.e., infection) from the normal healing process cannot be made unless serial scanning is performed and clearly demonstrates increasing reactive response. Lesions treated surgically in this fashion commonly require many months and even years to return to normal. Bone donor sites commonly return to normal far sooner than recipient sites (Fig. 13).

1. Osteoid Osteoma and Osteoblastoma

These benign bone forming tumors commonly produce lesions of rather intense uptake on radionuclide imaging (Fig. 13). Bone scanning proved extremely useful in the diagnosis of obscure but troublesome childhood osteoid osteomas where other diagnostic modalities had failed (Gilday, 1974). The increased level of uptake may be related as much to increased level of local perfusion as to neoplastic bone formation and adjacent osseous remodeling.

2. Chondroma

The benign lesions of cartilaginous origin commonly demonstrate increased levels of uptake on scanning although levels of uptake may not be as consistently high as commonly seen with the benign bone forming lesions. These lesions are equally well identified whether exophytic, as seen in multiple hereditary exophytic chondromatosis (Fig. 3), or intrinsically located as in enchondromas (Fig. 14d).

3. Giant Cell Tumor

The giant cell tumors show relatively marked affinity for bone seeking radionuclides (Fig. 14a). The bone scan cannot distinguish between the benign giant cell tumor and the lesion undergoing malignant degeneration.

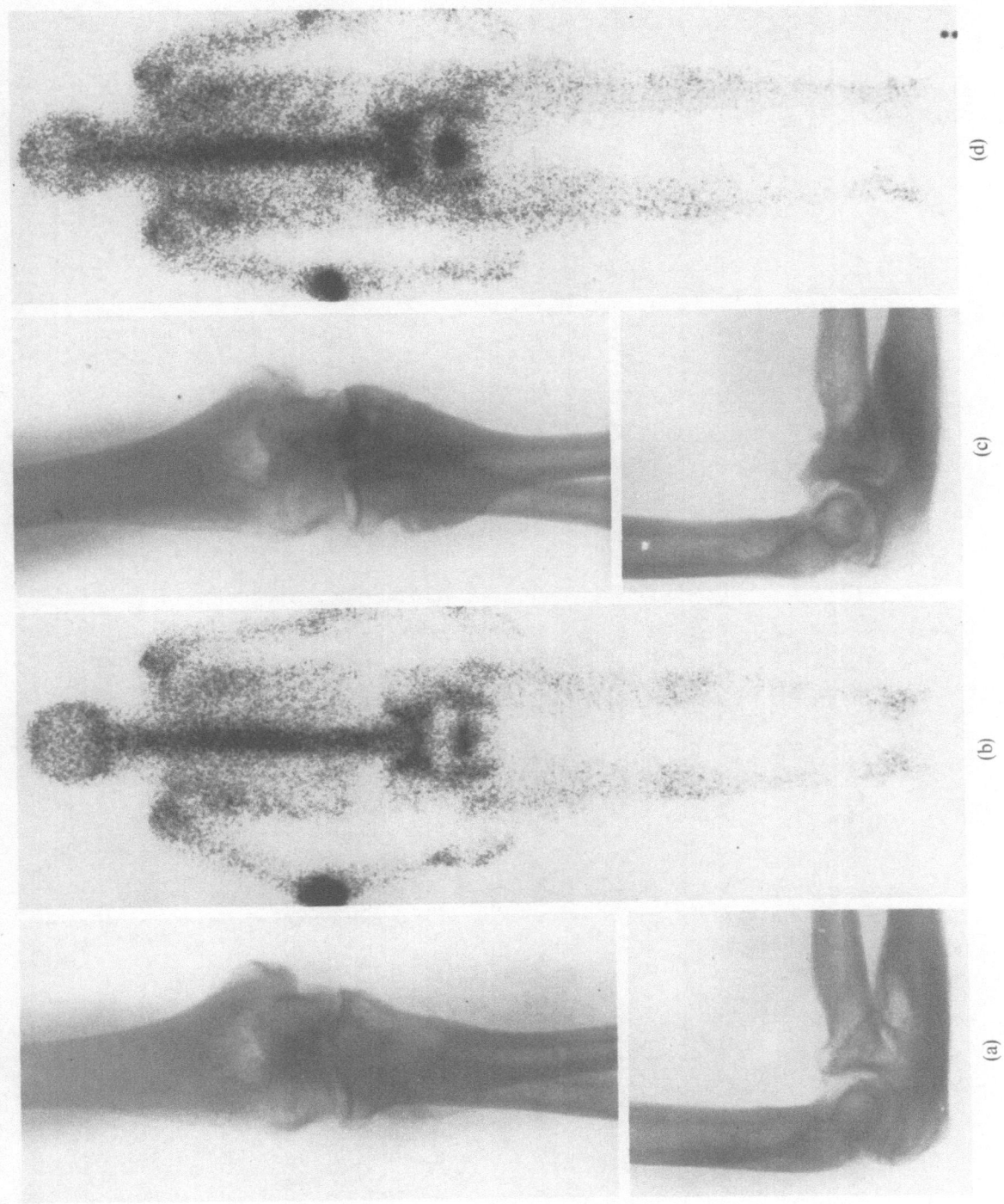

Fig. 13a–d. Osteoblastoma, pre- and postcurretage. (a) Preoperative roentgenography of 43-year-old male with painful right elbow demonstrates expanding lesion of proximal ulna with strikingly increased uptake on ^{18}F scan (b) and mild flexion deformity of right elbow. ^{18}F scan (d) 3 months after curettage demonstrates less flexion deformity with persistent uptake due to healing of lesion with implanted bone chips (c). Donor site (left ileum) has healed and is no longer apparent on scan

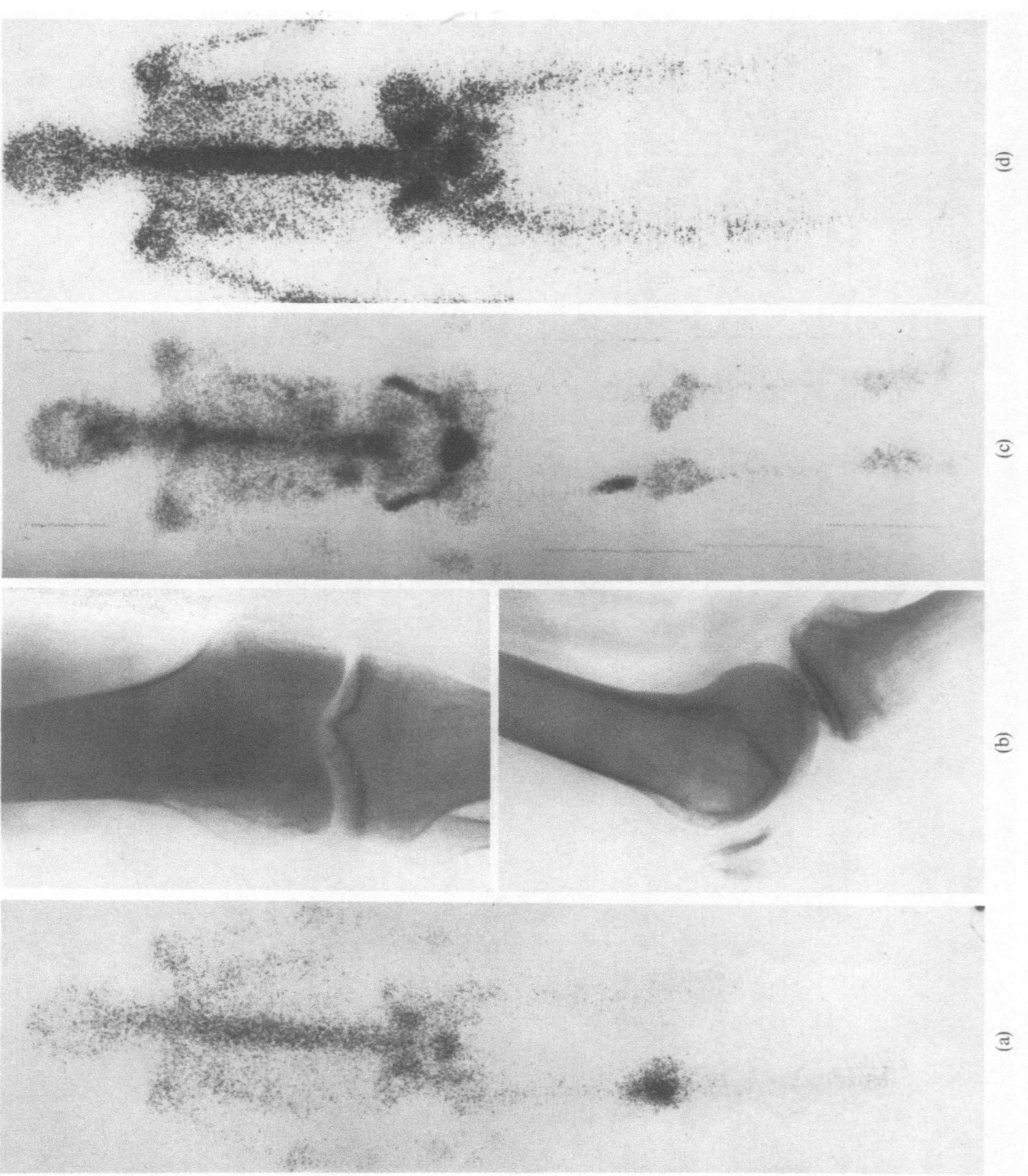

Fig. 14a–d. Benign bone lesions. (a) ^{18}F scan of patient with pain in right knee demonstrates monostotic lesion which proved to be giant cell tumor (b) on biopsy. ^{99m}Tc-EHDP scan (c) demonstrates monostotic lesion of distal femur which proved to be benign enchondroma on biopsy. Aneurysmal bone cyst of left ileum (d) shows rather mild degree of ^{99m}Tc-EHDP uptake

Fig. 15a–e. Fibrous dysplasia. Intense ^{18}F uptake in monostotic fibrous dysplasia of (a) mandible and (b) anterior floor of skull (indistinguishable from meningioma). ^{18}F scan (c) demonstrates polyostotic distribution of fibrous dysplasia in right lower extremity of patient suspected of monostotic disease. Fibrous dysplasia limited to one side of skull, facial bones, and mandible in patient with Albright's syndrome demonstrated by ^{18}F scan (d) and ^{99m}Tc-EHDP scan (e). Note better delineation of bones with ^{18}F in this obese patient. Thyroid uptake on ^{18}F scan is due to residual ^{131}I gland from treatment for hyperthyroidism

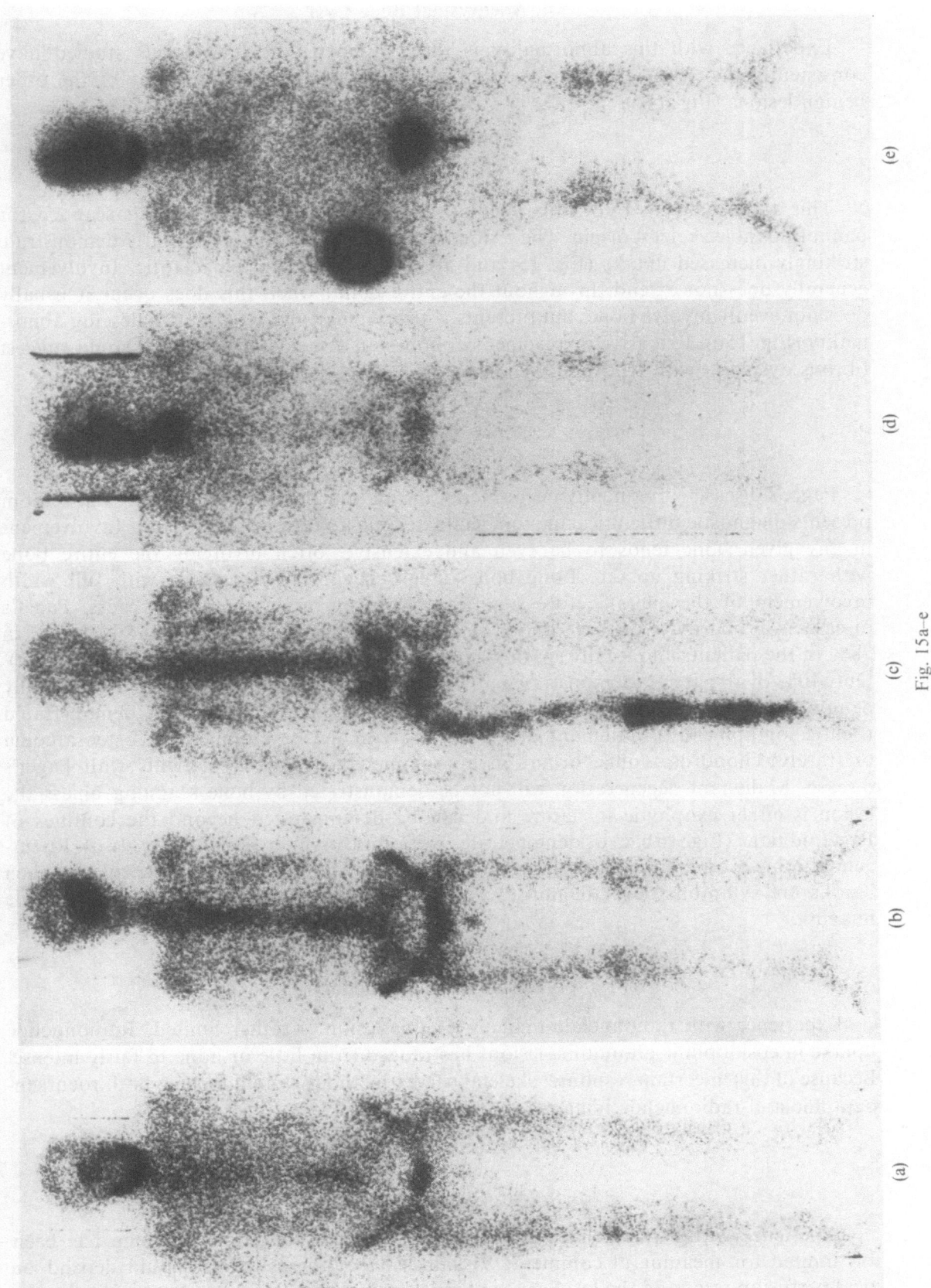

Fig. 15a–e

4. Aneurysmal Bone Cyst

Experience with this abnormality is rather limited; the few lesions studied have consistently shown increased uptake though not to levels seen with many of the other benign lesions (Fig. 14e).

5. Fibrous Dysplasia

This abnormality is frequently encountered incidentally and in patients scanned for pain of possible skeletal origin. The lesions of fibrous dysplasia consistently demonstrate strikingly increased uptake (Fig. 15) and are not infrequently polyostotic. Involvement generally does not extend throughout the entire bone; when this does occur it usually does not evenly involve bone, but presents with irregular, discrete, and coalescing abnormality (Fig. 15c). Extensive involvement of bones on one side of the body should suggest fibrous dysplasia with Albright's syndrome (Fig. 15d, e).

6. Paget's Disease

Paget's disease is frequently encountered in radionuclide skeletal imaging but seldom presents diagnostic difficulties due to a characteristic appearance (Fig. 16a). Involvement in any given bone tends to be even and extensive, often involving the entire bone with rather striking uptake. Long bone disease begins at the end(s) with full width involvement of the end(s) before significant involvement of the shaft occurs. Paget's disease is primarily a disease of the axial skeleton, involving pelvis and/or spine in 78% of the patients and totally sparing axial skeleton in only 2% (Shirazi et al., 1974c). Only 10% of all patients demonstrate monostotic involvement; the bone scan occasionally demonstrates polyostotic involvement when only monostotic disease was demonstrated roentgenographically. Malignant degeneration, with the development of osteosarcoma or (rarely) chondrosarcoma, occurs in approximately 3% of all patients with Paget's disease. Malignant degeneration will not be demonstrated by bone scanning unless the lesion is either exophytic in nature and can be demonstrated beyond the confines of Pagetoid bone (Fig. 16b, c) or demonstrates metastatic ossifying lesions (Fig. 16d). Roentgenographic examination is warranted in any case of Paget's disease, particularly when lesions are symptomatic or demonstrate any type of atypical pattern on radionuclide imaging.

7. Eosinophilic Granuloma

Experience with radionuclide imaging of this lesion is rather limited. Radionuclide uptake in eosinophilic granuloma lesions has ranged from little or none to fairly intense. Because of this uncertain response, skeletal survey methods should include both roentgenographic and radionuclide imaging.

8. Miscellaneous Lesions

Experience with other benign tumors and tumorlike conditions of bone has been too limited for meaningful comment. Visualization of these lesions should depend on local perfusion rates and the level of reactive and reparative osseous response in adjacent bone.

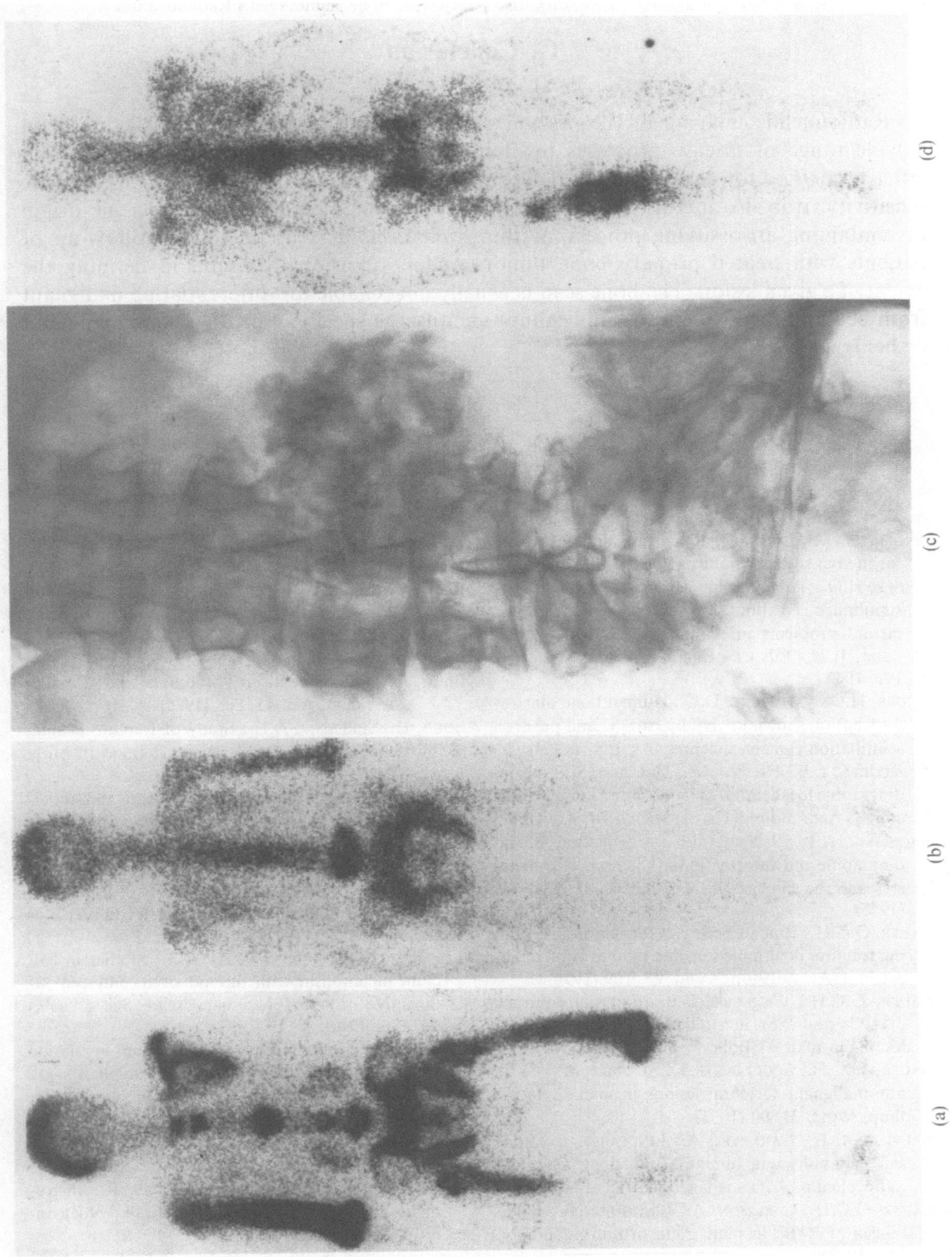

Fig. 16a–d. Paget's disease: Sarcomatous degeneration. (a) ^{99m}Tc-EHDP scan demonstrates classic configuration of uncomplicated Paget's disease with involvement of the six most common sites. ^{18}F scan (b) of patient with Paget's disease shows activity extending far beyond expected confines of L3–L4 due to sarcomatous degeneration (c) with exophytic chondrosarcoma. Irregular configuration of monostotic Paget's disease in distal right femur (d) suggests sarcomatous degeneration confirmed by additional metastatic osteosarcoma lesions in midfemur, pelvis, spine, and lungs

G. Conclusion

Radionuclide imaging of the osseous system has proved to be extremely useful in a wide range of disease processes involving bone. The bone scan is a practical and efficient method for demonstrating polyostotic disease, primarily because of an exquisite sensitivity. It is also useful for demonstrating soft tissue metastases of osteogenic origin or containing an ossifying process. Within limitations it is useful in the follow-up of patients with treated primary bone tumors and is occasionally useful in defining the extent of a given lesion. The bone scan is usually not reliable for differentiating malignant from benign processes and usually cannot identify the specific type of tumor, malignant or benign.

References

ANGER, H.O.: Use of a gamma-ray pinhole camera for in vivo studies. Nature (Lond.) 170, 200 (1949)

ANGER, H.O.: Tomographic gamma-ray scanner with simultaneous readout of several planes. In: Fundamental problems in scanning. GOTTSCHALK, A., BECK, R.N. (Eds.). Springfield: C.C. Thomas, p. 195, 1968

ANGER, H.O., VAN DYKE, D.C.: Human bone marrow distribution shown in vivo by Iron-52 and positron scintillation camera. Science. 144, 1587 (1964)

APPELGREN, L.E., NILSSON, A., ULLBERG, S.: Autoradiographic localization of strontium-85 in osteosarcomas. Acta radiol. [Ther.] (Stockh.) 1, 459 (1963)

BACHMAN, A.L., SPRONL, E.E.: Correlation of radiographic and autopsy findings in suspected metastases in the spine. Bull. N.Y. Acad. Med. 31, 146 (1955)

BAUER, G.C.H.: Rate of bone salt formation in a healing fracture determined in rats by means of radiocalcium. Acta orthop. scand. 23, 169 (1954)

BAUER, G.C.H., WENDEBERG, B.: External counting of ^{47}Ca and ^{85}Sr in studies of localized skeletal lesions in man. J. Bone Jt Surg. 41B, 558 (1959)

BAUER, G.C.H., SCOCCIANTI, D.: Uptake of ^{85}Sr in non-malignant vertebral lesions in man. Acta orthop. scand. 31, 90 (1961)

BAUER, G.C.H., CARLSSON, A., LINDQUIST, B.: Bone salt metabolism in humans studied by means of radiocalcium. Acta med. scand. 158, 143 (1957a)

BAUER, G.C.H., CARLSSON, A., LINDQUIST, B.: Metabolism of ^{140}Ba in man. Acta orthop. scand. 26, 241 (1957b)

BELLIN, J., LASZLO, D.: Metabolism and removal of ^{45}Ca in man. Science. 117, 331 (1953)

BERG, G.R., KALISHER, L., OSMOND, J.D., PENDERGRASS, H.P., POTSAID, M.S.: ^{99m}Tc-diphosphonate concentration in primary breast carcinoma. Radiology. 106, 393 (1973)

BLAU, M., NAGLER, W., BENDER, M.A.: Fluorine-18: A new isotope for bone scanning. J. Nucl. Med. 3, 332 (1962)

BLAU, M., LAOR, Y., BENDER, M.A.: Isotope scanning with ^{18}F for early detection of bone tumors. In: Medical isotope scintigraphy, Vol. III, Vienna, International Atomic Energy Agency, p. 341 (1968)

BLUM, T.: Osteomyelitis of Mandible and Maxilla. J. Amer. dent. Ass. 11, 805 (1925)

BOHR, H., SORENSEN, A.H.: Study of fracture healing by means of radioactive tracers. J. Bone Jt. Surg. 32a, 567 (1950)

BORAK, J.: Relationship between clinical and roentgenological findings in bone metastasis. Surg. Gynec. Obstet. 75, 599 (1942)

BROWER, A.C., CULVER, J.E., KEATS, T.E.: Histological nature of the cortical irregularity of the medial posterior distal femoral metaphysis in children. Radiology 99, 389 (1971)

CAMPBELL, W.W., GREENBERG, D.M.: Studies in calcium metabolism with the aid of its induced radioactive isotope. Proc. nat. Acad. Sci. (Wash.) 26, 176 (1940)

CARLSSON, A.: Metabolism of radiocalcium in relation to calcium intake in young rats. Acta pharmacol. (Kbh.) 7, Suppl. 1 (1951)

CARLSSON, A.: On the mechanism of the skeletal turnover of lime salts. Acta physiol. scand. 26, 200 (1952)

CASSEN, B., CURTIS, L., REED, C., LIBBY, R.: Instrumentation for ^{131}I use in medical studies. Nucleonics 9, 2, 46 (1951)

CASTRONOVO, F.P., JR., CALLAHAN, R.J.: A new bone scanning agent. ^{99m}Tc labeled l-hydroxy-ethylidene-l, l-disodium phosphonate. J. Nucl. Med. 13, 823 (1972)

CHARKES, N.D., SKLAROFF, D.M.: Early diagnosis of metastatic bone cancer by photoscanning with ^{85}Sr. J. Nucl. Med. 5, 168 (1964)

CHARKES, N.D., SKLAROFF, D.M.: The radioactive

strontium photoscan as a diagnostic aid in primary and metastatic cancer in bone. Radiol. Clin. N. Amer. **3**, 499 (1965)

CHARKES, N.D., SKLAROFF, D.M., YOUNG, I.: A critical analysis of strontium bone scanning for detection of metastatic cancer. Amer. J. Roentgenol. **96**, 647 (1966)

CHIEWITZ, O., HEVESY, G.: Radioactive indicators in the study of phosphorus metabolism in rats. Nature (Lond.) **136**, 754 (1935)

CONWAY, J.J.: Personal communication, 1975

COOKE, M.B.D., CLAYTON, G.D., KAPLAN, E.: Scanning scintillation camera with data storage and processing capacity. J. Nucl. Med. **11**, 309 (1970)

COOKE, M.B.D., KAPLAN, E.: Whole body imaging and count profiling with a modified Anger camera. I. Principles and applications. II. Implementation. J. Nucl. Med. **13**, 899 (1972)

CURIE, I., JOLIOT, F.: Physique nucléaire – Un nouveau type de radioactivité. C.R. Acad. Sci. (Paris) **198**, 254, 559 (1934)

DE NARDO, G.L.: ^{85}Sr scintiscan in bone disease. Ann. intern. Med. **65**, 647 (1966)

DE NARDO, G.L.: Clinical application of bone scintiscans. Clin. Med. **75**, 22 (1968)

DE NARDO, G.L., VOLBE, J.A.: Detection of bone lesions with ^{85}Sr scintiscan. J. Nucl. Med. **7**, 219 (1966)

DE NARDO, G.L., HORNER, R.W., LEACH, P.J., BOWES, D.J.: Radioisotope skeletal scanning. J. Amer. med. Ass. **200**, 121 (1967)

DUBRIDGE, L.A., MARSHALL, J.: Radioactive isotopes of Sr, Y and Zv. Physiol. Rev. **87**, 348 (1940)

DUDLEY, H.C.: Determination of gallium in biologic materials. J. Pharmacol. exp. Ther. **95**, 482 (1949)

DUDLEY, H.C., LEVINE, M.D.: Studies of the toxic action of gallium. J. Pharmacol. exp. Ther. **96**, 224 (1949)

DUDLEY, H.C., MADDOX, G.E.: Deposition of radio Gallium (^{72}Ga) in skeletal tissues. J. Pharmacol. exp. Ther. **96**, 224 (1949)

DURBIN, P.W., ASING, C.W., JOHNSTON, M.E., HAMILTON, J.G., WILLIAMS, M.H.: The metabolism of the lanthanons in the rat II. Time studies of the tissue deposition of intravenously administered radioisotopes. USAEC Report, Orins. **12**, 171 (1956)

DYKE, D. van, ANGER, H.O., YANO, Y.: Bone blood flow shown with ^{18}F and the positron camera. Amer. J. Physiol. **209**, 65 (1965)

ENGSTEDT, L., FRANZEN, S., JONSSON, L., LARSSON, L.G.: In vivo localization of colloidal ^{198}Au intravenously injected in polycythemia vera. Acta radiol. (Stockh.) **49**, 66 (1958)

ERF, L.A., PECHER, C.: Secretion of Radio-Strontium in milk of two cows following intravenous administration. Proc. Soc. exp. Biol. (N.Y.) **45**, 762 (1940)

FERRANT, A., RODHAIN, J., MICHAUX, L., PIRET, L., MALDAGUE, B., SOKAL, G.: Detection of skeletal involvement in Hodgkin's disease: A comparison of radiography, bone scanning, and bone marrow

biopsy in 38 patients. Cancer (Philad.) **35**, 1346 (1975)

FITZER, P.M.: ^{99m}Tc-polyphosphate concentration in a neuroblastoma. J. Nucl. Med. **15**, 905 (1974)

FLEMING, W.H., MC ILRAITH, J.D., KING, E.R.: Photoscanning of bone lesions utilizing ^{85}Sr. Radiology. **77**, 635 (1961)

FORDHAM, E.W., RAMACHANDRAN, P.C.: Radionuclide imaging of osseous trauma. Sem. Nucl. Med. **4**, 4, 411 (1974)

FRANKEL, R.S., JONES, A.E., COHEN, J.A., JOHNSON, K.W., JOHNSTON, G.S., POMEROY, T.C.: Clinical correlations of ^{67}Ga and skeletal whole body radionuclide studies with radiography in Ewing's sarcoma. Radiology. **110**, 597 (1974)

FRENCH, R.J., MC CREADY, V.R.: The use of ^{18}F for bone scanning. Brit. J. Radiol. **40**, 655 (1967)

GEIGER, H., MÜLLER, W.: Das Elektronenzählrohr. Wirkungsweise und Herstellung eines Zählrohrs. Physiol. Z. **29**, 839 (1928); Technische Bemerkungen zum Elektronenzählrohr. Physiol. Z. **30**, 489 (1929)

GENANT, H.K., BAUTOVICH, G.J., LATHROP, K.A., HARPER, P.V.: In vivo study of factors influencing skeletal uptake of bone seeking radionuclides. J. Nucl. Med. **15**, 493 (1974)

GERSON, B.D., DORFMAN, H.D., NORMAN, A., MANKIN, H.J.: Patterns of localization of ^{85}strontium in osteosarcoma. J. Bone Jt. Surg. **54A**, 817 (1972)

GHAED, N., THRALL, J.H., PINSKY, S.M., JOHNSON, M.C.: Detection of extraosseous metastasis from osteosarcoma with ^{99m}Tc-polyphosphate bone scanning. Radiology. **112**, 373 (1974)

GILDAY, D.L.: Diagnosis of obscure childhood osteoid osteomas with bone scan. J. Nucl. Med. **15**, 494 (1974).

GILLESPIE, P.J., ALEXANDER, J.L., EDELSTYN, G.A.: Changes in ^{87m}Sr concentrations in skeletal metastasis in patients responding to cyclical combination chemotherapy for advanced breast cancer. J. Nucl. Med. **16**, 191 (1975)

GIRAMES, G.M., JENSEN, C.: Abnormal bone scan in cerebral infarction. J. Nucl. Med. **14**, 941 (1973)

GOLDMAN, A.B., BRAUNSTEIN, D.: Augmented radioactivity on bone scans of limbs bearing osteosarcomas. J. Nucl. Med. **16**, 423 (1975)

GOLDMAN, A.B., BECKER, M.H., BRAUNSTEIN, P., FRANCIS, K.C., GENIESER, M.D., FIROOZNIA, H.: Bone scanning – osteogenic sarcoma. Correlation with surgical pathology. Amer. J. Roentgenol. **124**, 83 (1975)

GOTTSCHALK, R.G., ALLEN, H.C., JR.: Uptake of radioactive sulfur by chondrosarcomas in man. Proc. Soc. exp. Biol. (N.Y.) **80**, 334 (1952)

GREENBERG, D.M.: Studies in mineral metabolism with the aid of artificial radioactive tracers. VIII. Tracer experiments with radioactive calcium and strontium on the mechanism of vitamin D action in rachitic rats. J. biol. Chem. **157**, 99 (1945)

GYNNING, J., LANGELAND, D., LINDBERG, S., WALDESKOG, B.: Localization with ^{85}Sr of spinal metastasis in mammary cancer and changes in uptake after hormone and roentgen-therapy. A preliminary report. Acta radiol. (Stockh.) **55**, 119 (1961)

HARBERT, J.C., ASHBURN, W.L.: Radiostrontium bone scanning in Hodgkin's disease. Cancer (Philad.) **22**, 58 (1968)

HARPER, D.V., GOTTSCHALK, A., CHARLESTON, D.B.: Area scanning with Anger camera. The fundamental problems in scanning. Springfield: C.C. Thomas, p. 145, 1968

HOFFMAN, F.L.: Radium (Mesothorium) necrosis. J. Amer. med. Ass. **85**, 961 (1925)

HOSAIN, F., SYED, I.B., WAGNER, H.N.: Ionic ^{135m}Ba for bone scanning. J. Nucl. Med. **11**, 328 (1970)

JOLIOT, F., CURIE, I.: Artificial production of a new kind of ratio-element. Nature (Lond.) **133**, 202

JONES, H.B., CHAIKOFF, I.L., LAWRENCE, J.H.: Phosphorus metabolism of the soft tissues of the normal mouse as indicated by radioactive phosphorus. Amer. J. Cancer. **40**, 235 (1940)

KARSHER, H.: Der Calcium- und Phosphorstoffwechsel bei der normalen und gestörten Knochenbruchheilung sowie in frischen und konservierten Transplantaten. Ein Nachweis mit den radioaktiven Isotopen P^{32} and Ca^{45}. Arch. klin. Chir. **275**, 1 (1953)

KAYE, M., SILVERTON, S., ROSENTHAL, L.: Technetium ^{99m}-pyrophosphate: Studies in vivo and vitro. J. Nucl. Med. **16**, 40 (1975)

KNISELEY, R.M., ANDREWS, G.A., TANIDA, R., EDWARDS, C.L., KYKER, G.C.: Delineation of active marrow by whole body scanning with radioactive colloids. J. Nucl. Med. **7**, 575 (1966)

LANGE, R.C., TREVES, S., SPENCER, R.P.: ^{135m}Ba and ^{131}Ba as bone scanning agents. J. Nucl. Med. **11**, 340 (1970)

LARSON, S.M., NELP, W.B.: The radiocolloid bone marrow scan in malignant disease. J. surg. Oncol. **3**, 685 (1971)

LASA, E.D., PEREZ-MODREGO, S.: Detection of cartilaginous tumors with Selenium-75. Radiology. **85**, 149 (1965)

LAYTON, L.L.: Labelled inorganic sulfate in the diagnosis of cartilaginous tumors and their metastasis. Cancer (Philad.) **2**, 1089 (1949)

LEE, V.W., SANO, R., FREEDMAN, G.: Whole body gamma camera imaging using a moving table accessory. J. Nucl. Med. **14**, 830 (1973)

MARTLAND, H.S., CONLON, P., KNEF, J.P.: Some unrecognized dangers in the use and handling of radioactive substances. J. Amer. med. Ass. **85**, 1769 (1925).

MARTLAND, H.S., HUMPHRIES, R.E.: Osteogenic sarcoma in dial painters using luminous paint. Arch. Path. (Chicago) **7**, 406 (1929)

MARTY, R., HOFFMAN, H.C.: Bone Scannings: Its use in preoperative evaluation of patients with suspicious breast masses. J. Nucl. Med. **13**, 452 (1972)

MC LAUGHLIN, A.F.: Uptake of ^{99}Tc bone-scanning agent by lungs with metastatic calcifications. J. Nucl. Med. **16**, 322 (1975)

MC NEIL, B.J., CASSADY, J.R., GEISER, C.F., JAFFE, N., TRAGGIS, D., TREVES, S.: Fluorine 18 Bone scintigraphy in children with osteosarcoma or Ewing's sarcoma. Radiology. **109**, 627 (1973)

MC RAE, J., ANGER, H.O.: Bone imaging with multiplane tomographic scanner. J. Nucl. Med. **15**, 516 (1974)

MEYERS, W.G.: Radiostrontium-87m. J. Nucl. Med. **1**, 125 (1960)

MULRY, W.C., DUDLEY, H.C.: Studies of radiogallium as a diagnostic agent in bone tumors. J. Lab. clin. Med. **37**, 239 (1951)

NELP, W.B., LEWIS, R.J., LARSON, S.M.: Distribution of the erythron and the RES in the bone marrow organ. J. Nucl. Med. **7**, 366 (1966)

O'MARA, R.E., BRETTNER, A., DANIGELIS, J.A., GOULD, L.V.: ^{18}F uptake within metastatic osteosarcoma of the liver. Radiology. **100**, 113 (1971)

O'MARA, R.E., MC AFEE, J.G., SUBRAMANIAN, G.: Clinical experiences with rare earths as bone scanning agents. J. Nucl. Med. **10**, 363 (1969)

O'MARA, R.E., SUBRAMANIAN, G.: Experimental agents for skeletal imaging. Sem. Nucl. Med. **2**, 38 (1972)

PECHER, C.: Radio-calcium and radio-strontium. metabolism in pregnant mice. Proc. Soc. exp. Biol. (N.Y.) **46**, 86 (1941)

PECHER, C., PECHER, J.: Radio-calcium and Radio-strontium. Metabolism in Pregnant Mice. Proc. Soc. exp. Biol. (N.Y.) **46**, 91 (1941)

PENDERGRASS, H.P., POTSAID, M.S., CASTRONOVO, F.P.: The clinical use of ^{99m}Tc-diphosphonate. Radiology. **107**, 557 (1973)

PEREZ, R., COHEN, Y., HENRY, R., PANNECIERE, C.: A new radiopharmaceutical for ^{99m}Tc bone scanning. J. Nucl. Med. **13**, 788 (1972)

POULOSE, K.P., REBA, R.C., ECKELMAN, W.C., GOODYEAR, M.: Extra-osseous localization of ^{99m}Tc-Sn pyrophosphate. Brit. J. Radiol. **48**, 724 (1975)

RICHARDS, A.G.: Metastatic calcification detected through scanning with ^{99m}Tc polyphosphate. J. Nucl. Med. **15**, 1057 (1974)

ROSENFIELD, N., TREVES, S.: Osseous and extraosseous uptake of Fluorine-18 and Technetium-99m polyphosphate in children with neuroblastoma. Radiology. **111**, 127 (1974)

RUBIN, P., BRACE, K.C., GUMP, H., SWARM, R., ANDREWS, R.: The radiotoxic effects of ^{35}S in growing cartilage. Consideration of radioactive sulfur (^{35}S) as a possible radiotherapeutic agent in chondrosarcoma. Radiology. **69**, 711 (1957)

RUTHERFORD, E., GEIGER, H.: An electrical method of counting the number of α-particles from radioactive substances. Proc. roy. Soc. **A81**, 141 (1908)

SAMUELS, L.D.: Lung scanning with ^{87m}Sr in metastatic osteosarcoma. Amer. J. Roentgenol. **104**, 766 (1968)

SAMUELS, L.D.: Diagnosis of malignant bone disease with Strontium 87m scans. J. Canad. med. Ass. **104**, 411 (1971)

SARMIENTO, A.H., ALBA, J., LANARO, A.E., DIETRICH, R.: Evaluation of soft tissue calcifications in dermatomyositis with ^{99m}Tc phosphate compounds: Case report. J. Nucl. Med. **16**, 467 (1974)

SCHALL, G.L., ZEIGER, L., PRIMACK, A., DE LELLIS, R.: Uptake of ^{85}Sr by an osteosarcoma metastatic to lung. J. Nucl. Med. **12**, 131 (1971)

SCHLUNDT, H., BARER, H.H., FLINN, F.B.: The detection and estimation of radium and mesothorium in living persons. I. Amer. J. Roentgenol. **21**, 345 (1929)

SHARMA, S.M., QUINN, J.L.: Sensitivity of ^{18}F bone scans in search for metastasis. Surg. Gynec. Obstet. **135**, 536 (1972)

SHIRAZI, P.H., RAYUDU, G.V.S., FORDHAM, E.W.: Extraosseous osteogenic sarcoma of the small bowel demonstrated by ^{18}F scanning. J. Nucl. Med. **14**, 295 (1973)

SHIRAZI, P.H., RAYUDU, G.V.S., FORDHAM, E.W.: ^{18}F bone scanning: Review of indications and results of 1500 scans. Radiology. **112**, 360 (1974a)

SHIRAZI, P.H., RAYUDU, G.V.S., FORDHAM, E.W.: Review of solitary ^{18}F bone lesions. Radiology. **112**, 369 (1974b)

SHIRAZI, P.H., RYAN, W.G., FORDHAM, E.W.: Bone scanning in evaluation of Paget's disease of bone. CRC Crit. Rev. clin. Radiol. Nucl. Med. **5**, 523 (1974c)

SIMON, H.: Medial distal metaphyseal femoral irregularity in children. Radiology. **90**, 258 (1968)

SINGHER, H.O., MARINELLI, L.: Distribution of radioactive sulphur in the rat. Science. **101**, 414 (1945)

SKLAROFF, D.M., CHARKES, N.D.: Diagnosis of bone metastasis by photoscanning with ^{85}Sr. J. Amer. med. Ass. **188**, 1 (1964)

SNELL, A.H.: A new radioactive isotope of Fluorine. Physiol. Rev. **51**, 143 (1937)

SPENCER, R.P., LANGE, R.C., TREVES, S.: An intermediate-lived radionuclide for bone scanning. J. Nucl. Med. **11**, 95 (1970)

SPENCER, R.P., LANGE, R.C., TREVES, S.: Use of ^{135m}Ba and ^{131}Ba as a bone scanning agents. J. Nucl. Med. **12**, 216 (1971)

STAHELI, L.T., NELP, W.B., MARTY, R., GRIFFIN, J.T.: The early diagnosis of bone and joint infections in children by ^{87m}Sr scanning. J. Nucl. Med. **13**, 468 (1972)

STEWART, D.W., LAWSON, J.L., CORK, J.M.: Induced radioactivity in strontium and yttrium. Physiol. Rev. **52**, 901 (1937)

SUBRAMANIAN, G.: ^{135m}Ba: Preliminary evaluation of a new radionuclide for skeletal imaging. J. Nucl. Med. **11**, 650 (1970)

SUBRAMANIAN, G., MC AFEE, J.G.: A new complex of ^{99m}Tc for skeletal imaging. Radiology. **99**, 192 (1971)

SUBRAMANIAN, G., MC AFEE, J.G., BELL, E.G., BLAIR, R.J., O'MARA, R.E., RALSTON, P.H.: ^{99m}Tc-labeled polyphosphate as a skeletal agent. Radiology. **102**, 701 (1972a)

SUBRAMANIAN, G., MC AFEE, J.G., BLAIR, R.J., MEHTER, A., CONNOR, T.: ^{99m}Tc-EHDP: A potential radiopharmaceutical for skeletal imaging. J. Nucl. Med. **13**, 947 (1972b)

TILDEN, R.L., JACKSON, J., ENNEKING, W.F., DELAND, F.H., MC VEY, J.T.: ^{99m}Tc-polyphosphate: Histological localization in human femurs by autoradiography. J. Nucl. Med. **14**, 576 (1973)

TREADWELL, A.G., LOW-BEER, B.V.A., FRIEDELL, H.L., LAWRENCE, J.H.: Metabolic studies on neoplasm of bone with the aid of radioactive strontium. Amer. J. med. Sci. **204**, 521 (1942)

TUBIANA, M., ALBAREDE, P. NAHUM, H.: Study of radioactive phosphorus (^{32}P) distribution in man by external Bremsstrahlung measurements. In: Proc. Second Intern'l. Conf. Peaceful Uses of Atomic Energy. Vol. 26, p. 217. United Nations. Geneva 1958

TURNER, D.A., FORDHAM, E.W., RAMACHANDRAN, P.C., ALI, A., CZERWINSKI, B.: The Anger tomographic rectilinear scanner. Exhibit at the Society of Nuclear Medicine 21st Annual Meeting, San Diego, June, 1974 and the Radiological Society of North America 60th Annual Meeting, Chicago 1974

VOLKER, J.F., SOGNNAES, R.F., BIBBY, B.G.: Studies on the distribution of radioactive fluoride in the bones and teeth of experimental animals. Amer. J. Physiol. **132**, 707 (1941)

WANKEN, J.J., EYRING, E.J., SAMUELS, L.D.: Diagnosis of pediatric bone lesions: Correlation of clinical, roentgenographic, ^{87m}Sr scan and pathologic diagnosis. J. Nucl. Med. **14**, 803 (1973)

WEBER, W.G., DE NARDO, G.L., BERGIN, J.J.: Scintiscanning in malignant lymphomatous involvement of bone. Arch. intern. Med. **121**, 433 (1968)

WENZEL, W.W., HEASTY, R.G.: Uptake of ^{99m}Tc-Sn polyphosphate in an area of cerebral infarction. J. Nucl. Med. **15**, 207 (1974)

WERFF, J.TH. VAN DER: Clinical investigation on the use of radioactive gallium (^{66}Ga and ^{67}Ga) in bone diseases. Acta radiol. (Stockh.) **41**, 343 (1954)

WILKINSON, G.W., LEBLOND, C.P.: The deposition of radiophosphorus in fractured bones in rats. Surg. Gynec. Obstet. **97**, 143 (1953)

WOODBURY, D.H., BEIERWALTERS, W.H.: Fluorine-18 uptake and localization in soft tissue deposits of osteogenic sarcoma in rats and man. J. Nucl. Med. **8**, 646 (1967)

YANO, Y., MC RAE, J., VAN DYKE, D.C., ANGER, H.O.: ^{99m}Tc-labeled Sn(II) diphosphonate: A bone scanning agent. J. Nucl. Med. **13**, 480 (1972)

YANO, Y., MC RAE, J., VAN DYKE, D.C., ANGER, H.O.: ^{99m}Tc-labeled stannous ethane-l-hydroxy-l, l-diphosphonate: A new bone scanning agent. J. Nucl. Med. **14**, 73 (1973)

ZIMMER, A.M., ISITMAN, A.T., SCHMITT, G.H., HOLMES, R.A.: Enzymatic inhibition by diphosphonate: A proposed mechanism of tissue uptake. J. Nucl. Med. **15**, 546 (1974)

Angiography of Bone Tumors

by

Issa Yaghmai

A. Introduction

Arteriography has become an important and necessary procedure for the investigation of intracranial, intrathoracic, and abdominal disorders in today's modern medicine. The first experiments in arteriography concerned the differential diagnosis of bone neoplasms. The work of DOS SANTOS et al. (1932), CALDAS (1934), and FARINAS (1937) provided the major impetus in the development of modern selective arteriography. Despite the increasing use of arteriography in the study of intracranial, intrathoracic, and abdominal organs, the study of bone and soft tissues by arteriography has received relatively little attention due to the following reasons:

1. Primary bone lesions are uncommon.
2. These lesions are accessible to physical examination and biopsy.
3. It has been difficult to gain experience in the interpretation of arteriographic findings of bone lesions due to the limited number of investigations reported.
4. Conventional roentgenographic findings give adequate diagnostic information in most cases.

In some instances, however, the radiologist finds himself hard pressed to differentiate adequately between a benign and a malignant bone lesion. This difficulty, unfortunately, is not peculiar to radiologists, but often extends to pathologists as well, and the surgeon in such instances is left with the unhappy choice of performing a radical operation for what may turn out to be a benign lesion, or wait until unmistakable signs of malignancy appear.

Since primary malignant bone tumors constitute some of the most tragic cases, associated as they often are with the possibility of a mutilating operation and a poor prognosis, any contribution toward confirming or disproving their presence should be of value, provided such an investigation, like arteriography, causes little or no harm to the patient.

B. Vascular Anatomy

The present knowledge of anatomy and physiology of bone circulation is limited, because of difficulties in its investigation. The following description is based upon the observations of DRINKER et al. (1922), TILLING (1958), and DOAN (1922).

Arterial blood enters the long bone through three sources:

1. Nutrient arteries of the epiphysis and diaphysis
2. Periosteal and perichondral arteries
3. Epiphyseal and metaphyseal arteries.

I. Nutrient Arteries

The largest artery supplying a long bone is the nutrient artery of the diaphysis. The nutrient artery pursues a tortuous course obliquely through the cortex of the shaft before entering the medullary canal. In most instances after entering the medullary canal, it divides and contributes one or more branches to the metaphyses at either end of the bone. Along its course in the shaft, the nutrient artery gives off small branches, which pass to the inner surface of the cancellous bone through the horizontal canals known as Volkmann's canals. These vessels anastomose extensively with other small arterioles that enter the bone from the periosteum, and with a venous network comprised of very small vessels. The branches from central arteries become more numerous at the periphery of the bone, contributing to an extensive network of anastomoses between metaphyseal circulation and nutrient artery branches in the spongiosa. The only exception is in the head and neck of the femur, where in childhood, the nutrient artery supplies the entire vascular area of the metaphyseal aspect of the epiphyseal plate, in which endochondral ossification takes place. With increasing age, the nutrient artery and its branches become smaller because of the decreased blood demand in the diaphysis, due to replacement of the red marrow with less vascular fatty tissue, and to cessation of endochondral ossification at the metaphysis.

There are usually one or more nutrient arteries supplying the epiphysis. These vessels enter through nutrient foramen and pass to the central region of the epiphyses, from which branches radiate in different directions. These vessels anastomose with small peripheral arteries. During the period of enchondral ossification, branches of the nutrient artery of the epiphyses perforate the epiphyseal cartilaginous plates, and anastomose with the metaphyseal vessels.

II. Periosteal and Perichondral Arteries

Large periosteal arteries traverse the periosteum vertically, and branches arise at intervals and form rings around the circumference of the bone. These vessels provide numerous branches that supply the periosteum and enter the outer surface of the compact bone through the Volkmann's canals, and pass into the Haversian system. Generally, these vessels supply the periphery of compact bone and enter into extensive anastomosis with branches of the nutrient and metaphyseal arteries. The blood supply in the Haversian system is oriented in a vertical direction, with the vessels comprised mainly of arterioles, capillaries, and venules. Arteries similar to the large periosteal vessels arise from the perichondrium and enter the epiphyses.

III. Metaphyseal and Epiphyseal Arteries

Large and small branches from muscular and tendon arteries enter the epiphyseal and metaphyseal portions of the bone through numerous foramina in the bone. These vessels in the epiphyses and metaphyses maintain a separate vascular network, but anasto-mose freely. In the growing bone, the epiphyseal cartilage is perforated by arteries passing both from the epiphysis to the metaphysis and vice versa. The proximal end of the femur, however, is a notable exception.

In the spongiosa, arterioles divide extensively and enter large venous sinusoids. With the transition from red marrow to yellow fatty marrow, the sinusoids are replaced by capillaries that are similar in size and structure to capillaries elsewhere in the human body. The venous sinusoids are several times the caliber of capillaries and more numerous, but with walls of the same thickness as those of capillaries. Sinusoids are present in clumps in the red marrow, receive blood from different directions, and are the principal function-ing vascular bed for circulating blood. Capillaries are widely distributed in fatty marrow, and also contain most of the blood in compact bone.

Capillary blood converges with blood from the venous sinusoids to enter vessels that flow into larger venous trunks. All branches of the venous system are easily distin-guished from the corresponding arteries by their greater capacity, numerous branches, and larger lumens. The veins are thin-walled vessels in comparison with arteries of similar size. The course of veins is more tortuous, and sometimes may spiral around their companion artery. The intraosseous venous system does not have valves.

The veins draining tubular bones may be divided into the same three groups as the arteries: (1) The nutrient veins of the diaphysis and epiphysis; (2) periosteal and perichondral veins; and (3) metaphyseal and epiphyseal veins. The course of the veins in bone is roughly parallel to that of the corresponding arteries.

In living patients, attempts to follow roentgenographically the normal arterial and venous circulation through the bone have been unsuccessful due to the following reasons: (1) The narrow lumen of the nutrient arteries; (2) dilution effect created by the large pools of blood within bone; (3) greater bone density obscures the contrast material. The mineral content of bone obscures the normal vascular network, and indeed these can be seen only by special microangiographic techniques performed in vitro after decalci-fying normal bone.

IV. Arterial Supply of Bone Lesions

The periosteal and perichondral arteries are the main sources for blood supply in most bone lesions. The metaphyseal or epiphyseal vascular contribution will depend to some extent on the location of the bone lesion. In addition, most of the hypervascular bone neoplasms derive a blood supply from numerous large arteries arising from soft tissue surrounding the lesion. It is not clear whether this increased vascularity represents new vessel formation or increased utilization of pre-existing vascular channels. These arteries usually are not recognized in normal arteriograms, probably due to their narrow lumens. The superimposition of these arteries, when visualized, gives a reticular pattern to the lesion which is characteristic for hypervascular bone neoplasms. The nutrient artery of the diaphysis, which is the largest artery supplying the normal bone, is rarely involved. The greater density of the bone at the site of the foramen does not permit this artery to enlarge, except when the destructive process involves the foramen itself. In this case, the nutrient artery can be identified easily.

When a destructive lesion involves a bone, because of demineralization of the particu-lar area, the vascular network associated with the lesion becomes visible, disclosing abnormal vessels, displaced vessels, arteriovenous fistulae and areas of abnormal tissue staining. In cases of osteoblastic bone lesions, these findings are difficult to appreciate because of the increased bony density relative to contrast material. However, most bone lesions, especially malignant bone neoplasms, have associated soft tissue invasion and therefore arteriographic findings can be identified in the soft tissues around the bone. In cases of osteoblastic metastasis, interpretation of arteriographic findings is more difficult because of usual lack of soft tissue extension, and some authors believe that osteoblastic metastases are avascular (Schobinger, 1958). Also, subtraction is of great value for better visualization of the vascularity in most of these cases.

C. Arteriography

I. Technique

With the use of percutaneous arterial injection either by direct puncture or catheterization, lesions of any part of the skeleton may be demonstrated. Lesions of the head and neck can be visualized by injection into the common carotid, external carotid, or vertebral arteries. The upper extremities are studied by injection into the subclavian, axillary, or brachial arteries, and the lower extremities by injection into the external iliac or femoral arteries. The bones of the thorax, abdomen, and pelvis usually require aortography, or in some instances, selective arteriography by catheterization of the costocervical trunk, intercostal, lumbar, or hypogastric arteries. Depending on the site and size of the lesions, 15–30 cc of contrast material (Hypaque 50% or Renografin 60%) may be used. Hand injections are sufficient for excellent visualization of lesions involving the head and neck, lower extremity, upper extremities and in selective arteriograms.

Because some bone lesions are characterized by rapid circulation, abnormal arteriovenous communications, and prolonged tissue staining, it is desirable to demonstrate all these findings during arteriography. Roentgenograms should be obtained rapidly at first, then at intervals of 2 sec, and should be continued for 20 sec after the beginning of injection. In some cases, a 45 sec film is of great value in the differential diagnosis between benign hypervascular bone neoplasms and malignant bone lesions. Biplane arteriography will be of greater value than single plane studies.

II. Pharmacoangiography

During the past decade, a large number of drugs have been used in the hope of improvement in the angiographic diagnosis of benign and malignant lesions. Both vasoconstrictors and vasodilators have been examined experimentally and clinically. However, reports of the diagnostic value of pharmacoangiography have contradictory results.

In the evaluation of bone and soft tissue lesions, both vasoconstrictors (Ekelund and Lunderqvist, 1974) and vasodilators (Hawkins and Hudson, 1974) have been used. Vasoconstrictives that have been more extensively evaluated are angiotensin, vasopressin, and to a lesser extent, epinephrine and norepinephrine. Small intra-arterial doses of 10–20 mg angiotensin, depending on the size of the lesion, will cause constriction of the entire normal arterial system, but have no effect on abnormal vessels. Tumor vessels will be seen better than on the regular arteriogram in approximately 75% of the cases.

Several vasodilators have also been studied and the results of Priscoline (tolazoline hydrochloride) have been more extensively reported than others. An arterial dose of 25–50 mg of Priscoline in 10 ml of normal saline, depending upon the size of the patient and the size of the area to be studied, should be injected intra-arterially by infusion to obtain the best results. The injection of Renografin is usually made approximately 30 sec after the injection of Priscoline.

In the evaluation of bone and soft-tissue lesions, the results of vasodilators appear more informative than vasoconstrictive agents, especially in the diagnosis of malignant bone neoplasms with a low grade of vascularity.

III. Subtraction

This technique has been used increasingly in different kinds of angiography, and is of great value in bone angiograms, especially for the better evaluation of the intraosseous vascular pattern. Subtraction can be used in the ordinary fashion, or be modified to produce even better results in bone angiography by using the most informative film in the arterial phase as the mask and following the usual subtraction technique. The final subtraction film shows arteries white and veins dark against a gray background (Fig. 1 d). The anatomical relationship between arteries and veins is shown on one film, which can be especially advantageous in correlating normal and abnormal arteriovenous relationships. Finally, subtraction is of great value for the better visualization of the vascularity and especially the intraosseous tumor stain of osteoblastic bone lesions.

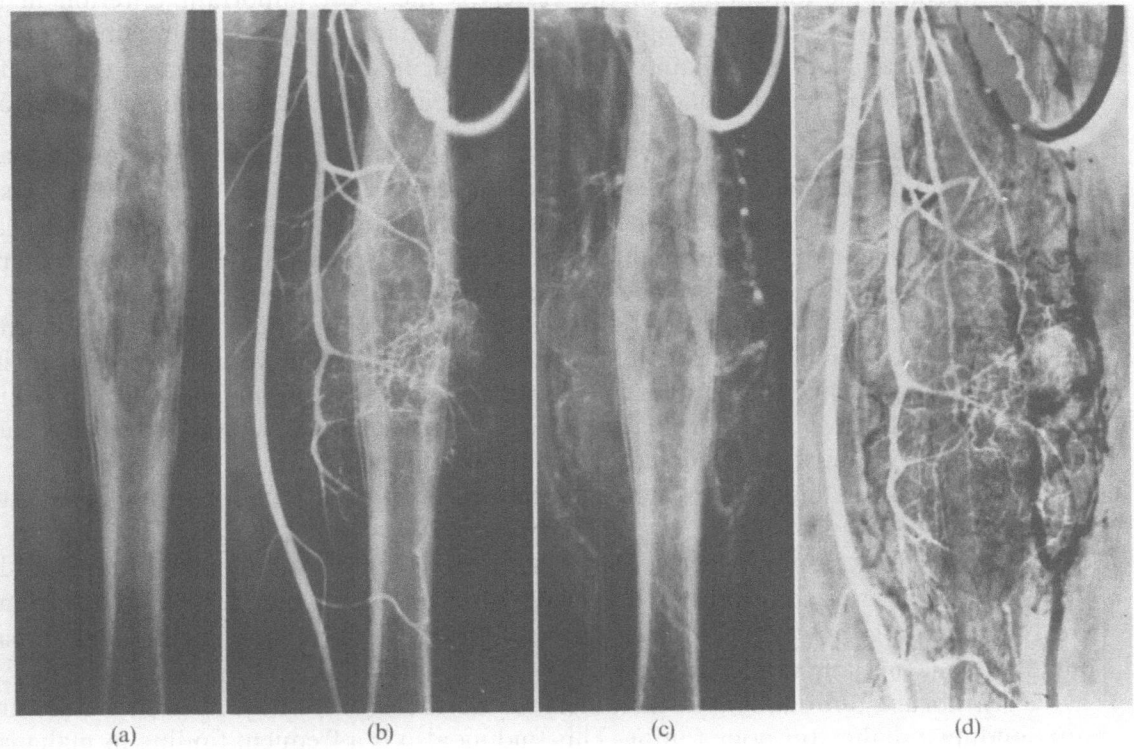

(a) (b) (c) (d)

Fig. 1a–d. Ewing's sarcoma in 15-year-old female with typical onion skin periosteal reaction, diaphyseal location, and permeative pattern for Ewing's sarcoma (a). Arteriogram reveals hypervascularity, soft-tissue invasion, abnormal veins, venous invasion compatible with an aggressive bone neoplasm (b, c). Modified subtraction film (d) reveals relation of arteries (white) to veins (black) in a gray background due to tumor stain

IV. Complications

The hazards of arteriography are well-known, and described in the literature. An additional theoretical objection to performing arteriograms of malignant lesions is the possibility of disseminating a localized lesion by the perfusion of a contrast medium in high concentration and pressure. This risk appears very minimal, and the advantages to be gained by performing arteriography are greater than the hazard involved. In addition, all these cases will sooner or later be biopsied, and dissemination by a surgical procedure is much greater than by arteriography.

V. General Roentgenographic Findings

The interpretation of arteriograms is based upon the visualization of the source and type of arterial supply, and the capillary and venous drainage of bone lesions. The evaluation of the course, number, contour, and caliber of the vessels is important in the differential diagnosis of these lesions, as well as evaluation of the dynamic flow in comparison with the normal. An abnormal staining of a lesion is occasionally encountered, consisting of an overall increase in density of the lesion for a prolonged period due to accumulation of contrast material in innumerable thin-walled, tortuous, irregular vascular channels in the case of malignant bone lesions, or prolonged contrast retention in cavity-like vessels in the giant cell tumor or aneurysmal bone cyst.

The morphologic appearance of the vessels is the most important criterion in the differential diagnosis between neoplastic and inflammatory lesions. In inflammatory lesions, the arterial channels remain orderly and taper in a normal fashion as they ramify in the tissues. In contrast, neoplastic lesions reveal pathologic vessels as described below.

1. Hypervascularity and new vessel formation in the area of the lesion is made up of pathologic vessels of variable size and shape (Fig. 2c, d). The pathologic vessels usually reveal small, deformed, tortuous vessels with irregularity in caliber, and alternate areas of narrowing and dilatation along the course of the vessels. The contrast material stays much longer in the pathologic vessels than in normal ones, perhaps because of the lack of elasticity of the vessel walls. At times, accumulation of these abnormal vessels causes a reticular pattern in the tumor area, and the vessels are often spiral in form. Their presence is an important factor in differentiating malignant from benign bone lesions. However, giant cell tumors and aneurysmal bone cysts may also show hypervascularity similar to hypervascular malignant bone lesions.

2. Arteriovenous shunts may be seen within the tumor in bone or in the soft tissues around the lesion (Fig. 3b).

3. Rapid circulation and early visualization of veins surrounding the tumor is due to dilated capillary arteriovenous connections or increased blood flow in the tumor area. This finding, however, has been observed in benign hypervascular bone neoplasms and sometimes inflammatory processes.

4. An abrupt termination to an otherwise normal artery may be seen in the area surrounding a malignant bone tumor. This finding also is a frequent finding in malignant bone lesions, and is due to local thrombosis or infarction in the tumor itself.

5. Avascular areas, usually in the center of the tumor, are related to tumor necrosis, arterial emboli, or hematoma. This information is important when biopsy, particularly needle biopsy, is planned to prevent unsatisfactory biopsy from necrotic areas of the tumors. In several of our cases of malignant hypervascular bone neoplasms, we observed

a nest of small vessels around the periphery of an area of relative avascularity which is presumably the mass of necrotic tumor. This sign has been observed only in cases of malignant bone neoplasms.

6. Soft-tissue extension outside the bone limits is a constant finding in malignant bone neoplasms (Fig. 2c, d). This sign is of greater diagnostic value, since it was not

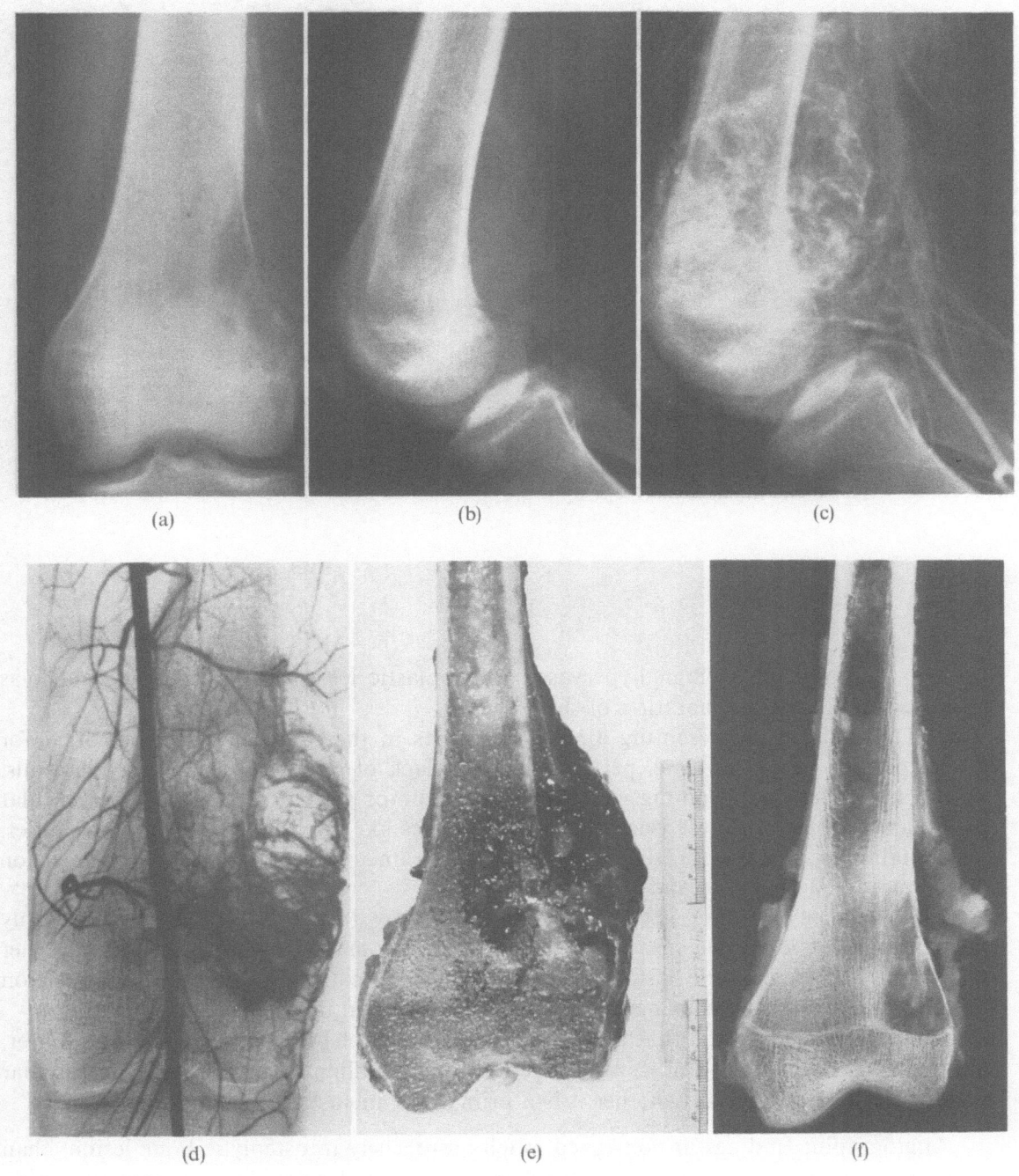

(a)   (b)   (c)

(d)   (e)   (f)

Fig. 2a–g. Osteolytic osteosarcoma in 16-year-old female. Angiogram reveals hypervascular tumor with early opacification of large draining veins. Intraosseous and soft-tissue extensions of tumor are well-demonstrated (c, d). Avascular area in upper part of tumor corresponds to location of hematoma seen on gross specimen (e, f). Histology: Undifferentiated osteosarcoma (g)

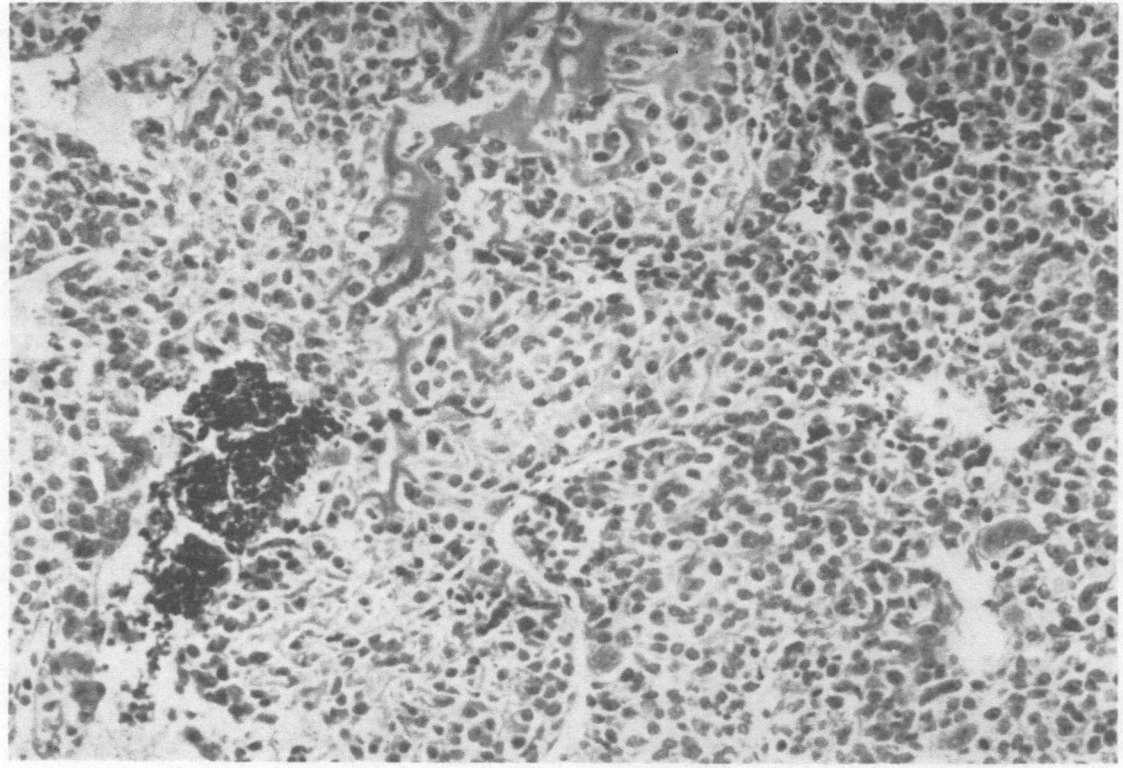

Fig. 2g

present in completely benign hypervascular neoplastic lesions, and when present, was a sign of malignant degeneration of these lesions.

7. Tumor lakes, representing amorphous areas in the tumor, remain opacified for a considerable period of time, perhaps due to a lack of elasticity in the vascular walls.

8. Large abnormal draining veins around the tumor were noted in all hypervascular malignant neoplasms. These veins do not have valves like normal veins of the extremities.

9. Staining was an useful sign in visualizing intramedullary and soft tissue extension of the tumors (Fig. 1b, c) and (Fig. 2c, d).

10. Direct invasion of great veins or arteries by tumor has been observed only in malignant bone neoplasms, especially in fibrosarcomas. However, sometimes other malignant or benign bone lesions, such as exostosis, can cause complete obstruction of veins and arteries by causing a pressure effect, not real invasion.

It must be remembered that all of these signs may not be present in any one tumor, although it is common to find several together in any malignant or benign hypervascular bone growth, regardless of whether it is a primary or metastatic tumor.

Angiographic findings are observed much more easily in osteolytic bone lesions than in osteoblastic ones, because of the considerable density of osteoblastic lesions obscuring the contrast material in blood vessels. However, the tendency for soft tissue invasion in all malignant neoplasms assists in the evaluation of the vascularity of these lesions, since the vascular detail is more readily appreciated in the soft tissues (Fig. 3b, c). Also, subtraction is of great help to visualize vascularity in these cases.

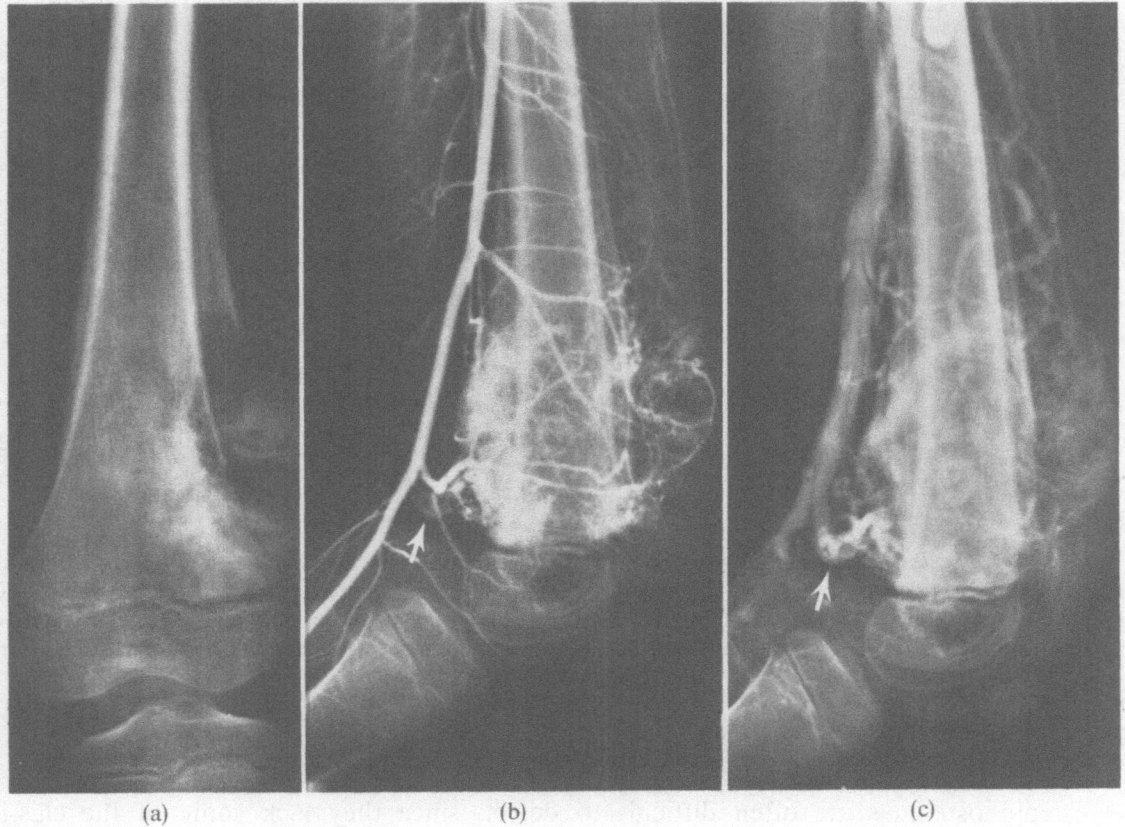

Fig. 3a–c. Mixed (osteolytic-blastic) osteosarcoma in 11-year-old male. This is a hypervascular tumor with rapid filling of veins due to arteriovenous shunting (*arrow*). Reticular angiographic pattern with large abnormal arteries and veins is typical for osteolytic or mixed osteosarcoma. Avascular areas in anterior portion of tumor was result of multiple small areas of tumor necrosis and arterial emboli (b, c)

D. Bone-Forming Tumors

I. Osteoma

These lesions are most frequently seen in the calvarium, especially in the frontal sinus area. Their vascularity is similar to normal bone and the supplying artery probably arises from intraosseous arteries, not soft tissues surrounding the tumor.

II. Osteoid Osteoma

Osteoid osteomas, considered a benign bone-forming neoplasm by most pathologists, are hypervascular, and angiographically characteristic. These lesions have an intense vascular stain only in the nidus area. The supplying artery or arteries of the nidus arise mainly from surrounding soft tissues. Complete opacification of the nidus is best appreciated in the subtraction film. There is usually no clinical indication for performing an arteriogram in such a patient, since the diagnosis is usually readily apparent by the history, physical examination, and routine roentgenograms. However, periarticular

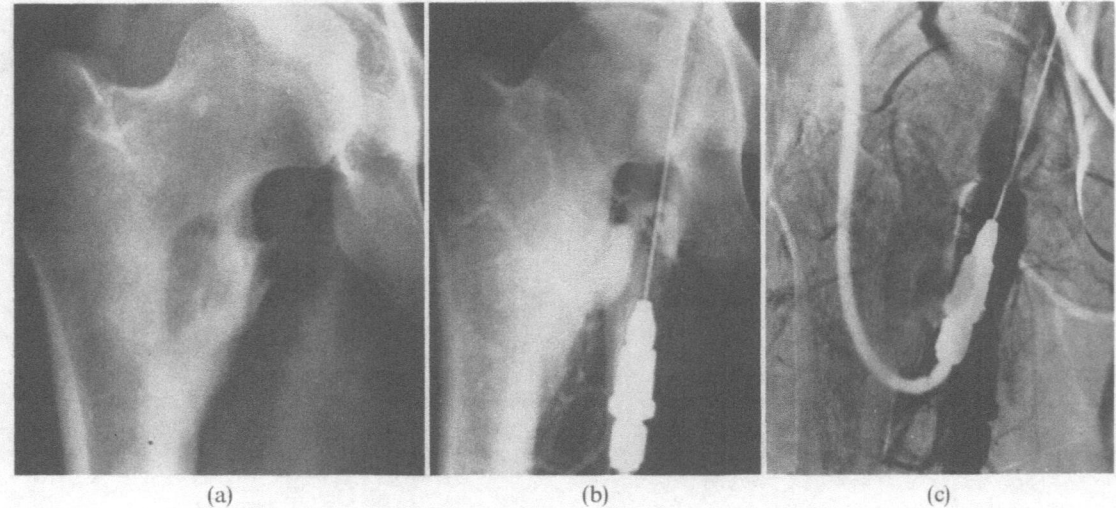

Fig. 4a–c. Osteoid osteoma in 23-year-old male suffering from pain and limping for the last 10 months. Conventional roentgenogram of right hip reveals large radiolucent lesion in lesser trochanter area, with considerable sclerotic reaction, suggestive of Brodie's abscess or atypical type osteoid osteoma (a). Angiography and subtraction films (b, c) reveal definite opacification of radiolucent area (nidus), a characteristic angiographic manifestation of osteoid osteoma

osteoid osteomas are often difficult to detect, since they lack some of the classical clinical and roentgenographic features seen in other locations. Such lesions may present little bone sclerosis, and the nidus may remain roentgenographically undetected. An arteriogram in this specific instance would prove its usefulness (Fig. 4a–c).

III. Benign Osteoblastoma

There is some variation in the angiographic manifestations of these lesions. However, there is usually moderate vascularity within the tumor, with feeding vessels arising from soft tissues adjacent to the lesion, but in contradistinction to osteosarcomas, there was no evidence of large abnormal veins, invasion of vessels, obstruction of veins, or a soft tissue mass around the lesion. Angiography can easily differentiate between benign osteoblastoma and osteosarcoma, regardless of their histopathologic similarity (Fig. 5c, d).

IV. Osteosarcoma

The difficulty in the interpretation of an osteosarcoma results from the great variability which exists in the histopathology and plain roentgenographic findings of these lesions. According to the majority of pathologists, the essential criteria for the diagnosis of an osteosarcoma are: (1) The presence of sarcomatous stroma, and (2) the direct formation of osteoid and bone within the tumor. Malignant counterparts of the following cell types have been seen in different cases of osteosarcomas, or in different sections of an osteosarcoma, namely, osteoblast, fibroblast, and occasionally giant cell, synovial cell, and undifferentiated mesenchymal cell.

In any one tumor, the predominant malignant cell type will usually determine the

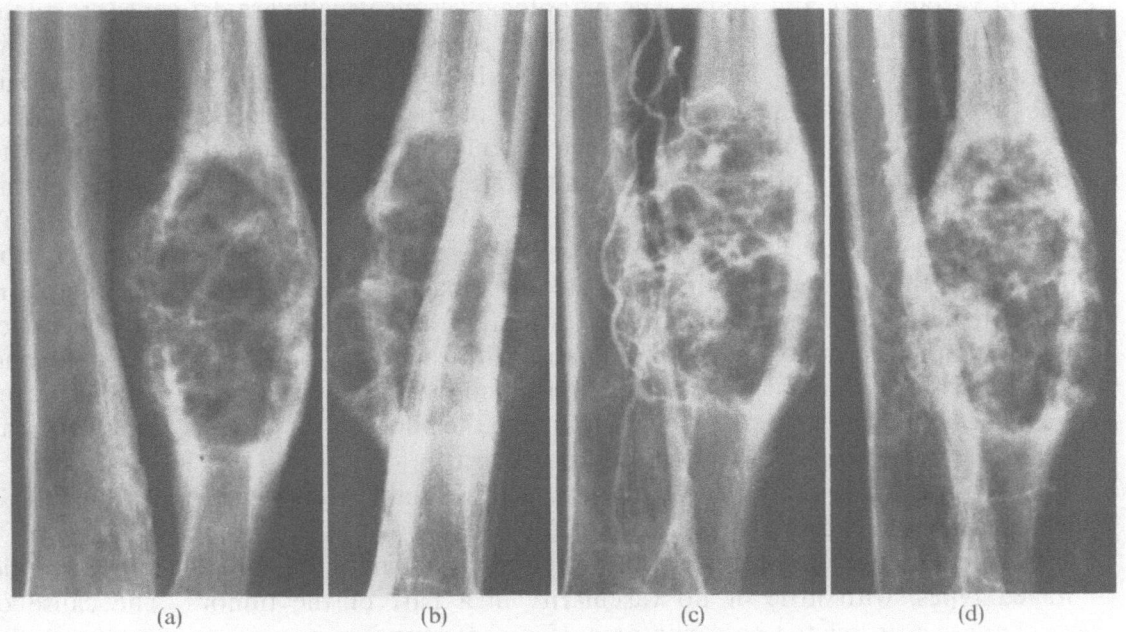

Fig. 5a–d. Benign osteoblastoma in 31-year-old male with history of trauma to right forearm 3 years ago and mild pain following trauma. There was evidence of gradual swelling over the last 1 year. Plain roentgenogram reveals a well-marginated mass with honeycombing and expansion of bone, suggestive of relatively slow growing bone neoplasm (a, b). Biopsy of lesion was reported as osteosarcoma. Angiography revealed only a few supplying arteries in tumor area with no evidence of soft tissue component (c, d). Repeat biopsy and later en bloc resection of distal radius proved the presence of a benign osteoblastoma

pathologic diagnosis. If osteoblasts are present, however, the lesion is always called an osteosarcoma because this is the most malignant and most vascular part, and clinically the tumor will act like an osteosarcoma. Based on these facts, these tumors fall into three different groups: (1) osteoblastic, (2) chondroblastic, and (3) fibroblastic, depending on the predominant histologic pattern. Histopathologic studies of the blood vessels of malignant bone neoplasms by LAGERGREN et al. (1961 b) revealed that osteoblastic tissues are the most vascular part of an osteosarcoma. Osteoblastic osteosarcomas, regardless of their plain roentgenographic findings (sclerotic, osteolytic, or mixed), are highly vascular. Chondroblastic osteosarcomas show much less vascularity, which is felt to be due to the peculiarity of osmotic intercellular nutrition of chondroid tissue. In cases of chondroblastic or fibroblastic osteosarcoma, the vascularity of these lesions is dependent on what percentage of tumor has been occupied by chondroid or fibroid tissue, and the degree of vascularity of these tumors also depends upon the degree of cell differentiation.

Angiographic manifestations: The arterial blood supply to the tumor was always derived from the arteries of the surrounding soft tissues rather than from the diaphyseal nutrient artery. This may be partly due to the fact that the majority of the tumors was in advanced stages, and extended beyond the normal bone limits. The caliber of supplying arteries was usually large, but they were never invaded by the tumor. Displacement of the artery was seen in the majority of these cases due to the mass effect. The second and third order branches commonly showed evidence of encroachment, direct invasion, or complete obstruction.

Neovascularity and hypervascularity were present in all instances, with pathologic vessels of variable size and shape. The pathologic vessels usually are deformed, tortuous vessels with irregularity of caliber, and alternate areas of narrowing and dilatation along the course of the vessels. The contrast material stays much longer in the pathologic vessels than in normal ones, perhaps because of the lack of elasticity of the vessel walls. Despite this prolonged stain, early venous drainage occurred in the majority of our cases, and was primarily the result of rapid circulation through parts of the tumor. Frank arteriovenous shunting was present in a few of our cases (Fig. 3b, c).

A tumor stain was related to the degree of vascularity of the osteosarcoma. It was evident from the angiograms that all osteosarcomas were well-demarcated and more vascular than the surrounding soft tissues. Several of the tumors were markedly heterogeneous in their vascularity and tumor stain, with some regions containing a myriad of wide vessels in an irregular reticular pattern, and in other areas, sparser, and narrower vessels. The highly vascular areas corresponded to the poorly differentiated zones, whereas in well-differentiated areas, there was less vascularity.

In our series of sclerotic osteosarcomas, we were able to see moderate to marked hypervascularity in each case.

Nonuniform angioarchitecture within the tumor was noted in some of our osteolytic or mixed types, with little or no vascularity in a part of the tumors. The cause of these changes was related to hematoma (Fig. 2d), tumor necrosis, fracture, and the presence of chondroblastic and well-differentiated fibroblastic tissues in an osteosarcoma (Fig. 6c, d).

The pathologic vessels and staining were best seen on subtraction films, particularly in sclerotic osteosarcomas (Fig. 7c). The draining veins were usually dilated. They showed evidence for displacement, direct invasion of the wall, or intraluminal extension of the tumor. These findings were responsible for obstruction of major veins in most of the cases. The presence of venous lakes was a distinct finding in the majority of osteolytic and mixed osteosarcomas (Figs. 2, 3). They were not detectable in osteoblastic tumors of this series.

The osteosarcoma had extended well beyond the confines of the host bone to involve adjacent soft tissues in all of our cases. The tumor stain was a highly reliable criterion for determining the extraosseous and intraosseous extent of the tumor.

The variability of osteosarcomas creates a spectrum of angioarchitecture, although a careful correlation of histology and angiography proved that all osteosarcomas were more vascular than surrounding soft tissues. Regardless of their plain roentgenographic appearance, 95% of our cases were classified as highly vascular tumors. Angiographic findings were observed much more easily in cases of osteolytic osteosarcoma than sclerotic ones, because the density of the sclerotic bone obscured the angioarchitecture in the latter group.

For this reason, most authors believe that sclerotic osteosarcomas are less vascular than osteolytic or mixed tumors, although our experience with subtraction films showed that sclerotic osteosarcomas are also hypervascular. In cases of sclerotic osteosarcoma with a sunburst periosteal reaction, the arteries arising from soft tissue surround the periphery of the tumor, and give rise to numerous large and small arterial branches which radiate toward the center of the tumor. The veins follow a similar course, draining from the center of the lesion toward its periphery. These vessels occupy the radiolucent space within the sunburst periosteal reaction. In other words, the sunburst periosteal reaction is seen around the arteries and veins supplying the sclerotic osteosarcoma (Fig. 7b, c). In osteolytic and mixed osteosarcomas, the vascular network of the tumor is more easily seen on the arteriogram, and because of superimposition of arteries, gives a reticular pattern to the lesion (Figs. 2, 3).

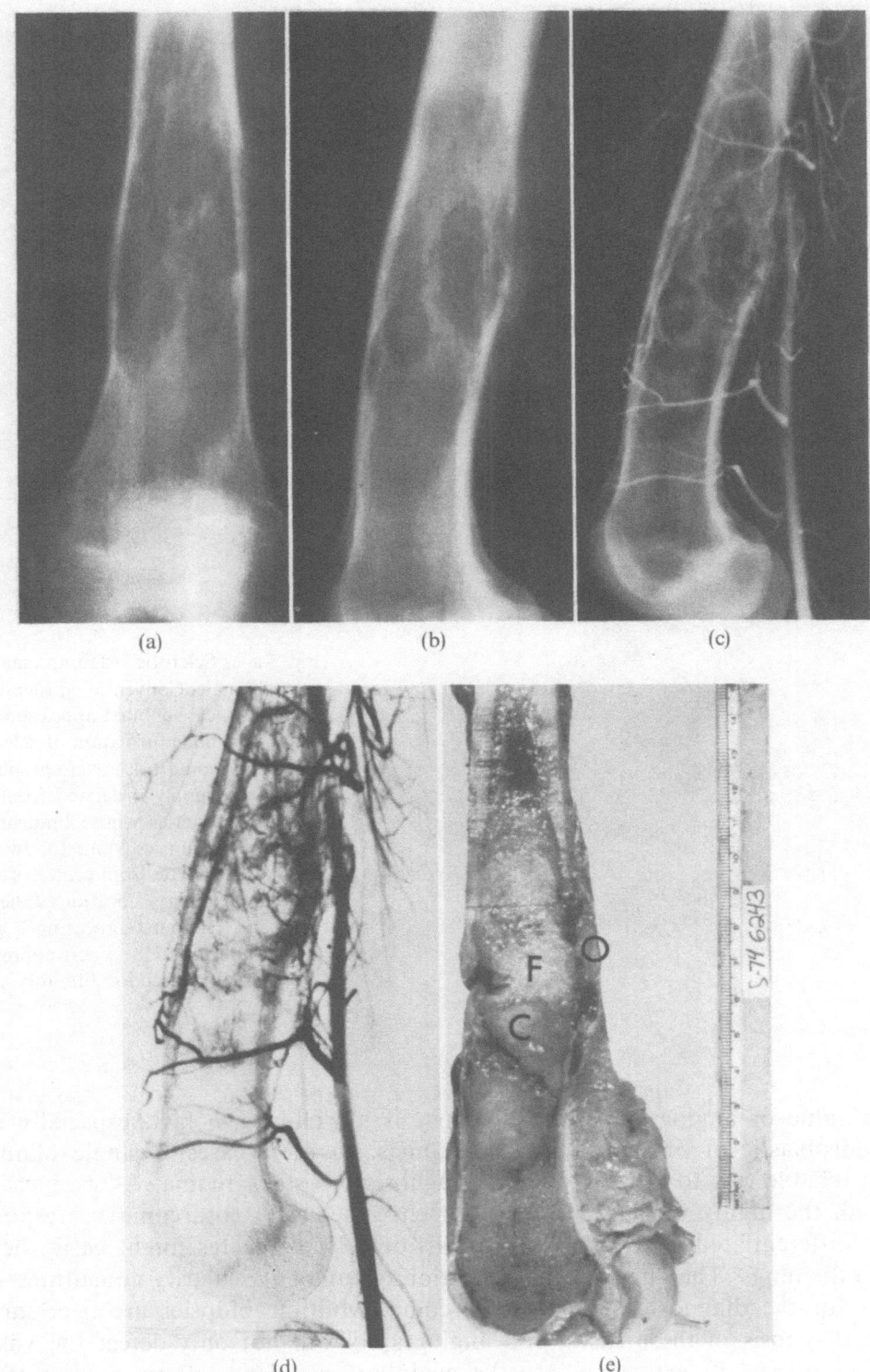

Fig. 6a–e. Fibroblastic-chondroblastic osteosarcoma. AP and lateral conventional roentgenogram reveals radio-lucent bone lesion involving medullary channel. Surprisingly, a tumor of this size reveals no great soft-tissue component (a, b). Arteriography reveals only a limited area of hypervascularity (c, d). Pathologically the tumor was polymorphic sarcoma containing minimal osteoid (*O*), and mainly chondroid (*C*) and fibroid (*F*) elements (e). The most vascular zone of tumor corresponds to osteoid tissue and least vascular to chondroid matrix

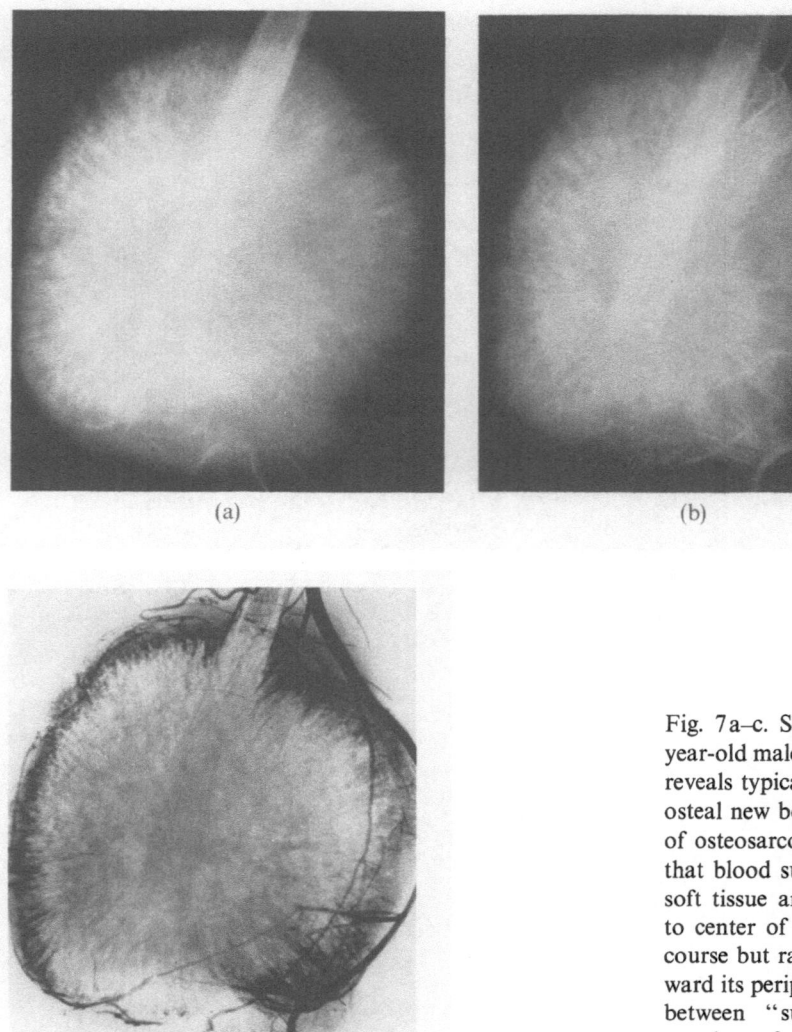

Fig. 7a–c. Sclerotic osteosarcoma in a 17-year-old male. Conventional roentgenogram reveals typical sunburst appearance of periosteal new bone formation of sclerotic type of osteosarcoma (a). Arteriography reveals that blood supply is derived from adjacent soft tissue arteries whose branches radiate to center of tumor. Veins follow a similar course but radiate from center of lesion toward its periphery. Location of these vessels between "sunburst-appearing" periosteal new bone formation is best appreciated on subtraction film (c)

The value of angiography before biopsy is a well-known fact, especially in cases of chondroblastic or fibroblastic osteosarcomas. In these cases, a single blind biopsy is not a reliable way to reach a definite diagnosis of osteosarcoma. As we have already discussed, the highly vascular part of a heterogeneous osteosarcoma corresponded to the less differentiated areas from which cells or cell aggregates might easily be carried away to the lungs. The angiographic detection of tumor vascularity constitutes valuable support for the diagnosis of an osteosarcoma. Multiple biopsies are necessary for a definite diagnosis in these cases, and angiography will not only detect the vascularity of the tumor and its extension into the medullary canal or soft tissue, but afford the opportunity to choose the best sites for biopsy.

Several benign bone lesions such as benign osteoblastoma, osteoid osteoma, callous formation, myositis ossificans circumscripta, osteomyelitis, and pseudotumors of hemophilia may occasionally have a similar pathologic and plain roentgenographic appearance to that of an osteosarcoma. In these instances, angiography is of great help in the differential diagnosis and should be used to prevent unnecessary mutilating operations.

V. Parosteal Osteosarcoma (Juxtacortical Osteosarcoma)

This highly differentiated tumor usually does not have any highly malignant or vascular component, resulting in a considerably more benign nature as compared to the ordinary osteosarcoma. The vascularity of these tumors, which is dependent upon the degree of their cell differentiation, is low to moderate, and supplying arteries arise from surrounding soft tissues (Fig. 8). JAFFE (1958) distinguishes two types of parosteal osteosarcoma, one of which has a more malignant course. Both revealed a low degree of vascularity within the tumor, and none of the angiographic findings of other osteosarcomas are usually seen. When angiography reveals a highly vascular region in such a tumor, it is probably of a more malignant type. This technique may be of value in the differentiation of types of parosteal osteosarcoma, and in making a prediction regarding their general prognosis (see chapter on parosteal osteosarcoma).

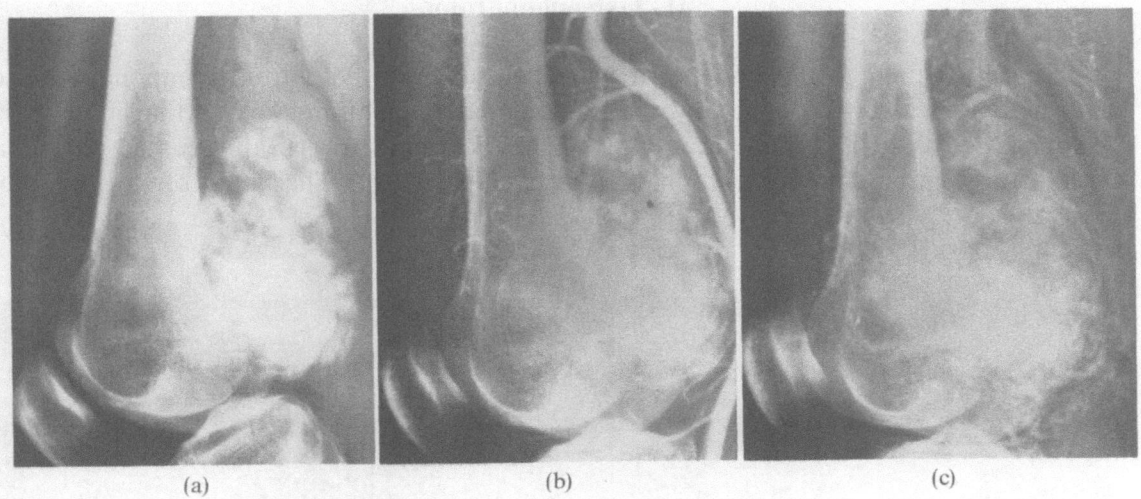

(a)   (b)   (c)

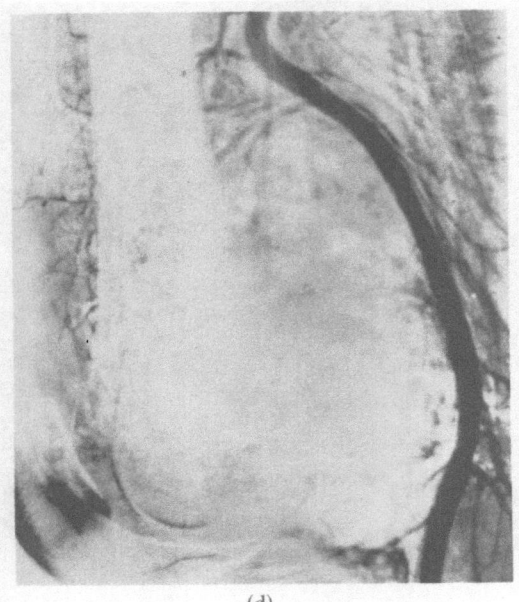

(d)

Fig. 8 a–d. Parosteal osteosarcoma in 38-year-old male with a history of tumefaction and pain for the last 10 years. Angiographic findings reveal relatively minimal vascularity in tumor area with no staining. These findings are best appreciated on subtraction film (d)

E. Cartilage-Forming Tumors

Cartilage tissue is avascular, and nutrition is via intercellular (osmotic) nutrition. The majority of benign and malignant cartilagenous tumors, except for the poorly differentiated chondrosarcoma or mesenchymal type of chondrosarcoma, are avascular. Avascularity or hypovascularity of some of the malignant cartilagenous tumors is the best explanation for their relatively better survival rate and prognosis.

I. Chondroma

The intramedullary and cortical types of chondromas are avascular tumors.

II. Osteochondroma

This is a benign bone lesion with mixed osteoid and chondroid components. The osseous part is always supplied by the intraosseous circulation. The cartilagenous part is sometimes avascular, but occasionally a few normal arteries are seen in the area without any pathologic angiographic findings (Figs. 9, 10). The value of angiography

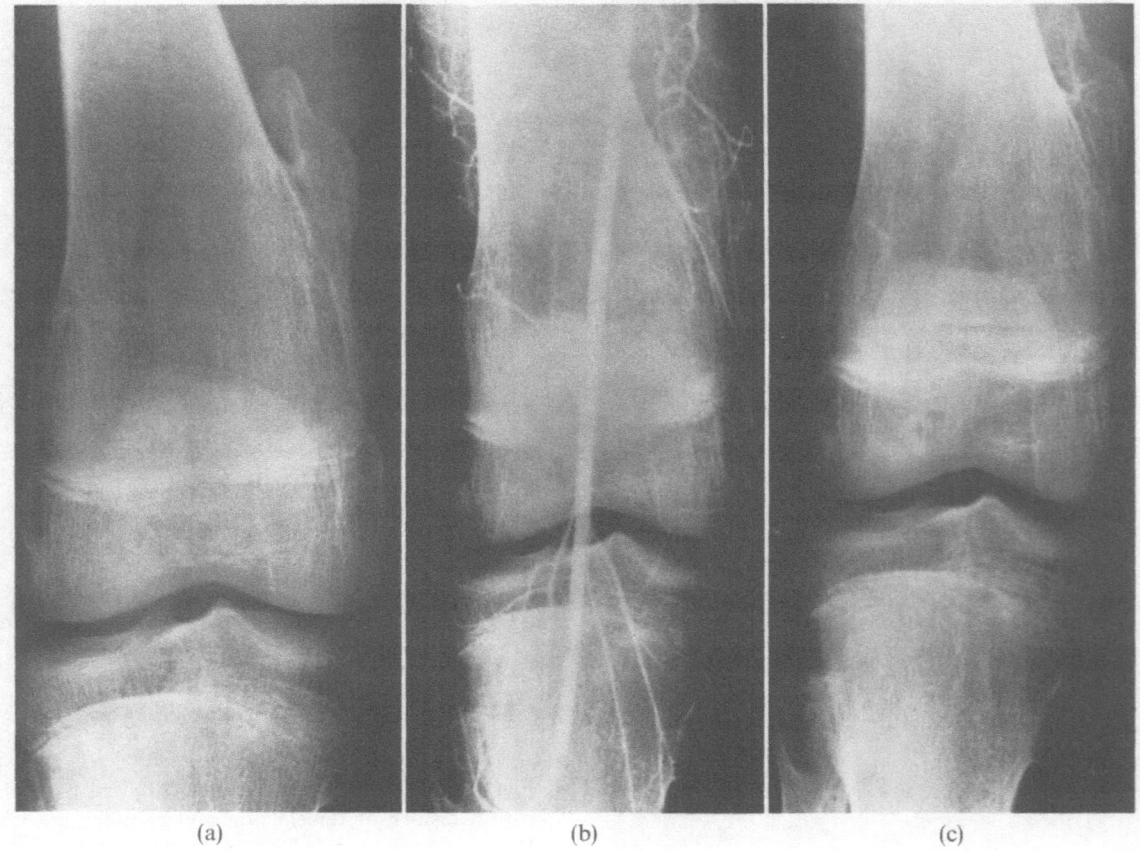

(a)   (b)   (c)

Fig. 9a–c. Osteochondroma (exostosis) involving distal femur with normal arteriogram (b, c)

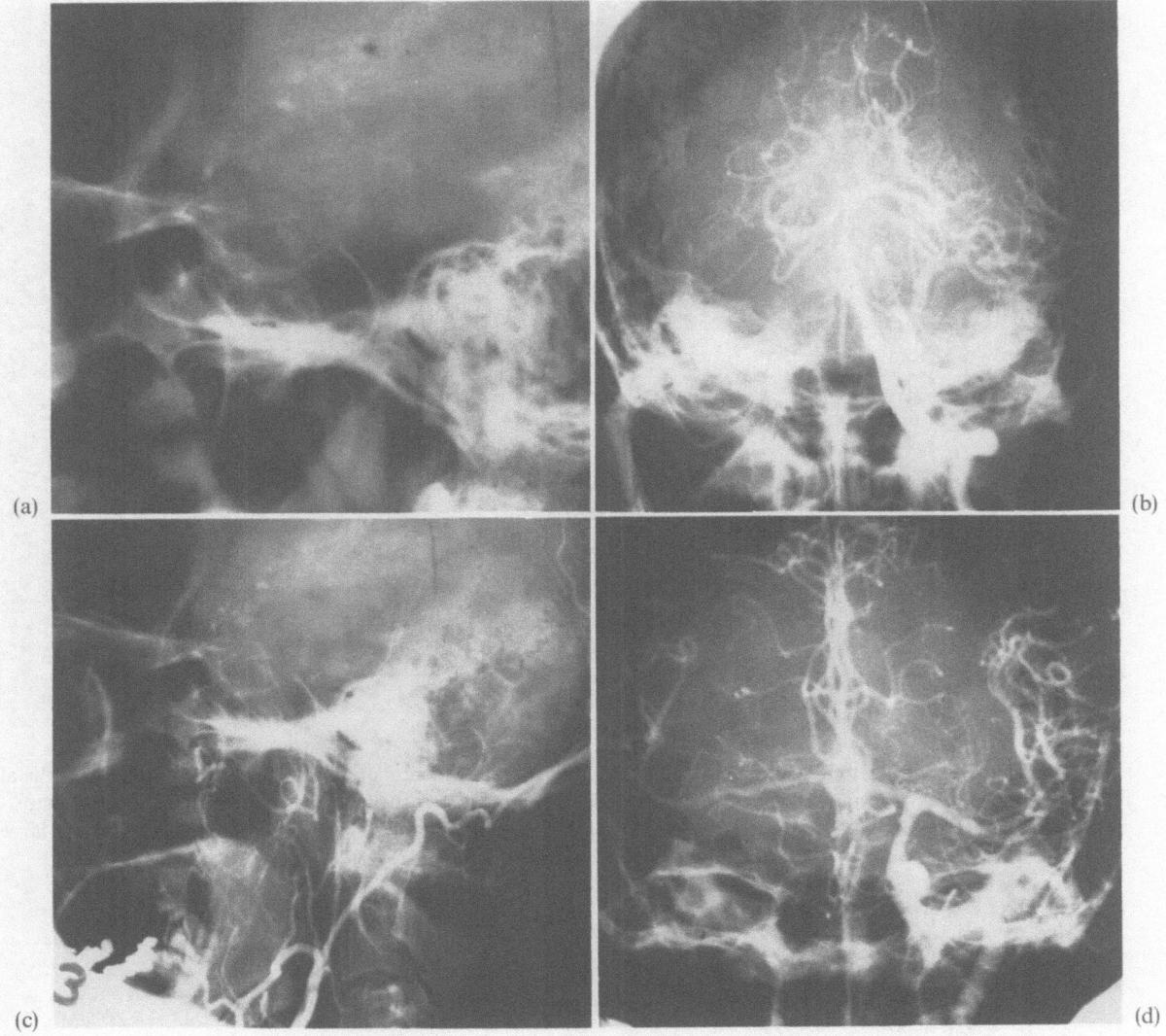

Fig. 10a–d. Osteochondroma involving sphenoid bone. Vertebral (b), internal (c), and external (d) carotid arteriograms reveal normal arteriograms

in the diagnosis of osteochondroma is limited. However, there is an indication for angiography in the evaluation of suspected malignant degeneration of osteochondroma to chondrosarcoma, especially in cases with rapid growth. There is no doubt that pathologists have difficulty in distinguishing between an osteochondroma and well-differentiated chondrosarcoma, especially in the axial skeleton where osteochondromas are more prone to undergo malignant degeneration. Angiography will enable us to assess the degree of vascularity, and possibly predict the aggressiveness of the lesion. Angiography is also applicable in the evaluation of large osteochondromas, especially in the shoulder or knee area, to rule out pressure or obstruction on adjacent arteries and veins, and to investigate the possibility of aneurysmal dilatation or hematoma in the tumor region (Fig. 11c, d).

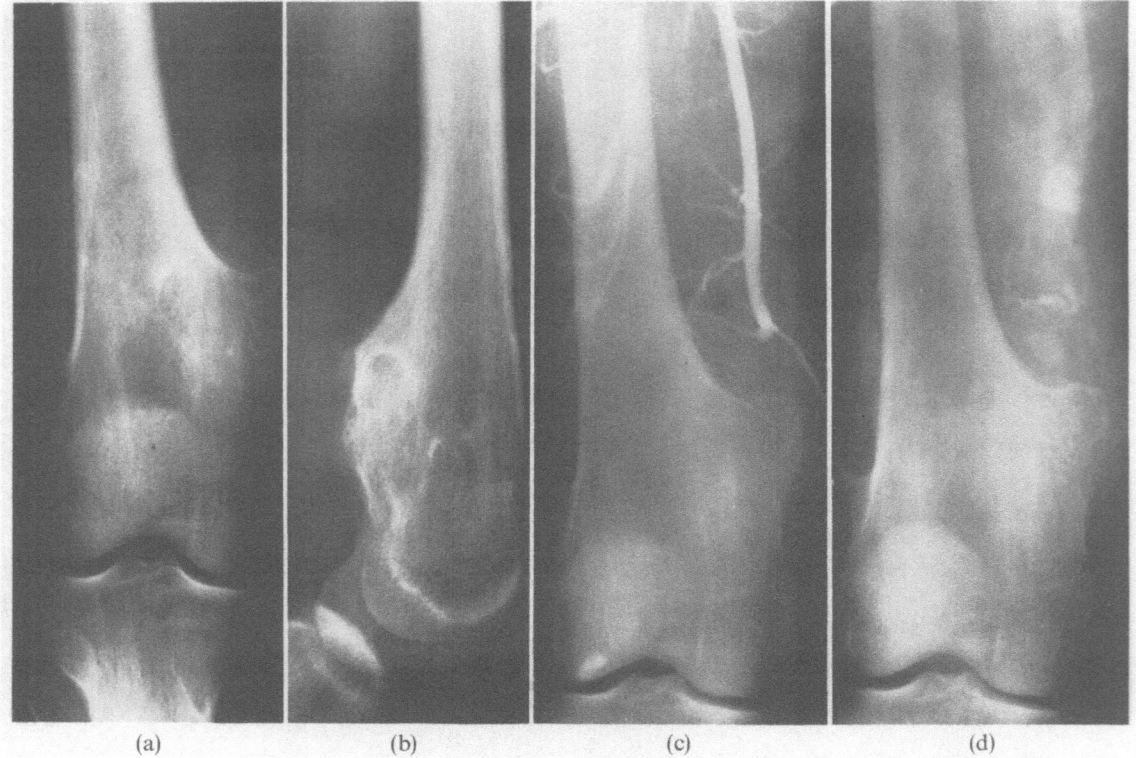

    (a)   (b)   (c)   (d)

Fig. 11a–d. AP and lateral views of left knee (a, b) reveal evidence of multiple exostoses involving distal femur, proximal tibia, and fibula. There was evidence of a large soft-tissue mass adjacent to large exostosis involving distal femur. Arteriogram reveals complete obstruction of superficial femoral artery by a large cartilaginous cup and hematoma in this region (b, c)

III. Chondromyxoid Fibroma

Like chondromas, these are avascular tumors. In cases of large chondromyxoid fibromas, with a more aggressive plain roentgenographic appearance, angiography may be of help in the differential diagnosis (Fig. 12b, c).

IV. Benign Chondroblastoma

These lesions are the most vascular of the benign cartilagenous tumors. The arterial supply arises from the surrounding bone. There is no evidence of pathologic vessels, involvement of veins, or soft tissue extension. A very light tumor stain is hardly recognizable on regular angiographic films, but can be seen on subtraction films. This is the main angiographic finding in these lesions (Figs. 13, 14).

V. Chondrosarcoma

A great spectrum of vascularity exists in chondrosarcomatous tissue, but the majority of them are either avascular or reveal a low degree of vascularity in comparison with

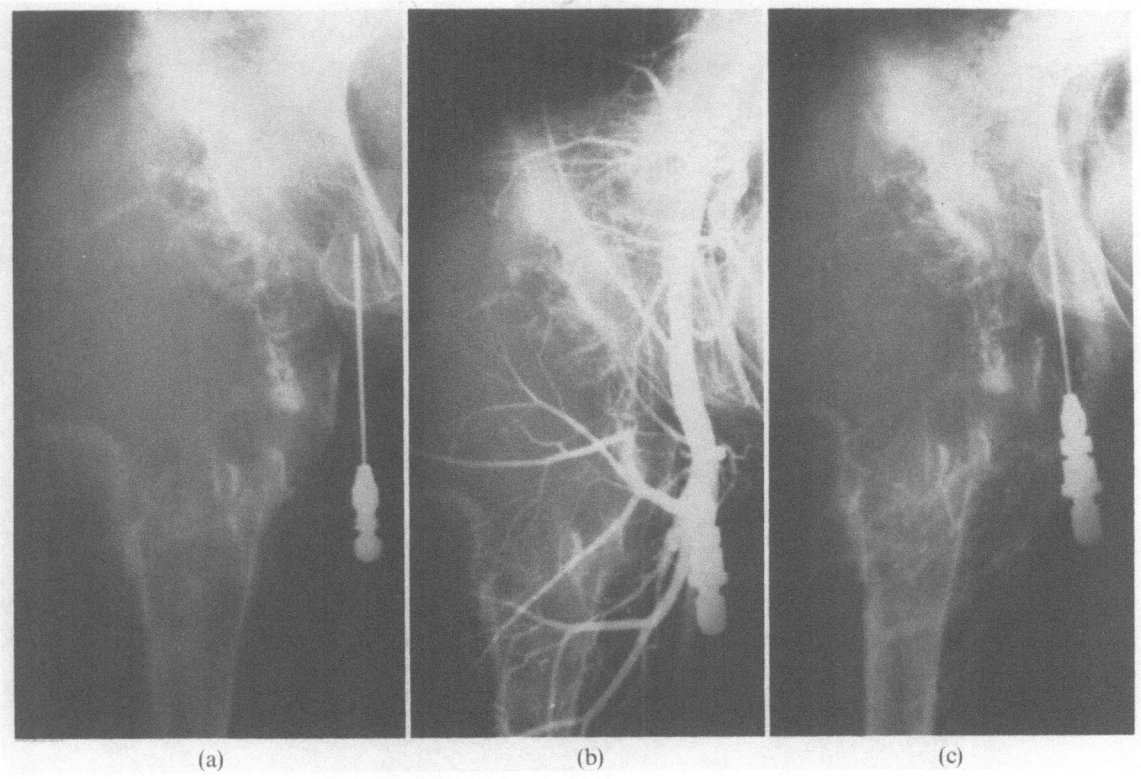

(a)   (b)   (c)

Fig. 12a–c. Chondromyxoid fibroma in an 18-year-old male suffering from mild pain and soft-tissue swelling over right upper femur for last 2 years. Conventional roentgenogram reveals apparent bone tumor with destruction in upper end of femur (a). Arteriography showed no neovascularity or stain in tumor area (b, c)

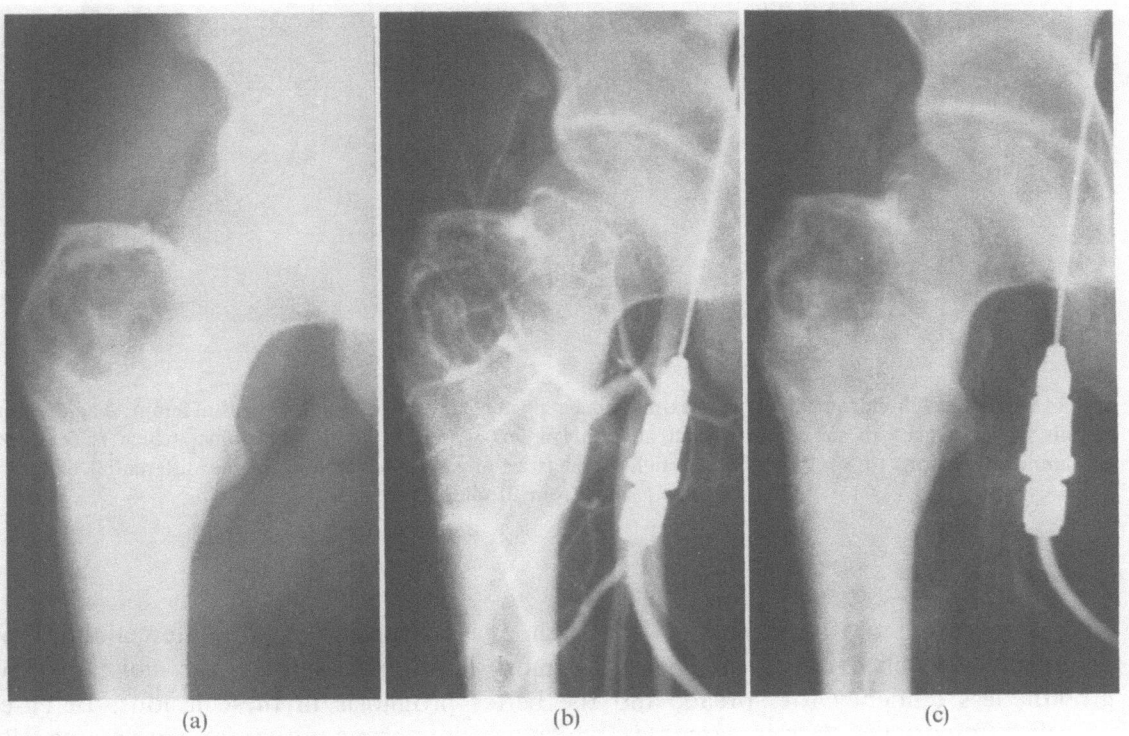

(a)   (b)   (c)

Fig. 13a–c. Benign chondroblastoma in 35-year-old male. Conventional roentgenography reveals a well-circumscribed, radiolucent lesion in greater trochanter area of right femur (a). Arterial and capillary phases demonstrate only a few arteries in tumor area with very light stain (b, c)

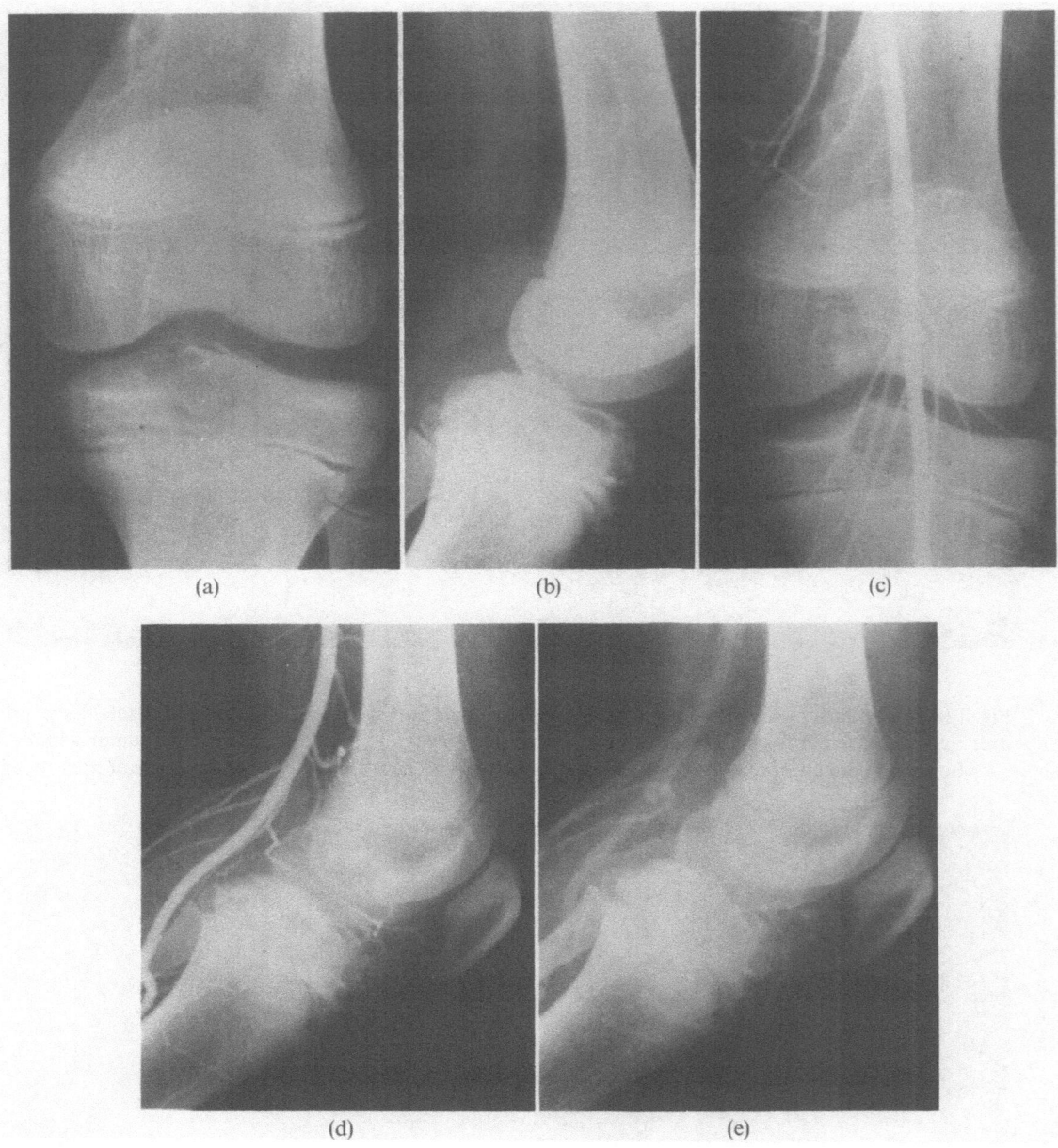

Fig. 14a–e. Benign chondroblastoma in proximal tibia and subcortical defect involving distal femur. Angiography reveals no vascularity in subcortical defect and only a few vessels in chondroblastoma, which is best seen on lateral projections (d, e). Presence of a light stain is an angiographic finding in the differential diagnosis of these lesions from Brodie's abscess

an osteosarcoma or fibrosarcoma. The main reason for this is the intercellular type of nutrition which exists in this type of tumor. This same factor is the cause of slow growth, less tendency for spread, and the better prognosis in these lesions. In cases of well-differentiated chondrosarcomas, which are slow growing tumors, patients usually are free of metastasis for many years, probably a result of avascularity or a low degree of vascularity in these lesions. The degree of vascularity of a chondrosarcoma, regardless of their location, is related to the differentiation of the cells (Figs. 15, 16). The poorly

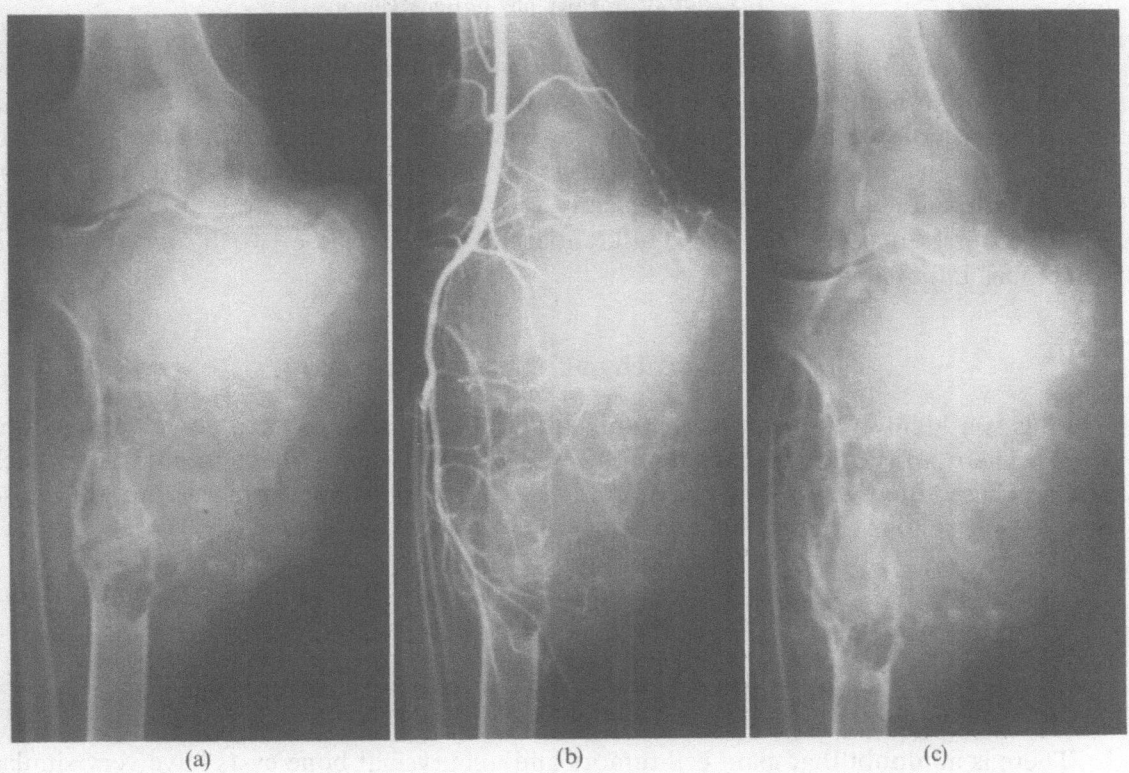

(a)   (b)   (c)

Fig. 15a–c. Chondrosarcoma (well-differentiated). Plain roentgenogram (a) reveals large osseous lesion involving proximal end of tibia with numerous calcifications in 65-year-old woman with a 15-year history of pain and slow growing mass in the same area. Arteriogram (b, c) reveals only a few supplying arteries in mass area without real evidence of staining. Pathology of this case was well-differentiated chondrosarcoma. These findings are seen in all well-differentiated chondrosarcomas. There is a close relation between differentiation of cells and number of vessels and malignant potentiality of chondrosarcoma

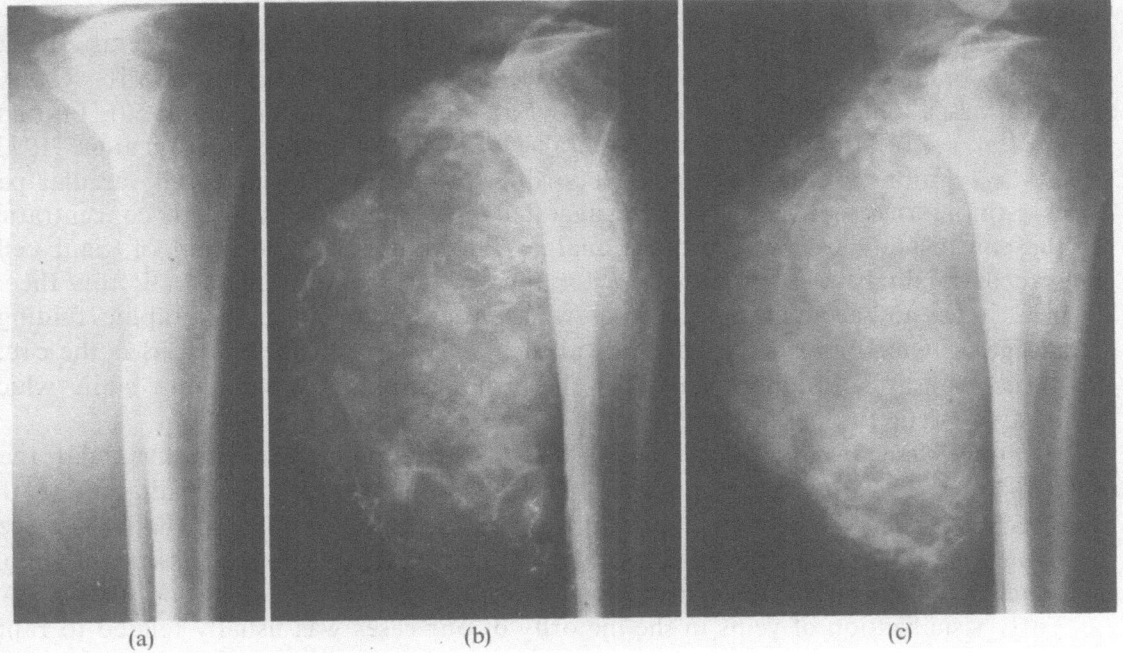

(a)   (b)   (c)

Fig. 16a–c. Periosteal chondrosarcoma in 22-year-old male suffering from pain and soft-tissue mass involving right leg for the last few months. Arteriogram reveals moderately vascular mass involving posterior aspect of right fibula and was diagnosed as chondrosarcoma arising from periosteum (b, c). Patient developed pulmonary metastasis after 8 months

differentiated tumor is the most vascular type of chondrosarcoma and carries the worst prognosis. The main difficulty in the interpretation of angiograms in these lesions is in distinguishing chondrosarcomas with normal or a low degree of vascularity from benign bone neoplasms. There is no difficulty in the angiographic diagnosis of the poorly differentiated type, which is usually very agressive in nature and have a similar clinical course to osteosarcomas. Differentiation between these two by angiography is sometimes impossible.

VI. Mesenchymal Chondrosarcoma

This is a highly vascular tumor, similar to grade III or IV fibrosarcoma or osteosarcoma. There are no unique angiographic signs to distinguish these tumors from each other. These tumors not only have similar angiographic appearances, but they also have a very similar clinical behavior and prognosis.

F. Giant Cell Tumor and Aneurysmal Bone Cyst

There is no doubt that giant cell tumors and aneurysmal bone cysts have very similar angiographic features, just as they also have very similar histopathologic and plain roentgenographic findings. Pathologists in some institutions now believe that the aneurysmal bone cyst is a variety of giant cell tumor. In our experience with angiography, we have had considerable difficulty in distinguishing these lesions from each other. At one time we tried to separate these lesions, but we had such confusing pathologic correlation that we now recognize that these lesions also have very similar and indistinguishable angiographic manifestations.

The angiographic features of these lesions have been described by several authors, including FARINAS (1937), DOS SANTOS (1950), SCHOBINGER and STOLL (1951), CALDAS (1951), LASSER and SCHOBINGER VON SCHOWINGEN (1955), STRICKLAND (1950), LINDBOM et al. (1961), ZUCCHI (1963), YAGHMAI et al. (1971), and BILLINGS and WERNER (1972). These descriptions are quite variable, reporting from normal to increased vascular patterns. SCHOBINGER and STOLL (1951) suggested that, since the degree of concentration of the contrast material was proportional to the number and location of giant cells, these cells might be the specific cause for these arteriographic findings. If this theory is true, it cannot account for the very wide variation in the arteriographic findings. The large distended and distorted thin-walled blood spaces in these lesions is the cause for the angiographic findings, especially the prolonged and uneven tumor stain, which is a characteristic finding in these lesions.

Arteriographic Manifestations. Over 90% of these lesions are more vascular than normal bone. The arteries are numerous, arising from the soft tissue adjacent to the involved bone. The vessels are smaller in caliber and shorter in length than those seen in malignant hypervascular neoplasms (Fig. 17b, c). Nevertheless, the vessels are abnormal and have the appearance of pathologic vessels.

Early visualization of veins in the majority of our cases was usually related to rapid capillary circulation, but in some there was evidence of arteriovenous shunting. Abnormal veins were primarily seen adjacent to the lesion, and only rarely in the mass of tumor (Fig. 18b, c). They were greater in number but smaller in size than those seen in malignant hypervascular neoplasms.

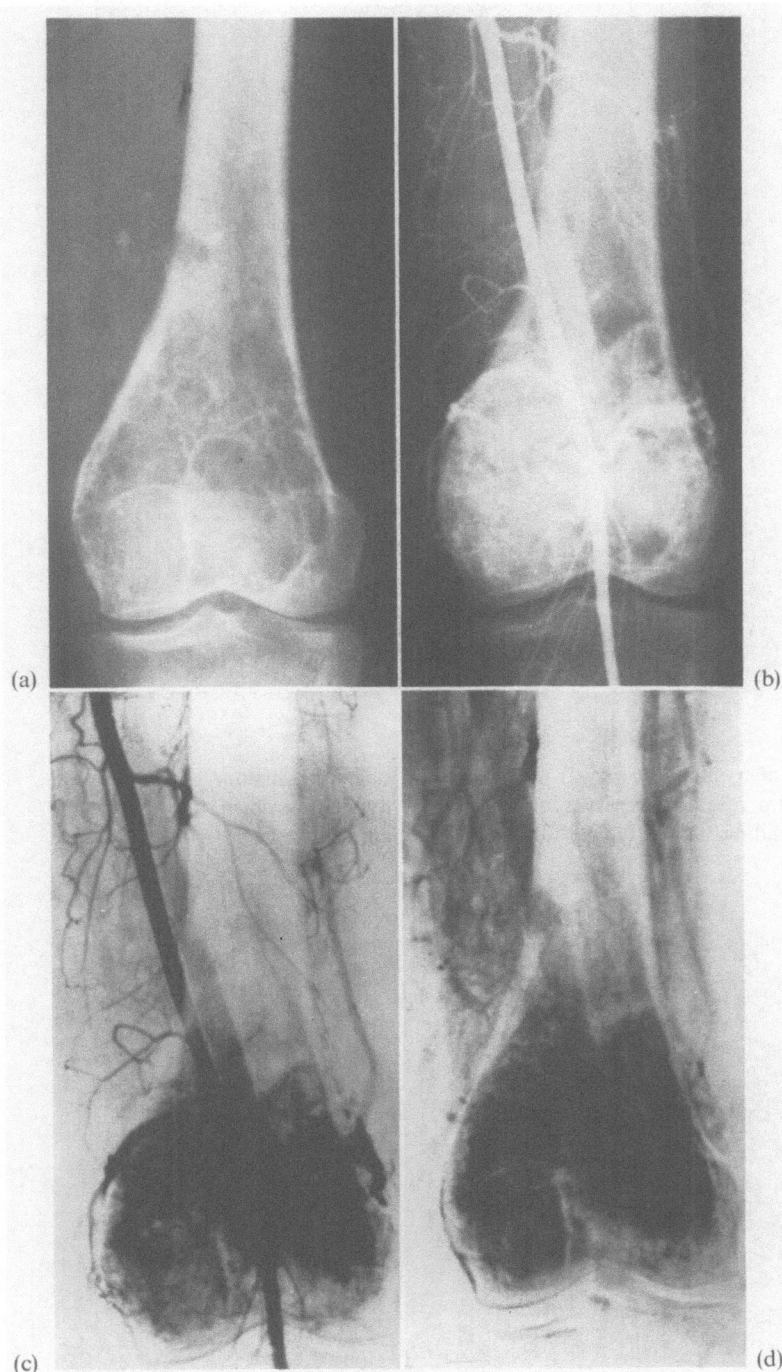

(a)

(b)

(c)

(d)

Fig. 17a–d. Giant cell tumor in 45-year-old female reveals typical roentgenographic pattern of giant cell tumor (a). Arteriogram (b, c) reveals highly vascular lesion with presence of A–V shunting due to rapid circulation through lesion. There was no evidence of soft-tissue invasion. Late venous phase (45 sec after injection) still reveals opacification of lesion, as a result of pooling of opaque material in cavitylike vessels in lesion area (d)

There was no involvement of normal arteries or veins close to the lesions, which usually is a frequent finding in hypervascular malignant bone lesions. In the majority of our cases, there was only displacement of these vessels.

A moderate, uneven, prolonged tumor stain limited to the bone lesion, and rarely extending to the soft tissue, is the result of accumulation of contrast material in the distended thin-walled blood spaces, resembling numerous cavities of different sizes. These cavities may contain contrast material for more than 60 sec after injection and are best

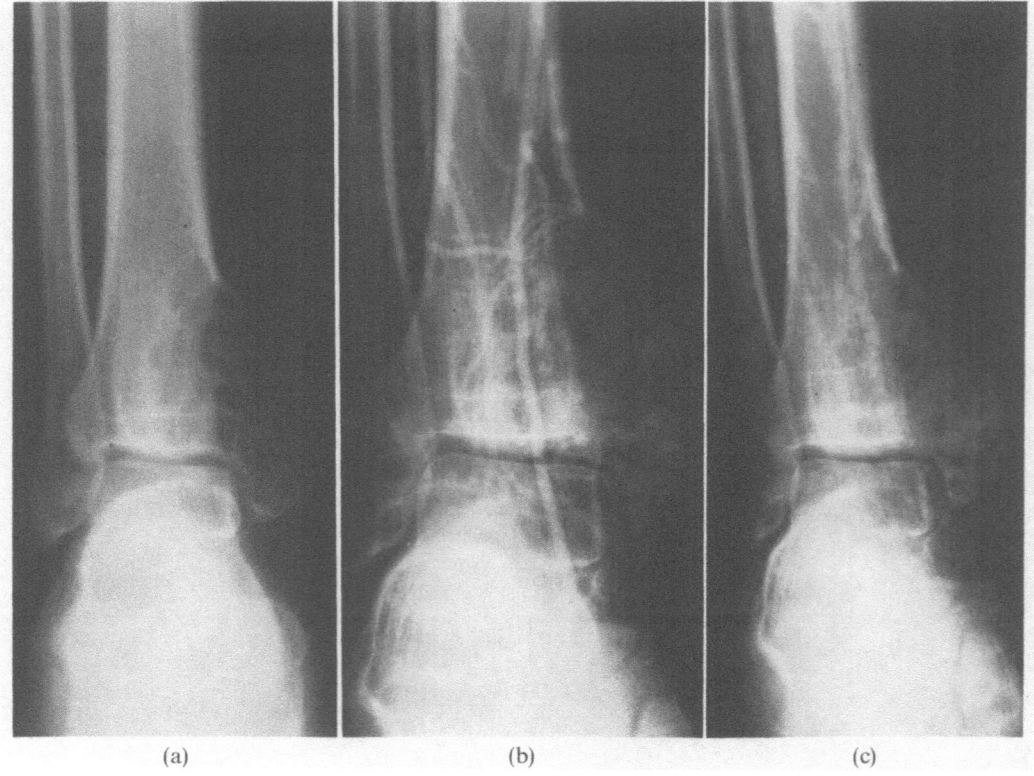

Fig. 18a–c. Cystic giant cell tumor (aneurysmal bone cyst) in 20-year-old male with history of trauma and pain involving right ankle. Arteriogram revealed hypervascularity and cavitylike vessels in tumor area (b, c). Uneven long-standing stain is typical for cystic-type giant cell tumor

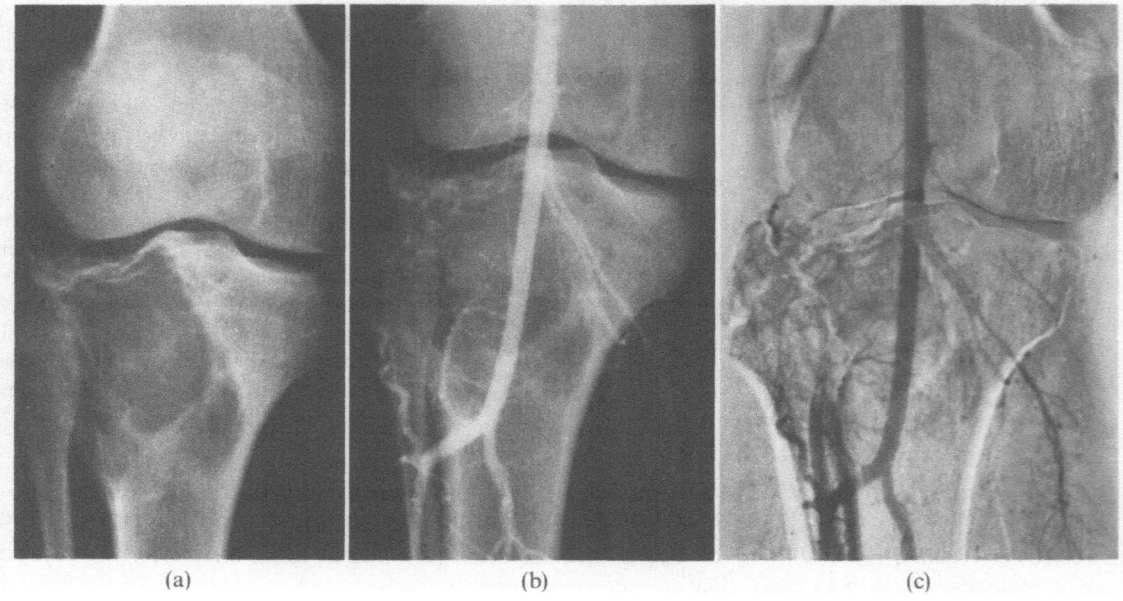

Fig. 19a–c. Giant cell tumor in 29-year-old female with pathologic fracture (a). Arteriogram reveals only a few vessels in lesion area with very light stain (b, c). The same lesion a few weeks before fracture was highly vascular and loss of vascularity is result of recent trauma

seen in subtraction films. Dos Santos (1934) reported that in cases of osteoclastomas (giant cell tumors), these cavities were opacified one or more months after the injection of thorotrast, probably the result of the selective fixation of thorotrast in the reticuloendothelial cells which may play a part in the genesis of giant cell tumors. This appearance was not observed in malignant bone neoplasms in his series. Finally, the most important finding in these lesions is the absence of soft-tissue invasion, which is a consistent finding in malignant hypervascular bone neoplasms. Although occasionally soft-tissue involvement may result from previous injury, this finding should strongly suggest malignant degeneration.

The findings described above have been noted to variable degrees in giant cell tumors and aneurysmal bone cysts. However, a few cases of giant cell tumors have been reported with normal arteriograms, and in these instances it is hard to reach a conclusive diagnosis. In our experience and review of literature, some giant cell tumors with minimal hypervascularity or normal vascularity were the result of postradiation effect, or an old fracture at the site of the tumor. Perhaps stress plays a role in causing some spontaneous healing of these lesions, with resulting avascularity (Fig. 19).

Angiography is of particular assistance in the differential diagnosis expanding osteolytic lesions, especially those involving the flat bones or vertebral column BILLINGS and WERNER (1972). In these areas it is usually hard to differentiate various types of lesions by plain roentgenographic findings.

G. Vascular Tumors

I. Hemangioma

This is a relatively common lesion of bone composed of thin-walled vascular channels. The majority of hemangiomas of bone may be classified as cavernous, and only a few cases of capillary hemangioma of bone have been reported.

The angiographic findings in hemangiomas are closely related to the caliber and number of vessels in the lesion. In cases of cavernous hemangiomas, there are typical angiographic findings which consist of large and tortuous feeding arteries. These lesions may possess large arteriovenous communications which cause a great amount of blood to be shunted from the arteries to the veins. The veins are of greater caliber than the arteries. Numerous sharply demarcated defects are present in the cortex of involved bones, the largest of which accommodate the vascular lakes. These findings are similar to those of soft tissue hemangiomas or arteriovenous fistulae (Figs. 20, 21). Frequently there are soft-tissue hemangiomas in combination with the bone hemangiomas. The arteriographic diagnosis in these cases is fairly certain. Capillary hemangiomas are usually less vascular and it is difficult to recognize vascularity in this type of bone lesion. In these instances, subtraction technique will be of help to see vascularity or staining in the lesion.

II. Lymphangioma

This lesion is rare and can be seen as single or multiple cystic lesions involving the bones. Angiography reveals no evidence of hypervascularity. In a few cases in the

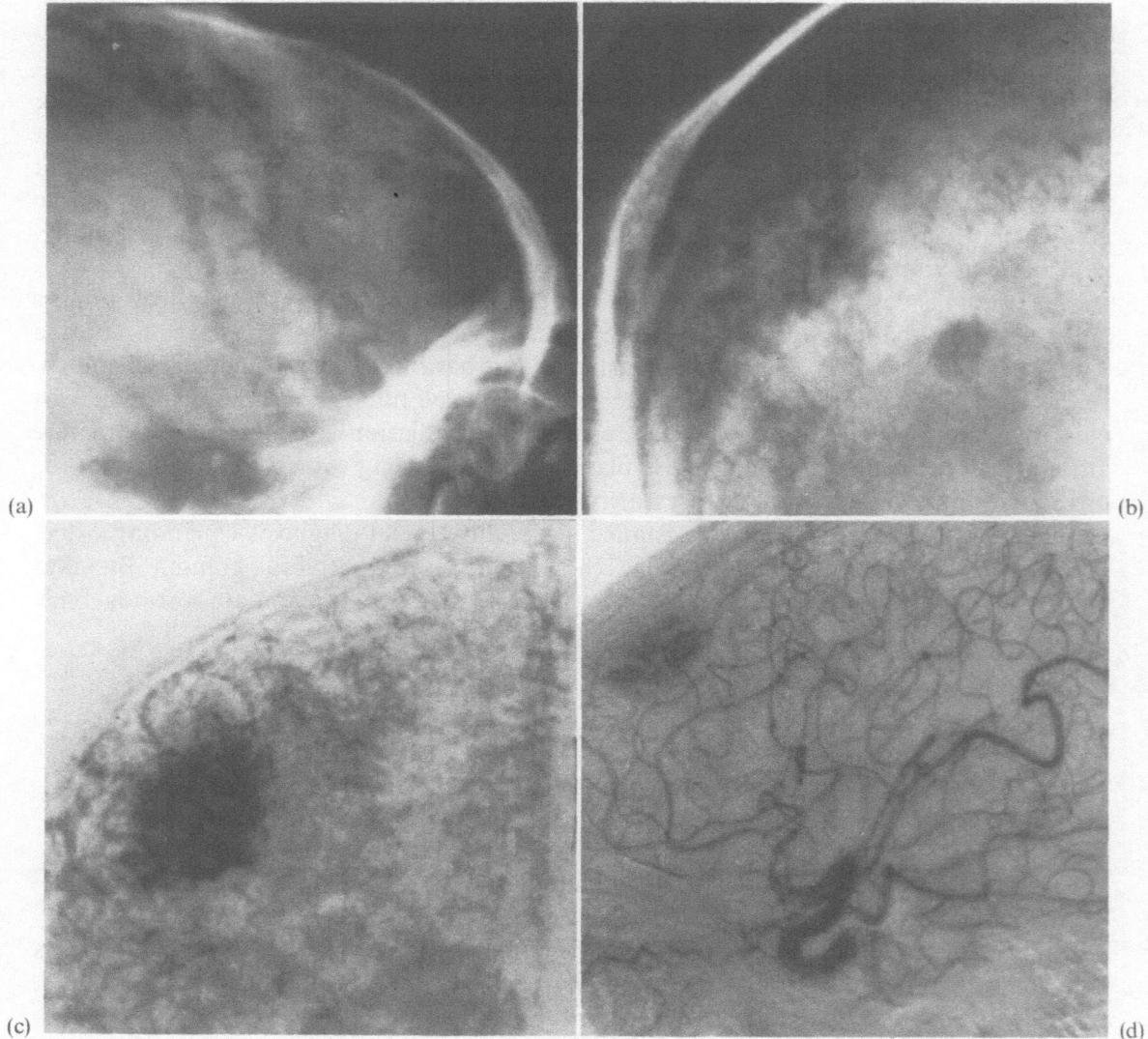

Fig. 20a–d. Hemangioma involving frontal bone (a, b). Arteriogram revealed hypervascular lesions with no soft-tissue component (c, d). On the basis of plain film and arteriographic findings, a diagnosis of meningioma was made. Pathology proved that this lesion was a hemangioma

literature there was opacification of the intraosseous cystic areas by lymphangiography (EDEIKEN and HODES, 1973), which is pathognomonic of lymphangiomas.

III. Hemangiopericytoma

This is a very rare bone lesion and only nine cases have been reported in the literature. The angiographic manifestations of soft-tissue hemangiopericytomas reported in the literature reveal that these lesions are hypervascular and well-defined, with evidence of rapid blood circulation through the tumor. We assume that the osseous form of these lesions has a similar angiographic appearance.

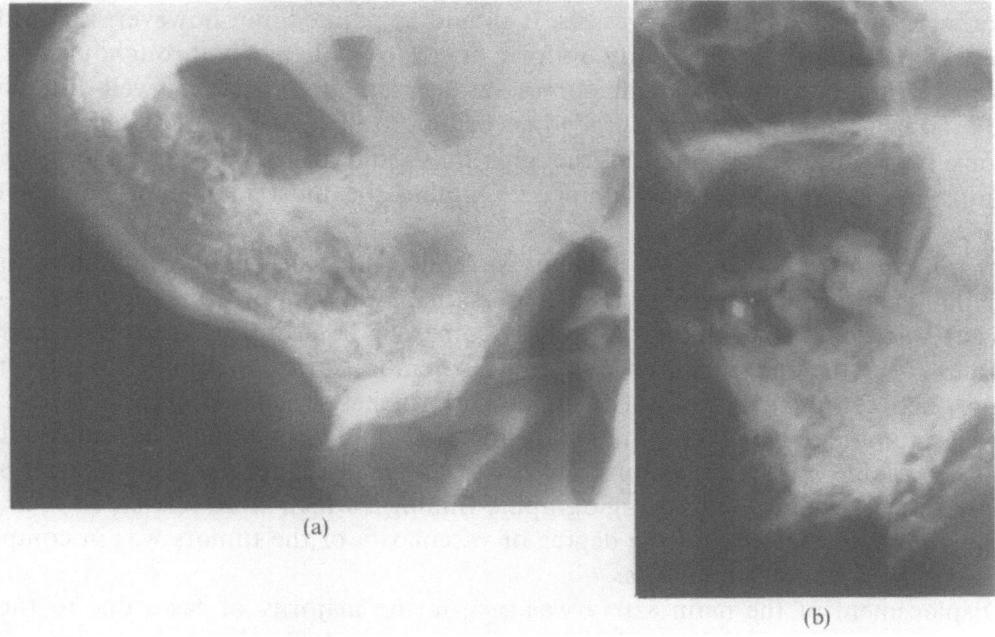

Fig. 21a and b. Arteriovenous malformation. Plain film (a) reveals evidence of slow growing lesion involving mandible with presence of soft-tissue component. Arteriogram (b) reveals evidence of intraosseous and extra-osseous av-malformation

H. Other Connective Tissue Tumors

I. Lipoma

This is a rare benign bone neoplasm and there is not a single case reported in the literature examined by arteriography. We would expect these lesions, like soft-tissue lipomas, to be avascular in nature.

II. Desmoplastic Fibroma

This is a rare lesion which is usually seen in soft tissue but rarely in bone, although secondary involvement of bone is frequently seen. These tumors are avascular, although they are aggressive and locally invasive. In our experience with only two cases of desmoplastic fibroma, only a few normal-looking arteries were seen in the lesion, but not more than the vascularity of normal surrounding soft tissues.

III. Fibrosarcoma

Fibrosarcoma is one of the malignant sarcomas which has been more extensively studied angiographically. Angiographic studies reported in the literature indicate that a great spectrum of vascularity exists in fibrosarcomatous tissues, whether they be of bone or soft-tissue origin. Some fibrosarcomas may appear to be hypervascularized, and others poorly supplied with vessels. It should be pointed out, however, that although fibrosarcomas usually show a fairly uniform degree of malignancy throughout the tumor, a more malignant focus may sometimes be seen in an otherwise, well-differentiated tumor. To insure that a tumor is graded according to its least differentiated part, several sections from different regions of the growth should be examined. For this reason, prebiopsy angiography is essential in determining the most malignant portion of the tumor.

Angiographic Manifestations: Primary osseous or periosteal fibrosarcomas, as with other malignant bone tumors, derive their main blood supply from the arteries of the adjacent soft tissue. In some large fibrosarcomas of bone in the knee area, numerous branches from the superficial as well as deep femoral arteries supply the tumor. The distance between the origin of these supplying branches sometimes exceeds 40 cm.

These tumors, like other tumors arising from undifferentiated mesenchymal cells, reveal a variable angioarchitecture. However, the majority of these neoplasms shared at least some of the following angiographic findings, which were related to their grade of malignancy. Assessment of the degree of vascularity of the tumors was in comparison to that of the surrounding tissues.

Displacement of the main artery was seen in the majority of cases due to the mass effect. Encroachment and direct invasion were seen in 48% of our cases, and of these, 50% revealed complete obstruction. The circulation to the limb distal to the site of obstruction was supplied by collateral circulation, frequently through the tumor itself. The second and third order branches commonly showed evidence of encroachment, direct invasion, or complete obstruction. Neovascularity and hypervascularity were present in all instances, although the most malignant tumors (grade IV) revealed more vascularity and demonstrated pathologic vessels of variable size and shape in comparison with the least malignant (grade I) fibrosarcomas (Fig. 23 b, c).

Early venous drainage occurred in the majority of hypervascular fibrosarcomas. Only a few of these cases, however, showed frank arteriovenous shunts.

A tumor stain was related to the degree of vascularity of the fibrosarcomas, and the majority of the tumors were markedly heterogeneous in their vascularity and tumor stain. Some regions contained a myriad of wide vessels in an irregular reticular pattern, other areas showed narrow vessels with a more normal pattern, and some areas were avascular. The highly vascular areas corresponded to the highly malignant part of the tumor, whereas in less malignant areas there was less vascularity (Fig. 23 b, c). The avascular areas usually corresponded to areas of tumor necrosis or hematoma.

The draining veins were usually dilated. They showed evidence of displacement, direct invasion of the wall, complete obstruction, and intraluminal extension of tumor. These findings were responsible for obstruction of major veins in the majority of cases (Fig. 22 c, d).

Extension of the lesion beyond the confines of the host bone into the adjacent soft tissue was noted in all cases of our series.

The ratio of the soft tissue component to bone was 3:1 in favor of soft tissue. This ratio was much greater in cases of the periosteal type of fibrosarcoma. The tumor margins were easily seen by a clear demarcation between tumor stain and surrounding soft tissue (Figs. 22, 23).

IV. Liposarcoma

This is a rare, malignant bone neoplasm. There have been only a few cases of primary liposarcoma of bone reported in the literature. Only one case has been studied

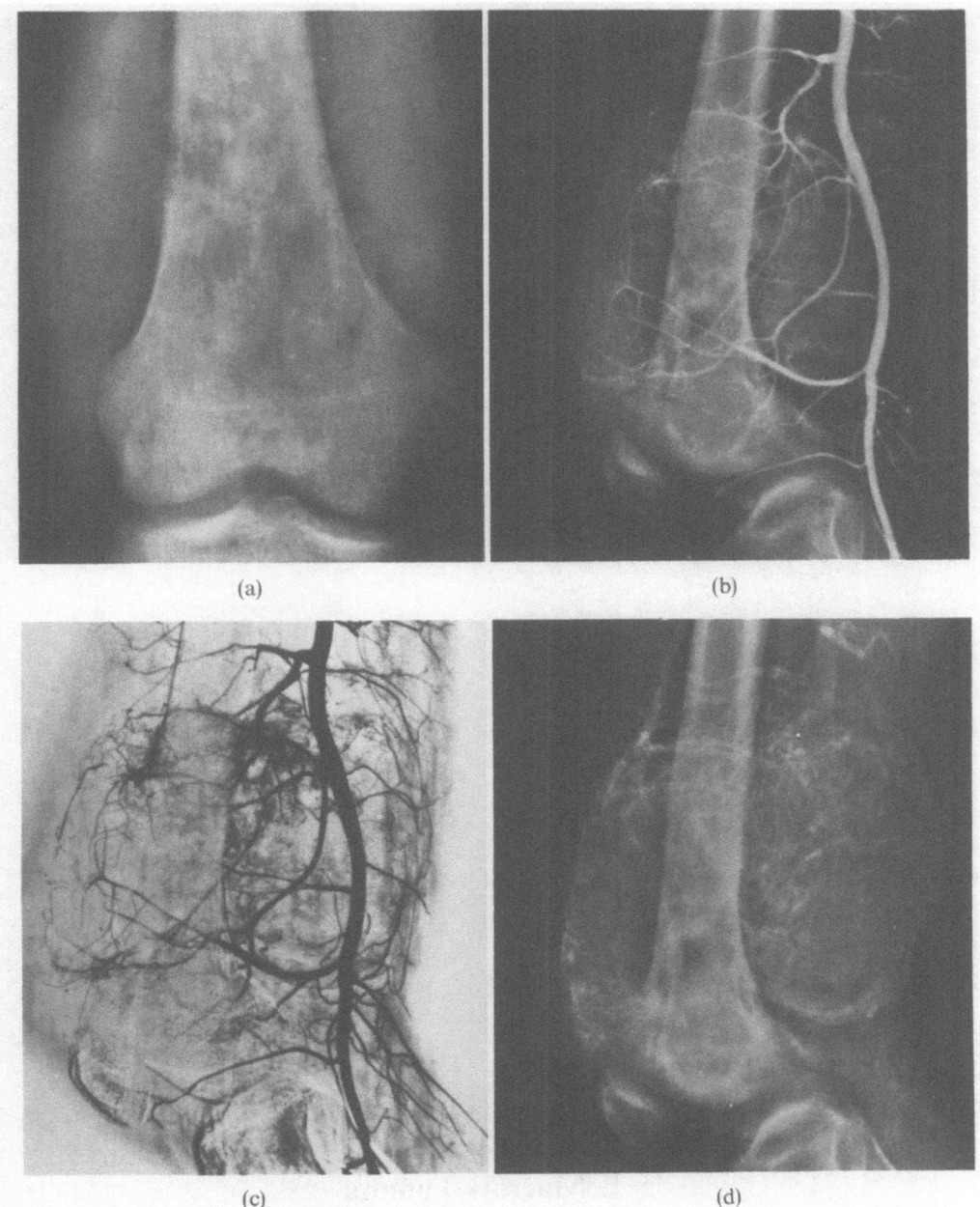

Fig. 22a–d. Fibrosarcoma (undifferentiated) in 19-year-old male. Arteriogram demonstrates hypervascularity with considerable large, well-defined soft-tissue component. There is posterior displacement of femoral arteries (b, c) and complete obstruction of femoral veins (d). The relatively less vascular area in anterior aspect of femur is a result of tumor necrosis

angiographically COHEN, (1968) and revealed a relative increase in vascularity at the tumor site. More experience is necessary before a definitive description of the angiographic findings in these tumors can be made. Our experience with liposarcomas of soft tissue has shown hypervascularity in these lesions, and maybe these lesions in bone have a similar angiographic appearance.

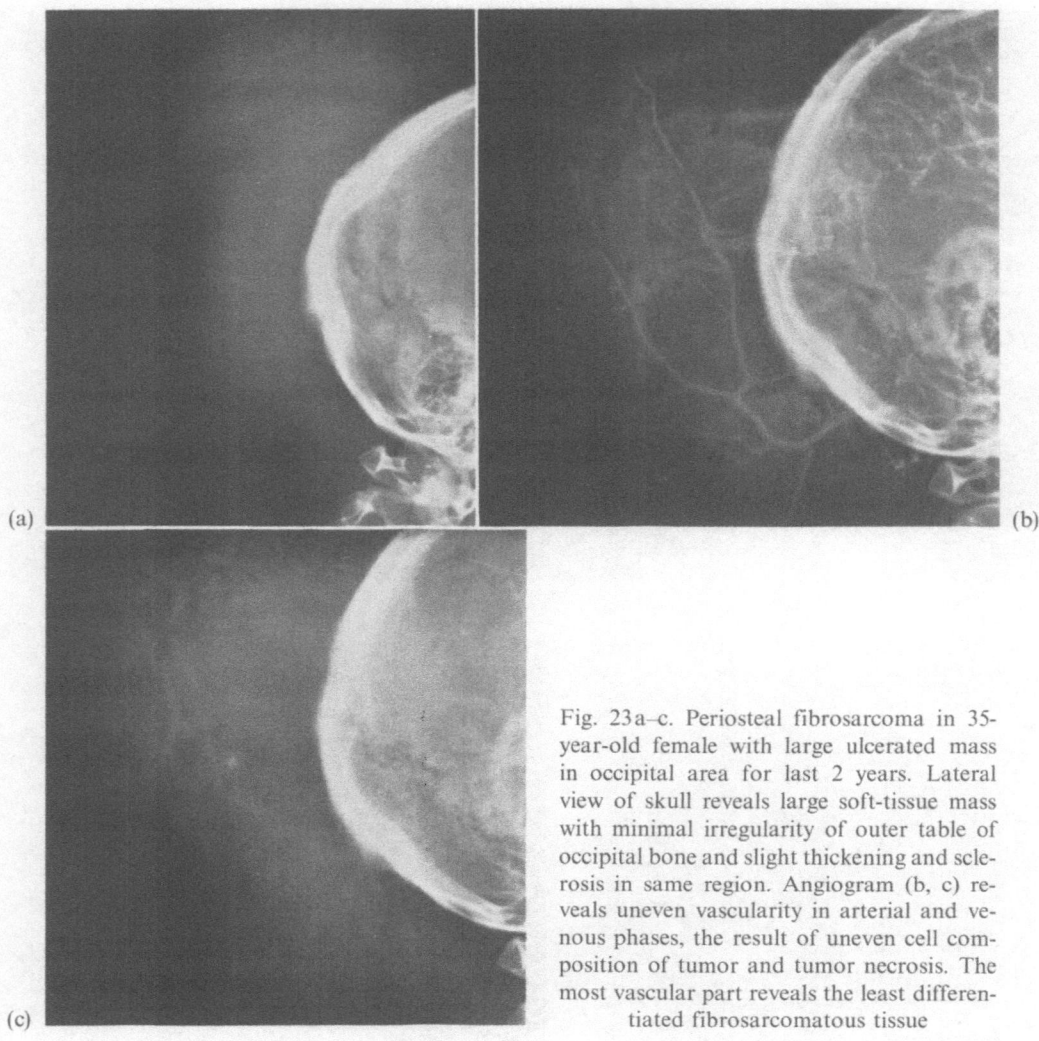

(a)

(b)

(c)

Fig. 23a–c. Periosteal fibrosarcoma in 35-year-old female with large ulcerated mass in occipital area for last 2 years. Lateral view of skull reveals large soft-tissue mass with minimal irregularity of outer table of occipital bone and slight thickening and sclerosis in same region. Angiogram (b, c) reveals uneven vascularity in arterial and venous phases, the result of uneven cell composition of tumor and tumor necrosis. The most vascular part reveals the least differentiated fibrosarcomatous tissue

I. Marrow Tumors

Marrow tumors are round cell tumors arising from bone marrow, including Ewing's sarcoma, reticulum cell sarcoma, and myeloma. The first two lesions have very similar vascular patterns. Because of this similarity, they will be discussed together.

I. Ewing's Sarcoma and Reticulum Cell Sarcoma

These sarcomas are vascular tumors and have the relatively typical angiographic features of malignant hypervascular bone lesions.

Angiographic Findings: Hypervascularity and the presence of pathologic vessels were noted in all reported cases, as well as in our series of Ewing's sarcoma and reticulum cell sarcoma (Figs. 1, 24). Numerous arteries arose from the soft tissue around the

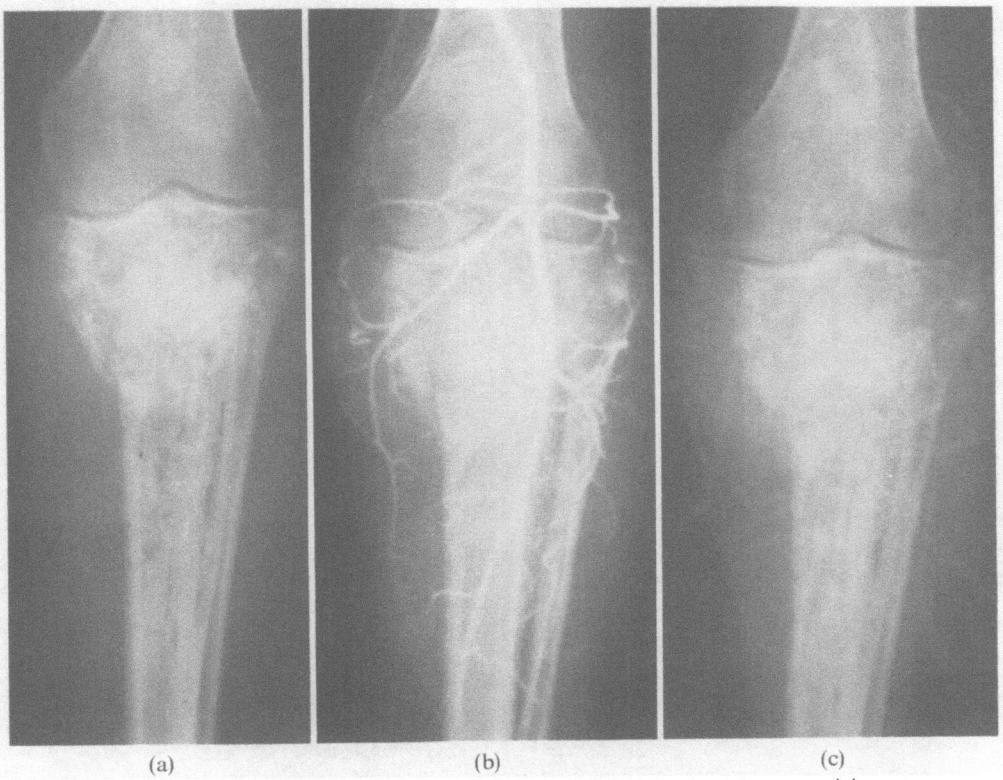

Fig. 24a–c. Reticulum cell sarcoma in 32-year-old female. A conventional radiograph (a) demonstrates pathologic fracture involving proximal end of tibia with permeative appearance and cortical destruction. Angiogram (b, c) reveals presence of hypervascularity and pathologic vessels in tumor area. Extension of soft-tissue involvement is best seen in venous phase, which also reveals relatively lighter stain than skeletogenic type of tumors. In our experience the angiographic pattern of Ewing's sarcoma and reticulum cell sarcoma is indistinguishable

lesion. The degree of vascularity varies, and some tumors tend to have a sparse vascular bed (Fig. 24c, d). Indeed, this has been the characteristic picture of these tumors in other studies. A relatively faint and moderately well-demarcated uniform tumor stain can often be seen in the late capillary phase. As a result of tumor necrosis, 12% of these cases showed poorly circumscribed areas of avascularity. The uniform stain probably is a result of the uniform cellularity of these tumors, and occasional avascular areas were the result of tumor necrosis or hematomas. As mentioned in the section on skeletogenic sarcomas, considerable variability in the angioarchitecture was not only related to tumor necrosis, but was also related to the variability of the cells in these tumors. An uniform vascularity and tumor stain, especially in larger tumors, was of great help in the differential diagnosis of myelogenic tumors from skeletogenic tumors.

Myelogenic tumors tend to penetrate the cortex of bone and form quite large and elongated extraosseous soft tissue masses around the tubular or flat bones. The extension of tumor was well delineated by the angiograms in every one of our cases. Displacement of large normal arteries by the tumor mass was a common finding, but involvement by way of encasement or obstruction was infrequently seen. Encasement of second and third order arteries was occasionally noted in far advanced cases. Abnormal veins, and obstruction of large normal veins at the site of the lesion, were seen frequently.

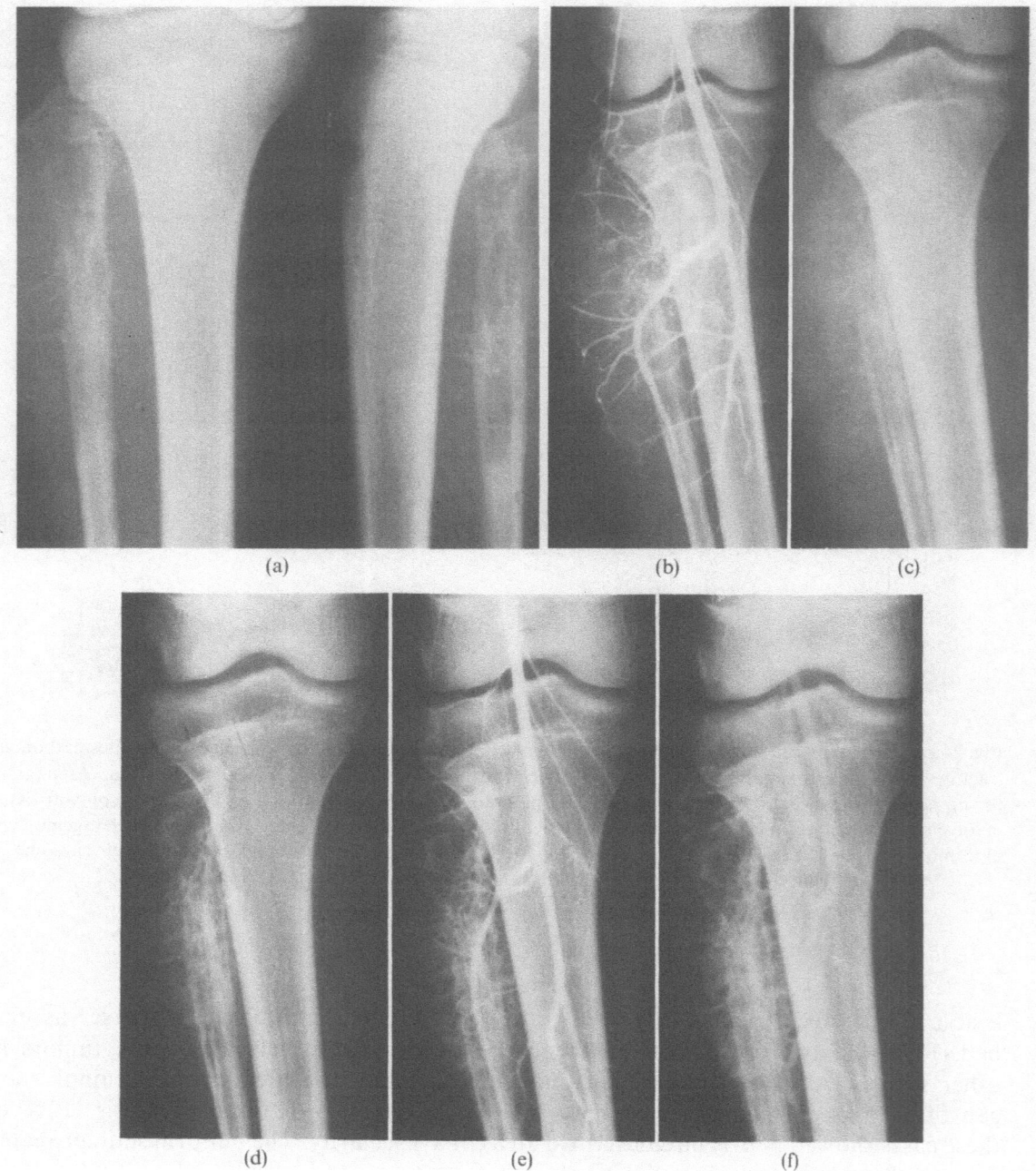

Fig. 25a–f. Ewing's sarcoma in 15-year-old female. AP and lateral views of left upper leg demonstrate a malignant pattern involving proximal end of fibula, which was interpreted as osteosarcoma. Arteriography reveals hypervascularity, exact extent of tumor in medullary channel and soft tissue. Tumor stain is relatively light in comparison to osteosarcoma (b, c). After 4500 rad tumor dose, tumor appears sclerotic (d) and arteriogram reveals relative avascularity in region of tumor. Size of tumor and soft-tissue mass is greatly reduced (e, f)

There is usually no clinical indication for performing angiograms routinely in these cases. However, in the following circumstances, arteriography will be of value:

1. When lesions arise from flat bones or vertebra, because of difficulty in plain roentgenographic interpretation, angiograms will be of value in seeing the vascularity

of the lesion as well as to indicate the exact extension of the tumor. This information not only is of great help in making the diagnosis, but also will be valuable for treatment planning, especially radiation therapy and surgery.

2. Pre- and postradiation or chemotherapy arteriograms in the majority of Ewing's and reticulum cell sarcoma not only will help to evaluate the effect of treatment by shrinkage of the arterial system of the tumor (Fig. 25), but is of great help in evaluating the recurrence of the tumor in very early stages. In these instances, revascularity of the lesion is due to progression of the tumor.

3. The differential diagnosis between acute osteomyelitis and Ewing's sarcoma on the basis of plain roentgenographic findings always creates a great difficulty for the radiologist. By performing an arteriogram, we can easily differentiate these two entities. There is no doubt that during certain phases in acute osteomyelitis, there is evidence of hypervascularity due to hyperemia, but in these instances the staining is uneven, ill-defined, and seems to penetrate into the soft tissues. In comparison, well-defined uniform staining is seen in cases of Ewing's sarcoma and reticulum cell sarcoma. In addition, invasion, encasement, or obstruction of normal arteries or veins around the lesion is rarely seen in cases of osteomyelitis, and is significant in the differential diagnosis.

II. Myeloma

In cases of solitary myeloma, we found somewhat different angiographic findings in comparison to Ewing's or reticulum cell sarcoma. These lesions were highly vascular with an even tumor stain. The tumor stain in some cases was very prolonged and resembled the staining of giant cell tumors, although the presence of soft tissue extension and major vessel encasement or obstruction was of great help in the differential diagnosis.

J. Other Tumors

I. Chordoma

These tumors are avascular lesions. In some instances, one or a few small supplying arteries with normal configuration are noted in the tumor area (Fig. 26c, d).

II. Adamantinoma of Long Bone

Adamantinoma of the limb bone is one of the rarer primary bone neoplasms. There are only 40 reported cases of adamantinoma in the world literature, and only 1 of them with angiographic features (ROSEN, 1966), revealing hypervascularity, pathologic vessels, and soft-tissue extension adjacent to the osteolytic bone lesion.

The angiographic features were similar to other hypervascular malignant bone neoplasms (Fig. 27c, d).

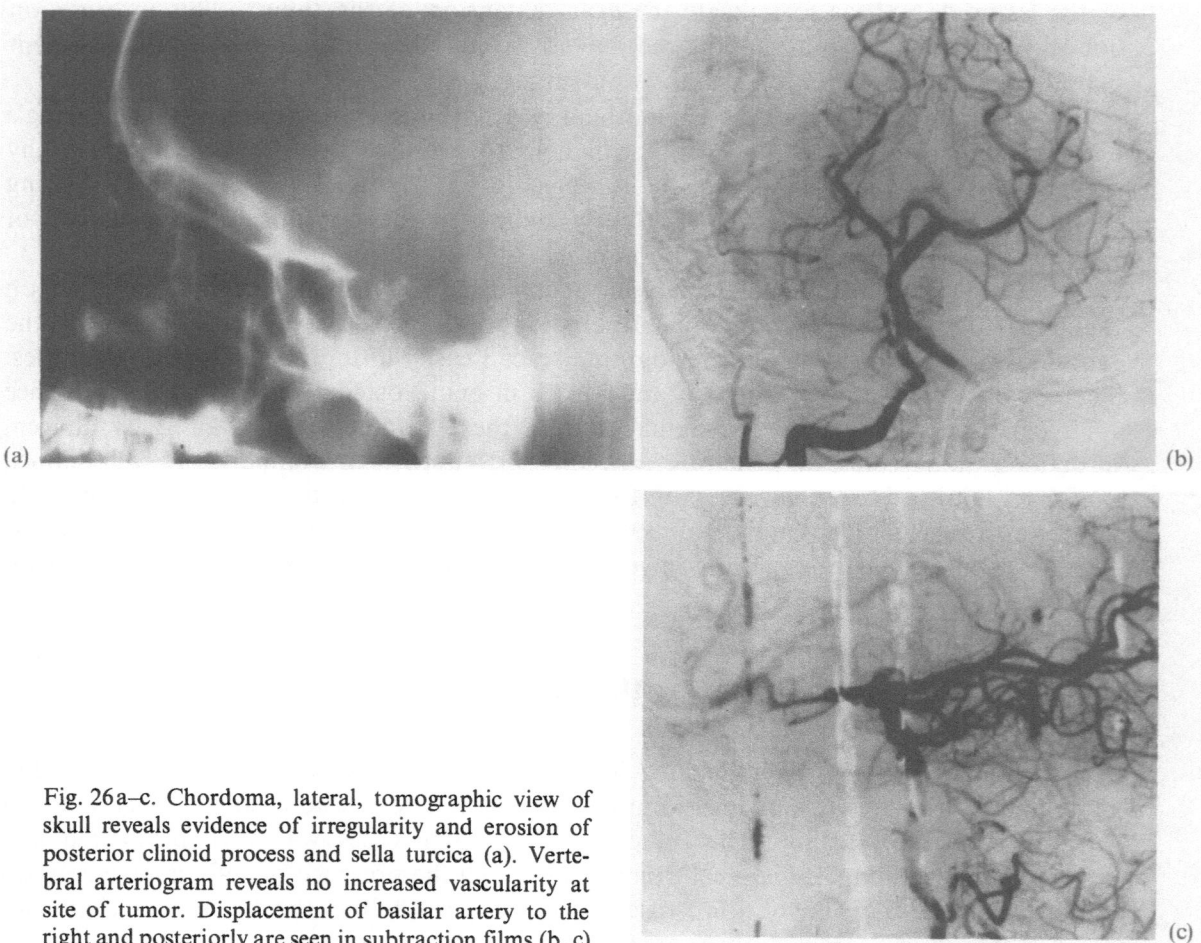

Fig. 26a–c. Chordoma, lateral, tomographic view of skull reveals evidence of irregularity and erosion of posterior clinoid process and sella turcica (a). Vertebral arteriogram reveals no increased vascularity at site of tumor. Displacement of basilar artery to the right and posteriorly are seen in subtraction films (b, c)

III. Neurolemmoma (Schwannoma, Neuronoma)

Soft-tissue neurolemmomas are hypervascular tumors, although we did not have an opportunity to study a neurolemmoma originating from bone. We assume these tumors, regardless of their location, are hypervascular.

K. Tumorlike Lesions

This group of bone lesions includes the solitary bone cyst (simple or unicameral bone cyst), juxta articular bone cyst (interosseous ganglion), eosinophilic granuloma, Brown tumor of hyperparathyroidism, metaphyseal fibrous defect (nonossifying fibroma), fibrous dysplasia, myositis ossificans, and aneurysmal bone cyst. These are benign bone lesions with a variety of angiographic manifestations. The first four lesions are avascular. Aneurysmal bone cysts are highly vascular lesions, and because of their angiographic similarity with giant cell tumor, were discussed previously. The remainder of the lesions of this group are moderately vascular and will be discussed below.

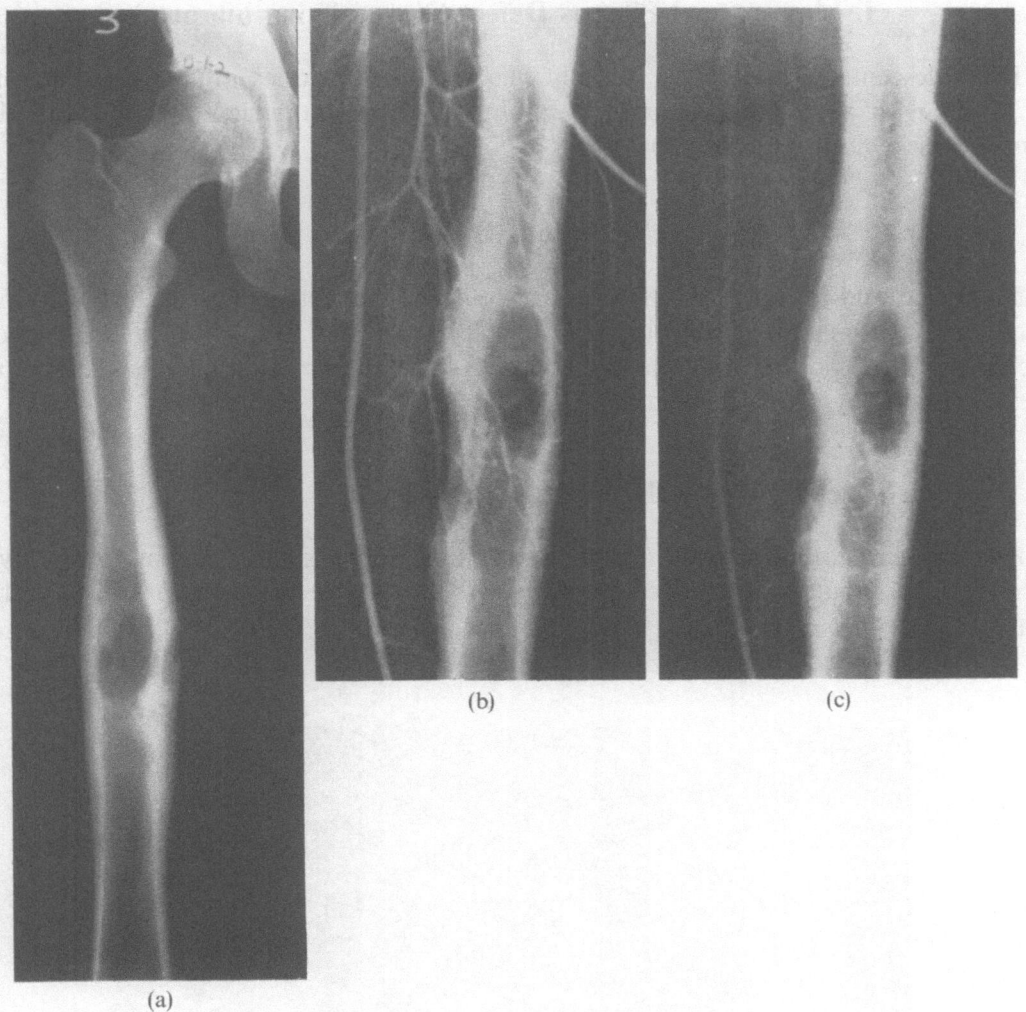

(a)

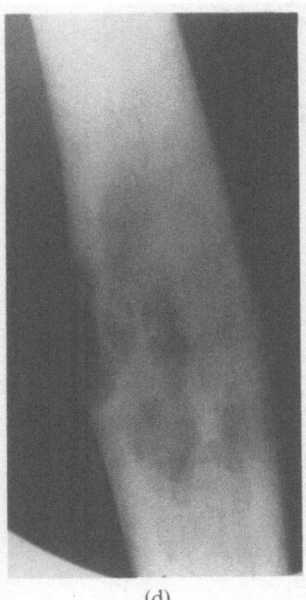

(d)

Fig. 27a–d. Adamantinoma involving shaft of the left knee in 16-
year-old female. Roentgenograms of femur show a cystic, slightly
expansile tumor within mid-portion of shaft (a, b). Late arterial
phase reveals well-defined vascular soft-tissue mass apparently contiguous with periosteum, with numerous abnormal vessels and tumor
stain in soft tissue and intraosseous portions of tumor. Courtesy
of Dr. Robert S. Rosen amer. J. Roentgenol. **97**, 1966

I. Metaphyseal Fibrous Defect (Nonossifying Fibroma)

In adolescents (active stage), usually one or a few arteries are seen at the site of the lesion with a very light tumor stain. In older patients, there was no vascularity seen in these lesions (Fig. 14c–e).

II. Fibrous Dysplasia

MARGULIS and MURPHY (1958) and SUTTON (1955) reported cases of fibrous dysplasia which were avascular bone lesions, although MUCCHI and COLUMELLA (1951) reported vascularity in the polyostotic type of fibrous dysplasia. Our experience has shown most cases of fibrous dysplasia to be avascular (Fig. 28).

III. Myositis Ossificans

Because this condition can superficially mimic more serious lesions, even by the pathologist, it should be evaluated carefully by all available means to prevent overtreatment.

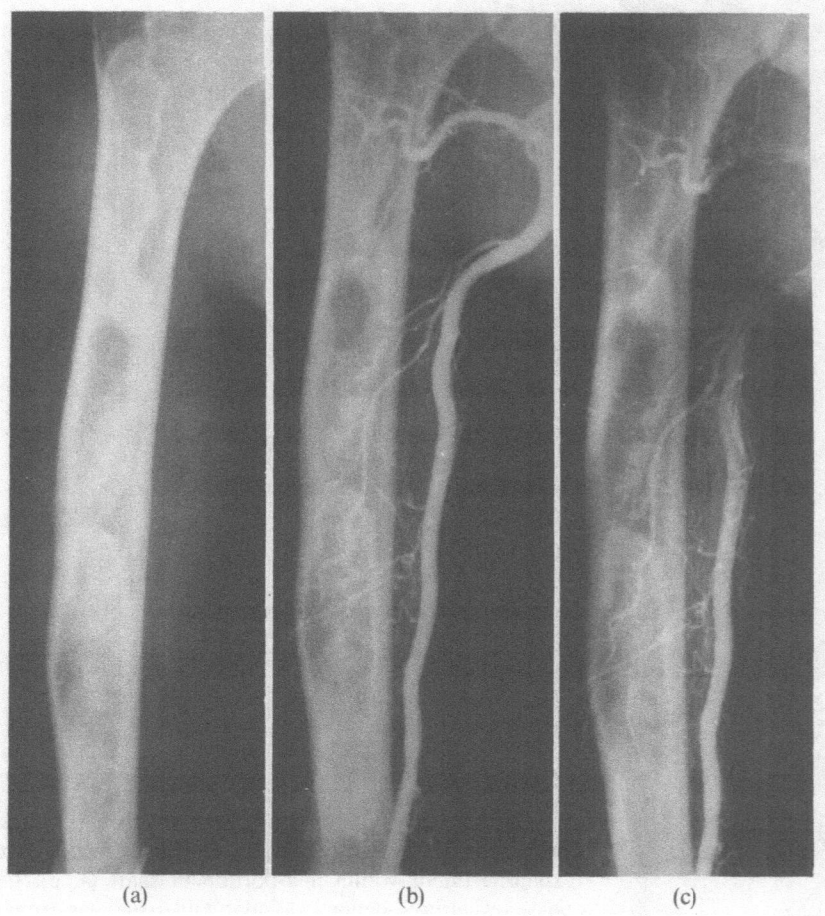

(a)   (b)   (c)

Fig. 28a–c. Fibrous dysplasia in 65-year-old female involving right humeral shaft. Arteriogram appeared normal (b, c)

The angiographic manifestations of myositis ossificans differ in various phases of the disease. In the active stage, these lesions are highly vascular with a heavy, ill-defined tumor stain, and should not be regarded as a sign of malignancy (HUTCHESON et al., 1972). To help distinguish these lesions from pathologically similar malignant tumors, there is an absence of arteriovenous shunts, invasion of large arteries or veins close to the lesion, venous lakes, or well-defined tumor stain.

In the inactive stage, there are usually only a few vessels in the area of the lesion and there is no difficulty in the differential diagnosis (Fig. 29).

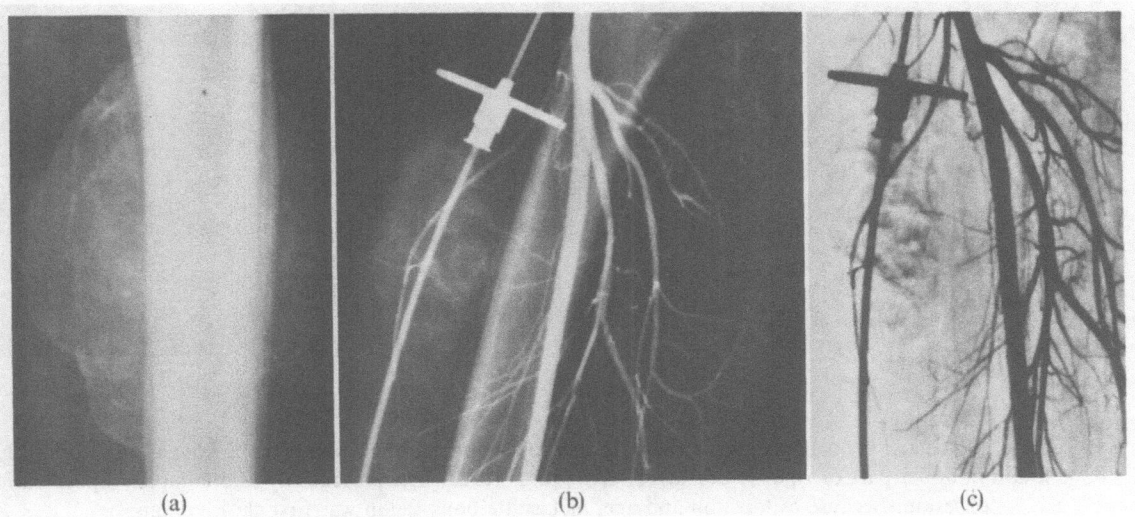

(a)   (b)   (c)

Fig. 29a–c. Myositis ossificans circumscripta in 14-year-old male. Conventional roentgenogram reveals large soft-tissue ossification around upper shaft of femur with presence of periosteal reaction. Biopsy was done and was reported as osteosarcoma. Angiogram revealed only a few small arteries in lesion area with no definite evidence of stain (b). Subtraction film (c) reveals only light stain, which was not apparent in regular angio film (b). These findings were uncomparable to angiographic manifestation of osteosarcoma (Figs. 2, 3, 7). Repeated biopsy proved presence of myositis ossificans. Courtesy of Dr. M. Tafazoli (Teheran, Iran)

L. Metastatic Bone Lesions

The most frequent malignant bone lesions are metastases. They are encountered in 16–35% of all patients dying of cancer. The malignant neoplasms most apt to metastasize to bone are those of the breast, prostate, thyroid, kidney, and lung. Other cancers also spread to bone, but less frequently. Several types of metastatic growth patterns may be seen in bone pathologically, including osteoblastic, osteolytic, subperiosteal, and intertrabecular. In the intertrabecular type of metastasis, the bone preserves its architecture regardless of the diffuse infiltration of tumor cells. This type, therefore, reveals no roentgenographic abnormality for long periods of time, but usually can be detected by isotope studies. The other types of bone metastases infrequently represent diagnostic problems, and explain the relative lack of literature dealing with the vascular supply of bony metastases. These lesions usually have an arteriographic pattern related to that of the primary tumor.

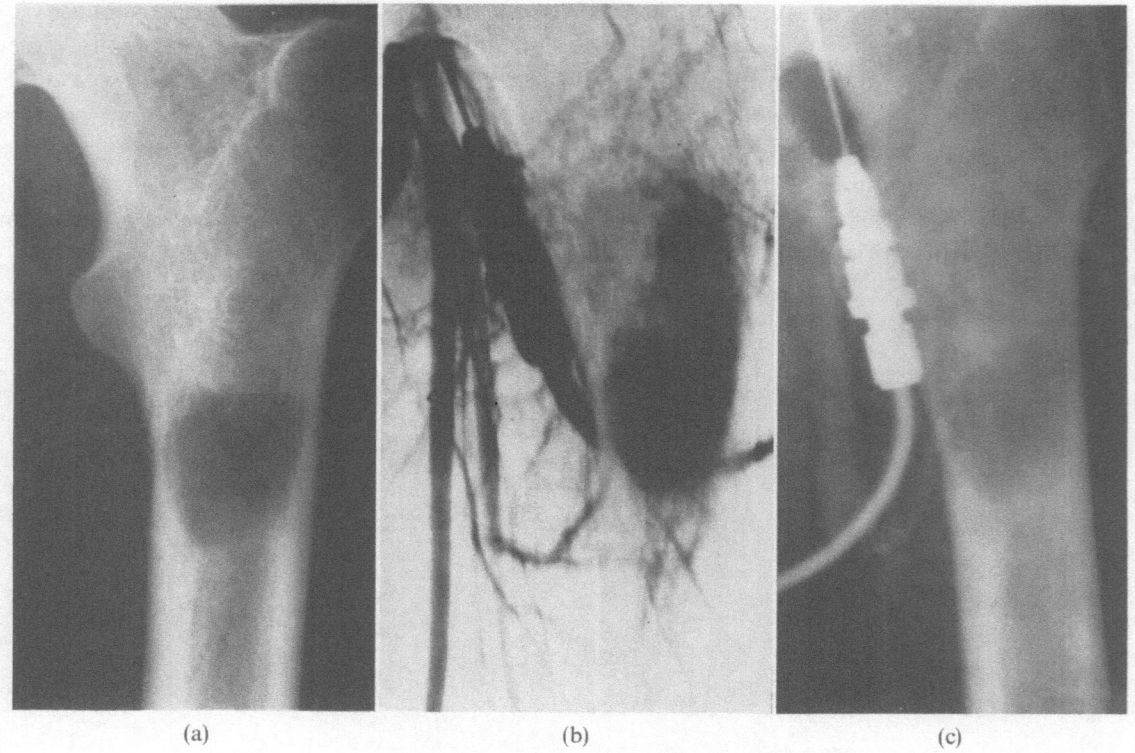

Fig. 30a–c. Metastatic bronchogenic carcinoma in 58-year-old male. Plain film reveals a punch-out radiolucent bone lesion in upper part of right femur (a). Arteriograms reveal hypervascularity and complete opacification of lesion. Because of location and age, metastatic bone lesion was first choice diagnosis

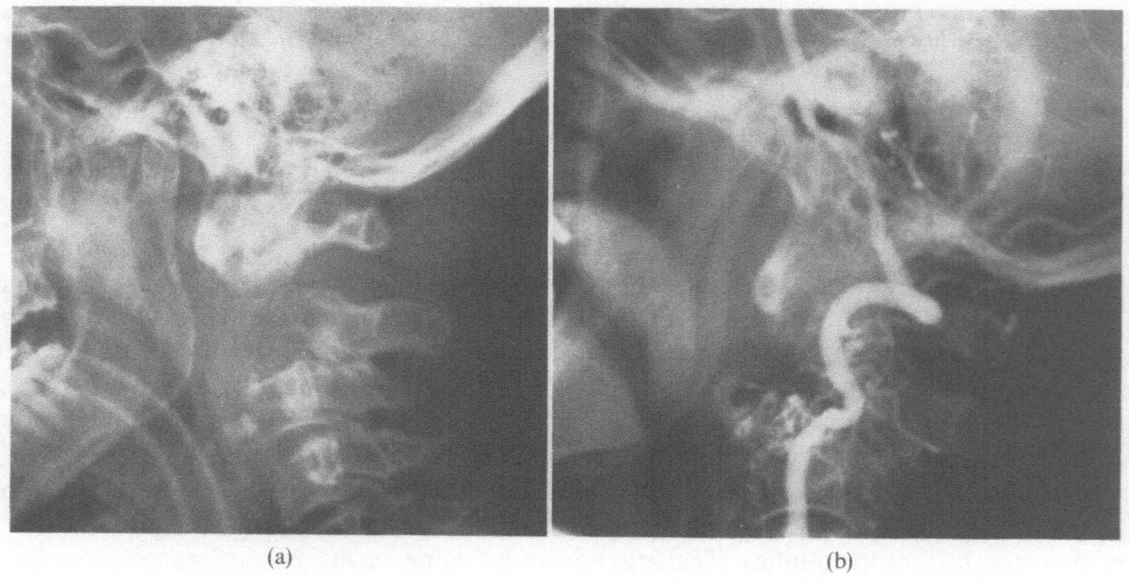

Fig. 31a and b. Metastatic hypernephroma in 49-year-old male involving 2nd cervical vertebrae. These tumors usually are highly vascular lesions

I. Osteolytic Metastasis

Osteolytic bone metastases may appear as multiple lucencies of intramedullary location, without disruption of the cortical boundaries. These lesions may fail to show any vascular abnormality, because the main supplying arteries arise from the intraosseous arterial system. Due to the considerable density of bone, the intraosseous arteries are not able to expand and deliver more blood to these lesions. The second group includes the larger osteolytic metastases with cortical disruption, which usually demonstrate abnormal vascular patterns because the main supplying arteries arise from the surrounding soft tissues. These lesions have all the criteria of malignant hypervascular neoplasms and usually are undistinguishable from that group (Figs. 30, 31).

II. Osteoblastic Metastasis

These lesions are usually less vascular than the osteolytic type of metastases. The majority of intramedullary osteoblastic metastases, especially from the prostate, are avascular, although in cases with cortical disruption, some degree of vascularity and tumor stain may be detected using the subtraction technique. Finally, the degree of vascularity of these lesions is closely related to the original lesion and the degree of their cell differentiation.

References

ABRAMS, H.L.: Angiography, 2nd ed. Boston: Little Brown, 1971

ACKERMAN, L.V.: Extra-osseous localized nonneoplastic bone and cartilage formation (so-called myositis ossificans): Clinical and pathological confusion with malignant neoplasms. J. Bone Jt Surg. **40-A**, 279–298 (1958)

AEGERTER, E.E., KIRKPATRICK, J.A., JR.: Orthopedic diseases: Physiology, pathology, radiology, 3rd ed. Philadelphia: Saunders 1968

BACIU, C., BROSTEANU, G., STANCIULESEU, P., BALENTY, P.V.: The value of arteriography in the differential diagnosis of bone tumors. Lyon chir. **59**, 206–212 (1963)

BEGG, A.C.: The vascular pattern as an aid to the diagnosis of bone tumours. J. Bone Jt Surg **37B**, 371–378 (1955)

BERK, M.E.: Arteriography in peripheral trauma. Clin. Radiol. **14**, 235–239 (1963)

BILLINGS, K.J., WERNER, G.L.: Aneurysmal bone cyst of the first lumbar vertebra. Radiology **104**, 19–20 (1972)

BRONDOLO, W. et al.: Angiographic pictures in primary bone tumors of extremities. Arch. Ortop. (Milano) **14**, 925–932 (1959)

BRUNELLI, B.: Arteriography in diagnosis of osseous tumors of the extremities. Minerva chir. (Torino) **14**, 925–932 (1959)

BRUNELLI, B. et al.: Arteriography in the diagnosis of bone tumors of the limbs. Panminerva med. **2**, 180–187 (1960)

CACDAC, M.A., MALIS, L., ANDERSON, P.: Aneurysmal parietal bone cyst (Case report). J. Neurosurg. **37**, 237–241 (1972)

CALDAS, J.P.: Radiodiagnosis of bone tumors by arteriography. Presented at the fourth International Congress of Radiology, Zürich (1934)

CALDAS, J.P.: Arteriographie des membres de l'aorte abdominale et des branches. J. Radiol. Electrol. **34**, 28–41 (1951)

CHIAPPA, S. et al.: Angiography in tumors of the bone and of the soft tissue of the extremities. Radiol. Electrol. **40**, 639–655 (1959)

COCKSHOTT, W.P., EVANS, K.T.: The place of soft tissue arteriography. Brit. J. Radiol. **37**, 367–375 (1964)

COHEN, G.: Primary liposarcoma of bone. The angiographic findings and doubts as to its intermedullary origin. Brit. J. Radiol. **31**, 442–444 (1968)

COLUMELLA, F., MUCCHI, L.: Biopsia o arteriografia nella diagnostica delle osteopatie degli arti? Chirurgia (Milano) **8**, 311–313 (1953)

DAHLIN, D.C.: Bone tumors. General aspects and data on 3987 cases, 2nd ed. Springfield, Ill.: Charles C Thomas 1967

DENNY, M.: Vascular pattern in tumors of the extremities. S. Afr. med. J. **27**, 27–30 (1956)

DENSTAD, T.: Arteriography in 2 cases of malignant

tumors; (melanoma and neurinoma). Acta radiol. (Stockh.) **35**, 309–312 (1951)

DIBBELT, W.: Über die Blutgefäße der Tumoren. Arch. path. Anat. Bakt. **8**, 114–117 (1912)

DOAN, C.A.: The circulation of the bone marrow. Contr. Embryol. Carney. Instn. **14**, 27–32 (1922)

DOS SANTOS, R.: L'artériographie dans les néoplasies des os et des parties molles. Bull. Soc. nat. Chir. **60**, 99–103 (1934)

DOS SANTOS, R.: Arteriography in bone tumours. J. Bone Jt Surg. **32-B**, 17–29 (1950)

DOS SANTOS, R., LAMAS, C., CALDAS, P.: Bull mém. Soc. nat. Chir. **48**, 635 (1932)

DRINKER, C.K., DRINKER, K.R., LUND, C.C.: The circulation in the mammalian bone marrow. Amer. J. Physiol. **62**, 1–12 (1922)

EDEIKEN, J., HODES, P.J.: Roentgen diagnosis of disease of bone, 2nd ed. Baltimore: Williams & Wilkins 1973

EKELUND, L., LUNDERQVIST, A.: Pharmacoangiography with angiotensin. Radiology **110**, 533–540 (1974)

FARINAS, P.L.: Differential diagnosis of bone tumors of the extremities by arteriography. Radiology **29**, 29–32 (1937)

FINE, G., STOUT, A.P.: Osteogenic sarcoma of the extraskeletal soft tissues. Cancer (Philad.) **9**, 1027–1043 (1956)

FONTAINE, R., WALTER, P., KIM, M., KIENY, R.: De l'utilité de l'artériographie pour le diagnostic des tumeurs des membres d'origine osseuse et extraosseuse. J. Radiol. Electrol. **305**, 165–168 (1954)

GILMER, W.S., ANDERSON, L.D.: Reactions of soft somatic tissue which may progress to bone formation: Circumscribed (traumatic) myositis ossificans. Sth. med. J. (B'gham, Ala.) **52**, 1432–1448 (1959)

HALPERN, M., FREIBERGER, R.H.: Arteriography in orthopedics. Amer. J. Roentgenol. **94**, 194–206 (1965)

HALPERN, M., FREIBERGER, R.H.: Arteriography as a diagnostic procedure in bone disease. Radiol. Clin. N. Amer. **8**, 277–288 (1970)

HAWKINS, I.F., JR., HUDSON, T.: Priscoline in bone and soft tissue angiography. Radiology **110**, 541–546 (1974)

HERZBERG, D., SCHREIBER, M.H.: Angiography in mass lesions f the extremities. Amer. J. Roentgenol. **111**, 541–546 (1971)

HEUL, R.O. VAN DER, VON RONNEN, J.R.: Juxtacortical osteosarcoma. Diagnosis, differential diagnosis, treatment, and an analysis of eighty cases. J. Bone Jt Surg. **49-A**, 415–439 (1967)

HIPP, A.: Possibilities and limitation in the use of angiography in the diagnosis of tumors of the bones and soft tissues. Acta chir. orthop. Traum. čech. **32**, 317–319 (1965)

HUDSON, T.M., HASS, G., ENNEKING, W.F., HAWKINS, I.F. JR.: Angiography in the management of mus-

culoskeletal tumors. Surg. Gyn. & Ostet. **141**, 11–21 (1975)

HURAJ, E.: Angiography in the tumors of the bones. Acta chir. orthop. Traum. čech. **32**, 235–238 (1965)

HUTCHESON, J., KLATTE, E.C., KREMP, R.: The angiographic appearance of myositis ossificans circumscripta (A case report). Radiology **102**, 57–58 (1972)

IMURA, S. et al.: Arteriography in bone tumors. Surg. Ther. (Osaka) **16**, 11–16 (1957)

INCLAN, A.: The possibilities of roentgenographic study of the arterial circulation in the early diagnosis of bone malignancy. J. Bone Jt Surg. **24**, 259–269 (1942)

JACOBS, J.B., HANAFEE, W.: The use of Priscoline in peripheral arteriography. Radiology **88**, 957–960 (1967)

JAFFE, H.L.: Tumors and tumorous conditions of the bones and joints. Philadelphia: Lea & Febiger 1958

KEATS, T.E.: Trends in peripheral arteriography. Radiol. Clin. N. Amer. **2**, 483–497 (1964)

LAGERGREN, C., LINDBOM, A.: Angiography of peripheral tumors. Radiology **79**, 371–377 (1962)

LAGERGREN, C., LINDBOM, A., SÖDERBERG, G.: Hypervascularization in chronic inflammation demonstrated by angiography (angiographic, histopathologic and microangiographic studies). Acta radiol. (Stockh.) **49**, 441–452 (1958)

LAGERGREN, C., LINDBOM, A., SÖDERBERG, G.: Vascularization of fibromatous and fibrosarcomatous tumors (histopathologic, microangiographic and angiographic studies). Acta radiol. (Stockh.) **53**, 1–16 (1960)

LAGERGREN, C., LINDBOM, A., SÖDERBERG, G.: The blood vessels of chondrosarcoma. Acta radiol. (Stockh.) **55**, 321–328 (1961 a)

LAGERGREN, C., LINDBOM, A., SÖDERBERG, G.: The blood vessels of osteogenic sarcoma (histologic, angiographic and microangiographic studies). Acta radiol. (Stockh.) **55**, 161–176 (1961 b)

LASSER, E.C., SCHOBINGER VON SCHOWINGEN, R.: Arteriography in bone tumors. A preliminary report. N. Y. St. J. Med. **55**, 3425–3430 (1955)

LESSMANN, F.P., SCHOBINGER VON SCHOWINGEN, R., LASSER, E.C.: Intra-osseous venography in skeletal and soft tissue abnormalities. Acta radiol. (Stockh.) **44**, 397–409 (1955)

LEVIN, D.C., WATSON, R.C., BALTAXE, H.A.: Arteriography in diagnosis and management of acquired peripheral soft-tissue masses. Radiology **103**, 53–58 (1972)

LICHTENSTEIN, L.: Aneurysmal bone cyst. A pathological entity commonly mistaken for giant-cell tumor and occasionally for hemangioma and osteogenic sarcoma. Cancer (Philad.) **3**, 279–289 (1950)

O.: Angiography of aneurysmal bone cyst. Acta radiol. (Stockh.) **55**, 12–16 (1961)

LINDBOM, A., LINDVALL, N., SÖDERBERG, G., SPJUT, J.: Angiography in osteoid osteoma. Acta radiol. (Stockh.) **54**, 327–333 (1960)

LINDBOM, A., SÖDERBERG, G., SPJUT, H.J., SUNNQVIST, retroperitoneal tumors. The role of the lumbar arteries. Radiology 104, 259–268 (1972)

LOWMAN, R.M., GRNJA, V., PECK, D.R., OSBORN, D., LOVE, L.: The angiographic patterns of the primary retroperitoneal tumors. The role of the lumbar arteries. Radiology 104, 259–268 (1972)

MARGULIS, A.R., MURPHY, T.O.: Arteriography in neoplasms of extremities. Amer. J. Roentgenol. 80, 330–339 (1958)

MARTINELLI, V., MICIELI, G., BIANCHI, M.: Arteriographic observations in certain osteopathies of the extremities. Ann. ital. Chir. 39, 311–332 (1962)

MUCCHI, L.: Arteriography in bone pathology. Arch. ital. Chir. 87, 463–472 (1961)

MUCCHI, L., COLUMELLA, F.: Arteriography in diseases of bone. J. Fac. Radiol. 3, 135–146 (1951)

MURPHY, T.O., MARGULIS, A.R.: Roentgenographic manifestations of congenital peripheral arteriovenous communications. Radiology 67, 26–33 (1956)

NEY, F.G., FEIST, J.H., ALTEMUS, L.R., ORDINARIO, V.R.: The characteristic angiographic criteria of malignancy. Radiology 104, 567–570 (1972)

NORMAN, A., DORFMAN, H.: Juxtacortical circumscribed myositis ossificans: Evaluation and radiologic features. Radiology 96, 301–306 (1970)

PAPE, R., SEYSS, R.: Zur Beurteilung des Mesenchyms bei malignen Prozessen unter Berücksichtigung arteriographischer Befunde. Fortschr. Röntgenstr. 75, 138–144 (1951)

RABAIOTTI, E., MALCHIODII, C.: Angiography in diagnosis of bone and soft tissue tumors. Ann. Radiol. diagn. (Bologna) 29, 352–369 (1956)

RATTI, A.: L'arteriografia e l'osteomedullografia nella diagnosi dei tumori delle ossa. Radiol. clin. 28, 263–275 (1959)

RATTI, A.: Die Osteomedullographie der Knochenerkrankungen mit besonderer Rücksicht auf die Tumoren. Röntgenblätter 14, 241–247 (1961)

ROSEN, R.S., SCHWINN, C.P.: Adamantinoma of limb bone, malignant angioblastoma. Amer. J. Roentgenol. 97, 727–732 (1966)

ROSENBERG, J.C.: The value of arteriography in the treatment of soft tissue tumors of the extremities. J. int. Coll. Surg. 41, 405–415 (1964)

SAKAI, N.: Angiographic study of bone tumors. Indications for the decision of surgery, with special reference to the hindquarter amputation. J. Jap. orthop. Ass. 41, 65–80 (1967)

SCHOBINGER, R.: The arteriographic picture of metastatic bone disease. Cancer (Philad.) 11, 1264–1268 (1958)

SCHOBINGER, R., LIN, R.R., MOSS, H.C.: Significance of venous phase in arteriographic studies of bone and soft tissue tumors. Cancer (Philad.) 11, 315–321 (1958)

SCHOBINGER, R., STOLL, H.C.: Arteriographic picture of benign bone lesions containing giant cells. J. Bone Jt Surg. 39-A, 953–960 (1951)

SHANOFF, L.B., SPIRA, M., HARDY, S.B.: Myositis ossificans: Evaluation to osteogenic sarcoma. Report of a histologically verified case. Amer. J. Surg. 113, 537–541 (1967)

SIEBERNS, H. et al.: Bone tumors in the angiographic pictures. Langenbecks Arch. klin. Chir. 311, 131–150 (1965)

SMITH, A.M., BECKER, J.A.: Malignant mesenchymoma of the retroperitoneum. Amer. J. Roentgenol. 104, 389–393 (1968)

SODYKLOV, A.G.: Experience with artrtiography in bone tumors. Khirurgiia (Moskva) 41, 99–103 (1956)

STABPLE, T.W., EVENS, R.G., STEIN, A.H., JR.: Arteriography in orthopedics. Arch. Surg. (Chicago) 97, 682–690 (1968)

STECKEL, R.J.: Usefulness of extremity arteriography in special situations. Radiology 86, 293–297 (1966)

STENER, B., WICKBOM, I.: Angiography in three cases of muscle rupture with organizing haematoma. Acta radiol. (Stockh.) 4, 169–176 (1966)

STRICKLAND, B.: The value of arteriography in the diagnosis of bone tumours. Brit. J. Radiol. 32, 705–713 (1959)

SUTTON, D.: Percutaneous arteriography with special reference to peripheral vessels. Brit. J. Radiol. 28, 13–25 (1955)

TEMPLETON, A.W., STEVENS, E., JANSEN, C.: Arteriographic evaluation of soft tissue masses. Sth. med. J. (B'gham, Ala.) 59, 1255–1295 (1966)

TILLING, G.: The vascular anatomy of long bones. Acta radiol. (Stockh.) Suppl. 161 (1958)

TILLMAN, B.P., DAHLIN, D.C., LIPSCOMB, R.E., STEWART, J.R.: Aneurysmal bone cyst. An analysis of 95 cases. Mayo Clin. Proc. 43, 478–495 (1968)

TRUETA, J.: The normal vascular anatomy of the human femoral head during growth. J. Bone Jt Surg. 39, 358–362 (1957)

VINIK, M.N., JR., FREED, T.A.: Retroperitoneal angiography. Sth. med. J. (B'gham, Ala.) 61, 645–650 (1968)

VOEGELI, M.D., UEHLINGER, M.D.: Arteriography in bone tumors. Skeletal Radiol. 1, 3–14 (1976)

VOGELSANG, H., WIEDENMANN, O.: Angiographic findings in giant cell tumors and benign osteoblastoma of the cervical spine. Fortschr. Röntgenstr. 110, 843–851 (1969)

VOGLER, E.: Results of angiography in disease of the bone. Radiol. Austria 12, 13–26 (1961)

VOGLER, E., DEU, W.: Wert der Angiographie in der Tumordiagnostik der Extremitäten. Fortschr. Röntgenstr. 83, 158–169 (1955)

YAGHMAI, I., SHAMSA, A.Z., SHARIAT, S., AFSHARI, R.: Value of arteriography in the diagnosis of benign and malignant bone lesions. Cancer (Philad.) 27, 1135–1147 (1971)

ZUCCHI, V.: Aneurysmal osseous cysts: Angiographic study. Arch. Ortop. (Milano) 76, 27–42 (1963)

ZUCCHI, V., ALLEGRINI, R.: Angiographic diagnosis in the eccentric subperiosteal variety of aneurysmal bone cyst. Atti. Accad. Med. Lombard. 22, 197–207 (1962)

High-Resolution Radiographic Techniques
for the Detection and Study of Skeletal Neoplasms

by

Harry K. Genant and Kunio Doi

An interdisciplinary approach to the diagnosis of skeletal neoplasms is essential. Such an approach requires the specialized training and expertise of the clinician, radiologist, and pathologist. Although, in this setting, the pathologist functions as the final arbiter, his decision is necessarily predicated upon clinical and radiographic features as well as specific gross and histologic changes in the tumor specimen (SPJUT et al., 1970; LICHTENSTEIN, 1972; DAHLIN, 1970; JAFFE, 1958; AEGERTER and KIRKPATRICK, 1975).

Careful radiographic analysis of a skeletal neoplasm provides useful information regarding location, shape, size, and extent of the lesion. Moreover, the aggressiveness of a neoplasm may be assessed frequently by careful study of the appearance of host response within the bone (JOHNSON, 1953; NORMAN and ULIN, 1969; EDEIKEN et al., 1966; MILCH and CHANGUS, 1956; LODWICK, 1965, 1971). Patterns of lysis, sclerosis, margination, periosteal reaction, or involvement of soft tissue provide helpful clues as to the biologic nature of the lesion. Internal characteristics, such as formation of matrix, may provide information regarding the type of histologic cell.

For accurate and detailed assessment of the subtle radiographic features, image quality may be of considerable importance (GENANT et al., 1975a; ROSSMANN, 1969; NORMAN and WU, 1966; GORDON et al., 1973; TAKAHASHI et al., 1966). To maximize diagnostic information, high-resolution radiographic techniques have been developed. The purpose of this chapter is to examine, quantitatively, the fundamental imaging properties and, qualitatively, the clinical applications of the conventional and newer high-resolution magnification techniques.

Magnification techniques in skeletal radiography have received increased attention in recent years (MALL et al., 1973a; MEEMA and SCHATZ, 1970; MEEMA and MEEMA, 1972; ISHIGAKI, 1973; WEISS, 1972; BERENS and LIN, 1969). This expansion of the technique has resulted from three factors; a) advances in roentgen technology; b) optimization of physical parameters and exposing factors; and c) delineation of the meaningful areas for clinical application. High-resolution magnification is achieved by two different techniques (DOI et al., 1976; GENANT et al., 1975a). The first is optical magnification of fine-grain films, and the second is direct radiographic magnification (Figs. 1a, b).

The optical magnification technique (GENANT et al., 1975a; MEEMA and SCHATZ, 1970; WEISS, 1972) consists of contact exposures obtained with conventional roentgen equipment and fine-grain industrial film, such as Kodak Type M. Clinical studies with this technique are not new. FLETCHER and ROWLEY (1951, 1952), in the early 1950's reported their experience when fine-grain film and photographic enlargement were employed for the study of peripheral arthritis. In a monograph published in 1969, BERENS

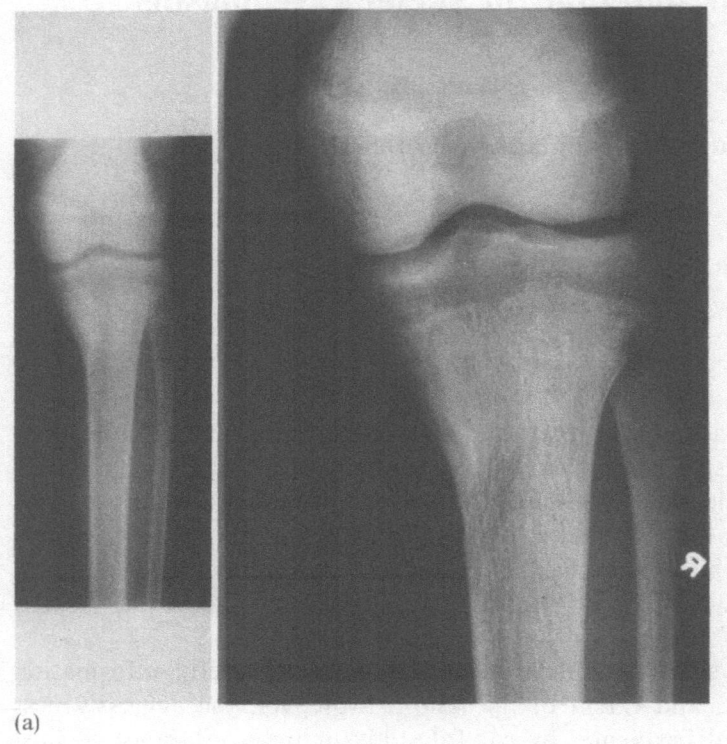

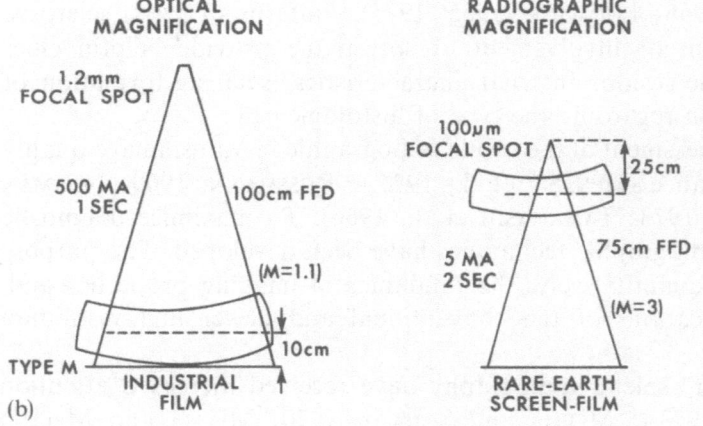

Fig. 1a and b. Optical and radiographic magnification techniques. (a) Image on left of knee was obtained with industrial Type M film and is optically magnified for interpretation. Image on right is direct radiographic magnification (3X), using microfocus tube and screen-film system. (b) The two techniques are compared schematically with optical magnification on left and direct magnification on right

and Lin reported their observations in rheumatoid arthritis with the use of industrial film and optical magnification. More recently, Meema and Schatz (1970), Meema and Meema (1972), Weiss (1972), Genant et al. (1973, 1975b, 1976) and Mall et al. (1973, 1974) have reported extensive experience with this technique in various metabolic and arthritic skeletal disorders. Thus, the clinical importance of the optical magnification technique for assessment of selected skeletal disorders appears established, although its application in the evaluation of bone tumors has been limited (Fletcher and Rowley, 1951; Fornasier and Horne, 1975).

　　Direct radiographic magnification for skeletal radiography has received far less attention than has optical magnification. Only with the recent development of roentgen tubes, whose very small focal spots are 50–100 μ in size and whose output for clinical examination is adequate, has this technique become available (TAKAHASHI et al., 1966; BOOKSTEIN and VOEGELI, 1971; DOI and ROSSMAN, 1974). Limited clinical experience with direct radiographic magnification of the skeleton has been reported by GORDON et al. (1973), ISHIGAKI (1973), DOI et al. (1976), and GENANT et al. (1975a). The initial results have been promising and applications for both thin and thick body parts are being established (GENANT et al., 1976).

A. Radiographic Techniques

The standard technique (GENANT et al., 1975a) for *optical magnification* employs Kodak industrial Type M film, which is exposed with approximately 50–60 kVp, 500 mA, and 0.5 sec at 100 cm focus-to-film distance. A conventional roentgen tube with a 1.2 mm focal-spot is used for these contact exposures and the inherent magnification for thin parts is low (approximately 1.01 to 1.04×, DOI et al., 1975a, 1976). Thus, for the peripheral skeleton, exposure times are relatively short, and geometric unsharpness is minimal because of the low degree of inherent magnification. The industrial film must be developed manually, or by means of an industrial processor. To achieve high contrast, the industrial film should be exposed fairly "dark" to an optical density of approximately 2. If industrial

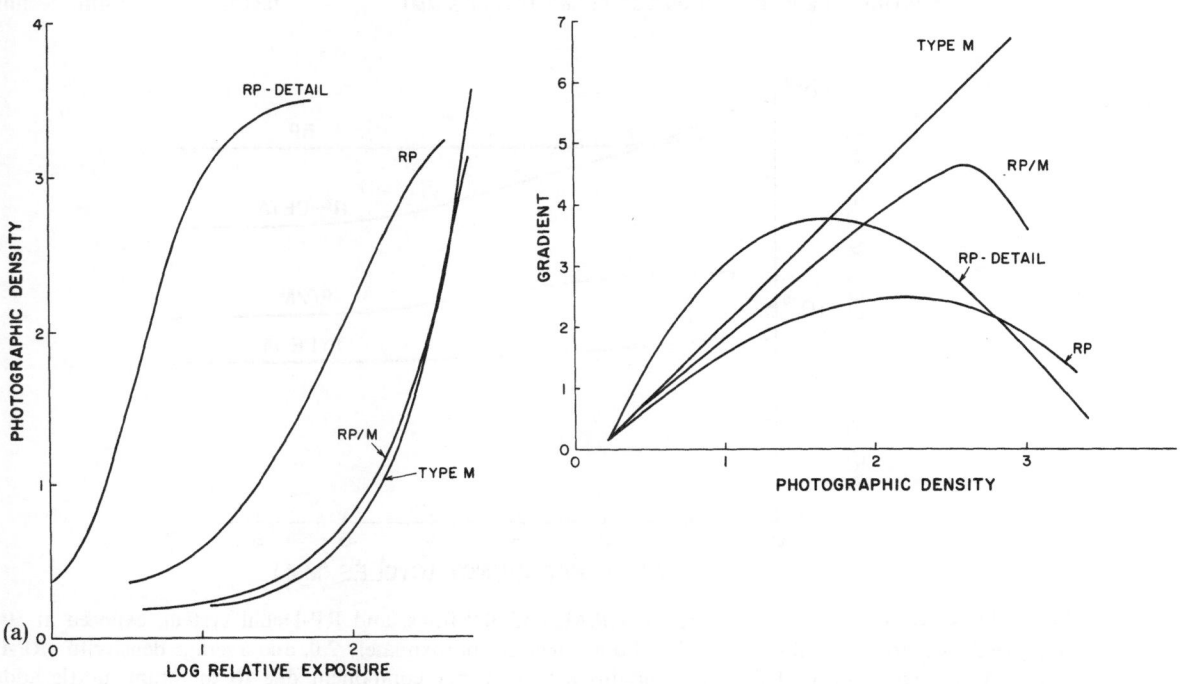

Figs. 2a and b. H & D curves and gradient curves for Type M, RP/M, and RP film, and RP-Detail system. RP film, exposed without screens, shows low contrast and slow speed compared with RP-Detail system. Type M film shows slightly higher contrast than does RP/M, and speed for Type M is nearly same as that of RP/M. The gradient of Type M film increases approximately in proportion to photographic density. The peak of gradient for RP-Detail is at photographic density slightly less than 2.0

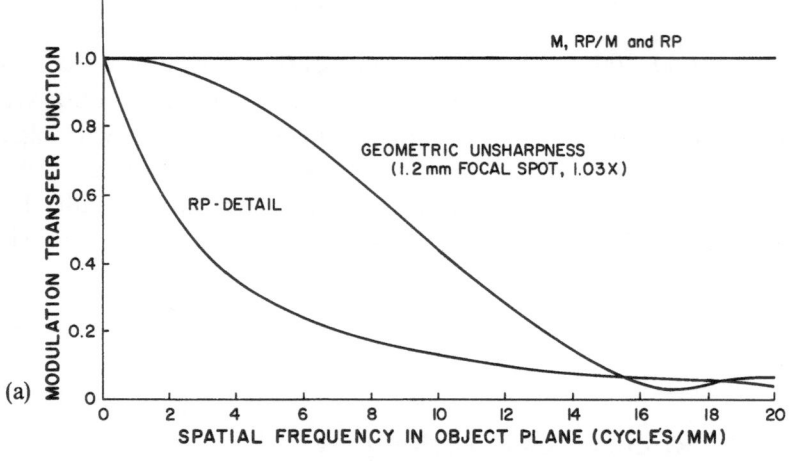

(a)

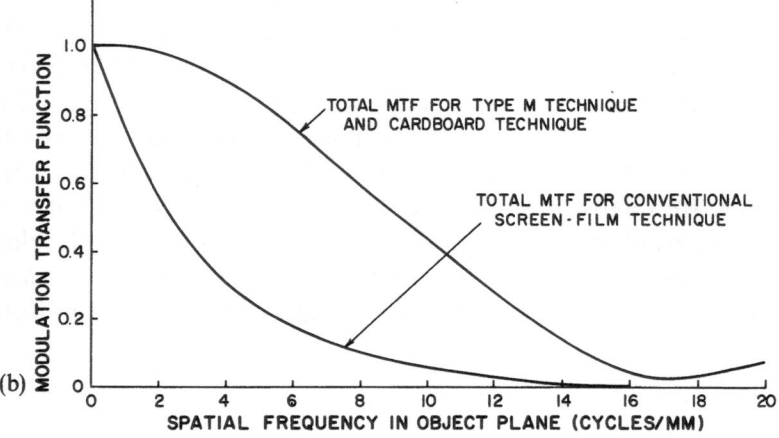

(b)

Fig. 3. (a) Modulation transfer functions (MTFs) of recording system and geometric unsharpness. MTFs of Type M, RP/M, and RP films are nearly perfect at spatial frequencies of less than 20 cyc/mm. By comparison, MTF of RP-Detail is quite poor. Geometric unsharpness, common to Type M technique and to conventional techniques, is caused by 1.2 mm focal-spot and 1.03X magnification. (b) Total MTFs for three techniques. Total MTF is derived as product of recording system MTF and geometric unsharpness MTF. Total MTF for Type M technique and cardboard technique is identical, and is considerably higher than total MTF for conventional screen-film technique. For Type M and cardboard techniques, geometric unsharpness is dominant factor that affects resolution, whereas screen-film unsharpness is determining factor for screen-film technique

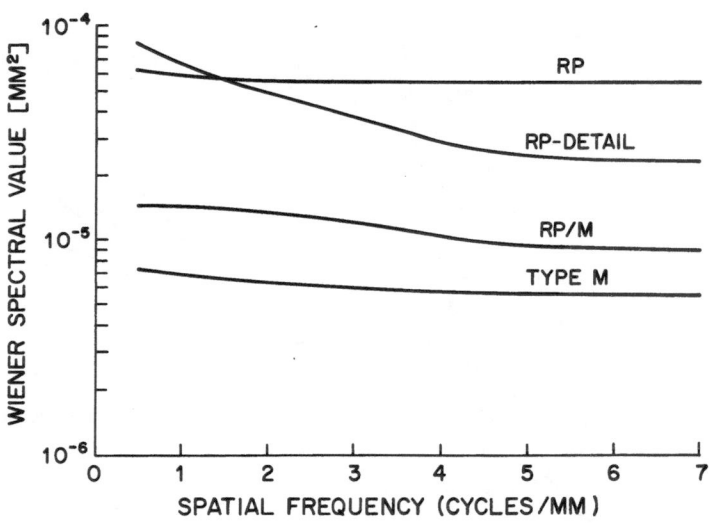

Fig. 4. Noise Wiener spectra for Type M, RP/M, and RP films, and RP-Detail system, exposed at 50 kVp. Average density for x-ray films exposed without screen is approximately 2.0, and average density for RP-Detail is 1.5. Wiener spectrum of RP-Detail contains low frequency component due to quantum mottle added to film graininess, whereas three x-ray films, RP, RP/M, and M, have rather uniform distribution over spatial frequency range measured. Noise in Type M is approximately one-tenth noise in RP medical film. Noise in RP/M is approximately twice noise in Type M film. Noise in RP with Detail screens and RP with direct exposure are more comparable. In higher frequency range, however, noise in RP is greater, possibly due to differing film response to direct x-ray exposure as compared to screen light exposure. Noise in these films with direct x-ray exposure decreases markedly with decreasing average density, whereas the noise in RP-Detail changes in a complicated manner. At average density of 2.0 for RP-Detail, noise in low frequency decreases slightly and noise in high frequency increases

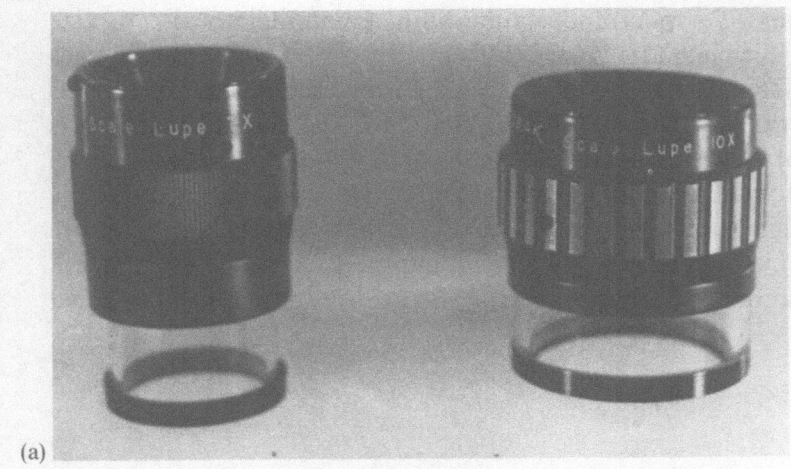
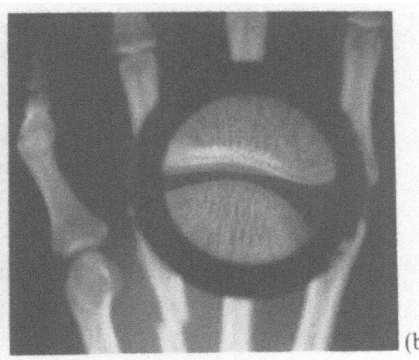
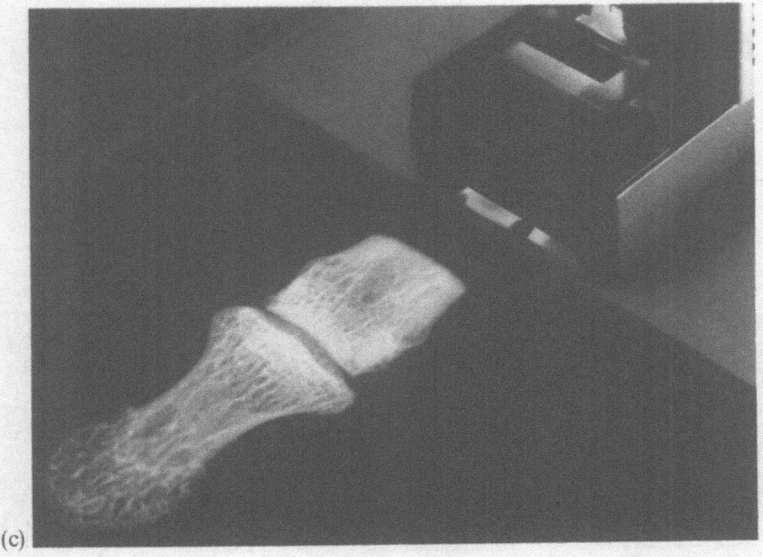

Fig. 5. (a) Typical lupes for optical magnification contain focusing eyepiece and magnify four to ten times. (b) Lupe is placed in direct contact with fine-grain industrial film and image thus viewed at close range. (c) For group-viewing, projector such as Leitz Macro Promar is used

film is underexposed, or "light," the contrast is poor (GENANT et al., 1975a). In practice the type M film is "sandwiched" together with a fine-grain rapid process film (Kodak RP/M) and the two are simultaneously exposed. The speed and resolution of Kodak RP/M film are approximately the same as those of the Type M film but the graininess is appreciably greater (Figs. 2–4). The RP/M film is developed immediately in a standard X-omat processor and is checked for quality. The Type M film is processed when convenient, and viewed for definitive interpretation. The completed industrial radiographs are surveyed without magnification initially, and then viewed with a hand-lens or a projector for optical magnification. Such magnification is important to take full advantage of the Type M film since fine bone structure may not be visible to the unaided eye. For individual viewing, a lupe or hand-lens (GENANT et al., 1975a; MEEMA and SCHATZ, 1970) is most convenient, whereas for demonstration or for group viewing, a projector (MALL et al., 1973; MEEMA, 1973) is most convenient (Figs. 5a–c).

The *radiographic magnification* technique (DOI et al., 1976; GENANT et al., 1975a; TAKAHASHI et al., 1966, 1974; ISHIGAKI, 1973) consists of direct geometric magnification of two to four times by means of a microfocus tube with a nominal focal-spot size of 50–100 μ (RSI MFT 1 or Siemens BI 125/3/50 RG roentgen tubes). The images are recorded onto recording systems of relatively high resolution, such as detail screens for the thin body parts, and rare-earth screen-film systems for the thicker body parts (GENANT et al., 1976). Typical exposure factors consist of 50–80 kVp, 3–5 mA (which is a maximum mA setting of several of the commercially available roentgen tubes), 0.5–2 sec and 50–80 cm focus-film distance (Fig. 1 b). Because of the relatively long exposure time, motion unsharpness is introduced unless careful immobilization is maintained. The films are processed in a standard X-omat processor and are viewed with the unaided eye.

B. Comparison of Images Using Magnification Techniques

I. Optical Magnification

A comparison of the imaging properties (GENANT et al., 1976) of the Type M film technique and two widely used conventional techniques for peripheral skeletal radiography are shown in Fig. 6. The Type M technique is compared with (1) a standard,

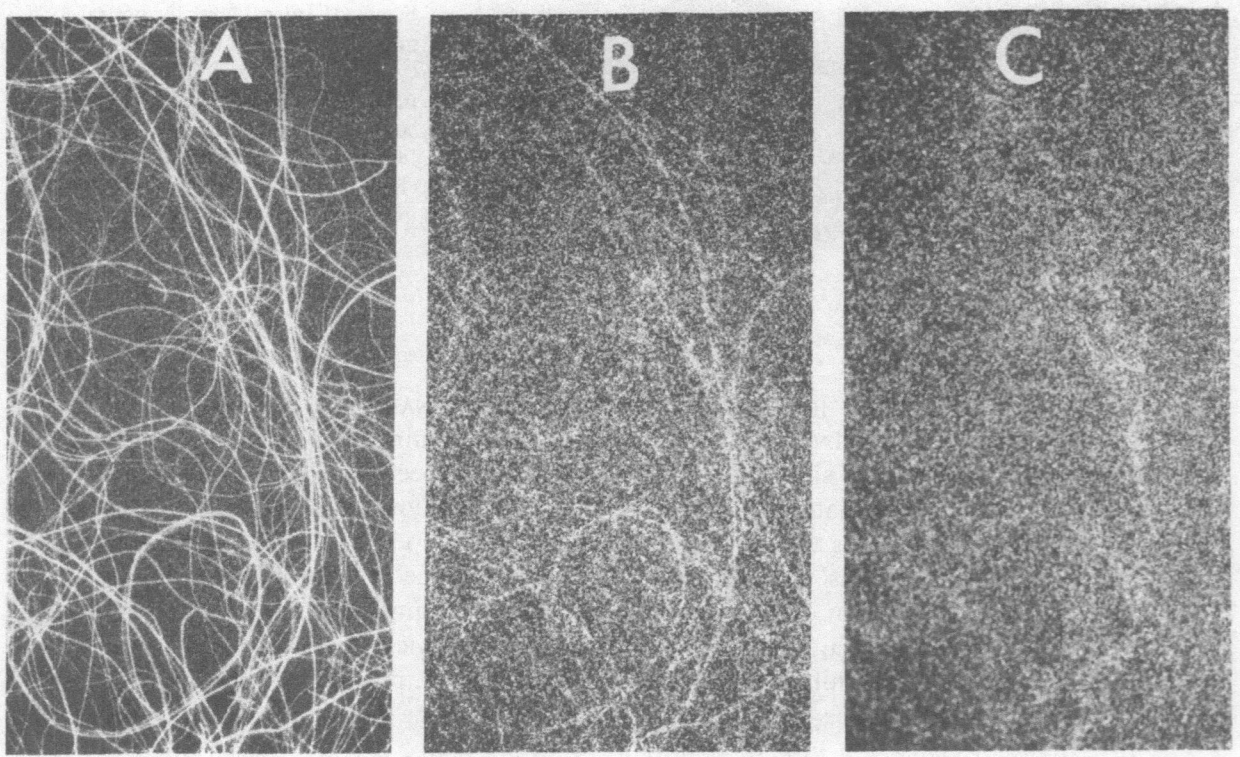

Fig. 6a–c. For qualitative comparison, fine steel wool has been radiographed with Type M technique (a), nonscreen cardboard technique with medical RP film (b), and fine screen-film system, RP-Detail (c). Type M technique affords higher resolution, greater contrast, and lower noise when compared with two standard techniques. Images in (b) and (c) are fairly comparable

nonscreen cardboard technique achieved with medical RP film and (2) a fine, screen-film system in which Dupont Detail screens and Kodak RP medical film are used. The small wire structures are best imaged with the Type M technique because of higher resolution, lower noise (or smoother background appearance), and greater contrast (Doi et al., 1976; GENANT et al., 1976). These imaging properties, i.e., resolution, noise, and contrast, are compared quantitatively by means of modulation transfer functions (MTFs), Wiener spectral analyses, and gradient curves, respectively (Figs. 2–4).

The MTF describes the signal-transmitting capability of the imaging system in the spatial frequency domain, which is often compared to the frequency response of a communication system. The MTF is defined as the ratio of the amplitude of the image to the amplitude of the sinusoidal object, expressed as a function of the spatial frequency. The higher the MTF value, the better the imaging system, i.e., the image obtained will resemble more closely the object. The ideal imaging system in regard to resolution is one that contains a flat MTF curve. The MTF may be measured by a number of methods (Doi and ROSSMANN, 1975; Doi et al., 1975b; and BATES, 1969) for imaging components such as the screen-film system and the roentgen tube focal-spot. The experimental data in this chapter were derived from the Fourier transformation of slit images. The Wiener spectral value of noise is plotted against the spatial frequency (Fig. 4). For Wiener spectra of similar shape, the higher the spectral value, the greater the noise level. The noise with a high-frequency component corresponds to the fine-noise pattern, whereas the noise at low frequencies corresponds to the coarse pattern. The Wiener spectra are determined by an electronic Fourier analysis method (Doi and ROSSMANN, 1975), in which the film is scanned circularly by a light-spot and fluctuating noise-signal in a photomultiplier that corresponds to the radiographic noise and is analyzed by an electronic wave-analyzer. The gradient is the slope of the characteristic (H & D) curve and is determined by the tangent at any point on the curve. It is taken as a measure of the inherent contrast of the recording system. The gradient curve is a plot of gradient against density. The H & D curve is measured by use of the roentgen inverse-square sensitometer.

Of the two conventional techniques quantified in Figures 2–4 and displayed in Figure 6, the cardboard technique has higher resolution and lower contrast than the fine screen-film system, and the noise is comparable. The over-all image quality for the cardboard and fine screen-film techniques is comparable, and far inferior to the Type M technique. Thus, the superior imaging properties of the Type M technique permit optical magnification of up to ten times for improved detection of subtle abnormalities. When the Type M technique and conventional techniques (Figs. 7–9), were compared in the peripheral skeleton, the delineation of bone destruction and host response was superior with the former technique. Radiation exposure is high, however, resulting in approximately 1 rad to the hand or foot, compared to $1/_3$ this dose for cardboard technique, and $1/_{70}$ this dose for Detail screens (GENANT et al., 1976). For this reason, the industrial film with optical magnification should be used *selectively* in those instances in which delineation of subtle abnormalities in the peripheral skeleton is important.

II. Optical Vs. Radiographic Magnification

More proximally from the peripheral skeleton, where skeletal neoplasms generally originate, the body parts become thicker and the optical magnification technique with Type M becomes less feasible. The limitations are attributed to the high radiation exposure

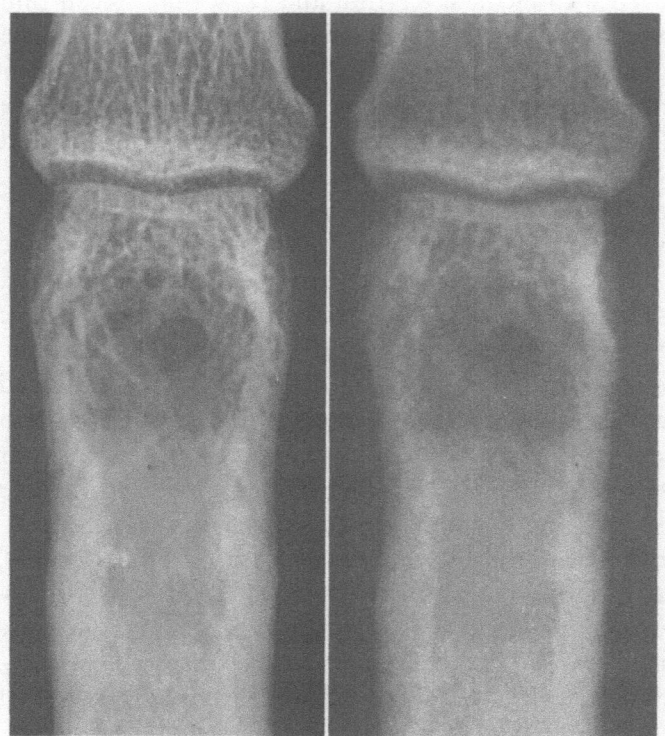

Fig. 7. Permeative lytic destruction with reticulated appearance in phalanx of patient with sarcoidosis. Subtle destructive changes are seen to advantage with Type M industrial film technique on left compared to cardboard technique with medical RP film on right

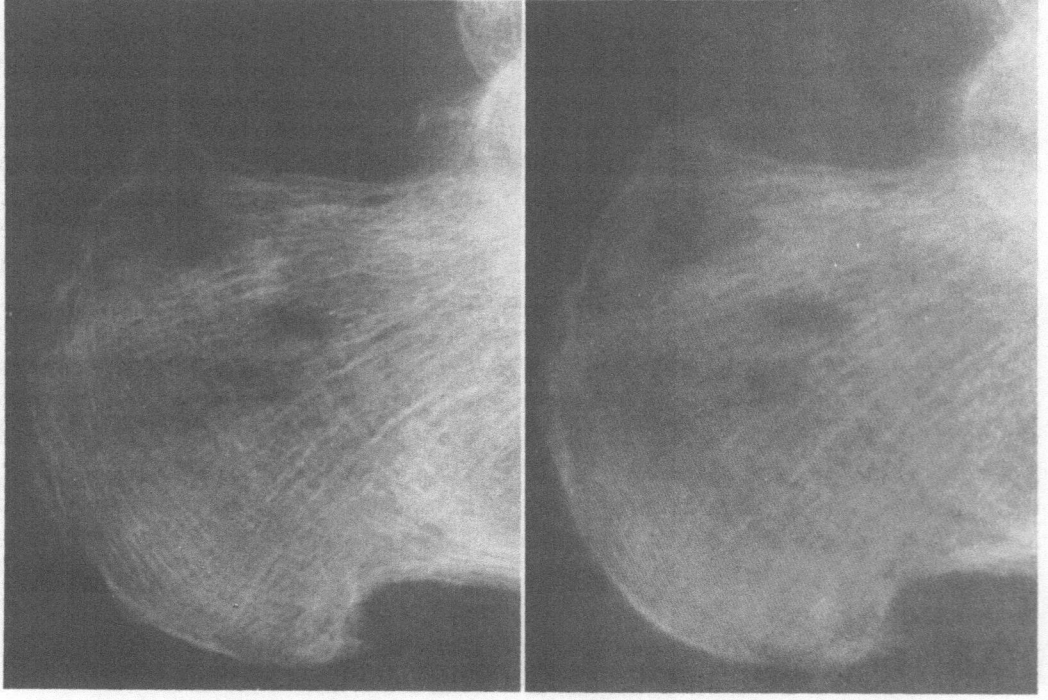

Fig. 8. Poorly defined, lytic destruction of cancellous bone in calcaneus and minimal reactive sclerosis in adjacent trabeculae in patient with metastatic uterine carcinoma. Type M industrial film on left clearly delineates destructive pattern, whereas Detail screen on right shows only gross changes

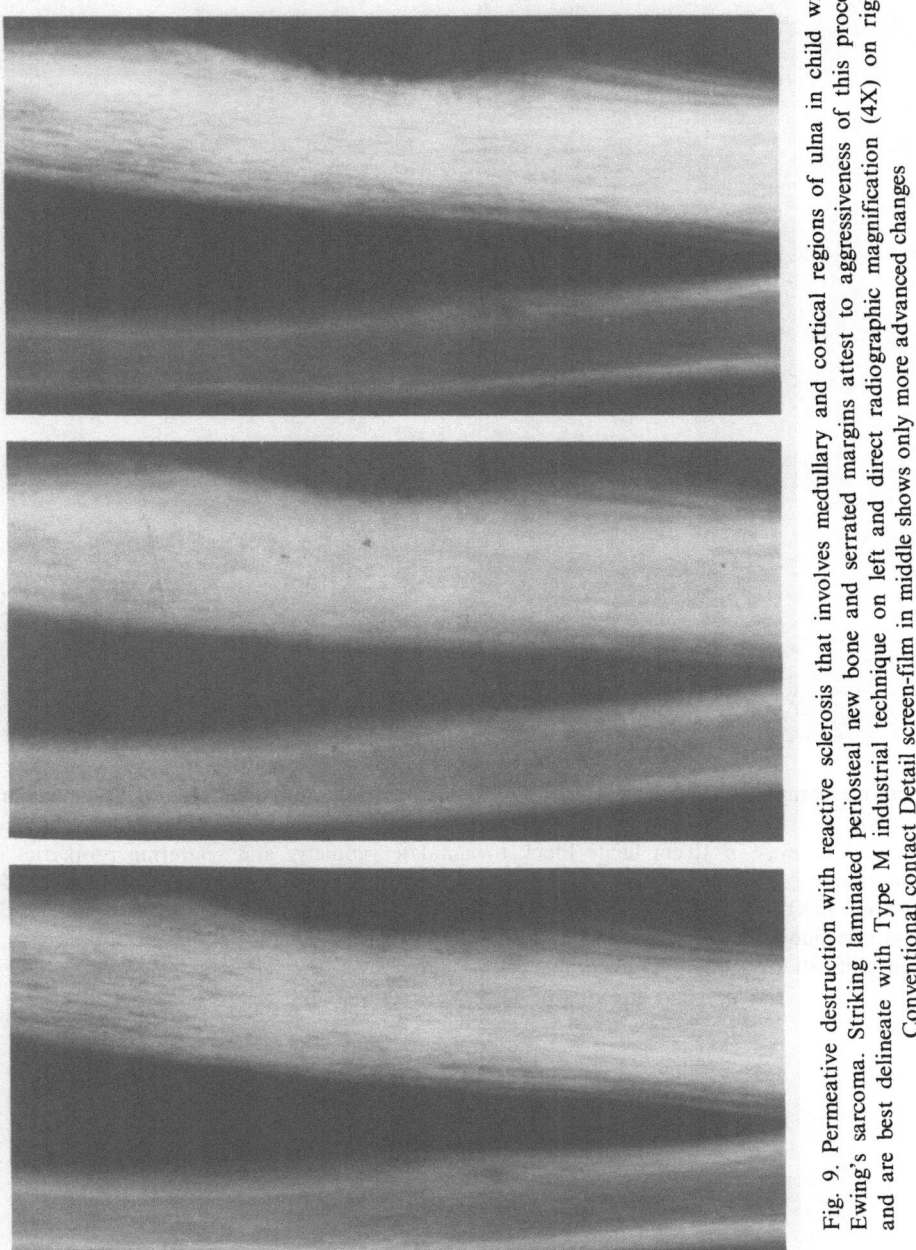

Fig. 9. Permeative destruction with reactive sclerosis that involves medullary and cortical regions of ulna in child with Ewing's sarcoma. Striking laminated periosteal new bone and serrated margins attest to aggressiveness of this process and are best delineate with Type M industrial technique on left and direct radiographic magnification (4X) on right. Conventional contact Detail screen-film in middle shows only more advanced changes

required and to the degradation of image quality related to increased geometric unsharpness, blurring by motion, and radiation scatter (DOI et al., 1976; GENANT et al., 1975a).

Direct radiographic magnification with the microfocus tube provides a reasonable alternative. In Figure 10, a comparison is shown of the imaging capability of the two high-resolution techniques – Type M and direct radiographic magnification – for a wire mesh test-object that simulates the geometry and scattering properties of the knee. As can be seen, the image obtained with the direct magnification is slightly superior to that of the Type M technique and results in approximately one-half to one-fourth the radiation exposure (DOI et al., 1976; GENANT et al., 1975a). These conclusions are supported quantitatively by means of the MTF and Wiener spectral data (Fig. 11).

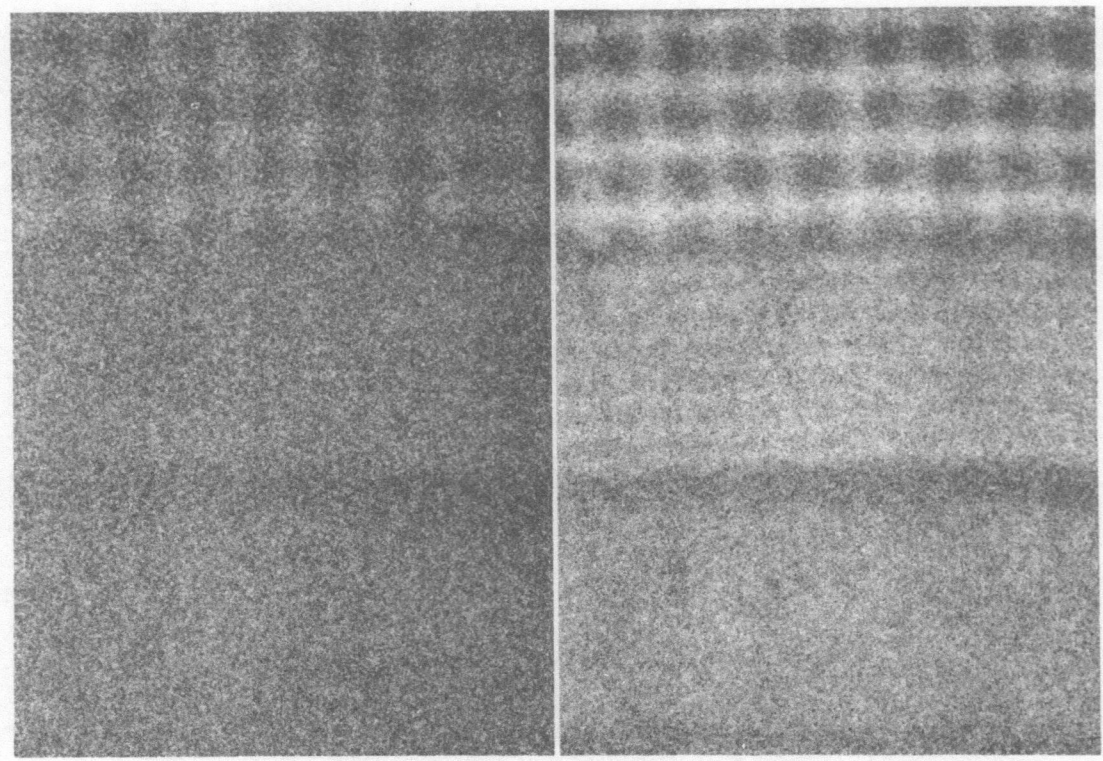

Fig. 10. Qualitative comparison between Type M technique on left and direct radiographic magnification technique on right. A wire mesh test-object, which has spatial frequencies of 4, 8, and 12 line pairs per mm was embedded midway in 10 cm lucite block to simulate geometry and scattering properties of knee. For Type M technique on left, a 1.2 mm focal-spot was used at focus-film distance of 100 cm (1.05X). For direct magnification (3X), nominal 100 μ focal spot was used at a focus-film distance of 65 cm. Radiographs are equalized in size photographically to facilitate visual comparison. Quality of image obtained with direct radiographic magnification on right is superior, yet radiation exposure for this image was approximately one-third that of Type M technique on left

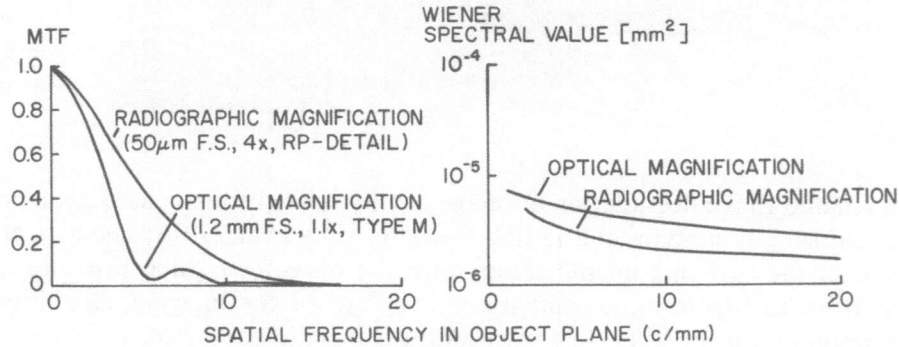

Fig. 11. Comparison of total MTFs and Wiener spectra for optical and radiographic magnification techniques for knee. Total MTF for radiographic magnification is higher than that for optical magnification, which is caused by increased geometric unsharpness for knee. Wiener spectrum for radiographic magnification is lower than that for optical magnification, mainly from effect of reduction of noise by radiographic magnification technique

Optical Vs. Radiographic Magnification 687

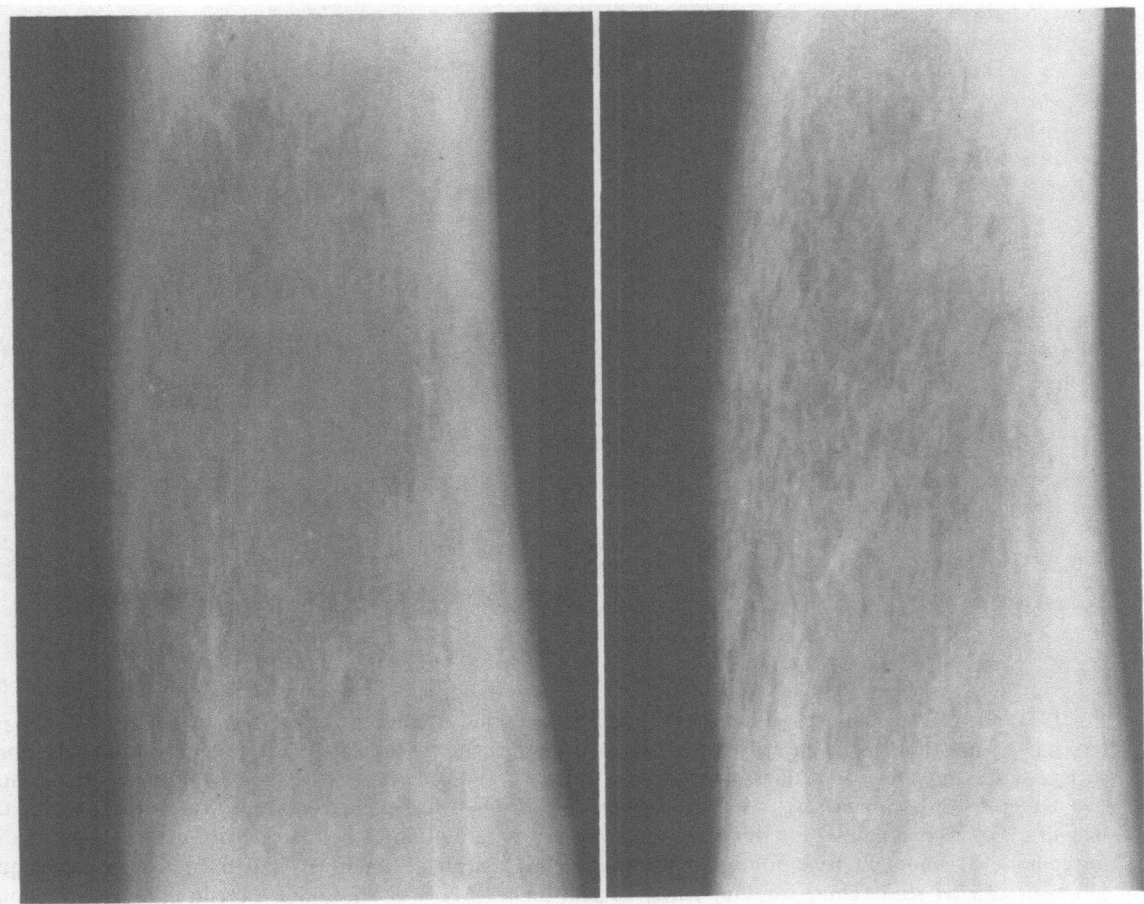

Fig. 12. Permeative destruction with reactive sclerosis that involves cortical and medullary region and is associated with periosteal new bone can be seen with both Type M technique on left and direct radiographic magnification (4X) on right. Quality of the image with the two techniques is fairly comparable, although magnification technique required approximately one-third radiation exposure to the patient

The total MTF, which is derived as the product of the MTF of the screen-film and geometric unsharpness, is lower for optical magnification than for radiographic magnification. The reason for this difference is that in optical magnification geometric unsharpness is considerable because of the increased thickness of the knee compared to a thin part, such as of hand. The Wiener spectrum for "effective" noise in radiographic magnification is lower than that in optical magnification, despite the greater inherent noise in the recording system for radiographic magnification. The effective noise, i.e., the noise in the recording system relative to the size of the original object, however, is reduced by radiographic magnification. This reduction is produced by the increased size of the input roentgen pattern to the screen-film system, with a resultant improvement in the effective noise. In clinical examples, in which optical *and* radiographic magnification were employed to view neoplasms of the appendicular skeleton similar diagnostic information was obtained with each for relatively thin body parts (Figs. 9, 12).

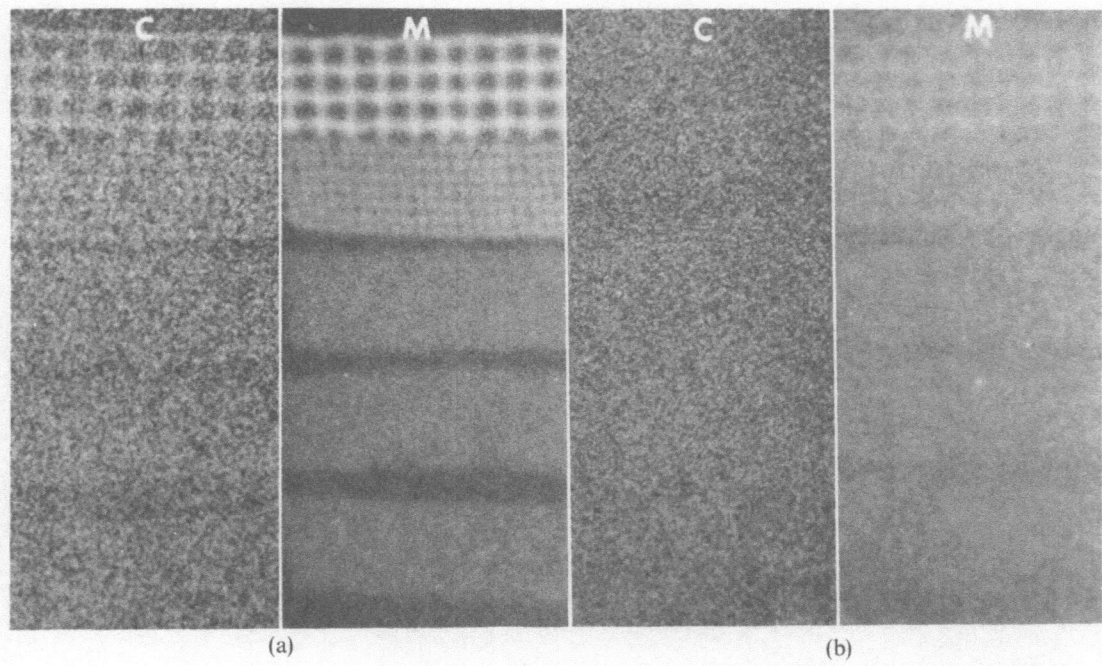

Fig. 13a and b. Wire mesh test-object that contains cyclic fine structures ranging from 4 to 20 line pairs per mm has been radiographed in appropriate thicknesses of lucite to simulate clinical conditions for thin part such as ankle (a) and for a thick part such as hip (b). (a) Conventional technique for thin parts, images two larger sets of wire meshes, which correspond to 4 and 8 line pairs per mm. Next to this image the magnification technique (M) for thin parts similarly shows resolution of two larger wire meshes. Appreciably lower noise or smoother background appearance, as well as greater contrast with magnification technique, however, can be seen. Thus, for thin parts, despite higher MTF or resolution of conventional technique, magnification technique is superior because of higher contrast and lower noise levels. (b) For thick parts with conventional technique (C), none of wire meshes are seen. With magnification technique (M), coarse wire mesh corresponding to 4 line pairs per mm can be seen. Again lower noise-level of magnification technique relative to conventional technique can be appreciated. (See Fig. 14 for corresponding physical data)

III. Radiographic Magnification

The direct radiographic magnification technique, then, unlike the optical magnification technique, may be applied readily to either thin or thick parts of the body. Insight into the value of the direct radiographic magnification compared with two widely used conventional techniques is provided by Figure 13, which was obtained as follows. For thin parts, the comparison techniques consist of 1) direct radiographic magnification (3×) onto a high resolution screen-film system (Dupont Lo-Dose) and 2) conventional contact (1.03×) exposure using nonscreen "cardboard" technique with Kodak RP medical film. For thick parts, the comparison consists of 1) direct magnification by means of a rare-earth screen-film system (3M Trimax Alpha 4-XD) and 2) contact exposure using a mid-speed screen-film system (Par-RP) with Bucky technique. These qualitative comparisons show the superiority of direct magnification compared with conventional techniques for both thin and thick parts.

These results are supported and clarified by quantitative analysis of resolution and noise (Figs. 14, 15). For the thin parts, the greatly lower noise with the radiographic

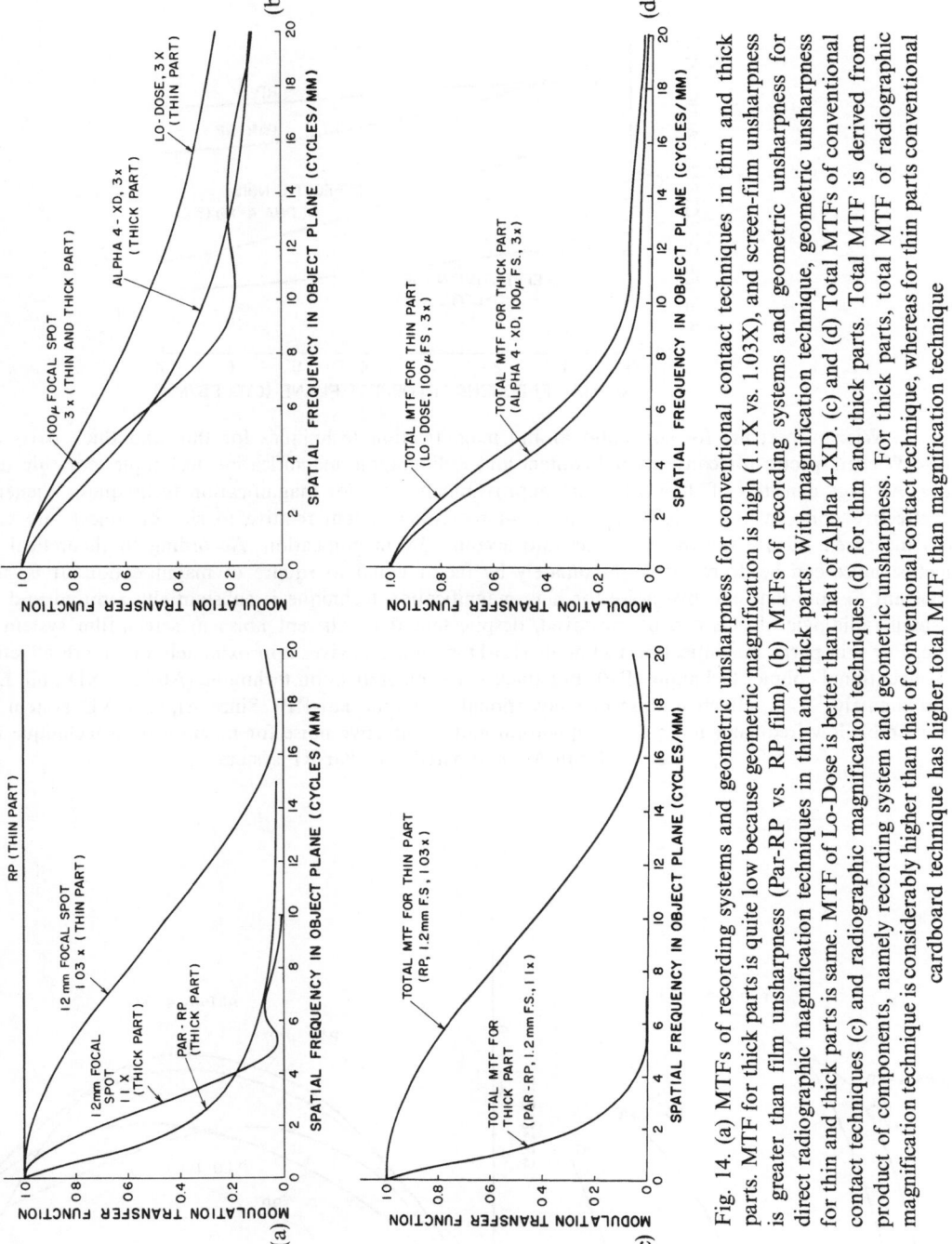

Fig. 14. (a) MTFs of recording systems and geometric unsharpness for conventional contact techniques in thin and thick parts. MTF for thick parts is quite low because geometric magnification is high (1.1X vs. 1.03X), and screen-film unsharpness is greater than film unsharpness (Par-RP vs. RP film). (b) MTFs of recording systems and geometric unsharpness for direct radiographic magnification techniques in thin and thick parts. With magnification technique, geometric unsharpness for thin and thick parts is same. MTF of Lo-Dose is better than that of Alpha 4-XD. (c) and (d) Total MTFs of conventional contact techniques (c) and radiographic magnification techniques (d) for thin and thick parts. Total MTF is derived from product of components, namely recording system and geometric unsharpness. For thick parts, total MTF of radiographic magnification technique is considerably higher than that of conventional contact technique, whereas for thin parts conventional cardboard technique has higher total MTF than magnification technique

magnification technique, accompanied by greater contrast due to the steeper film gradient and air-gap reduction of scatter, more than offset the slightly greater MTF for the cardboard technique. The relative speed of the four recording systems is shown in Figure 16. This figure provides a basis for approximating the relative radiation exposure in patients for the conventional contact and direct-magnification techniques. For thin and thick parts, magnification results in an approximate fourfold increase in exposure per surface area (skin dose), compared to conventional techniques when recording system speeds, air-gap, and grid are considered (GENANT et al., 1976). The size of the field with magnification is significantly reduced, however, which helps lower the total-body radiation (GENANT et al., 1976; TAKAHASHI et al., 1974).

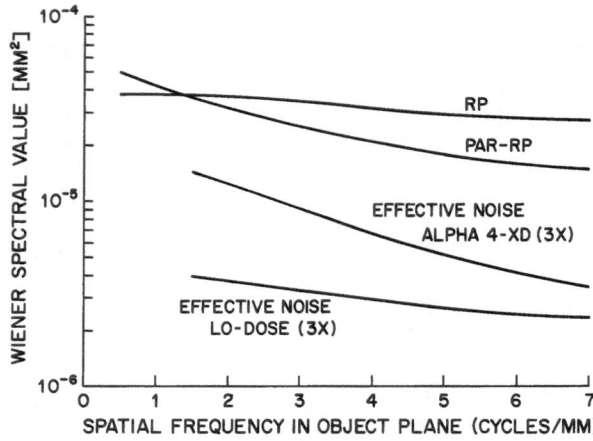

Fig. 15. Wiener spectrum for conventional and magnification techniques for thin and thick parts of body. Noise Wiener spectra for conventional contact and radiographic magnification techniques for thin and thick parts. Average densities of these films are approximately 1.5. For magnification techniques, Wiener spectra for effective noise, which is defined as noise in recording system relative to size of object, are calculated from measured Wiener spectra by taking into account 3X magnification. According to theoretical analysis effective noise can be decreased approximately by factor equal to square of magnification. It is, therefore important to note that effective noise for high magnification technique is substantially reduced and visibility of small radiologic objects can be improved, despite fact that inherent noise in screen-film system remains same. For thin parts, magnification technique (Lo-Dose and 3X) gives approximately one-tenth effective noise of conventional contact technique (RP). For thick parts, magnification technique (Alpha 4-XD and 3X) yields approximately $^1/_2$–$^1/_4$ effective noise of conventional technique Par-RP). Since Alpha 4-XD system contains considerable low frequency noise due to quantum mottle, effective noise for magnification technique increases at low frequency compared with Par-RP system

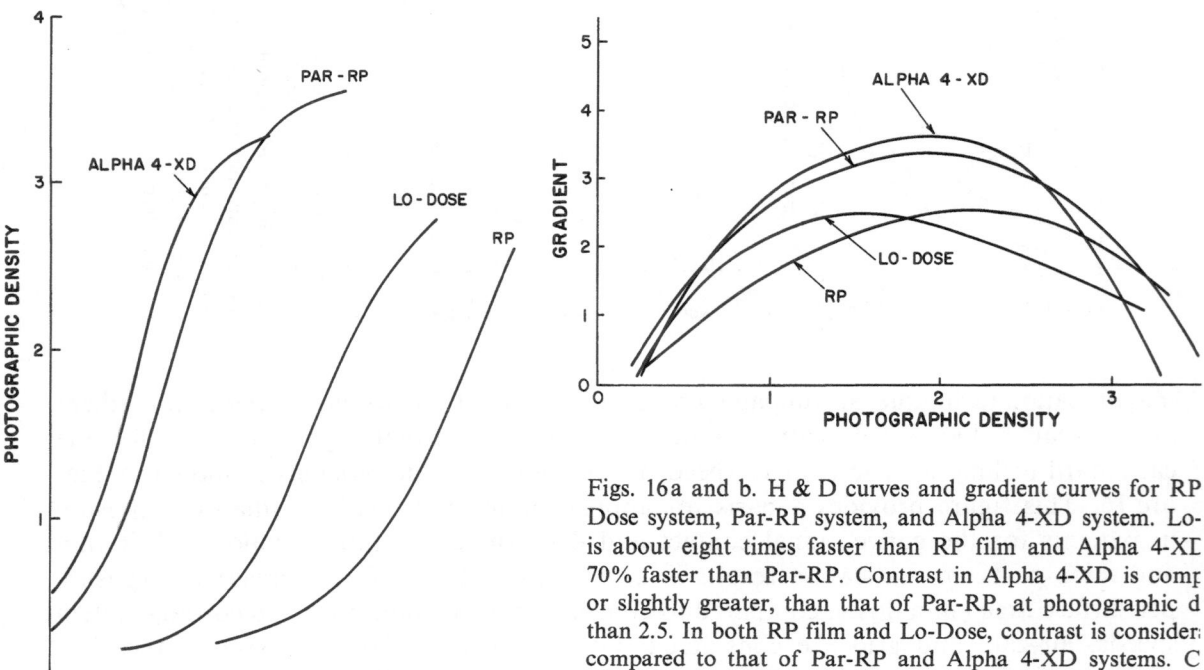

(a)

Figs. 16a and b. H & D curves and gradient curves for RP Dose system, Par-RP system, and Alpha 4-XD system. Lo- is about eight times faster than RP film and Alpha 4-XD 70% faster than Par-RP. Contrast in Alpha 4-XD is comp or slightly greater, than that of Par-RP, at photographic d than 2.5. In both RP film and Lo-Dose, contrast is consider compared to that of Par-RP and Alpha 4-XD systems. C Lo-Dose peaks at photographic density of about 1.5, whe of RP film is at about 2.2

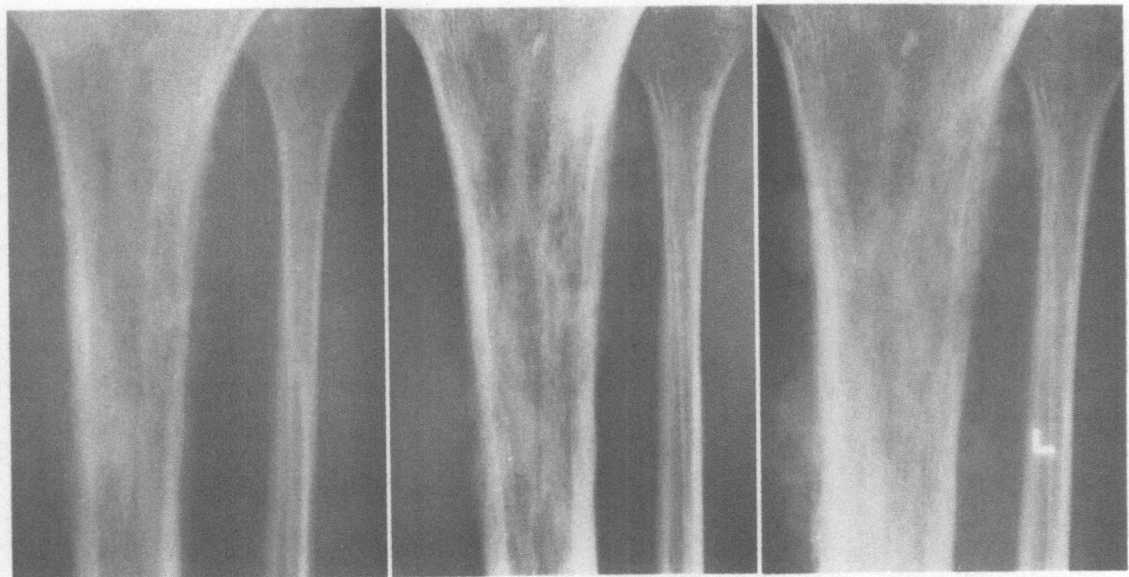

Fig. 17. Proximal tibia of patient with metastatic transitional cell carcinoma of bladder. Direct radiographic magnification film in center view demonstrates irregular lysis and sclerosis that permeates medullary space and cortex, and is associated with subtle periosteal reaction and bone formation in adjacent soft tissues. These important features are difficult to delineate with conventional technique on left, which employed contact exposure and mid-speed screen-film system. 4 weeks later serial magnification view (right) demonstrates remarkable increase in heterotopic bone formation

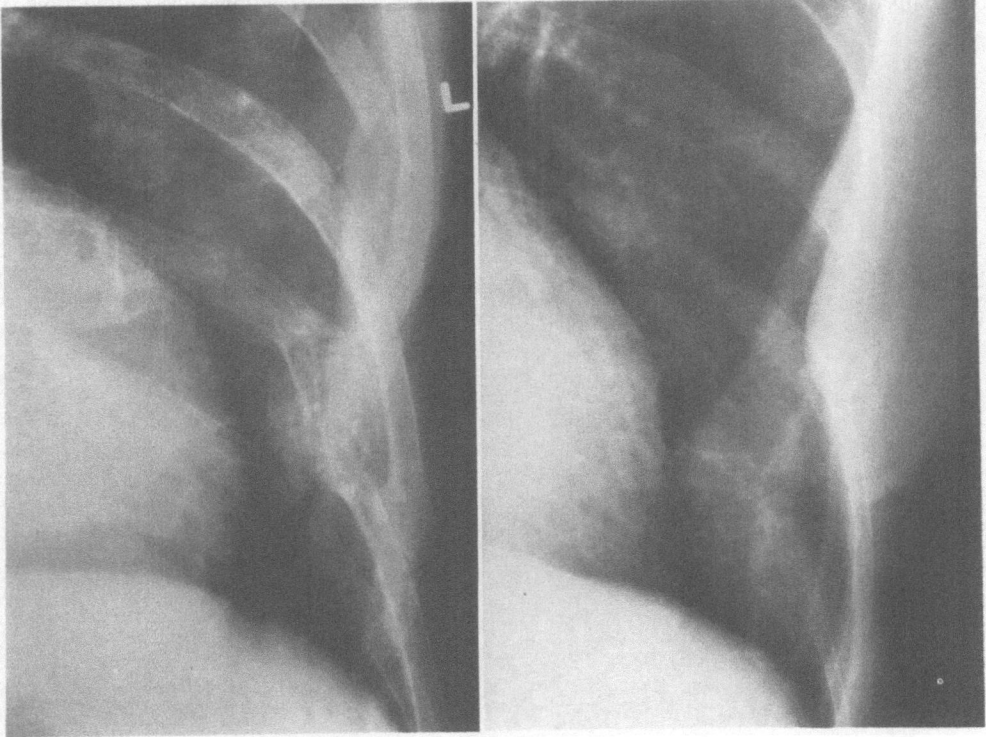

Fig. 18. Metastatic carcinoma of breast that involved ribs and produced mixed lytic and sclerotic destruction, as well as expansion. Conventional radiograph of chest (right) shows lateral soft-tissue mass and suggestion of rib destruction; however, extent of involvement is not well-defined. Direct magnification technique (left) is used frequently when rib lesions are suspected on conventional radiography of chest

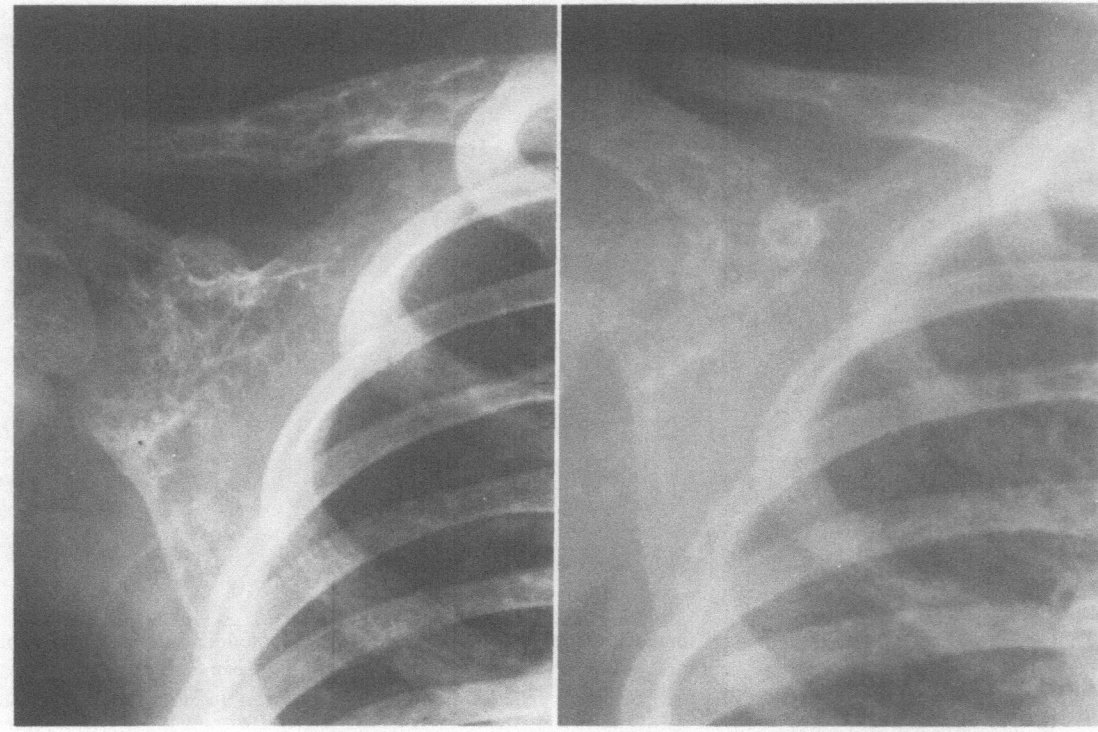

Fig. 19. Multiple well-defined cystic and lytic destructive lesions in scapula and clavicle in patient with hemangio-matosis of bone. Although larger lesions are seen with both techniques, evaluation of extent of involvement is far superior in magnification radiograph (left) compared with conventional chest radiograph (right)

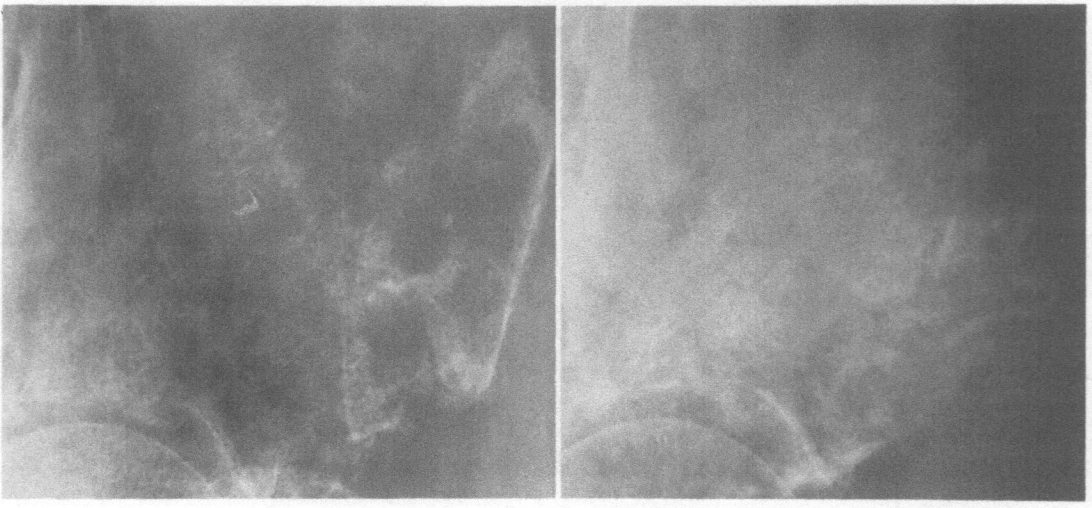

Fig. 20. Large areas of permeative destruction with adjacent reactive sclerosis in trabecular bone can be seen in magnification film (3X) on left and are not seen clearly with conventional Par-speed screen-film system on right in this patient with metastatic bronchogenic carcinoma to ilium

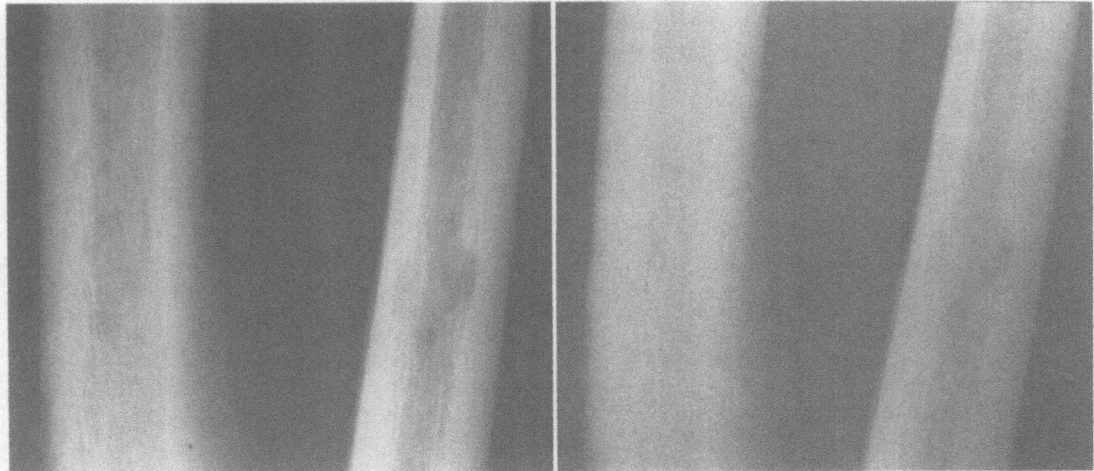

Fig. 21. Discrete areas of lytic destruction that involve medullary space and endosteal surface in patient with multiple myeloma. With cardboard technique, (right) only larger area of destruction is seen compared to magnification technique (3X) which shows multiple destructive sites (left)

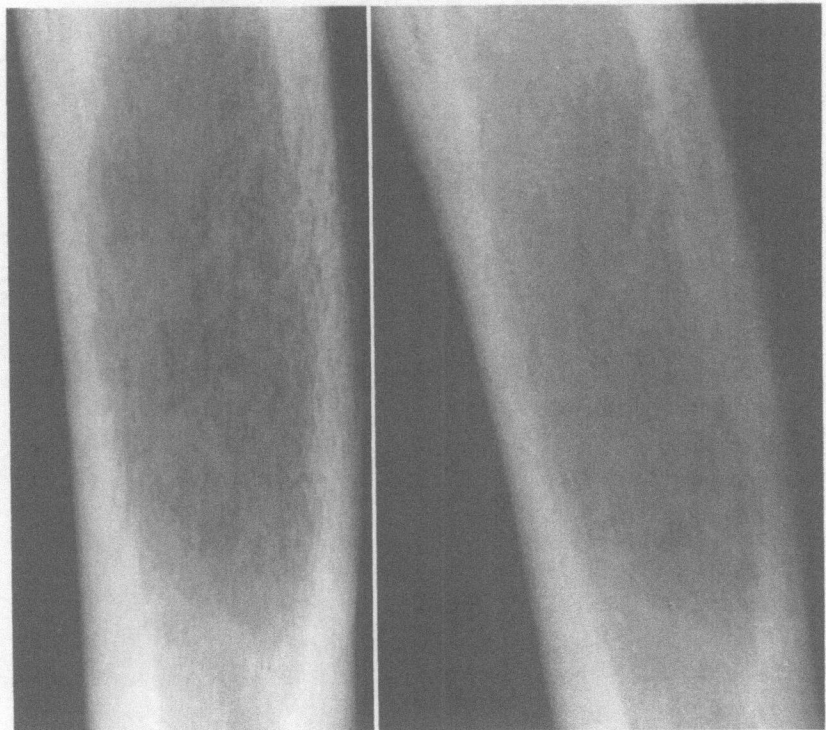

Fig. 22. Permeative destruction that involves endosteal surface and entire thickness of cortex with linear periosteal reaction in Ewing's sarcoma. These features are almost imperceptible on Detail screen technique on right when compared with magnification (4X) on left

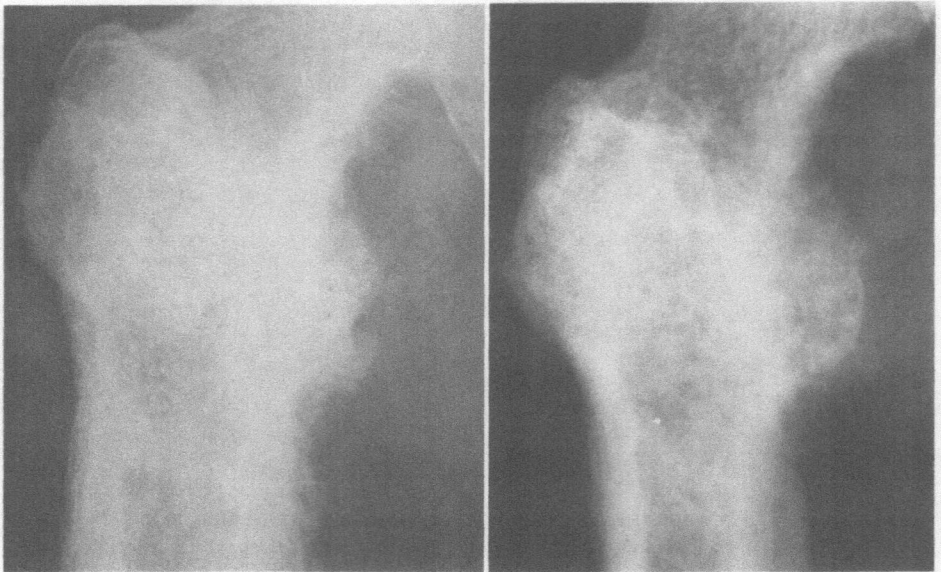

Fig. 23. Densely sclerotic metastatic lesion with both laminated and spiculated periosteal new bone in proximal femur of patient with uterine carcinoma. Gross cortical changes are seen with both techniques; however, fine periosteal changes, which attest to aggressiveness of this lesion, can be assessed only with magnification technique on left compared with conventional Par-speed screen-film system on right

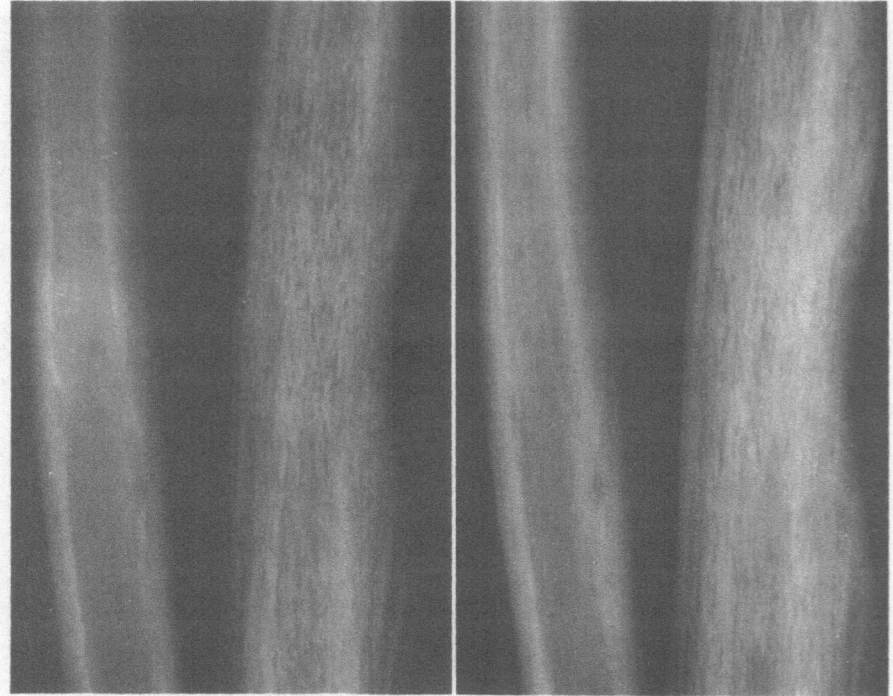

Fig. 24. Serial assessment of response to radiotherapy of Ewing's sarcoma, as viewed with direct magnification technique. On left, laminated periosteal new bone and serrated margins indicate aggressive, rapidly-evolving neoplasm. 6 weeks after radiation therapy, considerable sclerosis of lesion and consolidation of laminated periosteal new bone indicate healing response (right). Such serial assessment is enhanced by high-resolution techniques

A preliminary study in which the value of magnification for skeletal neoplasms was assessed, demonstrated that magnification was helpful in more than 50% of instances, but was essential in only 10% (GENANT et al., 1976).

Clinical examples in which the direct magnification technique was compared with conventional techniques in selected patients with skeletal neoplasms are shown in Figures 17–24. The examinations were largely of the thick body parts, such as ribs, pelvis, hips, spine, and femora. In some, the conventional radiographs appeared normal or equivocal, and magnification films served to delineate permeative, lytic destruction, or subtle periosteal reaction. In other instances, conventional radiography readily demonstrated the presence of the lesion; however, the character or pattern of host-response, and hence the aggressiveness, was best determined on the magnification view. Furthermore, serial assessment of progression of disease, or response to therapy was clearly enhanced. In some instances, the direct-magnification study was begun after a positive bone scan and conventional radiographs had provided inconclusive results. Direct radiographic magnification may be concluded to add useful information, but it is more difficult to perform than routine radiography and results in relatively high radiation exposure. It should be used selectively, therefore, when the diagnosis is uncertain or when symptoms or a positive bone scan strongly suggest a skeletal abnormality that is ill-defined or undetected on conventional radiographs.

Summary and Conclusions

As is apparent from the preceding discussion, magnification, both in our own experience and that of others, is helpful, or sometimes essential, in reaching an appropriate radiographic interpretation, or in serially studying skeletal neoplasms. For the thin parts of the peripheral skeleton, the choice lies between optical magnification of industrial film, or direct radiographic magnification. For the thick parts (where tumors generally originate), only the latter technique can be employed readily. With optical magnification, special processing and viewing are required; otherwise, conventional roentgen equipment can be used. With direct magnification, a special microfocus roentgen tube is necessary; however, conventional procedures of processing and viewing may be used. These advantages, along with the lower radiation exposure and the application for thick body parts, favor this technique over optical magnification in the study of skeletal neoplasms.

With further optimization of technical parameters, and with greater clinical experience, these newer high-resolution radiologic modalities may become diagnostic procedures of major importance.

References

AEGERTER, E., KIRPATRICK, J.A.: Orthopedic disease, 4th ed. Philadelphia: W.B. Saunders Co. 1975

BERENS, D.L., LIN, R.: Roentgen diagnosis of rheumatoid arthritis. Springfield: Charles C Thomas 1969

BOOKSTEIN, J.J., VOEGELI, E.: A critical analysis of magnification radiography; laboratory investigation. Radiology 98, 23–30 (1971)

CALENOFF, L., NORFRAY, J.: Magnification digital roentgenography: a method for evaluating renal osteodystrophy in hemodialysed patients. Amer. J. Roentgenol. 118, 282–292 (1973)

DAHLIN, D.C.: Bone tumors, 2nd ed. Springfield, Illinois: Charles C Thomas 1970

DOI, K., FROMES, B., ROSSMANN, K.: New device for accurate measurement of the x-ray intensity distribution of x-ray tube focal spots. Med. Phys. 2, 268–273 (1975b)

DOI, K., GENANT, H.K., ROSSMANN, K.: Effect of film

graininess and geometric unsharpness on image quality in fine-detail skeletal radiography. Invest. Radiol. 10, 35–42 (1975a)

Doi, K., Genant, H.K., Rossmann, K.: Comparison of image quality obtained with optical and radiographic magnification techniques for fine-detail skeletal radiography: effect of object thickness. Radiology 118, 189–195 (1976)

Doi, K., Rossmann, K.: The effect of radiographic magnification on blood vessel imaging with various screen-film systems. Med. Phys. 1, 257–261 (1974)

Doi, K., Rossmann, K.: Measurements of optical and noise properties of screen-film systems in radiography. In: Proceedings of the symposium of medical x-ray photo-optical systems evaluation. Palos Verdes Estates, California: Society of Photo-Optical Instruments and Engineers, 1975

Edeiken, J., Hodes, P.J., Caplan, L.H.: New bone production and periosteal reaction. Amer. J. Roentgenol. 97, 708–718 (1966)

Fletcher, D.E., Rowley, K.A.: Radiographic enlargements in diagnostic radiology. Brit. J. Radiol. 24, 598–604 (1951)

Fletcher, D.E., Rowley, K.A.: The radiological features of rheumatoid arthritis. Brit. J. Radiol. 25, 282–295 (1952)

Fornasier, V.L., Horne, J.G.: Metastases to the vertebral column. Cancer (Philad.) 36, 590–594 (1975)

Genant, H.K., Doi, K., Mall, J.C.: Optical versus radiographic magnification for fine-detail skeletal radiography. Invest. Radiol. 10, 160–172 (1975a)

Genant, H.K., Doi, K., Mall, J.C., et al.: Direct radiographic magnification for skeletal radiography: An assessment of image quality and clinical application. Radiology 123, April 1976

Genant, H.K., Doi, K., Mall, J.C.: Comparison of non-screen techniques (Medical versus industrial film) for fine-detail skeletal radiography. Invest. Radiol. 11, 486–500, Sept.-Oct. 1976

Genant, H.K., Heck, L.L., Lanzl, L.H., et al.: Primary hyperparathyroidism. A comprehensive study of clinical, biochemical and radiographic manifestations. Radiology 109, 513–524 (1973)

Genant, H.K., Kozin, F., Bekerman, C., et al.: The reflex sympathetic dystrophy syndrome. A comprehensive analysis using fine-detail radiography, photon absorptiometry, and bone and joint scintigraphy. Radiology 117, 21–32 (1975b)

Gordon, S.L., Greer, R.B., Wiedner, W.A.: Magnification roentgenographic technic in orthopedics. Clin. Orthop. 91, 169–173 (1973)

Ishigaki, T.: First metatarsal-phalangeal joint of gout-microroentgenographic examination in 6 times magnification. Nippon Acta. Radiology 33, 839–854 (1973)

Jaffe, H.L.: Tumors and tumorous conditions of the bones and joints. Philadelphia: Lea and Febiger 1958

Johnson, L.C.: A general theory of bone tumors. Bull. N.Y. Acad. Med. 29, 164–171 (1953)

Lichtenstein, L.: Bone tumors, 4th ed. St. Louis: C.V. Mosby Co. 1972

Lodwick, G.S.: A systemic approach to the roentgen diagnosis of bone tumors. In: Tumors of bone and soft tissue. Eighth clinical conference on cancer, 1963. Chicago: Year Book Medical Publishers, pp. 49–68, 1965

Lodwick, G.S.: The bones and joints, Chicago: Year Book Medical Publishers. Inc. 1971

Mall, J.C., Genant, H.K., Rossmann, K.: Improved optical magnification for fine-detail radiography. Radiology 108, 707–708 (1973)

Mall, J.C., Genant, H.K., Silcox, D.C., et al.: The efficacy of fine-detail radiography in the evaluation of patients with rheumatoid arthritis. Radiology 112, 37–42 (1974)

Meema, H.E.: Some preliminary in vivo microradioscopic-morphometric observations on bone resorption using a 70-mm roll-film enlarger ("Helio Contrastor"). Invest. Radiol. 8, 418–422 (1973)

Meema, H.E., Meema, S.: Comparison of microradioscopic and morphometric findings in the hand bones with densitometric findings in the proximal radius in thyrotoxicosis and in renal osteodystrophy. Invest. Radiol. 7, 88–86 (1972)

Meema, H.E., Schatz, D.L.: Simple radiologic demonstration of cortical bone loss in thyrotoxicosis. Radiology 97, 9–16 (1970)

Milch, R.A., Changus, G.W.: Response of bone to tumor invasion. Cancer (Philad.) 9, 340–351 (1956)

Norman, A., Ulin, R.: A comparative study of periosteal newbone response to metastatic bone tumor (solitary) and primary bone sarcomas. Radiology 92, 705–708 (1969)

Norman, A., Wu, J.: Enlargement tomography in the diagnosis of bone tumors and skeletal trauma—a preliminary study. Bull. Hosp. Jt Dis. (N.Y.) 27, 46–50 (1966)

Rao, U.V., Bates, L.M.: The modulation transfer functions of x-ray focal spots. Phys. in Med. Biol. 14, 93–106 (1969)

Rossmann, K.: Image quality. Radiol. Clin. N. Amer. 7, 419–433 (1969)

Spjut, H.J., Dorfman, H.D., Fechner, R.E., et al.: Tumors of bone and cartilage. Atlas of Tumor Pathology, 2nd Series, fasc. 5 Washington, D.C.: Armed Forces Institute of Pathology, 1970

Takahashi, S., Sakuma, S., Kaneko, M., et al.: Angiography at fourfold magnification with special reference to the examination of tumours. Acta. radiol. [Diag.] (Stockh.) 4, 206–216 (1966)

Takahashi, S., Sakuma, S., Ayakawa, Y., et al.: Radiation levels of microradiography. Radiology 112, 709–713 (1974)

Weiss, A.: A technique for demonstrating fine detail in bones of the hands. Clin. Radiol. 23, 185–187 (1972)

Author Index — Namenverzeichnis

Page numbers in *italics* refer to the references
Die *kursiv* gesetzten Zahlen beziehen sich auf die Literatur

les, A.B., Henderson, E.D. 480, *542*

Enterline, H.T., Culberson, J.D., Rochlin, D.B., Brady, L.W. 351, *353*

Enzinger, F.M., Shiraki, M. 171, 220, *238*

Enzinger, F.M., s. Wirth, W.A. 496, *548*

Epstein, B. 362, 369, 370, 376, 381, *415*, 484, *542*

Epstein, B.S. 589, 593, *600*

Epstein, M.J., s. Ben-Menachem, Y. 308, 309, 314, *332*

Erdheim, J. 529, *550*

Erf, L.A., Pecher, C. *631*

Erich, J.B., s. Kragh, L.V. *69*

Erlandson, R., s. Huvos, A. *9*

Erlandson, R.A., s. Huvos, A.G. 137, 142, 145, 148, 149, 152, 154, 155, 156, 179, *239*

Ernst, P. 203, *238*

Essammaa, E. *415*

Esterly, J.R., s. Gatewood, O.M.B. 496, *545*

Etchart, M., Viviani, G., Behn, K. *438*

Etter, L.E., Hurst, J.W. *544*

Evans, J. 491, 493, 511, *544*

Evans, J.A., s. Mujahed, Z. 329, *333*

Evans, K.T., s. Cockshott, W.P. *673*

Evans, R.D., s. Aub, J.C. *67*

Evans, W.R. 373, *416*

Evarts, C.M., s. Montoya, G. 494, *546*

Evens, R.G., s. Stabple, T.W. *675*

Evens, R.G., s. Stapel. T.W. 404, 405, *413*

Eversole, L.R., Sabes, W.R., Rovin, S. 490, 491, 497, *544*

Eversole, L.R., s. Daugherty, J.W. 453, *539*

Ewing, J. *68*, 136, *238*, 267, 268, 293, *304, 306*, 453, *539*

Eyre-Brook, A.L., Price, C.H.G. *11*, 344, 345, *353*

Eyring, E.J., s. Anderson, C.E. 202, *237*

Eyring, E.J., s. Wanken, J.J. 616, *633*

Faber, D.D., Wahman, G.E., Bailey, T.A., Flocks, R.H., Culp, D.A., Morrison, R.T. *601*

Fabricius, R., s. Sherman, M. 248, *257*

Fahey, F.F., O'Brien, E.T. 451, *536*

Fahmy, A., s. Vix, V.A. 165, *242*, 336, *354*

Fairbank, H.A.T. *8*, 128, 129, 130, *238*, 489, 491, 492, 493, 499, *544*

Fairbanks, T. *12*

Fairhall, L.T., s. Aub, J.C. 529, *550*

Fajans, S.S., s. Scurry, M.T. 496, *547*

Falconer, M.A., Bailery, I.C., Duchen, L.W. 365, 368, 374, 384, 389, 409, 411, *412*

Falconer, M.A., Cope, C.L., Robb-Smith, A.H.T. 490, 492, 493, 494, 496, *544*

Falconer, M.A., s. Nag, T.K. 108, 109, *240*

Falkmer, S., Tilling, G. *10*

Fanconi, G., Illig, R. 98, *238*

Farber, S. 479, *542*

Farber, S., s. Green, W.T. 479, 484, *542*

Farinas, P.L. 635, 656, *674*

Farman, J., s. Steiner, G.M. 324, *333*

Farman, J., s. Villiers, D.R. de 329, *332*

Farr. H.W., s. Highinbotham, N.L. 365, 374, 375, 376, 379, *416*

Farrow, J.H., s. Gibbons, J. 555, *601*

Faust, D.B., Gilmore, H.R., Mudgett, C.S. 365, 379, 381, *412*

Fawcett, K.J., Dahlin, D.C. 427, 428, 430, *440*

Fechner, R.E., Wilde, H.D. 138, 139, 140, *238*

Fechner, R.E., s. Dickson, J.H. 428, *440*

Fechner, R.E., s. King, J.W. 234, *239*

Fechner, R.E., s. Spjut, H.J. *12*, 85, 87, 96, 108, 118, 124, 135, 137, 138, 143, 144, 148, 150, 159, 161, 167, 170, 179, 215. 235, *241*, 248, 249, 250, 251, 256, *257*, 266, 278, 279, *304, 305*, 317, 330, *333*, 335, *354, 439*, 445, 455, 474, 475, 479, 480, 487, 498, 514, 525, 534, *538, 540, 541. 542, 543*, 554, 550, *551*, 677, *696*

Feintuch, T.A. 179, *238*, 496, *544*

Feiring, E.H., s. Feiring, W. 493, 496, *544*

Feiring, W., Feiring, E.H., Davidoff, L.M. 493, 496, *544*

Feist, J.H., s. Ney, F.G. *675*

Feketa, A., s. Rose, E.F. 90, 94, *241*

Feldman, F., Hecht, H.L., Johnston, A.D. 158, 159, 160, 161, 163, 165, 166, 167, 175, 176, *238*, 335, 336, 338, *353*

Feldman, F., Johnston, A. 466, 467, 468, *541*

Felson, B., s. Pratt, A.D. 501, *546*

Felson, B., s. Toomey, F.B. 577, 586, *602*

Fenni-Pearse, D., Olowu, A.O. 522, *549*

Fenyes, I., s. Zoltan, L. *416*

Ferguson, A.B., Jr., s. D'Ambrosia, R. 85, *238*

Fernandez, M.B., s. Gillison, E.W. 577, *601*

Ferrant, A., Rodhain, J., Michaux, L., Piret, L., Maldague, B., Sokal, G. 624, *631*

Fialho, F., Barcellos, J.M.P. 351, *353*

Fielding, J.W., Ratzan, S. 90, *238*

Fienberg, R., s. Smith, W.E. *11*, 349, *354*

Fievez, M., s. Mandard, J.C. *439*

Filippone, J.J. 176, *238*

Fine, G., Stout, A.P. *8*, 65, 68, 516, 525, *549, 674*

Finkelman, A., s. Shapiro, R. *354*

Finkelstein, J.Z., Ekert, H., Isaacs, H., Jr., Hoggins, G. 555, 556, *601*

Finkerl, A.J., s. Lucas, H.F. *70*

Finlayson, R. *68*

Finzi, O. 479, *542*

Firat, D., Stutzman, L. 490, 492, 496, *544*

Firooznia, H., s. Goldman, A.B. 618, *631*

Firooznia, H., s. Pinto, R.S. *412*

Firtel, S., s. Winter, A. *540*

Fischer, B. 417, 419, 420, 422, *438*

Fischer, B., Steiner *413*

Fischer, E.R., Vuzevski, V.D. 427, 429, *440, 441*

Fischer, I., s. Mourgues, G. de 443, 452, *537*

Fisher, R.G., s. Stough, D.R. *416*

Fitzer, P.M. 612, *631*

Fitzgerald, D.D., Sim, M.D. *8*

Fitzpatrick, B. 479, 480, *542*

Fitzpatrick, H.F., s. Bossart, R.A. 453, *538*

Fitzpatrick, Th.B., s. Benedict, P.H. 493, *543*

Leader, S.D., Grand, M.J.H. 489, *546*

Leavitt, D., s. Wirth, W.A. 496, *548*

Leblond, C.P., s. Wilkinson, G.W. 603, *633*

Lecoco, M. 494, *546*

Lederer, H., Sinclair, A.J. *11, 438*

Ledoux-Lebard, G. 494, *546*

Lee, E.B., s. Kinnmann, J.E.G. 493, *546*

Lee, J. 352

Lee, J., s. Lynn, M.D. 224, 228, *239*

Lee, K.W., Chin, T.C., Paul, G. *438*

Lee, S., s. Gillis, L. *68*

Leeds, N., Seaman, W.B. 491, 493, 505, 509, 510, *546*

Lee, V.W., Sano, R., Freedman, G. 610, *632*

Lefleur, R.S., s. Pinto, R.S. *412*

Legier, J.F., Tauber, L.N. *59,* 554, 580, 583, 586, *601*

Lehman, W.B., s. Ariel, I.M. 554, *600*

Lehrer, H.Z. 510, *546*

Lehrer, H.Z., Maxfield, W.S., Nice, C.M. *59, 69,* 580, 583, 586, *601*

Leiken, S., Puroganan, G., Frankel, A., Steerman, R., Chandra, R. 480, *542*

Lejeune, E., s. Ravault, P.P. 157, *240*

Lellis, R. De, s. Schall, G.L. 614, *633*

Leman, P., Cohaden, F., Cohaden, S. 370, *415*

Lemos, C., s. Schajowicz, F. *8*

Lent 6

Leonidas, J.C., s. Broder, M.S. *67*

Leopold, R.G., s. Hensinger, R.N. 129, *239*

Lepow, H., Schoenfeld, M.R., Messeloff, C.R., Chu, F. 555, *601*

Lessard, R., s. Aube, L. *67*

Lessman, F.P., Schobinger von Schowingen, R., Lasser, E.C. *674*

Lestrade, A., s. Argadu, M.R. *416*

Lettin, A.W.F. 160, *239*

Letts, R.W. 525, *549*

Levin, A.G., s. Marcove, R.C. *70*

Levin, B. 433, *442*

Levin, D.C., Watson, R.C., Baltaxe, H.A. *674*

Levine, A.N., Sheinkop, M.S. 597, 598, *601*

Levine, G., Bensch, K.M.D. *9*

Levine, G.D., Bensch, K.G. 137, 138, 206, *239*

Levine, M.D., s. Dudley, H.C. 606, *631*

Levy, B.M., s. Higgins, G.M. 179, *239*

Levy, W.M., Aegerter, E.E., Kirkpatrick, J.A., Jr. 108, 137, 177, *239*

Lewer, A.K., s. Danzinger, J. *415*

Lewer-Allen, K., Kerr, W.A. *415*

Lewis, H.H., Korbin, H.I. *441*

Lewis, M.M., Marshall, J.L., Mirra, J.M. 123, 230, *239*

Lewis, N.D.C. 363, 374, *414*

Lewis, R.J., Ketcham, A.S. 123, 128, *239*

Lewis, R.J., s. Nelp, W.B. 608, *632*

Lewitt, K., s. Jirout, J. 494, *545*

Li, J.K.H., s. Anderson, R.L. 92, 96, 206, *237*

Libby, R., s. Cassen, B. *630*

Liberman, U.A., Barzel, U., Vries, A. De, Ellis, H. 513, 514, 523, *549*

Lichtenstein, L. 6, *12, 69,* 95, 109, 112, 116, 122, 127, 137, 139, 144, 160, 168, 170, 173, 177, 178, 179, 181, 184, 195, 197, 198, 201, 203, 205, 224, 228, *239,* 243, 244, 248, 250, 251, 256, *257,* 335, 344, 345, 347, 348, *353,* 362, 363, 373, *412, 414,* 430, 432, *438, 441, 442,* 452, 453, 455, 458, 466, 473, 474, 475, 479, 480, 488, 491, *537, 539, 541, 542, 546, 674, 677, 696*

Lichtenstein, L., Bernstein, D. *9,* 158, 159, 205, 206, 227, *239*

Lichtenstein, L., Goldman, R.L. 159, 224, 226, 227, *239*

Lichtenstein, L., Hall, J.E. *9,* 132, 135, *239*

Lichtenstein, L., Jaffe, H.L. 127, 179, 184, 198, 201, 202, 203, *239,* 479, 489, 490, 492, 497, 499, *543, 546*

Lichtenstein, L., Sawyer, W.R. *8, 69*

Lichtenstein, L., s. Glynn, J.J. 32, *68*

Lichtenstein, L., s. Goldman, R.L. 235, *238*

Lichtenstein, L., s. Jaffe, H.L. *9, 69,* 118, 136, 137, 144, 148,

150, 154, 158, 159, 160, 168, 169, 170, 175, *239,* 243, 249, *256,* 335, 337, 342, *353,* 443, 444, 445, 447, 451, 452, 472, 475, 479, 480, 487, *537, 541, 542*

Lichtenstein, L., s. Jaffe, W.L. 453, *539*

Lichtensztajn, J.A., Golbert, Z.W. 453, *539*

Lichtman, H.M., s. Silver, C.M. 210, 230, *241*

Lidholm, S.O., Lindbom, A., Spjut, H.L. *10*

Liebegott, G. *539*

Lieberman, P.H., Jones, C.R., Dargeon, H.W., Begg, C.F. 480, *543*

Liebeskind, A.L., s. Schechter, M.M. 364, 365, 369, 376, 382, 384, 386, 387, 390, 391, 393, 409, *413*

Liebner, E.J. 66

Liedberg, G., Lindholm, K., Lindstedt, E., Lindstet, G. 69

Lignelli, G.J., s. Scott, M. 30, *71*

Lilienfeld, R.M., s. Agha, F.P. 428, 432, *440*

Lin, J.P., Goodkin, R., Chase, N.E., Kricheff, I.I. 505, *546*

Lin, J.P., s. Pinto, R.S. *412*

Lin, R., s. Berens, D.L. 677, *695*

Lin, R.R., s. Schobinger, R. *675*

Linck, A. *414*

Linck, A., Warstat, H. 359, *414*

Lind, O., Millerstrom, K. *69*

Lindberg, S., s. Gynning, J. 604, *631*

Lindbom et al. (1961) 656

Lindbom, A., Lindvall, N., Soderberg, G., Spjut, H. 32, *69, 674*

Lindbom, A., Soderberg, G., Spjut, H.J., Sunnqvist, O. *675*

Lindbom, A., Soderberg, O., Spjut, H.J., Sunnquist, O. 453, 458, 462, *539*

Lindbom, A., Soderberg, G., Spjut, H.J. *8, 70,* 179, *239*

Lindbom, A., s. Lagergren, C. 404, *412, 645, 674*

Lindbom, A., s. Lidholm, S.O. *10*

Lindenbaum, B., Gottes, N.I. 484, *543*

Lindgren, E., Chiro, G. Di 387, 409, *412*

Lindholm, K., s. Liedberg, G. *69*

Lindquist, B., s. Bauer, G.C.H. 604, 606, *630*

Lindstedt, E., s. Liedberg, G. *69*

Slager, U.T., Reilly, E.B. 555, *602*

Sloane, D., s. Wolfort, B. *440*

Slow, I.N., Stern, D., Friedman, E.W. 496, *547*

Slowick, F.A., Campbell, C.J., Kettelkamp, D.B. 453, *540*

Slulittel, J., s. Schajowicz, F. *8, 11*, 248, *257*, 479, 480, *543*

Slulittel, J.A., Schajowicz, F., Slulittel, J. 92, *241*

Slulittel, J., s. Slulittel, J.A. 92, *241*

Smith, A. 352,

Smith, A.G., Zavaleta, A. *354*, 491, *547*

Smith, A.G., s. Wrenn, R.N. 335, *354*

Smith, A.M., Becker, J.A. *675*

Smith, C.F., s. Smith, R.W. *537*

Smith, D.M., Zeman, W., Johnston, C.C., Deiss, W.P. 526, *550*

Smith, H.E., s. Gilman, W.S., Jr. 177, 179, *238*

Smith, I. 487, *543*

Smith, I., Schmaman, A. 491, *547*

Smith, I., s. Schmaman, A. 491, *547*

Smith, J. *71*

Smith, J.F. *354, 439*

Smith, J.L., s. Roca, A.N. *71*

Smith, J.R., s. Renner, R.R. 278, *305*

Smith, N.R. *537*

Smith, P.H., s. Albright, F. 489, 492, 494, 499, *543*

Smith, R., s. Russell, R.G. 528, *549*

Smith, R.J. 597, *602*

Smith, R.W., Smith, C.F. *537*

Smith, W.E., Fienberg, R. *11*, 349, *354*

Snapper, I., Kahn, A.I. 280, *305*

Snapper, I., Parisel, C. 489, *547*

Snapper, I., Turner, L.B., Moscovitz, H.L. *10*

Snarr, J.W., Abell, M.R., Martel, W. 31, *71*

Snell, A.H. 606, *633*

Snodgrass, G.J.A., s. Husband, P. *545*

Snook, T. *414*

Snyder, H.H., Jr., s. Habal, M.B. 184, *238*

Snyder, R.E., s. Sherman, R.S. 269, *305*

Sobarzo, V., s. Gutmann, J. 220, *238*

Soderberg, G., s. Lagergren, C. 404, *412*, 645, *674*

Soderberg, G., s. Lindbom, A. *674, 675*

Soderberg, O., s. Lindbom, A. 453, 458, 462, *539*

Sodyklov, A.G. *675*

Söderberg, G., s. Lindbom, A. *8, 32, 69, 70*, 179, *239*

Sognnaes, R.F., s. Volker, J.F. 606, *633*

Sokal, G., s. Ferrant, A. 624, *631*

Sokoloff, L., s. Carbone, P.P. 291, *305*

Solomon, L. 100, 108, *241*

Som, M., Peimer, R. 74, *82*

Sondag, Th. 579,

Sontag, L.W., Pyle, S.I. 472, 473, *542*

Soong, K.Y., s. McKenna, R.J. *8, 70*, 179, *240*

Soong, K.Y., s. Sherman, R.S. 261, *304*, 453, 458, *540*

Soren, A. 468, *541*

Sorensen, A.H., s. Bohr, H. 603, *630*

Soule, E.A., s. Allan, C.J. 67

Sowinski, J. *540*

Spady, H.A., s. McGavran, M.H. 480, *543*

Speed, J.S., s. Changus, G.W. *11*, 420, 423, *438*

Speiser, F. 119, *241*

Spence, K.F., Sell, K.W., Brown, R.H. 443, 451, 452, *538*

Spencer, J., s. Dresser, R. 293, *306*, 577, *600*

Spencer, R.P., Lange, R.C., Treves, S. 606, *633*

Spencer, R.P., s. Lange, R.C. 606, *632*

Spiess, H. 97, *241*

Spira, M., s. Shanoff, L.V. 525, *550, 675*

Spiro, R., s. Abrams, H.L. 553, 557, *600*

Spittle, M., s. Harmer, C.L. 556, *601*

Spjut, H., s. Lindbom, A. 32, *69*

Spjut, H.J. 90, 93, 96, *241*

Spjut, H.L., Dorfman, H.D., Fechner, R.E. 677, *696*

Spjut, H.J., Dorfman, H.D., Fechner, R.E., Ackerman, L.V. *12*, 85, 87, 96, 108, 118, 124, 135, 137, 138, 143, 144, 148, 150, 159, 161, 167, 170, 179, 215, 235, *241*, 248, 249, 250, 251, 256, *257*, 266, 278, 279, *304*,

305, 317, 330, *333*, 335, *354*, *439*, 445, 455, 474, 475, 479, 480, 487, 498, 514, 525, 534, *538, 540, 541, 542, 543, 547, 550, 551*

Spjut, H.J., Luse, S.A. *12*

Spjut, H.J., s. Ackerman, L.V. *67*, 73, 80, *81*, 117, 118, 179, 193, *237*, 348, *352, 440*

Spjut, H.J., s. Jakobson, E. 193, *239*

Spjut, H.J., s. King, J.W. 234, *239*

Spjut, H.J., s. Lidholm, S.O. *10*

Spjut, H.J., s. Lindbom, A. *70*, 179, *239*, 453, 458, 462, *539*, *675*

Spjut, H.L., s. Lindbom, A. *8*

Spjut, J., s. Lindbom, A. *674*

Spronl, E.E., s. Bachman, A.L. 614, *630*

Spouge, J.D. *439*

Spouge, J.D., Spruyt, C.L. *439*

Spranger, J.W., Langer, L.O., Wiedemann, H.R. 508, 511, *547*

Spratt, J.S., Jr. 83, *241*

Sproul, E.E., s. Bachman, A.L. 555, 587, *600*

Sproul, E.E., s. Gutman, E.B. 555, *601*

Spruyt, C.L., s. Spouge, J.D. *439*

Srivastava, K.K. *540*

Stabple, T.W., Evens, R.G., Stein, A.H., Jr. *675*

Städtler, F., s. Piepgras, U. 138, *240*

Stafne, E.C., s. Zimmerman, D.C. 491, *548*

Staheli, L.T., Nelp, W.B., Marty, R., Griffin, J.T. 604, *633*

Stalmann, A. 489, *547*

Stanciuleseu, P., s. Baciu, C. *673*

Stansfeld, A.G., s. Maudsley, R.H. 472, 473, *541*

Stapel, T.W., Evens, R.G., Stein, A.H. 404, 405, *413*

Staple, T.W., s. Debnam, J.W. 577, *600*

Staple, T.W., s. Forrest, J. 312, *332*

Staple, T.W., s. Reiter, F.B. 186, 188, *241*

Starr, P., s. Yettra, C.M. *548*

Stasney, R.J., s. Naji, A.F. 423, *439*

Stauffer, H.M., Arbuckle, R.K., Aegerter, E. 493, 496, *547*

Stavron, D. *442*

732 Author Index — Namenverzeichnis

Turner-Warwick, R.T., s. Thomson, A.D. *9,* 248, *257*
Tuttle, W.M., s. Sethi, R.S. 496, *547*
Tveteraas, E., s. Aarskog, D. 496, *543*
Twigg, H.L., s. Napoli, L.D. 577, 586, *602*
Tzamouranis, G., s. Berenbaum, S.L. 123, *237*

Uehlinger, E. *12, 72,* 293, *306*
Uehlinger, E., Botsztejn, Ch., Schinz, H.R. *10*
Uehlinger, E.A. *440*
Uehlinger, M.D., s. Voegeli, M.D. *675*
Ueno, L. *12*
Uhr, N., Churg, J. *416*
Ulin, R., s. Norman, A. 579, 580, 582, 586, *602, 677, 696*
Ullberg, S., s. Appelgren, L.E. 618, *630*
Unger, S.M., s. Sum, P.W. 577, *602*
Unni, K.K., Dahlin, D.C., Beabout, J.W., Ivins, J.C. 421, 423, 424, *440*
Unni, K.K., Ivins, J.C., Beabout, J.W., Dahlin, D.C. *10,* 329, 330, *333*
Urist, M.R., s. McLean, F.C. 530, *550*
Urist, M.R., s. Zaccaline, P.S. *550*
Utne, J.R., Pugh, D.G. 365, 370, 374, 376, 377, 379, 380, 381, 382, 384, 387, 395, 396, 397, 398, 405, 406, *413*
Uzel, A.R., s. Sherman, R.S. 138, 139, 140, 144, 145, *241*

Valderrama, J.A., Bullough, P.C. *10*
Valls, J., Ottolenghi, C.E., Schajowicz, F. 137, *242*
Valls, J., Polak, M., Schajowicz, F. 490, 497, 499, *548*
Vandenberg, H.J., Jr., Coley, B.L. 138, 153, 182, *242*
Vandenbussche, F., Donazzan, M., Carlier, G., Bonte, G. *440*
Vanderfield, G.K., s. Money, R.A. *412*
Vanderpool, D.W., s. King, J.W. 234, *239*
Vanneuville, G., s. Mercier, R. 327, 328, *333*
Vargas, H.A., s. Cornell, C.F. 433, 436, *441*

Varma, B.P., Gupta, I.M. 138, 147, 158, *242*
Vasilas, A., s. Mujahed, Z. 329, *333*
Vassar, P.S., s. Morton, K.S. *441*
Vaughan, V.C. III, s. Nelson 484, *543*
Vauzelle, J.L., s. Ravault, P.P. 157, *240*
Vellios, F., s. Samter, T.G. *11,* 430, *441*
Velvet, s. Pérochon *439*
Venerables, C. *550*
Venker, H. 493, *548*
Venturini, G., s. Forti, E. 365, *415*
Verbiest, H. 453, *540*
Verghese, A. 496, *548*
Verner, E.W., s. Stout, A.P. 220, 221, 222, *241*
Vernes, E., s. Oberling, C. *439*
Verocay, J. 427, *441*
Verstandig, C.C. *538*
Vetter, H., s. Johnson, L.C. 351, *353*
Vetter, J., s. Johnson, L.C. 444, *537*
Vey, J.T., s. Tilden, R.L. 612, *633*
Viallet, J.F., s. Mercier, R. 327, 328, *333*
Vianna, M.R., Horizonte, B. *540*
Vickers, C.W., Pugh, D.C., Ivins, J.C. 29, *72*
Vickers, R.A., Gorlin, R.J. *440*
Vicuna, R., s. Gutmann, J. 220, *238*
Vidoli, M.F., s. Copleman, B. *536*
Vieta, J.O., Friedell, H.L., Craver, L.F. 293, 294, 295, 297, 303, *306,* 577, *602*
Vietti, T., s. Perez, C.A. 86, 97, 98, *240*
Vignon, G., s. Ravault, P.P. 157, *240*
Villa, V.G., Laico, J.E., Banez, L.O.N. 435, *442*
Villiers, D.R. de, Farman, J., Campbell, J.A.H. 329, *332*
Vinardi, G., s. Natali, J. 327, 328, *333*
Viner Smith, K., s. Hirst, E. 455, *539*
Vines, R.H. 490, *548*
Vinik, M.N., Jr., Freed, T.A. *675*
Virchow, R. 85, 121, *242,* 365, *415,* 529, *548*
Virchow, R.L.L. 443, 446, *538*
Viswanath, C.K., s. Appalanarasayya, K. *67*

Vite, U. de, Guarino, M. *441*
Viriani, G., s. Etchart, M. *438*
Vix, V.A., Fahmy, A. 165, *242,* 336, *354*
Voegeli, E., s. Bookstein, J.J. 679, *695*
Voegeli, M.D., Uehlinger, M.D. *675*
Vogelsang, H., Weidenmann, O. *72*
Vogelsang, H., Wiedenmann, O. *675*
Vogler, E. *675*
Vogler, E., Deu, W. *675*
Volbe, J.A., s. Nardo, G.L. de 604, *631*
Volker, J.F., Sognnaes, R.F., Bibby, B.G. 606, *633*
Vore, D.T. de, Waldron, C.A. *441*
Vries, A. de, s. Liberman, U.A. 513, 514, 523, *549*
Vuzevski, V.D., s. Fischer, E.R. 427, 429, *440, 441*

Waddington, E.M. *415*
Wadsworth, T., s. Byers, P.D. 467, *541*
Waggener, J.D. 435, *441, 442*
Wagman, A.D., Weiss, E.K., Riggs, H.E. 510, *548*
Wagner, H.N., s. Hosain, F. 606, *632*
Wagner, J.E., s. Ebling, H. *539*
Wagner, R., s. Priesel, R. 489, *547*
Wahman, G.E., s. Faber, D.D. *601*
Waldenstrom, J. *10*
Waldeskog, B., s. Gynning, J. 604, *631*
Waldorn, C.A. 491, *540, 548*
Waldorn, C.A., Giansanti, J.S. *548*
Waldorn, C.A., Shafer, W.G. *540*
Waldron, C.A., s. Vore, D.T. de *441*
Waldron, R.L., Zeller, J.A. 317, 318, 319, *333*
Waldrun, C.A. *441*
Wallace, G.T., s. Dockerty, M.B. 494, *544*
Wallgren, A. 479, *543*
Wallis, L.A., Asch, T., Maisel, B.W. 316, 317, *333*
Walsh, W.S., s. Clarke, T.H. *416*
Walter, J. 125
Walter, P., s. Fontaine, R. *674*
Walters, P.J., s. Ellis, D.J. *539*

Subject Index

English-German

Where English and German spelling of a word is identical, the German version is omitted

742 Subject Index

Sachverzeichnis

Deutsch-Englisch

Bei gleicher Schreibweise in beiden Sprachen sind die Stichwörter nur einmal aufgeführt